Acta Neurochirurgica
Supplements

Editor: H.-J. Reulen
Assistant Editor: H.-J. Steiger

Brain Edema XI

Proceedings of the 11th International Symposium,
Newcastle-upon-Tyne, United Kingdom,
June 6–10, 1999

Edited by
A. D. Mendelow, A. Baethmann, Z. Czernicki, J. T. Hoff, U. Ito,
H. E. James, T. Kuroiwa, A. Marmarou, L. F. Marshall, H.-J. Reulen

Acta Neurochirurgica
Supplement 76

Prof. A. David Mendelow
Department of Neurosurgery, Newcastle General Hospital,
Newcastle-upon-Tyne, UK

Prof. Dr. Alexander Baethmann
Institut für Chirurgische Forschung,
Ludwig-Maximilians-Universität München, Germany

Prof. Dr. Zbigniew Czernicki
Department of Neurosurgery, Medical Research Center,
Polish Academy of Sciences, Warsaw, Poland

Prof. Dr. Julian T. Hoff
Section of Neurosurgery,
University of Michigan, Ann Arbor, MI, USA

Prof. Dr. Umeo Ito
Department of Neurosurgery,
Musashino Red Cross Hospital, Tokyo, Japan

Dr. Hector E. James
Pediatric Neurosurgery, San Diego, CA, USA

Dr. Toshihika Kuroiwa
Department of Neuropathology,
Medical Research Institute, Tokyo, Japan

Prof. Dr. Anthony Marmarou
Department of Neurosurgery, Medical College of Virginia,
Richmond, VA, USA

Prof. Dr. Lawrence F. Marshall
Division of Neurological Surgery,
San Diego Medical Research Center,
University of California, San Diego, CA, USA

Prof. Dr. Hans-Jürgen Reulen
Neurochirurgische Universitätsklinik, München, Germany

Typesetting: Asco Typesetters, Hong Kong
Printing: A. Holzhausen, A-1140 Wien
Binding: Fa. Papyrus, A-1100 Wien
Printed on acid-free and chlorine-free bleached paper
SPIN: 10783294

With 231 partly coloured Figures

CIP data applied for

ISSN 0065-1419
ISBN 3-211-83561-X Springer-Verlag Wien New York

A Brief Review of the Previous International Brain Oedema Symposia

The prevailing, unsatisfactory status of clinical management of brain edema (BE) has provided for some time an urgent need for an international symposium, to gain insight into some basic, underlying mechanisms and to obtain clues for the rational application of therapeutic measures. The first brain edema symposium was convened in *Vienna, September 11–13th in 1965 and was organized by I. Klatzo and F. Seitelberger.* There were 58 active participants in Vienna, who represented at that time the elite of clinicians, clinical neuropathologists and those who were experimentally engaged in illuminating some of the physiological, ultra-structural, and biochemical aspects of brain edema.

The existing confusion concerning the field was immediately apparent, and prompted the participants to take issue with some basic definitions and features of BE. It was apparent that neither the differentiation of BE into "edema" and "swelling", nor the classification according to etiologic aspects, was contributing to the elucidation of the basic mechanisms of BE, a search for which, consequently, drew the main focus and attention in the presentations and discussions.

The basic question as to where BE is located in brain tissue brought out differences between electron microscopists and physiologists as well as biochemists, the former localizing primarily edema in swollen glia cells (astrocytes), whereas the latter considered the enlargement of the extracellular space as the essential place and route of BE spreading. Since it was apparent that serum-proteins containing BE fluid derived mainly from "leaky" blood vessels, special attention was given to the blood-brain barrier. After dealing with various possible routes of passage through the endothelial barrier, three consecutive papers (presented by T. Broman and O. Steinwall; A. Lajtha *et al.* and G. Quadbeck and O. Hess) brought new, important findings on the active trans-endothelial transport, primarily, of glucose and amino acids, thus enhancing considerably the role of endothelium in BE. Socially, Vienna with its beautiful September weather was simply wonderful. The highlights were: The most dramatic staging of Tchaikovsky's "Queen of Spades" in the Vienna Opera, and a delightful evening in Grinzing enjoying Heuriger wine and typical Viennese music.

The second symposium organized by *K. Schuermann and H. J Reulen was held in Mainz, June 19–21, 1972* and testified to considerable progress in the understanding of some basic pathophysiological aspects of BE. There was a clear recognition of cytotoxic v. vasogenic edema as two main types, based on their distinctly different mechanisms of origin. The former is related to the intracellular accumulation of fluid in mostly irreversibly injured neurons, or in swollen astrocytes, which are normally involved in maintaining osmotic regulation within the environment, and in which fluid uptake can be reversible. On the other hand, vasogenic edema is related directly to increased vascular permeability, allowing escape into the extracellular space of scrum proteins, which tend to retain water, thus protracting the resolution of BE.

The symposium was heavily dominated by neurosurgeons and by their acute interest in the evaluation of the effect of steroids in the therapy of BE, and this was apparent from a great number of papers presented on the subject. An interesting pioneering paper, presaging the future focus of BE research on arachidonic acid cascades associated with cell membrane injury, was delivered by H. B. Demopoulos on the role of the free radicals and the effect of antioxidants in BE.

The meeting was certainly both a social as well as a scientific success and the highlight was a boat-cruise along the Rhine from Mainz to Bacharach for wine tasting. The "tasting" started in Mainz soon after boarding the ships, on the decks, with tables densely covered with open bottles of wine. Under gorgeous June weather, passing romantic castles and vineyards, the "tasting" continued after Bacharach on the way back. Next day, the participants were happy to discover that even the quite "hearty" consumption of white Rhine wine leaves amazingly little hangover.

The Montreal symposium organized by H. M. Pappius and W. Feindel in June 25–29th 1976 brought a remarkable enhancement in the further elucidation of some basic features of BE. Concerning the mechanisms of vasogenic edema, one full session was devoted to the function and dysfunction of the blood-brain barrier (BBB). With regard to the dynamics of this type of edema, the role of tissue pressure and bulk flow, as well as of serum proteins in the formation and resolution of vasogenic edema, was emphasized in several papers. A stimulating paper was given by K. G. Go, who draw attention to the significance of the changes in colloidal osmotic pressure between plasma and edematous tissue, which, according to the Starling equation, can significantly influence the dynamics of vasogenic edema.

Concerning cytotoxic edema, it was apparent that this type of edema plays a significant role in BE associated with ischemia, and therefore one whole session was devoted to the elucidation of this association. It was evident that in ischemic stroke both types of edema play a significant role, and this was clearly demonstrated in several papers, particularly by Hossmann, who used the electrical impedance assays for the determination of extracellular space. The clinical session revealed continuing interest in the steroid and osmotic therapies.

The highlight of the social events was a magnificent banquet in the City Hall and receptions at McGill University, allowing an opportunity to become acquainted with the impressive research program of the Montreal Neurological Institute.

As before, the interpretation of the main mechanisms of BE occupied the major attention of the fourth symposium organized by J. Cervos-Navarro and R. Ferszt in Berlin of 1980.

Among the new approaches, a fine estimation of water content by specific gravity measurements constituted unquestionable progress in the evaluation of this crucial indicator of BE. Considerable attention was given to "edema factors", such as glutamate, free radicals, arachidonic acid cascade, etc., observed in areas of vasogenic edema; however, the significance of these findings remained unclear, since it could not be determined whether the changes played a part in the induction of edema or were products of brain tissue injury. In the resolution of BE, the significance of serum proteins was emphasized, and their pinocytotic uptake by astrocytes was shown to correlate with a decrease in edema fluid. Otherwise, the dynamics of edema spreading and resolution directed towards the ependymal ventricular lining was presented convincingly by H. J. Reulen.

In evaluating therapeutic approaches, the effect of lowering the metabolic rate by barbiturates, or by endogenous CNS depressants was presented in several papers. The social event of the meeting was spectacular as the participants attended the new Berlin Opera to enjoy the ballet "Copelia", and sailed on Lake Wahnsee in lavish yachts provided by the organizers.

The fifth international symposium of brain edema was held in Groningen, Netherlands in 1982 and was hosted by K. G. Go and Jan Beks. There were several new areas of investigation introduced at this symposium. Among them, the complex interaction between cerebral blood flow, edema and metabolism as elucidated by positron emission tomography, which provided a unique insight into regional oxygen metabolism of edematous areas in human brain. Additional progress was made in identifying the hydrodynamics of the edema fluid and the conditions, which were required for drainage of fluid into the ventricular space. New methods of imaging edema by proton spin imaging and by prolongation of proton spin relaxation times were introduced. With regard to therapy, there was considerable attention paid to anti-inflammatory drugs, which interfered with prostaglandin synthesis and exerted a beneficial effect on the post-traumatic depression of cerebral glucose utilization. Equally important, an elegant study of oxygen availability was presented using an array of platinum electrodes in which the oxygen availability in edematous brain tissue was described. The social hallmark of this symposium was the opening of the symposium by Prince Klaus, the husband of Queen Beatrix, who was very charming and, above all, expressed a keen interest in our science. The banquet attended by all was equal to the royal standard of elegance and indeed was a memorable event.

In 1984 the sixth edema conference convened in Tokyo under the able guidance of Yutaka Inaba. This was the first time that the conference met in Asia in accordance with the recommendation by the organizers that we alternate from Europe, Asia and the West. Professor Inaba and his committee coordinated an extremely successful meeting and set a standard of hospitality that was hard to match. Scientifically, the meeting was exciting as workers reported on early results of non-invasive magnetic resonance techniques, which would eventually enable the measurement of brain water in patients non-invasively. The invited lecture by Bo Siesjo on membrane events leading to glial swelling and brain edema was of particular importance as it focused on Na/H and Cl/HCO3 exchangers and their alteration under pathological circumstances. Siesjo reported that these exchangers are also involved in intracellular pH regulation in such a way that acidosis triggers increased Na/H exchange with coupled influx of Cl via Cl/HCO3 antiporter and this underlies glial swelling in acidotic states. Studies of brain edema therapy continued to focus on dehydrating agents, free radical scavengers and steroids such as Glycerol, indomethacin and dexamethasone. No new breakthroughs in treatment were reported; however, the involvement of free radicals in the edematous process entertained new approaches to therapy.

On the social front, the meeting was extraordinary as many joined the "Tokyo by Night" and a smaller group enjoyed a spectacular dinner of "Shabu Shabu", to which two past Prime Ministers of Japan were also invited. Professor Inaba and his organizing committee could take heart in knowing that the first Edema in the Far East was truly a scientific and social success.

The seventh International Edema Conference held in 1987 moved to the United States in Baltimore Maryland under the able guidance of Donlin Long, Professor and Chairman of Neurosurgery at John Hopkins University. Don's interest in brain edema, particularly the vasogenic edema associated with contusion, extended over many years and his paper describing the cessation of edema progression following surgical excision of the lesion site remains a seminal contribution to the field. One of the highlights of the Baltimore meeting was the contribution to those working at the molecular level in defining the mechanisms responsible for glial swelling using in-vitro models and the importance of intracellular acidosis. The influence of the arachidonic cascade in lipid peroxidation and the forming of free radicals was also introduced. The keynote address was given by Hans Reulen, Professor and Chairman of Neurosurgery at Bern, Switzerland. Professor Reulen described the movement of fluid from the site of contusion using a novel CT imaging sequence, which was able to follow the movement of fluid over time. The influence of protein in the clearance of vasogenic edema was also elucidated. With regard to therapy, the effect of superoxide dismutase, a free radical scavenger, upon peritumoral edema was described. Several years later, this work combined with others formed the basis of a clinical trial in traumatic brain utilizing pegulated superoxide dismutase. After several days of focusing on brain water, the organizers arranged a trip to the natural waters of the Baltimore aquarium located in Baltimore's "Inner Harbor", which was truly spectacular.

The eighth symposium organized June 17–20th 1990 in Bern, Switzerland by H. J Reulen begun by memorializing Klaus Joachim Zuelch (1910–1988) for his outstanding contributions to understanding and research on brain edema. In the scientific sessions, the considerable interest was focused on the application of magnetic resonance for the evaluation of intra- and extracellular edema fluid. It was apparent that this approach can contribute most valuable information, both experimental and clinical, which could be used for interpretation of basic dynamics of BE, and in clinical management of patients. A special session was devoted to the clinically important entity of traumatic brain injury, commonly associated with BE. In the study of vasogenic edema related to changes in vascular permeability, a new approach was presented, namely, observations on the reactivity of cerebral endothelium, grown in tissue culture and exposed to various substances and factors which can affect the permeability of the BBB.

Social Events were blessed with most favorable weather and were simply magnificent. One day, there was a visit to an old castle, associated with a most enjoyable cruise on the lake Thun, with wine, yodeling and breathtaking scenery all around. The other highlight was a whole day excursion to Jungfrau, the highest mountain in Switzerland and second in altitude in the Alps. It was an unforgettable experience, although some people may have suffered from slight symptoms of mountain sickness. Most pleasant was also the closing banquet, with the band playing enticing to dancing, mostly American tunes.

Although the next symposium was to take place in Europe, the enthusiasm expressed by *Professor Umeo Ito convinced the advisory board to return to the Far East and the Ninth Edema Conference was held from May 16th–19th 1993 in Tokyo, Japan* under pleasant sunny skies. An entire session was devoted to glial swelling and the effect of mediators such as Glutamate and Bradykinin. Another major highlight was the work identifying differences in brain tissue characteristics identified by the degree of anisotropy, which colors the measurement of brain edema by NMR.

Thus, in the technology of NMR water measurement, the orientation of the fibre tracts was important. New advances in the differentiation of cytotoxic and vasogenic forms of edema were made as workers reported on the use of apparent diffusion coefficients (ADC). Positive changes in ADC signify a predominant vasogenic edema while reductions in ADC signify a predominant cytotoxic edema. This was the first time that a method for non-invasive identification of edema was presented. Another major highlight of this meeting was the introduction of NMDA antagonists for treatment of brain edema. It was postulated that NMDA antagonists would be effective in blocking the glutamate induced cell injury. This, along with other works, led the path to several clinical trials in traumatic brain injury employing competitive and non-competitive NMDA compounds. Unfortunately, all of these clinical trials have failed to show an effect on outcome. Finally, one must mention the utilization of mathematical modeling, which was a unique contribution to elucidating the process of edema formation and resolution in brain tissue. Japan is considered the land of the rising sun. The beauty of the sun over the horizon was epitomized by the spectacular sunset witnessed by the attendees during a memorable cruise along Yokahama harbor. The ships sailed quietly as we observed a sharp contrast between the old and the new. But this was nothing compared to the virtuoso cello performance given by none other than our organizer Umeo Ito. We left Tokyo with renewed scientific interest and admiration of Japan and its people.

The three-year lapse between meetings was held as the *tenth Edema conference met in San Diego California in October of 1996 under the leadership of Hector James.* At this meeting, the influence of mitochondrial damage was introduced as a mechanism for ischemic brain damage. It was reported that cumulative oxidative damage to mitochondrial deoxyribonucleic acid (DNA) with subsequent defects in oxidative phosphorylation reduced the ability of the brain to cope with stress and offered an explanation to the age related increase in cerebral infarct size documented with experimental MCA occlusion. The studies of diffusion weighted imaging (DWI) showed significant advance in the differentiation of edema types and strengthened the application of NMR technology and its application to studies of edema both in experimental and clinical settings. With regard to therapy, several papers focused on the protective effect of hypothermia on brain edema. Interestingly, the neuroprotection offered by hypothermia was reported in clinical studies in the sixties by lan Beks, Professor of Neurosurgery in Holland. Beks reported excellent results in the application of the technique for use in aneurysm surgery. It was interesting that the concept of neuroprotection by cooling the brain has passed through several cycles and is receiving increased attention once again. Further emphasis on the utilization of NMDA antagonists for treatment of brain edema and brain injury was evident in the San Diego Conference as well as the continuance of antioxidant therapy. As the meeting ended, we were treated to a magnificent evening at the Scripts Institute, observing the marine life and later having dinner on the terrace with the beautiful Pacific sunset. This followed a wonderful evening at the SAN DIEGO ZOOLOGICAL PARK where we witnessed a remarkable performance of trained birds who walked tight ropes, jumped through hoops and were simply amazing.

This brings us up to the present as we read in this volume the scientific contributions of investigators attending the *11th International Edema Symposium in Newcastle upon Tyne and ably hosted by David Mendelow.*

The progress in brain edema research must in large part be attributed to the organization of these international symposiums and the efforts by all of our hosts in all parts of the world. It is fitting that we honor them by this small tribute in documenting their contribution to the field of brain edema.

I. Klatzo and A. Marmarou

A Summary of the XIth International Brain Oedema Symposium Held in Newcastle Upon Tyne, England in June 1999

There were more than 150 submissions for the Newcastle meeting and the advisory board selected, chaired and coordinated their sessions. They have edited the papers that are collected in this book and have summarised their respective sections. The objective has been to review the important highlights of each section to allow the reader to have a quick and balanced overview of each topic. This represents a new way forward for conference proceedings of this nature. Hopefully they will make the book more valuable than simply a collection of unrelated papers.

These meetings provide a unique opportunity for the exchange of modern laboratory information with clinicians in practice because the individual delegates who attend the Brain Oedema meetings include basic and clinical scientists. The subject matter therefore ranges from molecular biology to prospective randomised controlled trials. It is important in this era of Evidence Based Medicine that the International Brain Oedema Society should be setting high standards that will lead to changes in clinical practice. Similarly, the most modern technology and laboratory methods are now being used for the clinical monitoring of patients as is demonstrated by the papers on microdialysis in head injury.

Perhaps the most important highlight of the Newcastle meeting was the demonstration of the effective use of Magnetic Resonance Imaging (MRI) in the detection of the nature of brain oedema experimentally and clinically. From the in-vivo quantification of N-acetyl aspartate (NAA) in rat brain by M R spectroscopy to the measurement of Apparent Diffusion Coefficients (ADC) with Diffusion Weighted Imaging (DWI) it is absolutely clear that MRI has become and will remain a very important clinical tool in the understanding and treatment of brain oedema.

The original classification into *Cytotoxic* and *Vasogenic* oedema, proposed by Klatzo and referred to in his review at the beginning of this volume, has been shown to stand the test of time. Although others (Betz and Ianotti) have suggested different nomenclature (open-barrier for vasogenic oedema and closed-barrier for cytotoxic oedema), the original terms are preferred and have been used predominantly in this volume. Other attempts to revise this nomenclature have simply led to confusion, so words like cellular oedema for cytotoxic oedema are best avoided. It is hoped that future generations will stick to the CYTOTOXIC/VASOGENIC differentiation described here by Klatzo and Marmarou.

There were many papers on trauma at this meeting and several on spinal trauma from the Uppsala group. The continuous monitoring of the chemical milieu in patients with head injury using microdialysis represents one of the potential great advances in head injury care. Low glucose and high glutamate levels were consistently reported in a total of 252 patients with severe head injury. This has confirmed previous views, based on experimental evidence, that ischaemia and glutamate neurotoxicity are important in the pathophysiology of neurotrauma.

New and promising neuroprotective agents are described. Growth factors and Cannabinoids are the latest additions to our potential therapeutic armamentarium.

The reader of this volume will discover that here is now no longer any doubt that brain oedema plays an important part in the pathophysiology of ischaemia, trauma and haemorrhage. Oedema is not just an epiphenomenon or marker of trauma/ischaemia, but rather plays an important role in the function, metabolism, regulation of blood flow and biology in relation to brain damage.

The Editors

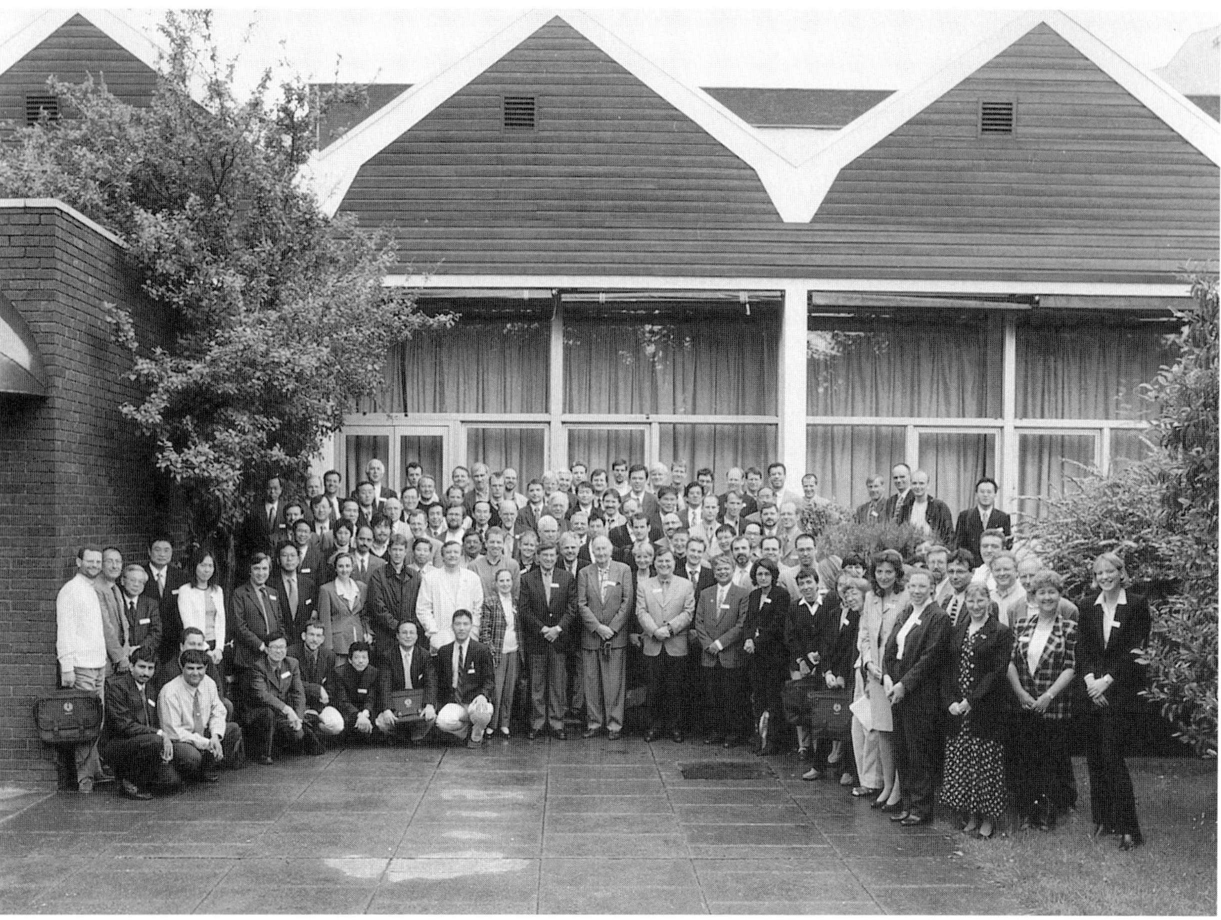

Contents

Listed in Current Contents

Imaging

Section on Imaging

The advances in imaging techniques have yielded significant inroads into the understanding of acute changes in the tissues following a variety of insults such as ischaemia, trauma, and with tumours. In this Section, we have articles that address the metabolic changes as defined by proton Magnetic Resonance Spectroscopy (MRS) both in patients as well as in experimental models. Pericontusional oedematous areas indicated by MRS are seen in the clinical setting in patients with mild head injury in the early and late stages. This had not been expected in the clinical course of mild head injury. The findings in patients are highlighted by the presentation in an experimental model in which the area of contusion as well as surrounding brain edema is noted by MRS to have increased two-fold in size within 24 hours. The significance of these findings are enhanced by the subsequent presentation of data demonstrating on MRI diffusion weighted imaging Apparent Diffusion Coefficients (ADC) in patients, in whom the dynamic changes in cerebral edema and swelling were documented by a capacity for oedema fluid accumulation to increase the central area of contusion, and at the same time swelling in the surrounding area which then creates an area of resistance for oedema fluid propagation. The combination of the oedema fluid accumulation and the swelling accounts for the mass effect seen with contusional oedema. The validity of this data was demonstrated further by another study comparing N-acetyl aspartate concentrations on MRS, using cerebral water as an internal reference standard, to accurately document the temporal changes of N-acetyl aspartate as a marker of neuronal death. The dynamic changes that imaging demonstrates as to the effects of trauma is highlighted in the works of Hoelper in monitoring regional cerebral blood flow (RCBF) in hemorrhagic and non-hemorrhagic contusions. These authors document that mixed contusions may evolve from hemorrhagic contusions with secondary increased periregional cytotoxic brain oedema, which then leads to reduced cerebral blood flow and further alterations of brain metabolism. The authors suggest that treatment of ICP may be individually modified by the measurement of intra and pericontusional cerebral blood flow.

Imaging has also allowed for a visualisation of what is to come with reference to the diagnosis of brain tumour malignancy by MRS. The work presented by Czernicki *et al.* in this Section compares the spectroscopy changes associated with malignant brain tumours, when compared to low grade meningiomas.

Acta Neurochir (2000) [Suppl] 76: 3–7

^{1}H-MR Spectroscopic Monitoring of Posttraumatic Metabolism Following Controlled Cortical Impact Injury: Pilot Study

M. U. Schuhmann[1], **D. Stiller**[3], **S. Thomas**[2], **T. Brinker**[2], and **M. Samii**[1,2]

[1] Department of Neurosurgery, Medical School Hannover, Germany
[2] Department of Neurosurgery, Nordstadt Hospital Hannover, Germany
[3] Leibnitz Institute of Neurobiology, Magdeburg, Germany

Summary

Proton magnetic resonance spectroscopy (^{1}H-MRS) has been increasingly utilised in experimental traumatic brain injury for characterisation of posttraumatic metabolic dysfunction. Following human brain injury pathological findings correlated with outcome measures. Combined with conventional T_2-weighted MR imaging MRS is a sensitive tool to evaluate metabolic changes in brain tissue following trauma. Studies have been restricted so far to diffuse axonal injury models and fluid percussion injury. Using a high resolution scanner at 4.7 T, MRI combined with ^{1}H-MRS was applied in a pilot study to the controlled cortical impact injury model of experimental brain contusion (CCII). Eight Sprague-Dawley rats were investigated, of which two served as controls. Four animals were injured 24 h after craniotomy, two investigated at 72 h post craniotomy. MRS/MRI indicated a transient brain oedema development and metabolic changes induced by the craniotomy itself. Following CCII MRI demonstrated that the area of contusion as well as the surrounding brain oedema increased twofold in size within 24 h ($p < 0.05$). MRS showed an immediate increase of N-acetylaspartate (NAA) and glutamate ipsilateral to the contusion and a drop of NAA on the contralateral side.

MRS/MRI investigations in the CCII model demonstrated a potential to further elucidate the pathophysiology following traumatic brain contusion.

Keywords: Traumatic brain injury; brain oedema; proton magnetic resonance spectroscopy; rats.

Introduction

Localised proton magnetic resonance spectroscopy (^{1}H-MRS) is a well-established technique for the in-vivo determination of metabolites in brain tissue [11, 12]. It permits to monitor neuronal damage and metabolic dysfunction following e.g. ischemia, trauma or neoplasm. MRS is per se combined with MR-imaging and therefore combines the advantages of an online metabolic monitoring with a precise visualisation of an anatomical region of interest. Since it can be arbitrarily repeated, the time-dependant metabolite kinetics of the same area as well as comparative investigations in different areas are possible. ^{31}P-MRS has been extensively used in experimental brain injury to characterise posttraumatic changes in various aspects of energy metabolism [4, 5, 9, 16]. In contrast ^{1}H-MRS has been used less frequently. In humans the results of neurochemical monitoring weeks or months after brain injury correlated with outcome [3, 12]. The few experimental studies were restricted to fluid percussion injury or diffuse axonal injury [1, 8, 13, 15]. Using ^{1}H-MRS we monitored in a model of brain contusion (controlled cortical impact injury – CCII) the time course of metabolic changes following application of a craniotomy and following impact trauma. Furthermore we determined the course of contusion and oedema development using T2-weighted MRI.

Materials and Methods

8 male Sprague Dawley rats weighting 330 ± 17 g were investigated. All animals were kept on a 12 h-light/dark cycle with free access to food and water. Two animals served as normal controls. Anaesthesia was induced with 5% Isoflurane in N_2O/O_2 ($2 \div 1$) and maintained with 1.5–2%. Animals were intubated and ventilated for surgical procedures or breathed spontaneously during MR investigations. With the head mounted in a stereotactic frame the left parietal bone was exposed via a midline incision. Using a high speed drill a left-sided 7 mm craniotomy was made with the centre 3 mm posterior and 4 mm lateral to bregma. After craniotomy the scalp was closed, animals extubated and returned to their cages. 24 h later baseline MR investigations were performed (n = 4). Afterwards animals were taken at 100% oxygen and received a controlled cortical impact injury (CCII) with a device similar to the development of Lighthall (7). Impact velocity was determined with a laser-optic system (optoNCDT, Mikro Epsilon Messtechnik, Ortenburg, Germany). A 5 mm flat impactor tip was accelerated to 3.93 ± 0.25 m/s

with a vertical deformation depth of 2.5 mm. Afterwards the animals were returned as fast as possible to the MR scanner. Investigations were done as early as possible (a.e.a.p. = 48 ± 10 min), at 2 h (2h05 min ± 14 min), 4 h (4h07 min ± 15 min) and 24 h (23h35 min ± 20 min) post injury. In 2 animals baseline examinations without trauma were performed 72 h after craniotomy. Body temperature was monitored with a rectal probe and kept between 36.5 and 37.5 °C.

MRI technique: We employed a Bruker Biospec 47/20 scanner at 4.7 running Paravision® software (Bruker GmbH, Ettlingen, Germany). For homogeneous exciation a 72 mm birdcage resonator and for detection an anatomically shaped 3-cm surface coil were used. Coronal T2-weighted RARE_8 sequences (TR 3100 ms, TE 79.4 ms, slice thickness 1.5 mm, FOV 3.2 cm, matrix 256^2) were generated for determination of contusion extension and visualisation of the surrounding oedema zone. For volume selective spectroscopy a PRESS-sequence (TR 2500 ms, TE 20 ms, 128 accumulations) was used. Voxel position (size 3 mm^3) was chosen right below the contused area covering the hippocampus and partly underlying thalamic structures. The corresponding contralateral position was taken as reference. In MR images the contusion volume and the volume of the surrounding oedema zone were determined by planimetry. MRS echoes were baseline corrected and exponentially filtered (LB 2 Hz), followed by zero filling before fast Fourier transformation. Metabolite spectra were manually phase corrected (0th and 1st order). Peak areas and intensities were determined by Lorentzian deconvolution algorithm (Bruker XWIN-NMR software package) for inositol (Ino), choline compounds (Cho), creatine + phosphocreatine (Cr), glutamate/glutamine (Glu), N-acetylaspartate (NAA), lactate (Lac), and -CH_3 of phospholipids (CH_3). A semiquantitative analysis was performed taking the creatine peak as reference point and calculating ratios for the remaining metabolites. Following CCII relative changes of ratios compared to pretrauma values (= 0) were calculated.

Results

25 MRI sequences and 55 ^{1}H-MRS investigations were performed.

Pre-trauma images 24 h post craniotomy showed dural/subdural changes and a zone of increased intensity consistent with localised brain oedema below the area of craniotomy. At 72 h post craniotomy, however, no signs of brain oedema were detected. The posttraumatic time course of increasing contusion and oedema volume is shown in Fig. 1. Early contusion volume measured 38.9 ± 10.5 mm^3 and increased to 79.3 ± 17 mm^3 at 24 h ($p < 0.01$). Oedema volume increased from 35.1 ± 11.1 mm^3 immediately after trauma to 78 ± 17.3 mm^3 at 24 h ($p < 0.01$).

^{1}H-MRS displayed differences between the hemispheres ipsi- and contralateral to the craniotomy for Ino/Cr, Cho/Cr and NAA/Cr 24 h post craniotomy compared to normal controls. These were not anymore apparent in animals after 72 h, however levels of Cho/Cr, NAA/Cr and Ch_3/Cr were determined slightly higher than in controls. Lactate was not detected in normal animals, however appeared bilaterally 24 h

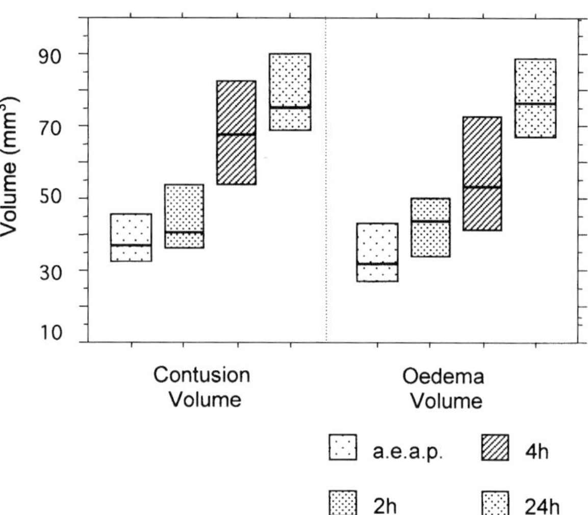

Fig. 1. The volume (mm^3) of the cerebral contusion as defined by MRI criteria following CCII increases over the first 24 hours. The biggest relative increase in contusion volume can be seen between the 2nd and the 4th hour. The volume of brain oedema surrounding the contusion core equals the contusion volume. It increases however steadily over time which results in the biggest relative increase between the 4th and the 24th hour; a.e.a.p. = as early as possible (48 ± 10 min)

post craniotomy and had not completely disappeared at 72 h.

^{1}H-MRS following CCII displayed a non-uniform pattern of relative changes in the metabolite ratios between the four animals. Therefore statistically significant changes in regard to the pre-trauma values or interhemispheric differences could not be calculated. Figure 2 shows relative changes post CCII for Cho/Cr, NAA/Cr, Glu/Cr, and Lac/Cr. For Cho/Cr exists a tendency to decrease bilaterally in the first 4 h following trauma to recover at 24 h. NAA/Cr dropped on the contralateral side in all animals and remained on this level. Ipsilaterally it increased immediately post trauma in 3 of 4 animals to decrease afterwards. In one animal it was low from the very beginning. Glu/Cr increased ipsilaterally in 3 of 4 animals immediately after CCII to decrease towards initial values within 24 h. One animal showed continuously depressed Glu/Cr values. Lac/Cr contralaterally remained decreased; ipsilaterally half of animals exhibited initial increases with a further increase in 3 of 4 animals at 24 hours.

Discussion

Controlled cortical impact injury (CCII) is a widely used contemporary model of experimental cerebral contusion. So far applications of MR techniques in

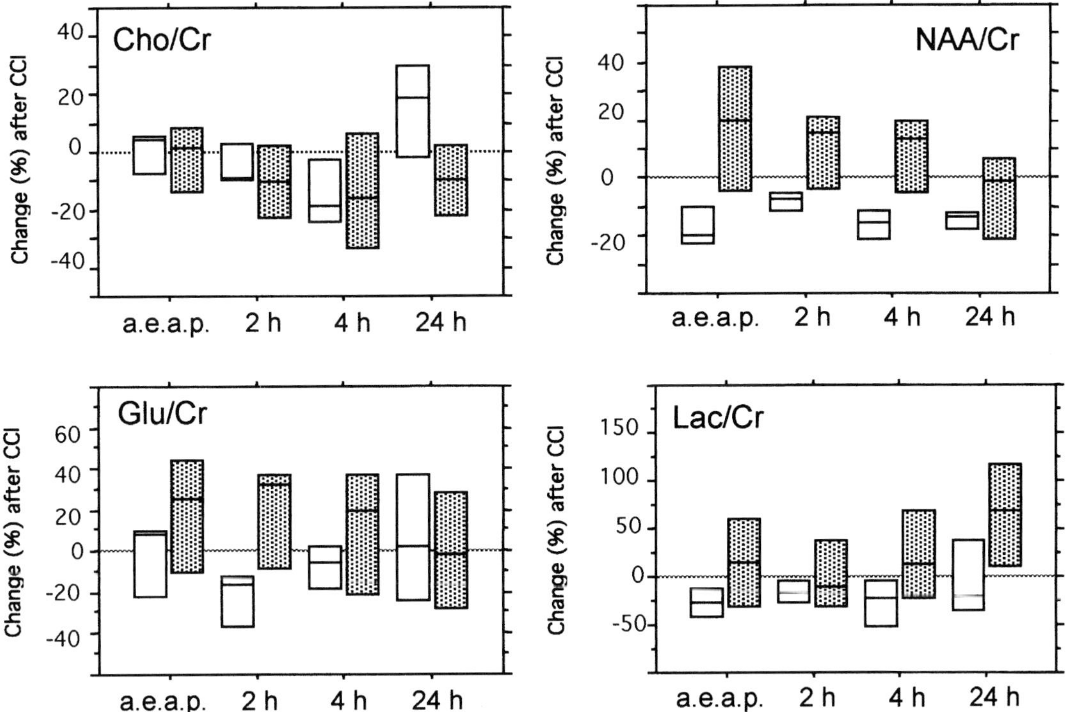

Fig. 2. The time course of the relative change of ratios compared to the value immediately before CCII is shown. For detail explanations see text. *Cho/Cr* Cholin – Creatine ratio; *NAA/Cr* N-acetylaspartate–Creatine ratio; *Glu/Cr* Glutamate – Creatine ratio; *Lac/Cr* Lactate–Creatine ratio; *a.e.a.p.* as early as possible (48 ± 10 min)

this model have focused on visualisation of contusion extension or brain oedema with T_2-weighted images and ADC maps, on demonstrating blood brain barrier damages or on measuring cerebral blood flow [2, 6, 15].

The used T_2-weighted RARE sequences in our study were very sensitive to monitor the increase in contusion and oedema volume within the first 24 h. In consistency with our results, previous studies in this model have demonstrated maximum oedema and hemispheric swelling at 24 h. MRI determination of contusion volume at 24 h [6] and oedema volume immediately post trauma and at 24 h [15] yielded results in a comparable range to our data. We observed a different time course in the increase of contusion volume versus oedema volume (see Fig. 1). Contusion volume defined as hypo- or isointense and anatomically distorted parenchyma below the craniotomy increased mostly between the 2nd and the 4th hour, probably as a result of rapidly progressive tissue transformation in the contusion core due to ischemia and necrosis. Oedema volume, defined as hyperintense parenchyma with normal structure surrounding the contusion, showed a rather steady increase over time.

Mainly phosphorous (^{31}P) and to a lesser amount proton (^{1}H) magnetic resonance spectroscopy have been extensively utilised in models of diffuse axonal injury of fluid percussion injury to monitor neuronal damage and metabolic dysfunction [1, 8, 13, 14, 18]. However, no previous investigation has applied the ^{1}H-MRS technique to the CCII model of focal brain contusion. For this pilot study which was undertaken without sham operated animals we assessed the influence of the craniotomy itself on the parameters detectable by MRI/MRS 24 h later. Although craniotomies were done with great crea and minimal manipulation of the dura, we observed signs of brain oedema and altered metabolite spectra ipsilaterally 24 h later which partly resolved at 72 h. This emphasises the sensitivity of MR techniques to detect changes following manipulation (vibrations of the drill, bone flap elevation, epidural blood collection) as the sensibility of the rat brain to these influences. These minor changes might not be detected by standard histological examinations on sham operated animals. As a result of the detected differences between craniotomised animals and normal controls, we calculated the posttraumatic changes as percent change to the value of the specific metabolite/Cr ratio determined immediately before CCII. NAA is a neuronal and axonal marker and a decrease is thought to indicate the chronic loss or damage of neurons or neuronal processes. To explain the acute drop of NAA seen immediately after fluid percussion injury, an increased utilisation for repair and regeneration was postulated since a reciprocal increase of acetate could not be seen [13]. In general the fall in NAA/Cr seen in otherwise normal appearing white matter soon after experimental trauma [14] or days to weeks after human traumatic brain injury [3, 12] is regarded as a sign of diffuse axonal injury. We saw a lower NAA/Cr ratio on the contralateral side and rather increased values in close neighbourhood to the impact. The lower levels on the contralateral side may therefore be indicative of diffuse injury. The immediate increase of NAA in tissue close to the impact might result from a release from disrupted cells or cell organs in or around severely damaged neurons which are not able to utilise it for reparative processes.

The increase in glutamate observed in 3 of 4 animals ipsilaterally is consistent with the known massive in-

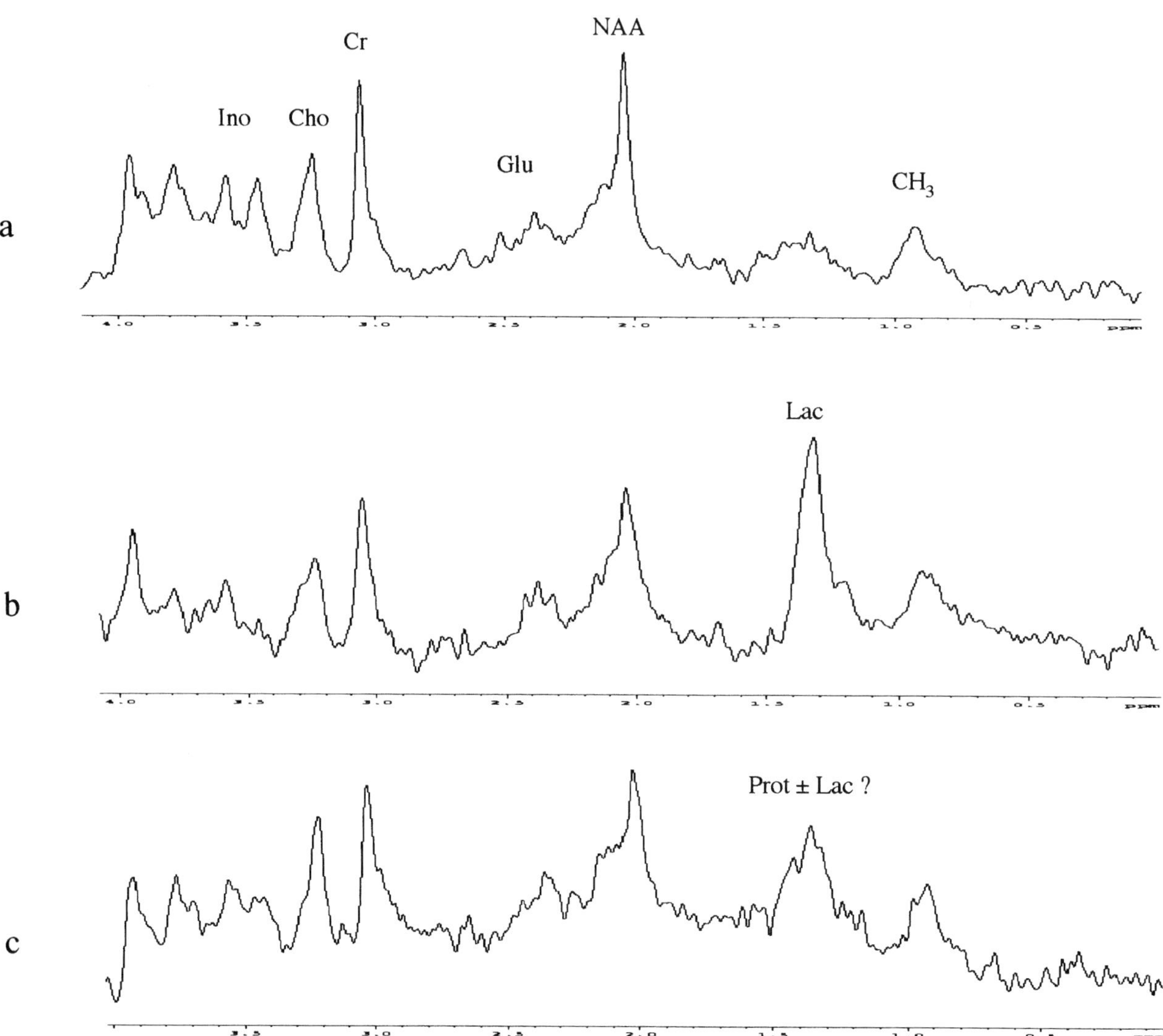

Fig. 3. Three ^{1}H magnetic resonance spectra are shown. (a) Demonstrates a normal spectrum with peak intensities as indicated without showing lactate at a chemical shift of 1.32 ppm. (b) Shows a spectrum of a normal animal the had died 10 minutes earlier due to hypoxia as a result of isoflurane overdose. A narrow and prominent peak intensity for lactate at 1.32 ppm is seen. (c) Is the spectra of an animal 4 h after CCII, demonstrating a broad hump in the lactate region which might be also due to accumulation of cytosolic proteins which have aminoacid side chains with a chemical shift very close and overlapping the intensity of lactate. Inositol *Ino*, choline compounds *Cho*, creatine + phosphocreatine *Cr*, glutamate/glutamine *Glu*, N-acetylaspartate *NAA*, lactate *Lac*, CH_3 of phospholipids *CH_3* and cytosolic proteins *Prot*

crease of interstitial excitatory aminoacids measured by microdialysis immediately following CCII [10].

The changes in the Lac/Cr ratio are difficult to interpret, since the chemical shift of lactate at 1.32 ppm is very close and partly overlapping to the chemical shift of amino acid side chains of cytosolic proteins at 1.39 ppm. All animals exhibited by the latest at 24 h not a narrow peak intensity at 1.32 ppm but a rather broad "hump" including the specific lactate shift (see Fig. 3). An intensity increase of the lactate region in water-suppressed, non-edited ^{1}H spectra following mild brain trauma has been demonstrated as a result of factors other than lactate accumulation [17]. On the other hand an acute rise in lactate paralleled by a decrease of pH was seen in a combined 31P and 1H MRS study with fluid percussion injury [8]. Consequently additional lactate editing techniques have to be applied in follow-up studies to clarify the question of lactate accumulation as a sign of disturbed energy metabolism following CCII.

The non-invasive MR techniques operating at a high field strength are an excellent tool for serial temporal monitoring of posttraumatic anatomic and metabolic changes in the rat, the most commonly used animal for experimental head injury. Although animals received comparable impacts according to the physical characteristics, we observed in this pilot study no uniformly consistent changes to be able to establish a statistical significance of the seen metabolic changes in the hippocampus regions bilaterally. Further studies with larger animal numbers and sham controls will help to clarify the metabolic changes following a type of injury which is thought to produce predominantly an unilateral brain contusion. The use of high resolution Chemical Shift Imaging might prove to be sensitive enough to clarify the extent of metabolic dysfunction with regard to the anatomical distance to the primary injury site.

References

1. Berry I, Moseley M, Germano IM, Ishige N, Nishimura MC, Bartkowski HM, Pitts LH, Brant-Zawadzki M (1986) Combined magnetic resonance imaging and spectroscopy in experimental regional injury of the brain. Ischemia and impact trauma. Acta Radiol [Suppl] (Stockh) 369: 338–349
2. Forbes ML, Hendrich KS, Kochanek PM, Williams DS, Schiding JK, Wisniewski SR, Kelsey SF, DeKosky ST, Graham SH, Marion DW, Ho C (1997) Assessment of cerebral blood flow and CO2 reactivity after controlled cortical impact by perfusion magnetic resonance imaging using arterial spinlabeling in rats. J Cereb Blood Flow Metab 17: 865–874
3. Friedman SD, Brooks WM, Jung RE, Chiulli SJ, Sloan JH, Montoya BT, Hart BL, Yeo RA (1999) Quantitative proton MRS predicts outcome after traumatic brain injury [In Process Citation]. Neurology 52: 1384–1391
4. Golding EM, Vink R (1995) Efficacy of competitive vs non-competitive blockade of the NMDA channel following traumatic brain injury. Mol Chem Neuropathol 24: 137–150
5. Heath DL, Vink R (1998) Neuroprotective effects of MgSO4 and MgCl2 in closed head injury: a comparative phosphorus NMR study. J Neurotrauma 15: 183–189
6. Kochanek PM, Marion DW, Zhang W, Schiding JK, White M, Palmer AM, Clark RS, O'Malley ME, Styren SD, Ho C (1995) Severe controlled cortical impact in rats: assessment of cerebral edema, blood flow, and contusion volume. J Neurotrauma 12: 1015–1025
7. Lighthall JW (1958) Controlled cortical impact: a new experimental brain injury model. J Neurotrauma 5: 1–15
8. McIntosh TK, Faden AI, Bendall MR, Vink R (1987) Traumatic brain injury in the rat: alterations in brain lactate and pH as characterized by 1H and 31P nuclear magnetic resonance. J Neurochem 49: 1530–1540
9. McIntosh TK, Vink R, Soares H, Hayes R, Simon R (1990) Effect of noncompetitive blockade of N methyl-D-aspartate receptors on the neurochemical sequelae of experimental brain injury: J Neurochem 55: 1170–1179
10. Palmer AM, Marion DW, Botscheller ML, Swedlow PE, Styren SD, DeKosky ST (1993) Traumatic brain injury-induced excitotoxicity assessed in a controlled cortical impact model. J Neurochem 61: 2015–2024
11. Prichard JW (1992) Magnetic resonance spectroscopy of the brain. Clin Chim Acta 206: 115–123
12. Ross BD, Ernst T, Kreis R, Haseler LJ, Bayer S, Danielsen E, Bluml S, Shonk T, Mandigo JC, Caton W, Clark C, Jensen SW, Lehman NL, Arcinue E, Pudenz R, Shelden CH (1998) 1H MRS in acute traumatic brain injury. J Magn Reson Imaging 8: 829–840
13. Rubin Y, Cecil K, Wehrli S, McIntosh TK, Lenkinski RE, Smith DH (1997) High-resolution 1H NMR spectroscopy following experimental brain trauma. J Neurotrauma 14: 441–449
14. Smith DH, Cecil KM, Meaney DF, Chen XH, McIntosh TK, Gennarelli TA, Lenkinski RE (1998) Magnetic resonance spectroscopy of diffuse brain trauma in the pig. J Neurotrauma 15: 665–674
15. Stroop R, Thomale UW, Pauser S, Bernarding J, Vollmann W, Wolf KJ, Lanksch WR, Unterberg AW (1998) Magnetic resonance imaging studies with cluster algorithm for characterization of brain edema after controlled cortical impact injury (CCII). Acta Neurochir [Suppl] (Wien) 71: 303–305
16. Vink R, Faden AI, McIntosh TK (1988) Changes in cellular bioenergetic state following graded traumatic brain injury in rats: determination by phosphorus 31 magnetic resonance spectroscopy. J Neurotrauma 5: 315–330
17. Vink R, McIntosh TK, Faden AI (1988) Nonedited 1H NMR lactate/n-acetyl aspartate ratios and the in vivo determination of lactate concentration in brain. Magn Reson Med 7: 95–99
18. Vink R, McIntosh TK, Weiner MW, Faden AI (1987) Effects of traumatic brain injury on cerebral high-energy phosphates and pH: a 31P magnetic resonance spectroscopy study. J Cereb Blood Flow Metab 7: 563–571

Correspondence: Martin U. Schuhmann, M.D., Neurochirurgische Klinik, Medizinische Hochschule Hannover, Carl-Neuberg-Str. 1, D-30625 Hannover, Germany.

Acta Neurochir (2000) [Suppl] 76: 9–12

Heterogeneous Mechanisms of Early Edema Formation in Cerebral Contusion: Diffusion MRI and ADC Mapping Study

T. Kawamata, Y. Katayama, N. Aoyama, and **T. Mori**

Department of Neurological Surgery, Nihon University School of Medicine, Tokyo, Japan

Summary

Severe cerebral contusion is sometimes associated with early edema formation within 24–48 hours post-trauma, and this frequently results in progressive ICP elevation and clinical deterioration. To investigate the underlying mechanisms of such severe contusion edema, diffusion imaging and ADC mapping were performed in 20 patients with cerebral contusion, employing 1.5 T echo planar MRI. Within 24 hours post-trauma, the diffusion images demonstrated a low intensity core in the central area and a high intensity rim in the peripheral area of contusion. The ADC value increased in the central area (ADC ratio (contusion/normal brain) = 1.13 ± 0.13) and decreased in the peripheral area (ADC ratio = 0.83 ± 0.13). This suggested that intra- and extracellular components underwent disintegration and homogenization within the central area, whereas cellular swelling was predominant in the peripheral area. A crescent-shaped zone of very high ADC value (ADC ratio = 1.38 ~ 1.61) was observed at the border between these two areas during the period of 24–48 hours post-trauma in some cases, apparently indicating that edema fluid was accumulated within a space formed by homogenization. The ADC values in the peripheral area shifted to an increase after 48–72 hours post-trauma. These findings imply that multiple mechanisms operate in early edema formation in cerebral contusion. It appears that the capacity for edema fluid accumulation increases in the central area and resistance for edema fluid propagation is elevated by cellular swelling in the peripheral area. We suggest that a combination of such events facilitates edema fluid accumulation in the central area and contributes, together with the cellular swelling in the peripheral area, to the mass effect of contusion edema. Diffusion MRI and ADC mapping represent powerful tools for investigating spatially as well as temporally heterogeneous mechanisms of contusion edema.

Keywords: Cerebral contusion; brain edema; diffusion image; ADC.

Introduction

Severe cerebral contusion is sometimes associated with early massive edema within 24–48 hours post-trauma. This often results in progressive intracranial pressure (ICP) elevation and clinical deterioration [7]. The precise mechanisms underlying such early contusion edema are not yet clearly understood. The early contusion edema, in contrast to delayed peri-contusion edema [3, 10, 11, 14], does not display the characteristics of vasogenic edema [5, 15]. Evaluations of the vascular permeability by 99mTc pertechnetate single photon emission CT [3], Gd-DTPA enhanced MRI [2, 7] and post-mortem immunohistochemical investigations [14] have failed to reveal any evidence of an increased vascular permeability within the area of contusion during the initial few days post-trauma. In contrast, diffusion images and apparent diffusion coefficient (ADC) mapping with echo planar MRI have provided data which are consistent with the idea that the early edema formation following traumatic brain injury (TBI) is, at least partially, cytotoxic in nature [6].

We previously proposed another mechanism for the early contusion edema; viz., that an elevated osmolality within the area of contusion necrosis, a direct consequence of mechanical impact (contusion necrosis proper [12]), plays an important role in edema formation in cerebral contusion [9]. The area of contusion necrosis is histopathologically evident at as early as 3 hours post-trauma [4]. The cellular elements in this well-demarcated area, both neuronal as well as glial, uniformly undergo shrinkage, and then disintegration, homogenation and cyst formation [8]. Unlike the cells in the area surrounding the contusion necrosis proper, they never exhibit swelling [12]. In the present study, we attempted to characterize the evolution of this area during the period of early contusion edema based on diffusion images and ADC mapping in patients with cerebral contusion.

Materials and Methods

A total of 20 patients with cerebral contusion were investigated during the period from April 1997 to December 1998. These patients were selected for the present study on the basis of the following criteria: GCS ≥ 9, no hypoxic episodes, no massive ICP increase, no massive intracerebral hematoma, no severe multiple injury and no severe systemic complications. The individuals selected with these criteria represented patients who had mild or moderate cerebral contusion with a relatively good clinical condition. The Glasgow Outcome Scale (GOS) at hospital discharge was MD in 9 patients and GR in 11 patients. No patients revealed a GOS of SD, VS, or D.

MRI (Siemens 1.5 T echo planar Magnetom Vision) was performed within 24 hours post-trauma in 4 cases, at 24–72 hours in 7 cases, and at 4–20 days in 9 cases. Following conventional T1- and T2-weighted imaging, diffusion images were obtained (TR: 0.8 ms, TE: 120 ms, matrix: 128×128, slice: 5 mm), and ADC mapping was computed from various b factor diffusion images. With reference to the T1- and T2-weighted, and diffusion images, several regions of interest (ROI) for ADC were defined in the central area and the peripheral area of cerebral contusion. When contusion hemorrhage was observed on the T1- and T2-weighted images, the area of hemorrhage was carefully excluded from the ROI. The ADC ratio (= ADC in contusion / ADC in normal brain) was calculated by dividing the ADC values in the ROI by a reference ADC value which was obtained from normal brain tissue of the contralateral side.

Results

The diffusion images during the early period (<48 hours post-trauma) demonstrated a low intensity core in the central area and a high intensity rim in the peripheral area of cerebral contusion (Fig. 1). This pattern was typically observed within 24 hours post-trauma. The ADC values increased in the central area (ADC ratio = 1.13 ± 0.13) and decreased in the peripheral area of contusion (ADC ratio = 0.83 ± 0.13) (Table 1). A crescent-shaped zone with very high ADC values (ADC ratio = $1.38 \sim 1.61$) developed at the border between the central and peripheral areas after 24 hours post-trauma, in 3 of 7 cases (43%) in which MRI was undertaken during the period of 24–72 hours post-trauma (Table 1). The crescent-shaped zone was always located in deep brain areas at the bottom of the cerebral contusion (Fig. 2). No case displayed such a crescent-shaped zone within 24 hours post-trauma. The crescent-shaped zone still existed at 2 weeks post-trauma in 3 cases (33%) (Fig. 3). The ADC values in the peripheral area shifted to an increase after 48–72 hours post-trauma (Table 1).

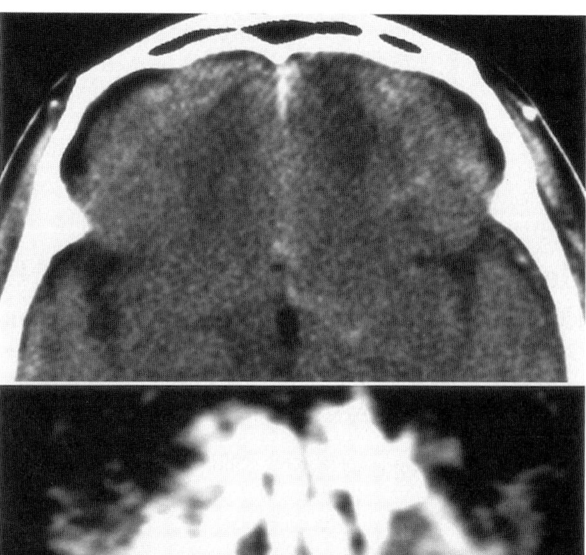

Fig. 1. Representative case of cerebral contusion in the acute phase, 36 hours post-trauma. (Upper) CT scan revealing a low density area in the bilateral frontal lobe. (Lower) Diffusion image demonstrating a low intensity core with a surrounding high intensity rim, which was the typical pattern of the diffusion images at the acute phase (<48 hours post-trauma) of cerebral contusion without massive hemorrhage. The ADC values were separately evaluated in the central and the peripheral area of contusion

Table 1. *ADC Values and Number of Cases Revealing with a Crescent-Shaped Zone with a High ADC Value at Each Time Point*

	<24 hr	24–72 hr	4–14 days
ADC ratio in central area	1.13 ± 0.13	1.31 ± 0.27	1.26 ± 0.22
ADC ratio in the peripheral area	0.83 ± 0.13	0.79 ± 0.18	1.16 ± 0.21
Crescent-shaped zone	0/4 = 0%	3/7 = 43%	3/9 = 33%

Discussion

The present study employing echo planar MRI with high spatial resolution confirmed a heterogeneous pathophysiology for cerebral contusion. An early histopathological investigation reported by Lindenberg *et al.* [12] demonstrated the presence of two components in cerebral contusion; one comprises the area of contusion necrosis proper and the other is the surrounding area in which microthrombosis and cellular swelling are observed. These two components are clearly separated by a line of demarcation. The central area of cerebral contusion which demonstrates high ADC values appears to correspond to the area of contusion necrosis proper, since cellular disintegration and homogeniza-

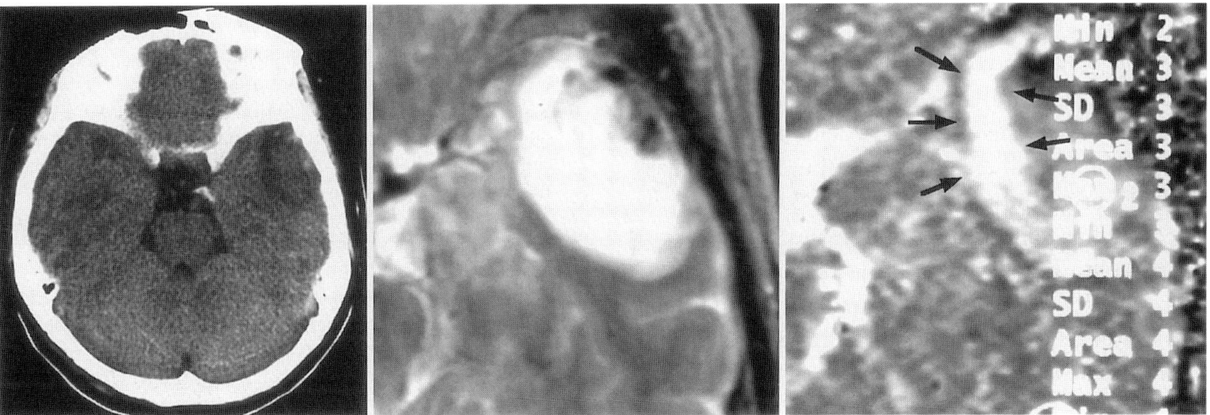

Fig. 2. Representative case of cerebral contusion in the temporal tip at 45 hours post-trauma. (Left) CT scan revealing a small LD area in the temporal tip. (Middle) T2-weighted MRI demonstrating a mixed intensity area in the core of contusion and surrounding edema formation. (Right) ADC mapping showing a crescent-shaped zone (arrows)

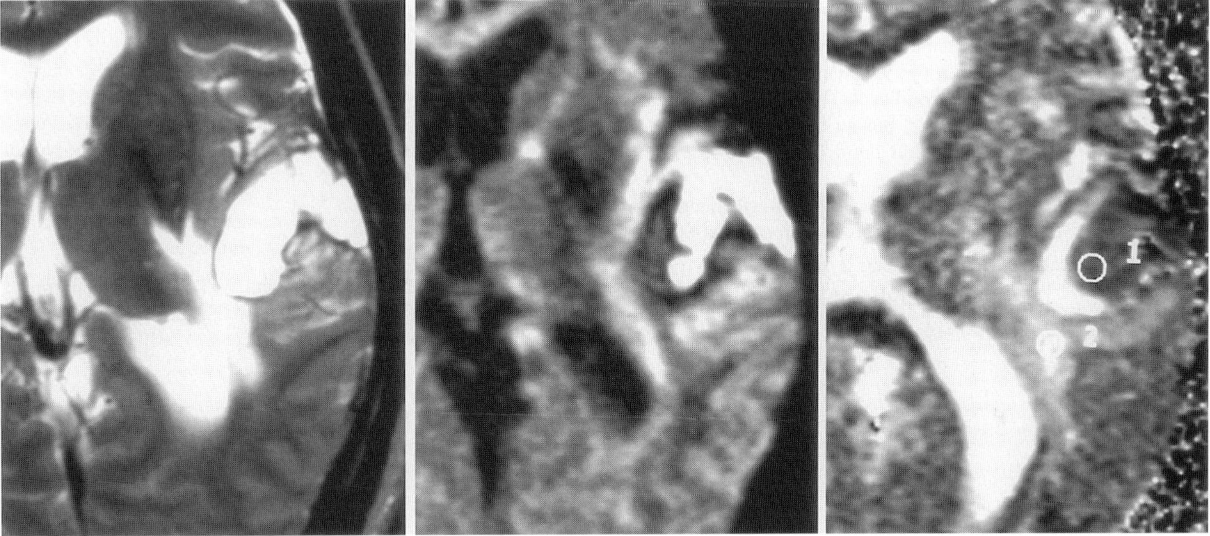

Fig. 3. Representative case of cerebral contusion in the subacute phase, 2 weeks post-trauma. (Left) T2-weighted image. (Middle) Diffusion image. (Right) ADC mapping. A crescent-shaped zone with a high ADC value still existed. The ADC value in the peripheral area of contusion increased, indicating that vasogenic edema became predominant

tion in this area would result in an expansion of the extracellular space [8]. The peripheral area of cerebral contusion in which the ADC values decrease, appears to correspond to the surrounding area, since cellular the swelling which is predominant in this area would result in a shrinkage of the extracellular space.

It appears that expansion of the extracellular space in the central area increases the capacity for edema fluid accumulation [8]. In contrast, the shrinkage of the extracellular space in the peripheral area increases the resistance for edema fluid propagation or resolution. Since the ADC values of the crescent-shaped zone at the border between the central and peripheral areas is very high, this zone may represent edema fluid accumulated within the area of contusion necrosis proper. We have demonstrated previously that a marked increase in tissue osmolality occurs within the area of contusion necrosis proper [9]. It is uncertain whether or not such a marked increase in osmolality is osmotically active and causes edema fluid accumulation. We hypothesize that the barrier formed by swollen cells in the peripheral area may prevent edema fluid propagation and also help to create an osmotic potential within the central area. Since blood flow is greatly decreased but is not completely interrupted in contused brain tissue [1], water is continuously supplied from the blood into the central area. We suggest that a combination of these events facilitates edema fluid accumulation in the central area and contributes to the mass effect of early contusion edema. In conclusion, the present findings imply that multiple mechanisms exist in early contusion edema. Diffusion images and ADC mapping offer powerful tools for investigating spatially as well as temporally heterogeneous mechanisms of contusion edema.

References

1. Alexander MJ, Martin NA, Khanna M *et al* (1994) Regional cerebral blood flow trends in head injured patients with focal contusions and cerebral edema. Acta Neurochir (Wien) s60: 479–481
2. Barzó P, Marmarou A, Fatouros P *et al* (1996) Magnetic resonance imaging-monitored acute blood-brain barrier changes in experimental traumatic brain injury. J Neurosurg 85: 1113–1121
3. Bullock R, Statham J, Patterson D *et al* (1990) The time course of vasogenic oedema after focal human head injury: evidence from SPECT mapping of blood brain barrier defects. Acta Neurochir (Wien) s51: 286–288
4. Eriskat J, Schurer L, Kempski O, *et al* (1994) Growth kinetics of a primary brain tissue necrosis from focal lesion. Acta Neurochir (Wien) s60: 425–427
5. Evans JP, Scheinker IM (1945) Histologic studies of the brain following head trauma. I. Post-traumatic cerebral swelling and edema. J Neurosurg 2: 306–314
6. Ito J, Marmarou A, Barzó P *et al* (1996) Characterization of edema by diffusion-weighted imaging in experimental traumatic brain injury. J Neurosurg 84: 97–103
7. Katayama Y, Tsubokawa T, Miyazaki S *et al* (1990) Oedema fluid formation within contused brain tissue as a cause of medically uncontrollable elevation of intracranial pressure in head trauma patients. Acta Neurochir (Wien) s51: 308–310
8. Katayama Y, Tsubokawa T, Kinoshita K *et al* (1992) Intraparenchymal fluid-blood levels in traumatic intracerebral hematomas. Neuroradiol 34: 381–383
9. Katayama Y, Mori T, Maeda T *et al* (1999) Pathogenesis of the mass effect of cerebral contusions: rapid increase in osmolality within the contusion necrosis. Acta Neurochir (Wien) (in press)
10. Kushi H, Katayama Y, Shibuya T *et al* (1994) Gd-DTPA enhanced magnetic resonance imaging of cerebral contusions. Acta Neurochir (Wien) s60: 472–474
11. Lang DA, Hadley DM, Teasdale GT *at al* (1991) Gadolinium DTPA enhanced magnetic resonance imaging in acute head injury. Acta Neurochir (Wien) 109: 5–11
12. Lindenberg R, Freytag E (1957) Morphology of cortical contusion. Arch Path 63: 23–42
13. Madsen FF (1990) Regional cerebral blood flow after a localized cerebral contusion in pigs. Acta Neurochir (Wien) 105: 150–157
14. Todd NV, Graham DI (1990) Blood brain barrier damage in traumatic brain contusion. Acta Neurochir (Wien) s51: 296–299
15. Tornheim PA, Prioleau GR, McLaurin RL (1984) Acute responses to experimental blunt head trauma: topography of cerebral cortical edema. J Neurosurg 60: 473–480

Correspondence: Tatsuro Kawamata, M.D., Ph.D., Department of Neurological Surgery, Nihon University School of Medicine, 30-1 Oyaguchi Kamimachi, Itabashi-ku, Tokyo 173-8610, Japan.

Acta Neurochir (2000) [Suppl] 76: 13–16

Metabolic Changes in Pericontusional Oedematous Areas in Mild Head Injury Evaluated by ^{1}H MRS

B. C. Son[1], C.-K. Park[1], B.-G. Choi[2], E.-N. Kim[2], B.-Y. Choe[2], K.-S. Lee[1], M.-C. Kim[1], and J.-K. Kang[1]

[1] Department of Neurosurgery, Kangnam St. Mary's Hospital, College of Medicine, The Catholic University of Korea, Seoul, Korea
[2] Department of Radiology, Kangnam St. Mary's Hospital, College of Medicine, The Catholic University of Korea, Seoul, Korea

Summary

In order to define metabolic brain changes associated with mild traumatic brain injury, proton magnetic resonance spectroscopy (MRS) was performed in patients with regional brain contusion and 13–15 of initial GCS score. The authors measured N-acetylasparta-te(NAA)/creatine(Cr) ratio and lactate signal on in vivo proton MRS, which indicated cell loss and ischaemic demage respectively, in pericontusional oedematous areas (region of interest; ROI) adjacent to trauamtic brain contusion on brain MRI to determine possible metabolic changes.

The metabolic ratio of NAA/Cr and lactate/Cr peaks was measured both in the ROI and a corresponding region of the contralateral hemisphere (ROC) in seven patients and twenty-five normal control.

In initial NAA/Cr ratios, the values of ROIs were significantly lower than those of the control ($p = 0.009$), but there was no difference either between ROI and ROC ($p = 0.410$) or between ROC of patients and the control ($p = 0.199$). In lactate/Cr ratios, the ROI in all seven patients and the ROC in two showed increased lactate signals. The lacate/Cr ratios of the ROIs were significantly elevated as compared to those of the ROCs ($p = 0.02$) and the control ($p = 0.015$). In 2-month follow up, lactate signals were absent or significantly reduced ($p = 0.015$). In no patients, clinical or radiological deterioration has been observed.

Our results demonstrate that there is significant neuronal dysfunction in pericontusional oedematous areas as indicated by NAA/Cr ratios in the patients with mild head injury at both early and late stages. And there are significant ischaemic changes as indicated by increase of lactate level in ROI at early stage. These findings suggest that pericontusional oedematous areas can be vulnerable to secondary brain insults even in the patients with mild head injury.

Keywords: Mild traumatic brain injury; proton magnetic resonance spectroscopy; brain contusion; secondary ischaemic insult.

Introduction

Proton MRS is a noninvasive method that allows us to assess in vivo brain tissue composition and metabolic process in neurologic disorders. The potential for obtaining good spatial localization and serial measurements with high resolution makes in vivo proton MRS an ideal investigative tool for brain function of biochemical interaction [2]. The prevention of secondary insult in traumatic brain injury has been emphasized especially in severe head injury patients wit GCS score <8. And there were several documents observing the metabolic changes in severe and acute stages of traumatic brain injury by proton MRS [1, 3, 4, 5, 8]. But there has been few reports dealing with metabolic changes in mild head injury patients (GCS 13–15). Brain contusion is common pathology in both mild and severe traumatic brain injuries and surrounding pericontusional oedematous area is suitable for voxel selection and studying metabolic changes in MRS, because this area could be vulnerable to secondary brain damage. The authors investigated the regional metabolic changes in mild head injury patients (GCS 13–15), by observing spatial and chronological changes of metabolic markers, NAA/Cr and lactate/Cr ratio of proton MRS in pericontusional oedematous areas.

Materials and Methods

During the period from June 1998 to January 1999, seven head injury patients with initial GCS 13–15 (3 males and 4 females: age range 15–65 years, mean age 33 years) and 25 normal controls (15 males and 10 females: age range 25–45) were included. Patients with ages under 15 and over 65 years and patients with combined subdural or epidural hematoma were excluded. Each patient presented definite haemorrhagic contusion on the initial CT scan and all had high signal oedematous area adjacent to haemorrhagic contusion on the T2-weighted MRI. There was no evidence of secondary insults such as hypotension or hypoxia. The patients' profile is described in table 1. Proton MRS study was done initially within 7 days after injury in all seven patients. Follow-up study was done at 2 months after injury in five patients. Control subjects were recruited from the fifteen Catholic University Medical Center staffs and ten other healthy volunteers.

Table 1. *Clinical Features of Patients*

Case no.	1	2	3	4	5	6	7
Age	60	45	32	15	18	25	52
Cause of TBI	MVA	FD	assault	FD	MVA	FD	FD
Initial GCS	15	14	13	14	13	14	13
Neurologic deficit	·	·	·	·	·	·	·
Episode							
– of hypoxia	·	·	·	·	·	·	·
– hypotension	·	·	·	·	·	·	·
Outcome (GOS)	GR	GR	GR	GR	GR	GR	GR

MVA Motor vehicle accident; *FD* fall down; *GR* good recovery.

All localized, water-suppressed in vivo ^{1}H MRS studies were performed on a 1.5T Siemens vision plus MRI/MRS system using a spin echo single voxel study. As a single voxel technique, $2 \times 2 \times 2$ cm^3 voxel was selected in pericontusional oedmatous area adjacent to contusion using spin-echo sequence (repetition time 1500 ms; echo time, 135–270 ms, number of aquisition 128–256). The ROI was noted in the frontal or temporal lobe, the prevalent site for contusion. Then the MRS voxel study was also carried out on the corresponding white-gray matter of the contralateral hemisphere (ROC) as a reference. Care was taken to avoid the contusion and normal brain around the ROI. Proton resonance in the spectra obtained from brain tissues was assigned on the basis of prior assignments [10]. Resonance peak assignments of major proton MRS were lactate, 1.30 ppm; CH3 of NAA, 2.01 ppm; N-CH3 of Cr, 3.00 ppm; N-(CH3)3 of Cho, 3.20 ppm. To obtain the relative metabolic ratios, Cr was used as a putative reference [11]. The metabolic ratios of NAA/Cr and lactate/Cr were compared between ROIs, ROCs and control values. In follow-up MRS studies, the value of the metabolic markers was taken from the same sites as in the initial studies.

Statistical analysis was performed using SPSS (SPSS for Windows, version 8.0, SPSS Inc., Chicago, IL). The data were analyzed with t-test, paired-sample t-tests, where $P < 0.05$ was considered significant.

Results

Figure 1 shows the typical voxel selection and proton MR spectra on the pericontusional oedematous area (ROI) and in the contralateral hemisphere (ROC). The results are presented in table 2. In normal brain, proton MR spectrum consists of three well-defined peaks, representing the concentration of choline, total creatine (creatine plus phosphocreatine) and NAA. Lactate is either not discernible as a peak, or presents in extremely small amount. Absolute concentrations were not calibrated, and concentrations of metabolites were expressed as a ratio of one metabolite (creatine) to another rather than absolute concentrations.

NAA/Cr ratios

The initial NAA/Cr ratios were compared with the control values. The values of ROIs were significantly lower than those of the control ($p = 0.0009$). But there was no difference either between ROIs and ROCs ($p = 0.410$) or between ROCs and the control ($p = 0.199$). In the comparison of ROIs between initial studies ($n = 7$) and 2-month follow up ($n = 5$), there was no significant difference either ($p = 0.263$).

Lactate/Cr ratios

The ROIs in all seven patients and the ROCs in two showed increased lactate signals. The lactate/Cr ratios of the ROIs were significantly elevated as compared to those of the ROCs ($p = 0.02$) and those of the control ($p = 0.015$). In 2-month follow-up ($n = 5$), lactate/Cr ratio of ROI became undetectable in two and reduced significantly in the remaining three ($p = 0.015$).

The clinical course was uneventful in all seven patients. There was neither neurologic nor radiologic deterioration. All the patients returned to pre-injury social activities.

Discussion

Over the past decades, the importance of secondary brain insults has become increasingly recognized in terms of patient outcome and possible therapeutic intervention. Cerebral ischaemia may be the single most important secondary event affecting outcome following severe traumatic brain injury (TBI) [7]. But the significance of secondary insult has not well known in mild head injury.

Proton MRS is an exellent in vivo technique for detecting neurochemical alterations associated with pathological conditions. There has been several documents observing biochemical changes using MRS in severe TBI [1, 3, 4, 5]. But there were few documents about the metabolic changes associated with mild head injury. So the authors evaluated the patients with focal

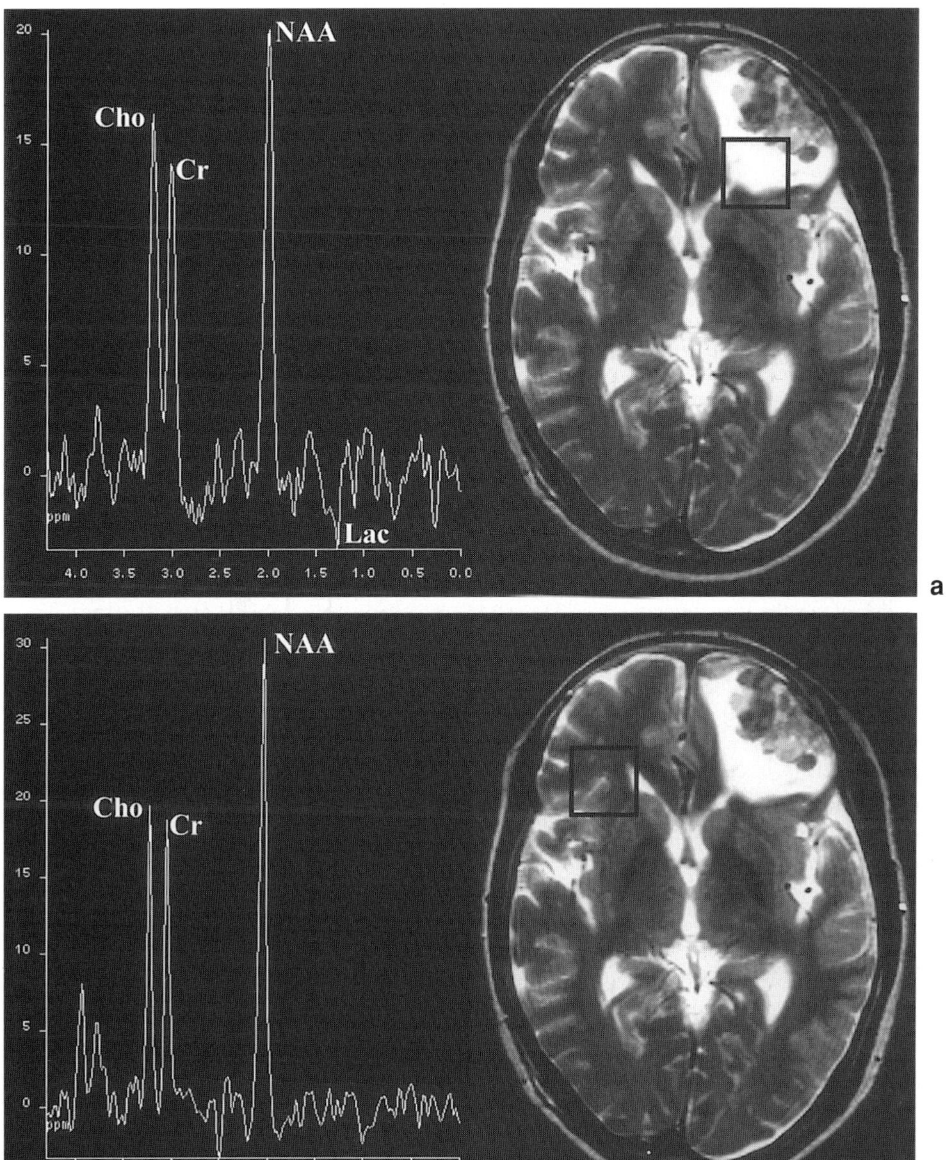

Fig. 1. Typical voxel sites for the pericontusional oedematous area (a: ROI) and the corresponding area in the contralateral hemisphere (b: ROC). Voxel of ROI was selected in the high signal oedematous area adjacent to contusion on T2 weighted image. There is typical lactate signal (Lac) on the spectrum of MRS in the pericontusional oedematous area in Fig. a (ROI)

brain contusion but high GCS score [13–15], especially focusing upon the pericontusional edematous areas, perhaps the only vulnerable area to secondary insult in this kind of patients.

NAA is located exclusively in neurons [8], and believed to be a neuronal marker [6]. It has been shown that the reduction in NAA peak was associated with pathological conditions of neuron, which strongly suggested that neuronal and axonal loss or dysfunction can be detected by proton MRS [3]. In the current study, the initial value of NAA/Cr ratios in ROI was significantly different from that in the control, but was insignificant when compared with that in ROCs and follow-up ROI value. These results indicate that some kinds of neuronal dysfunction might be present in the pericontusional areas even until 2 months postinjury. But it is hard to conclude that there is neuronal dysfunction in the contralateral hemisphere in spite of no difference in the values between ROI and ROC, because there was no difference in the value of NAA/Cr

Table 2. *Spectroscopic Data in Pericontusional Edematous Zone*

Case no.	Time after trauma	Location of cont.	NAA/Cr ratio		Lactate	
			ROI*	ROC*	ROI	ROC
Controls			1.92 ± 0.6692		0 (5.960E-02)	
1 – 1*	7 d	T	0.42	0.52	0.3	0
–2*	2 m	T	0.50	0.87	0.21	0
–3*	4 m	T	0.58	2.69	0	0
2 – 1	7 d	T	1.40	1.12	0.50	0
–2	2 m	T	1.38	1.50	0	0
3 – 1	7 d	F	1.36	1.87	0.21	0.13
–2	2 m	F	2.35	2.02	0	0
4 – 1	7 d	T	0.98	0.55	0.27	0
–2	4 m	T	1.05	0.94	0.01	0
5	5 d	T	1.68	1.68	0.19	0
6	7 d	T	1.65	1.58	0.28	0
7 – 1	2 d	T	0.67	3.27	0.51	0.28
–2	2 m	T	0.77	1.34	0.12	0.05

Cont. Contusion; *F* frontal; *T* temporal; *ROI* region of interest; *ROC* contralateral ROI; *d* days after trauma; *m* months after trasuma; *–1** initial values; *–2** values at 2-month follow up; *–3** values at 4-month follow up.

ratio between ROC and the control. Lactate, although not normally present, is detectable in ischaemia. Lactate accumulation characterizes energy production in the presence of inadequate oxygen supply, i.e. anaerobic glycolysis [4]. And lactate is generally thought as a marker of ischaemia. But there is still controversy about the origin and time course of lactate in TBI [4, 9]. In the current study, the initial lactate/Cr ratio in ROI was significantly elevated compared to that in ROC and the controls. In 2-month follow-up study, the lactate level of ROI declined significantly in three and absent in two patients. These findings suggest that there may be ischaemic changes in pericontusional oedematous areas in early stage after trauma and these changes gradually resolve with time.

Our results demonstrate that there is not only significant neronal dysfunction but also possible ischaemic change in pericontusional oedematous area in the patients of high GCS score with focal brain contusion. Even patients with mild head injury could be vulnerable to secondary brain insults as long as they have brain contusion.

References

1. Auld KL, Ashwal S, Holshouser BA, Tomasi LG, Perkin RM, Ross BM, Hinshaw DB Jr (1995) Proton magnetic resonance spectroscopy in children with acute central nervous system injury. Pediatr Neurol 12(4): 323–334
2. Bottomley PA (1989) Human in vivo NMR spectroscopy in diagnostic medicine: clinical tool or research probe? Radiol 170: 1–15
3. Cecil KM, Hills EC, Sandel ME, Smith DH, McIntosh TK, Mannon LJ, Sinson GP, Bagley LJ, Grossman RI, Lenkinski RE (1988) Proton magnetic resonance spectroscopy for detection of axonal injury in the splenium of the corpus callosum of brain-injured patients. J Neurosurg 88: 795–801
4. Condon B, Oluoch-Olunya D, Hardley D, Teasdale G, Wagstaff A (1998) Early 1H magnetic resonance spectroscopy of acute head injury: four cases. J Neurotrauma 15(8): 563–571
5. Holshouser BA, Ashwal S, Luh GY, Shu S, Kahlon S, Auld KL, Tomasi LG, Perkin RM, Hinshaw DB Jr (1997) Proton MR spectroscopy after acute central nervous system injury: outcome prediction in neonates, infants, and children. Radiol 202(2): 487–496
6. Miller BL (1991) A review of chemical issues in ^{1}H NMR spectroscopy: N-acetylaspartate, creatine and choline. NMR Biomed 4: 47–52
7. Miller JD (1985) Head injury and brain ischemia-Implications for therapy. Br J Anaesth 57: 120–130
8. Nadler JV, Cooper JR (1972) N-acetyl-L-aspartatic acid content of human neuronal tumors and bovine peripheral nervous tissues. J Neurochem 19: 313–319
9. Pellerin L, Magistretti P (1994) Glutamate uptake into astrocytes stimulates aerobic glycolysis: a mechanism coupling neuronal activity to glucose utilization. Proc Natl Acad Sci USA 91: 10625–10629
10. Petroff OAC, Spencer DD, Alger JR, Prichard JW (1989) High-field proton magnetic resonance spectroscopy of human cerebrum obtained during surgery for epilepsy. Neurol 39: 1197–1202
11. Ross B, Kreis R, Ernst T (1992) Clinical tools for the 90s: Magnetic resonance spectroscopy and metabolic imaging. Eur J Radiol 14: 128–140

Correspondence: Chun-Kun Park, M.D., Department of Neurosurgery, Kangnam St. Mary's Hospital, 505 Banpo-Dong, Seocho-Ku, Seoul, 137-040, Korea.

Acta Neurochir (2000) [Suppl] 76: 17–20

Malignancy of Brain Tumors Evaluated by Proton Magnetic Resonance Spectroscopy (^{1}H-MRS) in Vitro

Z. Czernicki[1], **D. Horsztyński**[1], **W. Jankowski**[3], **P. Grieb**[2], and **J. Walecki**[4]

[1] Department of Neurosurgery, Medical Research Centre, Polish Academy of Sciences, Warsaw, Poland
[2] Laboratory of Experimental Pharmacology, Medical Research Centre, Polish Academy of Sciences, Warsaw, Poland
[3] Department of Lipid Biochemistry, Institute of Biochemistry and Biophysics, Polish Academy of Sciences, Warsaw, Poland
[4] Department of Radiology, Medical Centre of Postgraduate Education, Warsaw, Poland

Abstract

Biopsies of 6 malignant gliomas (grade 3 or 4) and 11 low-grade meningiomas were extracted with perchloric acid or methanol/water, and the fully-relaxed ^{1}H-MRS spectra of the extracts containing water-soluble metabolites and a concentration and chemical shift standard were recorded at 11.4 T. The resonance signals assigned to inositol (Ino), glycerophospho- and phosphocholine (GPC + PC), choline (Cho), creatine and phosphocreatine (Cr + PCr), glutamate (Glu), acetate (Ac), alanine (Ala) and lactate (Lac) were integrated, and analyzed by two methods. First, the concentrations of the aforementioned substances in the bioptates were estimated from their resonance signals in the extracts. Second, these signals were normalized to the Cr + PCr resonance signal. The Mann-Whitney U-test was used to verify statistical significance between the data sets obtained for gliomas and meningiomas. When the first method of analysis was used, the only difference was in the Ala concentration, which in meningiomas was on average 4 times higher than in gliomas ($P < 0.01$). However, when the second method of analysis was applied, gliomas expressed lower normalized resonance signals of Ala and Glu ($P < 0.001$, ranges not overlapping), Lac ($P < 0.005$), as well as Ino and GPC + PC ($P < 0.05$). In proton MR spectra of brain tumor tissue extracts containing water soluble metabolites, the resonance signals normalized to that of total creatine may provide a very good discrimination between malignant gliomas and low-grade meningiomas.

Keywords: Glioma; meningioma; magnetic resonance spectroscopy; metabolite ratios.

Introduction

In vitro proton magnetic resonance (^{1}H MR) of extracts from intracranial tumor biopsies provide a complex qualitative and quantitative information concerning parent samples, which may possibly be used for automatic, objective classification of these tumors. Two most recent reports illustrate different approaches which may be employed to interpret the extracts' resonance spectra in terms of tumor classification. Maxwell *et al.* [4], without taking any *a priori* assumptions concerning metabolite importance for tumor biology, used pattern recognition techniques (factor analysis and neural networks) to establish complex features of the wide-range spectra of perchloric-acid (PCA) tissue extracts that would differentiate between the histological classes of the tumors. Prior to the analysis the resonance signals were normalized to the full-range spectrum integral (exclusive of lactate, which was not considered for technical reasons). Interestingly, over the 0–4.5 ppm range, data related only to very few compounds (creatine, glutamine, alanine and inositol) proved discriminative, while the use of more information just added noise to the classification. Sabatier *et al.* [6] have focused on the "choline peak" in the spectra of PCA extracts. When the resonance of choline-containing compounds was resolved into fractions assigned to glycerophosphocholine (GPC), phosphocholine (PC) and choline (Cho), highly significant differences were found between high- and low-grade gliomas, the former having lower GPC, but higher PC and Cho fraction, than the latter.

A major factor confounding the interpretation of the proton MR spectra in vitro may relate to the fact that tumor samples contain randomly variable proportions of viable and necrotic tissues, chemical composition of which is certainly different. Random changes in the relative contribution of necrotic compartment may distort the spectra and increase heterogeneity of the data. Necrotic areas may encounter the loss of creatine compounds. In the heart total tissue creatine content has been utilized as the measure of tissue necrosis, both in humans with the history of myocardial infarction and in an animal model of infarction [1]. On the other hand, viable tumor cells may keep Cr + PCr at a concentration relatively stable, and characteristic for a given histologic subtype and malignancy grade. No marker specific either for viable, or for necrotic tissues has been described. However, if a metabolite concentration in a tumor extract originates mainly from viable tumor cells, its resonance signal normalized to that of the total creatine may prove more discriminative in respect to tumor histology than its concentration in the parent sample.

In the present exploratory study we compare two methods of analysis of the proton resonance spectra of water-soluble metabolites extracted from a small number of biopsies taken from two extreme classes of intracranial tumors, high grade malignant gliomas and benign meningiomas, in respect to their relative power in discriminating between these two pathologies. In the first method the absolute metabolite concentrations in the parent sample, and in the second the ratios of resonance signals to that of creatine compounds were calculated.

Material and Methods

Biopsies from 17 intracranial tumors (weight range 83–1088 mg), obtained during routine surgery at two cooperating neurosurgical wards, were snap-frozen in liquid nitrogen within 3 min, and kept at −80 °C until processed. Tissue samples were pulverized and extracted either with 0.5 M perchloric acid (PCA) according to the protocol designed for the European multicenter trial [4], or by the Dual-Phase Extraction (DPE) method described by Tyagi *et al.* [7], in which water-soluble metabolites are recovered in the methanol-water phase. The extracts were freeze-dried and redissolved in 0.7 ml D_2O at pH 7.0 (uncorrected for the deuterium isotope effect) containing 1 nM 3-trimethylsilyl-2,2,3,3,-tetradeutero sodium propionate, TSP) as concentration and chemical shift reference standard. The fully relaxed proton MR spectra were collected at 25 °C using a Unity Plus spectrometer (500 MHz), 90° pulse, TR of 20 s, 120 acquisitions, and 8 kHz sweep width.

Resonance signals were assigned according to Remy *et al.* [5], as shown in the legend to Fig. 1, and integrated without curve fitting. For quantitation of tissue concentrations the integrals were normalized against that of DSP resonance, corrected for the number of protons contributing to each signal, and expressed in µmoles per gram of tissue wet weight. The ratios of resonance signals were calculated directly from the integrals.

Because the distributions of the data were not normal, statistical significance of differences between the two groups was evaluated with the nonparametric Mann-Whitney U test. $P < 0.05$ was considered significant. For comparison with data of other authors, in a few cases, including the sum of GPC + PC and Cho, the means and their standard errors, as well as the relative standard deviations (RSD = SD/mean) expressed in percent, have been calculated.

Results

Examples of the spectra are shown on Fig. 1. N-acetylaspartate (NAA) signal at 2.02 ppm was recorded from all extracts obtained from gliomas, but was absent in meningioma extracts.

The results of the two methods of analysis are shown in Tables 1 and 2. When the metabolites' concentrations in parent samples were estimated from their resonance signals, the only significant difference was in the tissue concentration of extractable alanine, which on average was more than four times higher in meningiomas than in gliomas. The results of the second analysis, in which the resonance signals of the metab-

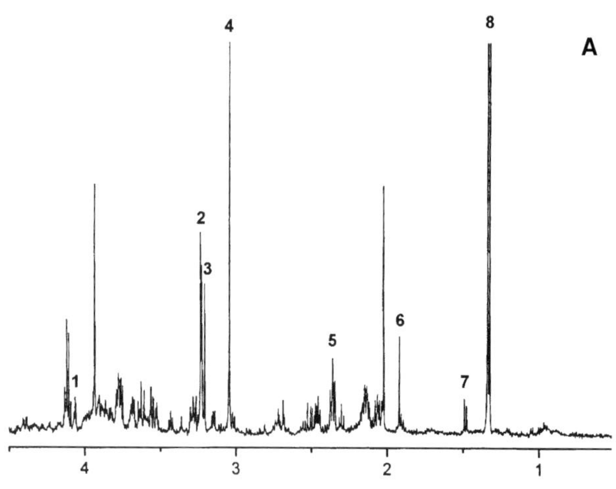

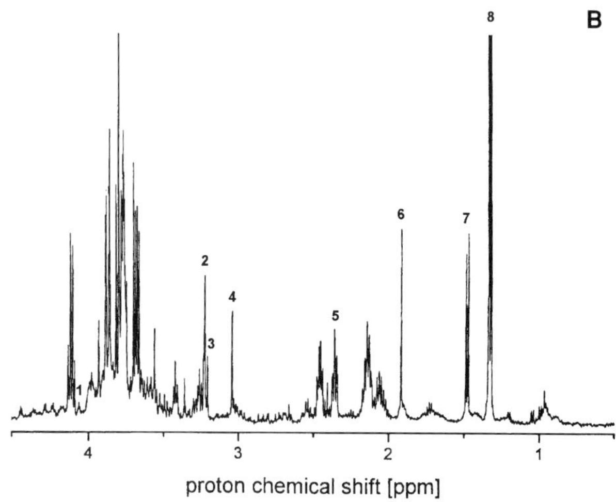

Fig. 1. Representative spectra of tissue extracts containing water-soluble compounds of intracranial tumors (not normalized). (A) Glioblastoma multiforme; (B) meningioma. Assignment of resonances for integration: *1* Ino (4.07 ppm); *2* GPC + PC (3.22 ppm); *3* Cho (3.19 ppm); *4* Cr + PCr (3.03 ppm); *5* Glu (2.35 ppm); *6* Ac (1.91 ppm); *7* Ala (1.48 ppm); *8* Lac (1.32 ppm)

Table 1. *Tissue Concentrations of the Metabolites in Tumor Samples [μmole/g wet Weight], Mean Values and Ranges (in Brackets)*

	Gliomas (n = 6)	Meningiomas (n = 11)	P
Ino	4.94 [1.77–7.60]	3.30 [0.96–11.30]	NS
GPC + PC	1.24 [1.11–3.63]	3.19 [0.41–6.04]	NS
Cho	1.19 [0.33–1.71]	0.73 [0.17–1.57]	NS
Cr + PCr	3.27 [1.36–9.54]	1.90 [0.30–7.40]	NS
Glu	5.99 [2.44–10.87]	13.04 [3.04–30.34]	NS
Ac	1.36 [0.60–5.20]	2.20 [0.70–13.60]	NS
Ala	1.96 [1.14–3.09]	8.79 [1.83–18.96]	<0.01
Lac	20.41 [10.76–26.84]	45.99 [6.57–96.10]	NS

Table 2. *Resonance Signals Normalized to that of Cr + PCr, Median Values and Ranges (in Brackets)*

	Gliomas (n = 6)	Meningiomas (n = 11)	P
Ino	0.54 [0.39–1.11]	1.20 [0.46–1.56]	<0.05
GPC + PC	1.84 [1.24–3.70]	5.14 [1.36–12.89]	<0.05
Cho	1.36 [0.54–2.16]	1.43 [0.84–4.27]	NS
Glu	1.31 [1.07–2.93]	4.57 [2.97–12.70]	<0.001
Ac	0.66 [0.19–5.51]	2.13 [0.77–17.94]	NS
Ala	1.07 [0.17–1.91]	4.27 [2.99–11.83]	<0.001
Lac	7.90 [3.44–18.84]	25.73 [13.90–55.73]	<0.005

olites were directly normalized to that of creatine compounds, revealed the significant difference between gliomas and meningiomas in 5 of 7 signal ratios analyzed. The highest level of significance was reached for Ala/Cr + PCr and Glu/Cr + PCr, where the ranges for gliomas and meningiomas do not overlap.

Discussion

Our data concerning the average metabolite concentrations calculated from the respective resonance signals seem to be somewhat higher than those reported by the others. For example, Usenius *et al.* [8] in PCA extracts of grade 3–4 astrocytomas (n = 24) have determined total creatine concentration of 2.37 ± 0.39 SE μmol/g wet weight, whereas our result is 4.12 ± 1.22 SE; their estimate of concentration of choline-containing compounds, 1.94 ± 0.29 SE (n = 24) was also lower compared to ours, 2.86 ± 0.53 SE for the sum of GPC + PC and Cho.

However, a large variability of metabolite concentrations in extracts of tissue specimens assayed by proton MR spectroscopy seems to be inevitable. Remy *et al.* [5], using a model of rat implantable C6 intracerebral glioma, estimated tumor tissue concentrations of Cr + PCr as 3.00 ± 1.37 SE, and Ala as 1.67 ± 0.28 SE (n = 5). It appears that, even in a well-standardized model based on implanting of an established tumor cell line, the scatter of individual results is considerable. Obviously, no reliable tumor classification can be based on the quantitation of metabolites' concentrations in tumor samples.

On the other hand, the results of the present study indicate that, in the analysis of proton MR spectra recorded from tumor tissue extracts containing water soluble metabolites, normalizing resonance signals of the chosen metabolites to the resonance signal of creatine compounds markedly decreases the scatter of individual results, and provides far better discrimination between malignant gliomas and benign meningiomas than that which would have been possible on the basis of estimates of tissue concentrations of extractable fractions of these metabolites in the bioptates. Similar conclusion may be drawn from the data of Usenius *et al.* [8] for astrocytomas grade 3–4, which, when recalculated, give the RSD values for total Cho and Cr concentration of 73% and 81%, respectively, while the RSD for Cho/Cr ratio is 42%. Our respective RSD values for gliomas are 45% and 73% for total Cho and Cr, and 29% for Cho/Cr ratio.

Our results differ from those reported by Maxwell *et al.* [4] in that their analysis indicated the critical value of glutamine and creatine signals for differentiation between gliomas and meningiomas (providing for 89% correct classification), whereas in the present study the information concerning alanine, glutamate and creatine, when expressed as metabolite ratios, seemed to provide full separation of malignant gliomas from meningiomas. A high discriminative power of total Cho/Cr and glycine/Cr ratios measured in vitro for differentiating anaplastic astrocytomas and glioblastomas has also been reported [2, 3]. It remains to be determined whether the use of metabolite/creatine ratios will prove useful when incorporated into pattern recognition techniques.

Acknowledgments

This work was supported by a grant no. 4 PO5B 054 14 p. 01 from the State Committee of Scientific Research (KBN). The authors thank dr. J. Wójcik from the Institute of Biochemistry and Biophysics, Polish Academy of Sciences, for acquiring and integrating the spectra.

References

1. Bottomley PA, Weiss RG (1999) Non-invasive magnetic-resonance detection of creatine depletion in non-viable infarcted myocardium. Lancet 351: 714–718

2. Carapella CM, Carpinelli G, Knijn A, Raus L, Caroli F, Podo F (1997) Potential role of in vitro ^{1}H magnetic resonance spectroscopy in the differentiation of malignancy grading of human neuroepithelial brain tumors. Acta Neurochir [Suppl] (Wien) 68: 127–132
3. Carpinelli G, Carapella CM, Palombi L, Raus L, Caroli F, Podo F (1996) Differentiation of glioblastoma multiforme from astrocytomas by in vitro ^{1}H MRS analysis of human brain tumors. Anticancer Res 16: 1559–1563
4. Maxwell RJ, Martinez-Perez I, Cerdan S, Cabanas ME, Arus C, Moreno A, Capdevila A, Ferrer E, Bartomeus F, Aparicio A, Conesa G, Roda JM, Carceller F, Pascular JM, Howells SL, Mazucco R, Griffiths JR (1998) Pattern recognition analysis of ^{1}H NMR spectra from perchloric acid extracts of human brain tumor biopsies. Magn Res Med 39: 869–877
5. Remy C, Arus C, Ziegler A, Sam Lai E, Moreno A, Le Fur Y, Decorps M (1994) In vivo, ex vivo, and in vitro one- and two-dimensional nuclear magnetic resonance spectroscopy of an intracerebral glioma in rat brain: assignment of resonances. J Neurochem 62: 166–179
6. Sabatier J, Gilard V, Malet-Martino M, Ranjeva J-P, Terral C, Breil S, Delisle M-B, Manelfe C, Tremoulet M, Berry I (1999) Characterization of choline compounds with in vitro ^{1}H magnetic resonance spectroscopy for the discrimination of primary brain tumors. Invest Radiol 3: 230–235
7. Tyagi RK, Azrad A, Degani H, Salomon Y (1996) Simultaneous extraction of cellular lipids and water-soluble metabolites: evaluation by NMR spectroscopy. Magn Reson Med 35: 194–200
8. Usenius J-PR, Kauppinen RA, Vainio PA, Hernesniemi JA, Vapalahti MP, Paljarvi LA, Soimakallio S (1994) Quantitative metabolite patterns of human brain tumors: detection by ^{1}H NMR spectroscopy in vivo and in vitro. J Comput Assist Tomogr 18: 705–713

Correspondence: P. Grieb, Laboratory of Experimental Pharmacology, Medical Research Centre, Polish Academy of Sciences, 5 Pawinskiego st., 02-106 Warsaw, Poland.

Acta Neurochir (2000) [Suppl] 76: 21–25

rCBF in Hemorrhagic, Non-Hemorrhagic and Mixed Contusions After Severe Head Injury and its Effect on Perilesional Cerebral Blood Flow

B. M. Hoelper[1,2], **M. M. Reinert**[1], **A. Zauner**[1], **E. Doppenberg**[1], and **R. Bullock**[1]

[1] Division of Neurosurgery, Medical College of Virginia, Virginia Commonwealth University, Richmond, Virginia, USA
[2] Clinic of Neurosurgery, City Hospital Fulda, Fulda, Germany

Abstract

Intracerebral contusions can lead to regional ischemia caused by extensive release of excitotoxic aminoacids leading to increased cytotoxic brain edema and raised intracranial pressure. rCBF mesurements might provide further information about the risk of ischemia within and around contusions. Therefore, the aim of the presented study was to compare the intra- and perilesional rCBF of hemorrhagic, non-hemorrhagic and mixed intracerebral contusions.

In 44 patients, 60 stable Xenon-enhanced CT CBF-studies were performed (EtCO2 30 ± 4 mmHg SD), initially 29 hours (39 studies) and subsequent 95 hours after injury (21 studies). All lesions were classified according to localization and lesion type using CT/MRI scans. The rCBF was calculated within and 1-cm adjacent to each lesion in CT-isodens brain.

The rCBF within all contusions (n = 100) of 29 ± 11 ml/100 g/min was significantly lower ($p < 0.0001$, Mann-Whitney U) compared to perilesional rCBF of 44 ± 12 ml/100 g/min and intra/perilesional correlation was 0.4 ($p < 0.0005$). Hemorrhagic contusions showed an intra/perilesional rCBF of 31 ± 11/44 ± 13 ml/100 g/min ($p < 0.005$), non-hemorrhagic contusions 35 ± 13/46 ± 10 ml/100 g/min ($p < 0.01$). rCBF in mixed contusions (25 ± 9/44 ± 12 ml/100 g/min, $p < 0.0001$) was significantly lower compared to hemorrhagic and non-hemorrhagic contusions ($p < 0.02$).

Intracontusional rCBF is significantly reduced to 29 ± 11 ml/100 g/min but reduced below ischemic levels of 18 ml/100 g/min in only 16% of all contusions. Perilesional CBF in CT normal appearing brain closed to contusions is not critically reduced. Further differentiation of contusions demonstrates significantly lower rCBF in mixed contusions (defined by both hyper- and hypodense areas in the CT-scan) compared to hemorrhagic and non-hemorrhagic contusions. Mixed contusions may evolve from hemorrhagic contusions with secondary increased perilesional cytotoxic brain edema leading to reduced cerebral blood flow and altered brain metabolism. Therefore, the treatment of ICP might be individually modified by the measurement of intra- and pericontusional cerebral blood.

Keywords: rCBF; severe head injury contusion.

Introduction

Intracerebral posttraumatic mass lesions such as contusions and intracerebral haematomas are common after severe head injury. An extensive release of excitotoxic aminoacids in such lesions leads to cytotoxic brain edema resulting in an increase of intracranial pressure (ICP) which might cause regional cerebral ischemia [7]. Elevated ICP caused by contusions might be treated with hyperventilation or with removal of the mass lesion. However, the measurement of regional cerebral blood flow (rCBF) within (intralesional) or around (perilesional) contusions can provide further information about injured brain tissue which might be still perfused and potentially vital. A profound reduction of rCBF in edematous brain tissue was shown by Schröder and coworkers together with glial and podocytic swelling in ultrastructural analysis [21]. McLaughlin and Marion [18] evaluated the rCBF within and around contusions in patients and found reduced rCBF in contusions, but the rCBF was below the ischemic level of 18 ml/100 g/min in only 21% of contusions. Until now, no study described differences in cerebral blood flow concerning hemorrhagic, non-hemorrhagic and mixed contusions. Therefore, the aim of the presented study was the evaluation of rCBF in these intracerebral lesions using the stable xenon-enhanced computed tomography (Xe-CT). This technique allows the measurement of rCBF in a reliable spatial resolution and it is safety for clinical use when administered with a constant arterial CO_2.

Table 1. *Regional Cerebral Blood Flow (rCBF, Mean ± Standard Deviation in ml/100 g/min) Classified According to the Anatomical Localization Frontal, Temporal and Others (Parietal, Occipital, Basal Ganglia) Measured in the Region of Interest (ROI) Within the Contusion (Intra) and in the CT-Isodense, Normal Appearing Brain 1 cm Adjacent to the Contusion (Peri)*

Contusion	Frontal $n = 52$		Temporal $n = 34$		Other $n = 13$	
ROI	intra	peri	intra	peri	intra	peri
rCBF	27.9 ± 11.9	42.9 ± 12.7	31.4 ± 10.4	45.8 ± 10.8	28.3 ± 11.9	42.4 ± 11.6

Patients and Methods

All studies were approved by the Committee for conduct of Human Research, at the Virginia Commonwealth University.

Patients

44 patients with severe head injury (Glasgow Coma Score ≤ 8), admitted to the Neuroscience Intensive Care Unit at the Medical College of Virginia (MCV) and older than 16 years were analyzed in this study. All patients were intubated, hemodynamically stabilized and received intracranial pressure (ICP) and cerebral perfusion pressure (CPP) directed treatment protocol.

Cerebral Blood Flow Measurement Studies

All stable xenon enhanced computed tomography studies (Xe-CT Enhancer 300 DPP Inc. Houston, TX) used for measuring cerebral blood flow were equipped with a xenon-gas delivery system and a matching software package capable to define certain regions of interest. The studies were performed by repeated CT scanning during the inhalation of a gas mixture containing 30% xenon, 30–60% oxygen and room air. The end tital ($EtCO_2$) was kept as near as possible to 30 mmHg during the Xe-CT study.

rCBF Measurement, Lesion Definition and Volume Calculation

All lesions were anatomically classified according to the localization and the lesion type was defined using CT and MRI scans. The intralesional rCBF was calculated by drawing a freehand region of interest around 1) a hemorrhagic contusion (HC) without visible edema in the CT scan, 2) a non-hemorrhagic contusion (NHC) and 3) a mixed contusion (hemorrhagic and non-hemorrhagic components) for both the hemorrhagic and the edematous component of the contusion. Furthermore, the rCBF was calculated 1-cm adjacent to each lesion in CT-isodens, normal appearing brain (perilesional rCBF). The global cerebral blood flow was calculated excluding areas of the brain where the rCBF of lesions was measured. The volume of each lesion was calculated according to an ellipsoid ($V = \pi abc/6$) [6].

Statistical Analysis

Mean and standard deviation of intra- and perilesional rCBF was determined at baseline $EtCO_2$ levels. Because data were not normally distributed, the significance in rCBF of different contusions and the volume was tested using the Spearman's rank test. Differences between different groups were calculated using the Whitney-Mann-U test.

Results

Xe-CT Cerebral Blood Flow Studies

In 44 patients, 60 stable Xenon-enhanced CT CBF-studies were performed by controlling the $EtCO_2$ to 30 ± 4 mmHg. 62 contusions were found in the initial 39 studies which were performed in average 29 hours after injury. In subsequent 21 studies (95 hours after trauma) 38 contusions were detected. 52 contusions were seen in the frontal lobe, 36 contusions in the temporal lobe and 12 contusions in other areas such as occipital and parietal lobe as well as basal ganglia (Table 1). Intralesional rCBF was less than 18 ml/100 g/min in 16%, between 18 and 33 ml/100 g/min in 53%, and rCBF higher than 33 ml/100 g/min in 31% of all contusions.

Intralesional and Perilesional rCBF

rCBF of 29 ± 11 ml/100 g/min within contusions ($n = 100$) was significantly lower ($p < 0.0001$, Mann-Whitney U) compared to perilesional rCBF of 44 ± 12 ml/100 g/min. The correlation between intralesional (Fig. 1) and perilesional (Fig. 2) rCBF was significant ($r = 0.4$, $p < 0.0005$). The intra/perilesional rCBF of hemorrhagic contusions (HC) was $31 \pm 11/44 \pm 13$ ml/100 g/min ($p < 0.005$) and of non-hemorrhagic contusions $35 \pm 13/46 \pm 10$ ml/100 g/min ($p < 0.05$) as shown in Table 2. The rCBF in mixed contusions was $25 \pm 9/44 \pm 12$ ml/100 g/min ($p < 0.0001$, Table 2). Comparing the different groups of lesions, a significantly lower intralesional rCBF was found for mixed contusions ($p < 0.02$) compared to hemorrhagic and non-hemorrhagic lesions, but no significant difference existed comparing the last two lesion types.

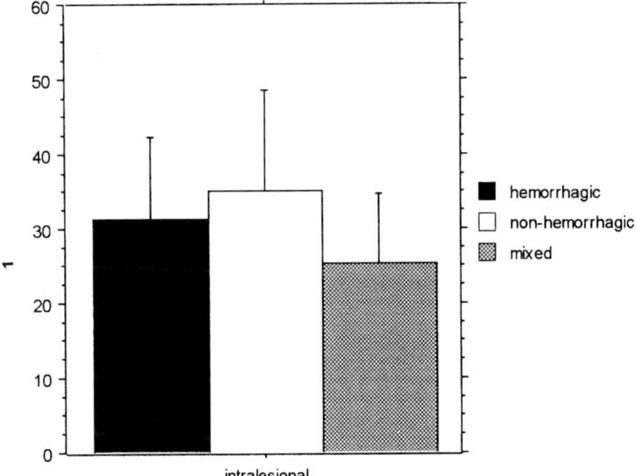

Fig. 1. Intralesional regional cerebral blood flow (rCBF, ml/100 g/min) displayed in mean ± standard deviation of hemorrhagic, non-hemorrhagic and mixed contusions. The intralesional rCBF of mixed contusions was significantly lower compared to hemorrhagic and non-hemorrhagic contusions ($p < 0.02$)

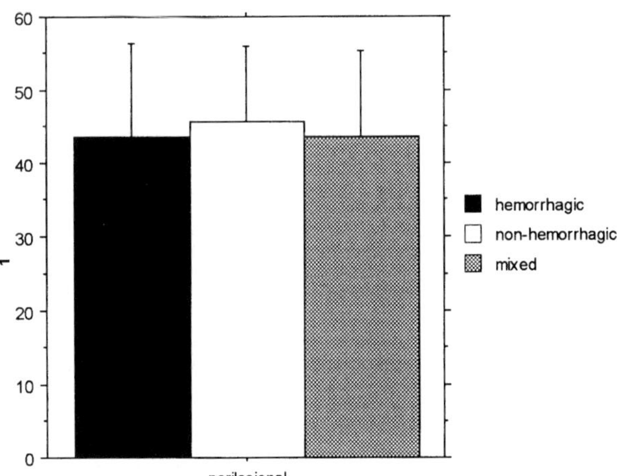

Fig. 2. No significant difference of perilesional regional cerebral blood flow (rCBF, ml/100 g/min) was found between hemorrhagic, non-hemorrhagic and mixed contusions when measured 1 cm adjacent to the contusion in CT-isodense, normal appearing brain

rCBF and Lesion Volume

The contusion volume (18 ± 22 ml) did not correlate to the rCBF within lesions or the perilesional rCBF. Furthermore, no correlation was found between the ratio of intra- and perilesional rCBF and the global cerebral blood flow taking into account interpatient differences of rCBF. Therefore, the rCBF does not directly correlate to the size of the lesion. Differentiating the lesion types (hemorrhage, non-hemorrhage and mixed contusions), there is also no correlation between lesion volume and rCBF within and around the lesions.

Discussion

Cortical contusions, which involve primarily the superficial cortical or subcortical are mostly not accordant to infarction, but are rather generated by brain tissue striking the skull during linear acceleration or deceleration and they appear therefore in areas of the brain adjacent to the floor of the anterior and middle cranial fossae [9, 10, 22, 23]. The CT density of cortical and subcortical hemorrhagic contusions which were found mostly in the frontal and temporal lobe was similar to the density of an intracerebral hemorrhage. A non-hemorrhagic contusion might be difficult to differentiate from a non-hemorrhagic infarction as seen in human middle cerebral artery occlusion, but contusions considered in this study were located in the superficial cortical or subcortical area without a distribution pattern of vascular supply thus implying a focal posttraumatic contusion. Mixed contusions, 46% of all contusions, either had a small hyper- and hypointense area or appeared as hemorrhagic contusions with a perifocal non-hemorrhagic rim. This study shows, that the cerebral blood flow within the contusion is reduced and also in the edematous perifocal brain the cerebral blood flow is impaired in mixed contusions, but the perilesional rCBF in brain tissue of normal CT density is not significantly reduced.

Table 2. *Regional Cerebral Blood Flow (rCBF, mean ± Standard Deviation in ml/100 g/min) of Hemorrhagic, non-Hemorrhagic and Mixed Contusions (Both Hyper- and Hypodense Areas in the CT-Scan) Measured in the Region of Interest (ROI, Intralesional (Intra), Perilesional (Peri), in the Hemorrhagic (hem) and non-Hemorrhagic (non-hem) Area of a Mixed Contusion)*

Contusion	Hemorrhagic n = 36		Non hemorrhagic n = 18		Mixed (hemorrhagic and non-hemorrhagic) n = 46			
ROI	intra	peri	intra	peri	intra	peri	hem	non-hem
rCBF	31.2 ± 11.2	43.6 ± 12.8	35.1 ± 13.4	45.7 ± 10.2	25.3 ± 9.3	43.6 ± 11.9	16.5 ± 7.9	26.3 ± 9.8

While different time-depending cerebral blood flow phases are defined following severe head injury [4, 5, 16], little is known about the intra- and perilesional cerebral blood flow of contusions. Perilesional areas are defined as contiguous low-density zones adjacent to the contusion by Schröder *et al.* [21], and McLaughlin and Marion defined pericontusional regions as a 1 cm rim of normal-appearing parenchyma [18]. We measured both CT-hypodense and CT-normodense appearing brain areas and defined perilesional rCBF according to McLaughlin and coworkers, while the rCBF in low-density zones was defined as intralesional (pericontusional) rCBF in edematous tissue of mixed contusions.

Interestingly, the rCBF within the contusions is below the ischemic threshold of 18 ml/100 g/min in only 16% of all lesions, which is consistent to findings of McLaughlin and Marion, who described in only 3 of 14 lesions ischemic cerebral blood flow of less than 18 ml/100 g/min [18] supporting the evidence that portions of posttraumatic contusions may be viable but might be vulnerable to ischemia. There is also evidence in animals that for edema formation cerebral blood flow must be reduced to a critical threshold and this threshold is almost twice the level at which homeostasis of ions is disrupted [1]. However, a lack of vascular supply precludes an increase of water within the tissue and cytotoxic brain edema is not associated with loss of cellular function [1].

Therefore, this study leads to the following four conclusions: 1) rCBF in mixed cerebral cortical and subcortical contusions might be lowered by various factors, but there is evidence that glial swelling with narrowing of the microvascular lumina due to massive podocytic process swelling supports microvascular compromise by vascular compression and occlusion which might lead to perilesional and intralesional hypoperfusion of edematous pericontusional and intracontusional tissue [7, 13, 21]. 2) Even if the intracerebral blood flow correlates to perilesional blood flow, the rCBF in perilesional CT-normodense brain tissue is not reduced to critical ischemic levels. These findings support descriptions of Marion and coworkers, who found no critical reduction of CBF in hemispheres with focal contusions [15]. 3) Brain metabolism depends on substrate delivery in regions with reduced CBF. 3) Brain metabolism depends on substrate delivery in regions with reduced CBF. Brain metabolism and CBF are coupled and both, a decrease and an increase of CBF and metabolism are described after brain trauma [2, 11, 17]. However, CBF and metabolism might be uncoupled when cerebral autoregulation is impaired and this might result in an increased risk for brain swelling and further reduced blood flow [3, 12, 14, 19, 20]. The therapeutical management by increasing the CPP in order to increase the cerebral blood flow might be limited by the CPP-independent cerebral vascular resistance, which correlates to the CBF and cerebral metabolism [8]. Therefore, cerebral metabolism might be less influenced by changes of CPP when CBF is maintained above the ischemic threshold. 4) Hyperemia was not found within contusions, which supports findings by Bullock *et al.*, who described focal zones of hyperaemia present in 42% of patients only within apparently normal tissue as judged by late MRI or CT, but not in damaged brain tissue [7].

Since it is known that critically low CBF or abnormal CO_2 vasoreactivity is not predictable on the basis of clinical examinations or CT findings [15], the measurement of rCBF might give further information concerning the risk of ischemia in the intra- and perilesional zone of a contusion which might result in treatment strategies specified for individual patients.

Conclusion

Intracontusional rCBF is significantly reduced to 29 ± 11 ml/100 g/min and reduced below ischemic levels of 18 ml/100 g/min in only 16%. Perilesional CBF in CT normal appearing brain close to contusions is not reduced to critical cerebral blood flow. Further differentiation of contusions demonstrates significantly lower rCBF in mixed contusions (both hyper- and hypodense areas in the CT-scan) compared to hemorrhagic and non-hemorrhagic contusions ($p < 0.02$). Mixed contusions may evolve from hemorrhagic contusions with secondary increased perilesional cytotoxic brain edema leading to reduced cerebral blood flow and altered brain metabolism. Therefore, the treatment of ICP might be individually modified by the measurement of intra- and pericontusional cerebral blood.

References

1. Bell BA, Symon L, Branston NM (1985) CBF and time thresholds for the formation of ischemic cerebral edema, and effect of reperfusion in baboons. J Neurosurg 62: 31–41
2. Bergsneider M, Hovda DA, Shalmon E, Kelly DF, Vespa PM, Martin NA, Phelps ME, McArthur DL, Caron MJ, Kraus JF,

Becker DP (1997) Cerebral hyperglycolysis following severe traumatic brain injury in humans: a positron emission tomography study [see comments]. J Neurosurg 86(2): 241–251

3. Bouma GJ, Muizelaar JP (1992) Cerebral blood flow, cerebral blood volume, and cerebrovascular reactivity after severe head injury. J Neurotrauma 9 [Suppl] 1: S333–348
4. Bouma GJ, Muizelaar JP (1993) Evaluation of regional cerebral blood flow in acute head injury by stable Xenon-enhanced computerized tomography. Acta Neurochir [Suppl] (Wien) 59: 34–40
5. Bouma GJ, Muizelaar JP, Choi SC, Newlon PG, Young HF (1991) Cerebral circulation and metabolism after severe traumatic brain injury: the elusive role of ischemia. J Neurosurg 75(5): 685–693
6. Bronstein IN, KA KAS, Musiol G, Mühling H (1995) Taschenbuch der Mathematik. Verlag Harri Deutsch
7. Bullock R, Sakas D, Patterson J, Wyper D, Hadley D, Maxwell W, Teasdale GM (1992) Early post-traumatic cerebral blood flow mapping: correlation with structural damage after focal injury. Acta Neurochir [Suppl] (Wien) 55: 14–17
8. Cruz J, Jaggi JL, Hoffstad OJ (1995) Cerebral blood flow, vascular resistance, and oxygen metabolism in acute brain trauma: Redefining the role of cerebral perfusion pressure? Neurol Crit Care 23(8): 1412–1417
9. Gentry LR, Godersky JC, Thompson B (1988) MR imaging of head trauma: review of the distribution and radiopathologic features of traumatic lesions. AJR Am J Roentgenol 150(3): 663–672
10. Gentry LR, Godersky JC, Thompson B, Dunn VD (1988) Prospective comparative study of intermediate-field MR and CT in the evaluation of closed head trauma. AJR Am J Roentgenol 150(3): 673–682
11. Jaggi JL, Obrist WD, Gennarelli TA, Langfitt TW (1990) Relationship of early cerebral blood flow and metabolism to outcome in acute head injury. J Neurosurg 72(2): 176–182
12. Kelly DF, Kordestani RK, Martin NA, Nguyen T, Hovda DA, Bergsneider M, McArthur DL, Becker DP (1996) Hyperemia following traumatic brain injury: relationship to intracranial hypertension and outcome. Neurosurg 85: 762–771
13. Kuroda Y, Bullock R (1992) Local cerebral blood flow mapping before and after removal of acute subdural hematoma in the rat. Neurosurg 30: 687–691
14. Marion DW, Bouma GJ (1991) The use of stable Xenon-enhanced computed tomograpic studies of cerebral blood flow to define changes in cerebral carbon dioxide vasoreactivity caused by a severe head injury. Neurosurgery 29(6): 869–873
15. Marion DW, Darby J, Yonas H (1991) Acute regional cerebral blood flow changes caused by severe head injury. Neurosurg 74: 407–414
16. Martin NA, Patwardhan RV, Alexander MJ, Africk CZ, Lee JH, Shalmon E, Hovda DA, Becker DP (1997) Characterization of cerebral hemodynamic phases following severe head trauma: hypoperfusion, hyperemia, and vasospasm. Neurosurg 87: 9–19
17. Mayevsky A, Weiss HR (1991) Cerebral blood flow and oxygen consumption in cortical spreading depression. J Cereb Blood Flow Metab 11: 829–836
18. McLaughlin MR, Marion DW (1996) Cerebral blood flow and vasoresponsivity within and around cerebral contusions [see comments]. J Neurosurg 85(5): 871–876
19. Nordström C-H, Messeter K, Sundbärg G, Schalen W, Werner M, Ryding E (1988) Cerebral blood flow, vasoreactivity, and oxygen consumption during barbiturate therapy in severe traumatic brain lesions. Neurosurg 6: 424–431
20. Obrist WD, Langfitt TW, Jaggi JL, Cruz J, Gennarelli TA (1984) Cerebral blood flow and metabolism in comatose patients with acute head injury. Relationship to intracranial hypertension. J Neurosurg 61(2): 241–253
21. Schröder ML, Muizelaar JP, Bullock MR, Salvant JB, Povlishock JT (1995) Focal ischemia due to traumatic contusions documented by stable xenon-CT and ultrastructural studies. J Neurosurg 82: 966–971
22. Teasdale E, Hadley DM (1997) Imaging the injury. In: Bullock R(ed) Head injury. Chapman & Hall, London, pp 167–207
23. Teasdale G, Teasdale E, Hadley D (1992) Computed tomographic and magnetic resonance imaging classification of head injury. J Neurotrauma 9 [Suppl] 1: S249–257

Correspondence: Ross Bullock, M.D., Ph.D., Division of Neurosurgery, Medical College of Virginia, Virginia Commonwealth University, Richmond, Virginia, USA.

Molecular Mechanisms

Molecular Mechanisms of Brain Injury and Oedema

Major topics were (a) the defence mechanisms of the blood-brain barrier, of endothelial cells, respectively with regard to glutathione homeostasis, (b) in-vivo quantification of cerebral of N-acetyl aspartate (NAA) levels by MR-spectroscopy, (c) the mediator role of bradykinin in disturbances of the cerebral microcirculation and ischemic brain damage, (d) the association of energy failure and infarct formation from ischaemia, (e) the activation of pro-inflammatory mechanisms from ischaemia and their therapeutic inhibition, (f) soluble adhesion molecules in the plasma of patients with subarachnoid haemorrhage, (g) activation of poly-ADP-ribose-polymerase (PARP) in traumatic brain injury, (h) effects of moderate hypothermia on cell volume control and on mediator-induced swelling of glial cells in-vitro. Obviously, the session had a wide spectrum of in-vivo and in-vitro approaches for elucidation of the cellular and molecular mechanisms of ischaemic and traumatic brain damage and the potential for their antagonism.

An important cellular defence against oxidative injury is the glutathione (GSH) system. The system was studied in endothelial cells from human brain as to its role in disruption of the blood-brain barrier from in-vitro ischaemia (hypoxia + substrate deprivation). This led to a reduction of GSH-Ievels while glutathione peroxidase was increased. The barrier enzyme gamma-glutamyltranspeptidase, which is metabolising GSH, was also reduced from in-vitro ischaemia. These changes may play a role during in-vivo breakdown of the blood-brain barrier. A technical contribution was concerned with in-vivo quantification of NAA in rat brain by MR-spectroscopy. N-acetyl aspartate can be nicely quantified by this procedure, although the significance of its pathophysiological concentration change is apparently not fully understood yet. On the other hand, the mediator functions of the kallikrein-kinin system, of bradykinin in particular, are well established leading to promising attempts at an inhibition, e.g. by receptor antagonism. A bradykinin B1/B2 receptor antagonist was studied as to its influence on leukocyte/endothelium interactions in animals with global cerebral ischaemia. Although the activation of leukocytes was widely inhibited thereby, protection against ischaemic brain damage was not afforded nor against deterioration of neurological function.

Short repeated episodes of cerebral ischaemia induce an intriguing pattern of disturbances of energy metabolism. The role of energy failure from ischaemia was analysed with regard to infarct formation in comparison with selective neuronal death. Whereas gross energy failure, particularly depletion of ATP was closely correlated with infarction, the delayed selective neuronal demise in vulnerable brain areas (e.g. hippocampus, infundibular cortex) was not attributable to disturbances of the energy state. Activation of inflammatory processes has been considered for quite a while to contribute to secondary damage from cerebral ischaemia. The role of the arachidonic acid cascade and of immunological mechanisms therein was studied by utilising indomethacin and cyclosporin A. Cyclosporin A is of particular interest as it blocks mitochondrial transition pores and thereby the release of toxic material into the cytosol. Both agents were inhibiting neutrophil chemotaxis from in-vitro ischaemia, most likely from inhibition of the expression of IL-8 and ICAM-1 by the ischaemically challenged cerebrovascular endothelial cells. The findings are complemented by corresponding in-vivo studies on soluble adhesion molecules in the plasma of patients with subarachnoid haemorrhage. Patients with and without delayed cerebral ischaemic deficits (DID) from vasospasm were compared as to the plasma levels of E-, P-, and L-selectin, which induce rolling along and adherence to the cerebrovascular endothelium of neutrophils in the microcirculation. Only patients with DID symptoms from subarachnoid haemorrhage had increased blood levels of P-selectin, while L-selectin was decreased, indicative of an activation of leukocyte/endothelial interactions in the brain under these circumstances.

The activation of poly-ADP-ribose-polymerase (PARP) was investigated with regard to higher CNS functions, such as cognition in experimental traumatic brain injury from a controlled cortical impact. For that purpose, knock-out mice with selective deletion of the PARP-gene were studied. These animals had a significantly better outcome from the standardised brain trauma than their wild types, which are activating PARP. As already known, PARP enhances energy failure from an increased NAD+-consumption and exhaustion of cellular ATP-levels. The present investigations on neurotrauma are important for the understanding of this system, as respective experiments have so far been limited mostly to cerebral ischaemia.

The chapter is an excellent example of the diversity of developments of scientific exploration of *brain oedema and injury* on cells at biological and molecular levels. Interestingly, the phenomena appear to be more frequently studied in *cerebral ischaemia* as compared to *brain trauma*. Further, many contributions make obvious the significance of *in-vitro models* to analyse these difficult processes in an organ as complex as the brain under the chaotic conditions of ischaemia or trauma. Accordingly, *in-vitro ischaemia, in-vitro blood-brain barrier, or in-vitro brain trauma*, among others are increasingly utilised in research laboratories all over the world. Our understanding of *leukocyte/endothelial interactions* in secondary brain damage from ischaemia or trauma is subjected to gradual modifications, indicating that the phenomenon elicited then may not necessarily contribute to brain damage.

Lafuente *et al.* present interesting results of chronic hypoxia on the expression of nitric oxide synthase in different structures of the brain. Two important conclusions are made: one that the adaptation plays a great role in adjustment of animals to difficult hypoxic conditions and the other – even more important – that there are local differences in the metabolic response to hypoxia. The studies of local metabolic differences are crucial for a better understanding of why brain structures respond with different resistance to hypoxia or ischaemia.

Rothoerl and co-workers tested the prognostic value of S-IOOB serum levels in clinical conditions. They found that S-IOOB concentration is a useful outcome indicator. Outcome prediction is a very important clinical problem and every clinician would be happy to see a reliable outcome prognostic factor. However S-100B studies need to be continued. The other problem that has not been addressed is how the patients can be compared if S100B is released rapidly after trauma. Its half-life time is only 2 hours and serum samples were taken from patients 1 to 6 hours after injury.

Haseldonckx and co-workers present a very interesting paper. Using a simple photochemical lesion the authors were able to produce a spectrum of brain damage grade from penumbra to tissue necrosis. This simple reproducible model of penumbra is especially promising. The study is well documented using histological, histochemical and electron microscope techniques.

Naruse and co-workers present the application of the brain infusion method originally developed by Marmarou. The authors used it to study spinal cord oedema. Spinal cord oedema is less known and, until now, investigated mostly in traumatic and ischaemic models, so the proposed procedure is promising.

In summary, the chapter demonstrates the continuing viability as well as necessity of experimental research of a clinically most relevant yet complex problem ~ *vasogenic and cytotoxic brain oedema* at the cellular and molecular level. The prospects are promising that these activities eventually provide clinically valuable interventions directed towards the ultimate goal to completely inhibit *secondary brain damage* from trauma and ischaemia.

Acta Neurochir (2000) [Suppl] 76: 29–34

Glutathione Homeostasis and Leukotriene-Induced Permeability in Human Blood-Brain Barrier Endothelial Cells Subjected to in Vitro Ischemia

A. Muruganandam, C. Smith, R. Ball, T. Herring, and **D. Stanimirovic**

Institute for Biological Sciences, National Research Council of Canada, Ottawa, Canada

Abstract

Ischemic alterations in the glutathione (GSH) redox system of the blood-brain barrier (BBB) may facilitate oxidative injury and formation of vasogenic brain edema. In this study, both the intra- and extracellular GSH contents of human cerebromicrovascular endothelial cells (HCEC) were reduced by 35% after exposing the cells to 4 h in vitro ischemia and 24 h-recovery. The intracellular/extracellular GSH ratio was not affected, indicating a constant rate of GSH efflux. The activities of the peroxide detoxifying enzymes, glutathione peroxidase and glutathione S-transferase, increased by 35%–50%, whereas the GSH regenerating enzyme, glutathione reductase, remained unchanged in ischemic HCEC. γ-glutamyl transpeptidase (GGTP), a GSH catabolizing enzyme enriched in brain capillaries, was reduced by 30–50% in ischemic HCEC. The effect of in vitro ischemia on HCEC permeability was assessed by measuring sodium fluorescein clearance across a compartmentalized in vitro BBB model. Sodium fluorescein clearance across HCEC monolayers exposed to leukotriene C_4 in the presence of the GGTP inhibitor, acivicin (1 μM), or after in vitro ischemia was increased by 60% and 30%, respectively, suggesting that oxidative stress and loss of GGTP may 'unmask' BBB permeabilizing actions of leukotrienes. These results indicate that oxidative stress and loss of GGTP activity in HCEC contribute to ischemic BBB disruption and vasogenic brain edema.

Keywords: Blood-brain barrier; glutathione metabolism; hypoxia; leukotrienes.

Introduction

Oxygen-derived free radicals have been implicated as mediators of both reperfusion injury and edema in various tissues including the brain [8]. During ischemia/reperfusion, cerebral endothelial cells (CEC) are exposed to free radicals originating from various sources including ischemic brain tissue and activated leukocytes [8]. Endothelial cells can generate significant amounts of free radicals in the arachidonic acid cascade [30] and/or *via* Ca^{2+}-dependent proteolytic conversion of xanthine dehydrogenase into xanthine oxidase [28].

Oxygen radicals have been shown to alter the reactivity of cerebral vessels to physiological regulators, to cause prolonged vasoconstriction or vasodilatation [11], and to increase permeability of the BBB for micro- and macromolecules [8, 30]. Furthermore, in vitro hypoxia has been shown to deplete endogenous CEC antioxidants including glutathione (GSH) [22, 23], thus increasing CEC susceptibility to oxidant injury. A redox imbalance in endothelial cells has also been shown to facilitate neutrophil-endothelial cell adhesion by up-regulating expression of adhesion molecules [18]. In the extreme, free radicals can cause damage to endothelial cells so severe that it results in the structural disorganization and a massive breach of the permeability barrier.

γ-glutamyl transpeptidase (GGTP), an enzyme highly enriched in mammalian brain capillaries [13], has been proposed to play a role in a biochemical pathway of GSH turnover and to function as an enzymatic barrier for peptidoleukotrienes [13]. In both tumor [2, 3] and ischemic tissues [1], in which leukotrienes are potent BBB permeabilizers, the affected cerebral capillaries were found to be depleted of GGTP activity [1–3]. Based on these observations, it has been suggested that in normal brain capillaries GGTP functions as an enzymatic barrier which rapidly degrades leukotriene C_4 (LTC_4) before it can affect the integrity of the BBB [3, 4].

In this study, we demonstrate that simulated in vitro ischemia causes a decrease in both GSH content and GGTP activity in human CEC (HCEC), leading to oxidative injury and increases in permeability of HCEC monolayers in response to leukotrienes.

Materials and Methods

Cell Culture

HCEC were isolated from human temporal cortex biopsies as previously described [25]. HCEC cultures were grown in media containing 65% medium M199 (Earle's salts, 25 mM Hepes, 4.35 g/l sodium bicarbonate and 3 mM L-glutamine), 10% fetal calf serum, 5% human serum, 20% murine melanoma cell (mouse melanoma, Cloudman S91, clone M-3, melanin producing cells)-conditioned media, 5 μg/ml insulin, 5 μg/ml transferrin, 5 ng/ml selenium, and 10 μg/ml endothelial cell growth supplement. Cultures of fetal human astrocytes were generously provided by Dr. Jack Antel of Montreal Neurological Institute. The procedures used in these experiments were approved by the National Research Council's and McGill University's Human Research Ethics Committees.

Simulated in Vitro Ischemia

HCEC were subjected to a combination of severe hypoxia (<2% O_2; anaerobic chamber equipped with a humidified, temperature-controlled incubator) and glucose and nutrient deprivation [glucose-free Krebs solution containing (in mM) 119 NaCl, 4.7 KCl, 1.2 KH_2PO_4, 25 $NaHCO_3$, 2.5 $CaCl_2$, 1 $MgCl_2$] for 4 hours followed by various periods of recovery (4–24 h) in ambient air (reoxygenation) and Krebs buffer containing 5 mM glucose [26]. Cell media were collected and cells harvested for simultaneous measurements of extra- and intracellular levels of glutathione and enzyme activities.

GSH Content

The intra- and extracellular contents of reduced glutathione (GSH) were measured using the method described by Juurlink *et al.* 1996 [17]. Control or ischemic HCEC were incubated with monochlorobimane (MCB; 100 μM) for 30 min at room temperature, media were then collected and cells were rinsed in PBS and scraped off. GSH-MCB adduct was extracted from cell pellets by sonication in the presence of 1% SDS in 50 mM Tris-HCl buffer (pH 7.5). In parallel, collected cell media were exposed to glutathione S-transferase (0.1 units/ml) for 60 min. GSH-MCB adduct was quantified spectrophotometrically (380 nm/470 nm) in both cell lysates and cell media. A standard curve was prepared using known concentrations of GSH incubated in the presence of glutathione S-transferase and MCB.

GSH Metabolizing Enzymes

Glutathione reductase (GR, EC 1.6.4.2) activity was determined in a kinetic enzyme reaction [7] initiated by the addition of HCEC extracts to an assay mixture containing (f.c.) 0.1 M phosphate buffer pH 7.0, 1 mM EDTA, 100 μM NADPH, and 1 mM GSSG. The NADPH utilization (i.e, decrease in absorbance at 340 nm) due to the enzymatic reduction of GSSG to GSH was monitored for 3 min at 30 °C. The specific activity of glutathione reductase was expressed in nmols of NADPH oxidized per minute per milligram protein.

Glutathione-S-transferase (GST, EC 2.5.1.18) activity was determined as the amount of S-2-4 dinitrophenylglutathione (ε_{340} = 9.6 mM^{-1} cm^{-1}) formed in the reaction initiated by the addition of HCEC extract to the solution containing 10 mM sodium phosphate buffer pH 6.5, 1 mM EDTA, 1 mM GSH and 1 mM 1-chloro-2, 4-dinitrobenzene at 30 °C [15]. Nonspecific activity was determined in the absence of HCEC sample. Enzyme activity was defined as the amount of enzyme that catalyzes the formation of 1 nmol of S-2-4 dinitrophenylglutathione per minute.

Glutathione peroxidase (GSHPx; EC 1.11.1.9) activity was determined in a coupled enzymatic assay in which HCEC sample (i.e., GSHPx) is used to catalyze formation of GSSG from GSH and a peroxide donor, and GSSG was then reduced to GSH in the presence of NADPH and glutathione reductase. The reaction mixture containing. 0.1 M potassium phosphate buffer (pH 7), 1 mM EDTA, 0.24 U glutathione reductase, 1 mM GSH, 0.1 mM NADPH, and 25 μl of HCEC extract was pre-incubated 10 min at 37 °C. NADPH (1.4 mM) was then added and the hydroperoxide-independent consumption of NADPH was allowed to take place for 3 min. The reaction was initiated by adding 100 μM t-butyl hydroperoxide solution for 5 min at 37 °C and NADPH utilization was monitored at 340 nm [12].

Activity of the cerebral-endothelium specific enzyme, γ-glutamyl transpeptidase (GGTP; EC 2.3.2.1) was determined using a previously described protocol [25]. Briefly, HCEC grown in 60 mm Petri dishes were scraped off the dishes and briefly sonicated. The membrane bound GGTP was extracted by the addition of 0.1% Triton X-100 to the extraction buffer. Aliquots of the suspension were used for parallel measurements of protein content [6] and GGTP activity. GGTP activity was measured as the amount of p-nitroaniline (diazotized by a modified Bratton-Marshall reaction) liberated in the 30 min reaction of HCEC suspensions with the GGTP substrate, 51 mM L-γ-glutamyl-p-nitroanilide and 1.1 mM glycylglycine.

Permeability Studies

HCEC are grown on a 0.5% gelatin coated Falcon tissue culture inserts (pore size-0.45 μm; surface area 0.83 cm^2) in 1 ml of growth medium. The bottom chamber of the insert assembly contained 2 ml of growth medium supplemented with the fetal human astrocyte (FHAS)-conditioned medium [1:1 (v/v) ratio]. The FHAS-conditioned medium was obtained by incubating confluent FHAS in a serum free M199 for 72 hrs. Paracellular passage of sodium fluorescein added to the upper chamber (25 μg/ml) across triplicate HCEC-layered membranes was determined from clearance values using previously described protocols [10, 21]. Samples were collected from the bottom chambers every 15 min over 180 min period. Clearance volume (μl) was calculated as:

$$\text{Clearance } (\mu l) = ([C]_A \times V_A)/[C]_L, \text{ where}$$

$[C]_A$ is the abluminal tracer concentration, V_A is the volume of the abluminal chamber, and $[C]_L$ is the initial luminal tracer concentration. The slopes of the clearance curves, representing permeability x surface area product (PS; μl/min), for membranes alone and membranes with cell monolayers were calculated using linear regression analysis. LTC_4 was added to differently treated cells at 60 min, and the effects on permeability were determined by comparing slopes of clearance curves prior to and after the LTC_4 addition.

Results

Effects of in Vitro Ischemia on GSH Levels and GSH Metabolizing Enzymes in HCEC

Intracellular levels of reduced glutathione (GSH) decreased by 35% in HCEC exposed to 4 h in vitro is-

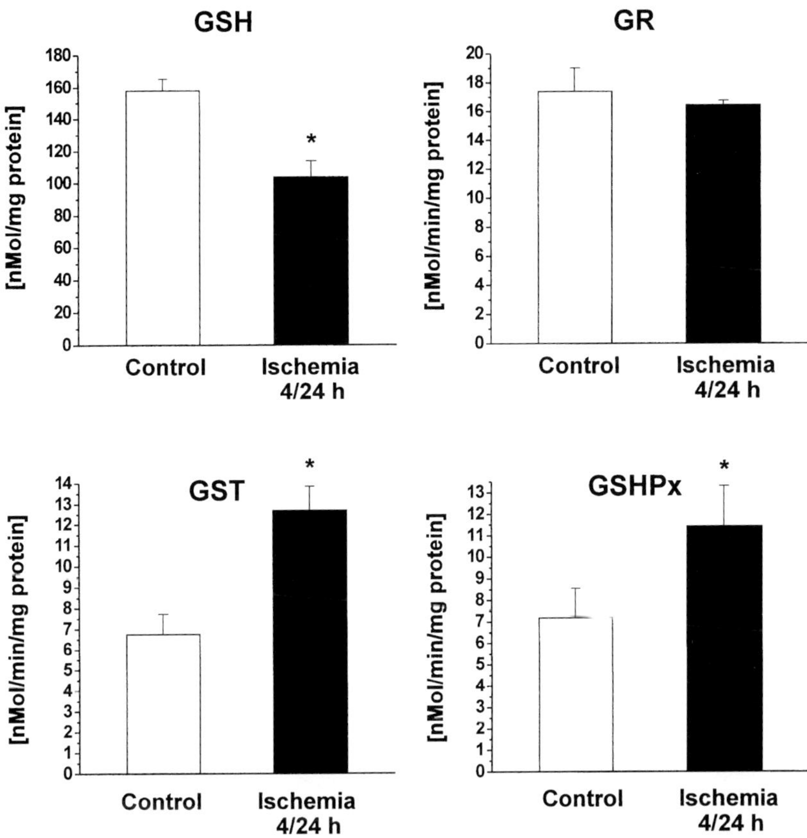

Fig. 1. Effects of simulated in vitro ischemia (4 h)/recovery (24 h) on the intracellular levels of reduced glutathione (*GSH*) and the activities of glutathione reductase (*GR*), glutathione-S transferase (*GST*), and glutathione peroxidase (*GSHPx*) in HCEC. HCEC were subjected to in vitro ischemia/recovery, and GSH and glutathione metabolizing enzyme activities were determined as described in Materials and Methods. Each bar represents the mean ± S.D. of four replicates in one representative experiment out of three yielding similar results. Asterisks indicate a significant difference ($P < 0.01$; ANOVA) from control values

chemia and 24 h recovery (Fig. 1). Extracellular GSH content, amounting to approximately 20% of total cellular GSH [(33 ± 2 vs. 191 ± 6) nmol/mg protein], was reduced by 25% after 4 h ischemia/24 h recovery (data not shown). Hence, intracellular/extracellular GSH ratio remained similar in control ($R = 4.75$) and ischemic ($R = 4.34$) HCEC.

The activity of glutathione reductase, an enzyme that recovers GSH from oxidized GSSG, was not affected by in vitro ischemia in HCEC (Fig. 1), whereas activities of glutathione S-transferase and glutathione peroxidase were stimulated by 50% and 35%, respectively (Fig. 1).

GGTP activity decreased initially at the end of in vitro ischemia (Fig. 2), and continued to decline during recovery period to levels below 40% of control activity at 24 h (Fig. 2). This reduction was reversible, since GGTP activity returned to near control levels (data not shown) 72 h after ischemia. GGTP activity was almost completely inhibited by 1 mM acivicin (Table 1).

Effects of Leukotriene C_4 (LTC_4) and in Vitro Ischemia on Paracellular Permeability of the in Vitro BBB Model

Clearance of the paracellular diffusion marker, sodium fluorescein, across semipermeable membranes (PSm = 15.4 ± 0.6 μl/min) was significantly restricted by the presence of HCEC monolayer (PSe = 3.95 ± 0.21 μl/min). Sodium fluorescein clearance across control HCEC monolayers was not affected by the addition of 1 μM LTC_4 (Table 1), but it increased by 60% in response to LTC_4 when HCEC were pretreated with the GGTP inhibitor, acivicin (Table 1). Acivicin alone did not affect HCEC permeability for sodium fluorescein (Table 1). Similarly, whereas simulated in vitro ischemia/recovery (4 h + 24 h) did not affect

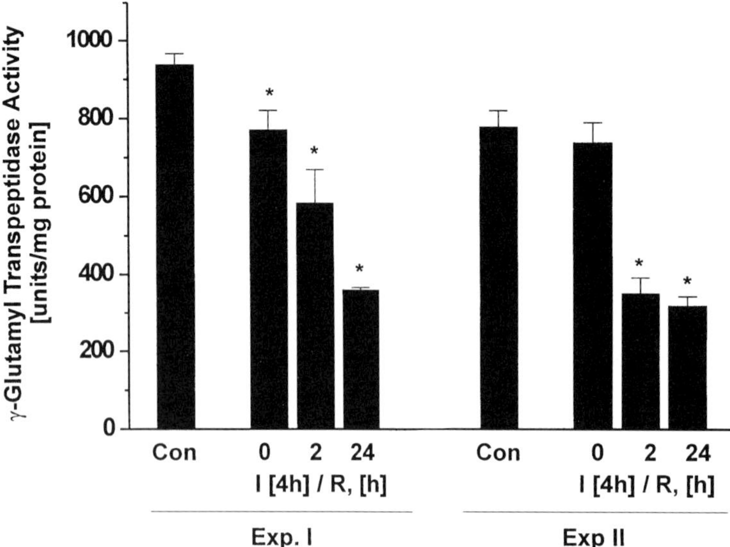

Fig. 2. Effects of simulated in vitro ischemia/recovery (*I*/*R*) on the activity of the BBB enzyme, GGTP. HCEC were exposed to a 4 h simulated in vitro ischemia and indicated periods of recovery, and GGTP activity was determined as described in Materials and Methods. Each bar represents the mean ± S.D. of six replicates in one experiment. Two experiments done in different cell isolations are shown. Asterisks indicate a significant difference ($P < 0.01$; ANOVA) from control values

Table 1. *Effects of Acivicin and Simulated in Vitro Ischemia on the GGTP Activity and Paracellular Permeability of the in Vitro BBB Model for Sodium Fluorescein*

	GGTP (units/min/mg protein)	PSe (μl SF/min)
Control	938.9 ± 37.6	3.95 ± 0.21
+1 μM LTC_4		3.84 ± 0.38
Acivicin, 1 mM	22.4 ± 3.2*	4.12 ± 0.65
+1 μM LTC_4		6.97 ± 0.42*#
Ischemia (4 h/24 h)	318.6 ± 40.2*	3.47 ± 0.24
+1 μM LTC_4		4.56 ± 0.31#

PSe—Slope of the clearance curves for sodium fluorescein (*SF*), representing permeability x surface area product. LTC_4 was added to cells 60 min after the start of the permeability study, and SF paracellular diffusion was monitored for additional 3 hours; PSe is derived from slopes of clearance curves before and after LTC_4 addition. PS for empty membranes was 12.4 ± 0.6 μl/min. Each value represents mean ± SD of three replicate samples/membranes in a representative experiment out of three to four experiments yielding similar results. Asterisks show a significant difference ($p < 0.01$; ANOVA) from control values. # shows a significant difference ($p < 0.01$; ANOVA) from values prior to the addition of LTC_4.

HCEC permeability for fluorescein (Table 1), the addition of 1 μM LTC_4 to ischemic HCEC caused a significant increase in PSe values (Table 1). Neither of the above experimental conditions affected PSe values for radiolabeled albumin (data not shown).

Discussion

This study shows that simulated in vitro ischemia/recovery in HCEC leads to: a) reduction in intracellular GSH levels without changes in GSH efflux; b) stimulation of the peroxide detoxifying enzymes, glutathione peroxidase and glutathione S-transferase, and c) reduction in the activity of GSH catabolizing enzyme, GGTP, accompanied by the 'opening' of the in vitro BBB by leukotrienes. These findings strongly suggest that HCEC subjected to in vitro ischemia experience oxidative and metabolic changes that significantly alter their response to otherwise nondisruptive pro-inflammatory mediators.

The major indicators of oxidative stress observed in HCEC subjected to in vitro ischemia are: a) reduced intracellular GSH levels, and b) increased activities of peroxide quenching enzymes, glutathione peroxidase and glutathione S-transferase. Although the loss of GSH could be attributed to an ischemia-induced depletion of ATP required for GSH synthesis, the observed ischemic induction of glutathione peroxidase and glutathione S-transferase along with the constant intra/extracellular GSH ratio, strongly suggest that intracellular GSH depletion is due to direct GSH oxidation and increased formation of GSH conjugates. Ischemically reduced GGTP may contribute to GSH depletion by failing to catabolise GSH conjugates and thus to recycle substrates for GSH synthesis.

In vitro studies on immortalized CEC have shown that decreased GSH levels increase the sensitivity of CEC to oxidative stress [16] and that exogenous glutathione can protect CEC from traumatic injury [14, 23]. In bovine CEC, hypoxia has been shown to increase both susceptibility to oxidative stress and the permeability of cell monolayers [22]. We have recently shown that oxidative stress exogenously applied to

CEC causes membrane lipid peroxidation, loss of Na, K-ATPase activity, and increased leakage of chromium-bound small molecules from CEC [27]. Both exogenously applied oxidative stress and in vitro ischemia have also been shown to result in arachidonic acid release from CEC [28].

Arachidonic acid is metabolized to pro-inflammatory leukotrienes through a 5-lipoxygenase pathway [24]. The first product in the cascade, an unstable epoxide leukotriene A_4 (LTA_4), is either enzymatically hydrolyzed to LTB_4 or is conjugated with GSH by the action of glutathione-S-transferase to yield LTC_4, which is further broken down by GGTP [24]. LTs play multiple roles as mediators of inflammation, allergy, and edema in various tissues [24]. The tissue levels of leukotrienes have been shown to increase in the brain during ischemia [20]. However, the putative role of these compounds in mediating BBB permeability and brain edema is still controversial.

In this study, LTC_4 was found to permeabilize an in vitro BBB model only when GGTP activity in HCEC is substantially inhibited by either an exogenous GGTP inhibitor, or by effects of in vitro ischemia. The study suggests that high levels of GGTP expressed in HCEC are important in neutralizing pro-inflammatory LTC_4 and that in vitro ischemia unmasks BBB permeabilizing actions of leukotrienes by reducing GGTP activity.

Several in vivo studies have also provided evidence that leukotrienes act as effective mediators of BBB opening only in the presence of other condition(s) that alter the BBB. Whereas in most studies, intracarotid injection, brain super-fusion, or intraparenchymal injection of higher than physiological (i.e., 10^{-9}–10^{-8} M) concentrations of peptido-leukotrienes failed to produce significant BBB disruption [29], intracarotid infusion of low doses of LTC_4 opened the BBB in peritumoral areas [4] and peritumoral edema was attenuated by lipoxygenase inhibitors [2, 5]. Similarly, a 3-fold increase in BBB permeability constants was observed when low doses of LTC_4 were administered 72 hours after permanent middle cerebral artery occlusion in rat [1].

It is still not clear whether CEC have the metabolic machinery to produce the peptidoleukotriene precursor LTA_4 in view of the reported lack of 5-lipoxygenase [19]. It has been suggested that precursor LTA_4 can be delivered to endothelial cells by neutrophils [9]. We have previously shown that in vitro ischemia/recovery induces the expression of adhesion molecules in HCEC and facilitates neutrophil adhesion to HCEC monolayers [26]. It is plausible to suggest that this interaction may enable neutrophils to deliver LTA_4 to HCEC where it is subsequently converted into LTC_4 and LTB_4. In addition, the demonstrated ischemic loss of GSH in HCEC may in part be due to an increased glutathione S-transferase-mediated GSH utilization for the leukotriene pathway. Since detoxifying GGTP is substantially reduced in ischemic HCEC, LTC_4 is allowed to accumulate and permeabilize BBB endothelium. During oxidative stress HCEC are damaged by both ischemia and activated neutrophils which most likely contributes to the BBB disruption. LTB_4 formed in this cascade is a potent neutrophil chemoattractant and may initiate neutrophil transmigration across the weakened BBB [9].

Even though many of the described molecular events are hypothetical, this study provides strong evidence that hypoxia/ischemia alters BBB properties of HCEC by inducing oxidative stress and by rendering the cells more vulnerable to permeabilizing actions of leukotrienes. These ischemia-induced changes are likely to underly the pathophysiology of both ischemic vasogenic edema and postischemic brain inflammation.

Acknowledgment

This study is supported by the grant (#ST2718) from the Heart and Stroke Foundation of Ontario.

References

1. Baba T, Black KL, Ikezaki K, Chen K, Becker DP (1991) Intracarotid infusion of leukotriene C_4 selectively increases blood-brain barrier permeability after focal ischemia in rats. J Cerebral Blood Flow Metab 11: 638–643
2. Baba T, Chio C-C, Black KL (1992) The effect of 5-lipoxygenase inhibition on blood-brain barrier permeability in experimental brain tumors. J Neurosurg 77: 403–406
3. Black KL (1995) Biochemical opening of the blood brain barrier. Adv Drug Delivery Rev 15: 37–52
4. Black KL, Baba T, Pardridge WM (1994) Enzymatic barrier protects brain capillaries from leukotrience C_4. J Neurosurg. 81: 745–751
5. Black KL, Hoff JT, McGillicuddy JE, Gebarski SS (1986) Increased leukotrience C_4 and vasogenic edema surrounding brain tumors in humans. Ann Neurol 19: 592–595
6. Bradford MM (1976) A rapid and sensitive method of quantification of microgram quantities of proteins utilizing the principle of protein dye binding. Anal Biochem 72: 248–254
7. Carlberg I, Mannervik B (1985) Glutathione reductase. Methods enzymol. In: Meister A (ed) Academic Press, New York, 113: 484–490

8. Chan PH, Schmidley JW, Fishman RA, Longar SM (1984) Brain injury, edema and vascular permeability changes induced by oxygen-derived free radicals. Neurology 34: 315–320
9. Claesson H-E, Haeggstrom J (1988) Human endothelial cells stimulate leukotriene synthesis and convert granulocyte released leukotriene A_4 into leukotrienes B_4, C_4, D_4, and E_4. Eur J Biochem 173: 93–100
10. Dehouck MP, Jolliet-Riant P, Bree F, Fruchart JC, Cechelli R, Tillement J-P (1992) Drug transfer across the blood-brain barrier: correlation between in vitro and in vivo models. J Neurochem 58: 1790–1797
11. delZoppo GJ (1994) Microvascular changes during cerebral ischemia and reperfusion. Cerebrovasc Brain Metab Rev 6: 47–96
12. Flohe L, Gunzler A (1984) Assays of glutathione peroxidase. Methods in enzymology. In: Packer L (ed) Academic Press, New York, 105: 114–121
13. Frey A (1993) Gamma-glutamyl transpeptidase: molecular cloning and structural and functional features of a blood-brain barrier marker protein. The blood-brain barrier cellular and molecular biology. In: Pardridge WM (ed) Raven Press, New York, pp 339–368
14. Gidday JM, Beetsch JW, Park TS (1999) Endogenous glutathione protects cerebral endothelial cells from traumatic injury. J Neurotrauma 16: 27–36
15. Habig EH, Pabst MJ, Jakoby WB (1974) Glutathione-S-transferases: the first enzymatic step in mercaptopuric acid formation. J Biol Chem 249: 7130–7139
16. Hurst RD, Heales SJ, Dobbie MS, Barker JE, Clark JB (1998) Decreased endothelial cell glutathione and increased sensitivity to oxidative stress in an in vitro blood-brain barrier model system. Brain Res 802: 232–240
17. Juurlink BHJ, Schultke, E, Hertz L (1996) Glutathione release and catabolism during energy substrate restriction in astrocytes. Brain Res 710: 229–233
18. Kokura S, Wolf RE, Yoshikawa T, Granger DN, Aw TY (1999) Molecular mechanisms of neutrophil-endothelial cell adhesion induced by redox imbalance. Circ Res 84: 516–524
19. Lindgren JA, Karnushina I, Clesson. H-E (1989) Role of brain microvessels and choroid plexus in cerebral metabolism of leukotrienes. Ann NY Acad Sci 559: 112–120
20. Moskovitz MA, Kiwak KJ, Hekimian K, Levine L (1984) Synthesis of compounds with properties of leukotriene C_4 and D_4 in gerbil brains after ischemia and reperfusion. Science 224: 886–888
21. Muruganandam A, Herx LM, Monette R, Durkin JP, Stanimirovic DB (1997) Development of immortalized human cerebromicrovascular endothelial cell line as an in vitro model of the human blood-brain barrier. FASEB J 13: 1187–1197
22. Plateel M, Dehouck M-P, Torpier G, Cecchelli R, Teissier E (1995) Hypoxia increases the susceptibility to oxidant stress and the permeability of the blood-brain barrier endothelial cell monolayer. J Neurochem 65: 2138–2145
23. Rabin O, Piciotti M, Drieu K, Bourre JM, Roux F (1996) Effects of anoxia and reoxygenation on antioxidant enzyme activities in immortalized brain endothelial cells. In Vitro Cell Dev 32: 221–224
24. Samuelsson B (1983) Leukotrienes: mediators of immediate hypersensitivity and inflammation. Science 220: 568–575
25. Stanimirovic D, Morley P, Ball R, Hamel E, Mealing G, Durkin JP (1996) Angiotensin II-induced fluid phase endocytosis in human cerebromicrovascular endothelial cells is regulated by the inositol-phosphate signaling pathway. J Cell Physiol 169: 455–467
26. Stanimirovic D, Shapiro A, Wong J, Hutchison J, Durkin J (1997) The induction of ICAM-1 in human cerebromicrovascular endothelial cells (HCEC) by ischemia-like conditions promotes enhanced neutrophil/HCEC adhesion. J Neuroimmunol 76(1–2): 193–205
27. Stanimirovic DB, Wong J, Ball R, Durkin JP (1995) Free radical-induced endothelial membrane dysfunction at the site of blood brain barrier: relationship between lipid peroxidation, Na, K-ATPase activity and ^{51}Cr release. Neurochem Res 20: 1417–1427
28. Strasser A, Stanimirovic DB, Kawai N, McCarron RM, Spatz M (1997) Hypoxia modulates free radical formation in brain microvascular endothelium. Acta Neurochir [Suppl] (Wien) 70: 8–11
29. Unterberg A, Schmidt W, Wahl M, Ellis EF, Marmarou A, Baethmann A (1991) Evidence against leukotrienes as mediators of brain edema. J Neurosurg 74: 773–780
30. Wei EP, Ellison M, Kontos HA, Povlishock JT (1986) O_2 radicals in arachidonate-induced increased blood-brain barrier permeability to proteins. Am J Physiol 251: H693–H699

Correspondence: Dr. Danica Stanimirovic, Cellular Neurobiology Group, Institute for Biological Sciences, National Research Council of Canada, Montreal Road Campus, Bldg. M-54, Ottawa, ONT, Canada, K1A 0R6.

Acta Neurochir (2000) [Suppl] 76: 35–37

Comparison of NAA Measures by MRS and HPLC

P. P. Fatouros[1], **D. L. Heath**[2], **A. Beaumont**[2], **F. D. Corwin**[1], **S. Signoretti**[2], **R. H. AL-Samsam**[2], **B. Alessandri**[2], **P. Lazzarino**[2], **R. Vagnozzi**[2], **B. Tavazzi**[2], **R. Bullock**[2], and **A. Marmarou**[2]

[1] Division of Radiation Physics, Medical College of Virginia, Virginia Commonwealth University, Richmond, VA, USA
[2] Division Neurosurgery, Medical College of Virginia, Virginia Commonwealth University, Richmond, VA, USA

Summary

This work investigates the accuracy of an in vivo estimation of absolute N-acetyl aspartate (NAA) concentrations by magnetic resonance spectroscopy (MRS) using cerebral water as an internal reference standard. Single-voxel, proton spectroscopy was carried out in two groups of rats (normal and diffuse head injury), using a PRESS sequence with TR = 3 s, TE = 135 ms. Fully relaxed water spectra and water-suppressed proton spectra were obtained from a $7 \times 5 \times 5$ mm^3 volume of tissue. MRI-based brain water content measurements were also performed. Following MRS, HPLC determinations of NAA were carried out. In the normal rats the MRS yielded 10.98 ± 0.83 mmol/kg w.w. vs 10.76 ± 0.76 for HPLC with a mean absolute difference of 0.8. In the injured rats the corresponding results were 9.41 ± 1.78 (MRS) and 8.16 ± 0.77 (HPLC) with a mean absolute difference of 1.66. The in vivo absolute method accurately documented the temporal NAA changes compared to the NAA/Cr approach.

Keywords: NAA quantification; MRS; proton spectroscopy.

Introduction

Reductions in NAA have been thought of as a marker of neuronal death. Non-invasive serial determinations of NAA are particularly important in situations where cell injury is expected such as in head injury as a means of assessing the metabolic state of the brain, initiating appropriate therapy and possibly arriving at a long-term prognosis. Currently, the majority of studies have by necessity reported results in the form of ratios of peak areas, typically NAA/Creatine or NAA/Choline. The use of relative concentrations is straightforward and easily implemented. However, it does assume constancy in the concentration of either Cr or Cho, a condition not necessarily correct in the presence of disease. Absolute determinations have used either internal or external standards, each with its own advantages and limitations. Investigators have used both approaches, making several assumptions and typically providing validations using solutions of known concentrations. A crucial assumption that is normally made is the use of tabulated values for brain water content, a situation clearly unsatisfactory because of differences in tissue type and the possibility of edema. The various assumptions have led to widely varying reported tissue NAA levels. In this work we have addressed these issues by using brain water as an internal standard. Brain water was have measured independently using an MRI-based non-invasive method and we compared our in vivo results with ex-vivo determinations by HPLC. The use of internal water as a reference standard avoids difficulties associated with inhomogeneities in the B_0 and B_1 fields which are inherent with the external standard approach. In addition to testing the accuracy of our approach we have investigated its sensitivity in detecting NAA changes following traumatic brain injury and have documented the temporal course of these changes whilst comparing them with the conventional NAA/Cr ratio method.

Materials and Methods

Animal Preparation and Injury Induction

All animals received humane care in compliance with the "Guide for the Care and Use of Laboratory Animals" (NIH Publication 86–23, 1989) and in compliance with the VCU Institutional Animal Care & Use Committee Regulations. Adult male Sprague-Dawley rats (350–400 gms) were housed in standard conditions, with food and water ad libitum before being initially anesthetized with Halothane 4% and a mixture of N_2O (66%) and O_2 (33%) in a ventilated anesthesia chamber. Animals were then trans-orally intubated and mechanically ventilated. Anesthesia was maintained with Halothane (1.5–2% during surgical procedures and 1% for duration of monitoring). A femoral arterial catheter (PE-50) facilitated hourly blood gas sampling and continuous mean arterial blood pressure monitoring (MABP) via a MacLab computer system. A midline scalp incision was made and the skin and periosteum reflected from the skull to the level of the temporalis muscles. All bleeding was controlled by electro-caurtery. Body temperature was monitored and maintained between 36.5–37.5 C during all surgical and magnetic resonance procedures.

Animals were randomly placed into one of two groups: sham injury (S/n = 4) or impact-acceleration followed immediately with 10 min hypoxia and hypotension (THH10/n = 5). All animals were placed prone and immobilized within a plastic cylinder; their head was rigidly supported within a specially designed MRI compatible stereotactic device that included both ear and mouth bars mounted inside the cylinder. Once surgically prepared, all animals were inserted into the magnet and baseline data as specified below was acquired for approximately one hour.

Following baseline MRI acquisition, all rats were removed from the magnet and the plastic cylinder. Animals subjected to trauma received a severe diffuse brain injury using the impact-acceleration model as previously described in detail [1]. Briefly, a stainless steel disc (10 mm in diameter and 2 mm in depth) was fixed to the skull centrally between lambda and bregma using rapid drying cyanoacrylic glue. Animals were then placed on a 10 cm deep foam bed and injury induced by dropping a 450 gm brass weight from a distance of two meters onto the stainless steel disc. Immediately following impact-acceleration injury the animal was repositioned in the magnet and a ten minute period of hypoxia and hypotension initiated. In the groups exposed to secondary insult, hypoxia was induced by reducing the oxygen content of the inspired gases ($FiO_2 = 12\%$), so that plasma PaO_2 was maintained at approximately 40 mmHg for 10 minutes. MABP was reduced by the influence of trauma, and hypoxia, but the inspired concentration of halothane was elevated by 2% to a mean of 3.5% in order to impair the vasopressor response to hypoxia. MABP was maintained at 30–40 mmHg. Animals were resuscitated by resetting anesthetic parameters to normal values while the animal was still within the magnet.

Immediately following the 4 h post injury MR schedule all animals were removed from the magnet and prepared for rapid brain tissue removal. Brain tissue correlating to the voxel studied by MR was extracted by performing a craniectomy. The bone was carefully removed ensuring the sinuses remained intact and that the animal's blood pressure was maintained. Guided by the transverse and sagittal MR images a scalpel blade was used to make two very quick incisions through the intact brain localizing the brain tissue measured by MR. The brain segment was then rapidly extracted and placed immediately into liquid nitrogen and stored for processing as described below.

Magnetic Resonance Studies

All magnetic resonance imaging (MRI) and spectroscopy (MRS) experiments were performed using a 2.35 T, 40 cm bore magnet (Biospec, Bruker Instruments, Billerica, MA) equipped with a 12 cm inner diameter actively shielded gradient insert. Proton RF excitation and reception was performed using a 5 cm saddle-shaped helmet coil. The PRESS single-voxel technique with water suppression, TR/TE 3000/135, 256 acq., $7 \times 5 \times 5$ mm^3 was used for acquiring NAA spectra. A fully relaxed water spectrum was obtained using the same technique with one acquisition. T_1 and T_2 measurements of brain tissue were performed using the PRESS sequence with variable TR and TE respectively.

Brain Water Measurements

Brain water was obtained by an MRI-based imaging technique previously described [2]. In brief, this method involves the generation of a pure T_1 image and its subsequent conversion to a water map by means of the following equation: $1/W = 0.907 + 0.407/T_1$.

HPLC Measurements

The amount of NAA in the extracted tissue sample was measured by HPLC. Frozen tissue samples were homogenised in acid conditions. NAA was separated using a buffer with the following composition: 2.8 mM tetrabutyl ammonium hydroxide (as the pairing reagent), 25 mM KH_2PO_4, 12.5% methanol, and pH 7.00 at a flow rate of 1 ml/min. A C-18, 250×4.6 mm, 5 um particle size column thermostated at 23 °C by a water jacket was used. The HPLC apparatus is composed by two pumps connected to a high sensitivity diode array detector set up between 200 and 300 nm wavelength. Acquisition and analysis of data is performed by a PC with a software package supplied by the HPLC manufacturer. Under these chromatographic conditions NAA is eluted with a retention time of 12.5 min (k' = 6.25). The lowest detection limit is 1 μM, i.e. 1000 times less than the level found in control brain. The concentration of NAA in tissue samples is calculated using the area under the NAA peak at 210 nm wavelength by comparison with the area of a sample of ultapure NAA of known concentration. The philosophy of this separation is to keep NAA bound to the column longer than all the uncharged or low charged compounds, generally present in tissue extract which may interfere with NAA. These are eluted and then NAA passes through the column in the absence of interfering molecules. This is necessary because NAA does not have any other characteristic absorbance apart from 210 nm wavelength, where many other compounds can absorb.

Results

In Vivo Rat Brain Relaxation Times

The measured normal rat brain relaxation times for NAA and water from variable TR and TE acquisitions yielded the following results (n = 7):

NAA (mean ± std dev): $T_1 = 1.58\ s \pm 0.31$
$T_2 = 297\ ms \pm 50$
Brain water (mean ± std dev): $T_1 = 1.19\ s \pm 0.08$
$T_2 = 78\ ms \pm 5$

Brain Water Content

The measured water content by MRI pre-injury and at 4 hrs post THH were 78.3% ± 0.9 and 78.8% ± 1.1 respectively.

NAA Concentrations

In the normal rats, the MRS and HPLC determined absolute NAA levels were 10.96 mmol/kg w.w. ± 0.83

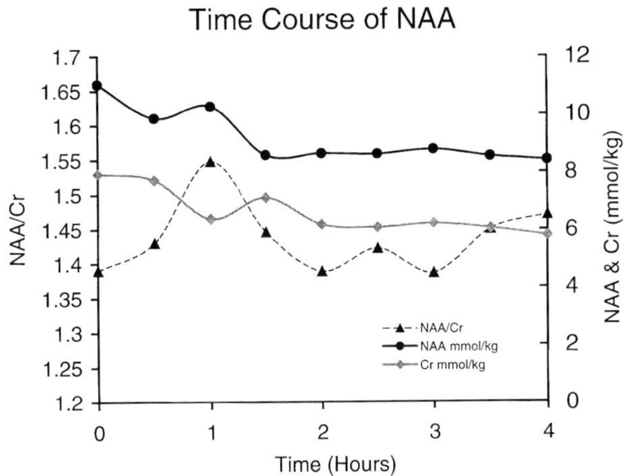

Fig. 1. The time course of NAA following traumatic brain injury for the NAA/Cr ratio, and the absolute concentration. The grey line indicates the calculated absolute creatine level from: [Cr] = [NAA]/[NAA/Cr]

and 10.76 mmol/kg w.w. ± 0.76, respectively with a mean absolute difference of 0.8 mmol/kg w.w. For the injured rats at 4 hrs the corresponding values were 9.41 mmol/kg w.w. ± 1.78 (MRS) and 8.16 mmol/kg w.w. ± 0.77 (HPLC) with a mean absolute difference of 1.66 mmol/kg w.w.

Temporal Course of NAA

The temporal course of absolute NAA changes in an injured animal is shown in Fig. 1 and is compared with the corresponding changes of the ratio NAA/Cr. Also plotted is the calculated creatine concentration from the equation: [Cr] = [NAA]/[NAA/Cr].

Discussion

The proposed in vivo method for determining absolute NAA metabolite concentrations was found to be in good agreement with the HPLC measurements in the normal animals with a mean absolute difference between the two methods of 0.8 mmol/kg w.w. and no statistical significant difference between the two sets of measurements. The agreement was less in the injured animals which at 4 hrs post injury exhibited a 24% average decrease in NAA concentration as measured by HPLC versus 14% as determined by MRS. The decrease in NAA following TBI was found to be statistically significant when compared to the normal group (t-test, $p < 0.001$) in the HPLC NAA measurements but not in the MRS-determined NAA levels. The mean absolute difference of 1.66 mmol/kg w.w. in this case was also higher. A possible reason for this discrepancy might be the presence of a fast-decaying water component which is not detectable by the commonly used long TE sequences. This issue is currently under investigation.

As seen from figure 1, the time-course of the absolute NAA concentration following TBI exhibits an expected monotonic decline, which was verified by the HPLC measurements. In contrast, the time-course of the NAA/Cr ratio shows wide fluctuations and a return to normal values at four hours, in disagreement with both the HPLC and absolute MRS measures. Hence one can conclude that the use of NAA/Cr ratio to document the temporal course of NAA changes might be misleading. This problem might be due to changes in the absolute creatine concentration which is usually assumed to remain constant.

References

1. Marmarou A, Abd-Elfattah Foda MA, van der Brink W *et al* (1994) A new model of diffuse brain injury in rats: part I: pathophysiology and biomechanics. J Neurosurg 80: 291–300
2. Fatouros PP, Marmarou A (1999) Use of magnetic resonance imaging for in vivo measurements of water content in human brain: method and normal values. J Neurosurg 90: 109–115

Correspondence: P. P. Fatouros, Ph.D., Medical College of Virginia/VCU, PO Box 980072, Richmond, VA 23298.

Acta Neurochir (2000) [Suppl] 76: 39–41

Influence of the Bradykinin B1/B2-Receptor-Antagonist B 9430 on the Cerebral Microcirculation and Outcome of Gerbils from Global Cerebral Ischemia

J. Lehmberg[1], **J. Beck**[1], **A. Baethmann**[1], and **E. Uhl**[2]

[1] Institute for Surgical Research, Klinikum of Ludwig-Maximilians-University Standort Großhadern, Munich, Germany
[2] Department of Neurosurgery, Klinikum of Ludwig-Maximilians-University Standort Großhadern, Munich, Germany

Summary

The influence of the bradykinin B1/B2 antagonist B 9430 on the cerebral microcirculation following global cerebral ischemia was investigated in a closed cranial window preparation in Mongolian gerbils by intravital fluorescence microscopy. Global cerebral ischemia (GCI) was induced by occlusion of both common carotid arteries for 15 min. Leukocyte-endothelium interactions, vessel diameters, and the segmental microvascular blood flow were observed by intravital microscopy before and up to three hours after global cerebral ischemia. Following the early reperfusion period the animals survived up to 4 days after ischemia. The neurological deficit and the body weight were assessed daily. On day 4 animals were subjected to perfusion fixation and the brain was removed. Nerve cell damage from ischemia was quantified histologically in cortex, hippocampus, and striatum. Animals with treatment received the bradykinin B1/B2 receptor antagonist B 9430 before (i.v.), during, and after ischemia (s.c.) until the end of the experiment. The frequency of leukocytes (cells/100 μm × min) rolling along the venular endothelium post ischemia was significantly decreased ($p < 0.05$) in treated animals as compared to untreated controls (33.0 ± 6.2 vs. 8.5 ± 2.3) as well as the number of leukocytes attached to the endothelial surface (7.2 ± 3.0 vs. 2.0 ± 1.0, n.s.). The neuroscore on day 4 (pre-ischemic control: 22 points) was reduced to 13.4 ± 3.2 in untreated animals, while to 4.7 ± 3.2 points in the treatment group. No differences between animals with and without treatment were found as to the number of viable neurons. Although bradykinin is released in the brain during global cerebral ischemia, its antagonisation does not improve outcome despite the effective inhibition of leukocyte-endothelium interactions.

Keywords: Leukocytes; endothelium; bradykinin antagonist; global cerebral ischemia.

Introduction

Kinin formation has been described in humans in cerebral ischemia and postischemic reperfusion [7]. Beside their effects on cerebral vessels, kinins are involved in the development of ischemic brain edema. It has been shown in peripheral tissues that the enzymes and factors of the kallikrein/kinin cascade are involved [4] in accumulation of neutrophils in acute inflammation [1]. Therefore it is surmised that the release of bradykinin following brain injury or cerebral ischemia contributes to the activation of leukocytes in affected brain tissue resulting in an enhancement of secondary brain damage. Therapeutical methods directed against activation of these cells may improve the outcome after stroke [5]. In a previous study we have shown, that selective antagonisation of bradykinin B1 and B2 receptors reduces leukocyte-endothelium interactions in global cerebral ischemia but does not affect the neurological deficit and neuronal damage from ischemia [6]. Aim of the present study was to examine whether blocking of both the B1 and B2 bradykinin receptor reduces leukocyte-endothelium interactions in cerebral vessels affording inhibition of secondary brain damage from ischemia and, thus, of the development of the neurological deficit.

Material and Methods

Male Mongolian gerbils (60–80 g b.w) were anaesthetised with halothane under spontaneous respiration. The animals were placed on a feedback controlled heating pad to maintain normothermia (37 °C). Catheters in the tail artery and the left femoral vein were used for continuous measuring of the arterial blood pressure and injection of fluorescent dyes and of the antagonist. The skulls of the animals were fixed in a stereotactic holder, and a closed cranial window of 5 × 5 mm was trephined over the left parietal cortex leaving the dura mater intact [3]. For intravital fluorescence microscopy the animals were placed on a microscopic stage equipped with a computer controlled moving device allowing repeated measurements of identical vessel segments over an extended period of time. Images were recorded by a highly sensitive SIT camera and stored on video tape for off-line evaluation. Rhodamine 6 G (0.03 μg/kg b.w. i.v., Sigma, Deisenhofen, Germany) was injected as in vivo marker for leukocytes. Contrast enhancement of microvessels was achieved by intravenous injection of FITC-Dextran (MW 150.000, 0.7 g/kg b.w., Sigma, Deisenhofen, Germany). Following a control period of 1 hour forebrain ischemia was induced by transient occlusion of both common carotid arteries with a 5-0 monofilament thread (Prolene, Ethicon, Norderstedt, Germany) for 15 min. Microvascular parameters including the frequency of leukocytes rolling along and firmly adhering (n/100 μm × min) to the venular endothelium, segmental microvascular perfusion, and venular and arteriolar diameters were assessed at 40, 20, and 5 min prior to ischemia and at 5, 20, 40, 60, 90, 120, and 180 min of reperfusion. Subsequently the skin was sutured over the cranial window, and animals were allowed to wake up. The animals were daily examined thereafter using a modified neuroscore as described by Mc Graw [8] up to day four of reperfusion. On day 4 the animals were perfused with 2% paraformaldehyde and the brains were removed for histomorphological evaluation. The density of vital neurons (n/mm^2) was quantified in the hippocampus (CA1–CA4), the striatum as well as in the parietal and frontal cortex using an image analysing program (Optimas 5.0, Seattle, Washington, USA) [9]. The bradykinin B1/B2-receptor antagonist B 9430 (Cortech Inc., Denver, Colorado, USA) was injected intravenously as a bolus of 18 μg/kg b.w. 15 min before ischemia followed by continuous subcutaneous administration of 300 ng/kg b.w. using a mini osmotic pump (Alza, Palo Alto, CA, USA).

Results

Leukocyte endothelium interactions were not observed in the control period before ischemia. Three hours after global cerebral ischemia the number of rolling and sticking leukocytes had increased to 33.0 ± 6.2 and to 8.5 ± 2.3 (cells/100 μm × min, mean ± SEM), respectively. Administration of the animals with B 9430 resulted in significant reduction ($p < 0.05$) of the number of rolling leukocytes to 3.7 ± 2.3 at 120 min and to 7.2 ± 3.0 at 180 min of reperfusion. Leukocyte adhesion was reduced to 2.0 ± 1.0 cells/100 μm × min at 180 min of reperfusion (n.s.). Vessel diameters and segmental microvascular blood flow did not differ significantly between controls and animals with the receptor blocker. 7/10 animals of the control group survived the four days of post ischemia but only 2/8 animals of the group with treatment ($p = 0.06$, Kaplan-Meier test). The neuroscore of control animals was steadily declining during the four days post ischemia from 22 points (pre-ischemic) to 13.4 ± 3.2 (mean ± SEM) points at day four. In treated animals the neuroscore declined even to 4.8 ± 3.2 points on day four, although this was not attaining statistical significance versus the untreated controls. Differences between the groups were not found as to the density of surviving neurons in the different brain areas.

Discussion

The present findings indicate that bradykinin is released during global cerebral ischemia, and that it is involved in the induction of leukocyte-endothelium interactions during the reperfusion period. Other microvascular parameters do not seem to be influenced by this mediator agent. This conclusion is based on the observation that blocking of bradykinin B1 and B2 receptors by the selective antagonist B 9340 reduces the number of leukocytes rolling along and adhering to the venular endothelium. Comparing these data with previous studies with separate blocking of B1 and B2 receptors, we could not observe additional effects [6]. Surprisingly, the inhibition of leukocyte-endothelium interactions by blocking bradykinin B1/B2-receptors did neither afford significant protection against nerve cell damage from ischemia, nor an improvement of functional outcome. This may indicate that leukocyte-endothelium interactions, at least during early reperfusion, have no influence on the survival of neurons after global cerebral ischemia. Whether blocking of leukocyte-endothelium interactions by the B1/B2 receptor antagonist has a negative influence on the functional outcome following such an incident remains uncertain. Our data may imply that the release of bradykinin even has a protective function. Yet, side effects of the B1/B2 antagonist enhancing the neurological deficit and lethal outcome from ischemia cannot be excluded.

References

1. Ahluwalia A, Perretti M (1996) Involvement of bradykinin B1 receptors in the polymorphonuclear leukocyte accumulation induced by IL-1beta in vivo in the mouse. J Immun 156: 269–274
2. Baatz H, Steinbauer M, Harris AG, Krombach F (1995) Kinetics of white blood cell staining by intravascular administration of Rhodamin 6G. Int J Microcirc 15: 85–91
3. Beck J, Stummer W, Lehmberg J, Baethmann, A, Uhl E (1997) Leukocyte-endothelium interactions in global cerebral ischemia. Acta Neurochir [Suppl] (Wien) 70: 53–55
4. Bhoola KD, Figueroa CD, Worthy K (1992) Bioregulation of kinins: kallikreins, kininogens, and kininases. Pharmacol Rev 44: 1–80
5. Kochanek PM, Hallenbeck JM (1992) Polymorphonuclear leukocytes and monocytes/macrophages in the pathogenesis of cerebral ischemia and stroke. Stroke 23: 1367–1379
6. Lehmberg J, Baethmann A, Uhl E (1998) Influence of the bradykinin B2-receptor-antagonist CP 0597 on the cerebral microcirculation and outcome on global cerebral ischemia. Cerebrovasc Dis 8 [Suppl] 4: 76
7. Makevnina LG, Lomova IP, Zubkov YuN, Semenyutin VB

(1994) Kininogen consumption in cerebral circulation of humans during brain ischemia and postischemic reperfusion. Brazilian J Med Biol Res 27: 1955–1963
8. McGraw CP (1977) Experimental cerebral infarction effects of pentobarbital in mongolian gerbils. Arch Neurol 34: 334–336
9. Stummer W, Weber DVM, Tranmer B, Baethmann A, Kempski O (1994) Reduced mortality and brain damage after locomotor activity in gerbil forebrain ischemia. Stroke 25: 1862–1869

Correspondence: Eberhard Uhl, M.D., Department of Neurosurgery, Klinikum of Ludwig-Maximilians-University Standort Großhadern, Marchioninistr. 15, D-81377 Munich, Germany.

Acta Neurochir (2000) [Suppl] 76: 43–46

Evolution of Energy Failure after Repeated Cerebral Ischemia in Gerbils

T. Kuroiwa[1], **U. Ito**[2], **Y. Hakamata**[3], **S. Hanyu**[4], **G. Mies**[5], and **D. Hermann**[5]

[1] Department of Neuropathology, Medical Research Institute, Tokyo Medical and Dental University, Tokyo, Japan
[2] Department of Neurosurgery, Musashino Red Cross Hospital, Tokyo, Japan
[3] Laboratory of Experimental Medicine, Jichi Medical School, Tochigi, Japan
[4] Department of Neurology, Jichi Medical School, Tochigi, Japan
[5] Max-Planck-Institute for Neurological Research, Cologne, Germany

Summary

We have examined the regional differences in the evolution of energy failure in experimental focal cerebral ischemia. In gerbil brain subjected to repeated unilateral common carotid artery occlusion, the tissue ATP content, pH and succinic dehydrogenase activity decreased at different rates after the circulation had been restored in various cerebral regions. Light microscopical infarction became apparent at different rates following the impairment of the energy metabolism in these regions. In brain cortex with selective neuronal necrosis, only minor alterations in energy metabolism were detectable over a 7-day period following the restoration of the circulation. The present data show that the rate of energy failure is significantly different in various cerebral regions after repeated periods of cerebral ischemia in the gerbil. A slowly evolving impairment of the cerebral energy metabolism after circulation of the brain has been restored appears to be indispensable for the delayed formation of infarction after transient cerebral ischemia.

Keywords: Repeated cerebral ischemia; energy failure; evolving infarction; selective neuronal necrosis.

Introduction

Cerebral infarction often evolves rapidly becoming apparent within several hours after the onset of ischemia. However, infarct formation may also be rather delayed, e.g. for a week after the circulation has been restored provided the ischemic episode was mild [1, 5]. Persistent energy failure has been documented as a cause of the rapid, irreversible infarct process often resulting from permanent vascular occlusion. The mechanisms of delayed infarct formation, however, remain unknown. In a previous study, we have observed that the cerebral energy metabolism was gradually failing over several days after restoration of the cerebral circulation in gerbil cortex with slowly evolving infarction [9]. In the current study, we have examined whether there are regional differences in the occurrence of energy failure with regard to infarct development after repeated episodes of focal cerebral ischemia. This paper is a summary of our recent studies [9, 10].

Materials and Methods

All animal experiments were performed in accordance with institutional guidelines for animal care and experimentation. Adult Mongolian gerbils weighing 60–80 g were anesthetized with halothane. The left common carotid artery (CCA) was occluded using a mini vascular clip, anesthesia was then discontinued. In animals that developed functional stroke symptoms [12], blood flow was restored after 10 min of occlusion. Five hours later, the animals were subjected to a second 10-min CCA occlusion under halothane anesthesia. The experiments were terminated at various time intervals after ischemia for determination of the tissue ATP and glucose contents, pH, activity of succinic dehydrogenase (SDH), and for light-microscopic tissue examination. For determination of the tissue ATP and glucose content by using a bioluminescence method, the animals' brains were frozen and removed from the skull in a cold-temperature cabinet. 20-μm coronal cryostat sections were prepared at −20 °C for quantitative imaging.

The regional tissue pH was measured quantitatively by the umbelliferone method. For determination of the tissue SDH activity, brains were removed rapidly under anesthesia and prepared for quantitative imaging [8]. For histological examination, the brain was subjected to transcardiac perfusion fixation with 4% buffered formalin under anesthesia, and the tissue was stained with hematoxylin-eosin and Kluever-Barrera. All values are presented as mean ± SD.

Results

The changes in post-ischemic energy metabolism in different cerebral regions were following different time courses. The tissue ATP content decreased to 50% of control at 5 h in the dorsolateral thalamus, after 1–2 days at the chiasmal level of brain cortex, and after 2–4 days in the caudate nucleus. In parallel with the reduction of the tissue ATP levels, the SDH activity was also decreasing at different rates. The SDH activity decreased to 50% of control at 5–12 h in the dorsolateral thalamus, after 1–2 days at the chiasmal level of brain cortex, and after 2–4 days in the hippocampal CA1 and CA3 sectors. The average brain tissue pH in the control group was 7.085 ± 0.189. The tissue pH decreased to 6.5 at 5–12 h in the dorsolateral thalamus, at 12 h–1 d in the caudate nucleus and at 2–4 d in the hippocampal CA1 and CA3 sectors. In the cortex at the infundibular level, which developed only disseminated selective neuronal necrosis, the tissue energy metabolism showed only minor changes during the various periods when the cerebral circulation was restored.

Cerebral infarction developed in the dorsolateral thalamus, dorsolateral caudate nucleus, hippocampal CA3 and CA1 sectors, and chiasmal level of cortex over a 5–48 h period after restoration of the cerebral circulation. Infarction became apparent at different time periods after energy failure in these regions. In brain cortex at the infundibular level, scattered eosinophilic neurons were observed with mildly shrunken and homogeneously stained cytoplasm, representing disseminated selective neuronal necrosis [3] over a 2–7-d period after restoration of the circulation. The neuropil showed very mild microvacuolation from 12 h to 7 d after restoration of circulation.

Discussion

We have observed that infarction develops in the same animal at different post-ischemic time intervals in various brain regions. The repeated induction of focal cerebral ischemia was associated with a deterioration in energy metabolism that was apparent before the manifestation of infarction. In contrast, in brain regions that developed selective neuronal necrosis, the disturbances of the energy metabolism were mild occurring in parallel with the appearance of neuronal necrosis.

Although cerebral infarction often develops rapidly in clinical cases, experimental as well as clinical data have shown that the injury process may take several days to weeks after an initial ischemic insult. Our results are indicating in addition that the rate of the infarction process may considerably vary in different cerebral regions.

Table 1. *Post-Ischemic Time Period Elapsing until the ATP Content and SDH Activity is Decreased to 50% Normal, the Tissue pH Reached 6.5, and the Glucose Content is 1.5 fold Increased in the Postischemic Brain. Note the Remarkable Variation Among Regions*

	ATP content	SDH activity	pH	Glucose content
Chiasmal level cortex	1–2 d	1–2 d	1–2 d	1–2 d
Caudate nucleus	2–4 d	12 h–1 d	12 h–1 d	12 h–1 d
Infundibular level cortex	–	–	–	–
CA 1 sector	–	2–4 d	2–4 d	2–4 d
CA 3 sector	–	2–4 d	2–4 d	2–4 d
Thalamus	5 h	5–12 h	5–12 h	5–12 h

It has been shown in previous studies that the ATP level in ischemic brain tissue rapidly declines to zero shortly after the onset of ischemia. This break-down of the energy metabolism, however, does not indicate irreversible tissue injury. In fact, after transient forebrain ischemia in gerbils, a temporary depletion of ATP has been observed in both ischemia-resistant and ischemia-vulnerable areas [11]. In our study, the regional ATP levels were decreasing at different rates in the post-ischemic brain. This decline occurred after restoration of the cerebral circulation only in those areas which were developing infarction in parallel with a decrease of mitochondrial enzyme activity. The observed decline is probably different from the well-known intraischemic ATP depletion. We assume that the observed disturbances of the energy metabolism are an important process that precedes slowly evolving infarction. Recently, it has been shown that the cellular bioenergetic state may partially recover followed by a subsequent secondary deterioration after transient middle cerebral artery occlusion in the rat [7]. Our findings agree with this finding and underline the importance of the progressive energy failure in the course of infarct formation. It has been shown that the injection of a specific and permanent inhibitor of SDH, 3-nitropropionic acid (3-NP), induces ischemic tissue injury in the brain [2]. A small dose of 3-NP, on the other hand, affords tolerance against subsequent ischemia [13]. Therefore, the duration and extent of the dysfunction of SDH appear to be crucial for both the development and prevention of ischemic cell injury.

The brain cortex at the infundibular level only developed selective neuronal necrosis that became light-microscopically evident 2–7 days after the onset of recirculation. This area revealed only a very mild decrease in tissue ATP levels and SDH activity, in con-

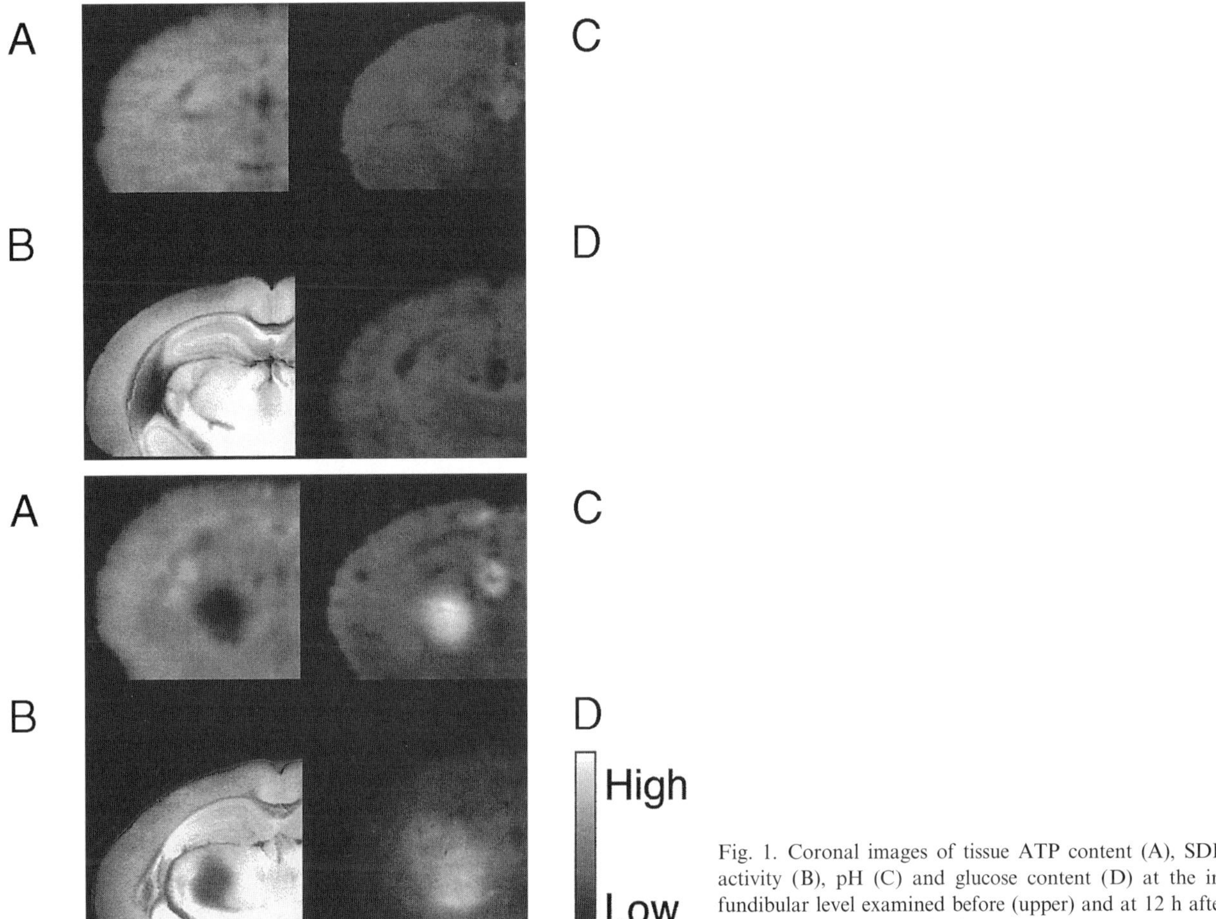

Fig. 1. Coronal images of tissue ATP content (A), SDH activity (B), pH (C) and glucose content (D) at the infundibular level examined before (upper) and at 12 h after repeated cerebral ischemia (lower)

trast to the changes in areas that developed infarction. It has been shown that the energy metabolism is preserved in the post-ischemic hippocampal CA1 sector during the recirculation period until delayed neuronal death of the pyramidal layer occurs [9, 11]. Post-ischemic impairment of the energy metabolism is probably not the primary factor for the development of selective neuronal death in either the cortex at the infundibular level or the hippocampal CA1 sector. Recent evidence that astrocytes in areas developing disseminated selective neuronal necrosis are swollen but preserve their cellular integrity [6] indicates that the energy metabolism of these astrocytes may have a crucial role in the prevention of infarction.

Using the same ischemia model, we have previously reported various genomic changes in regions developing selective neuronal necrosis and infarction [4]. Further studies are needed to examine the interaction between the genomic response and the development of energy failure in order to better understand the pathogenetic cascade leading to post-ischemic tissue injury.

References

1. Du C, Hu R, Csernansky CA, Hsu CY, Choi DW (1996) Very delayed infarction after mild focal cerebral ischemia: a role for apoptosis? J Cereb Blood Flow Metabol 16: 195–201
2. Hamilton BF, Gould DH (1987) Nature and distribution of brain lesions in rats intoxicated with 3-nitropropionic acid: a type of hypoxic (energy deficient) brain damage. Acta Neuropathol 72: 286–297
3. Hanyu S, Ito U, Hakamata Y, Yoshida M (1995) Transition from ischemic neuronal necrosis to infarction in repeated ischemia. Brain Res 686: 44–48
4. Hermann DM, Kuroiwa T, Ito U, Mies G (1998) Expression of c-jun, hsp-72 and gfap following repeated unilateral common carotid artery occlusion in gerbils – correlates of delayed neuronal injury. Brain Res 799: 35–43
5. Ito U, Spatz M, Walker JT, Klatzo I (1975) Experimental cerebral ischemia in Mongolian gerbils. I. Light microscopical observations. Acta Neuropathol 32: 209–223
6. Ito U, Hanyu S, Hakamata Y, Nakamura M, Arima K (1997) Ultrastructure of astrocytes associated with selective neuronal death of cerebral cortex after repeated ischemia. Acta Neurochir [Suppl] (Wien) 70: 46–49
7. Kuroda S, Katsura KI, Tsuchidate R, Siesjö BK (1996) Secondary bioenergic failure after transient focal ischemia is due to mitochondrial injury. Acta Physiol Scand 156: 149–150
8. Kuroiwa T, Terakado M, Yamaguchi T, Endo S, Ueki M,

Okeda R (1996) The pyramidal cell layer of sector CA1 shows the lowest hippocampal succinate dehydrogenase activity in normal and postischemic gerbils. Neurosci Lett 206: 117–120

9. Kuroiwa T, Mies G, Hermann D, Hakamata Y, Hanyu S, Ito U (1997) Maturation of mitochondrial dysfunction as a key recruitment process from neuronal necrosis into infarction. J Cereb Blood Flow Metabol 17 [Suppl] 1: 671
10. Kuroiwa T, Mies G, Hakamata Y, Hanyu S, Okeda R, Ito U (1999) Mitochondrial dysfunction and maturation phenomenon in ischemic gerbil cortex. Maturation phenomenon in cerebral ischemia III. Springer, Berlin Heidelberg New York Tokyo, pp 237–241
11. Mies G, Paschen W, Hossmann K-A (1990) Cerebral blood flow, glucose utilization, regional glucose and ATP content during the maturation period of delayed ischemic injury in gerbil brain. J Cereb Blood Flow Metab 10: 638–645
12. Ohno K, Ito U, Inaba Y (1984) Regional cerebral blood flow and stroke index after left carotid artery ligation in the conscious gerbil. Brain Res 297: 151–157
13. Riepe MW, Esclaire F, Kasischke K, Schreiber S, Nakase H, Kempski O, Ludolph AC, Dirnagl U, Hugon J (1997) Increased hypoxic tolerance by chemical inhibition of oxidative phosphorylation: "chemical preconditioning". J Cereb Blood Flow Metabol 17: 257–264

Correspondence: Toshihiko Kuroiwa, Department of Neuropathology, Medical Research Institute, Tokyo Medical and Dental University, Yushima 1-5-45, Bunkyo-ku. Tokyo 113-8510, Japan.

Acta Neurochir (2000) [Suppl] 76: 47–53

Indomethacin and Cyclosporin a Inhibit in Vitro Ischemia-Induced Expression of ICAM-1 and Chemokines in Human Brain Endothelial Cells

W. Zhang[1], **C. Smith**[1], **R. Monette**[1], **J. Hutchison**[2], and **D. B. Stanimirovic**[1]

[1] Institute for Biological Sciences, National Research Council of Canada, Ottawa, Canada
[2] Children's Hospital of Eastern Ontario, Ottawa, Canada

Abstract

Brain inflammation has been implicated in the development of brain edema and secondary brain damage in ischemia and trauma. Mechanisms involved in leukocyte infiltration across the blood-brain barrier are still unknown. In this study, we show that human cerebromicrovascular endothelial cells (HCEC) subjected to a 4 h in vitro ischemia (hypoxia + glucose deprivation) followed by a 4–24 h recovery express elevated levels of ICAM-1, IL-8, and MCP-1 mRNAs (semi-quantitative RT-PCR) and secrete increased amounts of the immunoreactive chemokines IL-8 and MCP-1 (ELISA). The ischemia-induced expression of ICAM-1 in HCEC, and the expression/release of IL-8 and MCP-1 in HCEC were abolished by the non-steroid anti-inflammatory drug, indomethacin (100–300 μM). The immunosuppressant cyclosporin A (50 μM) partially reduced the ischemia-stimulated IL-8 and MCP-1 secretion by HCEC. Both indomethacin and cyclosporin A also inhibited the ischemia-induced neutrophil chemotaxis elicited by HCEC media. The study indicates that in vitro ischemia augments the expression of adhesion molecules and leukocyte chemoattractants at the site of the BBB. This ischemic pro-inflammatory activation of HCEC may constitute a key event in initiating post-ischemic inflammation, and it can be suppressed by the anti-inflammatory drugs, indomethacin and cyclosporin A.

Keywords: Blood-brain barrier; chemokines; hypoxia; anti-inflammatory drugs.

Introduction

Secondary brain damage, a cell injury which is not apparent immediately after an insult, but develops after a delay of hours or days, has typically been observed after ischemia, trauma or subarachnoidal haemorrhage. Although the triggers and subsequent biochemical cascades leading to such damage are not clearly understood, recent discoveries implicate brain edema and inflammation as important components of this process [1, 3]. Neutrophils are commonly the first hemopoietic cells to infiltrate the brain following ischemia or trauma [3]. These blood cells may contribute to the development of secondary brain damage by causing capillary plugging, increasing blood-brain barrier (BBB) permeability, and by secreting a variety of injurious chemical mediators including activated oxygen species, cytokines, lipid-derived mediators (e.g., arachidonic acid, leukotrienes), and proteases [9]. The development of postischemic brain inflammation appears to be coordinated by the interactions of leukocytes and brain endothelial cells which are mediated by adhesion molecules and specific chemotactic gradients created in ischemic brain tissue [1, 17].The reduction of circulating neutrophils (i.e., neutropenia), [15], the administration of antibodies against endothelial or leukocyte derived adhesion molecules to experimental animals before and/or after ischemia [6], and the knock-out of the ICAM-1 gene [21], have all been shown to limit leukocyte infiltration into the brain and to reduce infarct size and brain edema. The importance of immunological processes in the development of secondary brain damage has recently been underlined by studies showing that the immunosuppressant drugs, cyclosporin A (CSA) and FK506, ameliorate brain damage after global [28] and focal cerebral ischemia [8] in vivo.

A family of 8-12kD chemokine peptides, [2], has been shown to mediate selective leukocyte recruitment at peripheral inflammation sites. Chemokines also play a role in the pathophysiology of brain injury accompanying autoimmune, post-traumatic and post-ischemic brain inflammation [17]. Increased levels of MCP-1, macrophage inflammatory protein-1 (MIP-1) [12], and IL-8 [14] have been detected in the ischemic brain. Systemic administration of anti-IL-8 antibody has been shown to reduce cerebral edema, blood-brain barrier (BBB) permeability, and infarct size in experimental models of stroke [14].

Leukocyte chemoattractants/chemokines released and presented by the BBB likely play a critical role in initiating and directing leukocyte transmigration into the ischemic brain. In this study we show that the exposure of human cerebromicrovascular endothelial cells (HCEC) to in vitro ischemia results in increased neutrophil adhesion, and stimulated expression and secretion of bioactive leukocyte chemoattractants. These processes are effectively suppressed by the non-steroid anti-inflammatory drug (NSAID), indomethacin, and by the immunophilin immunosuppressant, cyclosporin A.

Materials and Methods

Cell Culture

HCEC were isolated using a previously described protocol [23] from samples of human temporal cortex removed surgically for the treatment of epilepsy. HCEC cultures were maintained in growth media containing 65% medium M199 (containing Earle's salts, 25 mM Hepes, 4.35 g/l sodium bicarbonate and 3 mM L-glutamine), 10% fetal calf serum, 5% human serum, 20% murine melanoma cell (mouse melanoma, Cloudman S91, clone M-3, melanin producing cells)-conditioned media, 5 μg/ml insulin, 5 μg/ml transferrin, 5 ng/ml selenium, and 10 μg/ml endothelial cell growth supplement. The morphological, phenotypic, biochemical and functional characteristics of HCEC cultures derived by these procedures have been described in detail previously [23].

Simulated in Vitro Ischemia

The term 'simulated in vitro ischemia' is used in this study to describe an in vitro model of combined severe hypoxia (<2% O_2; anaerobic chamber equipped with a humidified, temperature-controlled incubator) and glucose- and nutrient-deprivation [glucose-free Krebs solution containing (in mM) 119 NaCl, 4.7 KCl, 1.2 KH_2PO_4, 25 $NaHCO_3$, 2.5 $CaCl_2$, 1 $MgCl_2$] that lacks the blood flow component of in vivo ischemia [24]. HCEC were subjected to simulated in vitro ischemia for 4 hours, and subsequently recovered in ambient air (reoxygenation) and media M199 containing 5 mM glucose (4–24 h). Cell media were collected and cells harvested for simultaneous measurements of chemokine mRNA expression and levels of chemokines released into the media.

RT-PCR

Total RNA was extracted from HCEC using TRI20L reagent (500 μl/35mm dish). Synthesis of single-stranded cDNA was performed by reverse transcription (42 °C, 1 h) in a reaction mixture (final volume 20 μl) containing 4 μl of 5× first strand buffer (Gibco BRL), 2 μl of 0.1 M DTT, 1 μl of 10 mM dNTP, 1 μl of 10 μM Oligo(dT), 100 units of RNase H^- reverse transcriptase (SuperScript™ II, Gibco-BRL), and 10 μl of DEPC-treated dH_20. The reverse transcriptase was inactivated by heating the reaction mixture at 70 °C for 15 min. Specific primers were designed according to published sequences of the human ICAM-1 (sense: 5′-ACAAGCCACGCCTCCCTGA-3′; anti-sense: 5′-CCATCAATCATGTCTTGAGTCTTG-3′) and chemokines IL-8 (sense: 5′-ATGACTTCCAAGCTGGCCGTG-3′; anti-sense: 5′-CTCCACAACCCTCTGCACCCA-3′) and MCP-1 (sense: 5′-GCTCGCTCAGCCAGATGCAAT-3′; anti-sense 5′-TGGGTTGTGGAGTGAGTGTTC-3′). The house-keeping genes, β-actin and β_2-microglobulin, were used as internal controls.

PCR amplifications were carried out in a final volume of 50 μl containing 1X reaction buffer (Promega; Madison, WI), 1.5 mM $MgCl_2$, 0.2 mM each of four dNTPs, 0.4 μM each of two pairs of the primers (primers for an internal control gene, and the primers for either IL-8 or MCP-1), 2.5 units Taq DNA polymerase (Promega), and 4 μl cDNA. All amplifications were done using a denaturation step at 94 °C for 30 seconds, annealing step at 55 °C for 45 seconds and polymerization step at 72 °C for 40 seconds, and were carried out for 45 cycles. Aliquots of the PCR (10 μl) and restriction digests were subjected to electrophoresis on a 1.5% agarose in a Tris-borate buffer containing 0.5 μg/ml ethidium bromide, and then photographed. PCR generated a 282bp DNA fragment for ICAM-1, a 289bp DNA fragment for IL-8, a 257bp DNA fragment for MCP-1, 504bp DNA fragment for β-actin, and 137bp DNA fragment for β_2-microglobulin.

ELISA

To quantify the levels of ICAM-1 expression in HCEC, cultures grown in 96-well microtiter plates (2×10^4 cells/100 μl/well) were sequentially incubated with a primary monoclonal anti-ICAM-1 antibody (2 μg/ml) for 1 h at 37 °C, followed by 1:500 diluted peroxidase-conjugated goat anti-mouse IgG in PBS for 45 min at 37 °C. Non-specific binding sites were blocked with 2% BSA in PBS for 30 min at 37 °C. Color was developed by the addition of the horseradish peroxidase substrate, 2,2′-azinobis (3 ethylbenzthiazoline-6-sulfonic acid) (ABTS). The optical density (O.D.) was read at 405 nm using a SpectraMAX (Molecular Devices, Menlo Park, CA) microplate reader.

The levels of IL-8 and MCP-1 released from variously treated HCEC were quantified by a 'sandwich' ELISA using commercially obtained ELISA kits, Quantikine human IL-8 kit (R&D System, Minneapolis, MN) and ID Elisa™ MCP-1 kit (ID Labs Biotechnology, London, ON). Aliquots of culture media were collected, centrifuged at 14,000 rpm for 5 min at 4 °C, and ELISA assays were carried out as instructed by the manufacturers.

Neutrophil Adhesion and Chemotaxis

Human neutrophils were isolated from fresh, EDTA-treated venous blood obtained from healthy adult volunteers. The neutrophil-containing band was separated on discontinuous polysucrose-sodium diatrizoate (Histopaque-1077 and -1119) gradients. Contaminating erythrocytes were removed by brief hypotonic lysis in ice-cold 0.15% NaCl. The neutrophils were labeled with 10 μM calcein-AM (Molecular Probe, Inc., OR, USA) in PBS for 20 min at 37 °C. Calcein-labeled neutrophils (5×10^4 cells/100 ul) were added to variously treated HCEC monolayers pre-labeled with the fluorescent dye, 3,3′-dipropylthiadicarbocyanine iodide [$DiSC_3(5)$] (1 μM, 20 min). Non-adherent neutrophils were removed by two rapid washes with PBS and fluorescent images were generated using a Zeiss LSM 410 (Carl Zeiss, Thornwood, NY) inverted laser scanning microscope (LSM) equipped with an Argon\Krypton ion laser and a Zeiss LD achroplan 20×, 0.4 NA objective. Alternatively, the intensity of the fluorescence remaining in each well was determined using a CytoFluor 2350 fluorescence microplate reader (Millipore Corp., Bedford, MA; 485/530 nm) and quantified against a standard curve generated from various numbers (1,000–100,000) of labeled neutrophils [24].

Chemotaxis of calcein-AM labeled neutrophils induced by media collected from variously treated HCEC was assessed by a quantitative in vitro assay using a ChemoTx # 101-5 (Neuro Probe, Inc., Gaithersburg, MD) assembly consisting of a 96-well plate and a polycarbonate filter membrane, as described by Junger *et al.* [10]. Briefly, the wells of the plates were loaded with media collected from variously treated cells or solutions containing known concentrations of chemoattractants, framed filter was positioned on top, 50,000 neutrophils suspended in 20 μl of matching non-conditioned media were applied on the top of each membrane/well, and the assembly was incubated for 90 min at 37 °C. The numbers of neutrophils transmigrated into wells of the 96-well plate were quantified by measuring intensity of fluorescence (excitation/emission: 485/530 nm) in a CytoFluor 2350 reader.

Results

Effects of in Vitro Ischemia on the Expression of ICAM-1 in HCEC and the Adhesion of Allogenic Neutrophils to HCEC

In vitro ischemia (4 h) followed by a 4 hour recovery resulted in a significant up-regulation of ICAM-1 mRNA in HCEC (Fig. 1A) persisting up to 24 h after ischemia. The levels of ICAM-1 quantified by ELISA were 3 times above control levels 24 h after in vitro ischemia (Fig. 1B). The same duration of ischemia/recovery caused a 2–3-fold increase in a number of allogenic neutrophils firmly adhering to HCEC monolayers as observed by confocal microscopy (not shown) and quantified by fluorimetry (Fig. 1B). The exposure of HCEC to IL-1β (100 u/ml) for 24 h caused a dramatic rise in ICAM-1 (10-fold above control) levels (Fig. 1B), and a 3–4 fold increase in the number of neutrophils adhering to HCEC (Fig. 1C).

A non-steroid anti-inflammatory drug, indomethacin (100–300 μM), inhibited both ischemia-induced ICAM-1 expression in HCEC (Fig. 1B) and ischemia-stimulated neutrophil adhesion to HCEC (Fig. 1C). The same concentrations of indomethacin have also been shown to inhibit both the IL-1β- and phorbol ester-stimulated ICAM-1 expression in HCEC and neutrophil adhesion to HCEC [24]. The immunophilin-binding immunosuppressant, cyclosporin A (CSA; 50 μM), inhibited both IL-1β-induced expression of ICAM-1 in HCEC (Fig. 1B) and neutrophil adhesion to HCEC (Fig. 1C). It also reduced the in vitro ischemia-induced ICAM-1 expression (not shown). Rapamycin, a calcineurin-independent immunophilin immunosuppresant, also reduced IL-1β-induced ICAM-1 expression in HCEC and neutrophil adhesion to HCEC, whereas the selective calcineurin inhibitor, the synthetic pyrethroid cypermethrin [16] (10 μM and 50 μM) was ineffective (not shown).

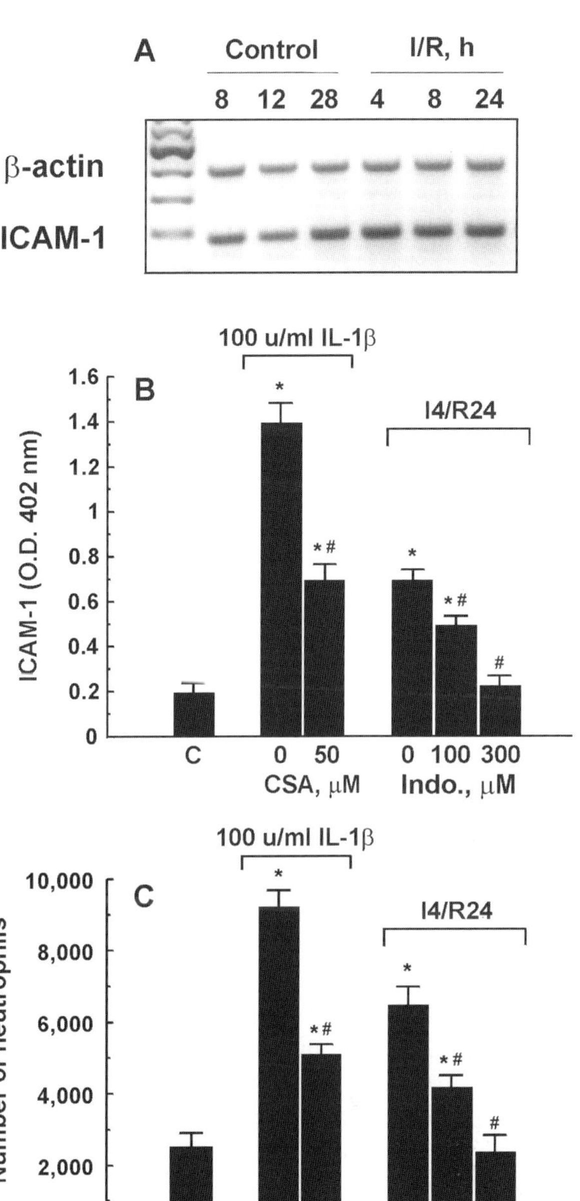

Fig. 1. Effects of in vitro ischemia/recovery (I/R) and IL-1β on the expression of ICAM-1 in HCEC and the adhesion of allogenic neutrophils to HCEC monolayers. ICAM-1 mRNA expression (A) was determined by RT-PCR, ICAM-1 levels (B) by ELISA, and neutrophil adhesion (C) was assessed by fluorescence confocal microscopy and fluorometry as described in Materials and Methods. Confluent HCEC monolayers were exposed to 4 h in vitro ischemia and indicated periods of recovery (4–24 h) (I/R), or to 100 u/ml of IL-1β for 24 h, in the presence or absence of the indicated concentrations of indomethacin (Indo) or cyclosporin A (CSA). Each bar represents the mean ± SD of six replicates and is representative of the results obtained in three separate experiments. Asterisks indicate significant differences ($p < 0.01$; ANOVA followed by the multiple comparisons among means) from control levels. #- Indicates significant difference ($p < 0.01$; ANOVA) from either 100 u/ml IL-1β or ischemia alone

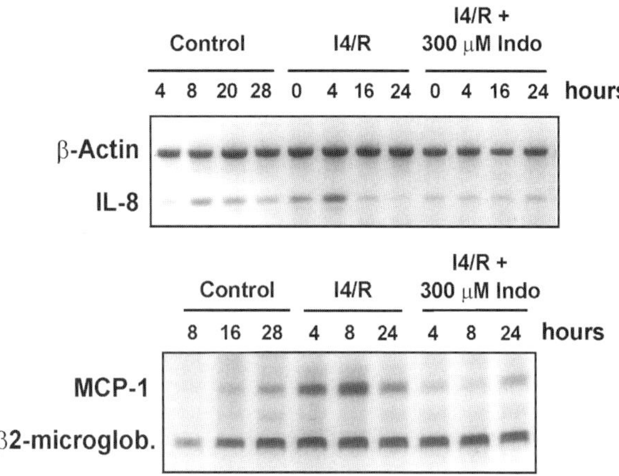

Fig. 2. Effects of indomethacin on the in vitro ischemia/recovery-induced expression of IL-8 and MCP-1 mRNA in HCEC. Confluent HCEC were exposed to 4 h in vitro ischemia and the indicated duration of recovery in the presence or absence of indomethacin (Indo; 300 μM). IL-8 and MCP-1 mRNA expression was determined by a semi-quantitative RT-PCR. The results shown are typical of at least four separate experiments

Effects of in Vitro Ischemia on the Expression/Secretion of Bioactive Chemokines in HCEC

The IL-8 mRNA was transiently up-regulated in HCEC at 4 h after in vitro ischemia (Fig. 2) whereas the MCP-1 mRNA was elevated at 4, 16 and 24 h after in vitro ischemia (Fig. 2).

The levels of immunoreactive IL-8 released into HCEC media increased significantly as early as 4 h after in vitro ischemia, and remained elevated (2.5-fold above control) up to 24 h (Fig. 3A). MCP-1 levels in HCEC media were also significantly elevated at 4 h and 24 h after in vitro ischemia (Fig. 3B).

IL-1β strongly up-regulated the expression of IL-8 and MCP-1 mRNA (not shown) and increased the secretion of IL-8 and MCP-1 in HCEC by 35 and 20 times, respectively (Fig. 3A and B).

Indomethacin inhibited both basal (not shown) and ischemia-induced IL-8 mRNA expression (Fig. 2), and basal (not shown) and ischemia-induced secretion of immunoreactive IL-8 in HCEC (Fig. 3A). Similarly, indomethacin diminished the ischemia-induced MCP-1 mRNA expression in HCEC (Fig. 2) and inhibited the ischemia-induced MCP-1 release at all time-points of post-ischemic recovery (Fig. 3B). CSA was found to significantly reduce both the ischemia-induced IL-8 (Fig. 3A) and MCP-1 (Fig. 3B) release from HCEC at 4 h and 24 h of recovery.

Media collected from HCEC subjected to control or ischemic conditions in the absence or presence of indomethacin or CSA, were tested for their ability to induce chemotaxis of freshly isolated human neutrophils. In vitro ischemia significantly increased the neutrophil chemoattractant capacity of cell media from HCEC (Fig. 3C). The neutrophil chemotactic activity was also markedly elevated in media of IL-1β-stimulated HCEC (Fig. 3C). Indomethacin (100–300 μM) completely inhibited the release of neutrophil chemoattractants in media of HCEC (Fig. 3C). CSA also significantly reduced the ability of ischemic HCEC media to elicit neutrophil chemotaxis (Fig. 3C).

Discussion

This study provides evidence that human BBB endothelial cells (HCEC) are an important source of neutrophil chemoattractants in brain ischemia. The study shows that HCEC subjected to in vitro ischemia express elevated levels of ICAM-1, IL-8 and MCP-1, exhibit increased adhesive properties, and secrete high levels of bioactive neutrophil chemoattractants.

We have previously reported that both cytokines and in vitro-ischemia stimulate the transcription of ICAM-1 mRNA in HCEC [24]. In both cases increased neutrophil adhesion to HCEC was blocked by a combination of anti-ICAM-1 and anti-CD18 antibodies [24]. In addition, this study shows that specialized BBB endothelium responds to in vitro ischemia by increasing the expression/secretion of the neutrophil chemokine, IL-8 and monocyte chemokine, MCP-1. The cytokine-induced release of chemokines [16] and hypoxic induction of IL-8 expression [11] have been previously reported in human peripheral endothelial cells. The up-regulation of IL-8 and MCP-1 expression in HCEC by in vitro ischemia is due to a stimulated transcription of these molecules. Nuclear factor κB (NF-κB), shown to mediate the transcription of cytokines and adhesion molecules in various cell types [7], and to be activated by hypoxia and oxidative stress [7], conceivably plays a role in the observed hypoxia-induced expression of these genes in HCEC. Alternatively and/or concomitantly, ischemia can induce secretion/release of factors that effect activation of cells through autocrine mechanisms. For example, hypoxia has been shown to induce IL-1 expression/release from peripheral human endothelial cells [19], which in turn may induce ICAM-1 or chemokines. Both autocrine and paracrine mechanisms of HCEC activation are likely to be important in cerebral ische-

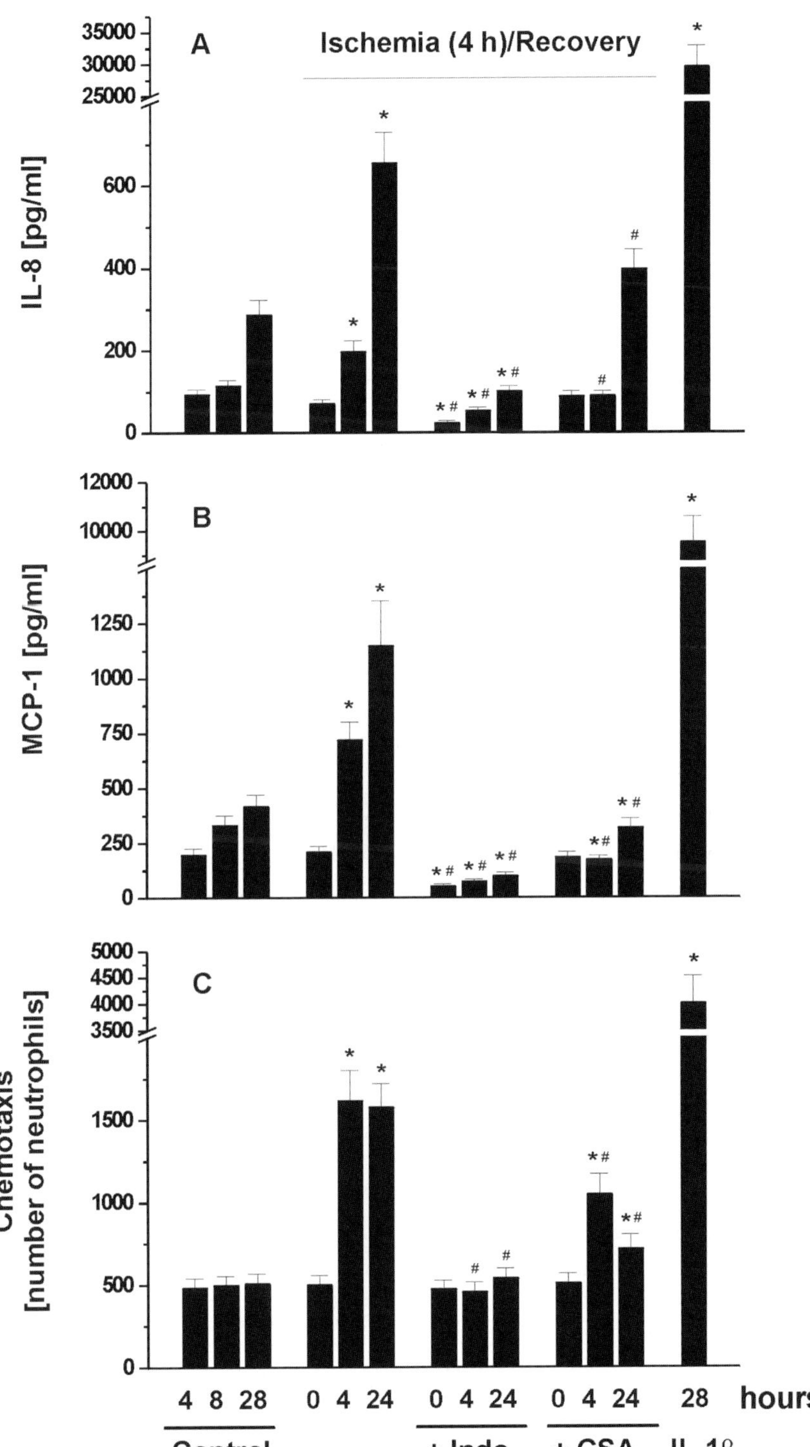

Fig. 3. Effects of in vitro ischemia/recovery and IL-1β on the secretion of immunoreactive IL-8 (A) and MCP-1 (B) into HCEC media and on chemotaxis of allogenic neutrophils enticed by HCEC media (C). HCEC were exposed to 4 h of in vitro ischemia and the indicated duration of recovery, in the absence or presence of 300 μM indomethacin (Indo) or 50 μM cyclosporin A (CSA), or to 100 u/ml of IL-1β. IL-8 and MCP-1 levels in media were determined by ELISA, as described in Materials and Methods. Same cell media were used to induce migration of fluorescently labeled allogenic neutrophils. Each bar represents the mean ± SD of six replicates and are representative of the results obtained in three separate experiments. Asterisks indicate significant differences ($p < 0.01$; ANOVA; followed by multiple comparisons of means) from time-controls. #-Indicates significant difference from ischemia/recovery alone

mia in vivo. For example, elevated message/levels of pro-inflammatory cytokines IL-1β [1] and TNFα [9] have been detected in the brain after both focal and global ischemia in animals, as well as in the cerebrospinal fluid of stroke patients [27], and HCEC have been shown to respond to cytokines IL-1β and TNFα by a pronounced up-regulation of the adhesion molecules ICAM-1, VCAM-1 and E-selectin [24, 25]. Cytokines have also been shown to stimulate the secretion of various vasoactive and pro-inflammatory mediators from HCEC, including prostaglandins [22] and endothelins [20].

The exact mechanisms by which neutrophils transmigrate across the BBB in ischemia and inflammation are not known. ICAM-1-mediated adhesion of neutrophils to cerebromicrovascular endothelial cells has been considered seminal step in this process [1, 17]. In addition, presentation of chemokines, such as IL-8 and MCP-1 by sentinel cells may be responsible for sustaining strong adhesive interactions between leukocytes and endothelium [2] and is probably a critical event in initiating leukocyte transmigration across the BBB.

The study further demonstrates the ability of the two anti-inflammatory drugs, indomethacin and CSA, to limit ischemia-induced pro-inflammatory responses in HCEC. Indomethacin virtually abolished the ischemia-induced induction of ICAM-1 and expression/secretion of IL-8 and MCP-1 in HCEC. The neuroprotective effect of indomethacin in a global model of cerebral ischemia has recently been attributed to the suppression of the inducible heat-shock protein 70 (iHSP 70) [4] and endothelial nitric oxide synthase (eNOS) [5] in brain vessels. We speculate that the neuroprotective effect of indomethacin in cerebral ischemia may also be due to the ability of the drug to suppress the pro-inflammatory activation of HCEC. It remains unclear from these studies, whether the inhibition of the ischemia-induced gene expression, including that of adhesion molecules and chemokines, by indomethacin is linked to the inhibition of cyclooxygenase activity or to other yet unknown action(s).

CSA was found to partially inhibit the ischemia- and cytokine-induced ICAM-1 expression, and the IL-8 and MCP-1 release from HCEC. Immunosuppressive actions of CSA have been attributed to the inhibition of the Ca^{2+}-dependent serine-threonine phosphatase, calcineurin (Marks, 1996). CSA has also been shown to inhibit NF-kB, although with much lower potency than the calcineurin-dependent activity of NF-ATc [13]. The study suggests that the mechanism(s) by which CSA inhibits HCEC-neutrophil interactions are calcineurin independent, since rapamycin, an immunosuppressant which does not inhibit calcineurin, was also effective in inhibiting IL-1β-induced ICAM-1 expression/neutrophil adhesion to HCEC. The selective inhibitor of calcineurin, cypermethrin failed to affect either process. In addition, the CSA effect(s) observed in this study may be explained by its reported ability to modulate autocrine effects of cytokine- or ischemia-induced endothelial mediators, such as nitric oxide and prostaglandins [18].

The neuroprotective properties of NSAID and immunophilin-binding immunosuppressants have recently been substantiated in studies demonstrating protective action(s) of indomethacin [4, 5] and CSA [8, 28] against ischemic brain damage in animal models of stroke. The evidence presented in this study implicates indomethacin and CSA as potentially important modifiers of HCEC activation by ischemia. Hence, we speculate that the neuroprotection afforded by these drugs in cerebral ischemia may originate in part from their ability to reduce pro-inflammatory activation of HCEC including synthesis/release of chemokines. Therefore, chemokines released/presented at the BBB may serve as attractive and accessible therapeutic targets to attenuate post-ischemic brain inflammation.

Acknowledgments

This project is supported by a grant (# ST2718) from the Heart and Stroke Foundation of Ontario. We thank Dr. Edith Hamel of Montreal Neurological Institute for providing human temporal lobe biopsies, and Mrs. Rita Ball for preparation of cell cultures.

References

1. Arvin B, Neville LF, Barone FC, Feuerstein GZ (1996) The role of inflammation and cytokines in brain injury. Neurosci Behav Rev 20: 445–452
2. Baggiolini M, Dewald B, Moser, B (1997) Human chemokines: an update. Ann Rev Immunol 15: 675–705
3. Barone FC, Hillegass LM, Price WJ, White RF, Lee EV, Feuerstein GZ, Sarau HM, Clark RK, Griswold DE (1991) Polymorphonuclear leukocyte infiltration into cerebral focal ischemic tissue: myeloperoxidase activity assay and histologic verification. J Neurosci Res 29: 336–348
4. Beasley TC, Bari F, Thore C, Thrikawala N, Louis T, Busija D (1997) Indomethacin attenuates early increases in inducible heat shock protein 70 after cerebral ischemia/reperfusion in piglets. Dev Brain Res 105: 125–135
5. Beasley TC, Bari F, Thore C, Thrikawala N, Louis T, Busija D (1998) Cerebral ischemia/reperfusion increases endothelial nitric oxide synthase levels by an indomethacin-sensitive mechanism. J Cereb Blood Flow Metab 18: 88–96
6. Clark WM, Madden KP, Rothlein R, and Zivin JA (1991) Reduction of central nervous system ischemic injury in rabbits using leukocyte adhesion antibody treatment. Stroke 22: 877–893
7. Collins T, Read MA, Neish As, Whitley MZ, Thanos D, Maniatis T (1995) Transcriptional regulation of endothelial cell adhesion molecules: NF-kB and cytokine-inducible enhancers. FASEB J 9: 899–909
8. Drake M, Friberg H, Boris-Moller F, Sakata K, and Wieloch T (1996) The immunosuppressant FK506 ameliorates ischaemic damage in the rat brain. Acta Physiol Scand 158: 155–159
9. Feuerstein GZ, Wang X, Barone FC (1997) Inflammatory gene expression in cerebral ischemia and trauma. Potential new therapeutic targets. Ann N Y Acad Sci 825: 179–193

10. Junger WG, Cardoza TA, Liu FC, Hoyt DB, Goodwin R (1993) Improved rapid photometric assay for quantitative measurement of PMN migration. J Immunol Meth 160: 73–79
11. Karakurum M, Shreeniwas R, Chen J, Pinsky D, Yan SD, Anderson M, Sunouchi K, Major J, Hamilton T, Kuwabara K (1994) Hypoxic induction of interleukin-8 gene expression in human endothelial cells. J Clin Invest 93: 1564–1570
12. Kim JS, Gautam SC, Chopp M, Zaloga C, Jones ML, Ward PA, Welch KM (1995) Expression of monocyte chemoattractant protein-1 and macrophage inflammatory protein-1 after focal ischemia in the rat. J Neuroimmunol 56: 127–134
13. Marks AR (1996) Cellular functions of immunophilins. Physiol Rev 76: 631–649
14. Matsumoto T, Ikeda K, Mukaida N, Harada A, Matsumoto Y, Yamashita J, Matsushima K (1997) Prevention of cerebral edema and infarct in cerebral reperfusion injury by an antibody to interleukin-8. Lab Invest 77: 119–125
15. Matsuo Y, Onodera H, Shiga Y, Nakamura M, Ninomiya M, Kihara T, and Kogure K (1994) Correlation between myeloperoxidase-quantified neutrophil accumulation and ischemic brain injury in rat: effects of neutrophil depletion. Stroke 25: 1469–1475
16. Parry GC, Martin T, Felts KA, Cobb RR (1998) Il-1beta-induced monocyte chemoattractant protein-1 gene expression in endothelial cells is blocked by proteasome inhibitors. Artherioscler Thromb Vasc Biol 18: 934–940
17. Ransohoff RM (1997) Chemokines in neurological disease models: correlation between chemokine expression patterns and inflammatory pathology. J Leuko Biol 62: 645–652
18. Rosenthal RA, Chukwuogo NA, Ocasio VH, and Kahng KU (1989) Cyclosporine inhibits endothelial cell prostacyclin production. J Surg Res 46: 593–596
19. Schreenewas R, Koga S, Karakurum M, Pinsky D, Kaiser E, Brett J, Wolitzky BA, Norton C, Ploconski J, Benjamin W (1992) Hypoxia-mediated induction of endothelial cell interleukin-1 alpha. An autocrine mechanism promoting expression of leukocyte adhesion molecules on the vessel surface. J Clin Invest 90: 2333–2339
20. Skopal J, Turbucz P, Vastag M, Bori Z, Pek M, deChatel R, Nagy Z, Toth M, Karadi I (1998) Regulation of endothelin release from human brain microvessel endothelial cells. J Cardiovasc Pharmacol 31 [Suppl] 1: S370–S372
21. Soriano SG, Lipton SA, Wang YF, Xiao M, Springer TA, Gutierrez-Ramos J-C, and Hickey PR (1996) Intercellular adhesion molecule-1-deficient mice are less susceptible to cerebral ischemia-reperfusion injury. Ann Neurol 39: 618–624
22. Stanimirovic DB, Bacic F, Uematsu S, and Spatz M (1993) Profile of prostaglandins induced by endothelin-1 in human brain capillary endothelium. Neurochem Int 23: 385–393
23. Stanimirovic DB, Morley P, Ball R, Hamel E, Mealing G, Durkin JP (1996) Angiotensin II-induced endocytosis in human cerebromicrovascular endothelial cells is regulated by the inositol-phosphate signaling pathway. J Cell Physiol 169: 455–467
24. Stanimirovic DB, Shapiro A, Wong J, Hutchison J, Durkin JP (1997a) The induction of ICAM-1 in human cerebromicrovascular endothelial cells (HCEC) by ischemia-like conditions promotes enhanced neutrophil/HCEC adhesion. J Neuroimmunol 76: 193–205
25. Stanimirovic DB, Wong J, Shapiro A, and Durkin JP (1997b) Increase in surface expression of ICAM-1, VCAM-1 and E-selectin in human cerebromicrovascular endothelial cells subjected to ischemia-like insults. Acta Neurochir [Suppl] (Wien) 70: 12–16
26. Steiner JP, Connolly MA, Valentine HI, Hamilton GS, Dawson TM, Hester L, and Snyder SH (1997) Neurotrophic actions of nonimmunosuppressive analogues of immunosuppressive drugs FK506, rapamycin and cyclosporin A. Nature Med 3: 421–428
27. Tarkowski E, Rosengren L, Blomstrand C, Wikkelso C, Jensen C, Ekholm S, Tarkowski A (1997) Intrathecal release of pro- and anti-inflammatory cytokines during stroke. Clin Exp Immunol 110: 492–499
28. Uchino H, Elmer E, Uchino K, Lindvall O, and Siesjo BK (1995) Cyclosporin A dramatically ameliorates CA1 hippocampal damage following transient forebrain ischaemia in the rat. Acta Physiol Scand 155: 469–471

Correspondence: Dr. Danica Stanimirovic, Cellular Neurobiology Group, Institute for Biological Sciences, National Research Council of Canada Montreal Road Campus, Bldg. M-54, Ottawa, ONT, Canada, K1A 0R6.

Acta Neurochir (2000) [Suppl] 76: 55–60

The Selectin Superfamily: The Role of Selectin Adhesion Molecules in Delayed Cerebral Ischaemia After Aneurysmal Subarachnoid Haemorrhage

J. J. Nissen, D. Mantle, A. Blackburn, J. Barnes, T. Wooldridge, B. Gregson, and **A. D. Mendelow**

Department of Neurosurgery, Newcastle General Hospital, Newcastle upon Tyne, UK

Summary

Cerebral ischaemia and reperfusion injury may be exacerbated by leukocyte recruitment and activation. Adhesion molecules play a pivotal role in leukocyte recruitment.

We report a prospective study of the potential role of the selectin family of adhesion molecules (E-, P- and L-selectin) in delayed cerebral ischaemia (DID) following aneurysmal subarachnoid haemorrhage.

In patients with good grade SAH, we have compared serum concentrations of E-, P- and L-selectin, between patients who do, and do not develop delayed cerebral ischaemia.

There was no difference in E-selectin concentration between the two groups (44.0 ng/ml vs. 37.4 ng/ml). Serum P-selectin concentration was significantly higher in patients with DID compared to those patients without DID (149.5 ng/ml vs. 112.9 ng/ml, $p = 0.039$). Serum L-selectin concentrations were significantly lower in patients with DID (633.8 ng/ml vs 897.9 ng/ml, $p = 0.013$).

We conclude that P- and L-selectin are involved in the pathogenesis of DID following aneurysmal subarachnoid haemorrhage. The results of this study do not elucidate the exact role of each selectin in DID.

Keywords: Subarachnoid haemorrhage; delayed cerebral ischaemia; adhesion molecule; selectin.

Introduction

The importance of leukocyte mediated tissue damage has been demonstrated in the pathogenesis of cerebral ischaemia and reperfusion injury in both animal and human studies [3, 10, 30, 31].

Recruitment of leukocytes from the circulation to areas of pathology involves Cellular Adhesion Molecules (CAM), a diverse set of macromolecules whose functions are pivotal in this process. Each step in the adhesion cascade [46] is mediated by one or more adhesion molecules interacting between white cell ligands and endothelial cells in response to activation of the endothelium. The steps involved in the cascade are initial "rolling" of leukocytes along the endothelial surface, subsequent activation and "firm adherence" to the endothelium and finally "transendothelial migration" of the leukocyte.

There are three families of adhesion molecules important in leukocyte-endothelial interaction; the Selectins (P-, E- and L-selectin) are transmembrane glycoproteins expressed on activated vascular endothelium (P- and E-), platelets (P-) and leukocytes (L-) and are involved in "rolling" and "activation" of leukocytes; the Immunoglobulin-like superfamily (intercellular adhesion molecules, ICAM-1,2,3, vascular cell adhesion molecule, VCAM-1, platelet-endothelial adhesion molecule, PECAM) are expressed by activated endothelium and act via binding to specific leukocyte transmembrane proteins, the Integrins. Immunoglobulin-Integrin interaction is pivotal in "firm adherence" and "transendothelial migration".

Adhesion molecules have been demonstrated in the pathogenesis of cardiac and renal transplant rejection [7, 24], atherosclerosis [40], malignancy and metastatic disease [26], rheumatoid disease [12] cardiac ischaemia [27], and a variety of central nervous system disorders including bacterial meningitis [19], encephalitis [50], multiple sclerosis [8] and cerebral ischaemia [9]. However, little work has been carried out to investigate the role of adhesion molecules in delayed cerebral ischaemia following subarachnoid haemorrhage (SAH).

Since leukocytes have been demonstrated in both the arteriopathy of "vasospasm" [11, 21, 25, 29, 38, 42, 47] and in brain infarction [9, 41], it may be postulated that potential roles for CAMs exist in the pathogenesis of delayed ischaemia after aneurysmal SAH.

We report a prospective study of the role of the Selectin family of adhesion molecules in delayed cerebral ischaemia after aneurysmal subarachnoid haemorrhage, by comparing serum levels of E-, P- and L-Selectin in patients without (group A) and with (group B) delayed cerebral ischaemia after aneurysmal subarachnoid haemorrhage.

Materials and Methods

Ethical approval for the study was obtained from the Joint Ethics Committee of the Newcastle and North Tyneside Health Authority.

Patient Selection

All consecutive patients refered to the Regional Neurosciences Centre at Newcastle General Hospital from July 1997 to November 1998 with CT scan or lumbar puncture proven WFNS grades 1 or 2 subarachnoid haemorrhage [15] treated with craniotomy and clipping of intracranial aneurysm were eligible for enrollment into the study.

In general, patients with WFNS grades 1 and 2 SAH undergo early angiography and surgery (within 48 of admission) and are given oral Nimodipine prophylaxis for delayed ischaemia from admission. Dexamethasone was not routinely used.

Delayed cerebral ischaemia was defined as a new focal neurological deficit not attributable to other causes, accompanied by an appropriate rise in middle cerebral arterial transcranial Doppler velocities to greater than 120 m/sec, or an MCA/ICA ratio ≥ 3. Angiography is not routinely used for diagnosis of delayed ischaemia. In general, patients with delayed ischaemia are treated with hypervolaemia and induced hypertension using inotropes where necessary. Non-symptomatic rises in Doppler velocities are not considered to be diagnostic of clinical delayed ischaemia.

Exclusion Criteria

Intercurrent medical conditions or nosocomial infection in which adhesion molecules may play a role, significant post-operative intracerebral haemorrhage.

Specimens

Informed written consent was obtained for all patients enrolled into the study. All blood samples were venous.

Initial samples were taken within 48 hrs. of admission (and always prior to craniotomy) and on alternate days thereafter until discharge. Specimens were allowed to coagulate and then centrifuged at 3,000 rpm for 12 minutes and the supernatants stored at $-40\,^{\circ}$C prior to analysis.

All adhesion molecule concentrations were assayed using commercially available enzyme-linked quantitative sandwich immunoabsorbent assay (ELISA) kits (R&D Systems, Abingdon, UK.) in accordance with the suppliers instructions. The assays involve the simultaneous reaction of sCAM (in sample or standard) with monoclonal antibody pre-coated on the walls of microtitre plate wells, and to an unbound second antibody directed against a different molecular epitope. The second antibody is conjugated with horseradish peroxidase. After removal of unreacted reagents, bound sCAM-HRP antibody conjugate is detected by reaction with a horseradish peroxidase specific substrate (tetramethylbenzidine) which yields a colored product, proportional to the concentration of CAM (determined relative to an appropriate standard curve). Absorbtion measurements were carried out at 450 nm (and correction wavelength of 650 nm to eliminate optical imperfections in the plate) using a microtitre plate reader (Dynatech MR5000). Serum samples were diluted 20–100 fold (depending on the analyte) prior to analysis.

Statistical Analysis

Mean sCAM values for each patient were compared between groups A and B. Un-paired t-tests (two-tailed) were used to assess the null hypothesis that the two groups would have identical levels of circulating adhesion molecules. A probability value less than 0.05 was used to indicate statistical significance.

Results

Forty-six patients were suitable for inclusion in the study. 10 were excluded, 8 with nosocomial infection and 2 with post-operative intracranial haemorrhage. 23 patients did not develop delayed ischaemia (group A) and 13 patients developed clinical delayed ischaemia (group B).

Mean levels of sE-selectin demonstrated no significant difference between groups A (44.0 ng/ml $\pm$ 4.3) and B (37.4 ng/ml $\pm$ 4.9), $p = 0.33$ (Fig. 1).

There was a significant rise in sP-selectin levels between groups A and B (112.9 ng/ml $\pm$ 8.14 vs. 149.5 ng/ml $\pm$ 17.0, $p = 0.039$) (Fig. 2). For sL-selectin, there was a significant fall in serum levels between groups A and B (897.9 ng/ml $\pm$ 53.6 vs. 633.8 ng/ml $\pm$ 93.7, $p = 0.013$), (Fig. 3).

Peripheral white cell count showed no significant difference (10.94 vs. 10.89), whereas mean platelet count demonstrated a significant rise between the groups A and B (262 ± 14.9 vs. 349 ± 30.8, $p = 0.008$).

Discussion

Overview of Selectins

Initial rolling of leukocytes along activated endothelium is mediated by members of the Selectin superfamily. The basic structure of the Selectins consists of an amino-terminal calcium-dependent lectin domain, an epidermal like growth factor region, between two and nine short consensus repeat units homologous to complement binding proteins, a membrane spanning region and a short cytoplasmic region [4]. E and P Selectins are expressed by endothelial cells and platelets (P-selectin) and L-selectin is constitutively expressed by leukocytes. E-selectin is synthesized in response to

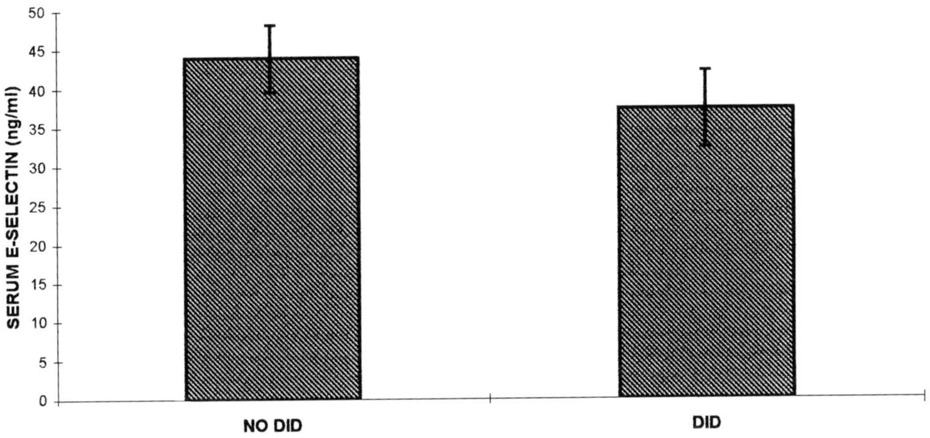

Fig. 1. Graph comparing serum E-selectin concentrations in patients without and with delayed ischaemia p = 0.33. Boxes represent mean of mean values. Bars denote standard errors of means. *DID* Delayed ischaemia

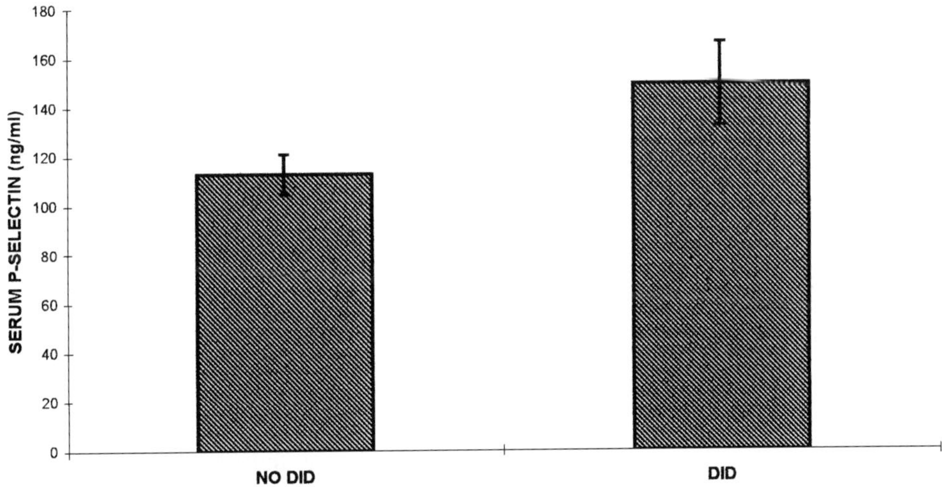

Fig. 2. Graph comparing serum P-selectin concentrations in patients without and with delayed ischaemia, p = 0.039. Boxes represent mean of mean values. Bars denote standard errors of means

endotoxin, IL-1 and TNF with peak expression at 4–6 hours after stimulation. In contrast, P-selectin is stored in platelet alpha granules and Weibel-Palade bodies of endothelial cells [32] and is redistributed to the cell surface in response to stimulation by histamine, thrombin and phorbol esters [23].

The selectins recognize cell surface glycoprotein bound carbohydrate ligands (sialyl Lewis X and related fucosylated lactosamines) which bind to the extracellular amino-terminal carbohydrate recognition domain (CRD) of the selectin molecule [4].

Adhesion Molecules and Ischaemia-Reperfusion Injury

The development of anti-adhesion therapy (oligosaccharide ligands to selectins or monoclonal antibodies (MAb) to adhesion molecules) has helped to elucidate the role of individual adhesion molecules in ischaemia-reperfusion injury.

Anti-Selectin antibodies have been demonstrated to attenuate ischaemic insults in cardiac ischaemia (L-selectin [28], P-selectin [49], E-selectin [1], intestinal ischaemia (P-selectin [13], and hepatic ischaemia (P-selectin [17]. In cerebral ischaemia, different lines of investigation have demonstrated that leukocytes and adhesion molecules may be involved in the pathogenesis of ischaemia and reperfusion injury. Firstly, animal studies have demonstrated that induced neutropenia by a variety of methods can protect against ischaemia/reperfusion injury [3, 10, 43, 44].

Secondly, in the study of adhesion molecules, Wang [48] has demonstrated increased E-selectin mRNA in

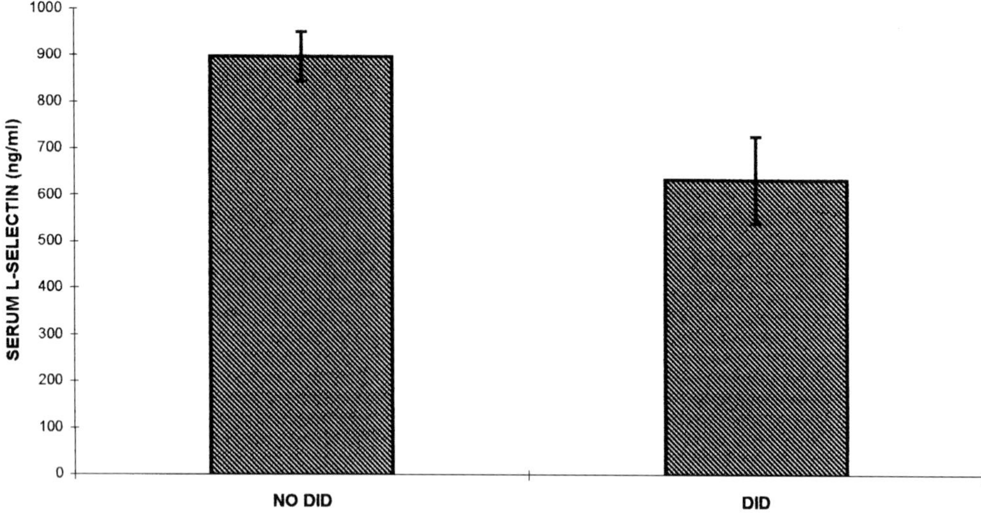

Fig. 3. Graph comparing serum L-selectin concentrations in patients without and with delayed ischaemia, p = 0.013. Boxes represent mean of mean values. Bars denote standard errors of means

ischaemic rat cortex compared to non-ischaemic cortex. E- and P-Selectin upregulation have been demonstrated in occlusion-reperfusion models [36, 51].

Thirdly, evidence for a role of the selectins in cerebral ischaemia has been demonstrated using anti-adhesion therapy. In an experimental model of transient cerebral ischaemia, the volume of ischaemic injury was reduced using a selectin oligopeptide [34].

Soluble Adhesion Molecules in Serum (sCAM)

Serum concentrations of adhesion molecules may not reflect local tissue levels but represent the balance between production, cleavage from cell membranes and clearance from the circulation [18]. However, a number of studies suggest that sCAM differ in disease states compared to controls and may correlate with outcomes in a variety of clinical circumstances. Elevated levels of sE-selectin were found on admission in critically ill patients and were further induced in non-surviving patients compared to survivors [6]. Raised E-selectin has also been demonstrated in septic shock [35]. In multiple sclerosis, elevated levels of sE- and sL-selectin have been demonstrated [14, 22], and McKeating demonstrated a reduction in sL-selectin after traumatic brain injury [33].

After acute ischaemic stroke, Frijns [16] demonstrated raised sE and sP-Selectin after 24 hrs, whereas Bitsch *et al.* demonstrated a fall in E-Selectin over 5 days [5].

Adhesion Molecules and Subarachnoid Haemorrhage

Despite the profuse literature on adhesion molecules and anti-adhesion therapy, few studies have investigated the potential roles of adhesion molecules and subarachnoid haemorrhage. Most studies have investigated the role of ICAM-1. Induction and ICAM-1 expression on the endothelial and medial layers has been demonstrated in rat basilar artery after cisternal injection of autologous blood [21]. There was a correlation between the degree and timing of spasm and leukocyte inflammatory response within the vessel. In a rat femoral artery model of vasospasm, Sills [45] demonstrated early induction of ICAM-1 on the endothelium and demonstrated direct correlation with an inflammatory response within the vessel wall. Using anti-ICAM-1 monoclonal antibodies given via an intraperitoneal route in the same rat femoral artery model, Oshiro [37] was able to demonstrate attenuation of both arterial narrowing and degree of inflammatory infiltrate within the periadventitia. Recently, Polin *et al.* [39] have demonstrated statistically significant elevated levels of ICAM-1, E-selectin and VCAM-1 in CSF in 17 patients with SAH having craniotomy, compared to 16 controls, and elevated (but not statistically significant) levels of L-selectin. Three patients developed "severe or moderate angiographically demonstrated vasospasm" and had higher levels of E-selectin than other patients with SAH. Bavbeck [2] demonstrated that after cisternal SAH in rabbits, cisternal administration of anti-ICAM-1 antibody or anti-CD18 antibody attenuated vasospasm. The effect was additive when given in combination.

We have demonstrated in a prospective study, significant differences in serum selectin concentrations between patients who do, and do not develop delayed cerebral ischaemia after aneurysmal subarachnoid haemorrhage. sE-selectin did not show any significant difference between the two groups, sP-selectin was significantly higher and sL-selectin significantly lower in those patients with delayed ischaemia.

Measurable sCAM will reflect the complex balance between production, shedding, and clearance [18]. Whilst we may postulate that the increase in P-selectin in patients with DID is consistent with the significant rise in peripheral platelet count, the reduction in L-selectin concentration may reflect reduced production or reduced availability in serum due to adhesion to counter receptor bearing cells. However, on the basis of serum concentrations of the selectins, we conclude that P- and L-selectins are involved in the pathogenesis of delayed ischaemia. From the results of this study, we are unable to determine whether adhesion molecules are involved in the pathogenesis of either the proliferative arteriopathy of vasospasm, or of brain ischaemia or infarction.

Further study is required to elucidate the relevance of serum concentrations compared to local cerebral concentrations and to determine whether anti-selectin therapy will attenuate delayed cerebral ischaemia after aneurysmal subarachnoid haemorrhage.

References

1. Altavilla D, Squadrito F, Ioculano M, Canale P, Campo GM, Zingarelli B, Caputi AP (1994) E-selectin in the pathogenesis of experimental myocardial ishaemia-reperfusion injury. Eur J Pharmacol 270: 45–51
2. Bavbeck M, Polin R, Kwan A, Arthur A, Kassell NF, Lee K (1998) Monoclonal antibodies against ICAM-1 and CD18 attenuate cerebral vasospasm after experimental subarachnoid haemorrhage in rabbits. Stroke 29: 1930–1936
3. Bednar MM, Raymond S, McAuliffe T, Lodge PA, Gross CE (1991) The role of neutrophils and platelets in a rabbit model of thrombo-embolic stroke. Stroke 22: 44–50
4. Bevilacqa MP, Nelson RM, Mannori G, Cecconi O (1994) Leukocyte-endothelial adhesion molecules in human disease. Annu Rev Med 45: 361–378
5. Bitsch A, Klene W, Murtada L, Prange H, Rieckmann P (1998) A longitudinal prospective study of soluble adhesion molecules in acute stroke. Stroke 29: 2129–2135
6. Boldt J, Wollbruck M, Kuhn D, Linke LC, Hempelmann G (1995) Do plasma levels of circulating soluble adhesion molecules differ between surviving and non-surviving critically ill patients? Chest 107: 787–792
7. Brockmeyer C, Ulbrecht M, Schendel DJ, Weiss EH, Hillebrand G, Burkhardt K, Land W, Gokel MJ, Riethmuller G, Feucht HE (1993) Distribution of cell adhesion molecules (ICAM-1, VCAM-1, ELAM-1) in renal tissue during allograft rejection. Transplantation 55: 610–615
8. Canella B, Raine CS (1995) The adhesion molecule and cytokine profile of multiple sclerosis lesions. Ann Neurol 37: 424–435
9. Clark WM, Lauten JD, Lessov N, Woodward W, Coull BM (1995) Time course of ICAM-1 expression and leukocyte subset infiltration in rat forebrain ischaemia. Mol Chem Neuropathol 26: 213–230
10. Connolly ES, Winfree CJ, Springer TA, Naka Y, Liao H, Yan SD, Stern DM, Soloman RA, Guitierrez-Ramos JC, Pinsky DJ (1996) Cerebral protection in homozygous null ICAM-1 mice after middle cerebral artery occlusion: Role of neutrophil adhesion in the pathogenesis of stroke. J Clin Invest 97: 209–216
11. Crompton MR (1964) The pathogenesis of cerebral infarction following the rupture of cerebral berry aneurysms. Brain 87: 491–510
12. Cronstein BN, Weissmann G (1993) The adhesion molecules of inflammation. Arthritis Rheum 36: 147–57
13. Davenpeck KL, Gauthier TW, Albertine KH, Lefer AM (1994) Role of P-selectin in microvascular leukocyte-endothelial interaction in splanchnic ischaemia-reperfusion. Am J Physiol 267: 622–630
14. Dore Duffy P, Newman W, Balabanov R, Lisak RP, Mainolfi E, Rothlein R, Peterson M (1995) Circulating, soluble adhesion proteins in cerebrospinal fluid and serum of patients with multiple sclerosis: correlation with clinical activity. Ann Neurol 37: 55–62
15. Drake CG, Hunt WE, Sano K, Kassell N, Teasdale G, Pertuiset B, Devilliers J (1988) Report of World Federation of Neurological Surgeons Committee on a universal subarachnoid haemorrhage grading scale. J Neurosurg 68: 985–986
16. Frijns CJ, Kappelle LJ, van Gijn J, Nieuwenhuis HK, Sixma JJ, Fijnheer R (1997) Soulble adhesion molecules reflect endothelial cell activation after ischaemic stroke and in carotid atherosclerosis. Stroke 28: 2214–2218
17. Garcia-Criado FJ, Toledo-Pereyra LH, Lopez-Niblina F, Philips ML, Paez-Rollys A, Misawa K (1995) Role of P-selectin in total hepatic ischaemia and reperfusion. Am J Coll Surg 181: 327–334
18. Gearing AJ, Newman W (1993) Circulating adhesion molecules in disease. Immunology Today 14: 506–512
19. Granert C, Raud J, Xie X, Lindquist L, Lindbum L (1994) Inhibition of leukocyte rolling with polysaccharide fucoidin prevents pleocytosis in experimental meningitis in the rabbit. J Clin Invest 93: 929–936
20. Handa Y, Kabuto M, Kobayashi H, Kawano H, Takeuchi H, Hayashi M (1991) The correlation between immunological reaction in the arterial wall and the time course of the development of cerebral vasospasm in a primate model. Neurosurgery 28: 542–549
21. Handa Y, Kubota T, Kaneko M, Tsuchida A, Kobayashi H, Kawano H, Kubota T (1995) Expression of intercellular adhesion molecule 1 (ICAM-1) on the cerebral artery following subarachnoid haemorrhage in rats. Acta Neurochir (Wien) 132: 92–97
22. Hartung HP, Reiners K, Archelos JJ (1995) Circulating adhesion molecules and tumour necrosis factor receptor in MS: correlation with MRI. Ann Neurol 38: 186–193
23. Hattori R, Hamilton KK, Fugate RD, McEver RP, Sims PJ (1989) Stimulated secretion of endothelial von Willebrand factor is accompanied by rapid redistribution to the cell surface of the

intracellular granule membrane protein GMP-140. J Biol Chem 264: 7768–7771
24. Herskowitz A, Mayne AE, Willoughby SB, Kanter K, Ansari AA (1994) Patterns of myocardial cell adhesion molecule expression in human endomyocardial biopsies after cardiac transplantation. Induced ICAM-1 and VCAM-1 related to implantation and rejection. Am J Pathol 145: 1082–1094
25. Hughes JT, Schianchi PM (1978) Cerebral artery spasm: a histological study at necropsy of the blood vessels in cases of subarachnoid haemorrhage. J Neurosurg 48: 515–525
26. Johnson JP (1991) Cell adhesion molecules of the immunoglobulin supergene family and their role in malignant transformation and progression to metastatic disease. Cancer Metastasis Rev 10: 11–22
27. Lefer AM, Lefer DJ (1996) The role of nitric oxide and cell adhesion molecules on the microcirculation in ischaemia-reperfusion. Cardiovascular Res 32: 743–751
28. Ma XL, Weyrich AS, Lefer DJ, Buerke M, Albertine KH, Kishimoto TK, Lefer AM (1993) Monoclonal antibody to L-selectin attenuates neutrophil accumulation and protects ischaemic reperfused cat myocardium. Circulation 88: 649–658
29. Mayberg MR, Okada T, Bark DH (1990) The significance of morphological changes in cerebral arteries after subarachnoid haemorrhage. J Neurosurg 72: 626–633
30. Matsuo Y, Kihara T, Ikeda M, Ninomiya M, Onodera H, Kogure K (1995) Role of neutrophils in radical production during ischaemia and reperfusion of the rat brain: effect of neutrophil depletion on extracellular ascorbyl radical formation. J Cereb Blood Flow Metab 15: 941–947
31. Matsuo Y, Onodera H, Shiga Y, Nakamura M, Ninomiya M, Kihara T, Kogure K (1994) Correlation between myeloperoxidase-quantified neutrophil accumulation and ischaemic brain injury in the rat. Effects of neutrophil depletion. Stroke 25: 1469–1475
32. McEver RP, Beckstead JH, Moore KL, Marshall CL, Bainton DF (1989) GMP-140, a platelet alpha-granule membrane protein, is also synthesized by vascular endothelial cells and is localised in Weibel-Palade bodies. J Clin Invest 84: 92–99
33. McKeating GF, Andrews PJ, Mascia L (1998) The relationship of soluble adhesion molecule concentrations in systemic and jugular venous serum to injury severity and outcome after traumatic brain injury. Anaesth Analg 86: 759–765
34. Morikawa E, Zhang S-M, Seko Y, Toyoda T, Kirino T (1996) Treatment of focal cerebral ischaemia with synthetic oligopeptide corresponding to lectin domain of selectin. Stroke 27: 951–956
35. Newman W, Beall LD, Carson CW (1993) Soluble E-selectin is found in supernatants of activated endothelial cells and is elevated in serum of patients with septic shock. J Immunol 150: 644–654
36. Okada Y, Copeland BR, Mori E, Tung MM, Thomas WS, del Zoppo GJ (1994) P-selectin and intercellular adhesion molecule-1 expression after focal brain ischaemia and reperfusion. Stroke 25: 202–211
37. Oshiro EM, Hoffman PA, Dietsch GN, Watts MC, Pardoll DM, Tamargo RJ (1997) Inhibition of experimental vasospasm with anti-intercellular adhesion molecule-1 monoclonal antibody in rats. Stroke 28: 2031–2038
38. Peterson JW, Kwun BD, Hackett JD, Zervas NT (1990) The role of inflammation in experimental vasospasm. J Neurosurg 72: 767–774
39. Polin RS, Bavbek M, Shaffrey ME, Billups K, Bogaev CA, Kassell NF, Lee KS (1998) Detection of soluble E-selectin, ICAM-1, VCAM-1 and L-selectin in the cerebrospinal fluid of patients after subarachnoid haemorrhage. J Neurosurg 89: 559–567
40. Poston RN, Haskard DO, Coucher JR, Gall NP, Johnson-Tidey RR (1992) Expression of intercellular adhesion molecule-1 in atherosclerotic plaques. Am J Pathol 140: 665–673
41. Pozzilli C, Lenzi CL, Argentino C, Carolei A, Rasura M, Signore A, Bozzao L, Pozzilli P (1985) Imaging of leukocyte infiltration in human cerebral infarcts. Stroke 16: 251–255
42. Ryba M, Jarzabek-Chorzelska M, Chorzelski T, Pastuszko M (1992) Is vascular angiopathy following intracranial aneurysm rupture immunologically mediated? Acta Neurochir (Wien) 117: 34–37
43. Schürer L, Grogaard B, Gerdin B, Afors KE (1990) Effects of neutrophil depletion and superoxide dismutase on postischaemic hypoperfusion of rat brain. Adv Neurol 52: 57–62
44. Shiga Y, Onodera H, Matsuo Y, Kogure K (1992) Cyclosporin A protects against ischaemia-reperfusion injury in the brain. Brain Res 595: 145–148
45. Sills A, Clatterbuck RE, Thompson RC, Tamargo RJ (1997) Endothelial cell expression of intercellular adhesion molecule 1 in experimental posthaemorrhagic vasospasm. Neurosurgery 41: 453–460
46. Talbott GA, Sharar SR, Harlan JM, Winn RK (1994) Leukocyte-Endothelial interactions and organ injury: The role of adhesion molecules. New Horizons 2(4): 545–554
47. Tanabe Y, Sekata K, Yamada Y (1978) Cerebral vasospasm and ultrastructural changes in cerebral arterial wall. J Neurosurg 49: 229–238
48. Wang X, Yue T-L, Barone FC, Feuerstein GZ (1995) Demonstration of increased endothelial-leukocyte adhesion molecule-1 mRNA expression in rat ischaemic cortex. Stroke 26: 1665–1669
49. Weyrich AS, Ma XY, Lefer DJ, Albertine KH, Lefer AM (1993) In vivo neutralisation of P-selectin protects feline heart and endothelium in myocardial icshaemia and reperfusion injury. J Clin Invest 91: 2620–2629
50. Wilcox CE, Ward AM, Evans A, Baker D, Rothlein R, Turk JL (1990) Endothelial cell expression of the intercellular adhesion molecule-1 (ICAM-1) in the central nervous system during acute and chronic relapsing experimental allergic encephalomyelitis. J Neuroimmunol 30: 43–51
51. Zhang RL, Chopp M, Zhang ZG (1996) E-selectin in focal cerebral ischaemia and reperfusion in the rat. J Cereb Blood Flow Metab 16: 1126–1136

Correspondence: J. J. Nissen, Department of Neurosurgery, Newcastle General Hospital, Westgate Road, Newcastle upon Tyne, NE4 6BE UK.

Acta Neurochir (2000) [Suppl] 76: 61–64

Traumatic Brain Injury in Mice Deficient in Poly-ADP(Ribose) Polymerase: A Preliminary Report

M. J. Whalen[1,5], **R. S. B. Clark**[1,2,5], **C. E. Dixon**[3,5], **P. Robichaud**[5], **D. W. Marion**[3,5], **V. Vagni**[5], **S. Graham**[4,5], **L. Virag**[6], **G. Hasko**[7], **R. Stachlewitz**[7], **C. Szabo**[7], and **P. M. Kochanek**[1,2,5]

[1] Department of Anesthesiology and Critical Care Medicine, University of Pittsburgh, Pittsburgh, PA
[2] Department of Pediatrics, University of Pittsburgh, Pittsburgh, PA
[3] Department of Neurological Surgery, University of Pittsburgh, Pittsburgh, PA
[4] Department of Neurology, Geriatric Research Educational and Clinical Center, VA Pittsburgh Health System, Pittsburgh, PA
[5] Safar Center for Resuscitation Research and the Brain Trauma Research Center, University of Pittsburgh, Pittsburgh, PA
[6] Department of Pathophysiology, Medical University of Debrecen, Debrecen, Hungary
[7] Inotek Corporation, Beverly, MA

Summary

Poly (ADP-ribose) polymerase (PARP) is a ubiquitous nuclear enzyme that, when activated by free-radical induced DNA damage, contributes to energy failure and cell death in models of central nervous system ischemia and reperfusion. PARP contributes to neuronal cell death in vivo after cerebral ischemia/reperfusion, however, the role of PARP in the pathogenesis of traumatic brain injury (TBI) is unknown. We hypothesized that, compared to wild type mice (+/+), mice deficient in PARP (−/−) would have reduced motor and cognitive deficits after TBI. Mice underwent controlled cortical impact (CCI) (6 m/s, 1.2 mm depth) and were tested for motor (d 1–5) and cognitive (d 14–18) function after CCI. PARP −/− mice demonstrated improved motor performance and improved cognitive function after CCI (both $p < 0.05$ compared to +/+). This is the first study to evaluate a role for PARP in functional outcome after TBI. The results suggest a detrimental role for PARP in the pathogenesis of TBI.

Keywords: Brain injury; poly(ADP-ribose) polymerase; controlled cortical impact; mice

Introduction

Poly (ADP-ribose) polymerase (PARP) is a nuclear enzyme involved in genomic surveillance, stability and repair of DNA damage [1]. PARP, activated by DNA strand breaks, such as those produced by oxygen radicals, catalyzes the addition of ADP-ribose units to nuclear proteins and PARP itself using nicotinamide adenine-dinucleotide (NAD^+) as substrate. Overactivation of PARP by extensive DNA damage can rapidly consume cellular NAD^+, deplete ATP, and cause cell death by energy failure [2].

Recent studies in experimental stroke demonstrate a key role for PARP in the pathogenesis of ischemic cell death in vivo [7, 9, 22, 23]. These and other studies [3, 4, 16, 25, 31] suggest that excitotoxicity and neuronal nitric oxide synthase activation contribute to peroxynitrite-induced DNA damage, PARP activation, and neuronal cell death. These studies have led to the hypothesis that PARP is central to the pathogenesis of CNS ischemia when energy failure mediates necrotic cell death [6, 9].

PARP activation has been implicated in the pathogenesis of CNS neurodegenerative diseases and traumatic spinal cord injury [13, 19], however, the role of PARP activation in the pathogenesis of TBI is unknown. ADP-ribosylation was detected in brain after fluid percussion in rats [14], and that PARP inhibition preserves neuronal electrophysiologic function in hippocampal slices after percussion TBI in vitro, suggesting that PARP activation might contribute to loss of neuronal function after TBI [24]. However, the role of PARP in the pathogenesis of functional or histopathologic outcome after TBI has not been elucidated yet. We have hypothesized that mice deficient in PARP (−/−) would have improved motor and cognitive function compared to wild type (+/+) mice after TBI induced by controlled cortical impact (CCI).

Materials and Methods

Mice

All experiments were approved by the University of Pittsburgh Institutional Animal Care and Use Committee and complied with the NIH Guide for the Care and Use of Laboratory Animals. Homozygous male (PARP −/−) and PARP +/+ wild type controls generated as previously described [26] were used at 12–13 wk of age (23–38 g).

Controlled Cortical Impact

A mouse CCI model that produces motor and cognitive deficits was used [28]. Mice were anesthetized with 2% isoflurane (Anaquest, Memphis TN), N_2O and O_2 (2:1) and brain temperature was monitored by a probe (0.009 in. diameter, Physitemp Corp., Clifton, NJ) in the left frontal cortex. CCI was produced at a brain temperature of 37–38 °C with a pneumatic cylinder (Bimba Co.) using a 3 mm flat-tip impounder, velocity 6.0 ± 0.2 m/s, and depth of 1.2 mm. Mice were recovered in oxygen then returned to their cages where they were given free access to food and water and 12 h day/night cycles.

Assessment of Motor Function

Gross vestibulomotor function was assessed at days 1–5 after injury using a beam balance test [5, 10]. Mice were suspended on a 1.0 cm wide wooden beam and the time the mouse remained on the beam for up to 60 seconds was recorded. Mice were trained before CCI in three trials during which baseline measurements of time on the beam were made.

Spatial Memory Acquisition Assessment

Spatial memory performance of mice was evaluated using the Morris water maze (MWM) task as previously described [11, 15]. A white pool (83 cm diameter, 60 cm deep) filled with water to 29 cm depth (24 °C) in a room with several highly visible extra-maze cues was used. A round (10 cm diameter), white goal platform located 1 cm below the water's surface was positioned approximately 15 cm from the southwest wall. The swimming movements of the mice were recorded with a video tracking system (Chromotrack 3.0, San Diego Instruments, San Diego, CA). MWM testing was performed on days 14–18 after CCI to ensure recovery from motor deficits. Each mouse was given 4 trials per day. For each trial, mice were placed in the pool facing the wall in one of 4 randomized locations (north, south, east, west) and released by the experimenter. If the mouse failed to reach the submerged platform by 120 seconds, it was placed on the platform by the experimenter and allowed to remain there for 30 seconds. Mice were warmed in a 37 °C incubator for 4 minutes between trials. Performance in the MWM was quantitated by latency to find the platform. Swim speeds of mice were determined on the first day of MWM testing by dividing the total distance that the mice swam during the 4 trials by the total swim time.

Statistical Analyses

Data are mean ± SD. Body weight, brain temperature, and swim speed were analyzed by t-test. Latencies for beam balance and MWM were analyzed by ANOVA for repeated measures (group × time). Between group differences were analyzed by post hoc tests at each timepoint, corrected for multiple comparisons. For each test, $p < 0.05$ was considered significant.

Results

Seventeen of the eighteen mice survived the 18 day trauma protocol. The body weight of mice prior to CCI did not differ between +/+ (29.6 ± 4.4 g) and −/− (30.6 ± 4.1 g).

Beam balance data on d 1 after CCI for both groups of mice are shown in Table 1. After TBI, wild type mice performed significantly worse than PARP −/− on the beam balance test ($p < 0.05$).

After injury, the latency to find the hidden platform in the MWM test was longer in +/+ versus −/− mice on d 16 and 18 of MWM testing ($p < 0.05$, Table 1). Swim speeds (cm/s) did not differ between +/+ (18.7 ± 1.1) and −/− (20.1 ± 1.0) mice.

Discussion

This is the first report of the effect of PARP on the functional outcome in an experimental model of TBI. Mice deficient in PARP exhibited protection from motor and cognitive deficits after severe CCI. The beneficial effect of PARP deletion on motor outcome was evident early (d 1) after TBI. In addition, the beneficial effects of PARP inhibition on cognitive function appear to be sustained, as PARP −/− mice had improved performance in the MWM at days 16 and 18 after injury vs. wild type. The data are not explained by differences in swim speed between +/+ and −/− mice.

Table 1. *Motor and Cognitive Function in PARP +/+ and −/− Mice after Controlled Cortical Impact*

Day of testing	1	2	3	4	5
Beam balance					
+/+	40.4 ± 7.2[a]	–	–	–	–
−/−	53.7 ± 3.3*	–	–	–	–
MWM					
+/+	59.2 ± 9.4	42.7 ± 8.2	48.1 ± 8.8	29.6 ± 7.4	30.8 ± 6.6
−/−	53.4 ± 30.4	30.4 ± 7.7*	18.1 ± 2.6	15.3 ± 2.4*	15.6 ± 2.8

[a] Values are latencies (sec); * $p < 0.05$ vs. +/+; *MWM* Morris Water Maze.

Studies in experimental cerebral ischemia, using PARP knockout mice or pharmacologic inhibition of PARP, have demonstrated a detrimental effect of PARP on motor function early after ischemia [9]. In addition, inhibition of PARP markedly reduces infarct size after experimental stroke [6, 8, 9]. Recent studies in rats have demonstrated PARP activation at 24 hours after spinal cord injury [20] and within 2 hours after fluid percussion brain injury [14], however histologic and functional outcome were not reported in these studies.

One mechanism by which inhibition of PARP could abrogate functional deficits in mice after TBI is by inhibition of posttraumatic energy failure. DNA damage occurs in injured brain early after TBI in rats [29], and DNA damage-initiated activation of PARP could lead to NAD+ consumption, depletion of ATP, and cell death by energy failure [18, 30]. This paradigm is supported by numerous studies that implicate PARP activation and energy failure in necrosis of neurons and other cell types exposed to excitotoxic or oxidizing agents in vitro, as inhibition of PARP prevents NAD+ depletion and cell death [4, 7, 21, 31]. Energy failure is an important component of the pathophysiology of both cerebral ischemia and TBI [12]. Mechanisms other than energy failure, such as inhibition of a variety of enzymes by ribosylation, may also play a role in PARP-mediated neural injury.

The finding of a detrimental role for PARP in the pathogenesis of TBI is in contrast to the lack of effects on functional outcome of other targeted mechanisms in the CCI model. No beneficial effect on functional outcome after CCI vs. wild type has been observed in studies by our group of mice deficient in intercellular adhesion molecule-1 (ICAM-1) [28], interleukin-8 receptor homologue [27], inducible nitric oxide synthase [17], or in P-selectin/ICAM-1 double knockout mice [32].

In conclusion, the results of this study suggest a powerful detrimental effect of PARP on functional outcome after TBI. Further studies are needed to examine the effect of PARP inhibition on motor and cognitive function in naïve (uninjured) mice, and to determine the effect of PARP inhibition on measures of histopathologic damage, such as contusion volume, after TBI. If the results of this study are confirmed by others, pharmacological inhibition of PARP could be investigated as a possible therapeutic strategy for reducing neurologic injury after TBI in the clinical setting.

References

1. Althaus FR, Richter C (1987) ADP-ribosylation of proteins. Enzymology and biological significance. Mol Biol Biochem Biophys 37: 1–237
2. Berger NA (1985) Poly(ADP-ribose) in the cellular response to DNA damage. Radiat Res 101: 4–15
3. Cookson MR, Ince PG, Shaw PJ (1998) Peroxynitrite and hydrogen peroxide induced cell death in the NSC34 neuroblastoma x spinal cord cell line: role of poly (ADP-ribose) polymerase. J Neurochem 70: 501–508
4. Cosi C, Suzuki H, Milani D, Facci L, Menegazzi M, Vantini G, Kanai Y, Skaper SD (1994) Poly(ADP-ribose) polymerase: early involvement in glutamate-induced neurotoxicity in cultured cerebellar granule cells. J Neurosci Res 39: 38–46
5. Dixon CE, Lyeth BG, Povlishock JT, Findling RL, Hamm RJ, Marmarou A, Young HF, Hayes RL (1987) A fluid percussion model of experimental brain injury in the rat. J Neurosurg 67: 110–119
6. Eliasson MJ, Sampei K, Mandir AS, Hurn PD, Traystman RJ, Bao J, Pieper A, Wang ZQ, Dawson TM, Snyder SH, Dawson VL (1997) Poly(ADP-ribose) polymerase gene disruption renders mice resistant to cerebral ischemia. Nat Med 3: 1089–1095
7. Endres M, Scott G, Namura S, Salzman AL, Huang PL, Moskowitz MA, Szabo C (1998) Role of peroxynitrite and neuronal nitric oxide synthase in the activation of poly(ADP-ribose) synthetase in a murine model of cerebral ischemia-reperfusion. Neurosci Lett 248: 41–44
8. Endres M, Scott GS, Salzman AL, Kun E, Moskowitz MA, Szabo C (1998) Protective effects of 5-iodo-6-amino-1,2-benzopyrone, an inhibitor of poly(ADP-ribose) synthetase against peroxynitrite-induced glial damage and stroke development. Eur J Pharmacol 351: 377–382
9. Endres M, Wang ZQ, Namura S, Waeber C, Moskowitz MA (1997) Ischemic brain injury is mediated by the activation of poly(ADP-ribose)polymerase. J Cereb Blood Flow Metab 17: 1143–1151
10. Feeney DM, Boyeson MG, Linn RT, Murray HM, Dail WG (1981) Responses to cortical injury: I. Methodology and local effects of contusions in the rat. Brain Res 211: 67–77
11. Hamm RJ, Dixon CE, Gbadebo DM, Singha AK, Jenkins LW, Lyeth BG, Hayes RL (1992) Cognitive deficits following traumatic brain injury produced by controlled cortical impact. J Neurotrauma 9: 11–20
12. Headrick JP, Bendall MR, Faden AI, Vink R (1994) Dissociation of adenosine levels from bioenergetic state in experimental brain trauma: potential role in secondary injury. J Cereb Blood Flow Metab 14: 853–861
13. Hivert B, Cerruti C, Camu W (1998) Hydrogen peroxide-induced motoneuron apoptosis is prevented by poly ADP ribosyl synthetase inhibitors. Neuroreport 9: 1835–1838
14. LaPlaca MC, Raghupathi R, Saatman KE, McIntosh TK (1998) Poly (ADP-ribose) polymerase activity following brain injury in the rat: An indicator of post-traumatic DNA damage? J Neurotrauma 15: 878
15. Long DA, Ghosh K, Moore AN, Dixon CE, Dash PK (1996) Deferoxamine improves spatial memory performance following experimental brain injury in rats. Brain Res 717: 109–117
16. Radons J, Heller B, Burkle A, Hartmann B, Rodriguez ML, Kroncke KD, Burkart V, Kolb H (1994) Nitric oxide toxicity in islet cells involves poly(ADP-ribose) polymerase activation and concomitant NAD+ depletion. Biochem Biophys Res Commun 199: 1270–1277
17. Sinz EH, Kochanek PM, Dixon CE, Clark RSB, Carcillo JA, Watkins SC, Schiding JK, Carlos TM, Billiar TM (1990) In-

ducible nitric oxide synthase is an endogenous neuroprotectant after traumatic brain injury in rats and mice. J Clin Invest 104: 647–656
18. Schraufstatter IU, Hyslop PA, Hinshaw DB, Spragg RG, Sklar LA, Cochrane CG (1986) Hydrogen peroxide-induced injury of cells and its prevention by inhibitors of poly(ADP-ribose) polymerase. Proc Natl Acad Sci U S A 83: 4908–4912
19. Scott GS, Hake P, Salzman AL, Szabo C (1998) Inhibition of poly(ADP-ribose) synthetase prevents the neurological development of experimental allergic encephalomyelitic. FASEB J 12: A753
20. Scott GS, Jakeman LB, Stokes BT, Szabo C (1999) Peroxynitrite production and activation of poly (ADP-ribose) synthetase in spinal cord injury. Ann Neurol 45: 120–124
21. Szabo C (1997) Role of poly(ADP-ribose) synthetase activation in the suppression of cellular energetics in response to nitric oxide and peroxynitrite. Biochem Soc Trans 25: 919–924
22. Takahashi K, Greenberg JH, Jackson P, Maclin K, Zhang J (1997) Neuroprotective effects of inhibiting poly(ADP-ribose) synthetase on focal cerebral ischemia in rats. J Cereb Blood Flow Metab 17: 1137–1142
23. Tokime T, Nozaki K, Sugino T, Kikuchi H, Hashimoto N, Ueda K (1998) Enhanced poly(ADP-ribosyl)ation after focal ischemia in rat brain. J Cereb Blood Flow Metab 18: 991–997
24. Wallis RA, Panizzon KL, Girard JM (1996) Traumatic neuroprotection with inhibitors of nitric oxide and ADP-ribosylation. Brain Res 710: 169–177
25. Wallis RA, Panizzon KL, Henry D, Wasterlain CG (1993) Neuroprotection against nitric oxide injury with inhibitors of ADP-ribosylation. Neuroreport 5: 245–248
26. Wang ZQ, Auer B, Stingl L, Berghammer H, Haidacher D, Schweiger M, Wagner EF (1995) Mice lacking ADPRT and poly(ADP-ribosyl)ation develop normally but are susceptible to skin disease. Genes Dev 9: 509–520
27. Whalen MJ, Carlos TM, Dixon CE, Schiding JK, Clark RSB, Baum E, DeKosky ST, Marion DW, Kochanek PM (1998) Traumatic brain injury in interleukin-8 receptor homologue-deficient mice. in Sixteenth Annual National Neurotrauma Society Meeting, Los Angeles, CA
28. Whalen MJ, Carlos TM, Dixon CE, Wisniewski SR, Schiding JK, Clark RSB, Baum E, MArion DW, Kochanek PM (1999) Effect of traumatic brain injury in mice deficient in intercellular adhesion molecule-1: assessment of histopathologic and functional outcome. J Neurotrauma 16: 299–309
29. Whalen MJ, Chen M, Clark RSB, Jin K, Kochanek PM, Marion DW, Graham SH (1999) DNA damage is temperature dependent early after traumatic brain injury in rats. in 28th Society of Critical Care Medicine Educational and Scientific Symposium, January 23–27 San Francisco, CA
30. Yamamoto H, Uchigata Y, Okamoto H (1981) Streptozotocin and alloxan induce DNA strand breaks and poly(ADP-ribose) synthetase in pancreatic islets. Nature 294: 284–286
31. Zhang J, Dawson VL, Dawson TM, Snyder SH (1994) Nitric oxide activation of poly(ADP-ribose) synthetase in neurotoxicity. Science 263: 687–689
32. Whalen MJ, Carlos TM, Dixon CE, Robichaud P, Clark RSB, Marion DW, Kochanek PM (2000) Reduced brain edema after traumatic brain injury in mice deficient in P-selectin and intercellular adhesion molecule-1. J Leuk Biol 67: 160–168

Correspondence: Patrick M. Kochanek, M.D., Safar Center for Resuscitation Research, 3434 Fifth Avenue, Pittsburgh, PA 15260.

Acta Neurochir (2000) [Suppl] 76: 65–68

Increased Immunolocalization of Nitric Oxide Synthases During Blood-Brain Barrier Breakdown and Cerebral Edema

S. Nag[1], **P. Picard**[2], and **D. J. Stewart**[2]

[1] Department of Pathology (Neuropathology), The Toronto Western Research Institute, Toronto, Canada
[2] Department of Medicine (Cardiology), St. Michael's Hospital, University of Toronto, Toronto, Canada

Summary

The role of nitric oxide (NO) in blood-brain barrier (BBB) breakdown and edema formation was investigated in the rat cortical cold injury model over a period of 10 min to 6 days post cold-injury by immunolocalization of fibronectin as a marker of BBB permeability alterations and endothelial (e) and inducible (i) nitric oxide synthases (NOS), which are markers of NO biosynthetic activity. BBB breakdown to fibronectin in lesion vessels was observed at 10 minutes post-injury, was maximal between 60 minutes and 3 hours and declined gradually thereafter, while perilesional vessels remained permeable up to 5 days. Increased eNOS immunoreactivity was observed in endothelium of perilesional permeable vessels starting at 12 hrs and was maximal between 4–6 days, after which immunoreactivity decreased reaching basal levels by 5–6 days. Immunoreactivity for iNOS was absent in normal brain and was first observed in polymorphonuclear leukocytes and endothelium of lesion vessels at 3 hrs. Maximal iNOS immunoreactivity was observed in endothelial cells and macrophages during the period of angiogenesis. Smooth muscle cells of overlying hyperplastic pial vessels showed iNOS immunoreactivity up to 6 days. The demonstration of increased NO synthases at the lesion site during BBB breakdown and edema formation and angiogenesis suggests that NO plays a role in these processes.

Keywords: Blood-brain barrier; nitric oxide; nitric oxide synthases; cerebral edema.

Introduction

The time course of blood-brain barrier (BBB) breakdown and edema formation and angiogenesis is well documented in the rat cerebral cortical cold-injury model [6]. Several vasoactive agents such as angiotensin II, epinephrine and norepinephrine [7], bradykinin [10], histamine [4], vascular endothelial growth factor [8] have been implicated in BBB breakdown. A few studies [1, 5] using inhibitors of nitric oxide synthases (NOS) suggest that nitric oxide may have a role in BBB breakdown in pathological states. The role of nitric oxide in the pathogenesis of blood-brain barrier (BBB) breakdown and cerebral edema was investigated by a time course immunohistochemical study of endothelial nitric oxide synthase (eNOS) and inducible nitric oxide synthase (iNOS) in the rat cerebral cortical cold injury model. Immunohistochemical demonstration of fibronectin was used as a marker of BBB permeability alterations in the same rats.

Materials and Methods

Male Wistar rats (100–120 g) were anesthetized by methoxyflurane inhalation. A cortical cold injury was produced as described previously [6]. Rats were sacrificed in groups of 5 along with 3 controls at 10, 30 and 60 min, 12 h and 1, 2, 3, 4, 5 and 6 days. At the time of sacrifice, rats were anesthetized with methoxyflurane and perfused with 3% paraformaldehyde in 0.1 M phosphate buffer as described previously [6]. A coronal slab of brain containing the cold injury site was processed for paraffin sectioning using standard techniques. Sections having a thickness of 5 μm were stained with hematoxylin and eosin and adjacent sections were used for immunohistochemistry.

The indirect streptavidin-biotin peroxidase method was used and paraffin sections were pretreated with 0.5% pepsin for 30 min at 37 °C prior to overnight incubation in primary antibody at 4 °C. Rabbit antibodies and the dilutions used were: eNOS (Transduction Labs) 1:50, iNOS (Santa Cruz Biotechnology, Inc) 1:1200 and Fibronectin (Gibco BRL) 1:700. In the case of eNOS, tyramide signal amplification was used to enhance the immunostaining.

The intensity of immunostaining was assessed semiquantitatively in a blinded manner by assigning the following scores: –, no change; 1+, mild increase; 2+, moderate increase; 3+, marked increase.

Results

Control Rats

Fibronectin: The pia-arachnoid membrane and the endothelial basement membranes of pial vessels showed marked fibronectin immunoreactivity. Mild immunoreactivity was present in the basement membrane of intracerebral vessels. Occasional poorly perfused vessels showed fibronectin immunoreactivity in the plasma proteins present in the vessel lumen. The BBB was intact and extravasation of plasma fibronectin from walls of intracerebral vessels was not observed.

NOS Immunoreactivity: Endothelium of both pial and intracerebral vessels showed mild eNOS immunoreactivity. iNOS immunoreactivity was not observed in brains of control rats.

Cold Injury Site

The morphological appearance of the cold injury was similar to previous observations [6, 8]. A central area of coagulative necrosis which extended into the 4th cortical layer was evident at 10 min. By day 3 most rats showed increased numbers of endothelial cells around viable vessels in the lesion. The cells then spread to occupy the entire lesion area. By 4 days neovessel profiles were apparent in the lesion site.

BBB Breakdown

The pattern of BBB breakdown to fibronectin was similar to our previous observations [8]. Extravasation of fibronectin from intracerebral arterioles (Fig. 1a) and microvessels in the lesion site was observed from 10 min post-injury. Fibronectin immunostaining was observed in the neuropil of the cold injury site and in continuity in the underlying white matter with extension into the white matter of the opposite hemisphere. At 2 days perilesional vessels showed fibronectin in their walls and in continuity in the surrounding neuropil. At 4 days, BBB breakdown was localized to the lesion site and fibronectin immunostaining surrounded individual endothelial cells forming a mesh-like pattern. At 5 and 6 days, increased fibronectin immunostaining was confined to the extracellular matrix in walls of neovessels at the cold injury site and in walls of pial vessels overlying the lesion site (Fig. 1b).

NOS Immunoreactivity

The endothelium of perilesional vessels showed a mild increase in eNOS immunoreactivity starting at 6 hrs post-lesion (Fig. 1c). Increased eNOS immunoreactivity was marked at 4 and 5 days when it was also observed in the endothelium of neovessels in the lesion site and in pial vessels overlying the lesion site (Fig. 1d).

Increased immunoreactivity for iNOS was first observed in polymorphonuclear leukocytes which were marginating in the pial vessels overlying the lesion site at 3 hrs post-lesion (Fig. 1e). Next, increased iNOS immunoreactivity was observed in the endothelium of viable lesion vessels and in macrophages. At 4 days, the proliferating endothelial cells at the lesion site showed iNOS immunoreactivity. At 5 and 6 days, iNOS immunoreactivity was only observed in the smooth muscle cells of hyperplastic pial arteries overlying the lesion and in occasional hyperplastic arterioles in the lesion site (Fig. 1f).

Discussion

This study demonstrates the temporal and spatial localization of both eNOS and iNOS protein at the cold lesion site during the period of BBB breakdown. The latter was demonstrated by fibronectin immunolocalization in the same brains. It is well known that immediate BBB breakdown is due to dissolution of cells in the vessel wall produced by the cold lesion [8]. Of interest are the factors responsible for sustained BBB barrier opening of lesion and perilesional vessels which persist up to 6 days post-injury.

Lesion and perilesional vessels with BBB breakdown to fibronectin also showed increased eNOS immunoreactivity. Similar to other reports in the literature [2, 3] immunolocalization of iNOS in this model was associated with the onset of the inflammatory response, and this enzyme was first demonstrable in polymorphonuclear leukocytes and then in macrophages. In addition, there was a marked increase in iNOS in the newly formed endothelial cells and smooth muscle cells of both lesional and overlying pial vessels. eNOS is known to produce NO phasically, while iNOS is reported to produce large amounts of NO for prolonged periods [9]. The increased immunolocalization of both these enzymes suggests that there is an increased production of nitric oxide at the lesion site and that it plays a role in BBB breakdown and cerebral edema in this model.

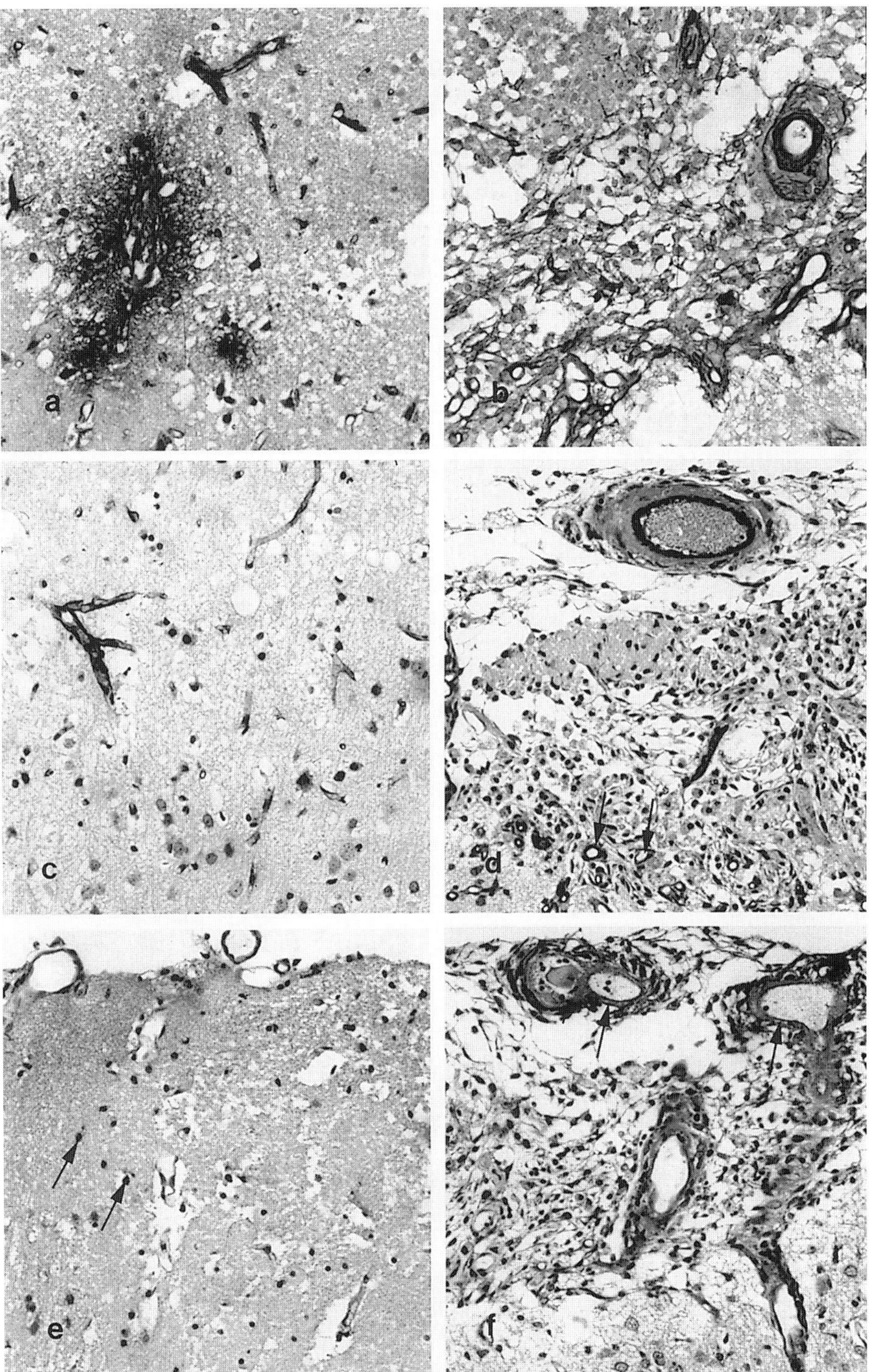

Fig. 1. Photomicrographs showing immunolocalization of fibronectin (a, b), eNOS (c, d) and iNOS (e, f) at the lesion site at 1 and 5 days post-injury. (a) At 1 day the cold injury site shows breakdown of the BBB with extravasation of fibronectin through vessel walls into the surrounding neuropil. (b) At 5 days, fibronectin immunoreactivity is localized to the extracellular matrix of vessel walls including the profiles of the neo-vessels. (c) At 1 day, a vessel near the margin of the lesion area shows mild increase in eNOS immunoreactivity as compared with the surrounding vessels. (d) At 5 days, the increase in eNOS immunoreactivity is marked in the pial artery overlying the lesion as well as in the neo-vessels (arrows) at the lesion site. (e) At 1 day, increased iNOS immunoreactivity is confined to the polymorphonuclear leukocytes (arrows) infiltrating the cold injury site. (f) At 5 days, iNOS immunoreactivity is marked in the smooth muscle cells of pial arteries overlying the cold injury site. a–f, ×250

References

1. Boje KMK (1996) Inhibition of nitric oxide synthase attenuates blood-brain barrier disruption during experimental meningitis. Brain Res 720: 75–83
2. Clark RSB, Kochanek PM, Schwarz, MA, Schiding JK, Turner DS, Chen M, Carlos TM, Watkins SC (1996) Inducible nitric oxide synthase expression in cerebrovascular smooth muscle and neutrophils after traumatic brain injury in immature rats. Pediatr Res 39: 784–790
3. De Groot CJA, Ruuls SR, Theeuwes JWM, Dijkstra CD, Van der Valk P (1997) Immunocytochemical characterization of the expression of inducible and constitutive isoforms of nitric oxide synthase in demyelinating multiple sclerosis lesions. J Neuropathol Exp Neurol 56: 10–20
4. Dux E, Joo F (1982) Effects of histamine on brain capillaries. Exp Brain Res 47: 252–258
5. Mayhan WG (1995) Role of nitric oxide in disruption of the blood-brain barrier during acute hypertension. Brain Res 686: 99–103
6. Nag S (1996) Cold-injury of the cerebral cortex: Immunolocalization of cellular proteins and blood-brain barrier permeability studies. J Neuropathol Exp Neurol 55: 880–888
7. Nag S, Harik SI (1987) Cerebrovascular permeability to horseradish peroxidase in hypertensive rats: effects of unilateral locus ceruleus lesion. Acta Neuropathol (Berl) 73: 247–253
8. Nag S, Takahashi JL, Kilty DW (1997) Role of vascular endothelial growth factor in blood-brain barrier breakdown and angiogenesis in brain trauma. J Neuropathol Exp Neurol 56: 912–921
9. Xie Q, Nathan C (1994) The high-output nitric oxide pathway: role and regulation. J Leukocyte Biol 56: 576–582
10. Raymond JJ, Robertson DM, Dinsdale HB (1986) Pharmacological modification of bradykinin induced breakdown of the blood-brain barrier. Can J Neurol Sci 13: 214–220

Correspondence: Dr S. Nag, Neuropathology, EW5-510, Toronto Western Hospital, 399 Bathurst Street, Toronto, On M5T 2S8, Canada.

Acta Neurochir (2000) [Suppl] 76: 69–72

Biological Functions of Extravasated Serum IgG in Rat Brain

E. Kadota[1], **Y. Muramatsu**[1], **K. Nonaka**[1], **M. Karasuno**[1], **K. Nishi**[1], **K. Dote**[1], and **S. Hashimoto**[2]

[1] Division of Pathology, Kishiwada City Hospital, Osaka, Japan
[2] Department of Pathology, Kinki University School of Medicine, Osaka, Japan

Summary

During blood-brain barrier opening serum IgG could be extravasated. The function of intraparenchymal IgG, however, is unknown. Its biological effects in the acute phase were currently investigated.

From rat autoserum IgG was purified and injected into the cortex. Similarly, IgG-Fab fragment was prepared and administered likewise. As for the control group, only vehicle was injected. Animals were sacrificed on days 1,2 and 4 after the infusion and were histologically evaluated.

On days 1 and 2, the infusion of IgG caused significant intraparenchymal infiltration of neutrophils which expressed LFA-1-alpha. It also induced CR3 up-regulation in microglia and endothelial ICAM-1 expression. On day 4, these findings had disappeared. HE stained brain sections and the TUNEL method did not reveal significant nerve cell death in IgG injected animals during the experiment as compared to the controls. IgG-Fab did not cause significant changes either.

Extravasated IgG has been viewed to have biochemical functions. Its Fc fragment seemed to cause microglial and endothelial activation, followed by leukocytic infiltration. This sequence itself was not neurotoxic. Therefore, it is suggested that extravasated IgG is one of the inducers that modulate cellular responses in the acute phase of brain damage.

Keywords: BBB; IgG extravasation; rat.

Introduction

Serum proteins are often used as conventional tracers for the detection of blood-brain barrier (BBB) opening. This method makes it unnecessary to administer exogenous tracers. And it could be utilized in both experimental approaches and in human pathology. Serum IgG(s) immunohistochemistry has provided reliable and reproducible results. There have been no reports, however, which are concerned with the biological function of extravasated serum IgG in the brain parenchyma. In this report, it was investigated whether extravasated serum IgG had any effect in the brain.

Materials and Methods

Male Wistar rats (body weight 250–320 g) were used. The animals were divided into 3 groups as follows. Group-1; their autosera were sampled, and the serum IgG concentrations were measured by immunoabsorbance. Thereafter, serum IgG was purified by using a ImmunoPure A/G IgG purification Kit (Pierce, USA). The IgG levels of the obtained IgG dissolved in physiological saline were measured. One week after the blood sampling, the IgG solutions were stereotactically infused into the right frontoparietal cortex using a glass micropipette (the external diameter of the tip; 100 micrometer) and a microinjection pump (CMA-100, BAS, Sweden, 100 micro/50 min). Group-2; IgG solutions were also obtained from autosera, and IgG-Fab fractions were purified by ImmunoPure Fab Preparation Kit (Piece, USA). The IgG-Fab solutions were also infused into the brain parenchyma. Group-3; blood sampling was performed as in Group-1 and -2. Only physiological saline was infused as control, however.

In each group, the animals were sacrificed at 1 day, 2 days and 4 days after the stereotactic injection by perfusion fixation using a 4% paraformaldehyde/PBS solution. The brains were carefully removed and histologically evaluated.

The sections were stained by routine HE, Bodian and luxol fast blue. The TUNEL method (ApoTagTM Peroxidase Kit, Oncor, USA) and immunohistochemistry using anti-CR3 antibody (MRC OX-42, Serotec, UK), anti-ICAM-1 antibody (TLD-4C9, Serotec, UK) and anti-LFA-1-alpha (WT-1, Serotec, UK) were also performed. In addition, electron-microscopic immunohistochemistry was done in some animals.

Results

In Group-1, the IgG concentrations in autosera were 298 ± 53.4 mg/dl (mean ± S.E., n = 5). Its level in the purified IgG-physiological saline solution was 197 ± 45.8 mg/dl (n = 5). Histologically, significant neutrophil infiltration was observed in HE stained sections at 1 day and 2 days after the brain infusions (Fig. 1). The neutrophil infiltration was wide-spread involving the ipsilateral frontoparietal cortex, subcortical white matter, hippocampus, subarachnoid

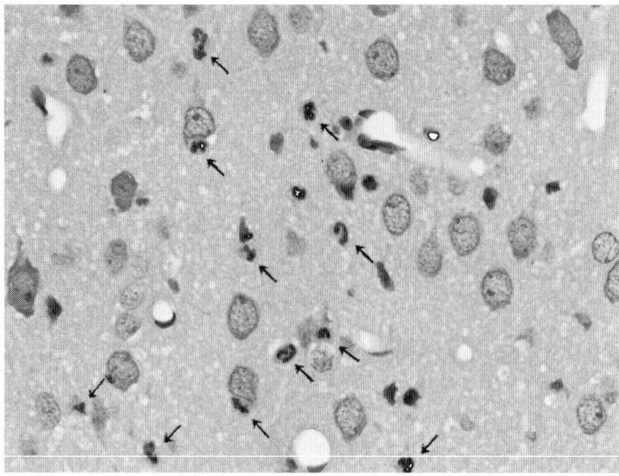

Fig. 1. Routine HE stained brain section of an animal of Group 1, at 1 day after cerebral IgG infusion. As seen, the IgG injection caused significant neutrophil infiltration (arrows). Yet, nerve cells do not show necrotic or degenerative changes

space, and the ventricular plexus. Even in the contralateral subcortical white matter, neutrophils were found to some extent. Yet, the affected brain tissue appeared histologically almost intact. The neuropil was not edematous and the nerve cells showed no major changes. There was no obvious degeneration or destruction of axons or of myelin in Bodian- or luxol fast blue stained sections. Immunohistochemistry revealed a significant up-regulation of CR3 in ramified microglia at 1 day and 2 days after injection (Fig. 2-A). The distribution of the CR3-up-regulation was almost coincident with that of the neutrophil infiltration. Pericytes showed also remarkable CR3 up-regulation in electron-microscopy. In addition, LFA-1-alfa was expressed on the cell membrane of the infiltrated neutrophils at 1 day and 2 days after the infusion (Fig. 2-B). Simultaneously, endothelial ICAM-1 expression was up-regulated in the brain parenchyma, subarachnoid space and in the choroid plexus (Fig. 2-C). Its distribuion coincided also with that of the neutrophil infiltration. Four days after the intracortical injection, the leukocytic infiltration and the immunohistochemically observed up-regulation had almost disappeared. Nerve cells, axons or myelin did not reveal any significant histological alterations.

Group-2 did not show significant differences in comparison with the control animals during the experiment (Fig. 3).

To evaluate the TUNEL-positive nerve cells, we were using the criteria of Sharov *et al.* (11). Accordingly, nerve cells with chromatin condensation form-

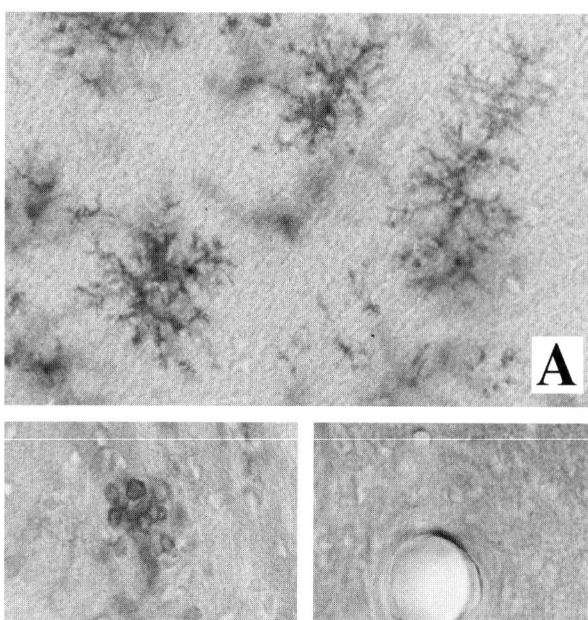

Fig. 2. Cerebral immunohistochemistry of an animal of Group 1, with 2 days survival after IgG infusion (A) CR3 immunohistochemistry revealing significant up-regulation in ramified microglia. (B) LFA-1-alpha immunohistochemistry demonstrating that the infiltrating leukocytes express LFA-1-alpha on their cell surface. (C) ICAM-1 immunohistochemistry showing up-regulation in endothelium

Fig. 3. CR3 immunohistochemistry of brain section of an animal of Group 2, at 2 days after cerebral IgG-Fab infusion. As shown, IgG-Fab failed to induce CR3 up-regulation in ramified microglia

ing patches or rings were considered as apoptotic. The numbers of positive nerve cells were counted in the frontal sections where the glass micropipette was inserted. Group-1 showed 1.71 ± 0.84 positive cells on day 1, 1.12 ± 0.73 on day 2, and 1.03 ± 0.57 on day 4 after injection. Group-2 showed 1.48 ± 0.78 positive cells, 1.62 ± 0.97, and 1.20 ± 0.88, respectively. Group-3 showed 1.52 ± 0.71, 1.68 ± 0.92, and 0.98 ± 0.71 positive cells. There were no statistically significant differences among these groups.

Discussion

It is concluded that extravasated serum IgG could induce microglial activation, followed by endothelial adhesion molecule expression, causing a marked leukocytic infiltration. On the other side, the IgG-Fab fragment did not induce any response at all. Consequently, the currently observed IgG function seemed to depend on its Fc fragment.

Serum IgG is in contact with monocytic and endothelial cells in the blood stream. It does not activate these cells, however, in such a condition. Hayashi *et al.* have reported that once the IgG-Fc fragment is restrictively cleared by an inflammatory SH protease, it becomes a strong chemokine for leukocytes [6]. It was, therefore, proposed that the extravasated IgG-Fc fragment was biologically active in brain parenchyma due to its enzymatic modification.

Microglia cells could express Fc receptors (FcRs) on their cell surface [12]. Vascular endothelium does also express FcRs under some circumstances [10]. Accordingly, the signal(s) from IgG-Fc or its metabolite(s) might be transduced by FcR(s). In addition, it has been reported that soluble FcR is present in the blood stream [12]. Hence, the blood-borne receptor(s) might be combined with the cell surfaces of microglia or endothelium following an acute BBB breakdown.

In common forms of brain damage, the tissue which is infiltrated by neutrophils shows obvious destructive changes. In spite of the significant leukocytic invasion, however, the cerebral parenchyma was almost intact in our study. Therefore, it is concluded that the chemotactically mobilized neutrophils are not neurotoxic by themselves under these circumstance. Presumably, additional stimulation of the cells by complement and/or cytokines must take place to induce leukocytic activation and release of reactive oxygen species, NO and/or cytokines, which seem to be required to confer neurotoxicity. It has been controversially discussed, whether neutrophils are neurotoxic or not. Many authors have reported that activated leukocytes are cytotoxic and induce brain damage [1, 5, 9], while some claim that these cells might be neuroprotective [2, 4]. This disparate view might be explained by different biochemical conditions contributing or not to an activation of leukocytes in a given experiment.

It has been emphasized that neuronal depolarization in acute injury followed by an increase of the extracellular potassium concentration and a K^+ ion influx into the microglial cytoplasm is a key event for the initial activation of microglial cells [7]. Barzo *et al.* reported however that BBB opening might occur during the acute phase of brain injuries [3]. It was therefore considered that in acute forms of brain damage, extravasation of serum IgG and of other blood-born active substances plays a considerable role in microglial and other inflammatory reactions. When brain tissue is damaged, general stress responses controlled by the hypothalamo-pituitary system could be triggered. It may result in marked changes of the body fluid milieu [8]. Further investigations of this aspect for an improvement of the body fluid management for neuroprotection are required.

References

1. Akopov S, Sercombe R, Seylaz J (1996) Cerebrovascular reactivity: role of endothelium/platelet/leukocyte interactions. Cerebrovasc Brain Metab Rev 8: 11–94
2. Aspey BS, Jessimer C, Pereira S, Harrison MJG (1989) Do leukocytes have a role in the cerebral no-reflow phenomenon? J Neurol Neurosurg Psychiatry 52: 526–528
3. Barzo P, Marmarou A, Fatouros P, Corwin F, Dunbar JG (1997) Acute blood-brain barrier changes in experimental closed head injury as measured by MRI and Gd-DTPA. Acta Neurochir [Suppl] (Wien) 70: 243–246
4. Beck J, Stummer W, Lehmberg J, Baethmann A, Uhl E (1997) Leukocyteendothelium interactions in global cerebral ischemia. Acta Neurochir [Suppl] (Wien) 70: 53–55
5. Del Zoppo GJ, Copeland BR, Harker LA, Waltx TA, Zyroff J, Hanson SR, Battenberg E (1986) Experimental acute thrombotic stroke in baboons. Stroke 17: 1254–1265
6. Hayashi H, Honda M, Mibu Y, Yamamoto S Hirashima M (1988) Natural mediators of leukocyte chemotaxis. In: Sabato GD (ed) Methods in enzymology. Academic Press, New York, pp 140–170
7. Koshinaga M, Fukushima M, Oshima H, Suma T, Takabata T, Katayama Y (1997) Rapid microglial activation induced by traumatic brain injury is independent of extravasated blood constituents as revealed by using selective cerebral perfusion model in rat. Adv Neurotrauma Res 9: 44–47
8. Kushner I (1982) The phenomenon of the acute phase response. Ann NY Acad Sci 389: 39–48
9. Okada Y, Copeland BR, Mori E, Tung MM, Thomas WS, del Zoppo GJ (1994) P-selectin and intercellular adhesion molecule-1 expression after focal brain ischemia and reperfusion. Stroke 25: 202–211
10. Sedmak DD (1991) Expression of IgG Fc receptor antigens in placenta and on endothelial cell in humans. Am J Pathol 138: 175–81

11. Sharov LY, Jiang VG, Zaloga C, Sabbah NH, Chopp M (1995) Ultrastructural and light microscopic evidence of apoptosis after middle cerebral artery occlusion in the rat. Am J Pathol 146: 1045–1051
12. Vedeler C, Ulvestad E, Grundt I, Conti G, Nyland H, Matre R, Pleasure D (1994) Fc receptor for IgG(FcR) on rat microglia. J Neuroimmunol 49: 19–23

Correspondence: E. Kadota, Division of Pathology, Kishiwada City Hospital, Osaka, Japan.

Acta Neurochir (2000) [Suppl] 76: 73–77

Possible Reverse Transport of β-Amyloid Peptide Across the Blood-Brain Barrier

R. Pluta[1], **A. Misicka**[2], **M. Barcikowska**[1], **S. Spisacka**[1], **A. W. Lipkowski**[2], and **S. Januszewski**[1]

[1] Department of Neuropathology, Medical Research Centre, Polish Academy of Sciences, Warsaw, Poland
[2] Neuropeptide Laboratory, Medical Research Centre, Polish Academy of Sciences, Warsaw, Poland

Summary

Our experiments were performed to test the hypothesis that human β-amyloid peptide 42 (βA) is able to enter and exit the brain parenchyma through the blood-brain barrier. In an effort to determine the effect of βA in an animal model, we have injected βA *i.v.* into rats following single and repeated brain ischemia. Rats were sacrificed at 3 and 12 months after injection and βA was localized by monoclonal antibody (mAb) 4G8. The present observations revealed an abundant presence of βA in the extracellular space of the brain, which appeared to be dilated, and a vigorous uptake of βA into the cytoplasm of endothelial and ependymal cells, pericytes, astrocytes and neurons. Some of the βA deposits were associated and/or had migrated to the vessels and to the ventricles, and by 3 months a significant amount of βA was directly associated with the vessels and was observed inside the ventricular space. Virtually no soluble and aggregating βA was found in brain tissue 1 year later. This suggests that phagocytic pericytes and astrocytes take up exogenous βA in an attempt to clear the peptide from the brain extracellular space and deliver it to the circulation. Further, direct removal of βA from the ventricles by the bloodstream is also possible. These observations suggest that a reverse transport of βA across endothelial cells of microvessels represents one of the possible mechanisms responsible for removal of extravasated βA. The findings of the present study indicate that in normal conditions βA is rapidly cleared from the cerebrospinal fluid and brain parenchyma, suggesting that irreversible changes in the physico-chemical properties of the cerebrovascular endothelial cell surface are involved in βA deposition in the brain in Alzheimer's disease (AD).

Keywords: Blood-brain barrier; amyloid; brain ischemia; Alzheimer's disease; disappearing plaques; immunization.

Introduction

The relationship between the extravasation of serum βA into the brain parenchyma and the dynamics of its deposition has recently been established in normal and pathological conditions [1–3]. Soluble βA forms are normally produced by constitutive proteolytic processing of parent amyloid precursor protein, and are present also in normal human cerebrospinal fluid (CSF). Recent evidence indicates that βA injected into CSF and brain in normal rats is rapidly cleared into blood and is appreciably accumulating by cerebral arteries [1]. Soluble βA is present at very low levels in normal brain [7], whereas in patient brain with AD a higher content of soluble βA can be isolated by direct extraction [7]. Such a rise in the amount of soluble βA could be attributable to overproduction, an increased transcapillary influx and/or a decreased clearance. Recent findings of Ghersi-Egea *et al.* [1] suggest that in normal brain soluble βA is rapidly cleared from CSF and brain parenchyma, and that a decreased elimination could be involved in amyloid deposition in AD.

Our own model to study the consequences of human βA deposition in brain [3, 4] was used to resolve these conflicting results on the possible role of both an elevated transcapillary influx and decreased elimination of human soluble βA in the pathogenesis of AD. Recently, we have shown that soluble human βA accumulates in the extra- and intracellular space in ischemic brain with repeated *i.v.* injection of protein for over 3 months [3, 4]. As in AD, there were multifocal and widespread diffuse amyloid plaques which predominated in hippocampus and cerebral cortex. This model closely mimics the condition of early AD pathology [3–6], and because of the long-term survival of rats, it offers the opportunity to study the dynamics of late βA deposition in the brain. Using this well defined model, we have currently addressed the issue, whether these diffuse plaques of human βA persist, and/or develop with time.

Materials and Methods

Female Wistar rats (n = 12; 150–180 g; 3 months old) under ether anaesthesia were subjected to a single 10 min *cardiac arrest* (CA) or to three repeated CA episodes [2–4]. All rats received synthetic human βA given in three injections per week of 1 mg each, into the femoral vein for 3 and 12 months [3, 4]. The dose of the first injection after all CA episodes was 5 mg. Controls were sham-operated (n = 6) with or without βA injections, or rats (n = 6) with single and repeated CA only [3, 4]. At 3 and 12 months following the acute experiment, animals were sacrificed and perfused transcardially with phosphate-buffered saline followed by buffered 2% paraformaldehyde [2–6]. For βA visualisation we used the human specific mAb 4G8 [3–6]. Control studies included omission of the primary antibodies and preabsorption of mAb 4G8 with an excess of our synthetic peptide [3, 4].

Results

Rats receiving βA during 3 months after CA demonstrated widespread and multifocal diffuse amyloid plaques in hippocampus and cerebral cortex (Fig. 1D). The brain stem was either unaffected or showed single, small deposits. Endothelial, pericyte, ependymal, neuronal and glial cell bodies were observed to contain βA (Fig. 1A–F). βA staining was mainly seen in undamaged cell bodies. Immunoreactivity was also extracellularly observed in perivascular areas (Fig. 1C). Perivascular βA deposits formed irregular, often asymmetric, well-delineated zones, which were usually located close to blood vessels, predominantly capillaries (Fig. 1C). These deposits frequently surrounded blood vessels, forming perivascular cuffs (Fig. 1C). In all rats studied, diffuse, weakly immunostained, non perivascular and perivascular βA areas could be encountered, predominantly in the cerebral cortex and hippocampus. βA was also present in the ependymal cells probably derived from cerebrospinal fluid (Fig. 1F). Rarely diffuse but rather faint immunoreactivity of βA was observed around the ventricles. The extravasation of βA increased in intensity with the frequency of the ischemic episodes (Table 1). No staining was noted in control brains. In a group surviving for 1 year no deposition of human βA was observed, either (Fig. 2). Extremely rare in this group βA was found in very small amounts as small dots dispersed around and in the wall of large blood vessels of the arachnoid.

Discussion

The brain of patients with AD contains diffuse and senile amyloid plaques. However, the source of these βA deposits is presently unknown. The factors responsible for the excessive accumulation and maturation of βA in AD have not been determined yet. The *in vivo* sequelae of βA deposition and/or the metabolism in brain tissue are not known owing to the lack of reliable and consistent experimental models. This has led us to study the role of βA in the aetiology of the disease in a rat model exhibiting early AD pathology [3–6]. These investigations indicated that diffuse amyloid plaques do not develop/mature with time, they simply disappear. Some of the βA containing phagocytic cells had migrated to the blood vessels and the ventricles, and by 3 months, a significant amount of βA was directly associated with the blood vessels and the ventricles. This suggests that phagocytes had taken up exogenous βA and were clearing the peptide from the central nervous system parenchyma. Our data support some indirect observation in patients with AD [10].

It can be assumed that besides uptake, digestion, and removal and/or transportation by the glial cells, especially by astrocytes and pericytes, the important part of removal of extravasated serum βA, leading to the resolution of diffuse amyloid plaques, takes place by other routes, such as blood vessel walls, CSF or lymphatic drainage.

Our previous observations have shown phagocytizing cells in the perivascular area which were integrated with the capillary wall and wrapped by the basement membrane shared with the endothelial cells (ECs) [9]. We have postulated that these phagocytes in cerebral capillaries play an important role in the process of perivascular in- and detoxication. Probably the phagocytes penetrate from the brain parenchyme into the lumen of capillaries [9]. All these observations strongly suggest that a reverse transport of βA across the endothelium of microvessels represent [8] one of the several mechanisms responsible for removal of extravasated βA. The transvascular pathway of βA removal from the extracellular space appears to begin at the basement membrane, from which the amyloid seems to be transported through endothelial cells from the abluminal side to the luminal surface [8]. Thus, only some and not a large fraction of the microvasculature (arterioles, capillaries, venules) seem to be engaged in the transportation of βA. Similar observations were reported by Ghersi-Egea at al. [1] who observed a reverse transport of intraventricularly injected βA across the wall of small arterioles. A change in the physico-chemical properties of the EC [8] surfaces both in capillaries and arterioles was indicated in the area of diffuse plaques.

Since most of the CSF is transported from the brain ventricles by the arachnoid vill *via* the subarachnoid space, βA in the CSF is probably also removed along

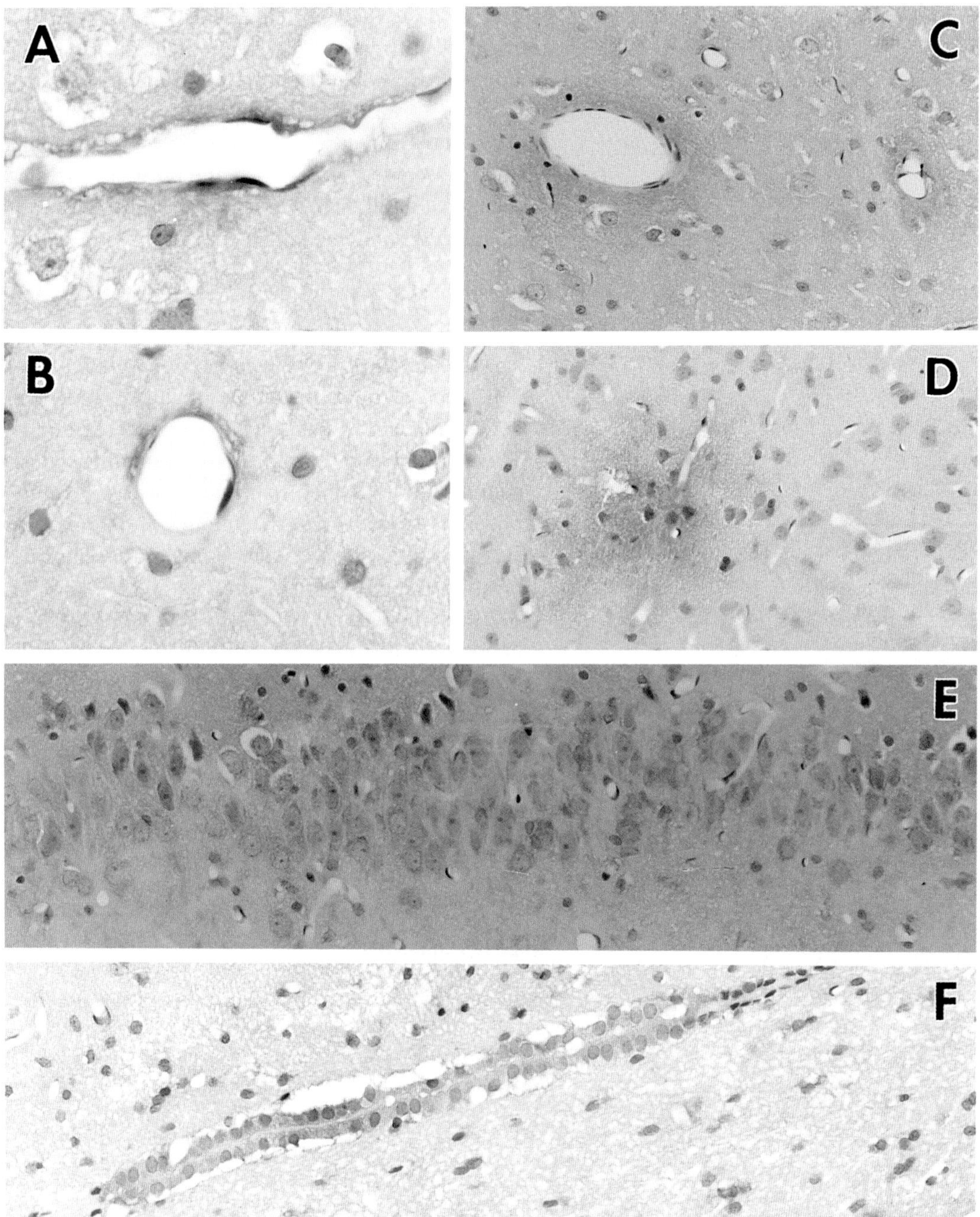

Fig. 1. Step by step movement of βA from circulation into brain parenchyma and cerebral ventricles. (A) Endothelial cells containing βA deposits. Repeated ischemia and βA injections. 3 months survival. Hippocampus. ×400. (B) βA depositions in pericytes. Repeated ischemia and βA injections. 3 months survival. Hippocampus. ×400. (C) Vessel surroundings showing expression of βA. Repeated ischemia and βA injections. 3 months survival. Cortex. ×200. (D) The cortex contains diffuse plaque. Repeated ischemia and βA injections. 3 months survival. Cortex. ×200. (E) Hippocampus showing disperse deposits of βA and neurons filled with βA. Single ischemia and βA injections. 3 months survival. Hippocampus. ×200. (F) Ependymal cells containing βA. Single ischemia and βA injections. 3 months survival. Area around lateral ventricle. ×200

this route. In addition, some βA could be absorbed from CSF by the choroid plexus. It is generally accepted that proteins penetrate from the ventricles into the brain parenchyma across the ependymal lining and from the subarachnoid space along the perivascular space. This leads to the conclusion that βA could be

Table 1. *Deposition of Human βA in Extra- and Intracellular and Intraventricular Space in rat Brain in Different Experimental Condition*

Groups and space	Survival in experiment (months)	
	3	12
Controls		
Extracellular space	–	–
Intracellular space	–	–
Intraventricular space	–	–
Single ischemia with βA		
Extracellular space	+	–
Intracellular space	++	–
Intraventricular space	+++	–
Repeated ischemia with βA		
Extracellular space	+++	–
Intracellular space	+++	–
Intraventricular space	+++	–

Deposits: –, no; +, single; ++, few; +++, multiple and widespread.

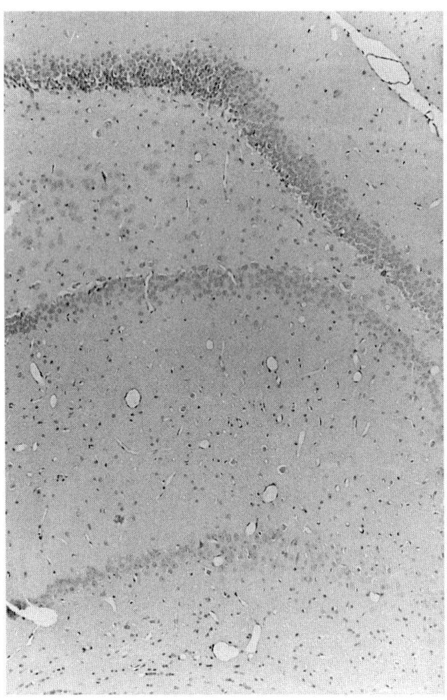

Fig. 2. βA was not identified in brain parenchyma. Repeated ischemia and βA injections. 1 year survival Hippocampus. ×200.

retrogradely transported from the ventricles directly into the blood by crossing vessel walls. Accordingly vessels close to the ventricles, which are directly exposed to βA in the extracellular space of the neuropil and also vessels deeper in the brain parenchyma are likely to contribute to the brain-to-blood transport of βA.

The observations reported in this paper confirm that retrograde transport of βA occurs in segments of the brain microvasculature. Immunohistochemical evidence is also presented that removal of protein from the ventricles directly *via* blood vessels is possible. Some βA becomes endocytosed and probably digested by phagocytic cells. Thus, phagocytes represent also a mechanism of βA removal.

Conclusions

- For the first time, we present data on a time dependent disappearance of diffuse amyloid plaques under experimental conditions.
- The data indicate that βA may not continue to accumulate during the Alzheimer's disease process, but rather support that the amount of βA observed at autopsy may reflect competing processes of deposition and resolution of amyloid.
- The findings of the present study suggest further that in normal individuals βA is rapidly cleared from the brain, raising the possibility that a decreased elimination could be involved in βA deposition in Alzheimer's disease.
- On the basis of the present data, we speculate that our model is useful to identify factors that prevent the assembly of diffuse amyloid plaques into mature plaques in the mammalian brain.

Acknowledgments

Supported by the CSR grant Nr 4.PO5A.091.12 and by PAS.

References

1. Ghersi-Egea JF, Gorevic PD, Ghiso J, Frangione B, Patlak CS, Fenstermacher JD (1996) Fate of cerebrospinal fluid-borne amyloid β-peptide: rapid clearance into blood and appreciable accumulation by cerebral arteries. J Neurochem 67: 880–883
2. Pluta R, Lossinsky AS, Mossakowski MJ, Faso L, Wiśniewski HM (1991) Reassessment of a new model of complete cerebral ischemia in rats. Method of induction of clinical death, pathophysiology and cerebrovascular pathology. Acta Neuropathol 83: 1–11
3. Pluta R, Barcikowska M, Januszewski S, Misicka A, Lipkowski AW (1996) Evidence of blood-brain barrier permeability/leakage for circulating human Alzheimer's β-amyloid-(1–42)-peptide. NeuroReport 7: 1261–1265
4. Pluta R, Misicka A, Januszewski S, Barcikowska M, Lipkowski AW (1997) Transport of human β-amyloid peptide through the rat blood-brain barrier after global cerebral ischemia. Acta Neurochir [Suppl] (Wien) 70: 247–249
5. Pluta R, Barcikowska M, Kida E, Zelamn I, Mossakowski MJ (1997) Late extracellular deposits of β-amyloid precursor pro-

tein in ischaemic rat brain show different immunoreactivity to the N- and C-terminal. Alz Res 3: 51–57

6. Pluta R, Barcikowska M, Mossakowski MJ, Zelman I (1998) Cerebral accumulation of β-amyloid following ischemic brain injury with long-term survival. Acta Neurochir [Suppl] (Wien) 71: 206–208
7. Tabaton M, Nunzi MG, Xue R, Usiak M, Autilio-Gametti L, Gambetti P (1994) Soluble amyloid β-protein is a marker of Alzheimer amyloid in brain but not in cerebrospinal fluid. Biochem Biophys Res Commun 200: 1592–1603
8. Vorbrodt AW, Lossinsky AS, Wiśniewski HM, Suzuki R, Yamaguchi T, Masaoka H, Klatzo I (1985) Ultrastructural observations on the transvascular route of protein removal in vasogenic brain edema. Acta Neuropathol 66: 265–273
9. Walski M, Celary-Walska R, Borowicz J (1991) Ultrastructure of phagocytizing cells of the rat hypothalamic neurosecretory nuclei in a remote period after the sustained clinical death. J Hirnforsch 32: 699–706
10. Yamaguchi H, Sugihara S, Ogawa A, Saido TC, Ihara Y (1998) Diffuse plaques associated with astroglial amyloid β protein, possibly showing a disappearing stage of senile plaques. Acta Neuropathol 95: 217–222

Correspondence: Ryszard Pluta, M.D., Ph.D., Department of Neuropathology, Medical Research Centre, Polish Academy of Sciences, 02-106 Warsaw, Pawińskiego 5 Str., Poland.

Acta Neurochir (2000) [Suppl] 76: 79–80

Reducing Conditions Produce a Loss of Neuroprotective Efficacy of Competitive but not non-Competitive Antagonists in a Model of NMDA-Mediated Excitotoxicity in Organotypic Hippocampal Slice Cultures

A. K. Pringle, J. Self, and **F. Iannotti**

Department of Clinical Neurological Sciences, University of Southampton, Southampton General Hospital, Southampton, UK

Summary

Experimental data indicate that NMDA receptor activation is strongly implicated in the pathogenesis of cerebral ischaemia. However, the results from in vivo studies are equivocal, with NMDA antagonists being active in only some models. It has recently been demonstrated that competitive and non-competitive NMDA antagonists behave differently under normal and ischaemic conditions. These studies have used organotypic hippocampal slice cultures to investigate whether this disparity is due to redox-modulation of the NMDA receptor which occurs in ischaemia. NMDA-mediated toxicity was concentration dependent with little damage occurring with less than 10 μM NMDA and maximal damage produced by 30 μM. NMDA toxicity was significantly enhanced by pre-treatment with 1 mM dithiothreitol, a reducing agent, such that damage occurred at 1 nM NMDA, and maximal damage was produced by 10 μM. The efficacy of MK-801 was not altered by reducing conditions, but the EC50 of the competitive antagonist APV was increased by 20-fold. These data strongly suggest that the neuroprotective efficacy of NMDA antagonists is significantly altered under ischaemic conditions, and that more beneficial effects will be obtained with antagonists having a higher affinity for the receptor in the reduced configuration.

Keywords: Cerebral ischaemia; NMDA; hippocampus; neuroprotection.

Introduction

NMDA receptor activation is strongly implicated in the cascade of events underlying ischaemia-induced neuronal death. Data from many in vitro studies have demonstrated that NMDA receptor antagonism provides significant neuroprotection against simulated ischaemia. However, data from in vivo studies is less clear, with NMDA antagonists having high efficacy in models of focal ischaemia but not global forebrain ischaemia [2]. Using an in vitro model of ischaemia based on organotypic hippocampal slice cultures, we have recently shown that MK-801, a non-competitive channel blocker, was highly neuroprotective whilst the competitive antagonist APV was completely inactive [4]. The mechanisms underlying this disparity are unclear, but a number of the modulatory sites on the NMDA receptor are influenced by the metabolic changes which occur under ischaemic conditions. In particular, the NMDA receptor is greatly influenced by changes in redox conditions [1], with significantly enhanced NMDA-induced neuronal damage occurring in reducing conditions simulating those which prevail during cerebral ischaemia [3]. We have therefore investigated how the efficacy of NMDA receptor antagonists is affected by changes in the redox environment using a model of NMDA-mediated excitotoxicity in organotypic hippocampal slice cultures.

Materials and Methods

Organotypic hippocampal slice cultures were prepared from 8–10 day old Wistar rat pups using a modification of the methods described by Stoppini [4, 5]. 400 μm hippocampal slices were cut on a McIlwain tissue chopper and 4 slices plated onto each Millipore-CM culture insert in a 6 well culture plate. Cultures were maintained at 37 °C in 5% CO_2 for 14 days with the medium changed every 3–4 days. Neuronal damage was determined using the fluorescence exclusion dye propidium iodide (PI), which is excluded from live cells, but enters damaged cells, intercalates into the DNA and becomes highly fluorescent. All experiments were performed in serum-free medium containing PI. Cultures were exposed to NMDA for 3 hours and damage was assessed after 24 hours recovery. Dithiothreitol (DTT-1 mM) was used as a reducing agent for 30 minutes prior to exposure to NMDA. APV (0.3–100 μM) or MK-801 (0.003–3 μM) were added simultaneously with the NMDA. Damage was assessed by determining the area of PI fluorescence above background in the CA1, CA3/4 and dentate gyrus cell layers, and expressing this as a percentage of the area of the cell layers measured from a light-transmission image [4].

Results

After 14 days in vitro, the pyramidal cell and dentate gyrus cell layers were clearly visible using light microscopy. Concentrations of NMDA below 10 μM did not produce significant toxicity under normal conditions. 10 μM NMDA produced a CA1 selective lesion, whilst 30 μM NMDA resulted in a non-selective lesion throughout the pyramidal cell layer. 1 mM DTT had no direct effect on neuronal survival, but dramatically increased the neurotoxic potency of NMDA. In DTT-treated slices, 10 μM NMDA produced damage throughout CA1 and CA3, and significant neuronal damage was evident in CA1 at 1 nM NMDA. The effects of DTT could be prevented by pre-oxidation with 2 mM DTNB (dithio-bis-2-nitrobenzoic acid), an oxidizing agent. Neuronal damage produced by 10 μM NMDA was antagonized in a concentration-dependent manner by both APV (EC50 = 1 μM) and MK-801 (EC50 = 0.02 μM). Reducing conditions produced by DTT had a differential effect on the two antagonists. Despite the enhanced neuronal damage, the EC50 for MK-801 was unaffected by DTT (EC50 = 0.06 μM), but the concentration-response curve for APV was significantly shifted such that the EC50 was increased to 20 μM. The loss of efficacy of APV was prevented by pre-oxidation of the DTT with DTNB.

Discussion

The influence of redox modulation on NMDA receptor function has been well documented in dissociated neuronal cell cultures [1, 3]. These studies extend previous work by demonstrating that modulation also occurs in the more anatomically complex organotypic slice cultures. The damage produced by very low concentrations of NMDA in the presence of DTT implies that in the ischaemic brain very low levels of glutamate will become significantly neurotoxic. Competitive and non-competitive antagonists behaved profoundly differently under reducing conditions. MK-801 was largely unaffected by DTT, with only a small change in the EC50. In contrast, the neuroprotective efficacy of APV was considerably reduced under reducing conditions. These data reflect our previous observations that MK-801, but not APV, is neuroprotective in a model of ischaemia [4], and support our hypothesis that the reducing conditions which occur during an ischaemic episode modify the pharmacological characteristics of the NMDA receptor. This has profound implications for the use of NMDA antagonists as therapeutic agents, as significantly higher concentrations of antagonist will be required for the prevention of ischaemic damage than would be predicted from affinity studies performed on receptors in the native configuration. As such an increase in dose will be associated with significant side-effects, it may be highly beneficial to develop compounds with high affinity for the reduced form of the receptor.

References

1. Aizenman E, Lipton SA, Loring RH (1989) Selective modulation of NMDA responses by reduction and oxidation. Neuron 2: 1257–1263
2. Gill R (1994) The pharmacology of alpha-amino-3-hydroxy-5-methyl-4-isoxazole proprionate (AMPA)/kainate antagonists and their role in cerebral ischaemia. Cerebrovasc Brain Metab Rev 6: 225–256
3. Levy DI, Sucher NJ, Lipton, SA (1990) Redox modulation of NMDA receptor-mediated toxicity in mammalian central neurons. Neuroscience 110: 291–296
4. Pringle AK, Iannotti F, Wilde GJC, Chad, JE, Seeley PJ, Sundstrom LE (1997) Neuroprotection by both NMDA and non-NMDA receptor antagonists in in vitro ischaemia. Brain Res 755: 36–46
5. Stoppini L, Buchs PA, Muller D (1991) A simple method for organotypic cultures of nervous tissue. J Neurosci Method 37: 375–380

Correspondence: Prof. Fausto Iannotti, Department Clinical Neurological Sciences, University of Southampton, LF73B, Level F, South Block, Southampton General Hospital, Tremona Road, Southampton SO16 6YD, UK.

Acta Neurochir (2000) [Suppl] 76: 81–86

Role of Nitric Oxide in Blood-Brain Barrier Permeability, Brain Edema and Cell Damage Following Hyperthermic Brain Injury. An Experimental Study Using EGB-761 and Gingkolide B Pretreatment in the Rat

H. S. Sharma[1], **K. Drieu**[2], **P. Alm**[3], and **J. Westman**[1]

[1] Laboratory of Neuroanatomy, Department of Medical Cell Biology, Biomedical Centre, Uppsala University, Uppsala, Sweden
[2] Institute Henri Beaufour-IPSEN, Paris, France
[3] Department of Pathology, University Hospital, Lund University, Lund, Sweden

Summary

The role of oxidative stress in hyperthermia induced upregulation of constitutive and inducible isoforms of nitric oxide synthase (NOS) in the central nervous system (CNS) was investigated using immunohistochemistry in a rat model. Exposure of rats to heat stress at 38 °C for 4 h resulted in marked upregulation of constitutive NOS (cNOS) and a mild but significant expression of inducible NOS (iNOS) in several brain regions exhibiting leakage of the blood-brain barrier (BBB), brain edema formation and cell injury. Pretreatment with the potent antioxidative compound EGB-761 or its constituent, Ginkgolide B significantly attenuated upregulation of cNOS and iNOS in the brain and also reduced the BBB permeability disturbances, brain edema and cell injury. These neuroprotective effects were most marked in the EGB-761 pretreated rats. Our observations strongly suggest that (i) EGB-761 and Ginkgolide B pretreatment offer significant neuroprotection in hyperthermic brain injury, (ii) upregulation of cNOS and iNOS are injurious to the cell and, (iii) oxidative stress plays an important role in NOS expression and cell injury.

Keywords: Hyperthermia; cNOS; iNOS; EGB-761; Ginkgolide B.

Introduction

Hyperthermia beyond 41 °C for few hours is associated with profound brain injury [9, 12, 19]. However, the molecular mechanisms of hyperthermia induced brain injury are still unclear. It appears that hyperthermia induces release of several neurochemicals and secondary injury factors which are quite similar to that observed in neural trauma [13]. These multiple injury factors play a significant role in the hyperthermia induced cell injury in the CNS.

Nitric oxide (NO) is shown to be involved in various forms of cell injury occurring in neurodegenerative diseases, excitotoxicity, ischemia, epilepsy, and acute or chronic brain injury [5, 14]. Recently, a role of NO in hyperthermia caused by bacterial endotoxin was described [5]. However, the involvement of NO in hyperthermic brain injury caused by systemic heat stress is still not well understood.

NO is a gaseous molecule which influences the neuronal communication by diffusing from one cell to the other within a very short time [5, 14, 15]. NO is synthesized by an enzyme, nitric oxide synthase (NOS) which occurs as constitutive (cNOS) and inducible (iNOS) isoforms [5]. Upregulation of cNOS or iNOS reflects an increased production of NO [14]. Expression of iNOS is associated with an abnormally high level of NO production for long time periods, whereas upregulation of cNOS is associated with a mild release of NO for a short period of time [5, 14]. Since specific blockers of different isoforms of NOS are still not available, the role played by NOS in the pathophysiology of brain injury is still speculative. Thus, it is not certain whether the upregulation of NOS is contributing to cell damage or cell survival. To understand the function of NOS in cell injury further studies are thus highly warranted.

Previously, our laboratory has shown an increased expression of cNOS following heat stress in several brain regions associated with breakdown of the blood-brain barrier (BBB), edema formation and cell injury [10, 11, 16]. NO is a potent free radical which can induce direct damage of the cell membrane if produced in abnormally high quantity within the biological system [5] indicating that production of NO is harmful to the cells. However, apart from cNOS expression, iNOS is also upregulated in regions associated with cell injury following traumatic or ischemic insults to the brain [5, 10].

There are reports that oxidative stress following trauma or ischemia is involved in nitric oxide production in the brain [5]. However, the detailed mechanisms of nitric oxide production in hyperthermia are still unknown. Since hyperthermic brain damage is associated with profound oxidative stress [1, 10, 16], the present study was undertaken to find out, whether EGB-761 [2, 8, 18], or one of its constituent, Ginkgolide B (BN 52021) (IHB-IPSEN, Paris, France) which both act as antioxidant and/or scavenger of free radicals, are able to attenuate cNOS or iNOS immunoreactivity, BBB permeability, brain edema formation, and cell injury following heat stress.

Materials and Methods

Animals

Experiments were carried out on 30 male Sprague Dawley rats (body weight 90–110 g, age 8–9 weeks) housed at controlled room temperature (21 ± 1 °C) with free access to food and tap water.

Heat Exposure

Rats (8–9 weeks) were exposed to 4 h heat stress at 38 °C in a biological oxygen demand (BOD) incubator (relative humidity 50–55%, wind velocity 20–25 cm/sec) [13, 17]. This experimental condition is approved by the Ethical Committee of Uppsala University, Uppsala, Sweden; Lund University, Lund, Sweden; and Banaras Hindu University, Varanasi, India. Rats kept at room temperature served as controls.

Pharmacological Treatments

We have used the two potent antioxidant substances EGB-761 and Ginkgolide B. EGB-761 is a standardised extract from Ginkgo biloba leaves. It contains flavonoids (24% of flavonol hetrosides and about 7% proanthocyanidins), and 6% terpene trilactones (Ginkgolides A, B, C and bilobalide) [10]. In a separate group of rats, EGB-761 (50 mg/kg, IBH-IPSEN, France) or Ginkgolide B (2 mg/kg, IPSEN-Medical, France) were administered *per os* in distilled water (0.3 ml/rat). This treatment was given daily for 5 days. One dose of the drugs was also administered 30 min before the onset of the heat stress experiments [10, 11]. Separate groups of EGB-761 or Ginkgolide B treated rats were used as drug treated controls and were not subjected to heat stress.

Perfusion and Fixation

Immediately after heat stress, animals were anaesthetised with Equithesin (0.3 ml/100 g, i.p.) and the chest was rapidly opened. The right auricle was cut and a 21 gauge butterfly needle was inserted into the left ventricle of the heart which was connected to the perfusion apparatus. About 50 ml of phosphate buffered saline (0.1 M, pH 7.0) was perfused for washout of the remaining blood. This was followed by perfusion of fixative containing 4% paraformaldehyde in 0.1 M phosphate buffered saline [10]. The perfusion pressure was effectively maintained at 90 torr throughout the perfusion process. After perfusion, the animals were wrapped in an aluminium foil and kept overnight in a refrigerator at 4 °C. On the next day, brain and spinal cord tissues were dissected out and kept in the same fixative at 4 °C for one week.

NOS Immunohistochemistry

The NOS immunoreactivity was examined using monoclonal antibodies directed against neuronal NOS (cNOS) [1, 14] and inducible NOS (iNOS, Calbiochem, USA) in several brain regions of the control, heat stressed rats, and EGB-761 or Ginkgolide B treated normal or heat stressed rats in parallel.

Immunohistochemistry of constitutive and inducible isoforms of NOS was examined on 40 μm thick vibratome sections obtained from the desired regions of the brain or spinal cord using standard procedures [14]. In brief, monoclonal antibodies against the constitutive isoforms of neuronal NOS (cNOS) were prepared as described earlier [10, 14]. The antibodies of nNOS or iNOS were diluted 1:5000 and applied to free floating vibratome sections for 48 h with continuous shaking at room temperature [10]. The immune reaction was visualised by using the peroxidase-antiperoxidase technique. NOS immunoreactivity was examined on vibratome sections obtained from control, heat stress, EGB-761 or Ginkgolide B treated normal and heat stressed rats. In few sections, the primary antibody step was omitted and the reaction product was developed as usual. The number of NOS positive immunostained cells in each group were counted in a blind fashion in all the animals [10, 11].

Blood-Brain Barrier Permeability

The BBB permeability was measured using Evans blue albumin and $^{[131]}$I-sodium extravasation as described earlier [13, 17]. In brief, both tracers were injected immediately after heat stress under Equithesin anaesthesia in the right femoral vein. The tracers were allowed to remain in the circulation for 5 min. The intravascular tracers were washed out by perfusion with 0.9% saline. The extravasation of Evans blue dye was measured colorimetrically [17]. The extravasation of radioactive iodine into brain tissue specimens was determined in a gamma counter [13].

Brain Edema Formation

Brain edema formation was determined in similar samples used for BBB permeability investigation to iodine. After counting the radioactive iodine the tissue samples were placed in an oven maintained at 90 °C for 72 h in order to determine the dry weight of the sample. The brain water content was calculated according to the difference in the wet and dry weight of the sample [13].

Statistical Analysis

The quantitative data were analysed using Student's unpaired t-test. The semiquantitative data were evaluated for statistical significance using Wilcoxon sum ranking test. A p-value less than 0.05 was considered to be significant.

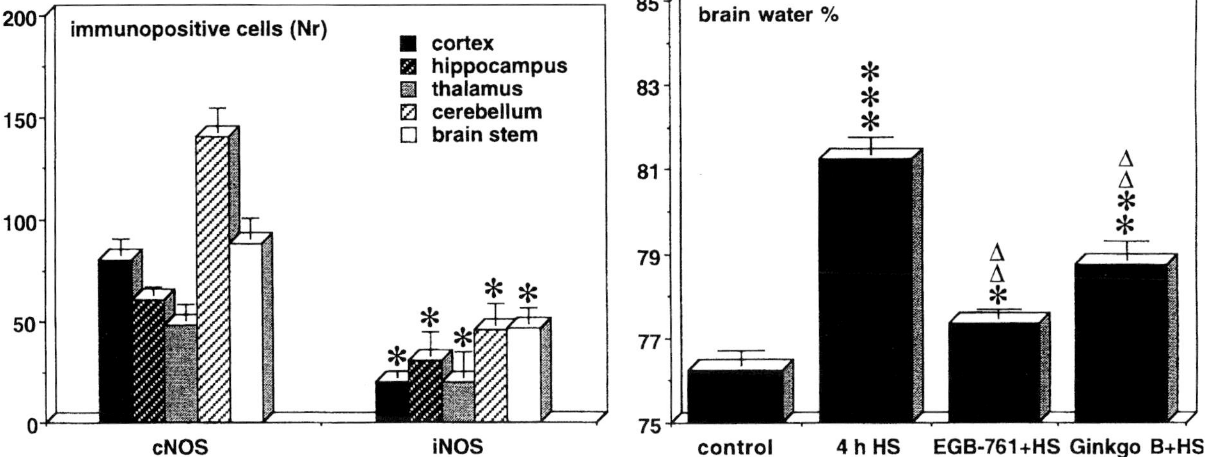

Fig. 1. Immunolabelling of cNOS and iNOS in several brain regions following heat stress (Left). * = $P < 0.01$, compared to cNOS expression (Wilcoxon sum ranking test). Brain edema in heat stress and its modification by EGB-761 or Ginkgolide B pretreatment (Right). *** = $P < 0.001$; ** = $P < 0.01$; * = $P < 0.05$, compared to control; △△ = $P < 0.01$ compared to 4 h heat stress (*HS*); Student's unpaired t-test

Results

Effect of EGB-761 and Ginkgolide B on NOS Immunoreactivity

Our results show that rats exposed to heat stress at 38 °C for 4 h exhibit a selective and specific upregulation of cNOS and iNOS expression in cerebral cortex, hippocampus, thalamus, hypothalamus, brain stem and cerebellum. However, expression of cNOS was much more widespread and pronounced in the above brain regions (Fig. 1). Normal rats did not show iNOS expression but few cNOS positive cells were seen in some areas in the brain. A representative example of cNOS and iNOS expression in the cerebral cortex from heat stress is shown in Fig. 2.

Pretreatment with EGB-761 (50 mg/kg/day, p.o. for 5 days) or Ginkgolide B (2 mg/kg/day, p.o. for 5 days) significantly attenuated the cNOS and iNOS expression in the brain following heat exposure (Fig. 2). The effect of EGB-761 on iNOS or cNOS expression was far more superior than that of Ginkgolide B pretreatment. The pretreatment with EGB-761 or Ginkgolide B alone did not influence NOS activity in normal rats (results not shown).

Effect of EGB-761 and Ginkgolide B on Brain Edema

Pretreatment with EGB-761 or Ginkgolide B significantly attenuated brain edema formation following heat stress (Fig. 1). This effect was most pronounced in animals which received EGB-761 as compared to Ginkgolide B administration. These drugs alone, however, did not influence the BBB permeability or brain water content in normal animals.

Effect of EGB-761 and Ginkgolide B on BBB Permeability

Our results show that heat stress significantly increases BBB permeability to Evans blue albumin (from 0.20 ± 0.06 to 1.48 ± 0.12 mg%, $P < 0.001$) and of radioactive iodine (from 0.30 ± 0.04 to 1.87 ± 0.10%, $P < 0.001$) in the brain. Pretreatment with EGB-761 (Evans blue 0.56 ± 0.12 mg%; iodine 0.64 ± 0.08%, $P < 0.01$) and with Ginkgolide B (Evans blue 0.68 ± 0.08 mg%; iodine 0.75 ± 0.12%; $P < 0.01$) significantly attenuated the permeability increase of the BBB following heat stress. However, the beneficial effects of EGB-761 on heat stress induced disruption of the BBB was more pronounced than the effect of Ginkgolide B pretreatment.

Discussion

The present results clearly show that heat stress is associated with profound upregulation of NOS activity in the brain which seems to play a crucial role in hyperthermia induced brain damage. Our results further show that both constitutive and inducible isoforms of NOS are upregulated following hyperthermia. However, the upregulation of cNOS was

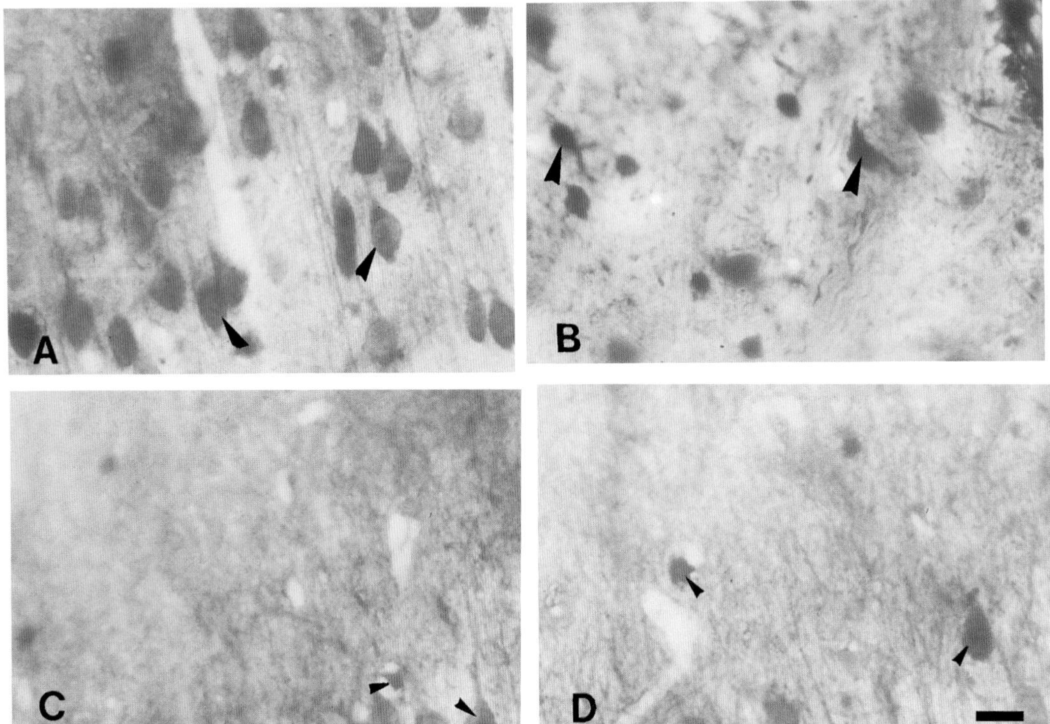

Fig. 2. Representative example of cNOS and iNOS expression in the cerebral cortex following heat stress and its attenuation by EGB-761 pretreatment. Many cNOS immunolabelled nerve cells (A) and few iNOS positive cells (B) (big arrow heads) can be seen in the untreated heat stressed rats. On the other hand, only a few nerve cells (small arrow heads) exhibit cNOS (C) and iNOS expression (D) in EGB-761 pretreated animals following heat stress. (bar = 100 μm)

more widespread than that of iNOS. To our knowledge, this study is the first to demonstrate an upregulation of iNOS in 4 h periods of heat stress in several brain regions. Expression of cNOS and iNOS was mainly seen in damaged and distorted nerve cells located in edematous regions. These observations strongly suggest that expression of NOS is involved in hyperthermia induced cell injury.

The salient new findings of the present investigation further demonstrate that pretreatment with the antioxidant EGB-761 or its constituent Ginkgolide B, significantly attenuates cNOS and iNOS upregulation in the brain following hyperthermia. This effect on NOS regulation was more prominent by EGB-761 pretreatment as compared to Ginkgolide B treatment. These observations clearly point out that oxidative stress associated with hyperthermia plays an important role in NOS induction in the CNS. Furthermore, the neuroprotective effect of EGB-761 appears to be far superior than Ginkgolide B pretreatment alone.

The molecular mechanisms of EGB-761 or Ginkgolide B pretreatment on NOS upregulation are not clear from this study. It appears that the antioxidant properties of both EGB-761 and Ginkgolide B play an important role [7, 18]. Biochemical evidence suggests that EGB-761 possesses powerful antioxidative effects [2, 11], and the compound responsible for most of the anti-oxidative properties of EGB-761 seems to be Ginkgolide B [6, 20]. This is supported by findings of in vitro experiments that Ginkgolide B scavenges free radicals [20]. However, the significantly less pronounced effect of this compound on NOS upregulation compared to EGB-761 in hyperthermia suggest that both Ginkgolide and bilobalide are needed to optimally affect the NOS regulation, a feature which requires additional investigation.

Oxidative stress associated with formation of free radicals is known to induce NO formation [2, 4, 5, 10, 14]. Increased expression of NOS and its attenuation by antioxidant compounds suggest that oxidative stress in heat stress also plays an important role in NO production. Increased production of free radicals may induce membrane damage and cell and tissue injury. Direct damage to the endothelial cell membrane is primarily responsible for the increased BBB permeability [4]. This hypothesis is supported by the data that pretreatment with EGB-761 or Ginkgolide B significantly reduced the breakdown of the BBB function in heat stress.

An increased production of NO induces direct damage eventually causing cell death via production of peroxynitrite and oxygen radicals [14]. Thus, it seems likely that in heat stress an abnormal production of NO in high quantities is related with cell injury. To further analyse this point, specific blockers of cNOS or iNOS are needed, an aspect currently under investigation in our laboratory.

The less pronounced protection of Ginkgolide B of the BBB permeability and against brain edema and cell injury can be understood in terms of its less effective inhibition of oxidative stress and production of free radicals as compared to EGB-761. However, it is known that the different constituents of EGB 761 act synergistically. Thus, Ginkgolide A also exhibits antioxidant activity, and bilobalide improves the respiratory cycle in mitochondria, limiting the release of free radicals and improving the formation of ATP [6]. Further, the bioavailability of pure compounds given orally appears to be less than that of total Ginkgo biloba extracts.

The breakdown of the BBB increases protein extravasation into the extracellular compartment of the brain [3]. An increased extracellular concentration of proteins may attract water from the blood compartment due to an altered colloid-osmotic pressure gradient between blood and brain enhancing formation of vasogenic edema [3, 13]. Obviously, the reduction in breakdown of the BBB is associated with a reduction in brain edema formation. Thus, it seems quite likely that both cNOS and iNOS are contributing to the damage of the BBB as a key factor of inducing edema formation and cell injury.

In conclusion, our observations strongly suggest that (i) hyperthermic brain injury is associated with upregulation of both cNOS and iNOS expression in a very selective and specific manner and (ii) the antioxidant compounds EGB-761 and Ginkgolide B are capable of attenuating both cNOS and iNOS expression. Taken together, these results suggest that both cNOS and iNOS upregulation in heat stress is injurious to the brain, and that the breakdown of the BBB permeability plays an important role in NOS upregulation, brain edema formation, and cell damage in hyperthermic brain injury.

Acknowledgments

This investigation is supported by grants from Swedish Medical Research Council nr. 2710 (JW, HSS), 11205 (PA/HSS); Göran Gustafsson Stiftelse (HSS), Sweden; IPSEN, France (HSS) and The University Grants Commission (HSS), New Delhi, India. The technical assistance to Kärstin Flink Kerstin Rystedt; Secretarial assistance of Gun-Britt Lind, Aruna Sharma; and photographic assistance of Frank Bittkowski are highly appreciated.

References

1. Alm P, Sharma HS, Hedlund S, Sjöquist P-O, Westman J (1998) Nitric oxide in the pathophysiology of hyperthermic brain injury. Influence of a new anti-oxidant compound H-290/51. Amino Acids 14: 95–104
2. Boveris AD, Puntarulo S (1998) Free-radical scavenging actions of natural antioxidants. Nut Res 18: 1545–1557
3. Bradbury MWB (1992) Physiology and pharmacology of the blood-brain barrier. Handb Exp Pharmacol 103: 1–450
4. Chen JX, Chen WZ, Huang HL, Chen LX, Xie ZZ, Zhu BY (1998) Protective effects of Ginkgo biloba extract against lysophosphatidylcholine-induced vascular endothelial cell damage. Acta Pharmacol Sinica 19: 359–363
5. Chiueh CC, Gilbert DL, Colton CA (1994) The neurobiology of NO· and ·OH. Ann NY Acad Sci 738: 1–471
6. Janssens D, Michiels C, Delaive E, Eliaers F, Drieu K, Remacle J (1995) Protection of hypoxia-induced ATP decrease in endothelial cells by Ginkgo biloba extract and bilobalide. Biochem Pharmacol 50: 991–999
7. Kim SY, Kwak JS, Shin JP, Lee SH (1998) The protection of the retina from ischemic injury by the free radical scavenger EGb 761 and zinc in the cat retina. Ophthalmologica 212: 268–274
8. Köse K, Dogan P (1995) Lipid peroxidation induced by hydrogen peroxide in human erythrocyte membranes. 1. Protective effect of Ginkgo Biloba extract (EGb 761). J Int Med Res 23: 1–8
9. Malamud N, Haymaker W, Custer RP (1946) Heat stroke: a clinicopathologic study of 125 fatal cases. Milit Surg 99: 397–449
10. Sharma HS (1999) Pathophysiology of blood-brain barrier, brain edema and cell injury following hyperthermia: New role of heat shock protein, nitric oxide and carbon monoxide. an experimental study in the rat using light and electron microscopy, Acta Universitatis Upsaliensis 830: 1–94
11. Sharma HS, Drieu K, Alm P, Westman J (1999) Upregulation of neuronal nitric oxide synthase, edema and cell injury following heat stress are reduced by pretreatment with EGB-761 in the rat. J Therm Biol 24: 439–446
12. Sharma HS, Westman J (1998) Brain Functions in Hot Environment, Progress in Brain Research, 115. Elsevier, Amsterdam, pp 1–516
13. Sharma HS, Westman J, Nyberg F (1998) Pathophysiology of brain edema and cell changes following hyperthermic brain injury. Brain Functions in Hot Environment. In: Sharma HS, Westman J (eds) Prog Brain Res 115: 351–412
14. Sharma HS, Alm P, Westman (1998) Nitric oxide and carbon monoxide in the pathophysiology of brain functions in heat stress. Brain Functions in Hot Environment. In: Sharma HS, Westman J (eds) Prog Brain Res 115: 297–333
15. Sharma HS (1998) Neurobiology of the nitric oxide in the nervous system (Editorial) Amino Acids 14: 83–86

16. Sharma HS, Westman J, Alm P, Sjöquist P-O, Cervós-Navarro J, Nyberg F (1997) Involvement of nitric oxide in the pathophysiology of acute heat stress in the rat. Ann NY Acad Sci 813: 581–590
17. Sharma HS, Dey PK (1987) Influence of long-term acute heat exposure on regional blood-brain barrier permeability, cerebral blood flow and 5-HT level in conscious normotensive young rats. Brain Research 424: 153–162
18. Shen JG, Wang J, Zhao BL, Hou JW, Gao TL, Xin WJ (1998) Effects of EGb 761 on nitric oxide and oxygen free radicals, myocardial damage and arrhythmia in ischemia-reperfusion injury in vivo. Biochim Biophys Acta 1406: 228–236
19. Sterner S (1990) Summer heat illnesses. Conditions that range from mild to fatal. Postgrad Med 87: 215–217.
20. Stücker O, Pons C, Duverger J-P, Drieu K (1998) Antioxidant effects of Ginkgolide B. Consequences on vascular regulation in rat cremastre muscle. Proc. 25th Eur. Conf. Microcirc. Paris, France, pp 319–323

Correspondence: Hari Shanker Sharma, Ph.D., Laboratory of Neuroanatomy, Department of Medical Cell Biology, Box 571, Biomedical Centre, Uppsala University, SE-75423 Uppsala, Sweden.

Acta Neurochir (2000) [Suppl] 76: 87–90

Extracts of Ginkgo Biloba and Panax Ginseng Protect Brain Proteins from Free Radical Induced Oxidative Damage in Vitro

M. S. Siddique[1], **F. Eddeb**[2], **D. Mantle**[2], and **A. D. Mendelow**[1]

[1] Department of Neurosurgery, Regional Neurosciences Centre, Newcastle General Hospital, UK
[2] Department of Neurochemistry, Regional Neurosciences Centre, Newcastle General Hospital, UK

Summary

Oxidative damage to normal human brain tissue was induced following exposure to hydroxyl ($OH^•$) or superoxide ($O_2^{-•}$) free radical species generated by CO^{60} irradiation in vitro. Both enzymic and cytoskeletal proteins showed substantial (dose dependent) oxidative damage following exposure to $OH^•$ or $O_2^{-•}$, as quantified by SDS-polyacrylamide gel electrophoretic analysis. Extracts of Ginkgo biloba or Panax ginseng showed a remarkable capacity to protect brain tissue proteins from oxidative damage in vitro, even at extreme (2000 kRads) dosage levels of $OH^•$ or $O_2^{-•}$. We suggest, therefore, that the beneficial effect of these plant extracts in preventing brain tissue damage in vivo (e.g. following ischemia-reperfusion) may result from their action in protecting brain proteins from oxidative damage, in addition to their previously reported capacity to reduce free radical induced lipid peroxidation.

Keywords: Free radicals; antioxidants; protein oxidation; brain tissue; medicinal plants; ginkgo biloba; panax ginseng.

Introduction

Free radicals are a highly reactive transient chemical species formed in all cells as unwanted by-products of normal aerobic metabolism. Cells are protected from free radical induced damage by a variety of radical scavenging antioxidant proteins, enzymes and chemical compounds. Cellular damage arising from an imbalance between free radical generating and scavenging systems ("oxidative stress") has been implicated in the pathogenesis of a wide range of human disorders, including cerebral ischaemic tissue injury following stroke/haemorrhage [10]. Recently, there has been an upsurge of interest in the potential use of medicinal plants in the treatment of such disorders [14], and it has been suggested that the beneficial effects of such plant extracts may result (at least in part) from their action as free radical scavengers [1]. Thus, extracts of Ginkgo biloba and Panax ginseng, which have a long history of use in traditional Chinese medicine for the treatment of neurological disorders, have been shown to prevent free radical induced CNS lipid peroxidation using isolated tissues in vitro, cultured cells, or animal model systems in vivo [4, 5, 6]. However, relatively little is known about free radical induced oxidative damage to brain proteins (arguably as important as lipid peroxidation in cell destruction), and the manner in which such oxidative damage may be prevented by antioxidants. The objective of the present investigation was, therefore, to determine whether extracts of Ginkgo biloba or Panax ginseng have antioxidant activity in protecting brain tissue proteins from oxidative damage induced by hydroxyl ($OH^•$) or superoxide ($O_2^{-•}$) radicals (the principal damaging species of physiological significance), generated radiolytically in vitro.

Methods

Samples of Ginkgo biloba (dried leaves) and Panax ginseng (Korean, dried root), obtained from G. Baldwin & Co., London, UK, were homogenized 1:10 (w/v) in 50% aqueous ethanol using a Waring blender (preliminary experiments established the above regimen as the optimum extraction conditions for subsequent determination of antioxidant activity). The plant extracts were centrifuged (3000 g, 10 min) to remove insoluble matter, and the supernatants retained for analysis.

Human brain tissue (cerebral cortex) was obtained at autopsy (within 15 h of death) from cases with no history of neurodegenerative disorders. Confirmation of the suitability of autopsy brain tissue for this type of investigation was established by comparison with fresh tissue obtained during surgery. This tissue was removed as a routine part of the operation (e.g. decompressive lobectomy following trauma) and would normally be discarded. The autopsy tissue samples were extracted via homogenization 1:10 (w/v) in 50 mM phosphate buffer pH 7.5 using an Ultra-Turrax homogeniser (2×10 sec at 5000 rev/min), and the homogenates centrifuged (5000 g, 15 min). After removal of the supernatants (comprising soluble, principally enzymic proteins), the pellets were washed (via rehomogenization/centrifugation) three times in extraction buffer, and reconstituted in the original volume of the latter buffer. Supernatant or reconstituted pellet (comprising principally structural cytoskeletal proteins) fractions were gassed to saturation with N_2O (for subsequent generation of $OH^\bullet$ radicals) or with O_2 (following addition of 20 mM sodium formate, for subsequent generation of $O_2^{-\bullet}$ radicals) immediately prior to irradiation (up to 40 hrs) using a Co^{60} irradiation source. The free radical dosage (equivalent to 100 kRads/hr) was determined by standard dosimetric techniques [8]. The theoretical and methodological aspects of generation of $OH^\bullet$ and $O_2^{-\bullet}$ by using irradiation have been described in detail previously [3]. Free radical induced oxidative damage to supernatant or pellet proteins in the absence or presence of extracts of the various plant species mentioned above (plant extract: brain extract 1:10 v/v) was assessed by SDS polyacrylamide gel electrophoresis (SDS-PAGE) as described previously [11], using a 5% stacking-gel and 5–20% linear acrylamide gradient in the separating gel. After staining, gels were scanned using an Alpha Multi Image Cabinet (with Alpha 3.3: software analysis) to determine quantitative oxidative damage (as% control band intensity lost) to individual proteins.

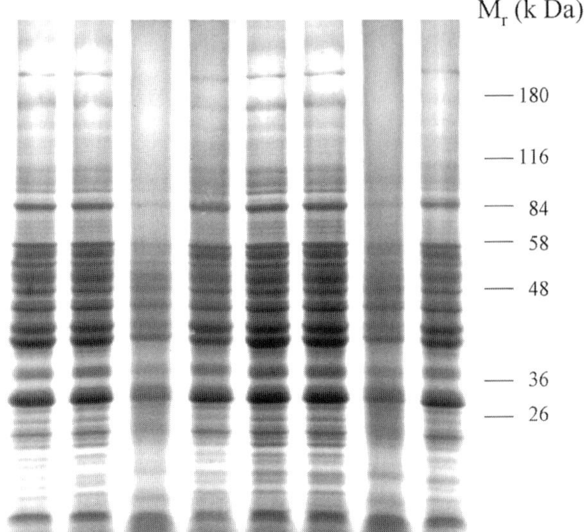

Fig. 1. Protection of brain soluble proteins from oxidative damage in vitro by extract of Panax Ginseng. The preparation of human brain tissue soluble protein extract and extract of Panax ginseng, exposure of brain proteins to $OH^\bullet$ or $O_2^{-\bullet}$ radical species in the presence or absence of plant extract, and subsequent analysis of protein oxidative damage via SDS PAGE are described under Methods. Brain extract gassed with O_2 without (lane 1, left-hand side) and with (lane 2) plant extract; Brain extract exposed to $O_2^{-\bullet}$ radicals without (lane 3) and with (lane 4) plant extract; brain extract gassed with N_2O without (lane 5) and with (lane 6) plant extract; brain extract exposed to $OH^\bullet$ radicals without (lane 7) and with (lane 8, light-hand side) plant extract

Results

The results of a typical experiment to determine the effects of free radical induced oxidative damage to brain tissue proteins in vitro are illustrated in Fig. 1; this shows substantial oxidative degradation of brain supernatant protein bands following exposure to equivalent doses (2000 kRads) of $O_2^{-\bullet}$ (lane 3) or $OH^\bullet$ (lane 7), compared to corresponding non-irradiated control tissue extracts (lanes 1 and 5 respectively). The overall SDS-PAGE protein fractionation pattern showed a general progressive loss in band staining intensities in a dose dependent manner, with essentially complete destruction of most protein species at 4000 kRads. The extent of protein damage by $OH^\bullet$ was greater than for $O_2^{-\bullet}$ (1.3–2.3 fold, depending on protein molecular mass) at equivalent irradiation dosages (Table 1). It was also evident (from densitometric analysis) that different protein species showed different relative susceptibility to oxidative damage by $OH^\bullet$ or $O_2^{-\bullet}$, with higher molecular mass proteins (>70 kDa) in general terms showing greater susceptibility to oxidative degradation (Table 1). There was no evidence for the formation of protein fragments or aggregates after exposure of brain extracts to $OH^\bullet$ or $O_2^{-\bullet}$, as previously reported following exposure of model proteins (lysosyme, haemoglobin) to free radicals generated radiolytically [7, 15]. Presumably the disappearance of protein bands induced by free radicals in the present study corresponds with the formation of either extremely large aggregates or very small peptides/free amino acids, which are not resolved by SDS-PAGE analysis. Broadly similar results were obtained to the above following exposure of brain cytoskeletal proteins to $OH^\bullet$ or $O_2^{-\bullet}$ in vitro (data not shown).

The addition of Panax ginseng extract (10-fold dilution of initial extract) to the brain supernatant fraction resulted in the substantial protection of all proteins from oxidative degradation by $O_2^{-\bullet}$ (lane 4) or $OH^\bullet$ (lane 8). The addition of Panax ginseng extract to non-irradiated brain supernatant samples did not result in any alteration of the SDS-PAGE fractionation pattern (lanes 2 and 6). The results of experiments to determine the capacity of extracts of Panax ginseng and Ginkgo biloba to prevent free radical induced oxidative damage to brain tissue soluble proteins (selected to cover molecular mass range 25–200 kDa) are summarised in Table 1.

Discussion

It is apparent from the data presented that extracts of both Ginkgo biloba and Panax ginseng provide a

Table 1. *Protection of Brain Soluble Proteins from Oxidative Damage in Vitro by Extracts of Panax Ginseng and Ginkgo Biloba*

Protein band molecular mass (kDa)	Protein band degradation (% non-irradiated control)					
	No extract		Panax ginseng		Ginkgo biloba	
	$OH^{\bullet}$	$O_2^{-\bullet}$	$OH^{\bullet}$	$O_2^{-\bullet}$	$OH^{\bullet}$	$O_2^{-\bullet}$
188	92 ± 8.2	80 ± 9.8	42 ± 6.5	27 ± 5.5	32 ± 8.1	25 ± 6.6
158	99 ± 5.1	97 ± 6.0	44 ± 6.9	30 ± 4.2	30 ± 5.8	31 ± 5.4
90	88 ± 9.4	80 ± 8.1	23 ± 7.1	27 ± 6.2	30 ± 3.8	28 ± 5.1
65	81 ± 5.9	63 ± 5.1	10 ± 4.7	18 ± 5.3	12 ± 4.4	24 ± 4.6
46	63 ± 7.5	44 ± 6.1	30 ± 3.9	10 ± 3.2	7.5 ± 3.2	11 ± 4.8
25	46 ± 5.4	20 ± 3.9	4.0 ± 3.1	11 ± 5.0	6.5 ± 2.5	12 ± 3.8

Data show the extent of protein band degradation (relative to non-irradiated control samples) following exposure of brain tissue to $OH^{\bullet}$ or $O_2^{-\bullet}$ in the absence or presence of plant extracts. Data (mean ± SD from 3 experiments) were derived from densitometric analysis of protein SDS-PAGE fractionation patterns.

remarkable degree of protection for soluble proteins against oxidative damage by both $OH^{\bullet}$ and $O_2^{-\bullet}$ species, even at the extreme free radical dosages employed (which are likely to be several orders of magnitude greater than those likely to pertain in tissues in vivo). Similar results to the above were obtained showing essentially complete protection of brain tissue cytoskeletal proteins from oxidative damage by $OH^{\bullet}$ or $O_2^{-\bullet}$ in vitro (2000 kRads) by extracts of Ginkgo biloba or Panax ginseng (data not shown).

There is evidence from clinical studies in human patients and from experimental studies using isolated tissues in vitro, cultured cells or animal model systems in vivo that extracts of Ginkgo biloba or Panax ginseng (or their specific constituent compounds) can reduce or prevent brain cell damage following ischaemia, and that this results from the efficiency of ginkgolide and ginsenoside compounds as free radical scavengers in preventing oxidative damage to lipids [2, 9, 12, 13, 16, 17, 18]. However, data obtained in the present investigation show extracts of Ginkgo biloba and Panax ginseng to have a remarkable capacity to protect brain proteins from oxidative damage in vitro, and we suggest that this phenomenon may be a major contributor to the beneficial action of these extracts in vivo.

Acknowledgments

This work was financially supported by, Newcastle University Hospitals Special Trustees, The Stroke Association and The Medical Research Council (MRC) UK.

References

1. Bors W, Heiser W, Michel C, Saran M (1990) Flavonoids as antioxidants: determination of radical scavenging efficiencies. Meth Enzymol 186: 343–355
2. Choi SR, Saji H, Iida Y, Magat Y, Yokoyama A (1996) Ginseng pretreatment protects against global cerebral ischemia in the rat: measurement of local cerebral glucose utilization by [^{14}C] deoxyglucose autoradiography. Biol Pharmaceut Bull 19: 644–646
3. Davies KJA (1987) Protein damage and degradation by oxygen radicals. I. General aspects. J Biol Chem 262: 9895–9906
4. Deby C, Deby-Dupont G, Dister M, Pincemail J (1993) Efficiency of Ginkgo biloba extract (EGB 761) in neutralizing ferryl ion induced peroxidation: therapeutic implications. Adv Ginkgo biloba Ext Res 2: 13–26
5. Dorman DC, Cole LM, Buck WB (1992) Effects of an extract of Ginkgo biloba on bromothalein induced cerebral lipid peroxidation and oedema in rats. Am J Vet Res 53: 138–142
6. Fotun A, Khalil A, Rousselot DB, Albert MG, Lepage MG, Lepage S, Delattre J, Lefaiz MTD. (1994) Effect of EGB 761 on the peroxidation of human low density lipoproteins inhibited by oxyradical generated by water dialysis. J Chim Phys 91: 1078–1084
7. Franzini E, Sellak H, Hakim J, Pasquier C (1993) Oxidative damage to lysosyme by the hydroxyl radical: comparative effects of scavengers. Biochim Biophys Acta 1203: 11–17
8. Fricke H, Hart EJ (1966) Radiation dosimetry. In: Roesch FH, Roesch WC (eds) Radiation dosimetry. Academic Press, New York, p 167
9. Garg RK, Nag D, Agrawal A (1995) A double blind placebo controlled trial of Ginkgo biloba extract in acute cerebral ischaemia. J Assoc Physic India 43: 760–763
10. Halliwell B, Gutteridge JMC (1990) Role of free radicals and catalytic metal ions in human disease – an overview. Meth Enzymol 186: 1–85
11. Laemli UK (1970) Cleavage of structural proteins during the assembly of bacteriophage T4. Nature 227: 680–685
12. Ni Y, Zhao B, Hou J, Xin W (1996) Preventive effect of Ginkgo biloba extract on apoptosis in rat cerebellar neuronal cells induced by hydroxyl radicals. Neurosci Lett 214: 115–118
13. Oyama Y, Chi Kahisa L, Ueha T, Kanemaru K, Noda K (1996) Ginkgo biloba extract protects brain neurons against oxidative stress induced by hydrogen peroxide. Brain Res 712: 349–352
14. Perry EK (1997) Cholinergic phytochemicals: from magic to medicine. Aging Mental Health 1: 23–32
15. Puchala M, Schuessler H (1993) Oxygen effect in the radiolysis of proteins and haemoglobin. J Radiat Biol 64: 149–156
16. Seif-El-Nasr M, El-Fattah AA (1995) Lipid peroxide, phospholipids, glutathione levels and superoxide dismutase activity in rat

brain after ischaemia: effect of Ginkgo biloba extract. Pharmacol Res 32: 273–278

17. Wang FZ, Ding AS, Liu ZW (1995) Effect of ginsenosides against anoxic damage of hippocampal neurons in culture. Chung-Kuo Yao Li Hsueh Pao. Acta Pharmacol Sinica 16: 419–422
18. Zhang YG, Liu TP (1996) Influences of ginsenosides Rb1 and Rg1 on reversible focal brain ischaemia in rats. Chung-Kuo Yao Li Hsueh Pao. Acta Pharmacol Sinica 17: 44–48

Correspondence: Dr. D. Mantle, Department of Neurochemistry, Regional Neurosciences Centre, Newcastle General Hospital, UK.

Acta Neurochir (2000) [Suppl] 76: 91–95

p-Chlorophenylalanine, an Inhibitor of Serotonin Synthesis Reduces Blood-Brain Barrier Permeability, Cerebral Blood Flow, Edema Formation and Cell Injury Following Trauma to the Rat Brain

H. S. Sharma[1], **T. Winkler**[2], **E. Stålberg**[2], **S. Mohanty**[3], and **J. Westman**[1]

[1] Laboratory of Neuroanatomy, Department of Medical Cell Biology, Biomedical Centre, Uppsala University, Uppsala, Sweden
[2] Department of Clinical Neurophysiology, University Hospital Uppsala, Sweden
[3] Department of Neurosurgery, Institute of Medical Sciences, Banaras Hindu University, Varanasi, India

Summary

The role of serotonin in trauma induced alterations in blood-brain barrier (BBB) permeability, cerebral blood flow (CBF), brain edema and cell changes were examined in a new model of cortical injury in the rat using a pharmacological approach. A longitudinal incision into the right parietal cerebral cortex (about 3 mm deep and 5 mm long) was associated with a profound increase in the BBB permeability to Evans blue and $^{[131]}$I-sodium, brain water content, and a reduction in the CBF in both the ipsilateral and contralateral hemispheres 5 h after trauma. Nissl staining showed a profound nerve cell reaction in the parietal cerebral cortex of both hemispheres. The intensity of these pathological changes was most pronounced in the traumatised hemisphere. Pretreatment with p-CPA, a serotonin synthesis inhibitor, significantly attenuated breakdown of the BBB permeability, brain edema and the CBF disturbances. Damaged and distorted nerve cells were markedly less frequent in p-CPA treated rats. This effect of the drug was most pronounced in the contralateral hemisphere. The observations strongly suggest that serotonin is one of the important neurochemical mediators of BBB permeability disturbances and brain edema formation in the trauma induced brain damage.

Keywords: Brain injury; serotonin; brain edema; cerebral blood flow.

Introduction

The blood-brain barrier (BBB) strictly regulates the composition of the extracellular fluid compartment to which neurons are exposed [1]. Therefore, any alterations in the fluid microenvironment of the brain may result in an abnormal brain function. The BBB permeability is severely compromised following traumatic, ischemic or hypoxic injuries to the brain, resulting in pathological cell reactions [1, 2], indicating that disturbances in the fluid microenvironment of the brain are an important factor in brain pathology. The breakdown of the BBB permeability results in vasogenic edema formation which in turn is associated with cell injury [19]. Thus, further details are needed to understand the possible mechanisms of the BBB breakdown in various forms of brain insults in order to attenuate the magnitude and severity of cell injury.

Several neurochemical mediators have been identified in the past which influence the BBB function and brain edema formation and the list is growing rapidly [1, 11]. Serotonin is one of the important neurochemical mediators of BBB dysfunction which has the capacity to induce brain edema when administered directly into the cerebral circulation [17, 18]. The amine is found in high quantity in the CNS and blood plasma including platelets [7]. The serotonergic nerve fibres emanating from the raphé nucleus located in the brain stem virtually project to almost all parts of the brain and spinal cord [3, 7]. Further, serotonergic receptors are present on neurons [3, 6, 7], cerebral microvessels, as well as on astrocytes [7].

Serotonin is mainly an inhibitory neurotransmitter, however, at some synapses in the CNS, the amine may act as an excitatory transmitter [3, 6, 7]. Serotonergic neurons often co-localise with other neurotransmitters or neuromodulators [7]. Thus, substance P and CGRP are known to be co-localised with serotonergic nerve fibers, indicating a profound neuromodulatory role of the amine in neural transmission [3, 7]. These observations suggest an important role of the amine in brain function. However, its involvement in CNS trauma is still not well understood in greater details.

Therefore, in the present investigations we have examined the potential contribution of serotonin to BBB permeability disturbances, edema formation, CBF changes, and cell injury following a localised cortical trauma in a rat model using a pharmacological approach. We have studied the influence of inhibition of the serotonin synthesis by p-CPA pretreatment on the trauma induced pathophysiology of brain injury in both ipsilateral and contralateral cerebral hemispheres.

Materials and Methods

Animals

Experiments were carried out on inbred Charles Foster rats (250–300 g) housed at controlled room temperature 21 ± 1 °C with 12 h light and 12 h dark schedule. The rat food pellets and tap water were supplied ad libitum.

Brain Injury

Under urethane anaesthesia (1.5 g/kg, i.p.) two burr holes were made in the right and left parietal bone (4 mm^2) of the skull with constant cooling of the skull surface by application of ice-cooled saline (4 °C). After opening of the skull, the dura mater was carefully removed on both sides. Traumatic brain injury was produced by making an incision into the right parietal cerebral cortex (about 3 mm deep and 3 mm long) [4, 5, 9, 10]. The deepest part of the lesion was mainly over the dorsal surface of the hippocampus [9]. The animals were allowed to survive 5 h after injury. The opening of the skull was covered by cotton soaked with saline in order to avoid a direct contact of the brain surface with air. Normal intact rats served as controls. The experimental protocol was approved by the Ethical Committee of the Uppsala University, Uppsala, Sweden and the Banaras Hindu University, Varanasi, India.

p-Chlorophenylalanine Treatment

In a separate group of 10 rats, p-CPA (Sigma Chemical Co., USA) was administered intraperitoneally (100 mg/kg/day) for 3 consecutive days [14]. On the fourth day, the animals were divided into two different groups. One group (n = 5) of animals was traumatised in the right parietal cerebral cortex, the remaining group of animals served as drug treated controls.

Blood-Brain Barrier Permeability

The BBB permeability in the cerebral cortex of both hemispheres was measured by using extravasation of Evans blue albumin (2% of a 3 ml/kg, i.v. solution) and ^{131}I-sodium as described earlier [13, 16, 17]. In brief, both tracers were administered 5 h after trauma through the right external branch of the jugular vein through a needle puncture [4, 5]. These tracers were allowed to circulate 5 min. The animals were perfused via heart with 0.9% saline for washout of the remaining intravascular tracer. Immediately before perfusion, about one ml of arterial blood was withdrawn via heart puncture for determination of the whole blood radioactivity. The BBB permeability to the radiotracer was determined as percent increase in radioactivity in the brain using the blood radioactivity as reference [15].

Brain Water Content

The brain water content of the right and left cerebral cortex was determined by the dry/wet weight method [4, 5, 15]. In brief, the right cerebral cortex and the left cerebral cortex were dissected out after perfusion and weighed immediately. The samples were then placed in an oven at 90 °C for 72 h or until the dry weight of the samples became constant in at least two determinations [15]. Swelling of the brain was calculated from the changes in the brain water content according to the equation of Elliott and Jasper (1955). In general, about 1% increase in the brain water is approximately equal to a 4% increase in the volume swelling of the brain [9, 10].

Cerebral Blood Flow

The blood flow was determined in cerebral cortex of both the traumatised and non-traumatised hemisphere using [125]Iodine labelled carbonised microspheres (15 ± 0.6 µm diameter) as described earlier [17]. In brief, about 10^6 microspheres were injected into the left atrium via a cannula implanted retrogradely towards the heart into the left common carotid artery. Timed peripheral arterial blood samples at 30 sec intervals were collected from the right femoral artery at a rate of 0.8 ml/min, beginning at 30 sec before the start of infusion of microspheres and continued until 90 sec after the end of the microsphere injection. The animals were decapitated and the cerebral cortex was removed. Tissue specimens of the cortex were weighed and counted in a 3-in well type Gamma counter at the energy window 25–50 KeV [17]. The CBF was calculated by the equation: CBF (ml/g/min) = C_B (CPM/g/brain tissue) × RBF ÷ CR (total counts in the reference) rate of withdrawal of the blood (0.8 ml/min) [17, 18].

Cell Injury

In a separate group of animals, the brain was fixed in situ using about 150 ml formaldehyde based fixative (4% paraformaldehyde in 0.1% cacodylate buffer in 0.1 M sodium phosphate buffer, pH 7.4 containing 0.25% picric acid) immediately after saline perfusion. After perfusion, the brain was dissected out and kept in the same fixative for 4 days at 4 °C. Small pieces of cortical tissues from the perifocal lesion site and the corresponding contralateral side were dissected out and embedded in paraffin or Epon for light and electron microscopy, respectively according to the standard protocol [13, 15, 16].

Statistical Analysis

Unpaired Student's t-test was used to evaluate the statistical significance of the data obtained. A p-value less than 0.05 was considered to be significant.

Results

Effect of p-CPA on BBB Permeability

The traumatic injury increased the permeability of the BBB to Evans blue and ^{131}I-sodium in both the traumatised and untraumatised cerebral cortex as compared to the intact control group (Fig. 1). The magnitude of these changes was most pronounced in the ipsilateral cortex as compared to the contralateral

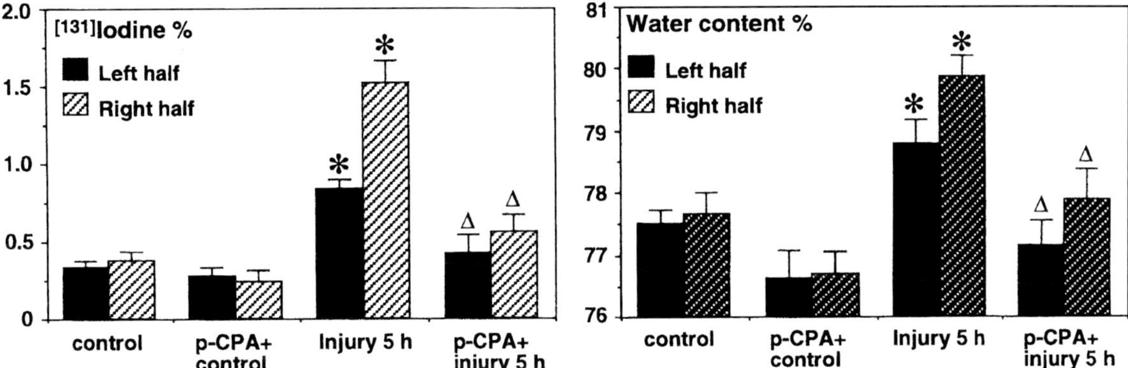

Fig. 1. Extravasation of radioactive iodine (left) and brain water content (right) in rats subjected to a focal cortical incision and their modification with p-CPA pretreatment. p-CPA, a serotonin synthesis inhibitor was administered (100 mg/kg/day, i.p.) for 3 days. The animals were traumatised 24 h after the last injection. * = $P < 0.001$ compared to the control group; Δ = $P < 0.001$ compared to the injured group, Student's unpaired t-test

side. Pretreatment with p-CPA significantly attenuated the extravasation of both tracers in the brain. This effect, however, was more pronounced in the contralateral hemisphere.

Effect of p-CPA on Brain Water Content

At 5 h after injury, the brain water content was increased significantly above the control group in both the traumatised and untraumatised cerebral cortex. The increase in brain water content was most pronounced in the ipsilateral hemisphere. The swelling in the traumatised and untraumatised cortex was reaching up to +4% and +12% as compared to the corresponding control group. The pretreatment with p-CPA significantly reduced the increase in brain water content. However, this beneficial effect was much more pronounced in the untraumatised left hemisphere (Fig. 1).

Effect of p-CPA on Cerebral Blood Flow

The measurements of CBF using radiolabelled microspheres show a profound reduction in blood flow in the traumatised as well as untraumatised hemisphere. The magnitude of flow reduction was maximal in the perifocal lesion site. The contralateral hemisphere also exhibited a mild but significant reduction in CBF as compared to the controls (Fig. 2). Pretreatment with p-CPA completely restored CBF in the contralateral hemisphere. The attenuation of flow disturbances in the traumatised half of the brain by the drug was also significant (Fig. 2).

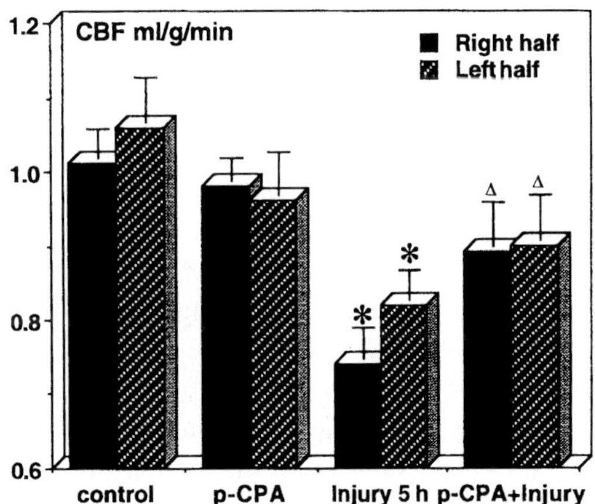

Fig. 2. Cerebral blood flow changes in traumatised rats and their modification by p-CPA pretreatment. * = $P < 0.001$, compared to the control group; $\Delta = 0.05$ compared to the injured group, Student's unpaired t-test

Effect of p-CPA on Cell Injury

The morphological investigations using Nissl staining of brain sections showed many distorted or degenerated neurons in the edematous region of the traumatised cerebral cortex. This effect was most marked in the vicinity of the lesion (Fig. 3). The ultrastructural studies revealed perivascular edema, collapsed vessels, membrane disruption, and synaptic damage in the ipsilateral as well as in the contralateral parietal cerebral cortex (results not shown). Pretreatment with p-CPA markedly reduced these nerve cell changes (Fig. 3). The ultrastructural changes were also considerably reduced in the p-CPA treated injured group (results not shown).

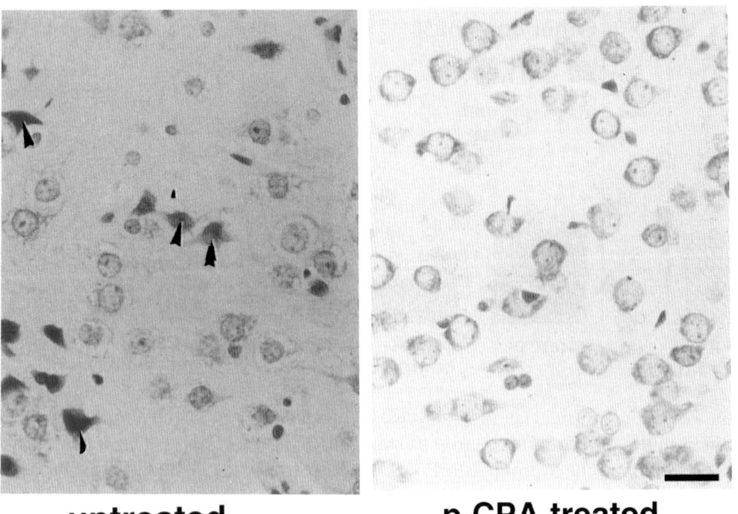

Fig. 3. Nissl stained nerve cells in the perifocal parietal cerebral cortex of the traumatised cortex with and without p-CPA pretreatment. Many distorted nerve cells (arrow heads) can be seen in the untreated rat. Distorted or damaged nerve cells were much less apparent in the p-CPA treated traumatised rat (bar = 200 μm)

Discussion

The salient new findings of the present study demonstrate that a focal lesion of cerebral cortex increases BBB permeability and induces brain edema formation in both the ipsilateral and contralateral cerebral hemispheres within the short period of 5 h. This observation indicates that edema fluid spreads quickly through the whole brain following a focal lesion, which may have serious consequences on the brain function within a relatively short period of time. The mechanisms underlying brain edema formation in the contralateral hemisphere are not known. It seems likely that the profound swelling of the contralateral hemisphere is due to a release of several chemical mediators following trauma into the circulation as well as to localised transport through the disrupted BBB around the lesion. Since the BBB was disrupted, neurochemicals may gain access to the circulation from the brain as well.

Trauma to the cerebral cortex induces physical damage of microvessels leading to haemorrhage in the cerebral compartment [15]. Thus, it is conceivable that serotonin released from damaged platelets had direct access to the cerebral parenchyma causing localised brain edema [8]. An additional amount of amine could be provided by endogenous release from cerebral cortex following trauma [7]. The accumulating serotonin in the brain could be transported to the other hemisphere via the cerebral circulation due to the disruption of the BBB as mentioned above [1, 2]. Alternatively, serotonergic transmission or release in the contralateral side could be directly induced by the trauma in the other hemisphere. However, to confirm this assumption, an immunohistochemical mapping of serotonin would be needed.

Serotonin has profound vasomotor effects in the brain [6, 13, 17]. An increased serotonin content of the tissue or in the circulation may induce constriction of cerebral microvessels [6]. The significant decrease in local CBF observed in this investigation suggests that a serotonin induced vasoconstriction was playing an important role following lesioning of the cerebral cortex. Mild but significant reduction in CBF was also present in the contralateral hemisphere. Thus, passage of serotonin via the cerebral circulation to the left hemisphere might have been involved.

An increased serotonin content of the tissue as well as in the circulation may induce a breakdown of the BBB [17]. Serotonin either directly or through stimulation of the endogenous prostaglandin synthesis in cerebral microvessels induces an increased synthesis of cAMP in the cerebral endothelium [17, 19, 20]. An increased synthesis of cAMP is associated with increased vesicular transport [17].

The most important evidence that serotonin is playing a crucial role in the formation of brain edema and ischemia caused by trauma is provided by the studies using p-CPA pretreatment. p-CPA is a potent serotonin synthesis inhibitor. In the dose used in this study it is able to inhibit serotonin synthesis for long-time periods [14–16]. The serotonin stores including platelets are significantly lowered [7]. Evidence is available that in p-CPA treated and serotonin depleted animals, trauma or other stress stimuli do not induce a serotonin release probably due to the depletion of the stores of the amine [6, 7]. Since in the p-CPA treated animals the trauma induced serotonin release was blocked, no breakdown of the BBB or edema formation could be observed. Obviously, in the absence of a BBB breakdown, vasogenic edema formation was inhibited affording less distortion of the neuropil as currently observed [12, 15]. Further, without release of serotonin, the microvessels did not constrict, explaining why no significant reduction in CBF in the p-CPA treated animals was seen following trauma [17]. Since the level of CBF reduction by the trauma itself was not sufficient to induce ischemic damage [18], a direct effect of ischemia on the nerve cell or on edema formation was unlikely.

The present study does not provide any information about the involvement of particular serotonin receptors in the breakdown of the BBB permeability, CBF disturbances and brain edema formation following trauma. Since serotonin has more than 7 receptors and multiple receptor subtypes [3, 6, 7], further studies are needed to elucidate the involvement of specific serotonergic receptors in brain edema formation.

In conclusion, our observations suggest that serotonin plays an important role in the pathophysiology of traumatic brain damage. Furthermore, our findings suggest that disruption of the BBB following trauma seems to be instrumental in causing brain edema and cell injury.

Acknowledgments

This investigation is supported by Grants from Swedish Medical research Council nr. 2710 (JW, HSS); 135 (ES); Alexander von Humboldt Foundation, Bonn, Germany (HSS); The University Grants Commission, New Delhi, India (HSS); The Indian Council of Medical research, New Delhi (HSS; SM); Indian Council of Scientific and Industrial research, New Delhi (HSS). The technical assistance of Kärstin Flink; Katjya Deparade; Franziska Drum and the secretarial assistance of Aruna Sharma; Gun-Britt Lind and Sigrid Pettersson is highly acknowledged with thanks.

References

1. Bradbury MWB (1979) The Concept of a Blood-Brain Barrier. Chicester, London
2. Cervós-Navarro J, Kannuki S, Nakagawa Y (1988) Blood-brain barrier (BBB): review from morphological aspect. Histol Histopathol 3: 203–213
3. Chaouloff F (1993) Physiopharmacological interactions between stress hormones and central serotonergic systems. Brain Res Rev 18: 1–32
4. Dey PK, Sharma HS (1984) Influence of ambient temperature and drug treatments on brain edema induced by impact injury on skull in rat. Indian J Physiol Pharmacol 28: 177–186
5. Dey PK, Sharma HS (1983) Ambient temperature and development of traumatic brain edema in anaesthetized animals. Indian J Med Res 77: 554–563
6. Edvinsson E, McKenzie ET (1977) Amine mechanisms in the cerebral circulation. Pharmacol Rev 28: 275–348
7. Essman W (1978) Serotonin in health and disease, vols. I-V. Spectrum, New York
8. Fernstrom JD, Wurtman RJ (1971) Brain serotonin content: physiological dependence on plasma tryptophan levels. Science 173: 149–152
9. Mohanty S, Dey PK, Sharma HS, Ray AK (1985) Experimental brain edema: role of 5-HT. Brain edema. In: S Mohanty, PK Dey (eds) Banaras Hindu University, Bhargava Bhushan Press, Varanasi, India, pp 19–27
10. Mohanty S, Dey PK, Sharma HS, Singh S, Chansouria JPN, Olsson Y (1989) Role of histamine in traumatic brain edema. An experimental study in the rat. J Neurol Sci 90: 87–97
11. Olesen SP (1989) An electrophysiological study of microvascular permeability and its modulation by chemical mediators. Acta Physiol Scand 136, Suppl 579: 1–28
12. Sharma HS, Westman J, Nyberg F (1997) Topical application of 5-HT antibodies reduces edema and cell changes following trauma to the rat spinal cord. Acta Neurochir [Suppl] (Wien) 70: 155–158
13. Sharma HS, Olsson Y, Dey PK (1995) Serotonin as a mediator of increased microvascular permeability of the brain and spinal cord. Experimental observations in anaesthetised rats and mice. New concepts of a blood-brain barrier. In: Greenwood J, Begley D, Segal M, Lightman S (eds) Plenum Press, New York, pp 75–80
14. Sharma HS, Olsson Y, Cervós-Navarro J (1993) p-Chlorophenylalanine, a serotonin synthesis inhibitor, reduces the response of glial fibrillary acidic protein induced by trauma to the spinal cord. Acta Neuropathol (Berlin) 86: 422–427
15. Sharma HS, Cervós-Navarro J, Gosztonyi G, Dey PK (1992) Role of serotonin in traumatic brain injury. An experimental study in the rat. The role of neurotransmitters in brain injury. In: Globus M, Dietrich WD (eds) Plenum Press, New York, pp 147–152
16. Sharma H S, Olsson Y (1990) Edema formation and cellular alterations following spinal cord injury in rat and their modification with p-chlorophenylalanine. Acta Neuropathol (Berlin) 79: 604–610
17. Sharma HS, Olsson Y, Dey PK (1990) Blood-brain barrier permeability and cerebral blood flow following elevation of circulating serotonin level in the anaesthetized rats. Brain Res 517: 215–223
18. Sharma HS, Dey PK, Olsson Y (1989) Brain edema, blood-brain barrier permeability and cerebral blood flow changes following intracarotid infusion of serotonin: modification with cyproheptadine and indomethacin. Pharmacology of cerebral Ischemia 1988. In: Krieglstein J (eds) CRC Press, Boca Raton, Florida, pp 317–323
19. Westergaard E (1980) Ultrastructural permeability properties of cerebral microvasculature under normal and experimental conditions after application of tracers. Adv Neurol 28: 55–74
20. Winkler T, Sharma HS, Stålberg E, Olsson Y, Dey PK (1995) Impairment of blood-brain barrier function by serotonin induces desynchronisation of spontaneous cerebral cortical activity. Experimental observations in the anaesthetised rat. Neuroscience 68: 1097–1104

Correspondence: Hari Shanker Sharma, Ph.D., Laboratory of Neuroanatomy, Department of Medical Cell Biology, Box 571, Biomedical Centre, Uppsala University, S-75123 Uppsala, Sweden.

Acta Neurochir (2000) [Suppl] 76: 97–100

S-100 Serum Levels and Outcome After Severe Head Injury

R. D. Rothoerl, C. Woertgen, and **A. Brawanski**

Department of Neurosurgery, University of Regensburg, Germany

Summary

S-100B a protein of astroglial cells is described as a marker for neuronal damage. Reliable outcome prediction from severe head injury is still unresolved. Clinical scores like the Glasgow Coma Score (GCS) and diagnostic scores like the Marshall CT Classification (MCTC) are well established and investigated, but there are still some concerns about these tools. The aim of this study was to investigate the predictive value of the initial serum level of S-100B. 44 patients with severe head injury (GCS < 9) were included. Blood samples were drawn within 1 to 6 hours of injury. After a period of 11 months their outcome was correlated using the Glasgow Outcome Scale. Patients with good outcome had significantly lower serum concentrations of S-100 on admission (0.96 μg/l versus 5.5 μg/l mean, $p < 0.0001$). In addition patients with a S-100 serum level below 2 μg/l showed a significant better rating on the GOS at follow-up (4 points versus 1.8 points mean, $p < 0.0001$). With this cut-off line it was possible to predict longterm outcome with a sensitivity of 75% and specitivity of 82%.

The serum level of S-100B calculated with one to six hours of a severe head injury is a useful additional outcome predictor.

Keywords: Severe head injury; S-100B.

Introduction

Reliable outcome prediction from severe head injury especially in the early stage is still unresolved [6, 7]. Predictions made during the first 24 hours after injury were correct only for 44 percent of these patients [7]. Clinical scores like the Glasgow Coma Score (GCS) and diagnostic scores like the Marshall CT Classification (MCTC) are well established and investigated, but there are still some concerns over these tools [6, 7, 8, 9, 11, 12]. Stein assumes that head-injured patients will need to be classified by a combination of clinical, radiographic and laboratory parameters [11]. In recent years serum markers such as Neuron Specific Enolase (NSE), CKBB, Myelin Basic Protein and S-100B were described as to give helpful information for outcome prediction after severe head injury, stroke, and subarachnoid hemorrhage [5, 13, 14, 15, 16, 17, 18, 19, 20, 21, 22, 23, 24]. Particularly the serum levels of a calcium binding protein of astroglial cells in the central nervous system, S-100B, are recognized to have statistically significant correlations to outcome after severe head injury [5, 23, 24]. The aim of this study was to investigate the predictive value of the initial serum level of S-100B to the longterm outcome after severe head injury.

Material and Methods

After obtaining the approval of our local ethics committee, we selected 44 patients after severe head injury Glasgow Coma Scale[8] (GCS) < 9 in our prospective study. Patients had been admitted within one to six hours of injury. The group consisted of 32 males and 12 females. The mean age was 35 years ranging from 16 to 79 years. The blood sample was drawn 2.6 hours after injury (mean) with a range from 1 to 6 hours. 28 patients had sustained isolated head injury. The remaining patients had a concomitant injury of the thorax and/or abdomen or rather extremities. We excluded patients after resuscitation or shock and with a known history of a neurological disease or spinal cord injury.

After separation, the serum was stored at −20 °C until analyzed for S-100B concentrations as described previously by using a commercially obtainable RIA (Byk-Sangtec®, Germany, Dietzenbach) [23]. Samples were analyzed in duplicate, the mean value of these probes was taken into account for further evaluations. S-100B concentrations of 0.5 μg/l or above were defined as being above normal. During the time of treatment of the patients the S-100B serum value was not known.

The outcome was calculated 11 months (mean) after trauma using the Glasgow Outcome Scale (GOS 1–3 unfavourable; GOS 4–5 favourable) [25]. The follow-up rate was 93%.

Statistical analysis was performed using the StatView® computer programme version 4.5 including Fisher's PLSD. The statistical significance was determined at a level of $p < 0.05$.

Results

51% of the patients had a favourable outcome (GOS 4–5). 42% died (GOS 1) and 7% were disabled (GOS

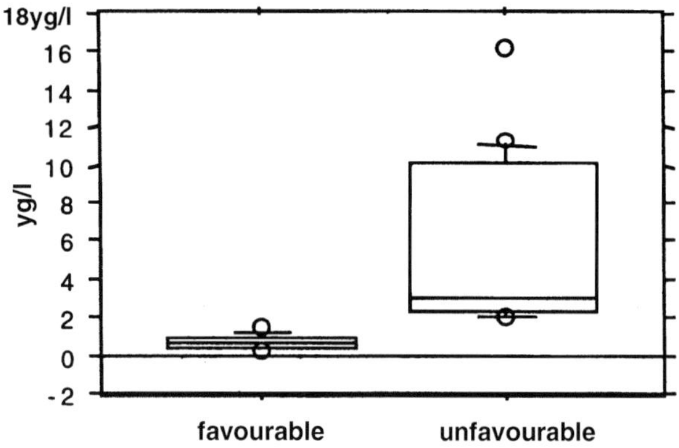

Fig. 1. Box plots of the S-100 serum levels on admission (n = 41) split up to Glasgow Outcome Scale (11 months after trauma, mean) significant difference: p < 0.0001

3). None of the patients remained in a vegetative state (GOS 4) 11 months (mean) after trauma.

Age correlated to outcome. Patients with an unfavourable outcome were significantly older than patients with a favourable outcome (42.7 years versus 28.9 years, mean, $p < 0.05$, Fisher's PLSD).

Following the GCS 45% of the patients scored three points. 57% of the patients were rated between 3 and 5 and 20% reached six points on the GCS. The remaining patients were scored to seven (14%) and 8 points (9%). The GCS showed a significant correlation to outcome after 11 months (mean). 70% of the patients with an unfavourable outcome scored between 3 and 5 on the GCS, 61.5% of the patients with a favourable outcome rated on the GCS between 6 and 8 ($p < 0.05$, Fisher's PLSD). See also Table 1.

77% of the patients showed an elevated S-100B serum level on admission (min. 0.25 μg/l,,max. 16.2 μg/l,). The S-100B serum levels correlated with outcome. Patients with an unfavourable outcome had a significantly higher S-100B serum level (5.55 μg/l, mean) than patients with a favourable outcome (0.96 μg/l, mean, $p < 0.0001$, Fisher's PLSD). In addition patients with a S-100 serum level below 2 μg/l showed a significant better rating on the GOS at follow-up (4 points versus 1.8 points mean, $p < 0.0001$).

The total misclassification rate of the GCS was 34%. 38% of the patients scoring between 3 and 5 on the GCS had a favourable outcome. 30% had a false negative prediction with this score system. The protein S-100B with 17% had a lower total misclassification rate. When compared with the GCS, the S-100B serum level on admission had a higher positive predictive value (95%) and negative predictive value (70%). For details see Table 2.

Discussion

Predicting outcome after severe head injury is of great interest for clinicians, especially in the early posttraumatic time course [6, 7]. It may provide a basis for therapeutic strategies and may be helpful to select different approaches [6]. Using different clinical and diagnostic tools it is possible to predict outcome with an accuracy rate of near 80% [6]. Predictions made during the first 24 hours after injury based solely on clinical findings were correct in only 44% [7]. Kaufmann *et al.* studied 100 patients with severe traumatic brain injury to determine the prognostic reliability of combined findings from neurological examinations and CT scans obtained during the first 24 hours after trauma. Here the accuracy rate was 59% [26]. Waxman found no correlation of outcome to the initial GCS score, because a substantial number of patients with initial GCS of three had a good recovery [27]. Our results regarding the predictive value of the Glasgow

Table 1. *Scoring on the Glasgow Coma Scale Split up to Outcome on the Glasgow Outcome Scale*

GCS, points			GOS 1–3		GOS 4–5	
	Count	Percent	Count	Percent	Count	Percent
3	20	45.5	13	65	6	28.6
4	3	7	1	5	1	4.8
5	2	4.5	0	0	1	4.8
6	9	20	1	5	8	38
7	6	14	3	15	3	14.3
8	4	9	2	10	2	9.5
Sum	44	100	20	100	21	100

GOS Glasgow Outcome Scale; *GOS 1–3* unfavourable; *GOS 4–5* favourable.

Table 2. *Predictive Values of Score Systems after Severe Head Injury*

(n = 41)	Favourable outcome[b] n = 21	Unfavourable outcome[b] n = 20	pos. predictive value	neg. predictive value	False pos.	False neg.
GCS 3–5[a]	38%[c]	70%[c]	62%	70%	38%	30%
S-100 > 2 μg/l	5%[d,e]	70%[e,f]	95%	70%	5%	30%

[a] *GCS* Glasgow Coma Score.
[b] Favourable outcome: Glasgow Outcome Scale *(GOS)* 4–5, unfavourable outcome: *GOS* 1–3, follow-up after 11 months (mean); neg.: negativ, pos.: positiv.
[c] Significant difference $p < 0.05$; according to Fisher's PLSD.
[d] S-100B: 0.96 μg/l (mean), f) S-100B: 5.55 μg/l (mean).
[e] Significant difference between d und f $p < 0.0001$; according to Fisher's PLSD.

Coma Scale are in the same range. The accuracy rate of the GCS was 65%.

When comparing this predictive value with the prognostic value of the serum marker S-100B, this marker collected between the first and sixth hours of trauma had a total misclassification rate of 17%, and an accuracy rate of 83%, respectively. Raabe studied S-100B serum levels in 44 patients with severe traumatic brain injury. A blood sample was drawn between 6 and 24 hours (median 12 hours). The follow-up examination was carried out after 6 months using the GOS [24]. S-100B serum values were significantly higher in patients with an unfavourable outcome than in patients with a favourable outcome (1.1 μg/l versus 0.3 μg/l) [24]. Using a cut-off value of 2 μg/l for S-100B the outcome could be predicted with a negative predictive value of 96% and a positive predictive value of 38% [24]. The GCS did not correlate to outcome in this study. The predictive values of the GCS were not calculated [24]. In our S-100B study (with the same cut-off line) we found a negative predictive value of 70% and a positive predictive value of 95%. The half-life for the protein S-100B in the serum of 2 hours is relatively short [28]. In our previous studies we found no significant secondary increase of S-100B serum levels during the first 5 days after trauma and a rapid release after trauma into the serum [5, 23]. Thus the collection period should be within a short time after trauma in order to obtain reliable S-100 serum reflecting the severity of trauma. This is probably the reason for the low positive predictive value of 38% in the study of Raabe [24].

Conclusion

The serum level of S-100B estimated one to six hours after severe head injury is a useful additional outcome predictor.

References

1. Hardemark HG, Ericsson N, Kotwica Z, Rundström G, Mendel-Hartwig I, Olsson Y *et al* (1989) S-100 protein and neuron-specific enolase in CSF after experimental traumatic or focal ischemic brain damage. J Neurosurg 71: 727–731
2. Ingebrigtsen T, Rommer B (1996) Serial S-100 protein measurements related of early magnetic resonance imaging after minor head injury. J Neurosurg 85: 945–948
3. Missler U, Wiesmann M (1995) Measurement of S-100 protein in human blood and cerebrospinal fluid: analytical method and preliminary clinical results. Eur J Clin Chem Clin Biochem 33: 743–748
4. Persson L, Hardemark HG, Gustafsson J, Rundström G, Mendel-Hartvig I, Esscher T *et al* (1987) S-100 protein and neuron-specific enolase in cerebrospinal fluid and serum: markers of cell damage in human central nervous system. Stroke 18: 911–918
5. Woertgen C, Rothoerl RD, Holzschuh M, Metz C, Brawanski A (1997) Comparison of serial S-100 and NSE serum measurements after severe head injury. Acta Neurochir (Wien) 139: 1161–1165
6. Choi SC, Barnes TY (1996) Predicting outcome in the head-injured patient. In: Narayan RK, Wilberger E, Povlishock JT (ed) Neurotrauma. McGraw Hill, New York San Franscisco, pp 779–792
7. Marion DW (1996) Outcome from severe head injury. In: Narayan RK, Wilberger E, Povlishock JT (ed) Neurotrauma. McGraw Hill, New York San Franscisco pp 767–777
8. Teasdale G, Jennett B (1974) Assessment of coma and impaired consciousness. A practical scale. Lancet 2: 81–84
9. Marion DW, Carlier PM (1994) Problems with initial Glasgow Coma Scale assessment caused by prehospital treatment of patient with head injuries: result of national survey. J Trauma 36: 89–95
10. Selladurai BM, Jayakumar R, Tan YY, Low HG (1992) Outcome prediction in early management of severe head injury: an experience in Malaysia. Brit J Neurosurg 6: 549–557
11. Stein SC (1996) Classification of head injury. In: Narayan RK, Wilberger E, Povlishock JT (ed) Neurotrauma. McGraw Hill, New York San Franscisco, pp 31–41
12. Report on the traumatic coma data bank, supplement to the journal of neurosurgery, vol 75, Nov 1991
13. Barone FC, Clark RK, Price J, White RF, Feuerstein GZ, Storer LS *et al* (1993) Neuron-specific enolase increase in cerebral and systemic circulation following focal ischemia. Brain Res 623: 77–82
14. Cunningham RT, Young IS, Winders J, O'Kane MJ, Kinstry S, Johnston C *et al* (1991) Serum neurone specific enolase (NSE)

levels as an indicator of neuronal damage in patients with cerebral infarction. Eur J Clin Investigation 21: 497–500
15. Hay E, Royds JA, Davies-Jones GAB, Lewtas NA, Timperley WR, Taylor CB (1984) Cerebrospinal fluid enolase in stroke. J Neurol Neurosurg Psychiatry 47: 724–729
16. Horn M, Seger F, Schlote W (1995) Neuron-specific enolase in gerbil brain and serum after transient cerebral ischemia. Stroke 26: 290–297
17. Marangos PJ, Schmechel D, Parma AM, Clark RL, Goodwin FK (1979) Measurement of Neuron-Specific (NSE) and Non-Neuronal (NNE) isoenzymes of enolase in rat, monkey and human nervous tissue. J Neurochem 33: 319–329
18. Nara T, Nozaki H, Nakae Y, Arai T, Ohashi T (1988) Neuron-specific enolase in comatose children. AJDC 142: 173–174
19. Prange HW (1994) Pathophysiologie, Therapie und Prognose des hypoxisch-ischämischen Hirnschadens. Z Kardiol 83: 127–134
20. Skogseid LM, Nordby HK, Urdal P, Paus E, Lilleaas F (1992) Increased serum creatine kinase BB and neuron specific enolase following head injury indicates brain damage. Acta Neurochir (Wien) 115: 106–111
21. Yamazaki Y, Yada K, Morii S, Kitahara T, Ohwada T (1995) Diagnostic significance of serum neuron-specific enolase and myelin basic protein assay in patients with acute head injury. Surg Neurol 43: 267–271
22. Waterloo K, Ingebrigtsen T, Romner B (1997) Neuropsychological function in patients with increased serum levels of protein S-100 after minor head injury. Acta Neurochir (Wien) 139: 26–32
23. Rothoerl RD, Woertgen C, Holzschuh M, Metz C, Brawanski A (1998) S-100 serum levels after minor and severe head injury. J Trauma 45: 765–767
24. Raabe A, Grolms C, Keller M, Döhnert J, Sorge O, Seifert V (1998) Correlation of computed tomography findings and serum brain damage markers following severe head injury. Acta Neurochir (Wien) 140: 787–792
25. Jennett B, Bond M (1975) Assessment of outcome after severe brain damage: a practical scale. Lancet 1: 480–484
26. Kaufmann MA, Buchmann B, Scheidegger D (1992) Severe head injury: should expected outcome influence resuscitation and first-day decisions? Resuscitation 5: 199–206
27. Waxman K, Sundine MJ, Young RF (1991) Is early prediction of outcome in severe head injury possible? Arch Surg 126: 1237–1241
28. Usui A, Kato K, Abe T, Murase M, Tanaka M, Takeuchi E (1989) S-100 a protein in blood and urine during open heart surgery. Clin Chem 35: 1942–1944

Correspondence: Ralf D. Rothoerl, M.D, Department of Neurosurgery, University of Regensburg, Franz Josef Strauß-Allee 11 93053 Regensburg, Germany.

Acta Neurochir (2000) [Suppl] 76: 101–104

A Microstructural Study of Spinal Cord Edema

H. Naruse[1], **K. Tanaka**[2], and **A. Kim**[3]

[1] Department of Neurosurgery, Higashisumiyoshi Morimoto Hospital, Osaka City, Japan
[2] University Medical School, Japan
[3] Moriguchi Ikuno Hospital, Japan

Summary

The experimental spinal cord edema was produced in a cat by the infusion method of Marmarou. Horseradish peroxidase (HRP) dissolved in autoserum of a cat was used as a tracer. After laminectomy, a 30-gauge needle was inserted into the intumescentia cervicalis. A total amount of 20 µl of a tracer was infused at a rate of 10 µl/hr. The structural features were studied immediately and 3 days after infusion.

Immediately after infusion, HRP was noted in the infused white and gray matters. Though the perivascular space in the white matter at the infused site was widely distended and filled with HRP, the space in the gray matter was not distended but filled with HRP. HRP which was observed along vessels led to the surface of the spinal cord. Swelling of astrocyte was not observed. Three days after infusion, the extracellular space and the perivascular space in the infused white matter were still expanded but were not filled with HRP.

The fine structural features were similar to the findings as seen in Marmarou's infusion type of brain edema. Using this model, it seems to be feasible to study the resolution process of spinal cord edema.

Keywords: Spinal cord edema; spinal cord injury; infusion model; extracellular space.

Introduction

Edema of the spinal cord has not been well understood because there have been only a few studies concerning experimental spinal cord edema [1, 2, 8]. We have previously reported that the fine structural features observed in the experimental spinal cord edema which was produced in a cat intumescentia cervicalis were similar to the findings which were seen in Marmarou's infusion type of brain edema [3, 4, 5, 6]. In order to investigate the resolution process of edema in the spinal cord, the infusion method was used. Horseradish peroxidase (HRP) dissolved in autoserum of a cat was used as a tracer. The animals were sacrificed by the perfusion technique immediately and 3 days after infusion. The morphological aspect of the spinal cord edema was investigated.

Materials and Methods

Animals and Anesthesia

A total of 6 cats were studied. Adult cats were anesthetized with intraperitoneal injection of pentobarbital (30 mg/kg), intubated and mechanically ventilated using halothane in a mixture of nitrous oxide and oxygen (1 : 1).

Production of Spinal Cord Edema

After laminectomy at levels of C4- C7, a 30-gauge needle, which was connected with the polyethylene tubing to the 1 ml syringe mounted on a variable speed infusion pump, was inserted into the right lateral faniculus of the intumescentia cervicalis at the position of 1/6th of the spinal cord width from its right lateral border. Twelve milligrams of horseradish peroxidase (HRP) dissolved in 1 ml of autoserum of a cat was used as a tracer. A total amount of 20 µl of a tracer was infused using the infusion pump at a rate of 10 µl/hr.

Morphological Study

Animals were sacrificed immediately (n = 2) and 3 days after infusion (n = 2). The animals were perfused by the transcardiac route with 0.9% saline for no longer than 2 min, followed with 4% paraformaldehyde in 0.1 M phosphate buffer solution at a pressure of 100 mmHg for about 10 min and finally with a mixture containing 4% paraformaldehyde and 0.5% glutaraldehyde in 0.1 M phosphate buffer solution for about 20 min. The spinal cord was removed and immersed in the same fixative for overnight and sliced in a horizontal direction with a vibratome. The slices were incubated for 30 min in 10 ml of 0.05 M Tris-HCl buffer containing 5.0 mg of 3,3′-diaminobenzidine (DAB) and 3 ml of 0.3% hydrogen peroxide.

In the group of microscopic study, the slices were air dried on glass slides after incubation of DAB and inspected microscopically.

In the group of electron microscopic study, small pieces of tissues were cut after incubation of DAB and postfixed in 1% osmium tetroxide in phosphate buffer for 2 hours and embedded in Epon after dehydration. Thin sections were prepared and examined with a transmission electron microscope (H-300, Hitachi).

Results

Neurologically, no paresis was observed at all in the animals sacrificed 3 days post-infusion.

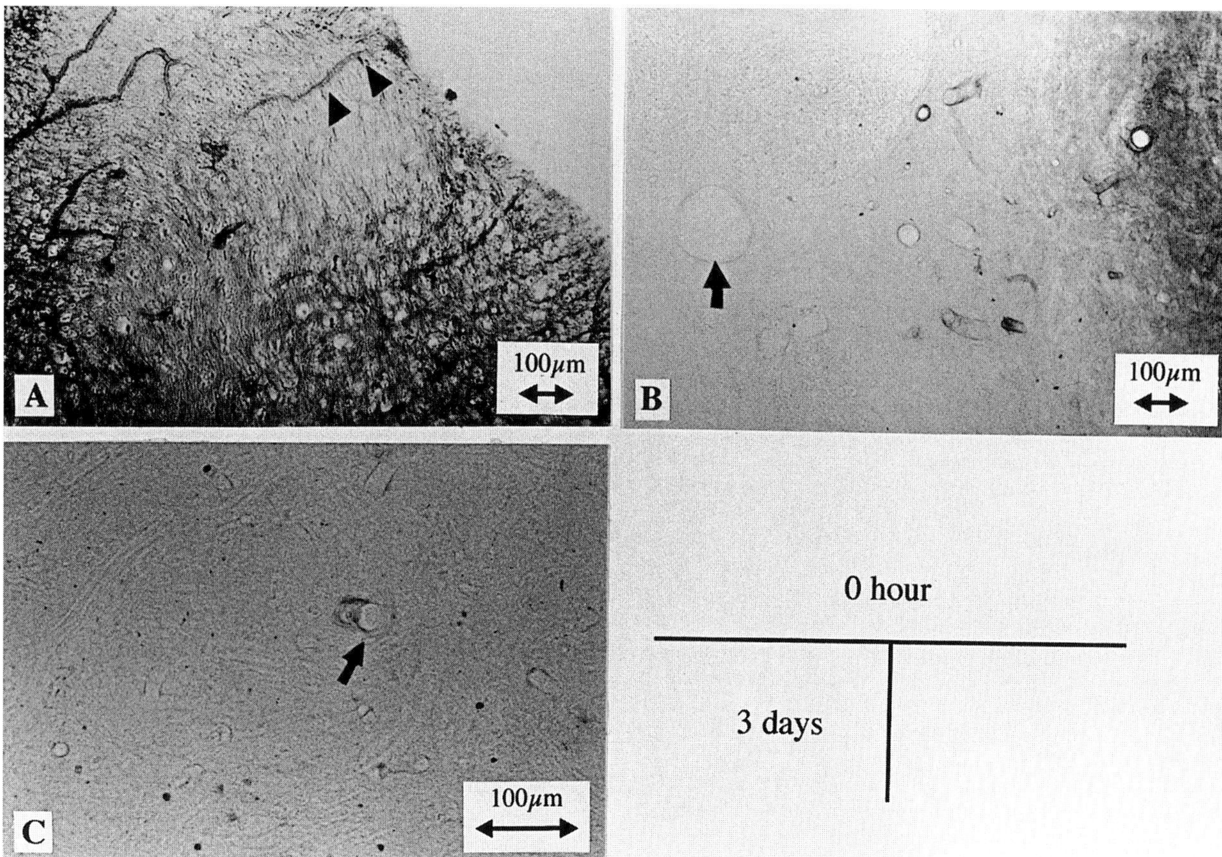

Fig. 1. Photographs of the spinal cord immediately and 3 days after infusion. (A) HRP reaction product was noted in the infused white matter and the surface of the infused site. HRP which was observed along vessels led to the surface of the spinal cord (arrow heads). (B) HRP was noted in the infused white and gray matters. HRP was not seen around central canal (arrow). Tissue necrosis was not observed. (C) HRP reaction product could be seen only around vessels (arrow)

Microscopic Observations

Dark staining indicative of the presence of HRP reaction product was noted in the infused white matter, gray matter and over the surface of the spinal cord at the infused site, immediately after infusion. HRP which was observed along vessels led to the surface of the spinal cord (Fig. 1A). HRP was not seen around central canal (Fig. 1B). Tissue necrosis was not observed. HRP reaction product could be seen only around vessels on the slices 3 days after infusion (Fig. 1C).

Electron Microscopic Observations

Changes Immediately After Infusion. The extracellular space was markedly distended and filled with electron-dense materials in the infused white matter immediately after infusion (Fig. 2A). The perivascular space was greatly expanded and filled with HRP reaction products (Fig. 2B). However, swelling of astrocyte was not observed.

Changes 3 Days After Infusion. In the infused white matter, the extracellular space was still widely expanded (Fig. 3A). However, the amount of dense material was markedly diminished. Cells around vessels contained large amounts of dense materials (Fig. 3B).

Discussion

There have been many reports of experimental models of brain edema. However, almost all of these models involve the processes of both formation and resolution at the same time because of tissue damages. In the infusion model of the experimental brain edema, the resolution process of edema can be separated from the formation process. There have been few reports of experimental spinal cord edema [1, 2, 8]. In the previ-

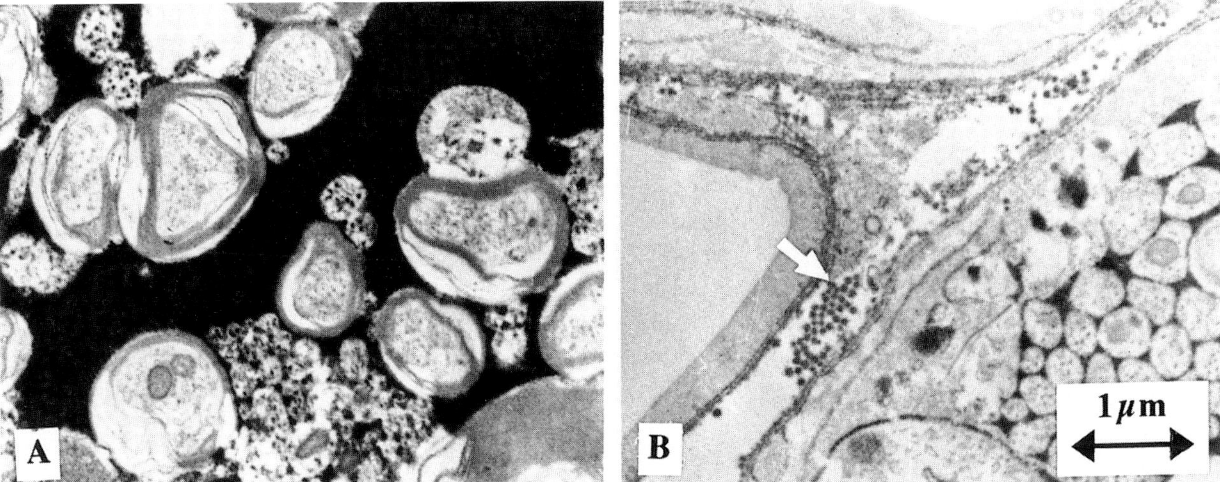

Fig. 2. Electronmicrographs immediately after infusion. (A) The extracellular space was markedly distended and filled with electron-dense materials in the infused white matter. (B) The perivascular space was greatly expanded and filled with HRP reaction products (arrow). However, swelling of astrocyte was not observed

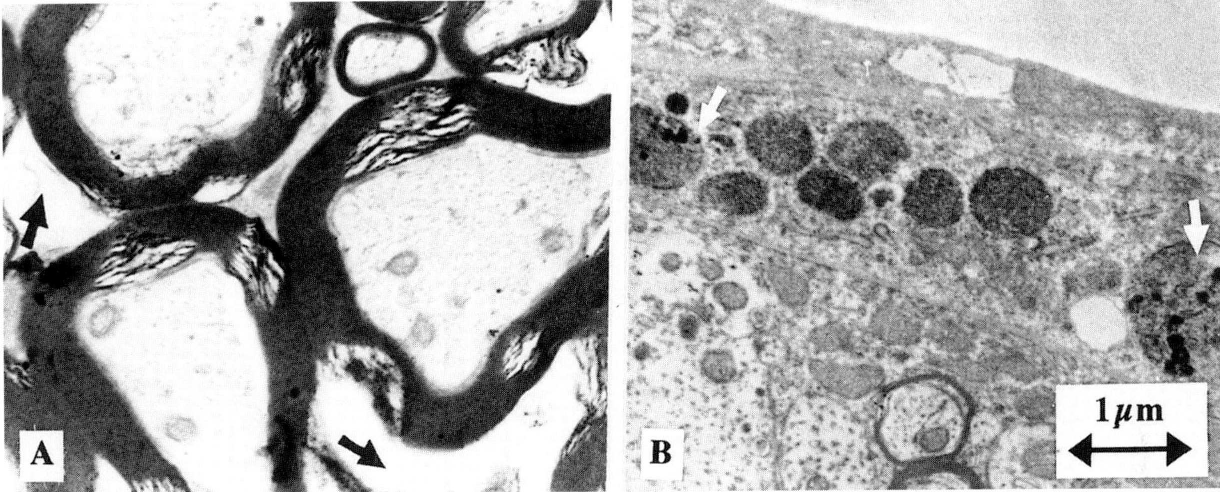

Fig. 3. Electronmicrographs 3 days after infusion. (A) In the infused white matter, the extracellular space was still widely expanded (arrows). However, the amount of dense material was markedly diminished. (B) Cells around the vessel contained large amounts of dense material (arrows)

ous studies, the experimental spinal cord edema was produced by injury which caused damage to the spinal cord, and involved formation and resolution processes of edema at the same time. Tissue necrosis was not observed in this experiment.

Using the total amount of 20 μl of tracers in this model, the infusate was observed mainly in the infused lateral faniculus and did not reach the midline. The tracer was also observed over the surface of the spinal cord. We have demonstrated that the extension of a tracer was obviously longer in longitudinal than in horizontal direction [5]. The spread of the spinal cord edema was directed mainly longitudinally. The extracellular space was markedly distended in the infused white matter. The structural features of the infused areas of the spinal cord were similar to the findings which were seen in Marmarou's infusion type of brain edema [3, 4, 6]. The major route for the expansion of the edema fluid seemed to be through the extracellular space.

No paresis was observed in the animals' behavior after surgery. We have reported that the spinal evoked potential did not show any significant change during infusion, while the water content around the infused white matter significantly increased [7]. Edema which was seen in this study might not cause major damages to the spinal cord.

This method of experimental spinal cord edema may produce reproducible spinal cord edema at any location according to the experimental purpose. Using this model, it seems to be feasible to study not only physiological aspects but also resolution processes of the spinal cord edema.

References

1. Balentine JD (1978) Pathology of experimental spinal cord trauma. I. The necrotic lesions as a function of vascular injury. Lab Invest 39: 236–253
2. Collins GH, West NR, Parmely JD, Samson FM, Ward DA (1986) The histopathology of freezing injury to the rat spinal cord. A light microscopic study. 1. Early degenerative change. J Neuropath Exp Neurol 45: 721–741
3. Hirano A, Marmarou A, Nakamura T, Inoue A (1984) The fine structural study of brain response to intracerebral infusion of serum in the cat. In: Inaba Y, Klatzo I, Spats M (eds) Brain edema. Springer, Berlin Heidelberg New York Tokyo, pp 32–39
4. Naruse H, Tanaka K, Nishimura S, Fujimoto K (1990) A microstructural study of oedema resolution. Acta Neurochir [Suppl] (Wien) 51: 87–89
5. Naruse H, Tanaka K, Kim A, Hakuba A (1997) A new model of spinal cord edema. Acta Neurochir [Suppl] (Wien) 70: 293–295
6. Tanaka K, Ohata K, Katsuyama J, Nishimura S, Marmarou A (1986) Effect of steroids on the resolution of edema, in Miller JD, Teasdale GM, Rowan JO *et al* (eds) Intracranial pressure VI. Springer, Berlin Heidelberg New York Tokyo, pp 611–619
7. Tanaka K, Kim A, Naruse H, Hakuba A (1998) The effect of experimental spinal cord edema on the spinal cord potential. Acta Neurochir [Suppl] (Wien) 71: 101–103
8. Wang R, Ehara K, Tamaki N (1993) Spinal cord edema following freezing injury in the rat: relationship between tissue water content and spinal cord blood flow. Surg Neurol 39: 348–354

Correspondence: Dr. H. Naruse, Department of Neurosurgery, Higashisumiyoshi Morimoto Hospital, 3-8-12, Nakano, Higashisumiyoshi-ku, Osaka, 546-0012, Japan.

Acta Neurochir (2000) [Suppl] 76: 105–109

Vasogenic Oedema and Brain Infarction in an Experimental Penumbra Model

M. Haseldonckx, D. van Bedaf, M. van de Ven, J. van Reempts, and **M. Borgers**

Department of Life Sciences, Neuropathology, Janssen Research Foundation, Beerse, Belgium

Summary

The aim of this study was to modify the photochemical stroke model of Watson *et al.* [23] so as to make possible microscopical investigation of the so-called penumbra, a tissue zone at risk that surrounds an infarction. The idea was to minimize photochemical challenge to endothelial membranes in such a way that thrombotic vascular obstruction is avoided but destabilization of the blood-brain barrier is still obtained. Morphological examination of the challenged area revealed open blood vessels, overt blood-brain barrier leakage over the entire area, severely swollen glial cells and structurally intact neurons. The lesion expanded over time due to progressive extravasation, formation of perivascular edema and consequent development of secondary ischemia through mechanical compression and microvascular congestion. In contrast to a photothrombotic infarct, in which the ischemic insult is more severe and blood vessels are completely congested by aggregated platelets, with this approach blood flow is partially preserved. In this way, an ischemic penumbra is created that mimics pathologic conditions secondary to stroke and trauma. The model may be useful in studying effects of drugs on pathologic phenomena that are characteristic of a penumbra, e.g. vasogenic and cellular edema, inflammation and infarction.

Keywords: Focal cerebral ischemia; edema; blood-brain barrier; histology.

Introduction

Traumatic brain injury and stroke are leading causes of death and morbidity in Western countries [3, 11]. Acute lesions such as infarcts and hemorrhagic contusions may become surrounded by areas of secondary flow reduction. This so-called penumbra region can be characterized as potentially salvageable and hence is a target for therapy [8, 16]. It consists of tissue zones in transition from a reversible to an irreversible state of damage, in which synaptic activity has ceased, ion homeostasis is jeopardized and cerebral blood flow is diminished [1, 13, 19]. Several animal models have been developed to mimic the neuropathological consequences of trauma [10] and stroke [6, 18], but no one model fulfils all the requirements of a good preclinical model [14]. Although substantial efforts have been made to test drugs in these models, no clinically successful drug has been found so far [15]. To discover a successful therapy it is essential to first understand the evolution of the disease. Therapy must be directed to specific aspects of the disease mechanism (the right drug at the right place) and delivered for an optimal period of time without interfering with normal function. The model presented in this paper is a modification of the photothrombotic stroke model of Watson *et al.* [23]. It is based on a moderate photochemical challenge of endothelial membranes in an attempt to destabilize the blood brain barrier (BBB), thereby preserving sufficient flow to facilitate induction of secondary progressive ischemia. The model has typical morphologic features of a penumbra (structurally intact neurons, open blood vessels and swollen astrocytes) [21], and enables study of secondary ischemic changes (cellular edema, inflammation, infarction) associated with the timely progression of stroke and trauma. The model may also be useful in investigating the effect of drugs interfering with these phenomena.

Materials and Methods

Animal housing and treatment conditions complied with European Union directive for Animal Welfare # 86/609, and were approved by the ethics committee on animal experiments of the Janssen Research Foundation. Male Wistar rats (n = 30) weighing 180–200 g were used. Tracheal intubation was performed under 4% halothane in a mixture of 30% O_2 and 70% N_2O (1000 ml/min). During the subsequent surgical procedure the halothane concentration was maintained at 1%.

The head of the rats was positioned in a stereotaxic apparatus and a scalp incision was made to expose the skull. The photosensitizing dye rose bengal was intravenously injected into the femoral vein. Illumination was performed with a Schott KL 1500 fiber optic light source equipped with an Osram Xenophot 150 watt lamp [22]. The light beam was limited to 2 mm by a diaphragm and positioned over the right hemisphere 2.5 mm lateral and 1.8 mm posterior to the bregma. Body temperature was kept at 37 °C with a rectal probe and a thermostatically regulated heating pad. Rats were divided into two groups: group 1 (n = 15) was subjected to penumbra conditions (10 mg/kg rose bengal, 2 min illumination at 50 kLux). Group 2 (n = 15) was given a thrombotic challenge (20 mg/kg rose bengal, 20 min illumination at 75 kLux) and served as a reference. Rats were sacrificed and the brains were fixed by transcardial perfusion with formalin 4% for 5 min at room temperature. Postoperative survival times for the two groups were either 10 min, 30 min, 1 h, 4 h or 24 h (n = 3 per condition).

To assess the stability of the BBB, 1 nm gold particles were intravenously administered (femoral vein) 2 min before the start of perfusion, as a tracer for extravasation [21].

The lesion was stereotaxically sampled. Alternating vibratome sections (50 μm) were prepared from the fixed rat brains and were either stained with azure eosine for histology [17] or silver-enhanced to visualize the gold particles [7], or reacted with diaminobenzidine (DAB) to display the catalase activity of erythrocytes [12]. Additional 300 μm vibratome sections of the same tissue were sliced at regular distances and postfixed with 2% osmium tetroxide, dehydrated in graded ethanol series and routinely embedded in epoxy resin.

The histological results were verified either on 2 μm Epon sections stained with toluidine blue or on ultrathin sections with electronmicroscopy (EM).

Results

The observed morphologic changes, as well as the aspect of extravasation and blood stasis were fully comparable to what has been described at the periphery of photothrombotic infarcts [21]. In group 1 substantial damage of the BBB was present already 10 min after onset of illumination (Fig. 1a). This could be inferred from the abundant dark spots, which represented leaking gold particles distributed all over the illuminated area. These spots coincided with histologically pale-stained areas.

Congestion of microvessels was limited, as indicated by the presence of a moderate positive catalase reaction of residual erythrocytes. Neurons remained intact but glial cells were severely swollen, particularly at perivascular sites. In group 2, however, at 10 min the majority of blood vessels were already congested. Tracer extravasation and early signs of edema were mainly situated at the margins of the thrombotic core (Fig. 1b). These results were confirmed by EM. Blood vessels in the lesion core of group 1, although compressed, remained open. Platelets were found only occasionally and perivascular glial end-feet were severely swollen. In contrast, blood vessels in the thrombotic core of group 2 were obstructed by platelets and erythrocytes. Perivascular swelling was limited.

In group 1, early signs of neurodegeneration became visible from 1 h. At the same time progressive congestion of red blood cells was observed, most probably due to extravasation and consequent formation of perivascular edema (Fig. 2a). In group 2, within 4 h the irradiated tissue was characterized by congested

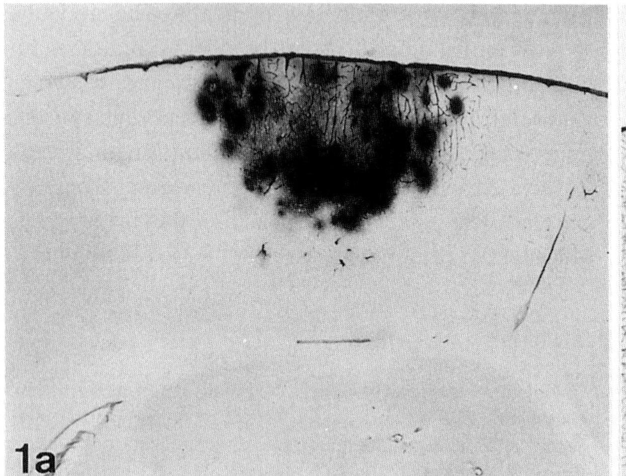

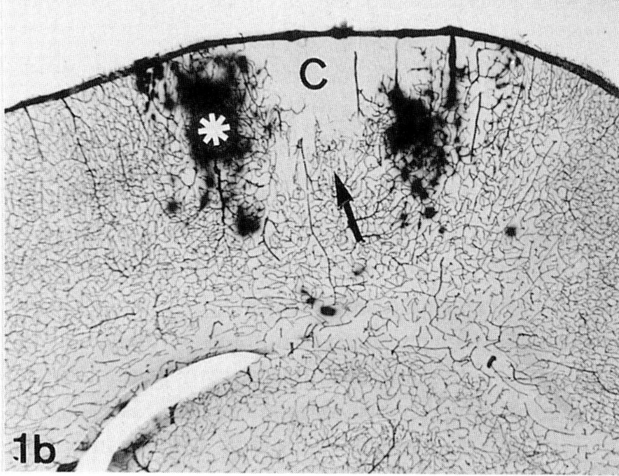

Fig. 1. Survey of silver-enhanced 50 μm vibratome section of cortical tissue injected with 1 nm gold tracer. At 10 min after induction of a photothrombotic penumbra (a) microcirculation is preserved as deduced by the presence of tracer in the entire illuminated area. The BBB is substantially damaged as indicated by the abundant dark spots of tracer extravasation. In rats subjected to photothrombotic challenge (b) no microcirculation is possible in the core, as shown by the absence of intravascular tracer (*C*). Flow is preserved at the periphery (arrow) and large amounts of tracer have penetrated the parenchyma (white asterisk) which indicates a disrupted BBB (×20)

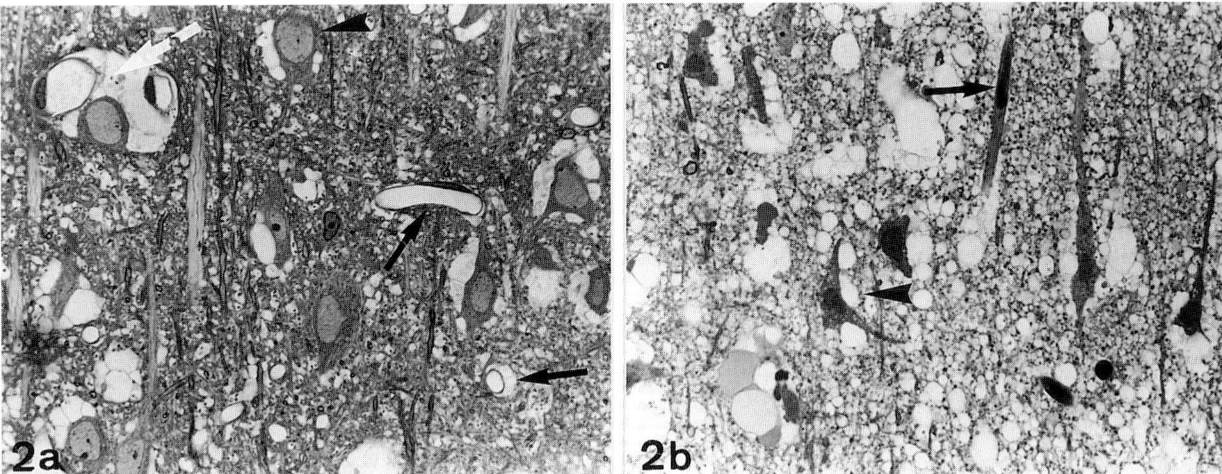

Fig. 2. Microscopic detail of the illuminated area 1–4 h after photochemical challenge. After mild challenge (a) the "penumbra aspect" is found in the core of the lesion. It is characterized by open vessels (black arrows), normal neurons (arrowhead), swollen astrocytes (white arrow) surrounded by a compact neuropil. After severe photothrombotic challenge (b), the core of the lesion shows congested blood vessels (arrow) and irreversibly damaged neurons (arrowhead) embedded in a spongeous parenchyma (2 μm epon section, toluidine blue-stained, ×520)

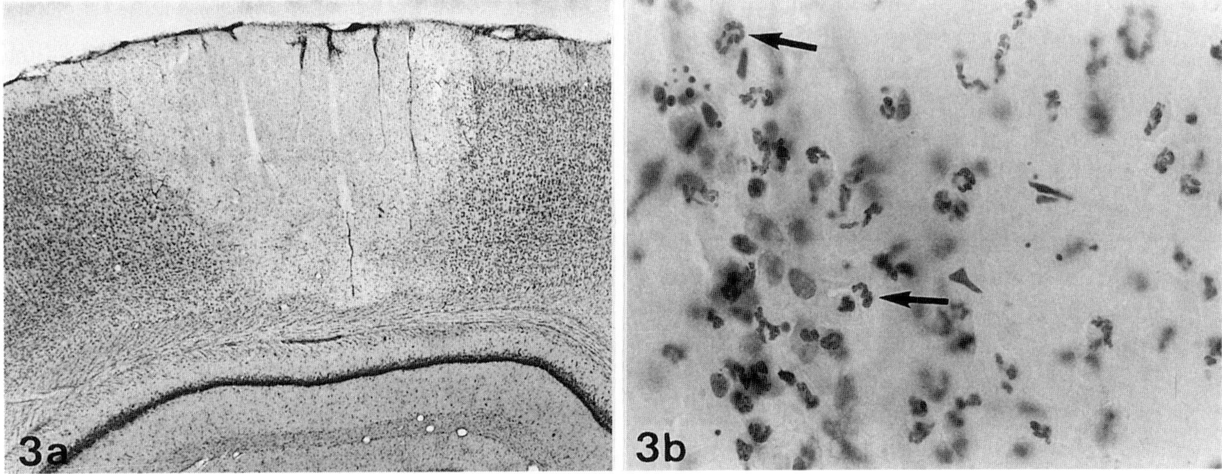

Fig. 3. Survey of a fully developed infarct with a characteristic pan-necrotic aspect 24 h after induction of a phototoxic penumbra (a). In contrast to photothrombotic challenge, in the phototoxic penumbra condition, invasion and migration of neutrophilic leukocytes (arrows) appears all over the infarcted area including the illuminated core (b) (50 μm vibratome sections, azure eosin-stained, a: ×20: b: ×520)

vessels, severely coagulated neurons, dilated glial cells and spongeous parenchyma (Fig. 2b). At 24 hours the infarct was fully developed in both groups. A cortical area of pannecrosis was found that was considerably larger than the initially illuminated region (Fig. 3a). Infiltration of macrophages and inflammatory polymorphonuclear leukocytes was observed in areas in which flow was transiently preserved, i.e. in the entire infarct in group 1 and at the margins in group 2 (Fig. 3b).

Discussion

In this study a modification of the photothrombotic stroke model [22, 23] is presented that makes it possible to produce focal infarcts without accompanying thrombotic occlusion. Photochemical aggression was radically limited, so that cortical flow was initially preserved and neurons remained intact. On the other hand, the BBB was sufficiently destabilized to induce extravasation and progressive glial swelling, which caused secondary ischemia, vascular congestion, inflammation and ultimately infarction. This pathologic picture is very similar to a penumbra condition that is typically found in a peri-infarct region or around hemorrhagic lesions after traumatic brain injury and from which damage may progressively expand as a result of vasogenic and cellular edema formation as well as inflammatory reactions [5, 6, 18]. The penumbra is an area at risk characterized by CBF conditions that balance between an upper flow threshold for electrical failure ($\pm 30\%$ of normal) and a lower threshold for structural degeneration ($\pm 15\%$ of normal) [1]. It occurs in humans suffering from stroke but also in experimental models that mimic the clinical situation of stroke and trauma. The penumbra may develop secondarily to a primary insult, which may be either a complete thromboembolic occlusion, intracerebral hemorrhage or partial reduction of flow in large arterial territories, e.g. the middle cerebral artery (MCA). But the primary insult itself may have characteristics of a penumbra situation e.g. MCA occlusion with collateral flow ranging from 15% to 30% of normal [4, 18]. In contrast to the photothrombotic ring model [24], in which a large penumbra zone is created secondary to thrombosis, in the present model cortical flow is partially preserved. This allows continuous supply from the microcirculation of edema substrates and inflammatory components, all of which may contribute to progressive deterioration [2, 9, 20]. A combination of an initial trigger (either ischemic, toxic, or mechanical) and BBB breakdown seems to be a prerequisite for final pan-necrotic damage, since neither global ischemia of short duration (ischemic tissue, intact BBB) nor hemorrhages induced by insertion of probes (normal tissue, BBB breakdown) lead to infarction.

The model in this investigation enables the separate study of isolated mechanisms that are part of a more complex pathogenetic evolution. Consequently, drugs with a profile corresponding to one of these mechanisms can be selected to evaluate possible neuroprotective effects. Interaction with BBB destabilization can be measured by analysis of the amount of tracer extravasation. Interaction with microvascular stasis or congestion can be measured by quantification of the DAB signal of residual erythrocytes or by means of a count of the number of immunostained migrating leukocytes. Since the model is simple and non-invasive, it might be useful in selecting active compounds before they are characterized in more complicated stroke or trauma models.

In summary, although the phototoxic penumbra model is not clinically relevant, it may provide a valid means of studying some of the complex and multifactorial mechanisms involved in the pathogenesis and secondary evolution of stroke and trauma.

References

1. Astrup J, Siesjo BK, Symon L (1981) Thresholds in cerebral ischemia: the ischemic penumbra. Stroke 12: 723–725
2. Betz AL, Iannotti F, Hoff JT (1989) Brain edema: a classification based on blood-brain barrier integrity. Cerebrovasc Brain Metab Rev 1: 133–154
3. Bonita R (1992) Epidemiology of stroke. Lancet 339: 342–344
4. Chen ST, Hsu CY, Hogan EL, Maricq H, Balentine JD (1986) A model of focal ischemic stroke in the rat: reproducible extensive cortical infarction. Stroke 17: 738–743
5. De Mulder G, van Rossem K, Van Reempts J, Van Deuren B, Borgers M, Verlooy J (2000) Validation of a closed head injury model for use in long-term studies. Acta Neurochir (2000) [Suppl] 76: 411–415
6. Dietrich WD (1998) Neurobiology of stroke. Int Rev Neurobiol 42: 55–101
7. Danscher G (1981) Histochemical demonstration of heavy metals. Histochem 71: 1–16
8. Fisher M (1997) Characterizing the target of acute stroke therapy. Stroke 28: 866–872
9. Gehrmann J, Banati RB, Wiessnert C, Hossmann KA, Kreutzberg GW (1995) Reactive microglia in cerebral ischaemia: an early mediator of tissue damage. Neuropathol Appl Neurobiol 21: 277–289
10. Gennarelli TA (1994) Animate models of human head injury. J Neurotrauma 11: 357–68
11. Goldstein M (1990) Traumatic brain injury: a silent epidemic. Ann Neurol 27: 327
12. Graham RC, Karnovsky MJ (1966) The early stages of absorption of injected horseradish peroxidase in the proximal tubules of mouse kidney: ultrastructural cytochemistry by a new technique. J Histochem Cytochem 14: 291–302
13. Hossmann KA (1994) Viability thresholds and the penumbra of focal ischemia. Ann Neurol 36: 557–565
14. Hunter AJ (1996) In vitro and in vivo models of cerebral ischaemia. Baillière's Clin Anaesthesiol 10: 391–408
15. Hunter AJ, Green RA, Cross AJ (1995) Animal models of acute ischemic stroke: can they predict clinically successful neuroprotective drugs? Trends Pharmacol Sci 16: 123–128
16. Lassen NA, Fieschi C and Lenzi GL (1990) Ischemic penumbra and neuronal cell death: comments on the therapeutic window in acute stroke with particular reference to thrombolytic therapy. Cerebrovasc Disorders 1 [Suppl] 1: 32–35
17. Lillie RD, Fullmer HM (1976) Histopathologic technic and practical histochemistry, 4th edn. McGraw-Hill, New York, pp 195–197
18. Mc Auley MA (1995) Rodent models of focal ischemia. Cerebrovasc Brain Metab Rev 7: 153–180
19. Obrenovitch TP (1995) The ischaemic penumbra: twenty years on. Cerebrovasc Brain Metab Rev 7: 297–323
20. Schroeter M, Jander S, Huitinga I, Witte O, Stoll G (1996) Phagocytic response in photochemically induced infarction of rat cerebral cortex. The role of resident microglia. Stroke 28: 382–386
21. Van Reempts J and Borgers M (1994) Histopathological char-

acterization of photochemical damage in nervous tissue. Histol Histopath 9: 185–195
22. Van Reempts J, Van Deuren B, Van de Ven M, Cornelissen F, Borgers M (1987) Flunarizine reduces cerebral infarct size after photochemically induced thrombosis in spontaneously hypertensive rats. Stroke 18: 1113–1119
23. Watson BD, Dietrich WD, Busto R, Wachtel MS, Ginsberg MD (1985) Induction of reproducible brain infarction by photochemically initiated thrombosis. Ann Neurol 17: 497–504
24. Wester P, Watson BD, Prado R, Dietrich WD (1995) A photothrombotic ring model of rat stroke-in-evolution displaying putative penumbral inversion. Stroke 26: 444–450

Correspondence: M. Haseldonckx, Department of Life Sciences, Neuropathology Janssen Research Foundation, Turnhoutseweg 30, B-2340, Beerse, Belgium.

Acta Neurochir (2000) [Suppl] 76: 111–113

Effects of Chronic Deep Hypoxia on the Expression of Nitric Oxide Synthase in the Rat Brain

J. V. Lafuente[1,2], **B. Adan**[1], and **J. Cervós-Navarro**[2,3]

[1] Department Neurosciences, University of the Basque Country, Leioa, Spain
[2] Inst of Neuropathol, Free University Berlin, Germany
[3] Inst of Neurological Sciences and Gerontology, International University of Catalonie, Barcelona, Spain

Summary

Experimental studies in extreme hypoxic conditions affecting the brain have been performed mainly in acute but not chronic models.

Twenty rats were housed and exposed to decreasing concentrations of oxygen (from 21% to 7% over 130 days) and ten normal rats were used as control. Paraffin slices from representative sections containing cerebral cortex, cerebellum, striatum, hippocampus, thalamus and hypothalamus were incubated with antisera against nitric oxide synthase.

Cortex and striatum showed small randomly distributed positive neurons with bipolar features, in greater numbers in the hypoxic group ($p < 0.02$). The granular layer of the cerebellum showed a strongly positive rim around some cell nuclei. Purkinje cells were immunopositive in hypoxic rats. Hipoccampal, thalamic and hypothalamic nuclei showed no quantitative differences in the number of positive neurons. The increased number of blood vessels and their dilation observed in some brain regions in hypoxic rats, mainly in ventral striatum, lead us to hypothesise that NOS may be overexpressed and act at these sites as vasomodulator and/or mediator of secondary cell injury affecting selective neuronal populations.

We conclude that prolonged periods of adaptation to deep hypoxia reduces the effect of hypoxia on the upregulation of NOS in the brain tissue.

Keywords: Nitric oxide; chronic hypoxia; cell injury; brain.

Introduction

Nitric oxide (NO) is a major mediator of cellular signals involved in vasorelaxation, neurotransmission and cytotoxicity. NO is synthesised by a cell-type specific enzym, the nitric oxide synthase (NOS). In the nervous system constitutive NOS (cNOS) may be activated in neurons and endothelial cells and has been shown to participate in the causation of cell damages in various neurological disease, ischaemia, epilepsy and several forms of acute and chronic CNS-injury. Inducible NOS (iNOS) activity also increases following exposure to cytokines or microbial products.

Experimental studies in extreme hypoxic conditions affecting the brain have been performed mainly in acute and subacute but not chronic models [3, 9]. Among the known effects of severe chronic hypoxia in the brain are atrophy [1], gliosis [11], vascular dilation and neoangiogenesis [9, 10]. Therefore, NOS should be a good candidate to be upregulated in this stress situation.

This work is aimed at elucidating the presence (enhancement or decrease of immunopositivity) of chronic normobaric hypoxia on constitutive NOS.

Materials and Methods

The experiments were carried out on 30 male adult Wistar rats, which were housed at constant environmental conditions, -temperature (22 + −1 C)), relative humidity (58–60%), air flow (30 l/min) and atmospheric pressure (759 + −4 Torr)- with 12 h dark schedule. At the beginning of the experiments, the body weight was 335 + −18 gr and the age of the animals 90 days. Food and tap water were available ad libitum. Twenty rats were exposed to decreasing concentrations of oxygen (from 21% to 7% in 130 days) whereas 10 controls were kept on breathing normal air. During cleaning of the cages and replenishing of food and water, at 2 days intervals, animals remained in hypoxic atmosphere.

For the tissue preparation, under anaesthesia (100 mg/kg body weight, Ketamine and 1 ml/kg xylazine) the chest was opened and the ascending aorta was cannulated via the left ventricle. The descending aorta was clamped and the right atrium was excised. The animals were perfused with about 300 ml of a 4% paraformaldehyde fixative solution in 0.01 M PBS buffer preceded by a brief saline rinse (0.9 NaCl). After transcardial perfusion, brains were immediatly removed and postfixed overnight in the same solution. Coronal sections were cut and embedded in paraffin. 4 μm thick slices from representative sections containing cerebral cortex, cerebellum, striatum, hippocampus, thalamus and hypothalamus were obtained, stained with cresyl violet and incubated with antisera against n-NOS (from rat and porcine brain) and antiserum against e-NOS (Alexis, 1/500,

1/2000, 1/2500). The reaction product was visualised with streptavidin-biotin-peroxidase complex (Vectastain Elite ABC Kit. Vector) using DAB as chromogen.

Results

Immunoreactive cell bodies and processes showed a widespread distribution in the brain in normal controls. Therefore, we only highlighted data from the comparison of both experimental groups.

Cortex and striatum showed small randomly distributed positive neurons with bipolar features in a lightly more significant amount in the hypoxic group ($p < 0.02$). Positive neurons were found mainly in neocortical layers III-IV and in the striatum within a network of positive fibres within the grey matter. This was more apparent in the dorsal putamen (Fig. 1). No differences were found with the two nNOS antibodies, although with the antiserum obtained against rat brain, more clearly positive fibre networks and higher numbers of neurons were found.

The granular layer of the cerebellum showed a strongly positive rim around the nuclei of numerous cells. Purkinje cells were immunopositive only in some hypoxic rats and, in the molecular layer, a network-like staining pattern was seen. In the hypocampus, thalamic and hypothalamic nuclei no quantitative differences in hypoxic vs. non-hypoxic rats were found.

An increase in the number of blood vessels was observed in some brain regions in hypoxic rats. Dilated vessel lumina were observed, but only exceptionally showed immunopositive endothelia for eNOS (Fig. 2). These vessels were mainly found in ventral striatum, a region with a remarkable positive fibre network and numerous positive neurons.

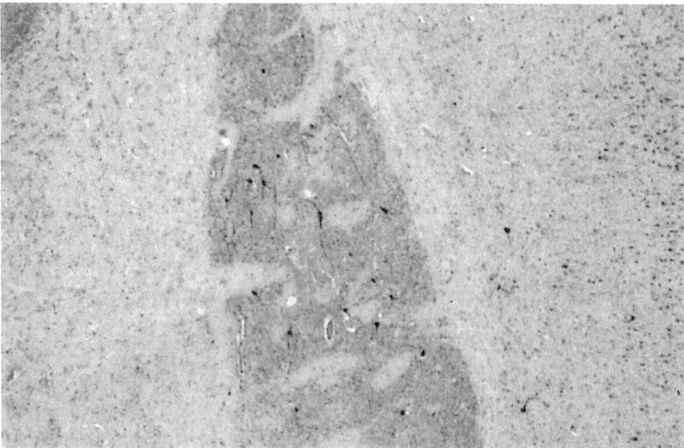

Fig. 1. Low magnification photomicrograph showing the presence of positive neurons and nerve fibres in the putamen, nNOS 35x

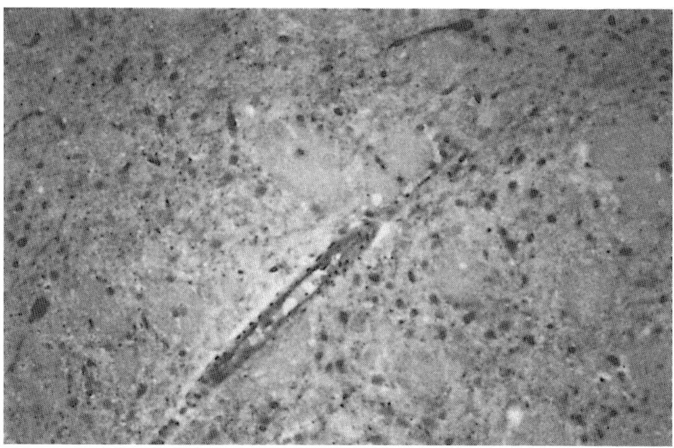

Fig. 2. Ventral striatum, vessel showing mild immunoreaction for eNOS surrounded by numerous neurons positive for nNOS, 85x

Discussion

Chronic hypoxia induces several adaptive changes in the brain [6], from dilation and neoformation of microvessels [9] to increase in glucose metabolism [4]. The issue of increase or decrease of NOS activity after hypoxia remains controversial. After acute severe hypoxia NOS activity is unaffected [2], although a significant decrease in NOS-activity in every region of the brain excluding the cortex has been reported [5]. The role of NO in different brain structures affected by chronic hypoxia is still not clarified although a protective mechanism has been postulated. We found no significant overexpression of NOS in a chronic severe hypoxic situation.

NOS positive neurons present in normal animals are supposed to be very resistant to various kinds of noxious insults. However upregulation of NOS following hypoxia-ischaemia in neurons may result in cell death. Thus induction of neuronal NOS is associated with cell injury. Combination of NO with superoxide could be extremely deleterious by forming peroxynitrites, which can cause DNA strand breaks [7].

The ventral striatum shows a special susceptibility to chronic severe hypoxia displaying a higher number of nNOS positive neurons, a compact fibre network and in addition regular presence of vessels with eNOS positive endothelial cell.

The increased number of blood vessels and their dilation observed in several brain regions in hypoxic rats [9] lead us to hypothesise that NOS may be overexpressed and acts at these sites as vasomodulator and/or mediator of secondary cell injury affecting selective neuronal populations.

The highest number of positive neurons after acute hypoxia was found mainly in CA3 and dentate gyrus [8] but after a progressive chronic adaptation only a moderate not significant increase could be observed.

Acute hypoxia induces drastic changes in NO concentration in brain tissue; however, the adaptive period to deep hypoxia led to compensation and little differences were observed with respect to the control animals in number and distribution of immunoreactive elements. This means that the adaptive period reduces the dramatical effects of hypoxia on brain tissue.

Studies in a purely hypoxic model may be interesting for further investigations e.g., altitude sickness, chronic obstructive pulmonary disease (COPD), but also for ischaemic cell injury (hypoxia and hypoglycaemia). It is still unclear how hypoxia participates in ischaemia; one way may be through the NO cascade.

In conclusion, acute hypoxia induces drastic changes in NO concentration in brain tissue, but a long period of adaptation to deep hypoxia also reduces the effect of hypoxia on the upregulation of NOS in the brain tissue.

Acknowledgment

Supported by Basque Government (Program P.&M. P.I. B1 1/97015).

References

1. Cervós-Navarro J, Sampaolo S, Hamsdorf G (1991) Brain changes in experimental chronic hypoxia. Exp Pathol 42 (4): 205–212
2. Groenendaal F, Mishra OP, McGowan JE, Hoffman DJ, Papadopoulos MD (1996) Cytosolic and membrane-bound cerebral nitric oxide synthase activity during hypoxia in cortical tissue of newborn piglets. Neurosci Lett 206: 121–124
3. Hamdorf G, Cervós-Navarro J, Müller R (1992) Increase of survival time in experimental hypoxia by Cytidine Diphosphate Choline. Arzneim-Forch/Drug Res 42 (4): 421–424
4. Harik SI, Behmand RA, LaManna JC (1994) Hypoxia increases glucose transport at blood brain barrier in rats. J Appl Physiol 77 (2): 896–901
5. Jiang K, Kim S, Murphy S, Song D, Pastuszko A (1996) Effect of hypoxia and reoxigenation on regional activity of nitric oxide synthase in brain of newborn piglets. Neurosci Lett 206: 199–203
6. LaManna JC, Vendel LM, Farrell RM (1992) Brain adaptation to chronic hypobaric hypoxia in rats. J Appl Physiol 72 (6): 2238–2243
7. MacManus JP, Linnik MD (1997) Gene expression induced by cerebral ischemia: An apoptotic perspective. J Cer Blood Flow Metab 17: 815–832
8. Matsuoka Y, Kitamura Y, Tooyama I, Kimura H, Taniguchi T (1997) In vivo hypoxia-induced neuronal damage with an enhancement of neuronal nitric oxide synthase immunoreactivity in hippocampus. Exp Neurol 146 (1): 57–66
9. Patt S, Sampaolo S, Janko A, Tscharirkini I, Cervós-Navarro J (1997) Cerebral angiogenesis triggered by severe chronic hypoxia displays regional differences. J Cer Blood Flow Metab 17: (801–806)
10. Patt S, Danner S, Théallier-Janko A, Breier G, Hottenrott G, Plate KH, Cervós-Navarro J (1998) Upregulation of vascular endothelial growth factor in severe chronic brain hypoxia of the rat. Neurosci Lett 252: 199–202
11. Zimmer C, Sampaolo S, Sharma HS, Cervós-Navarro J (1991) Altered glial fibrillary acidic protein immunoreactivity in rat brain following chronic hypoxia. Neurosci 40 (2): 353–361

Correspondence: J. V. Lafuente, Department Neurosciences, University of the Basque Country, Box 699, 48080-Bilbao, Spain.

Cellular Mechanisms

The mechanisms and treatment of post-taumatic brain oedema are the main focus of interest in this section. Although it has been documented that cytotoxic oedema can be responsible for post-traumatic brain edema, the role of vasogenic component has also been considered to be of importance. Beaumont *et al.* examined the time course of BBB opening in relation to the Apparent Diffusion Coefficients (ADC) changes in rats subjected to various types of traumatic brain injury. These authors showed that BBB permeability represents a passive component of post-traumatic oedema formation. When the barrier is open it acts as a low resistance pathway for oedema development. Beaumont *et al.* also demonstrated that dopamine – a vasopressor that can be clinically used to restore post-traumatic cerebral blood flow – may significantly worsen post-traumatic brain oedema. Thus there may be some situations in which vasogenic mechanisms greatly contribute to the formation of post-traumatic brain oedema.

Three papers in this section examined the effect of bradykinin B2 receptor antagonists on post-traumatic brain edema. Bradykinin, an active peptide of the kalikrein-kinin system, has been shown to enhance the vasogenic process of post-traumatic brain oedema. Shulz *et al.* examined the effect of a non-peptide bradykinin B2 receptor antagonist LF 16-0687 on oedema formation induced by a cortical cold lesion and cortical impact injury in rats. Stover *et al.* also investigated the effects in cortical impact injury. Both groups clearly showed that B2-receptor antagonists ameliorate post-traumatic brain oedema. A beneficial effect of another bradykinin B2 receptor antagonist HOE-140 was shown by Sharma *et al.* using a spinal cord trauma model. Sharma *et al.* also examined the neuroprotective effects of a new anti-oxidant compound H-290/51 in the same spinal cord trauma model. Their results indicated that the protective effect was mediated via the upregulation of a constitutive form of heme oxygenase (H0-2). Barth *et al.* demonstrated that more than 99% of the post-traumatic neuronal death was due to cell necrosis in rats after cortical cold injury.

Since many receptors involved in regulation of the BBB and CBF are localised on the cerebral endothelial cells, in vitro studies of the endothelial cell (the main constituents of the BBB and cerebral microvasculature) represent an essential approach for the understanding of blood-brain barrier functions under pathological and/or physiological conditions. There are two papers concerned with the functions of cultured human cerebrovascular endothelial cells. Chen *et al.* demonstrated that nitric oxide and endothelin-1 are closely linked in regulating [Ca2+] mobilisation and cytoskeletal actin reorganisation through activation of ETA receptors. The interaction between ET-1 and NO involves the cGGMP/PKG system. Adrenergic innervation derived from the locus ceruleus has been implicated in regulating BBB permeability and inflammatory responses associated with neurological disorders including stroke. Using the same in vitro model as Chen *et al.*, Ohara Y *et al.* demonstrated that adrenergic agents modulated the TNF-alpha stimulated ICAM-1 expression on human brain microvascular endothelial cells. Using a unique in vivo model using the stroke-prone spontaneously hypertensive rat (SHRSP) for investigation of hypertensive cerebrovascular injury, Ito *et al.* showed a decreased expression of ICAM-1 and amelioration of brain oedema by an angiotensin 1 receptor antagonist TCV-116. Their results indicated a pressure-independent mechanism involved in the amelioration of brain oedema. These two different models (in vitro and in vivo) are useful and important for further investigation to elucidate the pathophysiology of the human cerebromicrovascular compartment.

Another important topic in brain oedema research is the treatment of ischaemic oedema at the early cytotoxic phase prior to the exacerbation of the oedema formation by the vasogenic component. Hakamata *et al.* demonstrated that a Na+/H+ exchange inhibitor SM-20220 ameliorated early ischemic brain oedema. The effect was further enhanced by the combined use of an alkalising agent THAM presumably due to the buffering of tissue acidosis. These beneficial effects, however, disappeared when the treatment was initiated 48 hours post-ischaemia. Treatment applicable during the "therapeutic window" of post-ischaemic neuronal death would be attractive in the clinical field. There are a few methodological papers in this section concerned with ischaemia/trauma research. Soehle *et al.* showed the advantage of laser Doppler scanning over the single location assessment for reliable regional cerebral blood flow measurement. Bieberthaler *et al.* showed the influence of alcohol exposure on S-100b serum levels in patients with minor head trauma.

Acta Neurochir (2000) [Suppl] 76: 117–120

Adrenergic Mediation of TNFα-Stimulated ICAM-1 Expression on Human Brain Microvascular Endothelial Cells

Y. Ohara[1], **R. M. McCarron**[1], **T. T. Hoffman**[1], **H. Sugano**[1], **J. Bembry**[3], **F. A. Lenz**[2], and **M. Spatz**[3]

[1] Resuscitative Medicine Department, Naval Medical Research Center, Silver Spring, MD
[2] Department of Neurosurgery, JHU Medical School, Baltimore, MD
[3] Stroke Branch, NINDS, National Institutes of Health, Bethesda, MD

Summary

Adrenergic innervation derived from locus ceruleus has been implicated in regulating BBB permeability and inflammatory responses associated with neurological disorders. This report demonstrates that adrenergic agents attenuate the tumor necrosis factor-α (TNFα)-induced expression of intercellular adhesion molecule-1 (ICAM-1) on cerebral microvascular endothelial cells (HBMEC) derived from human brains. HBMEC were incubated with isoproterenol (1–10 μM) alone or in the presence of propranolol (10 μM) for 30 min followed by the addition of various concentrations of TNFα. ICAM-1 expression on cultured HBMEC was dose-dependently upregulated by TNFα. Incubation with isoproterenol significantly reduced levels of ICAM-1 expression indicating the possible involvement of adrenergic agents on ICAM-1 expression. Treatment with propranolol (β_1/β_2-adrenergic antagonist) and butoxamine (β_2-adrenergic antagonist), but not atenolol (β_1-adrenergic antagonist) reversed this inhibitory effect. Isoproterenol also dose-dependently stimulated cAMP production (assayed by RIA) by HBMEC; propranolol treatment abolished this effect. These data show that the β_2-adrenergic receptor/cAMP pathway may be partly involved in TNFα-stimulated ICAM-1 expression and indicate the possible involvement of adrenergic mediation of capillary function including BBB integrity.

Keywords: ICAM-1; HBMEC; TNFα; adrenergic agents.

Introduction

Vascular endothelial cells are localized at the interface between blood and tissues and they contribute to maintenance of vascular homeostasis under normal conditions. The anatomical location of these cells also indicates their potential involvement in inflammatory reactions at sites of injury. Capillary and microvascular endothelial cells have significant roles in regulating blood-brain barrier (BBB) properties. Their functions involve restricting access of circulating blood cells and other components to the central nervous system (CNS). Interestingly, these cells also possess the capacity to express HLA antigens and adhesion molecules, which permit or invite passage of cells across the BBB.

Extravasation of leukocytes from microvasculature at the sites of inflammation is controlled by a series of adhesion processes. These events rely on the expression of a range of adhesion proteins by vascular endothelial cells. In Multiple Sclerosis (MS), Experimental Allergic Encephalitis (EAE) and Stroke, adhesive interactions between endothelial cells and leukocytes are one of the steps involved in the pathogenic mechanism of the disease. Intercellular adhesion molecule-1 (ICAM-1) is a 90 kD surface glycoprotein, which is a member of the immunogloblin gene super-family. The relationship between ICAM-1 and EAE, MS and Stroke have previously been reported.

Tumor necrosis factor-alpha (TNFα) has also been implicated as one of the key factors in the pathogenesis of the above CNS diseases. It has been proposed that TNFα induces adhesion molecule expression on vascular endothelial cells and that this process facilitates leukocyte infiltration to the brain. In MS, TNFα is associated with progression of the disease [2]. In stroke, it has been shown that blocking TNFα activity with TNFα binding protein or anti-TNFα antibody reduces the ischemic lesion volume [6, 9].

It has been shown that adrenergic input participates in regulation of the BBB [3, 11]. Since adrenergic agents affect permeability of vessels [19], it is possible that adhesion molecule expression is likewise affected. In this study we investigated the effect of β-adrenergic agents on TNFα-induced ICAM-1 expression by human brain microvascular endothelial cells (HBMEC).

Materials and Methods

Endothelial Cell Cultures

HBMEC were isolated and cultivated as previously described [14]. All HBMEC cultures exhibited characteristic cobblestone appearance and determined to be >95% pure by immunocytochemistry using EC-specific anti-Factor VIII-related antigen (Accurate Chemical and Scientific Corp.; Westbury, NY). Cell cultures used for studies reported here were obtained from seven lines (6th–15th passage).

Chemicals and Treatment

HBMEC cultures were grown in 96-well microtiter plates for 24 hours at 37 °C in media alone or with indicated concentrations of recombinant TNFα (Endogen; Woburn, MA), isoproterenol (Research Biomedical International; Natick, MA), atenolol (Sigma; St. Louis, MO), butoxamine (Sigma) and propranolol (Research Biomedical International).

Enzyme-linked Immunosorbant Assay (ELISA)

ICAM-1 expression on HBMEC was quantified by enzyme-linked immunosorbant assay (ELISA), essentially as previously described [17]. Nonspecific binding sites were blocked using sheep IgG (Sigma) and cultures were sequentially incubated with 1:1000 anti-human ICAM-1 antibody (R&D Systems), 1:2000 biotinylated anti-mouse IgG (Sigma) and 1:3000 avidin-horseradish peroxidase (Sigma). All incubations were performed at 37 °C for 1 h and plates were washed 3 times with Dulbecco's phosphate buffer (PBS) containing 2% BSA after incubation with each of the above additions. The reaction was developed by adding phosphate-citrate buffer/0.004% O-phenylenediamine, 0.012% H_2O_2 25 °C, 30 min) and stopped by adding 4 N HCl. Background values (cells incubated with 2% BSA added PBS in lieu of primary antibody) for each condition were subtracted from experimental values (identical cultures incubated with primary antibody).

Assay of cAMP Production

Formation of cAMP were assayed as described by Karnushina *et al.* [5]. Briefly, the HBMEC harvested, homogenized and centrifuged. The supernatants were mixed with 10 mM phosphocreatine, 60 U/ml phosphocreatine kinase, 0.1 mM GTP, 2 mM $MgCl_2$ in 40 mM Tris HCl containing 2 mM NaCl and 1.5 mM 3-isobutylmethyl-1-xanthine (IBMX) and incubated at 37 °C. The reaction was initiated by adding 3 mM ATP and stopped after 10 min by heating samples to 95 °C for 10 min. cAMP was assayed in the supernatant using the cAMP-dependent regulatory subunit for protein kinase derived from beef heart in the presence of $[^3H]$cAMP. Protein was determined by the method of Lowry *et al.* [7].

Statistical Analysis

Results are presented as mean ± S.E.M. percent of control or percent above control. All data were analyzed by one-way analysis of variance (ANOVA) with Fisher's protected least squares difference (PLSD). $p < 0.05$ was considered to be a statistically significant difference. Statview 5 (Abacus Concepts, Berkeley, CA) was used for analysis.

Results

Effect of β-Adrenergic Agents on Constitutive ICAM-1 Expression

All HBMEC cultures constitutively expressed relatively low levels of ICAM-1. Various concentrations of isoproterenol [β-adrenergic receptor (AR) agonist], propranolol (non-specific β1/β2-AR antagonist), butoxamine (β2-AR antagonist) and atenolol (β1-AR antagonist) had no significant effect on constitutive ICAM-1 expression. This was true for all cultures incubated for different time intervals.

Effect of β-Adrenergic Agents on ICAM-1 Expression Induced by TNFα

Incubation with 10–200 U/ml TNFα dose-dependently increased ICAM-1 expression on cultured HBMEC as quantitated by ELISA. ICAM-1 expression was observed as early as 4–6 h after treatment with TNFα; maximal expression was seen after 24 h in the presence of 50 U/ml TNFα. Unless stated otherwise, these conditions were used to examine the effect of adrenergic agents.

In experiments investigating the effects of β-adrenergic stimulation on TNFα-induced ICAM-1 expression, HBMEC were treated with isoproterenol, propranolol, atenolol, and/or butoxamine for 30 min prior to the addition of TNFα. As shown in Fig. 1, isoproterenol (1 μM) significantly reduced ICAM-1 expression stimulated by 25 and 50 U/ml TNFα. Similar levels of inhibition were observed in cultures incubated with 10 μM isoproterenol. The concomitant treatment of these cultures with propranolol prevented the isoproterenol-induced down-regulation of ICAM-1 expression (Table 1). The same effect was observed with butoxamine but not with atenolol. Interestingly, the level of upregulated ICAM-1 expression on HBMEC stimulated with high doses of TNFα (i.e., 100 U/ml) were also inhibited by 10 μM isoproterenol (422 ± 32% vs. 357 ± 27%, respectively) but the differences were not statistically significant.

Effect of β-Adrenergic Agents on cAMP Production

Under normal conditions, cultured HBMEC produced varying levels of cAMP. Isoproterenol (1 μM) increased cAMP formation in HBMEC (2.5-fold above control). Incubation with either 10 μM propra-

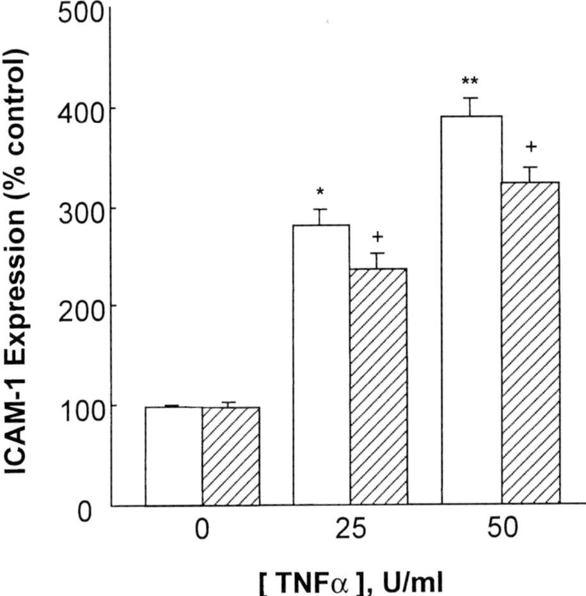

Fig. 1. The effect of isoproterenol on TNFα-induced ICAM-1 ex pression by human brain microvascular endothelial cells (HBMEC). HBMEC were cultured in the absence (open bars) or presence (hatched bars) of 1 μM isoproterenol for 24 h. ICAM-1 expressed was assessed by ELISA as described in the Methods section. Results are presented as mean ± S.E.M. percent of control (HBMEC incubated in media alone) from 8 to 10 experiments, performed in triplicate. All data were analyzed by one-way analysis of variance (ANOVA) with Fisher's protected least squares difference. * $p < 0.0001$ vs control; ** $p < 0.0005$ vs 25 U/ml TNFα; + $p < 0.005$ identical concentration of TNFα alone

Table 1. *Effect of β-Adrenergic Antagonists and Isoproterenol on TNFα-induced ICAM-1 Expression*

Treatment[1]	% Above control[2]	% Inhibition[3]
TNFα alone	161 ± 3	–
TNFα + ISO	128 ± 3	20.5 ± 1.7
TNFα + ISO + PRO	163 ± 4	−1.2 ± 2.5
TNFα + ISO + BTX	158 ± 6	1.9 ± 3.7
TNFα + ISO + ATN	121 ± 9	24.8 ± 4.9

[1] HBMEC cultures were incubated for 24 h in the presence of TNFα (50 U/ml) alone or with isoproterenol (ISO, 1 μM) and either propranolol (PRO, 10 μM), butoxamine (BTX, 10 μM), atenolol (ATN, 10 μM) or no addition.
[2] The data are presented as percent above control (% AC) according to the formula: [(OD exp – OD control)/OD control]×100 (%); control values for non-treated HBMEC were 0.640 ± 0.047 OD and for TNFα were 1.670 ± 0.057. All data represent the mean ± S.E.M. of 8 to 10 experiments, performed in triplicate.
[3] % Inhibition was calculated by the formula: [(% Above Control TNFα – (% AC exp)/% Above Control TNFα] × 100(%).

nolol or 25 U/ml TNFα did not significantly effect the levels of cAMP production. HBMEC cultures incubated in the presence of both isoproterenol and TNFα also exhibited high levels of cAMP (2-fold increase above control). These augmented levels of cAMP production in the presence of isoproterenol and TNFα were completely inhibited by pretreatment with propranolol (results not shown).

Discussion

As early as the 1970s, the noradrenergic (NA) innervation originating from locus ceruleus (LC) has been implicated in the regulation of cerebrovascular functions, including BBB permeability [11]. Recent research supports the anatomical association of NA innervation and intraparenchymal blood vessels [3]. Direct evidence indicating a relationship between BBB permeability and the LC was documented by Sarmento *et al.* [13]. In addition, these authors demonstrated that increased BBB permeability by stimulated LC could be augmented by pretreatment with β-adrenergic antagonists. The permeability of cultured cerebromicrovascular endothelium has also been shown to be affected by β_2-adrenergic agonists [1]. The data presented here demonstrate that pretreatment with isoproterenol modulated TNFα-induced ICAM-1 expression. This effect involved the β_2-adrenergic receptors and suggested that regulation BBB permeability and adhesion molecule expression may involve similar mechanisms.

It is known that endothelial β-adrenergic receptors coupled to adenyl cyclase via G-proteins affect cAMP production through activation of protein kinase A (PKA). Previous work reported the possible association of cAMP and PKA with expression of adhesion molecules. Jordan *et al.* reported that accumulation of cAMP in human umbilical vein endothelial cells (HUVEC) reduced ELAM and VCAM-1 (but not ICAM-1) expression induced by TNFα [10]. Treatment with dibutyryl cAMP, a cAMP analogue, enhanced ICAM-1 expression induced by IL-1 on rat heart endothelial cells [18]. In these studies, it was shown that a PKA inhibitor reduced the IL-1-upregulated expression of ICAM-1. In contrast, Sung *et al.* demonstrated that TNFα stimulated ICAM-1 expression on HUVEC was reduced by PKC inhibitor, but not PKA inhibitor [16]. Also, Renkonen *et al.* reported that cAMP did not induce ICAM-1 expression on HUVEC [12]. The discrepancies in these reports may be due to several factors including cell type and origin, cytokine treatment and kinetics. It is not surprising that similar cells obtained from different organs respond differently to identical treatment [8, 19]. Even cells derived from the same species and organ showed different events based on age [15] or vessel size [14].

In the experiments reported here, a difference was observed between the effect of isoproterenol on cells incubated in the presence or absence of TNFα. Pretreatment with isoproterenol reduced TNFα-induced ICAM-1 expression but had little or no significant effect on the constitutive level of ICAM-1 expression. These results indicated the possibility of different control systems for constitutive and TNFα-stimulated ICAM-1 expression. The mechanism(s) responsible for ICAM-1 expression are still unclear, but it has been reported that constitutive ICAM-1 expression occurs through a mechanism distinct from stress-induced ICAM-1 expression [4]. The present observation that isoproterenol increased cAMP production, regardless of the presence of TNFα, also suggests that the expression of constitutive and TNFα-induced ICAM-1 expression might be regulated by different pathways.

In conclusion, the data indicate the potential participation of the β_2-adrenergic receptor pathway in the regulation of TNFα-stimulated ICAM-1 expression on human brain microvascular endothelial cells. The findings also suggest a possible role for cAMP in this response. Most importantly, these results implicate adrenergic mediation in the regulation of microvascular endothelial responses, which includes the function of the BBB.

References

1. Borges N, Shi F, Azevedo I, Audus KL (1994) Changes in brain microvessel endothelial cell monolayer permeability induced by adrenergic drugs. Eur J Pharmacol 269: 243–248
2. Burger D, Lou J, Dayer JM, Grau GE (1997) Both soluble and membrane-associated TNF active brain microvascular endothelium: relevance to multiple sclerosis. Mol Psychiatry 2: 113–116
3. Cohen Z, Molinatti G, Hamel E (1997) Astroglial and vascular interactions of noradrenaline terminals in the rat cerebral cortex. J Cereb Blood Flow Metab 17: 894–904
4. Jahnke A, Van de Stolpe A, Caldenhoven E, Johnson JP (1995) Constitutive expression of human intercellular adhesion molecule-1 (ICAM-1) is regulated by differentially active enhancing and silencing elements. Eur J Biochem 228: 439–446
5. Karnushina I, Spatz M, Bembry J (1983) Cerebral endothelial cell culture II. Adenylate cyclase response to prostaglandins and their interaction with the adrenergic system. Life Sci 32: 1427–1435
6. Lavine SD, Hofman FM, Zlokovic BV (1998) Circulating antibody against tumor necrosis factor-alpha protects rat brain from reperfusion injury. J Cereb Blood Flow Metab 18: 52–58
7. Lowry OH, Rosenbough NU, Farr AL, Randall RJ (1951) Protein measurement with the folin phenol reagent. J Biol Chem 193: 265–275
8. McCarron RM, Wang L, Stanimirovic DB, Spatz M (1995) Differential regulation of adhesion molecule expression by human cerebrovascular and umbilical vein endothelial cells. Endothelium 2: 339–346
9. Nawashiro H, Tasaki K, Ruetzler CA, Hallenbeck JM (1997) TNF-alpha pretreatment induces protective effects against focal cerebral ischemia in mice. J Cereb Blood Flow Metab 17: 483–490
10. Pober JS, Slowik MR, De Luca LG, Ritchie AJ (1993) Elevated cyclic AMP inhibits endothelial cell synthesis and expression of TNF-induced endothelial leukocyte adhesion molecule-1, and vascular cell adhesion molecule-1, but not intercellular adhesion molecule-1. J Immunol 150: 5114–5123
11. Raichle M, Hartman BK, Echling JO, Sharpe LG (1975) Central noradrenergic regulation of cerebral blood flow and vascular permeability. Proc Nat Acad Sci (USA) 72: 3726–3730
12. Renkonen R, Mennander A, Ustinov J, Mattila P (1990) Activation of protein kinase C is crucial in the regulation of ICAM-1 expression on endothelial cells by interferon-gamma. Int Immunol 2: 719–724
13. Sarmento A, Borges N, Lima D (1994) Influence of electrical stimulation of locus coeruleus on the rat blood-brain barrier permeability to sodium fluorescein. Acta Neurochir (Wien) 127: 215–219
14. Spatz M, Kawai N, Merkel N, Bembry J, McCarron RM (1997) Functional properties of cultured endothelial cells derived from large microvessels of human brain. Am J Physiol 272: C231–239
15. Stins MF, Gilles F, Kim KS (1997) Selective expression of adhesion molecules on human brain microvascular endothelial cells. J Neuroimmunol 76: 81–90
16. Sung CP, Arleth AJ, Nambi P (1994) Evidence for involvement of protein kinase C in expression of intracellular adhesion molecule-1 (ICAM-1) by human vascular endothelial cells. Pharmacology 48: 143–146
17. Tanaka M, McCarron RM (1990) The inhibitory effect of tumor necrosis factor and interleukin-1 on Ia induction by interferon-gamma on endothelial cells from murine central nervous system. J Neuroimmunol 27: 209–215
18. Turunen JP, Ustinov J, Renkonen R (1993) Adhesion molecules involved in protein kinase A- and C-dependent lymphocyte adherence to microvascular endothelial cells. Scand J Immunol 37: 282–288
19. Zink S, Rosen P, Lemoine H (1995) Micro- and macrovascular endothelial cells in β-adrenergic regulation of transendothelial permeability. Am J Physiol 269: C1209–1218

Correspondence: Maria Spatz, M.D., National Institutes of Health, NINDS, Stroke Branch, 36 Convent Drive, MSC 4128, Bethesda, Maryland 20892-4128.

Acta Neurochir (2000) [Suppl] 76: 121–124

Time Course of Apoptotic Cell Death After Experimental Neurotrauma

M. Barth, L. Schilling, and **P. Schmiedek**

Department of Neurosurgery, Division of Neurosurgical Research, University Hospital Mannheim, Faculty of Clinical Medicine Mannheim, University Heidelberg, Mannheim, Germany

Summary

Traumatic or ischemic brain injury may give rise to the development of secondary brain damage. In the present study the time course of TUNEL staining which is widely used to delineate apoptotic reaction pattern was followed after experimental neurotrauma in order to test the hypothesis that apoptotic cell death may be involved in the development of secondary brain damage. Neurotrauma was induced in male Wistar rats by applying a cold probe to the exposed dura over the temporo-parietal cortex. Animals were sacrificed between 1 and 72 hours after trauma and coronal sections prepared from the lesioned area and adjacent tissue. The TUNEL staining was employed to detect DNA-fragmentation and conventional HE staining of sequential slices to delineate the extent of the lesion. Occurrence of positively stained cells was detected by a computer-based quantification system and stored on hard disk. TUNEL-positive nuclei were observed as early as one hour after lesion and peaked at 3 hours. There after, the number of cells detected decreased steadily. Histological examination revealed two different types of morphology in TUNEL-positive cells. A small proportion termed type I-cells displayed additional signs of apoptotic cell death such as nuclear condensation and fragmentation while type-II were considered to undergo necrotic cell death. Thus, TUNEL staining proved to be an unspecific marker of apoptotic cell death in the present study. Nevertheless, the data suggest that apoptotic cell death does not contribute substantially to the final extent of cold induced brain tissue damage.

Keywords: Apoptotic cell death; TUNEL staining; cold lesion; secondary brain damage.

Introduction

Traumatic brain injury may give rise to the development of secondary brain damage which reflects cell death occurring with a latency of hours or even days after trauma. Similar events may take place after brain ischemia. Although necrosis may be considered the most common avenue of cell death under these conditions [7], cells may also contribute to their own death when certain genetic programs become activated. This avenue called apoptosis is considered a physiological event in the developement of the central nervous system (for review see Naruse and Keino [13]). Interestingly, apoptotic cell death may also occur in adult brain under pathological conditions including ischemia [3, 8, 10] and trauma [14, 20]. However, the exact contribution of apoptotic cell death to secondary brain damage is still under discussion.

Apoptotic cell death differs from necrosis by reaction patterns resulting in DNA fragmentation [6, 11]. Several approaches to delineate apoptotic cell death are based upon the occurrence of DNA fragmentation. The TUNEL (terminal transferase mediated d-UTP nick end labeling) technique originally described by Gavrieli *et al.* [2] labelling the free 3‘ OH-ends of strand breaks has been widely used as an indicator of apoptosis. Additional approaches include detection of ultrastructural alterations by electron microscopy and biochemical techniques such as DNA-laddering [14, 20]. Among these approaches, TUNEL-staining is probably the most commonly used technique for investigating apoptotic cell death. In the present study this technique was adopted to follow the time course of apoptotic cell death using the standardized cold lesion model of brain trauma. This model has previously been shown to display a delayed growth of necrosis beween 12 and 24 h after injury [1].

Materials and Methods

Induction of Cold Injury

Cold injury was induced in male Wistar rats (250 g–300 g body weight [b.w.]) kept on a 12 h light/dark schedule. All experiments were performed in accord ance with the Institutional Animal Care and Use Guidelines. After induction of anesthesia (chloralhydrate, 3.6%; 1 ml/100 g b. w. i. p.), the head was fixed in a frame and a midline incision made over the skull. The exposed skullbone was cleared from adhering tissue over the right parietal cortex and a circular craniotomy (diameter, 6 mm) created by use of a high speed drill. Continuous cooling was performed by flushing with saline throughout drilling. The excised bone flap was removed with special care not to damage the dura and underlying cortex. Cold injury was produced by a copper probe (5 mm in diameter) cooled to −70 °C by a mixture of dry ice/acetone as described previously [5, 15]. The precooled probe was inflicted through the cranial burr hole to a depth 2 mm below the dural surface. After 10 sec the copper probe was removed, xylocaine 2% applied subcutaneously around the wound for local anaesthesia and the skin sutured. Animals were returned to their cages and allowed to recover with food and tap water available *ad lib.* Survival periods were 1, 2, 3, 6, 9, 12, 24, 36, 48 and 72 h, respectively.

Tissue Preparation

At the end of the survival periods animals were reanaesthetized with chloralhydrate and prepared for *in situ* perfusion fixation. Briefly, the abdominal aorta was exposed and cannulated with a polyethylene tubing (outer diameter, 1.27 mm). After disruption of the inferior vena cava perfusion with paraformaldehyde (PFA, 2%) dissolved in phosphate-buffered saline (PBS) was commenced. Initial perfusion pressure was set to 180 mmHg and decreased to 120 mmHg after 90 sec followed by another 180 sec perfusion period with 18% sucrose in PBS. Brains were then carefully removed and stored overnight in 18% sucrose solution at 4 °C for cryoprotection. Coronal tissue slabs (2 mm thickness) were obtained through the center of the lesion and in a distance of 2 and 4 mm in rostral and caudal directions, respectively. Tissues were frozen in prechilled isopentan and stored at −80 °C until use.

Histochemical and TUNEL Staining

From each tissue slab, sequential cryosections (5 μm thickness) were cut for standard haematoxylin/eosin (HE) and TUNEL staining. For the latter, sections were dried on air, rehydrated in 0.1% PBS and then incubated in a humid chamber for 1 h at 37 °C with a cocktail containing per brain slice: 36.4 μl sterile water (with 0.5% Triton X-100), 10 μl reaction buffer, 1 μl terminal transferase (25 U), 2 μl CoCl (25 mM), 0.3 μl fluorescein-11-dUTP (1 mM), 0.3 μl dATP (100 mM). After incubation sections were rinsed several times with Tris-buffer (10 mM) containing 1 mM EDTA followed by washes with PBS. Staining procedures with omission of terminal transferase or fluorescein-11-dUTP were performed for control and yielded negative results throughout (data not shown). Slices were then incubated with the TUNEL-POD kit according to the instructions supplied by the manufacturer, and visualisation of fluorescein-11-dUTP was achieved by addition of diaminobenzidine (DAB). Reaction was stopped by intensive rinsing with PBS, sections were dehydrated and coverslipped with Eukitt. Slices were viewed using a Leica microscope (DMRBG, Leica, Bensheim, Germany) with a ×10 magnification. Using a computer-controlled microscopical stage the slices were scanned and stored on hard disk. Detection of TUNEL-positive nuclei was performed using a threshold operator function supplied by the Quantimet Q600 system (Leica, Cambridge, England). The number of nuclei detected in each microscopic field was counted, stored in an extra file on hard disk and the total number calculated after scanning the total lesion area and the adjacent tissue.

Chemicals

Terminal transferase, reaction buffer, CoCl, TUNEL-POD kit from Boehringer Mannheim (Mannheim, Germany); Fluorescein-11-dUTP from Amersham (Little Chalfont, England); dATP and Triton X-100 from Sigma (Deisenhofen, Germany; St. Louis, USA.); Tris-buffer, EDTA and all other chemicals of analytical grade from Merck (Darmstadt, Germany).

Results

Screening of the slices revealed a strictly localized distribution of TUNEL-positive nuclei at each time point. Comparison with the sequential HE-stained slices showed accumulation of TUNEL-positive cells in and adjacent to the brain lesion. Occurrence of TUNEL-positive nuclei started as early as 1 h after lesion, increased dramatically and peaked at 3 hours after cold injury. Thereafter a steady decrease of the number of TUNEL-stained nuclei was observed (Fig. 1). Even at time points later than 3 days after trauma no secondary increase of the number of TUNEL-positive nuclei was observed (data not shown).

Careful histological examination of the TUNEL-positive cells strongly suggested the presence of two different types of morphological response. The Type-I cells displayed features of apoptotic cell death in addition to TUNEL staining, including nuclear condensation and fragmentation and occasionally formation of apoptotic bodies (Fig. 2, left). In contrast, Type-II cells were round, not condensated, and furthermore

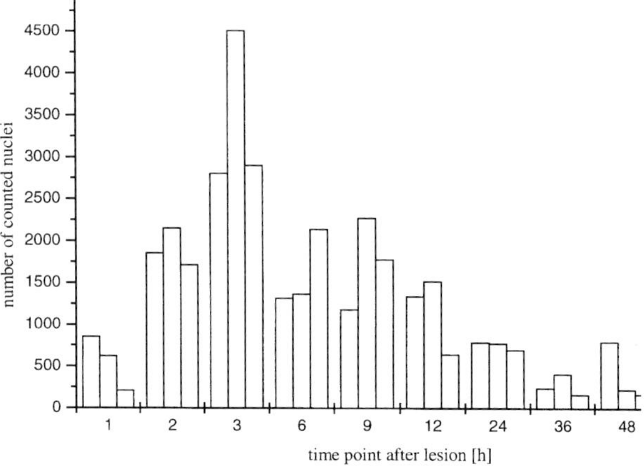

Fig. 1. Temporal distribution of TUNEL-stained nuclei from 1 to 72 h after cold-lesion. Coronal slices were cut through the center of each lesion and the TUNEL-positive nuclei detected by an individually adjusted threshold operator. Given is the total number of nuclei in the lesioned area. Each bar represents data obtained from an individual experiment.

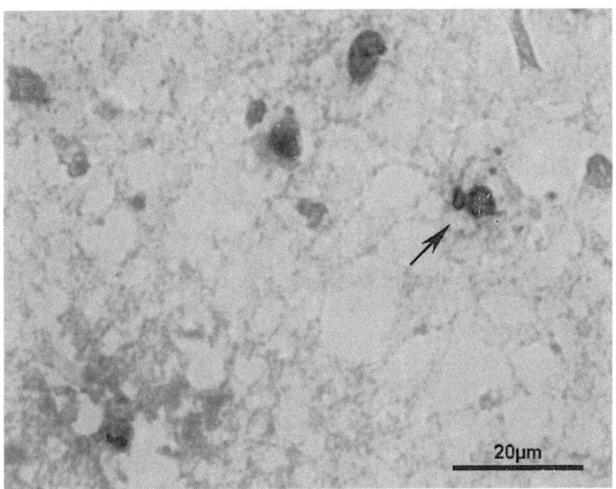

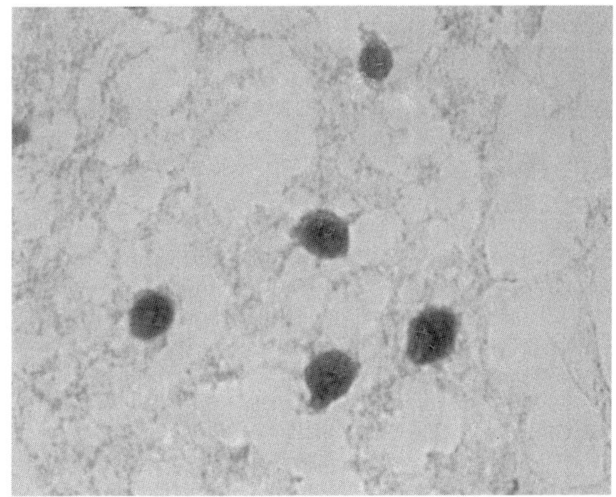

Fig. 2. Histological examination of TUNEL-stained slices after induction of cold-injury. In the section shown on the left side a TUNEL-stained cell exhibiting additional signs of apoptosis such as condensation and fragmentation of the nucleus is depicted. In the section on the right side TUNEL-stained cells which do not exhibit additional signs of apoptosis are shown. These cells are considered to undergo necrotic cell death.

did not show signs of fragmentation (Fig. 2, right). At all time points the relative amount of Type-I cells observed was very small, never exceeding 1% of all nuclei detected.

Discussion

In the present study cold injury inflicted directly to the exposed brain tissue was employed as an experimental model of brain trauma. The cold lesion model was introduced by Klatzo [9], and since then it has been widely used to study pathophysiological consequences of brain trauma including alterations of vasomotor responses [4, 18], occurrence and regression of brain edema [16] and the mechanisms underlying the development of secondary brain tissue damage as reviewed elsewhere [19]. Recently delayed growth of brain damage after cold lesion has been shown to occur between 12 and 24 h after trauma [1]. Using a different experimental model of brain trauma, Rink and coauthors [14] have previously provided evidence in favor of apoptotic cell death occurring in the cortex and subcortical regions after fluid percussion injury in rats. In this study, however, the peak of apoptotic activity appeared to occur beyond 24 hours after injury which is markedly later than the development of secondary brain damage observed beween 12 and 24 h after cold injury to the brain [1]. In the present study, occurrence of TUNEL-positive nuclei started as early as 1 h and displayed its maximum at 3 h after injury. Considering the discrepancy in the temporal profile of TUNEL staining and delayed growth of tissue necrosis [1] one may conclude that apoptotic cell death would not represent a major factor in the development of secondary brain damage.

However, the present results also show that two types of TUNEL-positive cells may be distinguished according to their morphological appearance. Type-I cells may be considered cells undergoing apoptotic death as suggested by nuclear condensation and fragmentation as well as by the presence of apoptotic bodies in addition to TUNEL-positive staining. In contrast, Type-II cells did not display any of these signs suggesting necrotic rather than apoptotic cell death taking place. A significant number of apparently necrotic cells detected by TUNEL staining has also been described by Rink *et al.* [14] and by Murakami and coworkers [12]. However, in the latter study cold injury was induced through the intact skull of mice. Similar to studies employing neurotrauma models, animal experiments in brain ischemia have also shown occurrence of TUNEL staining of necrotic cells. Thus, the meaning of TUNEL staining as a hallmark of apoptotic cell death has been questioned [12, 17].

In conclusion, TUNEL staining was found to be an unselective marker of apoptotic cell death in the present study. In addition, the results obtained indicate that apoptotic cell death may not be involved in the pathophysiological sequelae resulting in delayed neuronal cell death.

Acknowledgments

This paper contains data which are part of the dissertation of M. Barth.

References

1. Eriskat J, Schürer L, Kempski O, Baethmann A (1994) Growth kinetics of a primary brain tissue necrosis from a focal lesion. Acta Neurochir [Suppl] (Wien) 60: 425–427
2. Gavrieli Y, Sherman Y, Ben-Sasson SA (1992) Identification of programmed cell death in situ via specific labeling of nuclear DNA fragmentation. Cell Biol 119: 493–501
3. Gillardon F, Lenz C, Kuschinsky W, Zimmerman M (1996) Evidence for apoptotic cell death in the choroid plexus following focal cerebral ischemia. Neurosci Lett 207: 113–116
4. Görlach C, Benyó Z, Wahl M (1998) Reduced reactivity of the middle cerebral artery and its large branches after cold lesion. J Neurotrauma 15: 1067–1075
5. Görlach C, Sirén AL, Knerlich F, Feger G, Fricke A, Barth M, Schilling L, Ehrenreich H, Wahl M (1998) Delayed loss of ET_B receptor-mediated vasorelaxation after cold lesion of the rat parietal cortex. J Cereb Blood Flow Metab 18: 1357–1364
6. Hockenbery D (1995) Defining apoptosis. Am J Pathol 146: 16–19
7. Hutchins JB, Barger SW (1998) Why neurons die: cell death in the nervous system. Anat Rec 253: 79–90
8. Islam N, Aftabuddin M, Moriwaki A, Hori Y (1995) Detection of DNA damage induced by apoptosis in the rat brain following incomplete ischemia. Neurosci Lett 188: 159–162
9. Klatzo I, Piraux A, Laskowski EJ (1958) The relationship between edema, blood-brain barrier and tissue elements in a local brain injury. J Neuropathol Exp Neurol 17: 548–564
10. Li Y, Sharov VG, Jiang N, Zaloga C, Sabbah HN, Chopp M (1995) Ultrastructural and light microscopic evidence of apoptosis after middle cerebral artery occlusion in the rat. Am J Pathol 146: 1045–1051
11. Majno G, Joris I (1995) Apoptosis, oncosis, and necrosis. An overview of cell death. Am J Pathol 146: 3–15
12. Murakami K, Kondo T, Sato S, Li Y, Chan PH (1997) Occurrence of apoptosis following cold injury-induced brain edema in mice. Neuroscience 81: 231–237
13. Naruse I, Keino H (1995) Apoptosis in the developing CNS. Prog Neurobiol 47: 135–155
14. Rink A, Fung K-M, Trojanowski JQ, Lee VM-Y, Neugebauer E, McIntosh TK (1995) Evidence of apoptotic cell death after experimental traumatic brain injury in the rat. Am J Pathol 147: 1575–1583
15. Schilling L, Wahl M (1994) Effects of antihistaminics on experimental brain edema. Acta Neurochir [Suppl] (Wien) 60: 79–82
16. Stummer W, Götz C, Hassan A, Heimann A, Kempski O (1993) Kinetics of photofrin II in perifocal brain edema. Neurosurgery 33: 1075–1082
17. van Lookeren Campagne M, Gill R (1996) Ultrastructural morphological changes are not characteristic of apoptotic cell death following focal cerebral ischaemia in the rat. Neurosci Lett 213: 111–114
18. Vinas FC, Dujovny M, Hodgkinson D (1995) Early hemodynamic changes at the microcirculatory level and effects of mannitol following focal cryogenic injury. Neurol Res 17: 465–468
19. Wahl M, Schilling L, Unterberg A, Baethmann A (1993) Mediators of vascular and parenchymal mechanisms in secondary brain damage. Acta Neurochir [Suppl] (Wien) 57: 64–72
20. Xu RX, Nakamura T, Nagao S, Miyamoto O, Jin L, Toyoshima T, Itano T (1998) Specific inhibition of apoptosis after cold-induced brain injury by moderate postinjury hypothermia. Neurosurgery 43: 107–115

Correspondence: Lothar Schilling, M.D., Ph.D., Department of Neurosurgery, Division of Neurosurgical Research, University Clinic Mannheim, Faculty of Clinical Medicine Mannheim, University Heidelberg, Theodor Kutzer-Ufer 1-3, D-68135 Mannheim, Germany.

Acta Neurochir (2000) [Suppl] 76: 125–129

The Permissive Nature of Blood Brain Barrier (BBB) Opening in Edema Formation Following Traumatic Brain Injury

A. Beaumont[1], **A. Marmarou**[1], **K. Hayasaki**[1], **P. Barzo**[1], **P. Fatouros**[2], **F. Corwin**[2], **C. Marmarou**[2], and **J. Dunbar**[1]

[1] Division of Neurosurgery, Medical College of Virginia, Richmond, VA, USA
[2] Division of Radiation Physics, Medical College of Virginia, Richmond, VA, USA

Summary

The contribution of blood brain barrier opening to traumatic brain edema is not known. This study compares the course of traumatic BBB disruption and edema formation, with the hypothesis that they are not obligately related. Sprague-Dawley rats were divided into three groups: Group A ($n = 47$) – Impact Acceleration (IAM); Group B ($n = 104$) – lateral cortical impact (CCI); Group C ($n = 26$) – IAM + hypoxia & hypotension (THH). BBB integrity was assessed using iv markers (Evan's Blue, or gadolinium-DTPA). Edema formation was evaluated with gravimetry, and T1-weighted MRI.

In IAM, BBB opened immediately but closed rapidly, and remained closed for at least the next 36 hours whilst 24-hour hemispheric water content (HWC) rose by 0.9% ($p < 0.01$). In CCI, BBB opened in both hemispheres for up to 4 hours; four hour HWC in the uninjured hemisphere was indistinguishable from Sham, where HWC in the injured hemisphere rose by ~1.5% ($p < 0.005$). We distinguished two THH animals based on Apparent Diffusion Coefficient (ADC) recovery: in ADC-recovery animals 4 hour cortical water content (CWC) was 80.4 ± 0.6%, cf 81.4 ± 1.3% in ADC-non-recovery ($p < 0.05$). In all animals the BBB was open, however two populations of permeability were seen which likely related to flow-limited extravasation of gadolinium.

In IAM edema forms despite only brief BBB opening. Although there is diffuse BBB opening with lateral contusion, edema only forms in the injured hemisphere. In THH, edema formation in the face of a widely permeable barrier is driven by ADC changes or cell swelling. Edema formation clearly does not correspond with BBB opening and an open BBB is clearly not required for edema formation. However we hypothesize that a permeable BBB permissively worsens the process, by acting as a low resistance pathway for ion and water movement. These findings are consistent with our general hypothesis that edema formation after TBI is mainly cytotoxic.

Keywords: Traumatic brain injury; secondary insult; blood-brain barrier; cell swelling.

Introduction

The contribution of blood brain barrier leakage to cerebral edema formation following traumatic brain injury remains questionable. Recent studies in this laboratory have defined that cytotoxic swelling is the predominant type of edema following Impact Acceleration Injury [2] and other studies have shown similar results considering cortical contusion [9]. However it is important to recognise that movement of water into cells with cell swelling alone is insufficient to cause the increase in tissue water associated with edema formation. This phenomenon demands that water and ions enter the tissue from an external source. An increase in BBB permeability may therefore provide a route for fluid shifts to occur, where the driving force remains cellular swelling. In this case, BBB permeability would be a passive contributor to cytotoxic edema.

The aim of this study was therefore to compare the time-courses of BBB opening and edema formation in three models of TBI, and to draw conclusions about the role of the BBB in the swelling process, based on the pattern of observed relationships.

Methods

Adult male Sprague-Dawley rats weighing 340–400 g were divided into three groups. Group A ($n = 47$) were subjected to the Impact Acceleration injury; Group B ($n = 104$) were subjected to cortical contusion and Group C ($n = 26$) were subjected to Impact Acceleration with a 30 minute secondary insult of hypoxia and hypotension. An assessment of blood brain barrier integrity and edema formation was made at differing time points following trauma. All animals used received humane care in compliance with the "Guide for the Care and Use of Laboratory Animals" (NIH Publication No. 86-23, 1985).

Impact Acceleration was performed as described in detail previously [7]. Briefly, animals were anesthetised using 1–2% halothane in a mixture of 66% N_2O and 33% O_2. A 10 mm diameter, 2 mm deep stainless steel disk was mounted on the skull using rapid drying

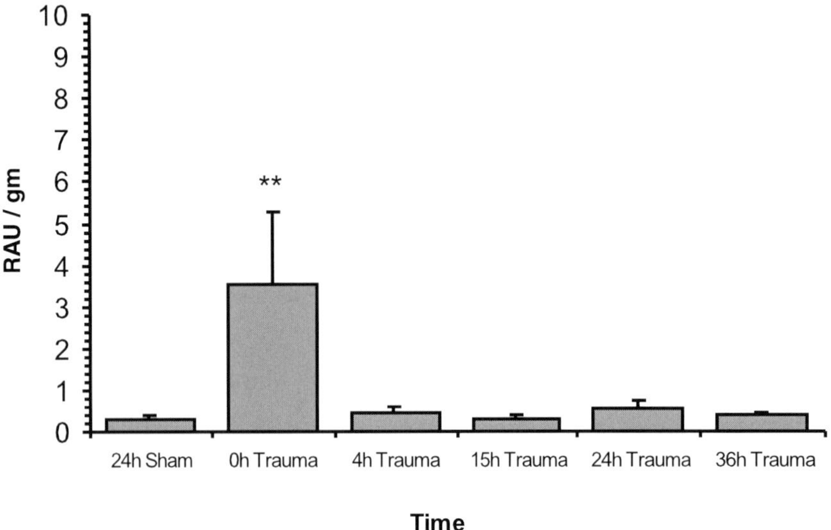

Fig. 1. Time course of blood brain barrier opening following Impact Acceleration Injury. All values are mean RAU/gm $\pm$ SEM. ** $p < 0.001$ cf sham injured animals

cyanoacrylic glue and a sectioned brass weight of 450 g was dropped from a height of 2 m onto the center of the disk.

Cortical contusion was performed as described in detail previously [3]. Briefly, animals were anesthetised using 1–2% halothane in a mixture of 66% N_2O and 33% O_2. A 10 mm craniotomy was prepared over the parietal cortex to the right of midline and cortical contusion was induced using a constrained stroke pneumatic impactor which delivered a controlled cortical impact, at 6.0 m/sec to a depth of 3 mm. Immediately after injury the craniotomy site was sealed with the bone flap, gelfoam and rapid drying cyanoacrylic glue.

In group C, secondary insult was induced by reducing FiO_2 to 12% following trauma, and increasing halothane to 2% above baseline, for 30 minutes. The reduction in FiO_2 caused hypoxia and hypotension, and the increased halothane served to prevent cardiovascular inotropic and chronotropic compensation. This insult yields a stable and reproducible reduction in mABP to 30–40 mmHg, and paO_2 of 40 mmHg as described previously [11].

Blood brain barrier dynamics in groups A and B were assessed using intravenous infusion of the azo dye Evan's Blue. At selected time points a 2% solution of Evan's Blue (Fisher Scientific E515, New Jersey) in 0.9% NaCl was administered intravenously in a dose of 7 ml/kg. Dye was allowed to circulate for 30 minutes prior to sacrifice after which dye was leached from cerebral tissue in pure formamide and absorbance of the solvent measured against a standard at 625 nm using a Shimadzu UV1600 Spectrophotometer (Shimadzu Instruments, Colombia, Maryland) [5]. The remaining brain tissue was then dried to constant weight in an oven at 95 °C. Data was then expressed as the relative absorbance (RAU) per gram of dry brain. BBB dysfunction was assessed in Group C using an intravenous injection of Gadolinium-DTPA (Omniscan, Nycomed, New Jersey), followed by MR assessment of T1 signal intensity, as described previously [1]. Baseline images were acquired prior to infusion, and post-infusion images were then evaluated as a change in signal intensity. Gd-DTPA was injected shortly after injury, and measurement continued for up to 60 minutes post-injury.

Tissue water content was established at various time points by either microgravimetric analysis as described elsewhere [8] (Group A), or MRI assessment, utilizing a calculation described previously [4, 6] (Groups B & C). Statistical significance was assessed using unpaired and paired student's t-tests.

Results

Following Impact Acceleration an immediate and uniform opening of the BBB occurred (3.55 ± 1.7 RAU/gm, $p < 0.001$ c.f. Sham), which rapidly closed and became indistinguishable from sham at 4 hours after injury (Fig. 1). Cortical and caudate water content at 24 hours was $79.5 \pm 0.39\%$ and $78.4 \pm 0.29\%$ (Table 1) compared with $78.6 \pm 0.17\%$ and $77.9 \pm 0.19\%$ respectively in the sham group ($p < 0.01$). This data is consistent with a modest degree of swelling over the 24 hours following injury. Furthermore this swelling occurred despite the presence of an intact BBB.

Following cortical contusion (Group B) the BBB opened rapidly in both the injured (8.06 ± 0.7 RAU/gm, $p < 0.001$ c.f. Sham) and non-injured hemispheres (5.75 ± 0.93 RAU/gm, $p < 0.01$ c.f. Sham) (Fig. 2a, b). Over 4 hours there appeared to be a steady decline in BBB permeability in both hemispheres. At 24 hours, 3 days and 7 days after injury, there was residual BBB damage only in the injured hemisphere ($p < 0.05$ c.f. Sham).

Edema formation as assessed at 4 hours was confined to the injured hemisphere (Table 1), where cortical water content had increased by ~1.5% ($p < 0.005$). In the uninjured hemisphere, water content remained constant at 78.25% both before and

Table 1. *Edema Formation with Three Models of TBI, at Varying Time-Points. Values Represent Mean Percentage of Tissue Water ± Standard Deviation. * Significant Difference from Baseline Group* ($p < 0.01$). $^{\psi}$ *Significant Difference from ADC-Recovery Group* ($p < 0.05$)

Model	Region	Baseline	1 hour	4 hours	24 hours
Impact acceleration	cortex	78.6 ± 0.17	–	–	79.5 ± 0.39*
	caudate	77.9 ± 0.19	–	–	78.4 ± 0.29*
Cortical contusion	right hemisphere	78.05 ± 0.79	–	79.45 ± 1.0*	–
	left hemisphere	78.25 ± 0.63	–	78.25 ± 0.67	–
Impact acceleration + 2nd insult	cortex ADC-Recovery	79.38 ± 0.57	80.27 ± 0.92*	80.42 ± 0.60	–
	cortex ADC-NonRecovery	79.2 ± 0.90	80.55 ± 0.84*	81.40 ± 1.30$^{\psi}$	–

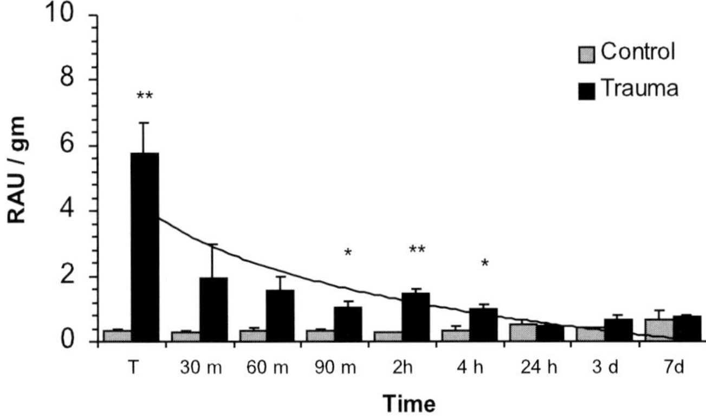

Fig. 2. Time course of blood brain barrier opening following unilateral cortical contusion, at varying time points (Trauma, 30 mins, 60 mins, 90 mins, 2 h, 4 h, 24 h, 3 d, 7 d). All values are mean RAU/gm ± SEM. Control values represent sham injured animals at each time point. (a) Ipsilateral hemisphere. (b) Contralateral hemisphere. * $p < 0.05$, ** $p < 0.01$, *** $p < 0.001$ cf sham injured animals

after injury. This occurred despite the marked opening in BBB observed in the contralateral hemisphere. Clearly, uninjured tissue can maintain a normal water content even in the face of a prolonged barrier opening.

In Group C (Impact Acceleration followed by secondary insult), two injury subgroups were observed based on the extent of recovery of early reductions in the Apparent Diffusion Coefficient (ADC). Water

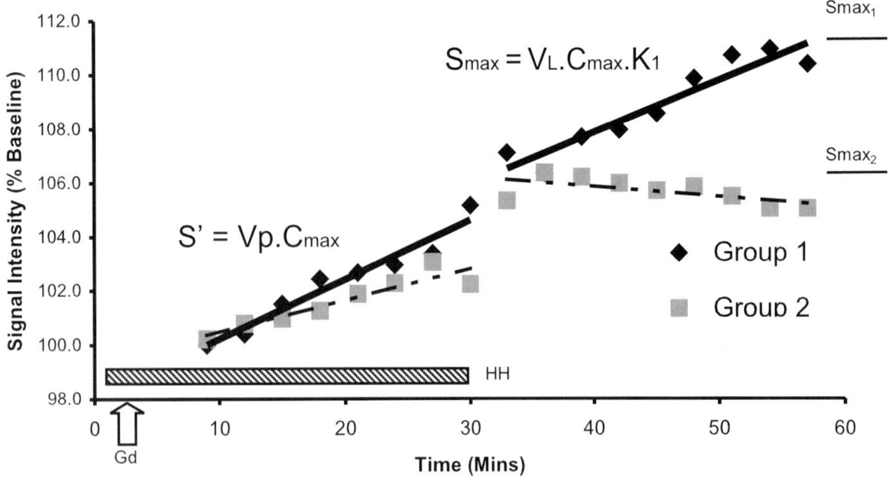

Fig. 3. Signal intensity changes in the presence of intravascular gadolinium-DTPA infused intravenously shortly after injury. Values expressed as a signal intensity percentage change. Lines represent regression lines calculated for the two distinct portions of gadolinium accumulation. S_{max} values are marked, as being the maximum signal intensity reached during testing. Annotated equations represent the interpretation of the kinetic analysis by Su *et al.* [10], where V_L is the leakage space of gadolinium, C_{max} is the peak plasma concentration reached, K_1 is the inward transfer coefficient for gadolinium (proportional to BBB permeability) and V_P is the volume of plasma for gadolinium distribution

content in the ADC-Recovery and ADC-Nonrecovery groups rose significantly and equally over the first hour after injury (Table 1, $p < 0.01$ c.f. control). Over the next three hours tissue water in the ADC-Nonrecovery group continued to increase, to a final value of $81.40\% \pm 1.30$ ($p < 0.05$ cf ADC-Recovery group) whereas the ADC-recovery group showed no further change.

IV infusion of gadolinium caused a marked increase in MR-T1-signal intensity, consistent with a deficient BBB (Fig. 3). There were two distinct populations of animals distinguishable based on the peak change in signal intensity; the slope of the initial signal intensity increase is approximately the same in both groups. Previous studies have determined that the initial slope is proportional to the product of plasma volume in the region of interest, and the peak plasma concentration of gadolinium [10]. The peak signal intensity increase is proportional to the product of the leakage volume, the peak plasma concentration of gadolinium and the transfer coefficient (a measure of BBB permeability). There are two possible explanations for the differences between the two groups. Firstly one group may have a much greater BBB permeability, and/or leakage space. However, it is notable that the changes in signal intensity coincide with the end of secondary insult, and restoration of cerebral blood flow (CBF). It is most likely that the transfer of gadolinium in this model is flow limited, and the differences between the groups represent a difference in the restoration of CBF. The only statement which can be made in this case is that barrier permeability is considerably greater than CBF.

If this assumption is correct, then BBB leakage is marked in both ADC-Recovery and ADC-Non-Recovery animals, and therefore the marked increase in tissue water seen in the ADC-NonRecovery group is a result of the difference in ADC values viz. a prolonged cellular swelling phase.

Discussion

This study has examined the time courses of BBB dysfunction and edema formation in three models of traumatic brain injury. In the first group (Impact Acceleration), BBB opening is brief and transitory, and yet over 24 hours there is a modest degree of edema formation. In the second group (Cortical Contusion), there is marked BBB dysfunction in both hemispheres; edema formation however is restricted to the hemisphere with contusion. Therefore edema does not accumulate in the uninjured hemisphere despite marked barrier permeability. In the third model (Impact Acceleration with Second Insult) water accumulation occurs to a greater extent in a subgroup showing a prolonged reduction in ADC. BBB disruption in this same model shows two groups of animals, with different kinetics of gadolinium movement. The differences in kinetics are likely related to flow limitations for gadolinium accumulation. Therefore despite BBB permeability, the cellular swelling is driving edema formation.

Considering the findings from these three models together, it is clear that increased BBB permeability is not a prerequisite for edema formation, although under such circumstances swelling is modest (viz. Impact acceleration). Equally the barrier can be open following injury, without a significant increase in tissue water (viz. contralateral hemisphere with cortical contusion). Finally, in the case of second insult where it appears there is widespread BBB permeability, then it is likely that the ADC changes and cellular swelling drives the swelling process.

These findings therefore suggest that BBB permeability represents a passive component of post-traumatic edema formation in these models of TBI. When the barrier is closed, than edema formation is modest. However when the barrier is open it acts as a low resistance pathway for the movement of water and ions into the tissue, probably driven by an increasing osmotic potential in the injured tissue as a result of breakdown of ionic homeostasis and cellular swelling.

References

1. Barzo P, Marmarou A, Fatouros P, Corwin F, Dunbar J (1996) Magnetic resonance imaging-monitored acute blood-brain barrier changes in experimental traumatic brain injury. J Neurosurg 85: 1113–1121
2. Barzo P, Marmarou A, Fatouros P, Hayasaki K, Corwin F (1997) Contribution of vasogenic and cellular edema to traumatic brain swelling measured by diffusion-weighted imaging. J Neurosurg 87: 900–907
3. Beaumont A, Marmarou A (1998) The effect of human corticotrophin releasing factor on the formation of post-traumatic cerebral edema. Acta Neurochir [Suppl] (Wien) 71: 149–152
4. Fatouros PP, Marmarou A, Kraft KA, Inao S, Schwarz FP (1991) In vivo brain water determination by T1 measurements: effect of total water content, hydration fraction, and field strength. Mag Res Med 17: 402–413
5. Ikeda Y, Wang M, Nakazawa S (1994) Simple quantitative evaluation of blood-brain barrier disruption in vasogenic brain edema. Acta Neurochir [Suppl] (Wien) 60: 119–120
6. Marmarou A, Fatouros P, Ward J, Appley A, Young H (1990) In vivo measurement of brain water by MRI. Acta Neurochir [Suppl] (Wien) 51: 123–124
7. Marmarou A, Foda MA, van den Brink W, Campbell J, Kita H, Demetriadou K (1994) A new model of diffuse brain injury in rats. Part I: pathophysiology and biomechanics. J Neurosurg 80: 291–300
8. Marmarou A, Poll W, Shulman K, Bhagavan H (1978) A simple gravimetric technique for measurement of cerebral edema. J Neurosurg 49: 530–537
9. Stroop R, Thomale UW, Pauser S, Bernarding J, Vollmann W, Wolf KJ, Lanksch WR, Unterberg AW (1998) Magnetic resonance imaging studies with cluster algorithm for characterization of brain edema after controlled cortical impact injury (CCII). Acta Neurochir [Suppl] (Wien) 71: 303–305
10. Su MY, Jao JC, Nalcioglu O (1994) Measurement of vascular volume fraction and blood-tissue permeability constants with a pharmacokinetic model: studies in rat muscle tumors with dynamic Gd-DTPA enhanced MRI. Mag Resonance Med 32: 714–724
11. Yamamoto M, Marmarou C, Stiefel M, Beaumont A, Marmarou A (1999) The neuroprotective effect of hypothermia on neuronal injury in diffuse traumatic brain injury coupled with hypoxia and hypotension. Neurotrauma (in press)

Correspondence: Anthony Marmarou, Division of Neurosurgery, P.O. Box, 508, MCV Station, Sanger Hall, Room 8004, 1101 E. Marshall Street, Richmond, Virginia 23298.

Acta Neurochir (2000) [Suppl] 76: 131–135

Endothelin-1 and Nitric Oxide Affect Human Cerebromicrovascular Endothelial Responses and Signal Transduction

Y. Chen[3], **R. M. McCarron**[1], **N. Azzam**[3], **J. Bembry**[3], **C. Reutzler**[3], **F. A. Lenz**[2], and **M. Spatz**[3]

[1] Naval Medical Research Center, Bethesda, MD
[2] Department of Neurosurgery, Johns Hopkins University School of Medicine, Baltimore, MD
[3] Stroke Branch, NINDS, NIH, Bethesda, MD

Summary

Endothelium plays a central role in regulating the vascular tone, blood flow and blood brain barrier (BBB) permeability. The experiments presented here examine the mechanisms by which nitric oxide (NO) and endothelin-1 (ET-1) may be involved in these processes. The findings indicate that ET-1-stimulated $[Ca^{2+}]_i$ accumulation occurs through activation of ET_A receptor. The capacity of NO to affect this response was indicated by results showing: 1) a two-fold increase in ET-1-stimulated $[Ca^{2+}]_i$ by L-NAME, the inhibitor of nitric oxide synthase, and 2) a dose-dependent decrease in $[Ca^{2+}]_i$ accumulation by pretreatment with Nor-1 (NO donor). Abrogation of this Nor-1 effect by ODQ (an inhibitor of guanylyl cyclase) or Rp-8-pCPT-cGMPS (an inhibitor of protein kinase G) and inhibition of ET-1 stimulated intracellular Ca^{2+} accumulation by 8-bromo-cGMP (a permeable, analog of cGMP) substantiate the involvement of interplay between ET-1 and NO in $[Ca^{2+}]_i$ accumulation in HBMEC. ET-1 treatment also increased thickness of F-actin cytoskeletal filaments in HBMEC. This effect was attenuated by pretreatment with NO; NO also rarefied F-actin filaments in control cultures. The findings support a linkage between NO and ET-1 in regulating microvascular tone, microcirculation and BBB permeability and indicate a role for cGMP/cGMP protein kinase system and cytoskeletal changes in responses of HBMEC.

Keywords: ET-1, NO, $[Ca^{2+}]_i$ mobilization; F-actin cytoskeleton.

Introduction

The vascular endothelium in central nervous system, as well as in the peripheral organs, plays a pivotal role in maintaining cerebrovascular functions. Through its capacity to produce and respond to various vasoactive substances, the endothelium possess an autocrine/paracrine ability to regulate cerebral blood flow, modulate vascular tone, and control blood brain barrier (BBB) permeability. Endothelin-1 (ET-1), the most potent vasoconstrictor produced by cerebromicrovascular endothelial cells [1] is found to be elevated in plasma and cerebrospinal fluid (CSF) in patients with ischemia, hypertension, head trauma, subarachnoid hemorrhage and vasospasm. In addition to ET-1, endothelium-derived nitric oxide (NO) is also an important mediator of vasodilation that controls vascular tone, cerebral blood flow and BBB permeability. Studies have shown that functional interaction between responses to both ET-1 and NO are involved in the overall response of the vasculature. *In vivo* administration of NO donors sodium nitroprusside or nitroglycerine through the CSF, rapidly reversed ET-1-induced cerebral vasoconstriction in rabbit basilar artery [18]. *In vitro* experiments, NO dissociates ET-1-receptor complex in CHO-ET cells and HBEC by reversibly modifying the affinity of the receptor to the ligand [5, 15]. Furthermore, it was shown that NO and ET-1 interaction involved calcium mobilization [12].

It is postulated that endothelial dysfunction in pathological conditions may be due to an imbalance between NO and ET-1 production. A possible consequence of such an imbalance may result in reduced concentrations of bioactive NO, thereby allowing the relatively unopposed actions of ET-1 to promote vasoconstriction. It is possible that such responses involve changes in cytoskeletal proteins. Enhanced actin polymerization during ischemic cell injury *in vivo* or in cell cultures has been described by many investigators [11]. However, more information is needed to fully understand the mechanisms regarding interaction of ET-1 and NO on intracellular signal transduction in cerebral endothelial cells. In this study, we utilized human brain microvascular endothelial cells (HBMEC) to characterize the ET-1-mediated signal transduction pathway leading to Ca^{2+} mobilization and the effect of NO on these responses. Additional experiments examined the effect of ET-1 and NO on cytoskeletal F-actin arrangements. The data indicate that the capacity of NO to prevent ET-1-stimulated $[Ca^{2+}]_i$ mobilization in HBMEC involves: 1) cGMP and cGMP-dependent protein kinase system; and 2) reorganization of cytoskeletal F-actin filaments.

Methods

Cell Culture

HBMEC used in this study were prepared as previously described [14]. Cultured cells were ≥98% Factor VIII-positive and virtually all cells incorporated acetylated low-density lipoprotein. Six cell lines (passages 7–15) derived from six different brains were grown to confluence on 1% gelatin-coated 24-well plates for 48 hours.

$[Ca^{2+}]_i$ Measurements

HBMEC were washed three times with solution containing NaCl (137 mM), KCl (5 mM), $MgCl_2$ (1 mM), sorbitol (25 mM), HEPES (10 mM), and $CaCl_2$ (3 mM), pH 7.0. After incubation of monolayers with 2.5 μM fluorescent probe Fluo-3/AM for 90 min at 37 °C, cells were washed three times. Fluorescence measurements were made using a fluorescence microplate reader (PerSeptive Biosystems, Framingham, MA, U.S.A.), with excitation wavelength 485 ± 10 nm and emission measured at 530 ± 10 nm. After recording the basal fluorescence value (F0), ET-1 was added and fluorescence was recorded at 30 sec. In some experiments, NOR-1 (NO donor, $T_{1/2} = 1.7$ min) was included for 1 min prior to the addition of ET-1. In indicated experiments, HBMEC were preincubated with ODQ or Rp-8-pCPT-cGMPs. Changes in $[Ca^{2+}]_i$ are expressed as fluorescence intensity ratio recorded as: [experimental fluorescence value (F) – basal fluorescence value (F0)]/F0 × 100%; ET-1-stimulated fluorescence change was taken as 100%.

F-Actin Staining

HBMEC cultured on coverslips were stimulated with ET-1 and/or NOR-1 as described above. After aspirating the medium, cell cultures were immediately fixed in 3.7% formaldehyde at room temperature for 10 min, and permeabilized by 0.1% Triton X-100 for 5 min. Cells were then incubated with 1% BSA for 20 min to block non-specific binding, followed by 1 unit of Texas Red-phalloidin for 20 min in the dark to stain F-actin; cells were washed three times with PBS between each step. The cells were viewed with a Zeiss Axioplan fluorescence microscope (Oberkochen, Germany).

Statistics

Each experiment was performed in quadruplicate with at least three separate cell cultures derived from two lines. Results were analyzed by Student's t test or one-way ANOVA followed by Fisher's protective least squares difference (PLSD) test. p-values < 0.05 were regarded as statistically significant.

Results

ET-1 Induces $[Ca^{2+}]_i$ Mobilization in HBMEC

ET-1 increased $[Ca^{2+}]_i$ in a dose-dependent manner (Fig. 1). A significant increase in $[Ca^{2+}]_i$ was seen with

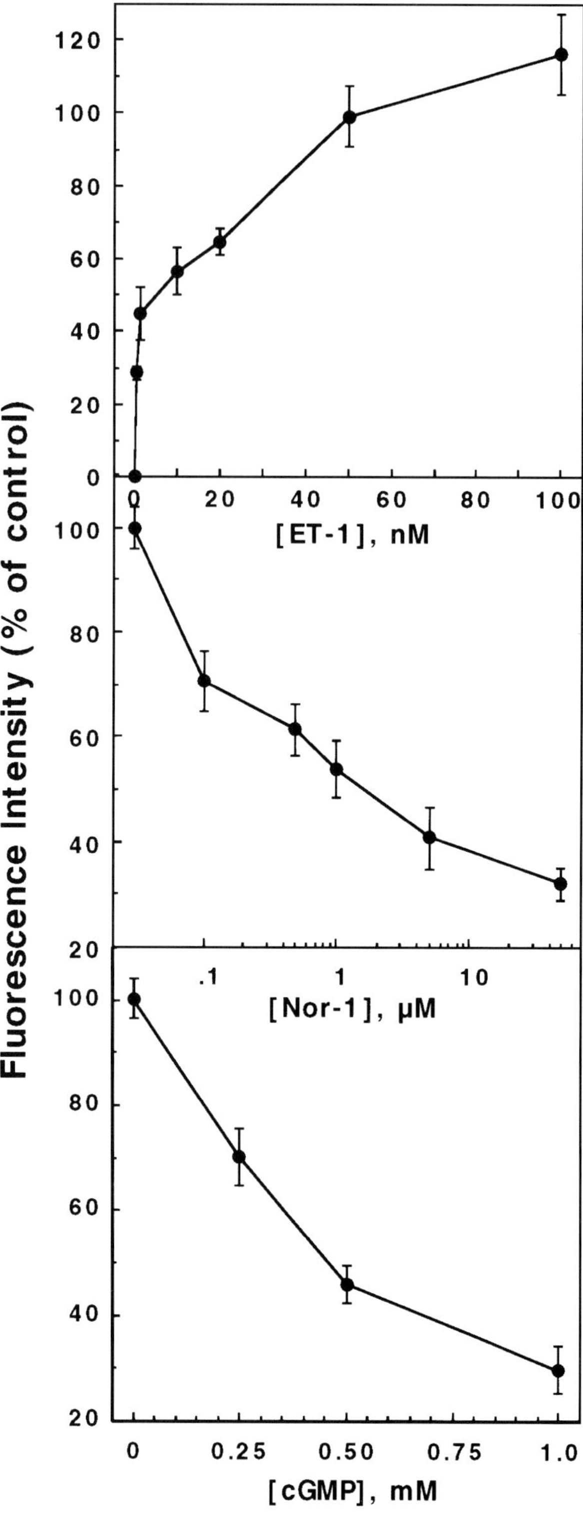

Fig. 1. Characterization of intracellular Ca^{2+} response in HBMEC. Cells were incubated with various concentrations of ET-1 alone (Upper panel), or in the presence of 20 nM ET-1 and pretreated (60 sec) with various concentrations of Nor-1 (Middle panel), or in the presence of 20 nM ET-1 and pretreated (100 sec) with various concentrations of cGMP (Lower panel). The data are means ± SEM of 3–36 experiments performed in quadruplicate

ET-1 concentration as low as 1 nM. The maximum effect of ET-1 was observed at a concentration of 100 nM resulting in an estimated EC_{50} of 20 nM. Endothelins are known to mediate vascular responses through activation of two receptors, ET_A and ET_B. Selective ET_A and ET_B receptor antagonists, BQ123 and BQ788, respectively were used to determine which subtype of receptor was responsible for ET-1-induced $[Ca^{2+}]_i$ mobilization. Treatment with BQ123 completely abolished the effects of ET-1, whereas BQ788 had no effect. In addition, the selective phospholipase C inhibitor, U73122, inhibited (60%) the ET-1-induced $[Ca^{2+}]_i$ mobilization, indicating that ET-1 induced $[Ca^{2+}]_i$ mobilization occurs through activation of ET_A receptor coupled to PLC.

Table 1. *Effect of Nor-1, ODQ or Rp-8-pCPT-cGMPs. Na on ET-1-Induced* $[Ca^{2+}]_i$ *Mobilization*

Addition		Fluorescent intensity
		(% of control)
–	–	100.0 ± 4.8
Nor-1	–	22.3 ± 3.3*
Nor-1	3 μM ODQ	45.4 ± 3.3*†
Nor-1	10 μM ODQ	78.2 ± 3.4*†Δ
Nor-1	40 μM Rp-8	61.2 ± 4.0*†
Nor-1	100 μM Rp-8	87.3 ± 11.1*†Δ

The data indicate Ca^{2+} mobilization in the presence of 20 nM ET-1 alone or with 50 μM Nor-1 ± the guanylyl cyclase inhibitor, ODQ or ± the protein kinase G inhibitor, Rp-8-pCPT-cGMPs. Na (Rp-8). Findings are presented as percent of control (20 nM ET-1 alone) ± SEM. * indicates significant difference from ET-1 alone; † indicates significant difference from Nor-1; Δ indicates significant difference from 3 μM ODQ or 40 μM Rp-8.

Nitric Oxide Inhibits ET-1-Induced $[Ca^{2+}]_i$ *Mobilization*

Pretreatment of cells with NOR-1 resulted in inhibition of ET-1-induced increases in $[Ca^{2+}]_i$ (Fig. 1). When L-arginine (a substrate for NO synthase) was added, ET-1-stimulated $[Ca^{2+}]_i$ mobilization was also decreased (50%). In contrast, administration of L-NAME (an inhibitor of nitric oxide synthase) doubled the ET-1-induced increases in $[Ca^{2+}]_i$ in the presence or absence of L-arginine. These results suggest that endogenous and exogenous NO inhibit ET-1-induced increases in $[Ca^{2+}]_i$ mobilization in HBMEC.

NO Signal Transduction Pathway

Preincubation with ODQ, a selective inhibitor of soluble guanylyl cyclase, dose-dependently prevented the inhibitory effect of NOR-1 on ET-1-induced $[Ca^{2+}]_i$ mobilization (Table 1). In contrast, pretreatment with the cell membrane permeable cGMP analog, 8-bromo-cGMP, inhibited $[Ca^{2+}]_i$ mobilization similar to that observed with NOR-1 (Fig. 1). The possible role of the cGMP-dependent protein kinase in NO-mediated changes in ET-1-induced $[Ca^{2+}]_i$ mobilization was evaluated by use of a selective inhibitor, Rp-8-pCPT-cGMPs. This compound dose-dependently prevented the reduction of ET-1-induced $[Ca^{2+}]_i$ mobilization induced by NOR-1 (Table 1). These data indicate that effects of NO on ET-1 induced $[Ca^{2+}]_i$ mobilization is regulated by cGMP/cGMP-dependent protein kinase system.

Effects of ET-1 and NOR-1 on Cytoskeletal Actin

ET-1 increased the number and density of the F-actin filaments in HBMEC as compared to untreated controls (Fig. 2). In contrast, pretreatment of ET-1-stimulated cells with NOR-1 reduced the number and length of F-actin filaments. A similar effect of NOR-1 was seen in controls.

Discussion

These studies demonstrate that ET-1 rapidly increased $[Ca^{2+}]_i$ in HBMEC through ET_A-receptor mediated activation of phospholipase C and G-protein. In addition, the prevention of ET-1-induced $[Ca^{2+}]_i$ mobilization by NOR-1 involves stimulation of guanylyl cyclase which converts guanosine triphosphate to the second messenger cGMP, which subsequently activates cGMP-dependent protein kinase. Studies have shown that NO can affect cellular Ca^{2+} via the targeting of various intracellular proteins. This may occur by nitrosylation of intracellular thiols [2] or reduction of thiol species [16]. Previous studies have also shown that exposure of HBMEC to NO donors modified both ET-1 receptor binding sites and ET-1-stimulated IP_3 formation [15]. Important roles in NO signal transduction have also recently been described for cGMP-dependent protein kinases [9]. Reduction of $[Ca^{2+}]_i$ by cGMP may be attributed to several mechanisms (*e.g.*, activation of Ca^{2+}-ATPase, inhibition of IP_3 formation, or direct effects on calcium channels). It should be added that mechanisms other than just cGMP-dependent protein kinases may certainly be in-

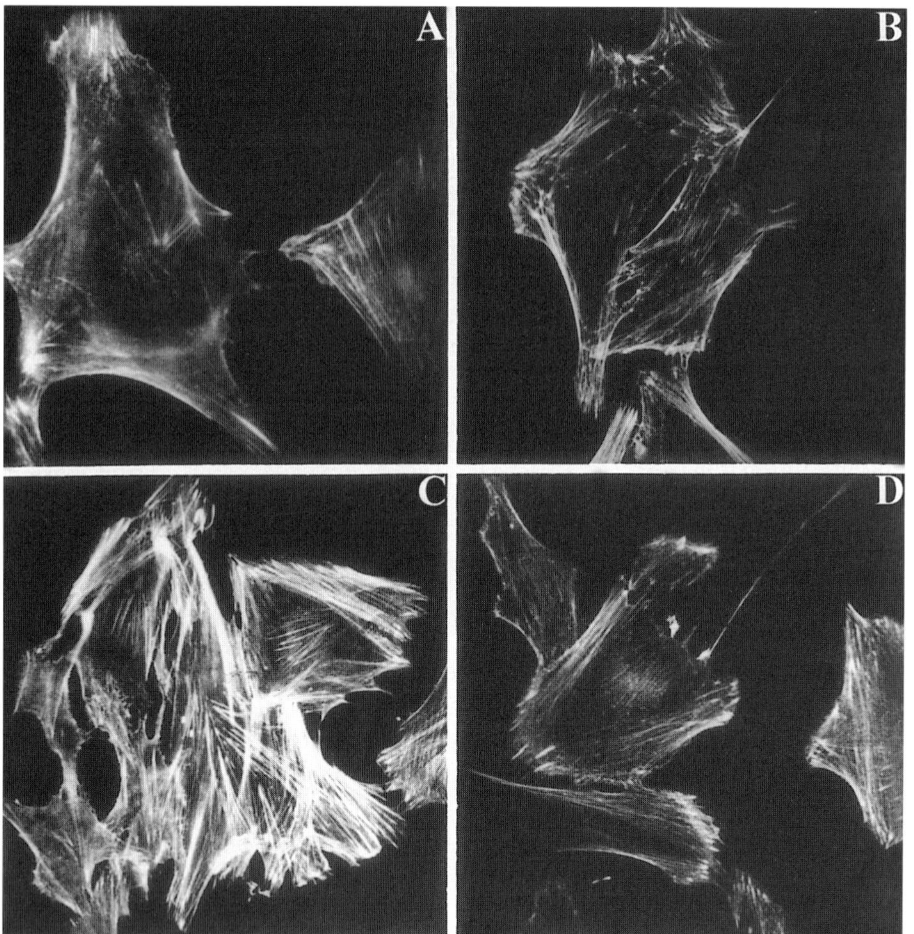

Fig. 2. Response of F-actin cytoskeleton in HBMEC to ET-1 and NOR-1. HBMEC grown on glass coverslips and processed as indicated in the methods were exposed to medium alone (A), NOR-1 (100 μM) for 60 sec (B), ET-1 (50 nM) for 30 sec (C), or NOR-1 (100 μM) for 60 sec followed by ET-1 (50 nM) for 30 sec (D). All cells were stained with phalloidin and examined with Zeiss Axioplan fluorescence microscopy (magnification × 63). (A) Control HBMEC display delicate (thin) longitudinal F-actin filaments which are more pronounced at the periphery. (B) HBMEC exposed to NOR-1 display rarified longitudinal filaments interposed by occasional granular-like filaments of F-actin. (C) HBMEC exposed to ET-1 for 30 sec contain numerous compacted F-actin filaments which are distributed throughout the entire cytoplasm. These filaments are more pronounced than those seen in control (A). (D) HBMEC pretreated with NOR-1 and exposed to ET-1 show delicate filaments that are thinner than those exposed to ET-1 alone (C) and are similar to those observed in (A) and (B)

volved in regulation of $[Ca^{2+}]_i$ (*i.e.*, cAMP and PKC) [13].

The findings presented here also indicate the effect of an interaction between NO and ET on cytoskeletal F-actin. The data indicate that ET-1 induced dramatic increases in cytoskeletal elements, whereas, NOR-1 modified this effect. Although ET-1-induced increases in $[Ca^{2+}]_i$ are responsible for many actions of ET-1, the role for these $[Ca^{2+}]_i$ increases in ET-1-induced effects on actin re-organization cannot be ascertained based on the present study. It has been suggested that transient increases in $[Ca^{2+}]_i$ may be involved in initiating actin polymerization in leukocytes [10]. In bovine brain pericytes, ET-1 induced increases in $[Ca^{2+}]_i$ were associated with the aggregation and realignment of F-actin into bundles [4]. However, Koyama and Baba have shown that ET-induced formation of actin stress fibers in cultured astrocytes involved GTPases [8] and was independent of changes in $[Ca^{2+}]_i$ [7]. Other studies showed that NO is associated with inhibition F-actin polymerization [3, 6, 17].

In conclusion, this study demonstrates that two biologically active molecules, ET and NO, are closely linked in regulating $[Ca^{2+}]_i$ mobilization and cytoskeletal actin reorganization in HBMEC. The findings may enhance our understanding of cerebromicrovascular biology and mechanisms underlying the active contribution of the endothelium to the function of the BBB.

References

1. Bacic F, Uematsu S, McCarron RM, Spatz M (1992) Secretion of immunoreactive endothelin-1 by capillary and microvascular endothelium of human brain. Neurochem Res 17: 699–702
2. Clancy RM, Levartpvsky D, Leszczynska-Piziak J, Yegudin J, Abramson SB (1994) Nitric oxide reacts with intracellular glutathione and activates the hexose monophosphate shunt in human neutrophils: evidence for S-nitrosoglutathione as a bioactive intermediary. Proc Natl Acad Sci USA 91: 3680–3684
3. Clancy R, Leszczynska J, Amin A, Levartpvsky D, Abramson SB (1995) Nitric oxide stimulates ADP ribosylation of actin in association with the inhibition of actin polymerization in human neutrophils. J Leukoc Biol 58: 196–202
4. Dehouck MP, Vigne P, Torpier G, Breittmayer JP, Cecchelli R, Frelin C (1997) Endothelin-1 as a mediator of endothelial cell-pericyte interactions in bovine brain capillaries. J Cereb Blood Flow Metab 17: 464–469
5. Goligorsky MS, Tsukahara H, Magazine H, Andersen TT, Malik AB, Bahou WF (1994) Termination of endothelin signaling: role of nitric oxide. J Cell Physiol 158: 485–494
6. Jun CD, Han MK, Kim UH, Chung HT (1996) Nitric oxide induces ADP-ribosylation of actin in murine macrophages: association with the inhibition of pseudopodia formation, phagocytic activity, and adherence on a laminin substratum. Cell Immun 174: 25–34
7. Koyama Y, Baba A (1994) Endothelins are extracellular signals modulating cytoskeletal actin organization in rat cultured astrocytes. Neuroscience 61: 1007–1016
8. Koyama Y, Baba A (1996) Endothelin-induced cytoskeletal actin re-organization in cultured astrocytes: inhibition by C_3 ADP-ribosyltransferase. Glia 16: 342–350
9. Lincoln TM, Komalavilas P, Cornwell TL (1994) Pleiotropic regulation of vascular smooth muscle tone by cyclic GMP-dependent protein kinase. Hypertension 23: 1141–1147
10. Marks PW, Maxfield FR (1990) Transient increases in cytosolic free calcium appear to be required for the migration of adherent human neutrophils. J Cell Biol 110: 43–52
11. Molitoris BA (1997) Putting the actin cytoskeleton into perspective: pathophysiology of ischemic alterations. Am J Physiol 272: F430–F433
12. Okishio M, Ohkawa S, Ichimori Y, Kondo K (1992) Interaction between endothelium-derived relaxing factors, S-nitrosothiols, and endothelin-1 on Ca2+ mobilization in rat vascular smooth muscle cells. Biochem Biophys Res Commun 183: 849–855
13. Reinhard M, Halbrugge M, Scheer U, Wiegand C, Jockusch BM, Walter U (1992) The 46/50 kDa phosphoprotein VASP purified from human platelets is a novel protein associated with actin filaments and focal contracts. EMBO J 11: 2063–2070
14. Spatz M, Kawai N, Merkel N, Bembry J, McCarron RM (1997) Functional properties of cultured endothelial cells derived from large microvessels of human brain. Am J Physiol 272: C231–C239
15. Spatz M, Yamamoto H, Yamamoto T, McCarron RM (1997) Effect of nitric oxide donors on ET-1 binding sites in human cerebrovascular endothelium. J Cereb Blood Flow Metab 17: S397
16. Stamler JS, Simon DI, Osborne JA, Mullins ME, Jaraki O, Michel T, Singel DJ, Loscalzo J (1992) S-nitrosylation of proteins with nitric oxide: synthesis and characterization of biologically active compounds. Proc Natl Acad Sci USA 89: 444–448
17. Sundqvist T, Forslund T, Bengtsson T, Axelsson KL (1994) S-nitroso-N-acetylpenicillamine reduces leukocyte adhesion to type I collagen. Inflammation 18: 625–631
18. Thomas JE, Nemirovsky A, Zelman V, Giannotta SL (1997) Rapid reversal of endothelin-induced cerebral vasoconstriction by intrathecal administration of nitric oxide donors. Neurosurgery 40: 1245–1249

Correspondence: Maria Spatz, M.D., National Institutes of Health, NINDS, Stroke Branch, 36 Convent Drive, MSC 4128, Bethesda, Maryland 20892-4128.

Acta Neurochir (2000) [Suppl] 76: 137–139

LF16-0687 A Novel Non-Peptide Bradykinin B2 Receptor Antagonist Reduces Vasogenic Brain Edema from a Focal Lesion in Rats

J. Schulz[1], **N. Plesnila**[1], **J. Eriskat**[1], **M. Stoffel**[2], **D. Pruneau**[3], and **A. Baethmann**[1]

[1] Inst. Surg. Res., Ludwig-Maximilians-University, Munich, Germany
[2] Department of Neurosurgery, University of Bonn, Germany
[3] Centre de Recherche, Laboratoires Fournier, Daix, France

Summary

Head injury world wide is still the most frequent cause of morbidity and mortality among the population under 45 years. Approximately 50% of patients dying from severe head injury have a therapy refractory intracranial pressure rise (Baethmann 1998). Traumatic brain edema, e.g. resulting from disruption of the blood-brain barrier is viewed as an important factor of the increased intracranial pressure. Bradykinin, an active peptide of the kallikrein-kinin system is considered to enhance brain edema formation which is attributed to its permeabilizing effect on the blood-brain barrier and on dilation of arterial blood vessels in the brain mediated by B2-receptors facilitating extravasation.

Currently, LF16-0687, a novel non-peptide bradykinin B2 receptor antagonist was experimentally tested as to its therapeutical potential on vasogenic brain edema from a cortical focal lesion. Following trephination of the skull in anaesthesia, male Sprague-Dawley rats were subjected to a focal cold injury of the left parietal cortex. Animals of two experimental groups were receiving either LF16-0687 as high or low dose, whereas one group of untreated animals with trauma was treated with 0.9% NaCl as continuous infusion beginning 10 min before until 24 h after lesion. 24 h after trauma the brain was removed from the skull, and the cerebral hemispheres were separated in the median plane for gravimetric assessment of hemispheric swelling.

No significant reduction of hemispheric brain swelling ($+7.4 \pm 2.9\%$) was found in animals receiving high-dose LF16-0687 as compared to the untreated controls. Brain swelling, however was significantly attenuated by the low-dose treatment, i.e. to $+6.4 \pm 1.3\%$; vs. $+9.3 \pm 1.1\%$ found in the controls, ($p < 0.05$). The current data confirm that blocking of bradykinin B2-receptors by LF16-0687 is significantly attenuating vasogenic brain edema from a focal cold lesion. The therapeutical properties of the antagonist on brain edema formation cannot be attributed to a lowering of the blood pressure. Rather, specific blocking effects of B2-receptors in the brain appear to be involved.

In conclusion, the understanding of secondary brain damage including brain edema in head injury has been markedly enhanced by the discovery of pathophysiologically active mediator compounds playing a role in its various manifestations. The current data confirm a pathophysiological function of bradykinin in vasogenic brain edema mediated by activation of B2-receptors. Currently it is studied whether LF16-0687 also reduces brain swelling when given after an insult.

Keywords: Bradykinin; B2-receptor antagonist; vasogenic brain edema.

Introduction

Head injury continues to represent world wide the most frequent cause of mortality and morbidity up to an age of 45 years [1]. Brain trauma, cerebral ischemia, or cerebral haemorrhage often is followed by an opening of the blood-brain barrier with formation of brain edema [2]. The primary brain damage acutely induced by the traumatic insult can be separated from the subsequently evolving sequelae collectively summarised as secondary brain damage. The primary irreversible lesion, e.g. a traumatic contusion directly produced by the dynamic impact cannot be influenced by the medical treatment in contrast to the secondary brain damage, resulting e.g. from edema and brain swelling raising intracranial pressure. Nevertheless, a specific drug treatment of traumatic brain edema which is inhibiting underlying mechanisms is not yet available for patients, and it must further be noted that approximately 50% of patients dying from severe head injury have a refractory intracranial pressure rise [3, 7].

The kallikrein-kinin system has been identified as a mediator of secondary brain damage [10, 13]. Administration of bradykinin, the active peptide of the kallikrein-kinin system, to the intact brain raises the blood-brain barrier permeability [6] and dilates cerebral arteries thereby increasing the transmural pressure gradient in capillaries and venules which facilitates extravasation of edema fluid [11, 12]. Bradykinin exerts its pathophysiological effects upon binding to specific receptors, of the B1- and B2-type [5, 8]. The B2-receptor appears to mediate most of the acute pharmacological and pathophysiological effects and bradykinin in the brain, respectively [11].

Therefore, blocking of bradykinin B2-receptors can be considered as a therapeutically promising approach to inhibit vasogenic brain edema formation. The novel non-peptide bradykinin B2-receptor antagonist LF16-0687 was developed for that purpose.

Material and Methods

The experiments were performed by utilising 24 male Sprague-Dawley rats of 250 g to 300 g body weight. The animals were intubated by the oro-tracheal route and mechanically ventilated. For anaesthesia 0.8% halothane and a mixture of 70% N_2O_2 and 30% O_2 were administered. The tail artery was cannulated by a polyethylene catheter for permanent blood pressure monitoring and blood gas assessment. A second catheter was inserted into the right jugular vein for continuous (24 h) drug (or saline) infusion. The body temperature was measured by a rectal probe and kept at 37.5 °C to 38.5 °C, using a feedback controlled heating pad. The skull was fixed in a stereotactic frame for trephination above the left parietal cortex. The preparation of a 5-mm ϕ cranial window of the left parietal skull between the lambda suture and the bregma was carried out by a water-cooled high-speed dental drill. The dura mater remained intact. The cold lesion of the brain (Klatzo *et al.* 1958) was induced by stereotactic attachment of a (ϕ 4.5 mm) copper cylinder onto the exposed brain for 15 s. The metal cylinder contained a mixture of acetone and dry ice cooled to −68 °C. The precise timing of lesioning as well as the exact placement of the probe was accomplished by a stereotactic device with a computer-controlled stepper motor to which the probe was attached. After trauma, the animals where maintained in anaesthesia for another 40 minutes for wound closure and monitoring followed by wake up and delivery to their cages. 24 h after trauma the animals were sacrificed in anaesthesia by decapitation. Blood was collected, e.g. for the assessment of LF-levels. The brain was carefully removed from the skull, and the cerebral hemispheres were separated in the median plane. The fresh-weight of both hemispheres and of plasma samples were gravimetrically determined. The brain tissue was dried then for 24 h at 110 °C for the assessment of the tissue water content by the dry/wet-weight ratio.

For the current experimental studies, the animals were randomised in three groups (n = 8 each) and treated with 10 µg/kg/min, or 100 µg/kg/min LF16-0687, untreated control animals with trauma received 0.9% NaCl infused into the right jugular vein. The infusion started 10 min prior to trauma and was continued up to 24 h post trauma.

Results

Cold injury of the brain in untreated animals receiving saline resulted in an increase of the hemispheric water content to 81.4 ± 0.3% as compared to 80.0 ± 0.2% of the contralateral control side ($p < 0.001$). Brain edema led to an increase in weight (swelling) of the exposed hemisphere of +9.3 ± 1.1% of the contralateral control hemisphere ($p < 0.05$). In animals with high-dose LF the increase of the water content of the traumatised hemisphere was limited to 80.8 ± 0.8%. Yet the high-dose protocol was also lowering the water content of the contralateral control hemisphere to 79.5 ± 0.6%. Thereby the difference in weight between the traumatised and the contralateral control hemisphere was affected, resulting in swelling of the exposed hemisphere of +7.4 ± 1.3% (ns. vs. control). Animals with low-dose LF16-0687 treatment, however, had a significant attenuation of hemispheric brain swelling to +6.4 ± 1.3% ($p < 0.05$%; vs. swelling in untreated controls). The corresponding water content of the exposed hemisphere in this group was reaching up to 81.3 ± 0.6% (ns. vs. control; of Table 1).

The blood pressure remained stable throughout the monitoring period of 10 min prior to lesion and 40 min thereafter. Thus blood pressure was neither influenced by the trauma, nor by the drug during the first 50 min of administration (Table 2).

Discussion

The present findings provide further evidence for a mediator role of the kallikrein-kinin system, bradykinin, the active principle, as mediator in secondary brain damage from trauma [6, 9, 10, 11]. In addition,

Table 1. *Cerebral Water Content and Increase in Weight (Brain Swelling) of the Traumatised Hemispheres (Mean ± SEM) Over the Corresponding Contralateral Hemispheres of Animals with and Without Treatment (n = 8 per group)*

	Hemispheric water content		Hemispheric swelling
	Left	Right	
Control	81.4 ± 0.26%	80.0 ± 0.2%	9.3 ± 1.1%
Low-dose LF160687	81.3 ± 0.63%	80.1 ± 0.53%	6.4 ± 1.3%
High-dose LF160687	80.8 ± 0.75%	79.5 ± 0.59%	7.4 ± 2.9%

Table 2. *Mean Arterial Blood Pressure (Mean ± SEM) of Animals Prior and after Trauma*

Exp. groups	10 min pre trauma	Post trauma	30 min post trauma
Control	77 ± 10 mmHg	79 ± 9 mmHg	78 ± mmHg5
Low dose	79 ± 13 mmHg	77 ± 8 mmHg	77 ± 5 mmHg
High dose	71 ± 11 mmHg	78 ± 11 mmHg	78 ± 8 mmHg

the therapeutical efficacy of inhibition of bradykinin B2-receptors by the novel non-peptide agent LF16-0687 raises expectations for the usefulness of this drug for clinical treatment protocols. As known, neither traumatic nor ischemic brain damage in patients has been shown so far in clinical trial procedures to benefit from any pharmacological drug treatment. Even at the closure of the millennium the medical care of head injury patients liable to be at risk from the development of secondary brain damage is restricted to the general procedures of the emergency and intensive care management. These include the symptomatic methods of lowering the increased intracranial pressure, or to prevent intracranial hypertension, respectively [3].

The discovery of the kallikrein-kinin system as a powerful mediator of secondary brain damage in trauma or ischemia is a case in point for expectations concerning a breakthrough to enrich the clinical treat ment protocol by more specific methods. With regard to potential side effects of the novel non-peptide antagonist, the current findings do not provide any evidence, as for example on reduction or increase of the systemic blood pressure which both would adversely affect the clinical course in patients with severe head injury [3]. Another point, of course, is concerned with the permeability of the drug through the intact blood-brain barrier, notwithstanding that in a severe head injury producing focal lesions (i.e. contusions) the blood-brain barrier may be disrupted providing access of the drug to the brain parenchyma. Yet, there are further neuropathological manifestations in head injury, such as the diffuse axonal injury, where apart from microscopic lesions gross blood-brain barrier opening does not seem to occur. Therefore, diffuse axonal injury unlikely is a target for the treatment by bradykinin receptor antagonists, which rather are influencing the development of traumatic brain edema evolving in and around contused brain tissue.

The present mechanism of inhibition of traumatic brain edema from the focal lesion by the receptor antagonist may be explained by both restriction of barrier opening after trauma – which is facilitated by the release of bradykinin and the antagonisation of arteriolar dilation and venular constriction [9]. The latter is particularly effective to enhance fluid extravasation into the brain parenchyma from the resulting increased transmural pressure gradient, particularly if the blood-brain barrier is broken [11].

It must be emphasized, however, that the conclusions drawn from the present data have to be limited. In fact, it is currently only shown that the B2-receptor antagonist is in principle effective in traumatic brain edema no more no less. In order to have optimal experimental conditions the drug was administered *prior* to the induction of the lesion. As a next step it should be tested whether LF 16-0687 is exerting its therapeutical potential also when the treatment is initiated *after* the insult but not before. Since activation of the kallikrein-kinin system is likely to continue after trauma for a while resulting in an ongoing release of kinins in a pathologically deranged brain parenchyma, it is conceivable that B2-receptor antagonisation is also effective, if administration of the drug commences post insult. This laboratory is presently involved in respective experiments.

References

1. Statistisches, Bundesamt Wiesbaden, (1993–1995) Sterbefälle beim Schädel- Hirntrauma durch Schädelfraktur (ICD800–804) und intrakranielle Verletzungen (ICD 850–854), Fachserie 12, Gesundheitswesen Reihe 4
2. Baethmann A (1978) Pathophysiological and pathochemical aspects of cerebral edema. Neurosurg Rev 1: 85–100
3. Baethmann A, Eriskat J, Stoffel M, Chapuis D, Wirth A, Plesnila N (1998) Special aspects of severe head injury-recent develepements. Curr Opinion Anaesthesiol 11: 193–200
4. Baethmann A, Kempski O (1997) Pathophysiologie des Hirnödems. Anästhesiol. Intensivmed 38: 347–356
5. Hall JM (1992) Bradykinin receptors: pharmacological properties and biological roles. Pharmacol Ther 56: 131–190
6. Maier-Hauff K, Baethmann A, Lange M, Schürer L, Unterberg A (1984) The kallikrein-kinin system as mediator in vasogenic brain edema, part 2. J Neurosurg 61: 97–106
7. Miller JD, Becker DP, Ward JD, Sullivan HG, Adams WE, Rosner MJ (1977) Significance of intracranial hypertension in severe head injury. J Neurosurg 47: 503–516
8. Regoli D, Barabe J (1980) Pharmacology of bradykinin and related kinins. Pharmacol Rev 32: 1–46
9. Unterberg A, Wahl M, Baethmann A (1984) Effects of bradykinin on permeability and diameter of pia vessels in vivo. J Cereb Blood Flow Metabol 4: 574–585
10. Unterberg A, Baethmann A (1984) The kallikrein-kinin system as mediator in vasogenic brain edema. Part 1, cerebral exposure to bradykinin and plasma. J Neurosurg 61: 87–96
11. Wahl M, Whalley ET, Unterberg A, Schilling L, Parsons AA, Baethmann A, Young AR (1996) Vasomotor and permeability effects of bradykinin in the cerebral microcirculation. Immunopharmacology 33: 257–263
12. Wahl M, Young AR, Edvinsson L, Wagner F (1983) Effects of bradykinin on pial arteries and arterioles in vitro and in situ. J Cereb Blood Flow Metabol 3: 231–237
13. Whittle IR, Piper IR, Miller JD, (1983) The role of bradykinin in the etiology of vasogenic brain edema and perilesional brain dysfunction. Acta Neurochir (Wien) 115: 53–59

Correspondence: Nikolaus Plesnila, Institute for Surgical Research, Klinikum Großhadern, Ludwig- Maximilians Universität, Marchioninistr. 15, 81366 München, Germany.

Acta Neurochir (2000) [Suppl] 76: 141–145

AT1 Receptor Antagonist Prevents Brain Edema Without Lowering Blood Pressure

H. Ito, K. Takemori, J Kawai, and **T. Suzuki**

Department of Pathology, Kinki University School of Medicine, Osaka, Japan

Summary

In order to investigate the role of Angiotensin II (AII) for the vasogenic cerebral edema, the AT1 receptor antagonist (TCV-116) was administered to 19-week-old stroke-prone spontaneously hypertensive rats (SHRSP) for 2 weeks at a dosage which did not decrease the blood pressure. Although no remarkable changes were found in blood pressure after treatment, the average brain weight of the treated group was relatively lower as compared to that of control SHRSP and no edematous changes were found in any brains. The immunohistochemical expression of intercellular adhesion molecule-1 (ICAM-1) was less and the glucose transporter-1 (GLUT-1) expression was much more intense in the endothelial cells of the micro vessels in the cerebral cortex of the treated group. Fibrinogen expression around micro-vessels was also remarkably reduced in the treated group. A decreased expression of ICAM-1 in the treated group was confirmed by RT-PCR analysis. These results indicate that the AT1 receptor blockade ameliorates hypertensive cerebral injury in a blood pressure-independent manner and suggest that AII may have an important role for endothelial injury in severe hypertension.

Keywords: Angiotensin II; AT1 receptor antagonist; adhesion molecule; brain edema.

Introduction

It is well known that hypertension is the major risk factor for various kinds of vascular injury. As an animal model, Okamoto *et al.* [11] developed a stroke-prone spontaneously hypertensive rat strain (SHRSP), spontaneously showing severe hypertension, and over 95% of these rats suffered from cerebrovascular injury. Using these rats, many experimental studies were conducted to elucidate the pathogenesis of hypertensive cerebral injury (See the review article by Ito H. and Suzuki T [4]). In this model, two types of cerebral changes were identified, i.e. cerebral stroke (softening and/or hemorrhage) and cerebral edema; thus, SHRSP is the most suitable model for the study on vasogenic cerebral edema. Although it has been reported that cerebral stroke could be caused by fibrinoid necrosis of a small artery (angionecrosis), the pathogenesis of a cerebral edema is still unknown. Undoubtedly, cerebral edema is caused by the increase of vascular permeability due to endothelial injury of brain micro-vessels. With regard to endothelial changes in SHRSP, we revealed that the endothelial cells of the SHRSP aorta were more vulnerable to free radical intoxication as compared to those in normotensive Wistar-Kyoto rats (WKY) [5]. Among the many risk factors for endothelial changes (except for high blood pressure itself), we focused on Angiotensin II (AII), because it is one of the major humoral factors for blood pressure regulation, and it exerts its vasoconstrictory and trophic actions on endothelial cells as well as smooth muscle cells via AT1 receptors (See the review article by Pulyo and Michel [12]). In the present study, the effects of AT1-receptor blockade were investigated with special reference to the vascular permeability in brain micro-vessels, in order to elucidate the causative role of AII on vasogenic edema in severe hypertension.

Materials and Methods

Male SHRSP from the original Okamoto strain were maintained in our animal center and used at 19 weeks of age. Age-matched WKY rats were used as a control. The AT1-receptor antagonist (TCV-116, Takeda, Osaka, Japan) was administered to 7 SHRSP at a dosage of 1 mg/kg/day, p.o., for 2 weeks. Another 7 SHRSP and an equal number of WKY were used as a control. In the preliminary study, it was confirmed that this dose of TCV-116 did not decrease the blood pressure of SHRSP. The blood pressure and body weight were measured before the TCV-116 administration and once a week after administration. At the end of the experiment, the rats were sacrificed by decapitation under light ether anesthesia and the brain was immediately removed.

Immunohistochemical Examination

Sections from occipital lobe of each brain were frozen in dry ice-isopenthan (−80 °C) and kept at −20 °C for preparation. Using a cryostat, 10 μm sections were obtained and mounted on slide glass. Immunohistochemical staining for Intercellular adhesion molecule-1 (ICAM-1, ligand in endothelial cells for Mac-1 in leukocytes), Glucose transporter-1 (GLUT-1, as a marker of blood-brain barrier) and fibrinogen (marker of vascular permeability) were performed using specific antibodies by the ABC methods. Positively stained cells for ICAM-1 and GLUT-1 and positive vessels for fibrinogen in the cerebral cortex were counted under a microscope at a magnification of ×400 by 3 different pathologists without any information of the experiment. The average cell number from 5 portions in one cerebral cortex were estimated as positive cells per high power field (HPF).

Reverse-Transcription and Polymerase Chain Reaction (RT-PCR) Analysis

RT-PCR analysis on ICAM-1 expression was carried out using the left cortex of each brain. Total RNA was isolated using ISOGEN (NIPPON GENE Co.), redissolved in water, and then determined photometrically at a wave length of 260 nm. The synthetic primers, sense and antisense, were designed specifically for rat ICAM-1 and rat β-actin, as follows: for ICAM-1, 5′-CTGGAGAGCACAAACA GCAGAG-3′ and 5′-AAGGCCGCAGAGCAAAAGAAGC-3′; for β-actin, 5′-TGTTTGAGACCTTCAACACC-3′ and 5′-TCAGGCAGCTCATAGCTCTT-3′. Base pair positions were those given in the published cDNA sequences for rat ICAM-1 and rat β-actin. RT-PCR were performed using the mRNA selective PCR Kit (Ver. 1.1, TaKaRa BIOCHEMICALS Co. Tokyo) according to Manufacturer's instructions. The amplification profile involved reverse transcription at 50 °C for 25 min, denaturation at 85 °C for 30 sec, annealing at 55 °C for 30 sec, and extension at 72 °C for 30 sec for 30 cycles. The final extension was carried at 72 °C for 7 min. The PCR products were separated by electrophoresis in 1.5% agarose gel, stained with ethidium bromide, and located by UV light fluorescence. Bio Max 1D TM1.5.1 (Kodac) was used to quantitate the band intensities of the PCR band. The ICAM-1 signal was normalized to the corresponding β-actin signal from the same RNA.

Results

Blood pressure of the control group was 215 ± 3 mmHg and the TCV group was 216 ± 4 mmHg before TCV administration. In the control group, blood pressure gradually increased with advancing age and reached 213 ± 3 mmHg at the end of the experiment, whereas it was slightly decreased in the TCV group, being 203 ± 4 mmHg. Although blood pressure of the TCV group was significantly lower than the control group at the end of the experiment, it was still over 200 mmHg. No significant differences were found in body weight between the two groups either before or after the experiment. In the control group, the average brain weight was slightly, but not significantly, heavier than the TCV group (1.904 ± 0.018 g in the former and 1.882 ± 0.048 g in the latter). Some of the brains in the control group showed a mild edematous change, whereas no pathological changes were found in the TCV group either macroscopically or microscopically. Figure 1 shows the typical example of immunohistochemical staining of ICAM-1 (A and B) and GLUT-1 (C and D) in the cerebral cortex. As clearly shown in this figure, there are many positive cells for ICAM-1 in the control group (A) and remarkably few in the TCV group (B). On the other hand, the numbers of GLUT-1 positive cells were higher in TCV-group (D) than in the control group (C). Positive cells were counted at 5 different sites in the cerebral cortex, and the average cell numbers were compared between the two groups. For ICAM-1, the positive cell number was 21.5 ± 2.7 in the control and 10.5 ± 5.0 in the TCV group ($p < 0.01$). For the GLUT-1, the positive cell number was 22.2 ± 1.0 in the control group and 27.0 ± 3.0 in the TCV group ($p < 0.05$). Furthermore, the positive vessel count for fibrinogen was 8.45 ± 2.0 in the control group and 5.45 ± 2.03 in the TCV group ($p < 0.05$). Figure 2 shows the electrophoretic pattern of PCR products for ICAM-1 and β-actin. There was a single band at 334 bp for ICAM-1 (lane 4–6) and at 298 bp for β-actin (lane 1–3) in the three groups. To estimate the difference of ICAM-1 expression among the three groups, the electron density of ICAM-1 was normalized by that of β-actin. For ICAM-1, the ratio of ICAM-1/β-actin were 1.82 ± 0.03 in the control group, 0.27 ± 0.02 in WKY and 0.21 ± 0.01 in the TCV group ($p < 0.05$, one way analysis of variance (ANOVA)). Although the ICAM-1 expression was significantly higher in SHRSP than in WKY, it was lower in the TCV-treated group as compared to the control SHRSP ($p < 0.01$).

Discussion

In the present study, it was clearly demonstrated that functional changes of endothelial cells in SHRSP cerebral cortex, such as increased expression of ICAM-1 and decreased expression of GLUT-1, were ameriolated by the TCV-116 administration. Since it is well recognized that ICAM-1 is an adhesion molecule against Mac-1 of leukocytes and that GLUT-1 makes the blood brain barrier in endothelial cells in brain micro-vessels, the data obtained in the present study suggest that the increased adhesion of leukocyte-endothelial cell and the disruption of the blood brain barrier could occur in the cerebral cortex of control SHRSP. This was supported by the findings showing

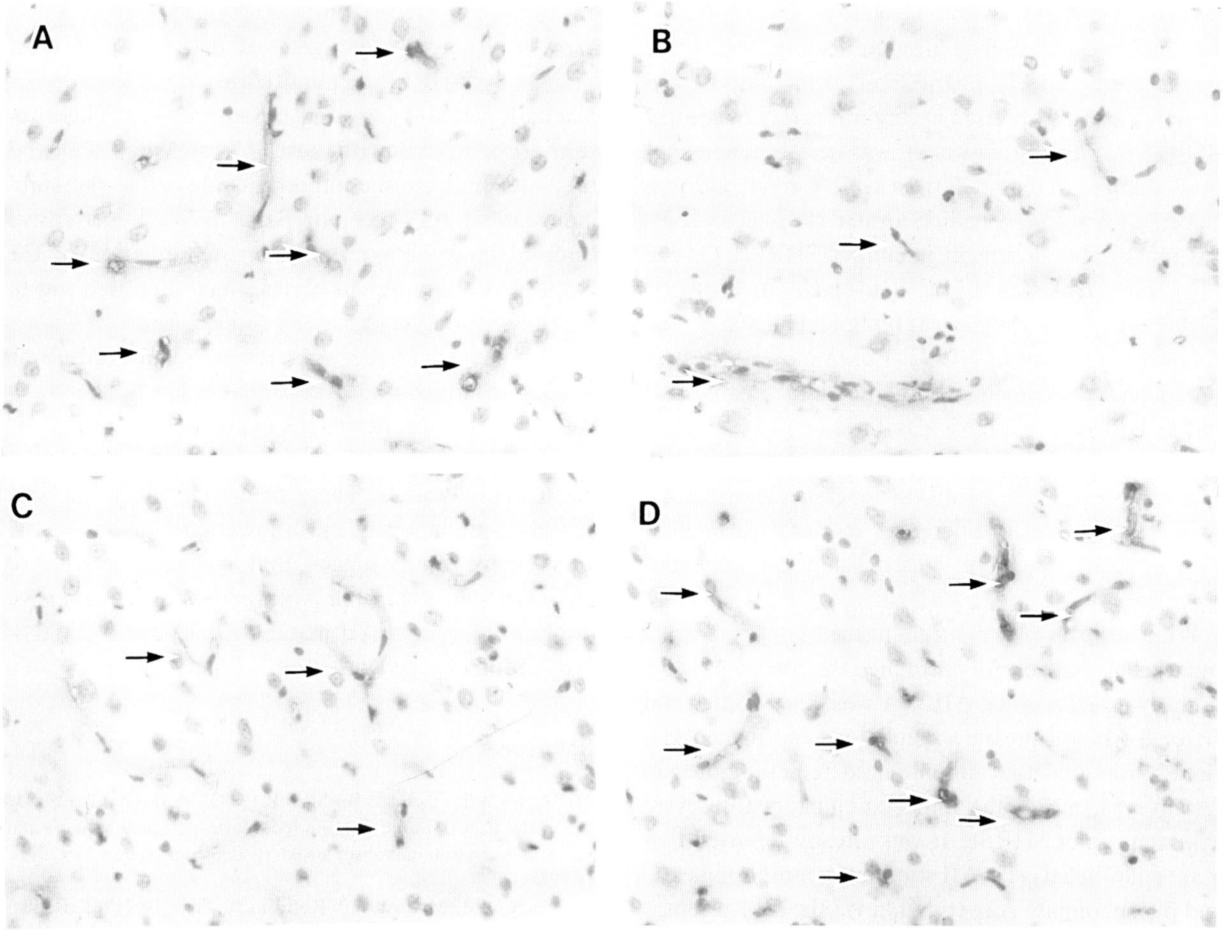

Fig. 1. Immunohistochemical expression of ICAM-1 and GLUT-1 in cerebral cortex. Positive cells are indicated by arrows. (A) ICAM-1, control group, (B) ICAM-1, TCV-treated group, (C) GLUT-1, control group, (D) GLUT-1, TCV-treated group

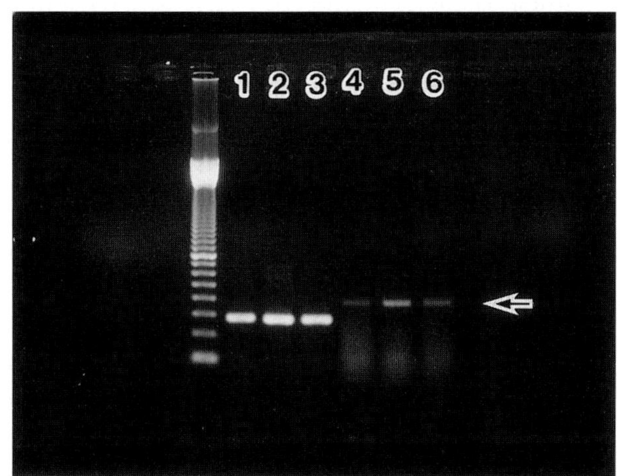

Fig. 2. Electrophoresis of PCR-products by polyacryl amide gel. *Lane 1–3*: β-actin (*1*) WKY, (*2*) control, (*3*) TCV, *Lane 4–6*: ICAM-1 (*4*) WKY, (*5*) control, (*6*) TCV

decreased extravasation of fibrinogen in TCV-treated group. However, we do not have direct evidence about the correlation between leukocyte adhesion and the disruption of the blood brain barrier in brain micro vessels.

Although there have been no reports regarding the expression of ICAM-1 in the brain of SHRSP, it has been reported that ICAM-1 expression was identified in the carotid artery of SHRSP and SHR, but not in WKY, and monocyte-endothelial cell adhesion was much more intense in SHRSP than in SHR [8]. Up-regulation of ICAM-1 is well documented in ischemia-reperfusion injury in rat brain [7, 16, 17] and such cerebral damage was prevented by anti-ICAM-1 administration [1, 2, 18]. In ischemia and reperfusion model using rat mesenteric venules, a positive correlation between leukocyte adhesion and albumin leakage was found, and monoclonal antibodies against CD18,

CD11b, and ICAM-1 and L-selectin reduced leukocyte adherence as well as albumin leakage [6]. In the present study, GLUT-1, a marker of the blood-brain barrier, was less expressed in cerebral cortex of control SHRSP, in which brain weight was heavier and edematous changes were found, than in TCV-treated group. Indeed, fibrinogen expression around the micro vessels was remarkably dominant in control SHRSP. On the other hand, McCall *et al.* [10] have investigated GLUT-1 expression in the rat brain and have reported the over expression of GLUT-1 in micro vessels after global cerebral ischemia. Similarly, Urabe *et al.* [14] and Gehart *et al.* [3] have also found an over expression of GLUT-1 in the cerebral cortex after ischemia or reperfusion. These results do not coincide with ours. This may be due to differences in the experimental model, such as severe hypertension or ischemia-reperfusion.

With regard to the mechanisms of hypertensive endothelial changes, we postulated the role of AII as a causative factor, since AII is a well known humoral factor for blood pressure regulation, and it has been already reported that an enhanced renin-angiotensin system was one of the important factors for severe hypertension of SHRSP. It was already reported that in rat endothelial cells, AII stimulates phospholipase C and phospholipase A2 activation via the AT1 receptor and also stimulates the tyrosine phosphorylation of several proteins [12]. Although few reports are available on the effects of AT1-receptor blockade, Vacher *et al.* [15] examined the effects of losartan on cerebral arteries and reported the beneficial effects on vascular morphology and function, i.e. losartan limited the increases in cerebral arterial wall thickness and the wall: lumen ratio, and it also limited the cerebrovascular contractility impairment and age-related alteration of the endothelium-dependent relaxation of cerebral arteries. As a result, losartan prevents stroke and improves the cerebral artery's smooth muscle and endothelial cell functions. Furthermore, Strawn *et al.* [13] investigated the effects of losartan on endothelium-monocyte interactions using hypertensive transgenic rats [TGR(mRen2)27] and found that losartan significantly decreased the number of activated circulating and endothelium-adherent monocytes. Based on the results in their experiment, they indicated that the recruitment and infiltration of leukocytes into the sub-endothelium associated with renin-angiotensin system-induced hypertension is partly mediated by the pressure-independent AT1-receptor pathway. In the present study, we showed the down-regulation of ICAM-1 expression and the up-regulation of GLUT-1 expression in the SHRSP cerebral cortex by AT1-receptor blockade without lowering blood pressure. These results are coincident with those of Strawn *et al.* [13], and they also indicate the important role of the pressure-independent AT1-receptor pathway for hypertensive cerebral injury. Regrettably, an investigation of the pathophysiology of leukocytes was not carried out in the present study and remains to be clarified.

In conclusion, the AT1-receptor blockade was shown to ameliorate the enhanced expression of ICAM-1 and the decreased expression of GLUT-1, and it thus prohibited the vascular permeability of brain micro vessels. These beneficial effects of AT1 blockade are independent of lowering blood pressure. Thus, these results suggest that leukocytes may have an important role in the pathogenesis of hypertensive cerebral injury and AII may be a mediator for leukocyte-endothelial cell adhesion.

References

1. Bowes WP, Zivin JA, Rothlein R (1993) Monoclonal antibody to the ICAM-1 adhesion site reduces neurological damage in a rabbit cerebral embolism stroke model. Exp Neurol 119: 215–219
2. Clark WM, Madden KP, Rothlein R, Zivin JA (1991) Reduction of central nervous system ischemic injury by monoclonal antibody to intercellular adhesion molecule. J Neurosurg 75: 623–627
3. Gerhart DZ, Leino RI, Taylor WE, Borson ND, Drewes LR (1994) GLUT-1 and GLUT-3 gene expression in gerbil brain following brief ischemia: an in situ hybridization study. Brain Res Mol Brain Res 25: 313–322
4. Ito H, Suzuki T (1994) Pathophysiological overview of M-SHRSP. Progress in Hypertension, vol 3. In: Satio H *et al* (eds) VSP, Utrecht Tokyo, pp 1–19
5. Ito H, Torii M, Suzuki T (1995) Comparative study on free radical injury in the endothelium of SHR and WKY aorta. Clin Exper Pharmacol Physiol [Suppl] 1: S157–S159
6. Kurose I, Anderson DC, Miyasaka M, Tamatani T, Paulson JC, Todd RF, Rusche JR, Granger DN (1994) Molecular determinants of reperfusion-induced leukocyte adhesion and vascular protein leakage. Circ Res 74: 336–343
7. Liu T, Clark RK, McDonnell PC, Young PR, White MS, Barone FC, Feuerstein GZ (1994) Tumor necrosis factor – expression in ischemic neurons. Stroke 25: 1481–1488
8. Liu Y, Liu T, McCarron RM, Spatz M, Feuerstein G, Hallenbeck JM, Siren AL (1996) Evidence for activation of endothelium and monocytes in hypertensive rats. Am J Physiol 270: H2125–H2131
9. Matsuo Y, Onodera H, Shiga Y, Shozuhara H, Ninomiya M, Kihara T *et al* (1994) Role of cell adhesion molecule in brain injury after transient middle cerebral artery occlusion in the rat. Brain Res 656: 344–352
10. McCall AL, Van Bueren AM, Nipper V, Moholt-Siebert M, Downes H, Lessov N (1996) Forebrain ischemia increases Glut1

protein in brain microvessels and parenchyma. J Cereb Blood Flow Metab 16: 69–76
11. Okamoto K, Yamori Y, Nagaoka A (1986) Establishment of stroke-prone spontaneously hypertensive rat (SHR). Circ Res 34&35 [Suppl] I: I-143–I-153
12. Pueyo ME, Michel JB (1997) Angiotensin II receptors in endothelial cells. Gen Pharmacol 29: 691–696
13. Strawn WB, Gallagher PE, Tallant EA, Ganten D, Ferrario CM (1999) Angiotensin II AT1-receptor blockade inhibits monocyte activation and adherence in transgenic (mRen2) 27 rats. J Cerdiovasc Pharmacol 33: 341–351
14. Urabe T, Hattori N, Nagamatsu S, Sawa H, Mizuno Y (1996) Expression of glucose transporters in rat brain following transient focal ischemic injury. J Neurochem 67: 265–271
15. Vacher E, Richer C, Giudicelli JF (1996) Effects of losartan on cerebral arteries in stroke-prone spontaneously hypertensive rats. J Hypertens 14: 1341–1348
16. Wang X, Sieren AL, Liu Y, Barone FC, Feuerstein GZ (1994) Upregulation of intercellular adhesion molecule 1 (ICAM-1) on brain microvascular endothelial cells in rat ischemic cortex. Mol Brain Res 26: 61–68
17. Wang X, Yue TL, Barone FC, Feuerstein GZ (1995) Demonstration of increased endothelial-leukocyte adhesion molecule-1 mRNA expression in rat ischemic cortex. Stroke 26: 1665–1669
18. Zhang RL, Chopp M, Li Y, Zaloga C, Jiang N, Jones ML *et al* (1994) Anti-ICAM-1 antibody reduces ischemic cell damage after transient middle cerebral artery occlusion in the rat. Neurology 44: 1747–1751

Correspondence: H. Ito, Department of Pathology, Kinki University School of Medicine, Osaka-sayama, Osaka, Japan.

Acta Neurochir (2000) [Suppl] 76: 147–151

The Effects of Dopamine on Edema Formation in two Models of Traumatic Brain Injury

A. Beaumont[1], **K. Hayasaki**[1], **A. Marmarou**[1], **P. Barzo**[1], **P. Fatouros**[2], and **F. Corwin**[2]

[1] Division of Neurosurgery, Medical College of Virginia, Richmond, VA, USA
[2] Division of Radiation Physics, Medical College of Virginia, Richmond, VA, USA

Summary

The risk of vasopressors worsening cerebral edema has been raised. Previously we have reported that dopamine was able to restore cerebral blood flow in a model of monotonically rising intracranial pressure. In this study the effects of dopamine on cortical contusion and diffuse injury with secondary insult are examined. Adult male rats were divided into two groups: group 1 ($n = 32$) – Impact Acceleration Injury (IAM) with 30 minutes hypoxia and hypotension; group 2 ($n = 12$) – controlled cortical impact (6.0 m/sec, 3 mm depth). Dopamine was administered 2 hours post-injury (10–60 μg/kg/min iv). Cerebral water content and apparent diffusion coefficients (ADC) values were measured at baseline and four hours post-injury using MRI. Preinjury water content was the same in each group. Group 1 was subdivided into Groups 1A & 1B based on the ADC profile. Post-injury water content in Group 1A did not differ between saline or dopamine treated animals. Water content was higher in Group 1B-dopamine ($83.4 \pm 1.1\%$) than Group 1B-saline animals ($81.4 \pm 1.3\%$, $p = 0.006$). Contusion caused significant edema formation, however there was no significant difference between the dopamine treated or untreated group when considering either ipsilateral or contralateral cortex. Dopamine however significantly worsened edema in ipsilateral and contralateral hippocampus and both temporal cortices. ADC remained unchanged except in the contralateral hippocampus where both water content and ADC rose with dopamine suggesting precipitation of a vasogenic edema. In this study dopamine clearly worsened edema formation in two models of traumatic brain injury, and we conclude that there may be analogous clinical situations; therefore pressors should not be considered a 'blanket' therapy for all patients with a low cerebral perfusion pressure.

Keywords: Traumatic brain injury; cerebral perfusion pressure; dopamine; edema.

Introduction

Management of Cerebral Perfusion Pressure (CPP) is of critical importance for the severely head injured patient. CPP represents the driving force for blood to perfuse the brain and cerebral ischemia has been identified as an adverse determinant of outcome following traumatic brain injury [2, 3]. Advocates of pressor therapy propose that the necessity for maintaining CPP is more complex than can be explained by the continued delivery of blood to the tissue. It is thought that maintenance of CPP within a range which permits autoregulation allows vascular reactivity to control intracranial pressure (ICP) [12].

Previous studies [10, 11, 13] have shown that uncontrolled hypertension in damaged brain can exacerbate edema and increase intracranial pressure. A recent experimental study demonstrated that elevating CPP with pressors can increase contusional volume [7]. Rosner *et al.* (1995) [12] however have demonstrated that CPP could be iatrogenically elevated in patients by inducing systemic hypertension without potentiating mortality.

The aim of this study was therefore to assess the effects of administering dopamine on edema formation and the apparent diffusion coefficients (ADC) in two models of traumatic brain injury.

Materials and Methods

All animals received humane care in compliance with the "Guide for the Care and Use of Laboratory Animals" (NIH Publication 86-23, 1989). Forty-eight adult male Sprague Dawley rats, weighing 350 to 380 g, were separated into two groups, A & B. All animals were anesthetised animals using 1–2% halothane in a mixture of 66% N_2O and 33% O_2. Group A ($n = 32$) experienced Impact Acceleration Injury followed by a 30 minute secondary insult of hypoxia and hypotension. Group B animals ($n = 12$) were exposed to the controlled cortical impact model of cortical contusion.

The Impact Acceleration Model was performed according to methods described in detail elsewhere [9]. Briefly a 10 mm diameter, 2 mm deep stainless steel disk was mounted on the skull using rapid drying cyanoacrylic glue. A brass weight of 450 g was then dropped from a height of 2 m onto the center of the disk. A secondary insult

Table 1. *Cortical Water Content (Percent) and ADC Values ($\times 10^{-3}$ mm^2/sec) Before and 4 h After Diffuse TBI with Secondary Insult Either Treated with Dopamine, or Untreated. Values are Means $\pm$ Standard Deviation.* $^{+}p < 0.05$ *vs. ADC-Recovery Group,* $^{*}p < 0.01$ *vs. Untreated Group*

Group	Baseline	4 h Post-trauma untreated	4 h Post-trauma + dopamine
Cortical water			
ADC-recovery	79.38 ± 0.57	80.42 ± 0.60	81.13 ± 0.7
ADC-nonrecovery	79.20 ± 0.90	81.40 ± 1.30^{+}	83.4 ± 1.10*
Cortical ADC			
ADC-recovery	0.66 ± 0.07	0.64 ± 0.07	0.59 ± 0.02
ADC-nonrecovery	0.68 ± 0.05	0.49 ± 0.08	0.40 ± 0.01*

of hypoxia and hypotension was induced by reducing the FiO_2 to 12%, which in previous studies has been shown to reduce the PaO_2 to 40 mmHg [15]. During this time mABP fell to 30–40 mmHg, and cardiovascular inotropic and chronotropic responses were abolished by elevating halothane levels to 2% above baseline.

Animals in group B were exposed to a controlled cortical impact, the methods for which have been described more fully elsewhere [1, 4]. Briefly, after baseline assessment, a 10 mm craniotomy was prepared over the parietal cortex to the right of midline, and a constrained-stroke pneumatic impactor was set to deliver a blow at 6 m/s to a depth of 3 mm. Immediately after injury the craniotomy site was sealed with the bone flap, gelfoam and rapid drying cyanoacrylic glue.

Dopamine treatment began 2 hours following trauma in both groups A & B, administered as a continuous infusion titrated to maintain mABP above 100 mmHg. Although the use of MRI precluded simultaneous ICP measurement, this mABP was known from previous studies to maintain CPP sufficiently.

Animals in groups A and B were assessed using MRI for tissue water content as described elsewhere [5, 8], and for changes in the Apparent Diffusion Coefficient using methods described more fully by Ito *et al.*, (1996) [6]. All data are presented as means ± SD. Statistical significance was assessed using paired and unpaired student t-tests.

Results

Group A was divided into ADC-Recovery and ADC-NonRecovery subgroups based on the profile of ADC change. Water content at 4 hours in the Non-Recovery group was 81.4 ± 1.3%, whereas in the recovery group it was 80.4 ± 0.6% ($p < 0.01$). In the non-recovery group of animals dopamine caused a significant increase in water content as compared with the untreated group (83.4 ± 1.1%, $p < 0.01$). ADC was unaffected by dopamine treatment (Table 1).

In group B water content was assessed both before and 4 hours after injury. In the ipsilateral hemisphere, water content rose markedly (4.7 ± 2.0%) in the site of contusion, and to lesser degrees in other regions. Dopamine did not influence edema formation in the site of the contusion. However, water content in both the adjacent temporal cortex and underlying hippocampus was markedly increased by dopamine (Fig. 1). ADC values in these regions were unaltered by the administration of dopamine, suggesting that treatment exacerbates pre-existing cell swelling (Fig. 3 a–c).

In the contralateral hemisphere, cortical water also increased (0.8 ± 1.65%), but this increase was unaffected by dopamine (Fig. 2). In the untreated group brain water content in the contralateral hippocampus was unchanged from baseline, and in the temporal cortex it actually fell over the four hours (1.1 ± 1.29% drop in water content). With dopamine treatment water content in both these regions rose markedly (0.8 ± 0.68%, 1.27 ± 1.05% respectively). ADC values remained unaltered, except for the contralateral hippocampus however, where dopamine caused an increase in ADC suggesting initiation of a vasogenic swelling process (Fig. 3 e–f).

Discussion

This study has demonstrated that dopamine is capable of worsening edema formation in two models of traumatic brain injury. In the subgroup of Impact Acceleration Injury with no recovery of ADC, tissue water content after two hours of dopamine treatment was significantly higher compared with an untreated group. ADC values were unaffected by the treatment, suggesting an exacerbation of cellular swelling. Following cortical contusion, dopamine also markedly increased tissue water content in sites remote from the contusional area, and in this case ADC values in all but one region were unaltered by treatment; in the contralateral hippocampus, ADC values rose, suggesting a shift to vasogenic edema.

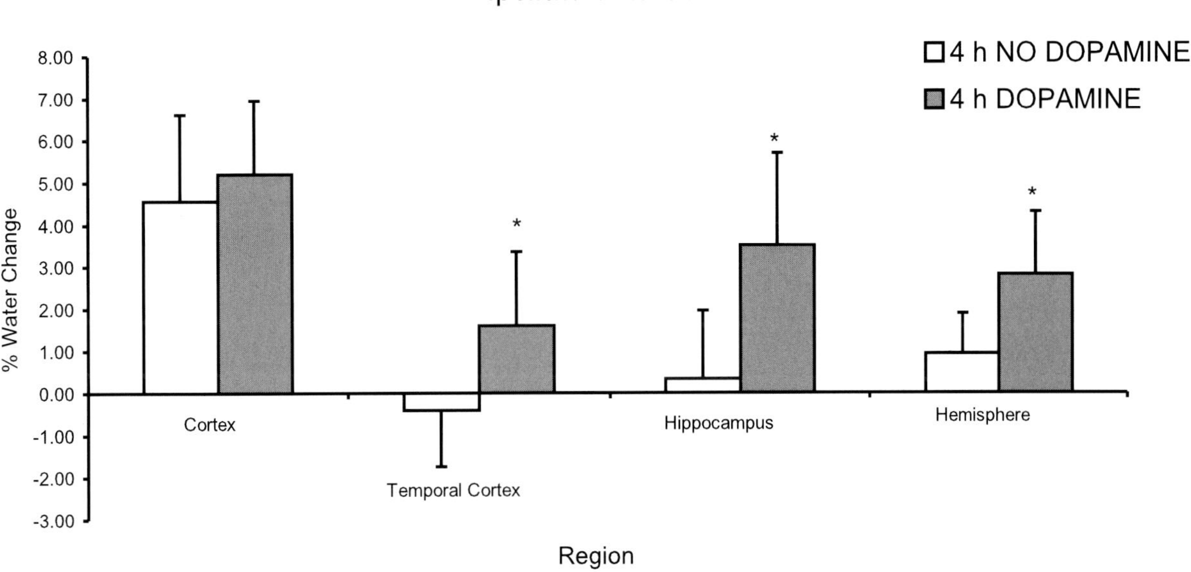

Fig. 1. Graph depicting the change in water content over 4 h of different anatomical regions of the brain ipsilateral to a cortical contusion, calculated by MR. The maximal site of swelling is in the site of the injury, and dopamine has little effect on water accumulation in this region. However edema formation in remote regions is lower, and dopamine in these areas causes a marked increase in water as compared with the untreated animals. $*p < 0.05$ cf untreated group

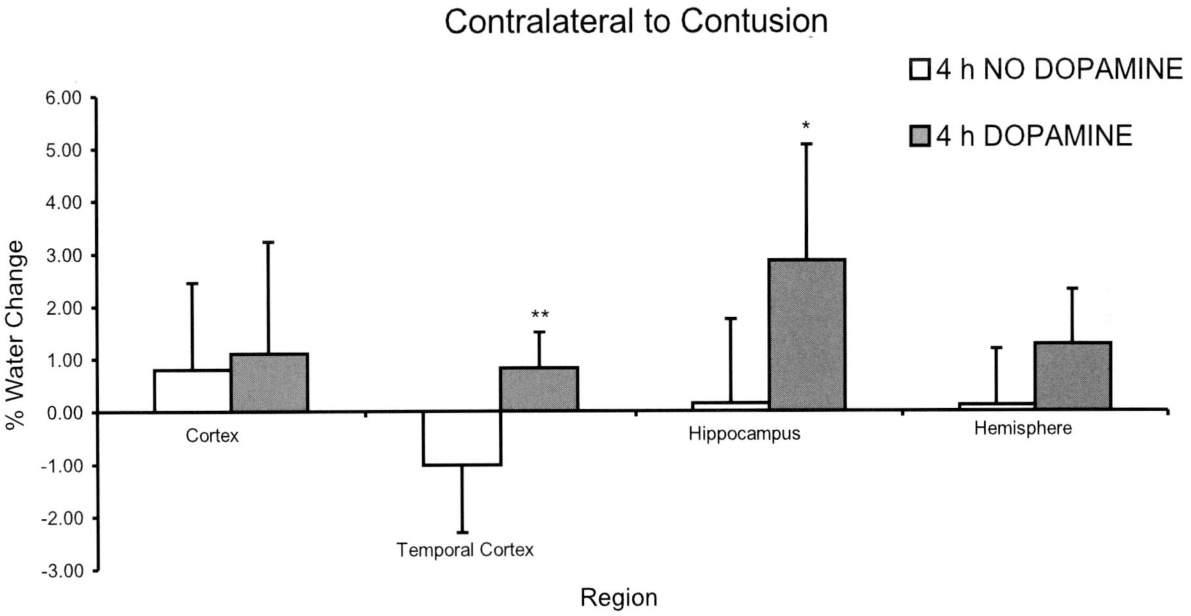

Fig. 2. Graph depicting the change in water content over 4 h of different anatomical regions of the brain contralateral to a cortical contusion, calculated by MR. There was a slight increase in cortical water content, but all other regions were characterised by minimal increases or even decreases in tissue water. In the presence of dopamine these same regions of the brain showed large increases in tissue water content. $*p < 0.05$; $**p < 0.005$ cf untreated group

Management of Cerebral Perfusion Pressure (CPP) is of critical importance for the severely head injured patient. CPP represents the driving force for blood to perfuse the brain and cerebral ischemia has been identified as an adverse determinant of outcome following traumatic brain injury [2, 3].

Pressor therapy is one clinical route by which CPP can be enhanced, however previous studies have sug-

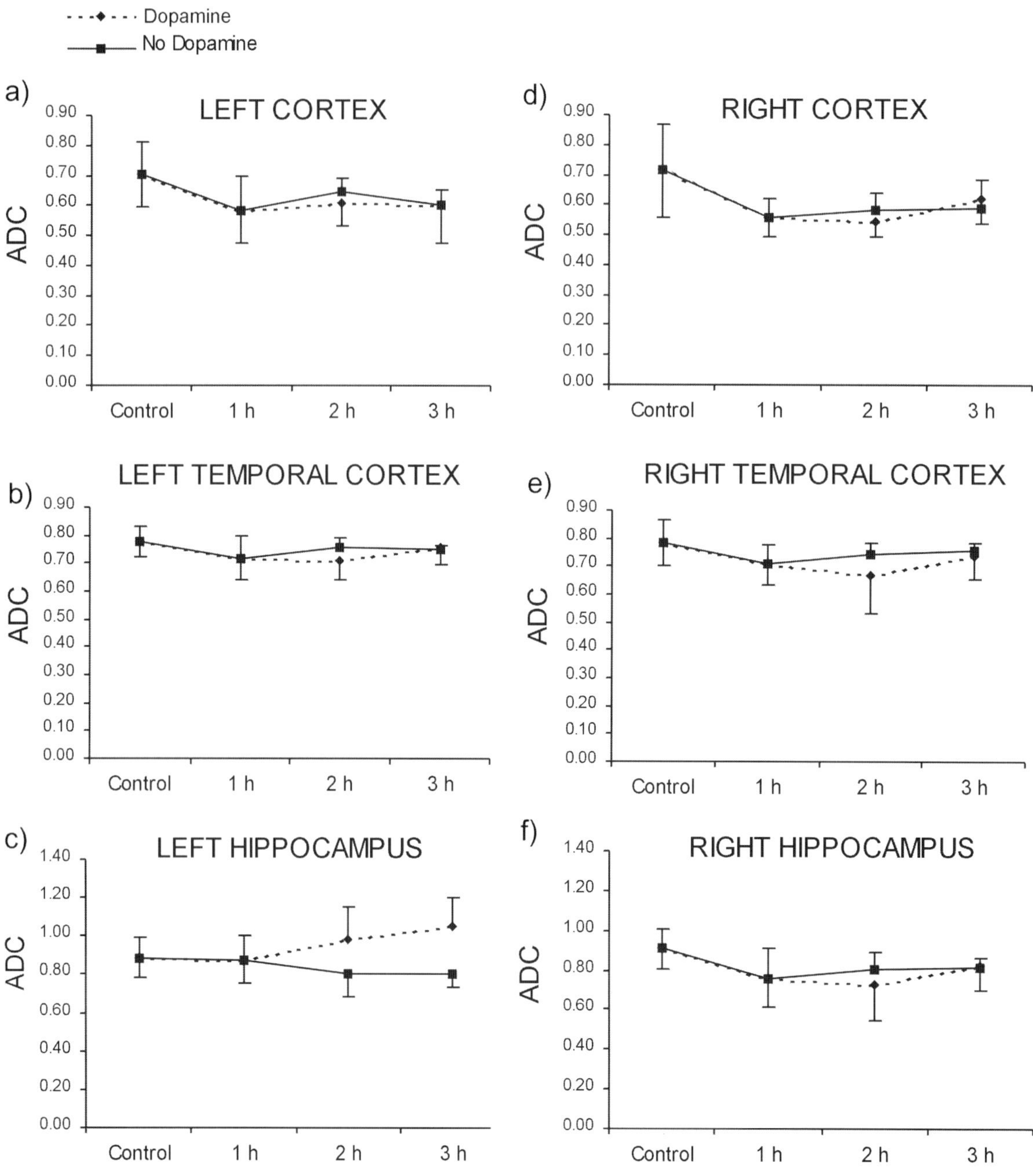

Fig. 3. Graphs showing the ADC values in six different anatomical regions of the contused brain, and the effects on ADC value of administering dopamine at 2 h post-injury. In all cases except one, ADC is diminished with injury, and dopamine does not cause any change despite worsening edema. In the contralateral hippocampus there is initially no change in ADC, but with dopamine administration the ADC value rises markedly (c), suggesting the onset of a vasogenic swelling process. (All ADC values are expressed in units of 10^{-3} mm^2/sec). $^*p < 0.01$ cf untreated group

gested that uncontrolled hypertension in damaged brain may exacerbate edema [10, 11, 13]. In a recent study dopamine was shown to increase experimental contusion volume [7]. Rosner *et al.* [12], however demonstrated that CPP in severely head injured patients could be iatrogenically elevated by inducing systemic hypertension without potentiating mortality. It is thought that maintenance of CPP within a range which permits autoregulation, allows vascular reactivity to control ICP.

The mechanism by which dopamine worsens edema in this study is not known. There are two possible pathological explanations: either a pressure passive circulation or an increase in hydrostatic pressure across an open blood brain barrier. It is interesting that in the case of contusion, dopamine worsens edema in sites remote from the contusion, but not the contusion itself. This may relate in part to regions of very high capillary resistance or "zero-flow" with CCI. In the majority of regions where dopamine worsens edema, the ADC value is unaltered suggesting that dopamine exacerbates pre-existing pathology. The increase in ADC seen in the contralateral hippocampus is however interesting – it suggests that dopamine stimulates a vasogenic edema. This apparent discrepancy can be resolved if one assumes that dopamine will always extravasate water from the capillary bed, but the destination of this water will depend on the state of the tissue. In gross cellular injury water will exit the blood vessel and pass straight into cells, (no change in an already low ADC). However in regions of the brain with a damaged BBB, and relatively intact cells, fluid will exit the blood vessel and lodge in the extracellular space (causing an increase in ADC, viz. contralateral cortex).

Having shown that dopamine is capable of enhancing edema formation the logical progression of this work is in two directions. Firstly, it is possible that the greater tissue water content is an epiphenomenon of dopamine treatment, where improved CBF and neuronal survival far outweigh this problem. Therefore the effects of dopamine on histological damage in these models should be assessed. Secondly, and most importantly, there should be careful consideration of whether or not there exists a subgroup of patients in whom dopamine may not be beneficial, and if so by what means the physician can identify them in advance of therapy.

Acknowledgments

We thank Jana Dunbar, M. S. and Christina Marmarou, B. S., for their expert technical assistance.

References

1. Beaumont A, Marmarou A (1998) The effect of human corticotrophin releasing factor on the formation of post-traumatic cerebral edema. Acta Neurochir [Suppl] (Wien) 71: 149–152
2. Bouma GJ, Muizelaar JP, Choi SC, Newlon PG, Young HF (1991) Cerebral circulation and metabolism after severe traumatic brain injury: the elusive role of ischemia. J Neurosurg 75: 685–693
3. Chesnut RM, Marshall LF, Klauber MR, Blunt BA, Baldwin N, Eisenberg HM, Jane JA, Marmarou A, Foulkes MA (1993) The role of secondary brain injury in determining outcome from severe head injury. J Trauma 34: 216–222
4. Dixon CE, Clifton GL, Lighthall JW, Yaghmai AA, Hayes RL (1991) A controlled cortical impact model of traumatic brain injury in the rat. J Neurosci Meths 39: 253–262
5. Fatouros PP, Marmarou A, Kraft KA, Inao S, Schwarz FP (1991) In vivo brain water determination by T1 measurements: effect of total water content, hydration fraction, and field strength. Mag Res Med 17: 402–413
6. Ito J, Marmarou A, Barzo P, Fatouros P, Corwin F (1996) Characterization of edema by diffusion-weighted imaging in experimental traumatic brain injury. J Neurosurg 84: 97–103
7. Kroppenstedt SN, Kern M, Thomale UW, Schnerider GH, Lanksch WR, Unterberg AW (1999) Effect of cerebral perfusion pressure on contusion volume following impact injury. J Neurosurg 90: 520–526
8. Marmarou A, Fatouros P, Ward J, Appley A, Young H (1990) In vivo measurement of brain water by MRI. Acta Neurochir [Suppl] (Wien) 51: 123–124
9. Marmarou A, Foda MA, van den Brink W, Campbell J, Kita H, Demetriadou K (1994) A new model of diffuse brain injury in rats. Part I: pathophysiology and biomechanics. J Neurosurg 80: 291–300
10. Marshall WJ, Jackson JL, Langfitt TW (1969) Brain swelling caused by trauma and arterial hypertension. Hemodynamic aspects. Arch Neurol 21: 545–553
11. Miller JD, Garibi J, North JB, Teasdale GM (1975) Effects of increased arterial pressure on blood flow in the damaged brain. Neurol Neurosurg Psych 38: 657–665
12. Rosner MJ, Rosner SD, Johnson AH (1995) Cerebral perfusion pressure: management protocol and clinical results. J Neurosurg 83: 949–962
13. Schutta HS, Kassell NF, Langfitt TW (1968) Non-necrotising cortical trauma as a factor in cerebral swelling induced by arterial hypertension. J Neuropath Exp Neurol 27: 130–132
14. Simard JM, Bellefleur M (1989) Systemic arterial hypertension in head trauma. Am J Cardiol 63: 32C–35C
15. Yamamoto M, Marmarou C, Stiefel M, Beaumont A, Marmarou A (1999) The neuroprotective effect of hypothermia on neuronal injury in diffuse traumatic brain injury coupled with hypoxia and hypotension. J Neurotrauma (*in press*)

Correspondence: Anthony Marmarou, Division of Neurosurgery, P.O. Box 508, MCV Station, Sanger Hall, Room 8004, 1101 E. Marshall Street, Richmond, Virginia 23298.

Acta Neurochir (2000) [Suppl] 76: 153–157

A New Antioxidant Compound H-290/51 Attenuates Upregulation of Constitutive Isoform of Heme Oxygenase (HO-2) Following Trauma to the Rat Spinal Cord

H. S. Sharma[1], **P. Alm**[2], **P.-O. Sjöquist**[3], and **J. Westman**[1]

[1] Laboratory of Neuroanatomy, Department of Medical Cell Biology, Biomedical Centre, Uppsala University, Uppsala, Sweden
[2] Department of Pathology, University Hospital, Lund, Sweden
[3] Pharmacology CV, Astra Zeneca, Mölndal, Sweden

Summary

Influence of a new antioxidant compound H-290/51 on carbon monoxide (CO) production following spinal cord injury was examined using immunohistochemistry of the constitutive isoform of heme oxygenase-2 (HO-2) in a rat model. Subjection of rats to 5 h spinal cord injury by making an incision into the right dorsal horn of the T10–11 segments resulted in upregulation of HO-2 in the injured and adjacent T9 and T12 segments. At this time, disruption of the blood-spinal cord barrier (BSCB) permeability, edema formation and cell injury were more pronounced. Pretreatment with H-290/51 (50 mg/kg, p.o., 30 min before trauma) significantly attenuated the HO-2 immunoreactivity along with breakdown of the BSCB permeability, edema and cell injury. These results for the first time demonstrate that the antioxidant compound H-290/51 is capable of attenuating HO-2 expression and thereby influencing CO production. Furthermore, our observations indicate that oxidative stress is involved in CO production, as reflected by HO-2 expression, which is injurious to the cord and H-290/51 exerts powerful neuroprotective effects in spinal cord injury.

Keywords: Spinal cord injury; H-290/51; heme oxygenase-2; carbon monoxide.

Introduction

Carbon monoxide (CO) is a gaseous molecule which influences neuronal communication within the central nervous system (CNS) [1, 4, 11, 14, 18]. However, its involvement in cell injury following brain or spinal cord trauma is still unclear [3, 6, 9, 11]. CO is synthesised by the enzyme, heme oxygenase (HO), a microsomal enzyme responsible for cleaving heme to produce CO, biliverdin and iron [1, 4, 18]. This enzyme is present in two isoforms, i.e. HO-1 and HO-2 which corresponds to the inducible and constitutive isoforms respectively [1, 4]. Recent reports suggest that traumatic brain injury, ischemia or haemorrhagic insult to the CNS induces upregulation of HO-1 in the nervous system [3, 6, 7, 17]. However, upregulation of HO-2 in such forms of injury is not known. HO-2 is constitutively expressed in normal animals and a few positive neurons in the spinal cord can be seen using immunohistochemistry [2, 5, 13].

Upregulation of HO-2 is associated with increased production of CO which will influence neuronal function [2]. Increased formation of CO may disrupt membrane function and augment cell injury [1, 4, 13]. This idea is in line with our previous observations exhibiting profound increase in HO-2 expression following hyperthermia-induced brain injury in areas associated with edema formation and cell distortion [11, 13]. The mechanisms of cell injury caused by either hyperthermia, trauma, ischemia or hypoxia are basically similar in nature [12, 13, 15, 20]. Thus, if CO is harmful in brain injury caused by hyperthermia, similar function of this gaseous molecule may be seen in the pathophysiology of spinal cord injury.

Previous observations from our laboratory show that a focal spinal cord injury is associated with microhaemorrhages, leakage of serum proteins, edema and abnormal cell reaction in the perifocal segments [8, 10, 20]. These pathological changes were significantly reduced by pretreatment with a potent antioxidant compound H-290/51 [15, 20]. This indicates that oxidative stress plays important role in the pathophysiology of cell injury and further suggests a potential neuroprotective effect of H-290/51 in spinal cord injury.

The present investigation was undertaken to find out whether CO plays any role in cell injury caused by spinal trauma by studying expression of HO-2 in the cord using immunohistochemistry. In addition, the contribution of oxidative stress on CO formation and its involvement in cell injury was examined using H-290/51 pretreatment.

Materials and Methods

Animals

Experiments were carried out on 20 male Sprague Dawley rats (220–250 g) housed at controlled room temperature (21 ± 1 °C) with 12 h light and 12 h dark schedule. These animals were supplied tap water and food pellets *ad libitum*.

Spinal Cord Injury

Under Equithesin anaesthesia (3 ml/kg, i.p.) one segment laminectomy was performed on the T10–11 segments. Spinal cord injury was made by making an incision on the right dorsal horn (about 2 mm deep and 5 mm long). The wound was covered with cotton soaked in saline [8, 12]. Animals were allowed to survive 5 h after injury. Normal rats under anaesthesia served as controls. This experimental condition was approved by the Ethical Committee of Uppsala University, Uppsala, Sweden and Banaras Hindu University, Varanasi, India.

H-290/51 Treatment

In a separate group of rats H-290/51 (Astra-Zeneca, Mölndal, Sweden) was given orally (50 mg/kg) as suspension in distilled water 30 min before injury. One group of treated rats was used as drug-treated control group and no injury was made in these animals. These animals were sacrificed 5.5 h after the drug administration [20].

Perfusion and Fixation

At the end of the experiments, animals were perfused with about 50 ml phosphate buffer saline (0.1 M, pH 7.0) to wash out blood from the body via heart. This was followed by 150 ml of fixative containing 4% paraformaldehyde in the phosphate buffer saline. After the perfusion animals were wrapped in aluminium foil and kept overnight in a refrigerator at 4 °C. On the next day, the desired portion of the spinal cord was removed comprising T9 to T12 segments, divided into three parts (T9, T10–11 and T12) and kept in the same fixative at 4 °C for another 48 h [10, 12].

HO-2 Immunoreactivity

HO-2 immunostaining using monoclonal HO-2 antiserum (StressGene Laboratory, Canada) on 40 µm thick vibratome section was done as described earlier [9, 11]. Immunohistochemistry on spinal cord tissues obtained from control, spinal cord injured, H-290/51 treated normal and spinal cord injured rats were done in parallel and examined in a blind fashion by two independent observers.

Spinal Cord Edema

In separate group of rats, spinal cord water content was examined in the T9, T10–11 and the T12 segments of the cord by using differences in wet and dry weight of the samples. For this purpose, immediately after the experiments, the spinal cord samples were dissected out, weighed and placed immediately in an oven maintained at 90 °C. The samples were dried in this oven for 72 h. The water content was calculated as follows: Wet weight of the sample (mg) – dry weight of the sample (mg)/wet weight of the sample (mg) × 100 [8, 20].

Blood-Spinal Cord Barrier Permeability

The BSCB permeability was examined using Evans blue albumin (2% of a 3 ml/kg, i.v. solution) and $^{[131]}$I-sodium (100 µCi/Kg, i.v.) [10–12]. In brief, both the tracers were administered into the right femoral artery via needle puncture at the end of the experiment. These tracers were allowed to circulate for 5 min. The intravascular tracers were washed out by a brief saline rinse through heart. Immediately before the saline perfusion, one ml blood was withdrawn from the heart for later determination of the blood radioactivity [13]. The BSCB permeability was calculated as percentage of spinal cord tissue radioactivity over the blood iodine counts [8].

Statistical Analysis

Unpaired Student's t-test was used to evaluate statistical significance of the data obtained. A p-value less than 0.05 was considered significant.

Results

Effect of H-290/51 on HO-2 Immunohistochemistry

Only a few HO-2 positive cells can be found in the spinal cord of normal rats. Subjection of rats to a focal spinal cord injury profoundly increased HO-2 immunostaining in the nerve cells located within the injured as well as in the adjacent spinal cord segments (Fig. 1). This upregulation of HO-2 was mainly confined within the damaged or distorted neurons located in the edematous region of the spinal cord. The HO-2 immunoreactivity was most pronounced in the vicinity of the lesion site.

Pretreatment with H-290/51 significantly attenuated HO-2 immunoreactivity in the spinal cord following trauma (Fig. 1). Thus, only a few HO-2 positive cells can be seen in the spinal cord of H-290/51 treated animals compared to the untreated traumatised rats (Fig. 1). In untreated animals, general sponginess, edematous expansion and cellular distortion of the spinal cord is apparent following trauma. These cell changes are considerably reduced in H-290/51 treated injured animals.

Effect of H-290/51 on the Blood-Spinal Cord Barrier Permeability

The BSCB permeability was significantly increased to Evans blue albumin and radioactive iodine following trauma. Pretreatment with H-290/51 significantly

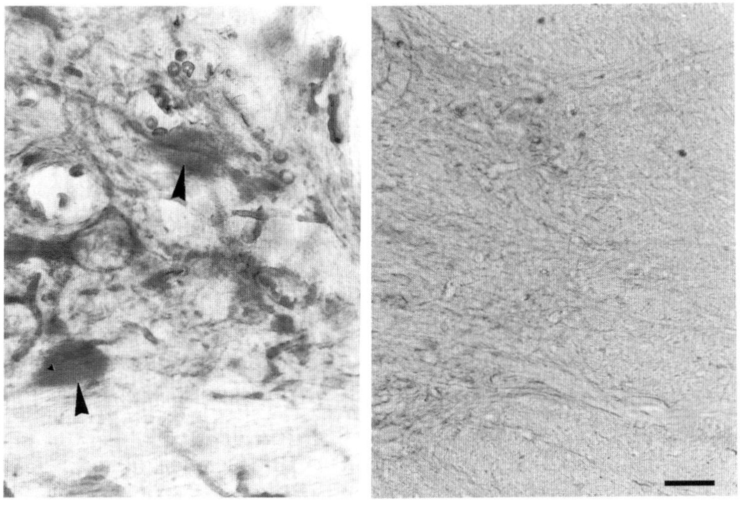

Fig. 1. Upregulation of HO-2 in the T9 segment of the spinal cord in one rat following 5 h after an incision in the right dorsal horn of the T10–11 segment (left). The HO-2 expression is mainly seen in the nerve cells (arrow heads) and the dendrites. General expansion of the cord and distortion of the nerve cells are apparent. Pretreatment with H-290/51 markedly attenuated the expression of HO-2 in the T9 segment of the cord (right). In this drug treated rat, nerve cell distortion and general expansion of the cord are considerably reduced (bar = 60 μm)

reduced the extravasation of Evans blue and $^{[131]}$I-sodium tracers in the spinal cord (Fig. 2). However, pretreatment with H-290/51 alone did not influence the BSCB permeability to either tracers compared to the control group.

Effect of H-290/51 on Spinal Cord Edema Formation

Subjection of rats to a focal spinal cord trauma resulted in profound edema formation (Fig. 2). Pretreatment with H-290/51 resulted in significant reduction in the edema development at the end of 5 h after injury. The compound given in normal rats did not influence spinal cord water content.

Discussion

Our results for the first time show that spinal cord injury has the capacity to induce an increased formation of CO as evident from the marked upregulation of its constitutive isoform of heme oxygenase (HO-2) enzyme. Furthermore, the present investigations clearly demonstrate that pretreatment with the new antioxidant compound H-290/51 significantly attenuated the expression of HO-2 indicating that oxidative stress plays an important role in the upregulation of CO following spinal cord injury, not reported earlier.

Involvement of biological gases, like nitric oxide (NO) and CO in the pathophysiology of cell injury is

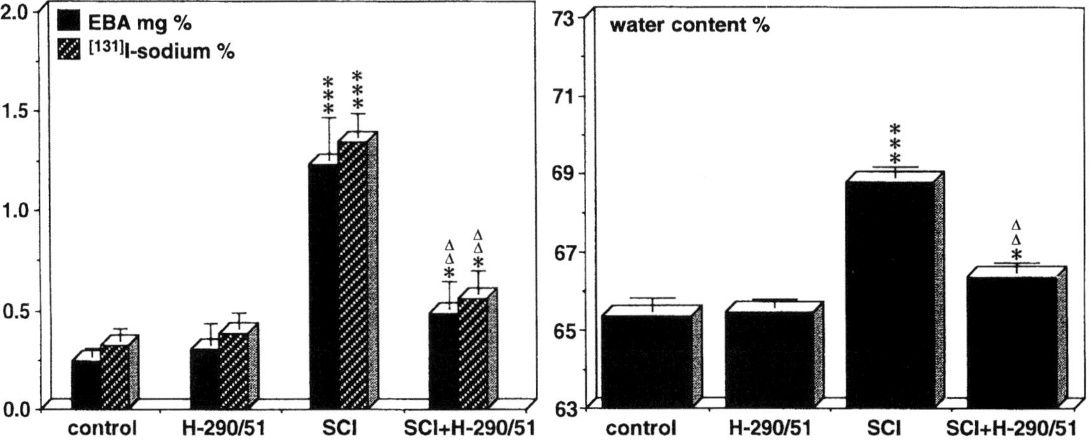

Fig. 2. Blood-spinal cord barrier (*BSCB*) permeability (left) and spinal cord water content (right) in the T9 segment of the spinal cord following trauma and their modification with H-290/51 pretreatment. *** $P < 0.001$, * $P < 0.05$, compared to the control; ΔΔ $P < 0.01$, compared from spinal cord injury (SCI); student's unpaired t-test

still controversial [11, 13, 14, 18]. One reason for this discrepancy is due to the fact that CO, like NO will influence neurotransmission by diffusing from one cell to the another cell in a relatively very short time [14]. Thus, CO does not require the classical synaptic machinery to influence neurotransmission. Therefore, to understand the function of CO in cell injury expression of its synthesising enzymes HO-1 or HO-2 have been used by several workers in the past employing various animal models. However, the results so far obtained are contradictory.

There are reports that upregulation of HO reflects the increased production and release of CO in the biological system [14, 18]. Previously, upregulation of HO-1 is reported in the glial cells after several days to weeks after brain trauma [3]. In this study, HO-1 is present in glial scars which are known to be involved in the mechanisms of regeneration and tissue repair [6]. Thus, increased expression of HO-1 in the brain following trauma is considered to be beneficial in nature [6, 7]. However, further evidences are needed to support this assumption. On the other hand, upregulation of HO-2 following trauma is not known and thus, the role of HO-2 expression in the cell injury is still unclear.

Only a few HO-2 positive nerve cells can be found in the normal spinal cord indicating that small production of CO from HO-2 positive cells is important for normal spinal cord function [11, 13]. However, it seems likely that abnormal production of CO following upregulation of HO-2 in nerve cells not normally exhibiting this activity is injurious to the cell [9, 11, 13]. Increased CO production may induce a direct disruption of the cell membrane or inhibit its metabolism leading to cell injury.

That the abnormal production of CO is injurious to the cord is further supported by the results of the present investigation. In the present study, HO-2 positive cells are found in the regions exhibiting profound edema and breakdown of the BSCB permeability. Although, increased expression of any enzyme in the region associated with cell injury does not necessarily reflect the harmful effects of that particular substance on cells. However, our results obtained with H-290/51 pretreatment strongly indicate that the increased HO-2 activity in spinal cord trauma is associated with cell injury. This is evident with the fact that pretreatment with H-290/51 significantly attenuated the upregulation of HO-2 expression, edema formation and breakdown of the BSCB permeability.

A reduction in HO-2 expression as the cause or effect of the neuroprotection offered by the compound H-290/51 following trauma is not clear from this study. The fluid microenvironment of the spinal cord is less perturbed in H-290/51 treated traumatised rats compared to the untreated injured animals. This could be one of the important factors in less expression of HO-2 in the drug-treated injured animals. Taken together, these observations clearly suggest that secondary injury factors such as oxidative stress, edema formation and breakdown of the BSCB permeability play important roles in HO-2 expression [12, 20].

The neuroprotective effects of H-290/51 on spinal cord edema formation and breakdown of the BSCB permeability indicate that oxidative stress is playing a major role in the pathophysiology of spinal cord injury. H-290/51 is a known compound which effectively inhibits the formation of free radicals [16] and probably act as a chain-breking antioxidant [19]. Since oxidative stress and formation of free radicals disrupt membrane integrity and induce breakdown of the BBB permeability and brain edema formation [15], it seems reasonable to assume that pretreatment with H-290/51 which reduces the formation of free radicals, will exert a powerful neuroprotection in spinal cord injury. Obviously, a less expression of HO-2 in drug treated animals is mainly due to a lack of generation of free radicals and/or oxidative stress following trauma.

In conclusion, our results suggest that H-290/51 pretreatment effectively inhibited HO-2 expression, breakdown of the BSCB permeability and edema formation. This indicates that disturbances in the fluid microenvironment of the cord and extravasation of proteins or edema fluid in the extracellular compartment are potential biological signals for upregulation of HO-2 expression. Alternatively, oxidative stress and formation of free radicals may have a direct effect on HO-2 expression, a subject which require additional investigation.

Acknowledgments

This work is supported by grants from the Swedish Medical Research Council nr. 2710 (JW/HSS); (PA-11205); Astra Zeneca, Mölndal (HSS), Sweden; Alexander von Humboldt Foundation (HSS), Bonn, Germany; The University Grants Commission (HSS), New Delhi, India. The expert technical assistance of Kärstin Flink; Katja Deparade; Elisabeth Scherer and Kerstin Rystedt; and the secretarial assistance of Aruna Sharma, Gun-Britt Lind and Angela Ludwig are highly appreciated with thanks.

References

1. Abraham NG, Drummond GS, Lutton JD, Kappas A (1996) The biological significance and physiological role of heme oxygenase. Cell Physiol Biochem 6: 129–168
2. Dore S, Takahashi M, Ferris CD, Hester LD, Guastella D, Snyder SH (1999) Bilirubin, formed by activation of heme oxygenase-2, protects neurons against oxidative stress injury. Proc Natl Acad Sci USA 96: 2445–2450
3. Fukuda K, Richmon JD, Sato M, Sharp FR, Panter SC, Noble LJ (1996) Induction of heme oxygenase-1 (HO-1) in glia after traumatic brain injury. Brain Res 736: 68–75
4. Maines, MD (1988) Heme oxygenase: function, multiplicity, regulatory mechanisms and clinical applications. FASEB J 2: 2557–2568
5. McCoubrey K, Maines MD (1994) The structure, organisation and differential expression of gene encoding rat heme oxygenase-2. Gene 139: 155–161
6. Panahian N, Yoshiura M, Maines MD (1999) Overexpression of heme oxygenase-1 is neuroprotective in a model of permanent middle cerebral artery occlusion in transgenic mice. J Neurochem 72: 1187–1203
7. Rajdev S, Fix AS, Sharp FR (1998) Acute phencyclidine neurotoxicity in rat forebrain: induction of heme oxygenase-1 and attenuation by the antioxidant dimethylthiouria. Eur J Neurosci 10: 3840–3852
8. Sharma HS, Olsson Y, Dey PK (1990) Early accumulation of serotonin in rat spinal cord subjected to traumatic injury. Relation to edema and blood flow changes. Neuroscience 36: 725–730
9. Sharma HS, Alm P, Westman J (1997) Upregulation of hemeoxygenase-II in the rat spinal cord following heat stress, Thermal physiology. In: Nielsen-Johanssen B, Nielsen R (eds) The August Krogh Institute, Copenhagen, pp 135–138
10. Sharma HS, Nyberg F, Westman J, Gordh T, Alm P, Lindholm D (1998) Brain derived neurotrophic factor and insulin like growth factor-1 attenuate upregulation of nitric oxide synthase and cell injury following trauma to the spinal cord. Amino Acids 14: 121–129
11. Sharma HS, Alm P, Westman J (1998) Nitric oxide and carbon monoxide in the pathophysiology of brain functions in heat stress. Prog Brain Res 115: 297–333
12. Sharma HS, Nyberg F, Gordh T, Alm P, Westman J (1998) Neurotrophic factors attenuate neuronal nitric oxide synthase upregulation, microvascular permeability disturbances, edema formation and cell injury in the spinal cord following trauma, Spinal cord monitoring. Basic principles, regeneration, pathophysiology and clinical aspects. In: Stålberg E, Sharma HS, Olsson Y (eds) Springer, Wien New York, pp 181–210
13. Sharma HS (1999) Pathophysiology of blood-brain barrier, brain edema and cell injury following hyperthermia: New role of heat shock protein, nitric oxide and carbon monoxide. an experimental study in the rat using light and electron microscopy, Acta Universitatis Upsaliensis 830: 1–94
14. Snyder SH, Jaffrey SR, Zakhary R (1998) Nitric oxide and carbon monoxide: parallel roles as neural messengers. Brain Res Rev 26: 167–175
15. Stålberg E, Sharma HS, Olsson Y (1998) Spinal cord monitoring. Basic principles, regeneration, pathophysiology and clinical aspects. Springer, Wien New York, pp 1–527
16. Svensson L, Börjesson I, Kull B, Sjöquist P-O (1993) Automated procedure for measuring TBARS for in vitro comparison of the effect of antioxidants on tissues. Scand J Clin Lab Invest 53: 83–85
17. Takizawa S, Hirabayashi H, Matsushima K, Tokuoka K, Shinohara Y (1998) Induction of heme oxygenase protein protects neurons in cortex and striatum, but not in hippocampus, against transient forebrain ischemia. J Cereb Blood Flow Metab 18: 559–569
18. Verma A, Hirsch DJ, Glatt CE, Ronnett GV, Snyder SH (1993) Carbon monoxide: a putative neural messenger. Science 295: 381–384
19. Westerlund Ch, Östlund-Lindqvist A-M, Sainsbury M, Shertzer HG, Sjöquist P-O (1996) Characterization of novel indenoindoles. Part I. Structure-activity relationships in different model system of lipid peroxidation. Biochem Pharmacol 51: 1397–1402
20. Winkler T, Sharma HS, Stålberg E, Westman J (1998) Spinal cord bioelectrical activity, edema and cell injury following a focal trauma to the rat spinal cord. An experimental study using pharmacological and morphological approaches. Spinal cord monitoring. Basic principles, regeneration, pathophysiology and clinical aspects. In: Stålberg E, Sharma HS, Olsson Y (eds) Springer, Wien New York, pp 283–364

Correspondence: Hari Shanker Sharma, Ph.D., Laboratory of Neuroanatomy, Department of Medical Cell Biology, Biomedical Centre, Box 571, Uppsala University, SE-75123 Uppsala, Sweden.

Acta Neurochir (2000) [Suppl] 76: 159–163

A Bradykinin BK_2 Receptor Antagonist HOE-140 Attenuates Blood-Spinal Cord Barrier Permeability Following a Focal Trauma to the Rat Spinal Cord

An experimental study using Evans blue, ^{131}I-sodium and lanthanum tracers

H. S. Sharma

Laboratory of Neuroanatomy, Department of Medical Cell Biology, Biomedical Centre, Uppsala University, Uppsala, Sweden

Summary

The role of bradykinin in breakdown of the blood-spinal cord barrier (BSCB) permeability following a focal lesion to the cord was examined using a potent bradykinin BK_2 receptor antagonist, HOE-140 in a rat model. Spinal cord injury was produced by an incision into the right dorsal horn of the T10–11 segment. In a separate group of rats HOE-140 (1 mg/kg) was administered intravenously 30 min before injury. A focal trauma to the cord markedly increased the extravasation of Evans blue and ^{131}I-sodium tracers in the cord at 5 h. Pretreatment with HOE-140 significantly attenuated the extravasation of these tracers in the spinal cord. At ultrastructural level, lanthanum was seen within the endothelial cell cytoplasm, in vesicular profiles as well as in the basal lamina in the untreated traumatised rats. In HOE-140 treated rats, the lanthanum was mainly confined within the lumen. These observations strongly suggest that bradykinin is involved in the breakdown of the BSCB permeability probably via bradykinin BK_2 receptors, not reported earlier.

Keywords: Bradykinin; spinal cord injury; HOE-140; blood-spinal cord barrier permeability.

Introduction

Spinal cord fluid microenvironment is strictly regulated by the blood-spinal cord barrier (BSCB) [8, 11, 17, 18]. Although the permeability properties of the BSCB are not examined in greater details, there are reasons to believe that the physiochemical properties of the BSCB under normal and in pathological conditions are very similar to that of the blood-brain barrier (BBB) [9, 18]. The BSCB is characterised by endothelial cells connected with tight junctions [8, 9, 11] and contains a very low level of pinocytotic vesicles [8]. A focal trauma to the spinal cord is associated with breakdown of the BSCB permeability which is mainly characterised by an increase in the transendothelial cell transport either caused by an increased number of the vesicular profiles or increased endothelial cell membrane permeability without disrupting the tight junctions [8, 11].

The molecular mechanisms of trauma induced breakdown of the BSCB permeability is not well known. It appears that release of neurochemicals and secondary injury factors play important roles in breakdown of the BSCB [8, 12, 17, 18]. Extravasation of serum proteins following breakdown of the BSCB will lead to vasogenic edema formation and initiate several biochemical, molecular, ionic and immunological disturbances leading to cell injury [9, 11, 18]. Thus maintenance of the BSCB permeability seems to be vital for the normal spinal cord function.

There are several neurochemical mediators identified in the brain which are involved in the BBB permeability and the brain edema formation [9, 19]. It seems likely that these chemical mediators are also involved in the BSCB permeability and spinal cord edema formation. Previous reports from our laboratory suggest that serotonin, prostaglandins, opioid peptides, histamine and catecholamines are involved in disruption of the BSCB permeability following trauma to the rat spinal cord [8, 11, 14, 18]. These observations clearly show that breakdown of the BSCB permeability is a complex phenomena and many neurochemical mediators are involved in this process.

Almost all neurochemical receptors are localised on the cerebral endothelial cells in both luminal and in abluminal side of the microvessels within the CNS [1, 9, 19]. Thus, a possibility exists that release of neurochemicals will influence selective receptor mediated events and signal transduction mechanisms in order to increase the permeability of the microvessels in a specific way. However, involvement of specific neurochemical receptors in BSCB permeability is still a new subject and requires further investigation.

Recently, bradykinin (BK) has been identified as a mediator of the BBB permeability and brain edema formation following several noxious insults to the brain [1]. However, its involvement in the BSCB permeability is still unknown. Bradykinin receptors known as BK_1 and BK_2 have been identified in both neural and non neural cells in the CNS [1, 4]. There are some reports which indicate that blockade of BK_2 receptors or both BK_1 and BK_2 receptors attenuate bradykinin induced breakdown of the BBB permeability [4]. However, the role of BK receptors in modifying the BBB permeability is still controversial. Since the role of bradykinin and its receptors in BSCB permeability is still unknown, the present investigation was undertaken to find out whether BK plays any role in the breakdown of the BSCB following a focal spinal trauma using one selective BK_2 receptor antagonist HOE-140 pretreatment.

Materials and Methods

Animals

Experiments were carried out on 20 male Sprague Dawley rats (200–300 g) housed at controlled room temperature at $21 \pm 1\,^{\circ}C$ with 12 h light and 12 h dark schedule. The commercial rat food pellets and tap water were supplied ad libitum.

Spinal Cord Injury

Spinal cord injury was produced under urethane anaesthesia (1.5 g/kg, i.p.) by making an incision on the right dorsal horn of the T10–11 segment (about 2 mm deep and 4 mm long) following one segment laminectomy over the T10–11 segments [10, 13]. The wound was covered with cotton soaked saline in order to prevent a direct exposure to the air. The animals were allowed to survive 5 h post injury. Normal intact rats were used as controls. This experimental condition was approved by the Ethical Committee of Uppsala University, Uppsala, Sweden and Banaras Hindu University, Varanasi, India.

Pretreatment with HOE-140

In a separate group of 10 rats BK_2 receptor antagonist HOE-140 (Hoechst Pharmaceuticals, Germany) was administered 1 mg/kg, intravenously. In 5 rats spinal cord injury was produced 30 min after the drug administration. The remaining 5 rats were used as drug-treated controls.

Blood-Spinal Cord Barrier Permeability

The BSCB permeability was examined using Evans blue albumin (0.3 ml/100 g body weight, i.v.) and $^{[131]}$I-sodium (10 μCi/rat) tracers [16]. In brief, both tracers were administered into the right femoral vein after needle puncture and allowed to circulate for 5 min. At the end of 5 min following tracer injection, the animals were perfused with 0.9% saline through the heart in order to remove the intravascular tracers followed by perfusion with 4% paraformaldehyde in 0.1% cacodylate buffer containing 2.5% lanthanum hydrochloride. Immediately before the onset of saline infusion, one ml whole blood was withdrawn from the left ventricle through cardiac puncture in order to determine the whole blood radioactivity. To determine the spinal cord radioactivity, small tissue pieces of the spinal cord comprising T9 and T12 segments were dissected out, weighed and counted in a 3-in Gamma counter at the energy window of 500–800 KeV [9, 16]. The extravasation of the radiotracer was assessed as percentage of the radioactivity over blood activity.

After counting the radioactivity of spinal cord samples, the extravasation of Evans blue in these spinal cord segments was first assessed by naked eye inspection. Then the dye entered into the cord was extracted using a salt saturated butanol solution at pH 6.4 and extravasation was measured colorimetrically [9, 16].

Ultrastructural Studies on the BSCB Permeability Using Lanthanum Tracer

Some tissue pieces were post fixed in osmium tetraoxide and embedded in Epon for routine ultrastructural examination. Lanthanum, an electron dense tracer, could be easily visualised at transmission electron microscopy as dark black particles. The distribution of lanthanum across the microvessels was examined in 250 vascular profiles from 5 animals in the dorsal horn of the T9 segment [9, 11, 16].

Statistical Treatment of the Data

Unpaired Student's t-test was used to examine the statistical significance of the data obtained between control, experimental and drug treated normal or traumatised spinal cord using standard procedures. A p-value less than 0.05 was considered significant.

Results

Effect of HOE-140 on the BSCB Permeability to Evans Blue and $^{[131]}$-Iodine

A focal spinal cord trauma to the T10–11 segments significantly increased the BSCB permeability to Evans blue albumin and $^{[131]}$I-sodium tracers in the perifocal T9 segment (Fig. 1). Pretreatment with HOE-140 significantly attenuated the trauma induced breakdown of the BSCB permeability (Fig. 1). However, the extravasation of tracers in HOE-140 treated rats remained significantly elevated from the control group. HOE-140 alone did not alter the BSCB permeability in normal rats.

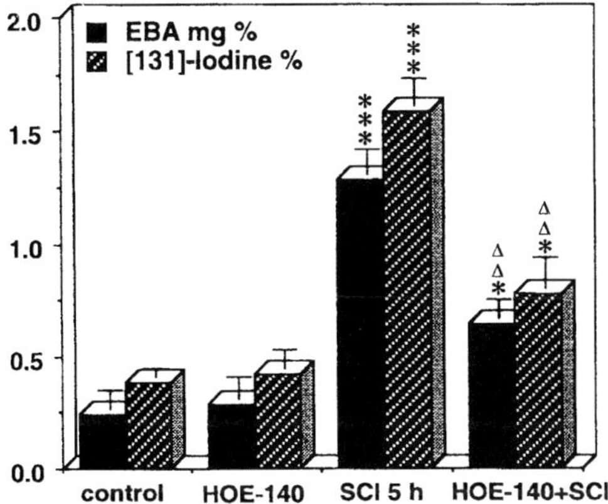

Fig. 1. Blood-spinal cord barrier (*BSCB*) permeability to Evans blue and $^{[131]}$I-sodium in spinal cord injury and its modification with bradykinin BK_2 receptor antagonist, HOE-140. The compound HOE-140 was administered intravenously (1 mg/kg) 30 min before spinal cord trauma (for details see text). * $P < 0.05$; *** $P < 0.001$ compared with control; ΔΔ $P < 0.01$, compared with spinal cord injury (SCI), Student's unpaired t-test

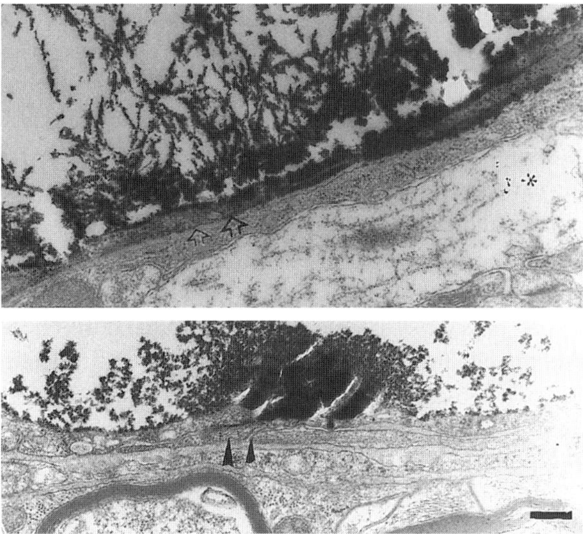

Fig. 2. Extravasation of lanthanum across one microvessel in one untreated spinal cord injured rat (upper panel). Lanthanum infiltration can be seen within the endothelium (blank arrows). Pretreatment with HOE-140 did not result in lanthanum exudation within the endothelium following spinal cord trauma (lower panel). Lanthanum, however, can be seen within the vesicular profile in the drug treated rat. The tight junction is completely normal in appearance (bar = 500 nm)

Effect of HOE-140 on the BSCB Permeability to Lanthanum

In normal rats, lanthanum was mainly confined within the lumen of the endothelial cells often seen as attached particles on the luminal side of the endothelium. Presence of lanthanum in the vesicular profile or infiltration of the tracer within the spinal cord endothelium was completely lacking in normal animals.

However, in spinal cord traumatised rats, lanthanum infiltration within the endothelial cell cytoplasm was a common finding (Fig. 2). Lanthanum extravasation in the endothelial cell was however, seen in a specific and selective manner. Thus one endothelium may be completely infiltrated with lanthanum tracer while the adjacent endothelial cell appears to be completely devoid of lanthanum. In large superficial vessels, lanthanum was often localised within the vesicular profiles of the endothelial cell cytoplasm. However the tight junctional permeability remained intact. In some vascular profiles, lanthanum was seen in the basal lamina.

In HOE-140 treated and traumatised rats, only a few vesicular profiles contained lanthanum within the endothelial cell cytoplasm. However, infiltration of lanthanum within the endothelial cell or the presence of endothelial cell in the basal lamina was mainly absent (Fig. 2). The tight junctions appear normal in HOE-140 treated traumatised rats.

Discussion

The present results clearly demonstrate that bradykinin is involved in the breakdown of the BSCB permeability following trauma. This is evident from the fact that blockade of bradykinin BK_2 receptors by HOE-140 significantly attenuated the leakage of Evans blue albumin and radioactive iodine tracers across the microvessels of the cord following a focal spinal trauma. These results for the first time show that BK_2 receptors are involved in the BSCB permeability disturbances in the cord following trauma.

Extravasation of serum protein across the endothelial cell is mainly responsible for the formation of vasogenic edema formation which in turn is related with the development of cell injury [9]. Thus it seems quite likely that breakdown of the BSCB permeability is associated with edema formation and cell injury indicating a potential therapeutic role of BK_2 receptor antagonists in spinal trauma, a feature which requires further investigation.

We have used two protein tracers to study the permeability of the BSCB following trauma. Evans blue and radioactive iodine when introduced into the circulation will bind to the serum proteins [15, 16]. These tracers mainly bind to serum albumin followed by gamma globulin and fibronectin. However, there are some minor differences in their protein binding capacity into the circulation. Evans blue is about 68% bound to serum albumin whereas iodine is only bound to 50% to serum albumin [15]. This difference in protein binding capacity into the circulation may account for some minor differences in the extravasation of these tracers across the spinal cord microvessels seen in the present study following trauma.

The passage of tracers across the spinal cord endothelial cells following trauma is not known in detail. Previous observations in our model suggest that tracer extravasation is mainly due to increased endothelial cell permeability [8, 11]. This is supported by the fact that increase in intracellular vesicular profiles containing lanthanum or infiltration of lanthanum within the endothelial cell cytoplasm are quite common after spinal trauma in our model. Widening of spinal cord endothelial tight junctions is absent in incision induced trauma model [11]. Thus it seems quite likely that a focal spinal cord trauma influences the BSCB permeability by transendothelial cell transport. The present results are in good agreement with our previous findings and further confirm this idea.

We have seen a selective increase in lanthanum permeability within the spinal cord microvessels. The mechanism of a selective increase of lanthanum permeability in some specific endothelial cells in one microvessel leaving the adjacent endothelial cell completely intact is not well understood. Specific receptor mediated increase in the permeability of the BSCB via neurochemical mediators seems to be primarily responsible for this phenomenon. This idea is further supported by the results obtained with bradykinin BK_2 receptor antagonist compound HOE-140. Thus, in HOE-140 treated animals, infiltration of lanthanum was mainly absent in the endothelial cell following trauma. This observation clearly suggests that some endothelial cells may possess BK_2 receptors which are selectively distributed in a particular manner. Blockade of BK_2 receptors with HOE-140 in endothelial cell is mainly responsible for absence of lanthanum infiltration. To further confirm this, binding studies using radiolabelled BK_2 receptors are needed, which require additional investigation. We did not find a reduction in vesicular profile containing lanthanum in the HOE-140 treated group or alterations in the tight junctional permeability following trauma. These observations suggest that BK_2 receptors mainly influence endothelial cell membrane permeability.

The biochemical pathways and related signal transduction mechanisms responsible for the increased BSCB permeability by bradykinin after its binding to the BK_2 receptors are not clear from this investigation. It seems likely that bradykinin may stimulate cAMP within the endothelial cell which may induce membrane permeability increase probably through transendothelial mechanisms [5, 6, 15]. Other possibilities may include bradykinin induced increased synthesis of prostaglandins, histamine and/or nitric oxide within the endothelial cells [2, 7]. These compounds alone or in combination are well known to enhance endothelial cell permeability in the CNS [11, 12, 15, 18]. However, bradykinin induced stimulation of other chemical mediators is a new subject and require additional investigation.

Bradykinin is a mediator of brain edema and has the capacity to disrupt the BBB [19]. An increased production and release of bradykinin occurs following brain trauma [3, 20] and bradykinin infusion into the brain increases the BBB permeability and induces brain edema formation [1]. Our results for the first time show that bradykinin is also a mediator of the BSCB permeability. Pretreatment with HOE-140 in identical doses attenuated spinal cord water content (HS Sharma, unpublished observation) indicating that bradykinin is also a potential mediator of spinal cord edema formation following trauma.

Bradykinin acts on the CNS tissues through BK_1 and BK_2 receptors [1, 4]. Previously, drugs with mixed BK_1 and BK_2 receptor antagonist properties exerted some beneficial effects in brain trauma [1]. Our investigations suggest that blockade of BK_2 receptor is beneficial in spinal cord injury. It has been shown that low doses of BK receptor antagonists may provide neuroprotection whereas high dose of the compound may in fact act as bradykinin agonist [5]. Thus, dose of the BK receptor antagonists is crucial in determining the effects. We have used a moderately low dose of the compound HOE-140 (1 mg/kg, i.v.,) [4] which in our series attenuated the BSCB permeability. However, a dose response study is needed to understand the optimal dose of the compound in spinal cord trauma. Recently many new compounds have been added to the list of BK receptor antagonist. Thus further studies are needed to find out the role of BK_1 and BK_2 receptors separately in BSCB permeability disturbances in spinal cord trauma. These investigation are currently underway in our laboratory.

In conclusion, our results demonstrated that blockade of bradykinin BK_2 receptors attenuate the BSCB permeability to Evans blue, radioactive iodine and lanthanum tracers following trauma. These observations for the first time suggest that BK_2 receptors are involved in the trauma induced breakdown of the BSCB permeability in vivo. Our results further indicate that bradykinin is a mediator of the BSCB permeability and play an important role in the pathophysiology of spinal cord injuries, not reported earlier.

Acknowledgments

This work is supported by grants from the Swedish Medical Research Council nr. 2710; Alexander von Humboldt Foundation, Bonn, Germany; The University Grants Commission, New Delhi, India. The expert technical assistance of Kärstin Flink; Katja Deparade; Elisabeth Scherer and Kerstin Rystedt and the secretarial assistance of Aruna Sharma and Angela Ludwig are highly appreciated with thanks.

References

1. Bartus RT (1999) The blood-brain barrier as a target for pharmacological modulation. Curr Opin Drug Discov Devlop 2: 152–167
2. Bogar LJ, Bartula LL, Parkman HP, Myers SI (1999) Enhanced bradykinin-stimulated prostaglandin release in the acutely inflamed guinea pig gallbladder is due to new synthesis of cyclooxygenase 1 and prostacyclin synthase. J Surg Res 84: 71–76
3. Bhoola KD, Figueroa CD, Worthy K, (1992) Bioregulation of kinins: kallikreins, kininogens, and kininases. Pharmacol Rev 44: 1–80
4. Black KL (1995) Biochemical opening of the blood-brain barrier. Adv Drug Del Rev 15: 37–52
5. Cloughesy T, Black K, Gobin Y, Farahani K, Nelson G, Villablanca P, Kabbinavar F, Vinuela F, Wortel C (1999) Intraarterial Cereport (RMP-7) and carboplatin: a dose escalation study for recurrent malignant gliomas. Neurosurgery 44: 270–278
6. Hurst RD, Clark JB (1998) Alterations in transendothelial resistance by vasoactive agonists and cyclic AMP in a blood-brain barrier model system. Neurochem Res 23: 149–154
7. Nakai S, Furuya K, Miyata S, Kiyphara T (1999) Intracellular Ca^{2+} responses to nucleotides, amines, amino acids and prostaglandins in cultured pituicytes from adult rat neurohypophysis. Neurosci Lett 266: 185–188
8. Olsson Y, Sharma HS, Pettersson CÅV (1990) Effects of p-chlorophenylalanine on microvascular permeability changes in spinal cord trauma. An experimental study in the rat using ^{131}I-sodium and lanthanum tracers. Acta Neuropathol (Berlin) 79: 595–603
9. Sharma HS, Westman J, Nyberg F (1998) Pathophysiology of brain edema and cell changes following hyperthermic brain injury. Prog Brain Res 115: 351–412
10. Sharma HS, Olsson Y, Westman J (1995) A serotonin synthesis inhibitor, p-chlorophenylalanine reduces the heat shock protein response following trauma to the spinal cord. An immunohistochemical and ultrastructural study in the rat. Neuroscie Res 21: 241–249
11. Sharma HS, Olsson Y, Pearsson S, Nyberg F (1995) Trauma induced opening of the blood-spinal cord barrier is reduced by indomethacin, an inhibitor of prostaglandin synthesis. Experimental observations in the rat using ^{131}I-sodium, Evans blue and lanthanum as tracers. Restorative Neurol Neuroscie 7: 207–215
12. Sharma HS, Olsson Y, Nyberg F, Dey PK (1993) Prostaglandins modulate alterations of microvascular permeability, blood flow, edema and serotonin levels following spinal cord injury. An experimental study in the rat. Neuroscience 57: 443–449
13. Sharma HS, Olsson Y (1990) Edema formation and cellular alterations following spinal cord injury in rat and their modification with p-chlorophenylalanine. Acta Neuropatholo (Ber) 79: 604–610
14. Sharma HS, Olsson Y, Dey PK (1990) Early accumulation of serotonin in rat spinal cord subjected to traumatic injury. Relation to edema and blood flow changes. Neuroscience 36: 725–730
15. Sharma HS, Olsson Y, Dey PK (1990) Blood-brain barrier permeability and cerebral blood flow following elevation of circulating serotonin level in the anaesthetized rats. Brain Res 517: 215–223
16. Sharma HS (1987) Effect of captopril (a converting enzyme inhibitor) on blood-brain barrier permeability and cerebral blood flow in normotensive rats. Neuropharmacology 26: 85–92
17. Stålberg E, Sharma HS, Olsson Y (1998) Spinal cord Monitoring. Basic principles, regeneration, pathophysiology and clinical aspects. Springer, Wien New York, pp 1–527
18. Winkler T, Sharma HS, Stålberg E, Westman (1998) Spinal cord bioelectrical activity, edema and cell injury following a focal trauma to the spinal cord. An experimental study using pharmacological and morphological approach. Spinal cord monitoring. In: Stålberg E, Sharma HS, Olsson Y (eds) Springer Wien New York, pp 281–348
19. Wahl M, Unterberg A, Baethmann A, Schilling L (1988) Mediators of blood-brain barrier dysfunction and formation of vasogenic brain edema. J Cereb Blood Flow Metab 8: 621–634
20. Xu J, Hsu CY, Junker H, Chao S, Hogan EL, Chao J (1991) Kininogen and kinin in experimental spinal cord injury. J Neurochem 57: 975–980

Correspondence: Hari Shanker Sharma, Ph.D., Laboratory of Neuroanatomy, Department of Medical Cell Biology, Biomedical Centre, Box 571, Uppsala University, SE-75123 Uppsala, Sweden.

Acta Neurochir (2000) [Suppl] 76: 165–169

Combined Therapy Utilizing a Novel Na^+/H^+ Exchange Inhibitor (SM-20220) and THAM for Ischemic Brain Edema

Y. Hakamata[1], **U. Ito**[2], **T. Kuroiwa**[3], **S. Hanyu**[4], **N. Ohashi**[5], and **I. Nakano**[4]

[1] Laboratory of Experimental Medicine, Jichi Medical School, Tochigi, Japan
[2] Department of Neurosurgery, Musashino Red Cross Hospital, Tokyo, Japan
[3] Department of Neuropathology, Medical Research Institute, Tokyo Medical and Dental University, Tokyo, Japan
[4] Department of Neurology, Jichi Medical School, Tochigi, Japan
[5] Sumitomo Pharmaceuticals Research Center, Osaka, Japan

Summary

We investigated in the gerbil model whether the therapeutic effect of a novel Na^+/H^+ exchange inhibitor SM-20220 on ischemic brain edema could be enhanced by improving the decreased intracellular pH with an alkalizing agent, tris (hydroxymethyl) aminomethane (THAM). The left carotid artery of the animals was occluded twice for 10 min at a 5 hr interval. Ischemia-positive animals were selected and classified into the SM-20220- (0.5 mg/kg, ip), THAM- (2.0 ml/kg, iv, 0.3M-THAM), combination of SM-20220 (0.5 mg/kg, ip) and THAM (2.0 ml/kg, iv), and vehicle- (0.9% saline, ip) treatment groups. Each agent was administered at 0, 6, 12 and 36 hr after recirculation following the 2nd episode of ischemia. The brain water, sodium and potassium contents were measured at 12, 24, and 48 hr after recirculation. The water content of the ischemic hemisphere 12 hr after recirculation was significantly lower in the combination-treated group (79.02%; $P < 0.05$) than in either the SM-20220- (79.28%) or THAM-treated group (79.32%). At 24 hr after recirculation the water content was significantly lower in the combination-treated group (79.83%, $P < 0.05$) than in the vehicle group (80.95%). At 48 hr after recirculation there were no significant differences in the water content between the vehicle group and any of the other treatment groups. The changes in brain water (ΔH_2O) and sodium plus potassium ($\Delta Na + \Delta K$) content in the ischemic hemisphere showed a significant correlation in each group. The combined treatment with the novel Na^+/H^+ exchange inhibitor SM-20220 and THAM is more effective on ischemic brain edema than treatment with a single agent. The results of this study indicate that improvement of intra- and extracellular acidosis by THAM infusion enhanced the activity of the NHE inhibitor SM-20220.

Keywords: Na^+/H^+ exchange inhibitor, THAM; brain edema; cerebral ischemia.

Introduction

We have demonstrated the temporal profiles of brain edema in the cerebral cortex associated with disseminated selective neuronal necrosis (DSNN) and impending focal infarction after repeated ischemia in gerbils [1]. In the early period after repeated induction of ischemia, only cytotoxic edema develops in both the areas of progressive DSNN and those of impending infarction. Later, vasogenic edema, in addition to cytotoxic edema, develops in areas of infarction with disruption of the blood brain barrier (BBB). Ultrastructural examination of astrocytes reveals that the glial cells in areas of cytotoxic edema are viable, and that they swell and accumulate glycogen granules [4]. Cytotoxic edema is recognized as a reaction of glial cells acting as housekeepers of the neuronal environment [7, 15]. Investigations in cultured C6 glioma cells have shown that glial cells exchange intracellular H^+ and HCO_3^- for extracellular Na^+ and Cl^- by cell-membrane-bound ion-channels, such as a Na^+/H^+ exchanger, Cl^-/HCO_3^- exchanger, and Na^+/HCO_3^- cotransporter, to restore intracellular pH due to lactacidosis after ischemic insults, and consequently that the cells swell up [8, 9, 15, 16]. This cell swelling is inhibited by a Na^+/H^+ exchange (NHE) inhibitor (amiloride).

The novel NHE inhibitor SM-20220 inhibits the NHE of cultured glial cells more selectively than amiloride [5], and it has also been found to reduce brain edema and infarction volume after cerebral ischemia in rats in a middle cerebral artery (MCA) occlusion model [5, 10]. However, it is possible that the recovery of lactacidosis is delayed by inhibition of extrusion of the intracellular H^+ by the NHE inhibitor. The present study investigated whether the therapeutic effect of the novel NHE inhibitor SM-202220 on ischemic brain edema could be enhanced by improving the intracellular pH with an alkalizing agent THAM.

Materials and Methods

Under 2% halothane anesthesia, the left carotid artery of adult Mongolian gerbils was occluded twice for 10 min in each time, with a 5-hr interval between the occlusions. Ischemia-positive animals were selected during the first 10-min period of ischemia [14]. In this model, focal infarction evolves 24 hr following the 2nd 10-min episode of ischemia in the cerebral cortex, basal ganglia and thalamus after the development of cytotoxic edema associated with DSNN [1, 3]. The ischemic animals were assigned to the following groups: the SM-20220-treated (0.5 mg/kg, ip, Sumitomo Co., Japan), THAM-treated (2.0 ml/kg, iv, 0.3M-tris[hydroxymethyl] aminomethane), SM-20220 (0.5 mg/kg, ip) and THAM (2.0 ml/kg, iv) combination-treated, and vehicle-treated (0.9% saline) groups. Each agent was administered at 0, 6, 12, 24, and 36 hr after recirculation following the 2nd episode of ischemia under anesthesia. Animals were sacrificed at 12, 24, and 48 hr after recirculation, and the ischemic left hemisphere was cut into 3 blocks, at the chiasmatic and infundibular levels. The water content of the middle block, which included the cerebral cortex, basal ganglia, and thalamus, was measured by a wet and dry tissue method; and the sodium and potassium content was measured by flame photometry (Corning Medical 480, USA) after extraction with concentrated nitric acid. Tissue pH was measured 24 hr after recirculation using a pH meter with a needle-type antimony electrode (TN-98054; outer diameter 0.5 mm; Unique Medical, Japan) streotaxically inserted into the ischemic hemisphere under anesthesia ($n = 5$, in each treatment group). Another six animals were used as a normal control group. Statistical evaluation was performed with one-way analysis of variance (ANOVA) and Fisher's PLSD. The linear regression line between ΔH_2O and $\Delta Na + \Delta K$ in the ischemic hemisphere was calculated by linear regression analysis. AP level <0.05 was accepted as indicating statistical significance. The data were presented as means ± SD.

Results

The water content of the ischemic hemisphere at 12 hr after the 2nd 10-mm episode of ischemia was significantly lower in both the SM-20220- (79.28 ±0.28%, $P < 0.05$) and THAM-treated groups (79.32 ± 0.24%, $P < 0.05$) than in the vehicle group (79.73 ± 0.21%, Fig. 1). The water content was significantly lower in the combination-treated group (79.02 ± 0.41%, $P < 0.05$) than in either the SM-20220-treated or the THAM-treated group. At 24 h after the 2nd 10-min episode of ischemia, the water content of the ischemic hemisphere was lower in both the SM-20220-treated group (80.32 ± 0.52%, $P < 0.06$) and the THAM-treated group (80.41 ± 0.58%, $P < 0.11$) than in the vehicle group (80.95 ± 0.71%), and the water content was significantly lower in the combination-treated group (79.83 ± 0.60%, $P < 0.05$) than in the vehicle group. At 48 hr after the start of the recirculation there were no differences in the water content between any of the treatment groups and the vehicle group.

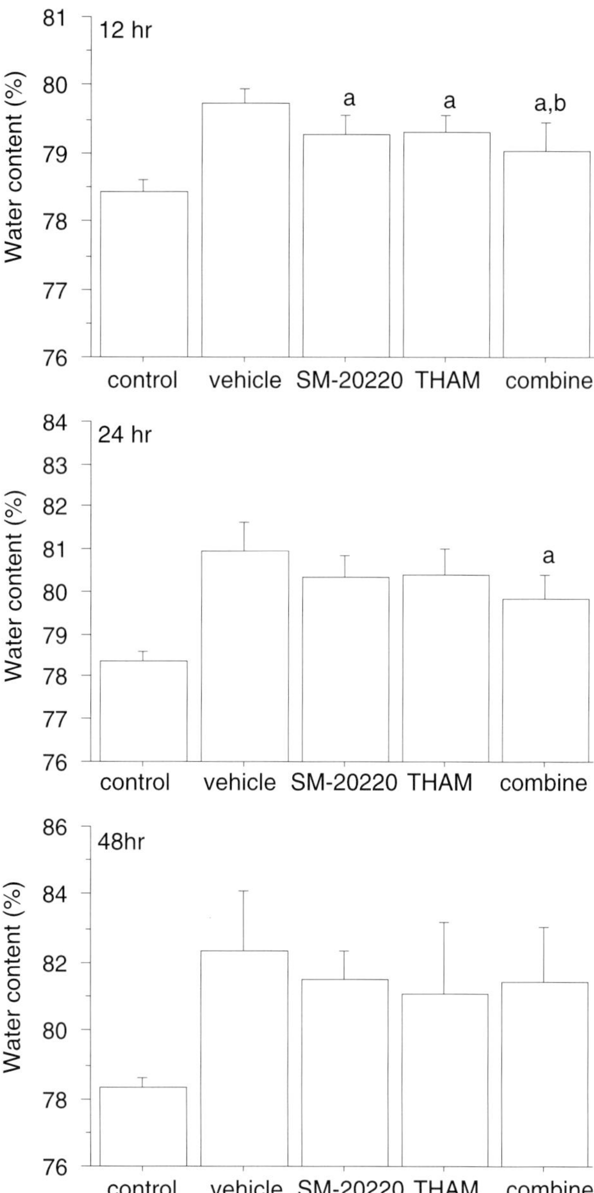

Fig. 1. Changes in the water content of ischemic hemisphere at 12 hr (top), 24 hr (middle) and 48 hr (bottom) after recirculation following repeated cerebral ischemia in the SM-20220-, THAM-, combination of SM-20220 and THAM-, and vehicle-treated groups. Data are shown as means ± SD of 6–7 animals. *a* $P < 0.05$ indicates a statistically significant difference from the vehicle group. *b* $P < 0.05$ indicates a statistically significant difference from each single-agent treatment group

ΔH_2O and $\Delta Na + \Delta K$ in the ischemic hemisphere were calculated on the basis of differences in the brain water, Na, and K levels between the ischemic and nonischemic hemisphere in each animal. There was a significant correlation in each of the treated groups

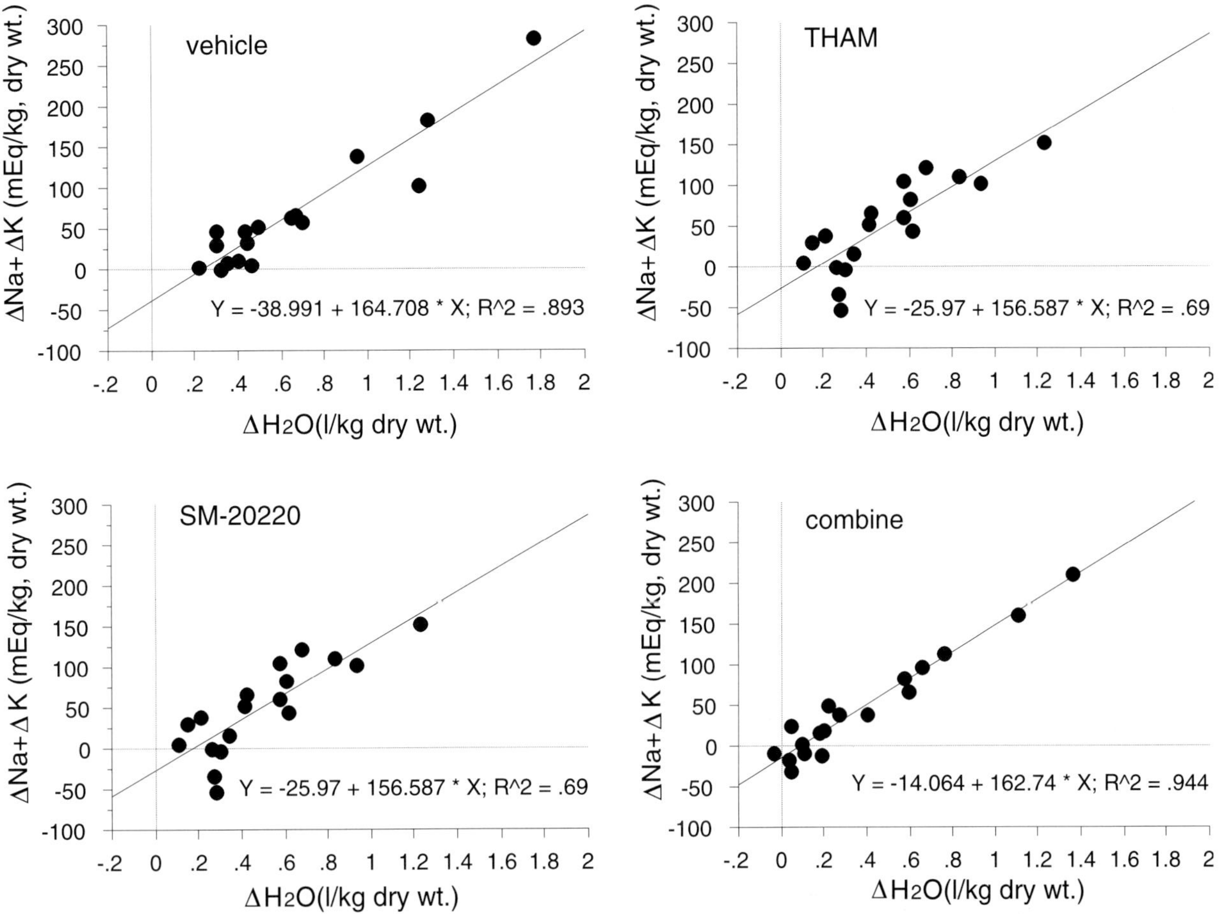

Fig. 2. Scatterplots of the water shifts (ΔH_2O) and sodium plus potassium shifts ($\Delta Na + \Delta K$) in the ischemic hemisphere after recirculation following repeated cerebral ischemia in each of the treated groups. Each point represents changes in the water content and the sodium plus potassium shift calculated from differences in content between the ischemic and nonischemic hemispheres

between the increase in the water content (ΔH_2O) and the sum of the increase or decrease in the sodium and potassium content ($\Delta Na + \Delta K$) in the ischemic hemisphere ($P < 0.01$, Fig. 2). The mean ΔH_2O was significantly smaller in the combination-treated group than in the vehicle-treated group ($P < 0.05$).

Tissue pH at 24 hr after recirculation was significantly lower in the SM-20220 group (7.22 ± 0.08) and vehicle group (7.25 ± 0.05) than in the control group (7.42 ± 0.06, $P < 0.05$, Fig. 3). The pH levels in the THAM-group (7.42 ± 0.10) and combination-treated group (7.45 ± 0.05) were significantly higher than those in thc SM-20220 group and vehicle group, and the same as in the control group.

Discussion

The repeated ischemia model in gerbils in this study can reproducibly induce disseminated selective neuronal necrosis (DSNN) and focal infarction after cerebral ischemia [3]. Cytotoxic edema develops in areas where DSNN progresses, while vasogenic edema, in addition to cytotoxic edema, develops in areas where focal infarction evolves [1]. At 12 hr after the 2nd 10-min episode of ischemia, cytotoxic edema develops in areas of progressing DSNN and areas of impending focal infarction [1]. Astrocytes swell during this period, but remain viable [4]. Vasogenic edema develops in the impending infarcted foci from 24 hr to 48 hr after recirculation [1]. In this study we measured water, Na, and K content of the middle block between the chiasmatic and infundibular levels where focal infarction evolved in the progressing DSNN, and examined the therapeutic effects of an NHE inhibitor on brain edema after repeated cerebral ischemia.

In the present study, the novel NHE inhibitor SN-20220 inhibited cytotoxic edema at 12 hr after recirculation. SM-20220 has been demonstrated to

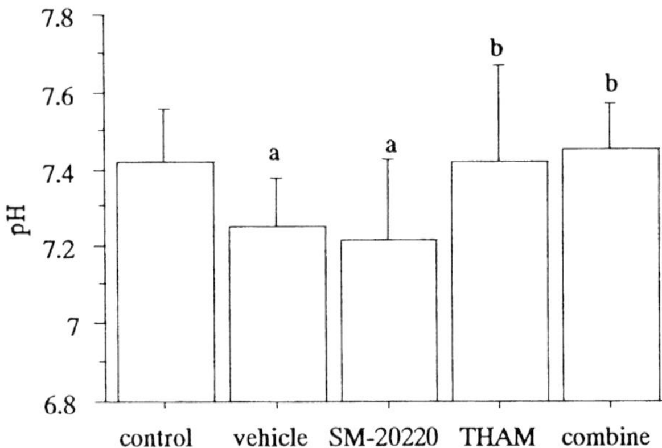

Fig. 3. Tissue pH of the ischemic hemisphere at 24 hr after recirculation following repeated cerebral ischemia in each of the treated groups. Data are means $\pm$ SD of 5 animals. *a* $P < 0.05$ indicates a statistically significant difference from the control group. *b* $P < 0.05$ indicates a statistically significant difference from the vehicle and SM-20220 treated group

provide more effective inhibition than the previously reported amiloride, and to selectively block the glial swelling induced by lactacidosis [5]. Furthermore, it reduces brain edema and infarction after cerebral ischemia in vivo [5, 10]. Glial cells actively remove extracellular H^+ and glutamate, free radicals, K^+, and some mediators that are produced after ischemic insults, thereby acting as housekeepers of the neuronal environment. In vitro examinations of cultured glial cells have revealed that they exchange intracellular H^+ and HCO_3^- for extracellular Na^+ and Cl^- via an Na^+/H^+ exchanger, a Cl^-/HCO_3^- exchanger, and an Na^+/HCO_3^- cotransporter to compensate for the decreasing in intracellular pH due to lactacidosis after ischemic insults [8, 9, 15, 16]. Consequently the cells swell up, and the swelling can be inhibited by the NHE inhibitor. The results of this study indicate that NHE inhibitors can reduce cytotoxic edema.

While the NHE inhibitor blocks the influx of Na^+ into the cell, intracellular pH is thought to be kept low due to accumulation of intracellular H^+. This indicates that the NHE inhibitor can not improve lactacidosis after ischemic insults. THAM improves the acidosis in the area of the peri-infarct penumbra, and it reduces the production of lactate, brain edema, and infarct volume [11–13]. We hypothesized that the therapeutic effect of the NHE inhibitor on ischemic brain edema could be enhanced by improving the decrease in intracellular pH with THAM. Combined treatment with the NHE inhibitor and THAM in this study is more effective than treatment with either of the single agents. It is concluded that the improvement of intra- and extracellular acidosis by THAM infusion enhanced the activity of the NHE inhibitor.

The effect of the NHE inhibitor on brain edema decreased 24 hr after recirculation. The NHE inhibitor seems to have little effect in the infarcted area where the all cell membranes are disrupted. THAM is reported to have no therapeutic effect on the ischemic core area, and to affect only the area of the peri-infarct penumbra [13]. In this study the changes in brain water (ΔH_2O) and sodium plus potassium ($\Delta Na + \Delta K$) in the ischemic hemisphere showed a significant correlation in each group. The ΔH_2O was significantly lower in the combination-treated group than in the vehicle group. It suggests that the NHE inhibitor also acts on the Na^+/H^+ exchanger of the endothelial cells in the cerebral capillaries, and not only that of the glial cells. The NHE inhibitor seems to fail to act on the Na+/K+ exchanger of the BBB which is disrupted in the infarcted focus [6].

The suggested strategy for ischemic edema thus consists of the combined therapy with SM-20220 and THAM for cytotoxic edema, and oncotic therapy using albumin [2] for vasogenic edema which develops in the infarcted area.

In conclusion, the novel NHE inhibitor SM-20220 is effective against cytotoxic edema after ischemic insults, and its effect is enhanced by combined treatment with the alkalizing agent THAM.

References

1. Hakamata Y, Ito U, Hanyu S, Kuroiwa T (1997) Brain edema associated with progressing selective neuronal death or impending infarction in cerebral cortex. Measurement of specific gravity. Acta Neurochir [Suppl] (Wien) 70: 20–22
2. Hakamata Y, Ito U, Hanyu S, Yoshida M (1995) Long-term high colloid oncotic therapy to ischemic brain edema in gerbils. Stroke 26: 2149–2153
3. Hanyu, S, Ito U, Hakamata Y, Nakano I (1997) Topographical analysis of cortical neuronal loss associated with disseminated selective neuronal necrosis and infarction after repeated ischemia. Brain Res 767: 154–157
4. Ito U, Hanyu S, Hakamata Y, Nakamura M, Arima K (1997) Astrocytic swelling associated with progressing selective neuronal death or impending infarction in cerebral cortex. Acta Neurochir [Suppl] (Wien) 70: 46–49
5. Itoh N, Kuribayashi Y, Ohashi N (1998) Effect of SM-20220, a novel Na+/H+ exchanger inhibitor, on cerebral ischemia. Jpn J Pharmacol 76: 251P
6. Kempski O, Behmanesh S (1997) Endothelial cell swelling and brain perfusion. J Trauma 42: S38–40
7. Kempski O, Volk C (1994) Neuron-glial interaction during injury and edema of the CNS. Acta Neurochir [Suppl] (Wien) 60: 7–11

8. Kempski O, Staub F, Jansen M, Schodel F, Baethmann A (1988) Glial swelling during extracellular acidosis in vitro. Stroke 19: 385–392
9. Kempski O, Staub F, von Rosen F, Zimmer M, Neu A, Baethmann A (1988) Molecular mechanisms of glial swelling in vitro. Neurochem Pathol 9: 109–125
10. Kuribayashi Y, Horikawa N, Itoh N (1999) Delayed treatment with SM-20220, a potent Na+/H+ exchange inhibitor attenuates the brain damage following focal ischemia in rats. Jpn J Pharmacol 79: 229P
11. Kuyama H, Kitaoka T, Fujita K, Nagao S (1994) The effect of alkalizing agents on experimental focal cerebral ischemia. Acta Neurochir [Suppl] (Wien) 60: 325–328
12. Marmarou A (1992) Intracellular acidosis in human and experimental brain injury. J Neurotrauma 9: S551–561
13. Nagao S, Kitaoka T, Fujita K, Kuyama H, Ohkawa M (1996) Effect of tris-(hydroxymethyl)-aminomethane on experimental focal cerebral ischemia. Exp Brain Res 111: 51–56
14. Ohno K, Ito U, Inaba Y (1984) Regional cerebral blood flow and stroke index after left carotid artery ligation in the conscious gerbil. Brain Res 297: 151–157
15. Staub F, Winkler A, Haberstok J, Plesnila N, Peters J, Chang RC, Kempski O, Baethmann A (1996) Swelling, intracellular acidosis, and damage of glial cells. Acta Neurochir [Suppl] (Wien) 66: 56–62
16. Staub F, Baethmann A, Peters J, Weigt H, Kempski O (1990) Effects of lactacidosis on glial cell volume and viability. J Cereb Blood Flow Metab 10: 866–876

Correspondence: Yoji Hakamata, Laboratory of Experimental Medicine, Jichi Medical School, Tochigi, Japan, 3311-1 Yakushiji, Minamikawachi-machi, Kawachi-gun, Tochigi 329-0498, Japan.

Acta Neurochir (2000) [Suppl] 76: 171–175

Bradykinin 2 Receptor Antagonist LF 16-0687Ms Reduces Posttraumatic Brain Edema

J. F. Stover, N.-K. Dohse, and **A. W. Unterberg**

Charité – Department of Neurosurgery, Berlin, Germany

Summary

Activation of the kallikrein-kinin system contributes to traumatic brain edema formation. Inhibition of bradykinin 2 (B_2) receptors has been shown to successfully reduce brain edema formation. The purpose of this study was to investigate the protective effect of the novel nonpeptide B_2 receptor antagonist LF 16-0687Ms in brain-injured rats.

Contusion was produced in forty rats by controlled cortical impact injury. Five minutes after trauma rats received a single dose of 0, 3, or 30 mg/kg of LF 16-0687Ms. After 24 hours brain swelling and hemispheric water content were determined.

Brain swelling was significantly decreased by 25% in the low and 27% in the high dose group compared to controls ($p < 0.03$). Water content of the traumatized hemisphere tended to be decreased (80.2 ± 0.1 vs. $80.4 \pm 0.1\%$) while water content of the non-traumatized hemispheres tended to be increased after administering LF 16.0687 Ms (79.3 ± 0.1 vs. $79.0 \pm 0.1\%$).

Single administration of the novel nonpeptide B_2 receptor antagonist LF 16-0687Ms significantly reduces brain swelling. The missing significant reduction in water content of the traumatized hemisphere, however, could be related to an unspecific increase in water content due to LF 16.0687Ms as suggested by increased water content in the non-traumatized hemisphere.

Keywords: Bradykinin receptor; brain edema; controlled cortical impact injury; neuroprotection.

Introduction

Following traumatic brain injury cerebral edema formation is crucial in influencing neurological outcome of brain-injured patients. Any increase in brain water content due to vasogenic or cytotoxic brain edema augments intracranial pressure and reduces cerebral perfusion, possibly resulting in secondary damage related to ischemia.

Since primary traumatic damage cannot be influenced therapeutically it is important to define pharmacological targets to reduce evolving secondary damage. Secondary damage is related to compromised functional and structural integrity of astrocytes, neurons, and endothelial cells which among others is caused by glutamate-mediated excitotoxicity, lipid peroxidation, free radicals, disturbed energetic and ionic homeostasis [16], and activation of tissue and plasma mediators as, e.g., bradykinin [4, 25]. These changes are responsible for evolving posttraumatic vasogenic and cytotoxic brain edema formation and necrosis [5, 10] and are believed to explain secondary growth of contusion following focal traumatic brain injury [24].

To date, the majority of neuroprotective drugs are directed towards attenuating cellular damage and reducing cytotoxic edema formation [17]. Only few drugs have been used to attenuate blood-brain barrier damage and to reduce vasogenic brain edema formation as, e.g., aminosteroids [6] and bradykinin B_2 receptor antagonists [12, 22]. B_2 receptor antagonists have successfully reduced brain damage and edema formation following ischemia [12, 22] and cryogenic brain damage [27]. The observed neuroprotection is thought to be mediated by the inhibition of constitutive B_2 receptors [21] located on cerebral endothelial cells, on smooth muscle of cerebral arterioles and postcapillary venules [30], astrocytes [7] and neurons [20]. Thus, administration of a B_2 receptor antagonist should counteract the action of the endogenous B_2 receptor agonist bradykinin. Bradykinin is a potent mediator of vasogenic brain edema formation [25, 29, 31] as it increases blood-brain barrier permeability [3, 26, 31] and causes arteriolar dilatation and venous constriction [11, 26, 28].

LF 16-0687 Ms is a novel nonpeptide kinin B_2 receptor antagonist which potently binds to the human B2 receptor giving a k_i value of 0.67 nM [19]. In the present study the protective potential of LF 16-0687Ms was evaluated in a rat model of focal traumatic brain injury.

Materials and Methods

For the present study a total of forty male Sprague-Dawley rats (250–350 g) (Charles River, Germany) were used. Animals were accustomed to the laboratory for approximately 24 hours before the study was performed.

Anesthesia

Anesthesia was induced and maintained with isoflurane and N_2O/O_2 in all animals. After induction, anesthesia was tapered to maintain stable mean arterial blood pressure (MABP) values between 80 and 90 mmHg (isoflurane: 1.0–2.5 vol%; N_2O: 0.5 l/min, O_2: 0.3 l/min). Animals were kept breathing spontaneously. Anesthesia was maintained during surgery, trauma, drug application and the first 20 minutes following drug application. Anesthesia was performed again 24 hours after trauma to allow recording of MABP, intracranial pressure (ICP), cerebral perfusion pressure (CPP), blood sampling and brain removal. Intracranial pressure was measured with a Codman ICP microsensor (Johnson & Johnson Medical Ltd. Berkshire, United Kingdom).

Surgery and Trauma

Within 10 minutes after beginning of anesthesia an arterial catheter was implanted in the right femoral artery and mean arterial blood pressure (MABP) was recorded throughout the study. Thereafter, the rats were positioned in a stereotaxic holder and a left parieto-temporal craniotomy was performed within the anatomical barriers outlined by the saggital, lambdoid and coronal sutures and the cygomatic arc. Brain trauma was performed with the controlled cortical impact injury device [14] using an 8 mm bolt which was pneumatically driven at a velocity of 7 m/sec (100 p.s.i.), a depth of 2 mm, and a contact time of 0,3 sec. After trauma the scalp was sutured and rats were returned to their cages where they remained until brain removal.

Drug Dosage and Substance Application

LF 16-0687Ms was given in a low (3 mg/kg body weight) and a high dose (30 mg/kg body weight). Control animals received identical amounts of physiological saline (1 ml). The drug LF 16.0687Ms was dissolved in physiological saline 10 minutes before its administration. A volume of 1 ml of LF 16-0687Ms (3 mg/kg or 30 mg/kg) or physiological saline was injected subcutaneously at 5 minutes following trauma. MABP was recorded for 25 minutes after drug administration. Therafter, rats were returned to their cages where they remained until brain removal.

Determination of Arterial Blood Gases

Arterial blood gases were assessed 10 minutes before trauma, 20 minutes after drug administration and immediately before brain removal (24 hours after trauma).

Determination of Brain Swelling and Hemispheric Water Content

All animals were killed 24 hours after trauma and drug application by exsanguination. Upon removal of the brains the hemispheres were dissected along the interhemispheric line. Both hemispheres were weighed to assess wet weight (WW) and dried for 24 hours at 104 °C to determine dry weight (DW). Based on wet and dry weight swelling of the traumatized hemisphere and water content of both, the traumatized and non-traumatized hemispheres were calculated:

(1) Brain swelling [%]: $(WW_{traumatized} - WW_{non\text{-}traumatized})/WW_{non\text{-}traumatized} \times 100$

(2) Hemispheric water content [%]: $(WW - DW)\ WW \times 100$.

Statistical Analysis

Results are presented as mean ± standard error of the mean. Investigated variables were compared for significant differences between the different groups using one-way analysis of variance (ANOVA) for pairwise multiple comparison. Differences between the groups were rated significant at a probability error less than 0.05.

Results

Arterial Blood Gases

Arterial blood gases remained within physiological ranges in all animals at all time points. There were no differences between the groups (data not shown).

Changes in MABP, ICP, and CPP

MABP remained within narrow limits at all time points in all animals. There was no difference between the different groups at any investigated time point. Administration of LF 16-0687Ms did not result in any adverse effects on MABP as MABP remained stable (Table 1).

At the time point of brain removal ICP and CPP were within the same range in all animals (Table 1). There were no significant differences between the groups.

Brain Swelling

Swelling of the traumatized hemisphere was significantly decreased in animals receiving the low ($5.6 \pm 0.6\%$; $n = 12$) and high dose ($5.5 \pm 0.5\%$; $n = 12$) of LF 16-0687Ms s.c. compared to control animals ($7.5 \pm 0.5\%$; $n = 14$; $p < 0.03$) (Table 2). These observed findings correspond to a decrease by 25% and 27%, respectively. Administration of high dose LF 16-0687Ms did not decrease brain swelling any further.

Hemispheric Water Content

At 24 hours after brain trauma and drug administration water content of the traumatized hemisphere

Table 1. *Changes in Mean Arterial Blood Pressure (MABP) Before and after Drug Application, and Before Brain Removal. Intracranial Pressure (ICP), and Cerebral Perfusion Pressure (CPP) were Recorded Before Removal of Brains at 24 Hours after Trauma and drug Administration. Data are Shown for Animals Receiving no, low, or High Dose of LF 16-0687Ms*

LF 16-0687Ms	MABP (mmHg)			ICP (mmHg) 24 h after drug application	CPP (mmHg) 24 h after drug application
	Before drug application	25 min. after drug application	24 h after drug application		
0 mg/kg	84 ± 1	84 ± 1	84 ± 1	12 ± 1	73 ± 1
(range)	(77–93)	(76–95)	(79–90)	(8–19)	(67–80)
3 mg/kg	87 ± 1	87 ± 2	85 ± 1	11 ± 1	75 ± 2
(range)	(77–105)	(72–105)	(79–96)	(6–20)	(68–86)
30 mg/kg	84 ± 2	85 ± 2	86 ± 2	12 ± 1	74 ± 2
(range)	(74–100)	(75–102)	(78–94)	(5–21)	(63–84)

Table 2. *Changes in Brain Swelling and Hemispheric Water Content in Rats Receiving no, low or high Dose of LF 16-0687Ms. Differences in Brain Swelling Between the Groups are Significant $p < 0.03$ (§). Differences in Hemispheric Water Contents Between Traumatized and non-Traumatized Hemispheres are Significant at $p < 0.05$ (#)*

LF 16-0687Ms	Brain swelling	Hemispheric water content	
		Traumatized hemisphere	Non-traumatized hemisphere
0 mg/kg (n = 12)	7.5 ± 0.5%	80.4 ± 0.2%#	79.0 ± 0.15%
3 mg/kg (n = 12)	5.5 ± 0.6%§	80.2 ± 0.1%#	79.3 ± 0.1%
30 mg/kg (n = 14)	5.5 ± 0.5%§	80.2 ± 0.1%#	79.2 ± 0.1%

was significantly increased compared to the non-traumatized hemisphere (Table 2). In rats receiving the low and high dose of LF 16-0687Ms water content of the traumatized hemisphere tended to be decreased compared to control animals. In the non-traumatized hemisphere water content tended to be increased in rats receiving the low and high dose of LF 16-0687Ms compared to controls (Table 2). There was no difference between the low and high dose group.

Discussion

Posttraumatic subcutaneous administration of a single dose of the nonpeptide kinin B_2 receptor antagonist LF 16-0687Ms successfully reduced brain edema formation following controlled cortical impact injury in rats. These results are consistent with a previous study showing that LF 16-0687 Ms markedly reduced cerebral edema in a rat model of closed head trauma [18].

Kallikrein-Kinin-System and Brain Edema

The physiological role of the kallikrein-kinin-system which is widely distributed within the central nervous system (CNS) remains unclear. The kallikrein-kinin-system is believed to "process precursors of neuronal cell growth factors that maintain the integrity of transmitters and synaptic function" [2]. Under normal conditions, activation of the kallikrein-kinin-system is tightly regulated as precursor proteins (tissue and plasma kininogens) and specific tissue and plasma enzymes (kallikreins) are only present in their inactive form [2] requiring enzymatic cleavage to enable activation of these enzymes with subsequent production of kinins as e.g., bradykinin. Furthermore, spontaneous activation of this system is prevented by a variety of endogeneous inhibitors, such as C1-esterase inhibitor, α_2-macroglobulin, α_1-antitrypsin, and antithrombin, demonstrating an interrelationship between blood clotting, complement, and kinin activation [23]. Under normal circumstances, bradykinin is only present in very low concentrations and its very short biological half-life (<30 sec) [13] is explained by fast deactivation through specific enzymes (kininases) [2].

Under pathological conditions, however, the role of the kallikrein-kinin-system has been characterized more closely. Traumatic and ischemic brain damage are associated with the activation of the kallikrein-kinin-system resulting in sustained production of bradykinin as kallikreins mediate cleavage of kinins as e.g., bradykinin from precursor tissue and plasma kininogens [2]. It is widely accepted that the actions of released bradykinin is mainly mediated by the activation of constitutive B_2 receptors. These bradykinin receptors are widely distributed within the CNS and are present on the luminal and abluminal side of endothelial cells [8, 30], on smooth muscle cells of cerebral arterioles and postcapillary venules [30], astrocytes [7] and neurons [20].

Activation of these G-protein coupled B_2 receptors results in activation of intracellular second messenger systems, leading, among others, to an increased uptake and mobilization of calcium, sustained activation of phospholipase A_2 and C, and increased production of nitric oxide [2].

Activation of these second messenger systems, in turn, results in production of prostaglandins and leukotrienes and is associated with intracellular release of calcium [2]. These endogenous substances, in turn, are well-known mediators of cell damage. Bradykinin has been shown to cause and aggravate vasogenic brain edema formation by causing arteriolar vasodilatation and venous vasoconstriction, and breakdown of the blood-brain barrier [29]. This, in turn, leads to sustained extravasation of proteins and plasma into brain tissue, the hallmarks of vasogenic edema formation. Furthermore, it is believed that the activation of the second messenger systems mediate and aggravate cytotoxic edema formation. In this respect, bradykinin has been shown to release excitatory amino acids such as glutamate and aspartate from astrocytes [9].

Reduction of Brain Edema Formation with B_2 Receptor Antagonists

Successful reduction of brain edema formation by blocking B_2 receptors underlines the contribution of the kallikrein-kinin-system within the pathophysiology of brain damage. At present the exact targets addressed by the administered B_2 receptor antagonist within the focal contusional lesion cannot be defined. It remains to be answered whether there is a decrease in blood-brain barrier damage, a decrease in number of necrotic cells, a decrease in cellular edema formation, and ameliorated perfusion within the vicinity of the contusion. Histological and functional analysis is warranted to address these different potential targets, which are important denominators in influencing secondary growth of cerebral traumatic lesions [5].

At present it remains unclear why cerebral water content tends to be higher in the non-traumatized hemisphere of rats treated with the B_2 receptor antagonist LF 16-0687Ms. In a closed head trauma model LF 16-0687Ms tended to reduce and not increase water content of the uninjured hemisphere [18]. Injury to the contralateral hemisphere can be excluded as it appears normal in histological studies [14]. Furthermore, at 24 hours after trauma blood-brain barrier of the contralateral hemisphere remains intact as assessed by extravasation of Evans Blue [1]. Systemic reasons, as e.g., hypoxemia and insufficient cerebral perfusion seem unlikely as all animals survived and did not show any abnormal blood pressure or arterial blood gas values 20 minutes after drug administration and before brain removal (24 hours after injury).

Eventually, administration of this drug could lead to an unspecific increase in cerebral water content by influencing normal regulatory mechanisms.

Further detailed investigations using histologic, laser doppler and microdialysis studies should follow to elucidate the exact mechanisms of the B_2 receptor antagonist LF 16-0687Ms following traumatic brain injury.

Acknowledgments

Lf 16-0687 Ms was a kind gift by Dr. Pruneau of Laboratoires Fournier, Daix, France.

References

1. Baskaya MK, Rao AM, Dogan A, Donaldson D, Dempsey RJ (1997) The biphasic opening of the blood-brain barrier in the cortex and hippocampus after traumatic brain injury in rats. Neurosci Lett 226: 33–36
2. Bhoola KD, Figueroa CD, Worthy K (1992) Bioregulation of kinins: kallikreins, kininogens, and kininases. Pharmacol Rev 44: 1–80
3. Butt AM (1995) Effect of inflammatory agents on electrical resistance across the blood-brain barrier in pial microvessels of anesthetized rats. Brain Res 696: 145–150
4. Ellis EF, Chao J, Heizer ML (1989) Brain kininogen following experimental brain injury: evidence for a secondary event. J Neurosurg 71: 437–442
5. Eriskat J, Schürer L, Kempski O, Baethmann A (1994) Growth kinetics of a primary brain tissue necrosis from a focal lesion. Acta Neurochir [Suppl] (Wien) 60: 425–427
6. Hall ED, McAll JM, Means ED (1994) Therapeutic potential of the lazaroids (21-aminosteroids) in acute central nervous system trauma, ischemia and subarachnoid hemorrhage. Adv Pharmacol 28: 221–268
7. Hösli E, Hösli L (1993) Autoradiographic localization of binding for neuropeptide Y and bradykinin on astrocytes. Neuroreport 4: 159–162
8. Homayoun P, Harik SI (1991) Bradykinin receptors of cerebral microvessels stimulate phosphoinositide turnover. J Cereb Blood Flow Metab 11: 557–566

9. Jeftinija S, Jeftinija KV, Stefanovic G, Liu F (1996) Neuroligand-evokde calcium-dependent release of excitatory amino acids from cultured astrocytes. J Neurochem 66: 676–684
10. Kochanek PM, Marion DW, Zhang W (1995) Severe controlled cortical impact in rats: assessment of cerebral edema, blood flow, and contusion volume. J Neurotrauma 12: 1015–1025
11. Kamitani T, Little MH, Ellis EF (1985) Evidence for a possible role of the brain kallikrein-kinin system in the modulation of the cerebral circulation. Circ Res 57: 545–552
12. Kamiya T, Katayama Y, Kashiwagi F, Terashi A (1993) The role of bradykinin in mediating ischemic brain edema in rats. Stroke 24: 571–575
13. Kariya K, Yamauchi Am Hattori S, Tsuda Y, Okada Y (1982) The disappearance rate of intraventricular bradykinin in the brain of the conscious rat. Biochem Biophys Res Comm 107: 1561–1466
14. Kroppenstedt S-N, Kern M, Thomale U-W *et al* (1999) Effect of cerebral perfusion pressure on contusion volume following impact injury. J Neurosurg 90: 520–526
15. Maier-Hauff K, Baethmann AJ, Lange M, Schürer L, Unterberg A (1984) The kallikrein-kinin system as mediator in vasogenic brain edema. Part 2: studies on kinin formation in focal and perifocal brain tissue. J Neurosurg 61: 97–106
16. Mclntosh TK, Smith DH, Meaney DF *et al* (1996) Neuropathological sequelae of traumatic brain injury: relationship to neurochemical and biomechanical mechanisms. Lab Invest 74: 315–342
17. Mclntosh T, Juhler M, Wieloch T (1998) Novel pharmacologic strategies in the treatment of experimental traumatic brain injury: 1998. J Neurotrauma 15: 731–769
18. Pruneau D, Chorny J, Benkowitz V *et al* (1998) LF 16-0687, a new nonpeptide bradykinin B_2 receptor antagonist, reduces cerebral edema in a rat model of closed head trauma. Kinin'98 Nara, The 15th International Conference on Kinins, October 19–24, 1998, Nara, Japan
19. Pruneau D, Paquet JL, Luccarini JM *et al* (1999) Pharmacological profile of LF 16-0687, a new potent non peptide bradykinin B_2 receptor antagonist. Immunopharmacology (*in press*)
20. Raidoo DM, Ramchhurren N, Naidoo Y *et al* (1996) Visualization of bradykinin B2 receptors on human brain neurons. Immunopharmacology 33: 104–107
21. Regoli D, Alogho SN, Rizzi A, Gobeil FJ (1998) Bradykinin receptors and their antagonists. Eur J Pharmacol 348: 1–10
22. Relton JK, Beckey VE, Hanson WL, Whalley ET (1997) CP-0597, a selective bradykinin B_2 receptor antagonist, inhibits brain injury in a rat model of reversible middle cerebral artery occlusion. Stroke 28: 1430–1436
23. Schachter M (1980) Kallikrein (kininogenases)- a group of serine proteases with bioregulatory actions. Pharmacol Rev 31: 1–17
24. Stover JF, Morganti-Kossmann MC, Lenzlinger PM *et al* (1999) Glutamate and taurine are increased in ventricular cerebrospinal fluid of severely brain-injured patients. J Neurotrauma 16: 135–142
25. Unterberg A, Baethmann A (1984) The kallikrein-kinin system as mediator in vasogenic brain edema. Part 1: cerebral exposure to bradykinin and plasma. J Neurosurg 61: 87–96
26. Unterberg A, Wahl M, Baethmann A (1984) Effects of bradykinin on permeability and diameter of pial vessels in vivo. J Cereb Blood Flow Metab 4: 574–585
27. Unterberg A, Dautermann C, Baethmann A, Müller-Esterl W (1986) The kallikrein-kinin system as mediator in vasogenic brain edema. Part 3: Inhibition of the kallikrein-kinin system in traumatic brain swelling. J Neurosurg 64: 269–276
28. Wahl M, Young AR, Edvinsson L, Wagner F (1983) Effects of bradykinin on pial arteries and arterioles in vitro and in situ. J Cereb Blood Flow Metab 3: 231–237
29. Wahl M, Unterberg A, Baethmann A, Schilling L (1988) Mediators of blood-brain barrier dysfunction and formation of vasogenic brain edema. J Cereb Blood Flow Metab 8: 621–634
30. Wahl M, Whalley ET, Unterberg A *et al* (1996) Vasomotor and permeability affects of bradykinin in the cerebral microcirculation. Immunopharmacology 33: 257–263
31. Whittle IR, Piper IR, Miller JD (1992) The role of bradykinin in the etiology of vasogenic brain edema and perilesional brain dysfunction. Acta Neurochir (Wien) 115: 53–59

Correspondence: John F. Stover, M.D., Department of Neurosurgery, Charité- Virchow Medical Center, Augstenburger Platz 01, D-13353 Berlin.

Acta Neurochir (2000) [Suppl] 76: 177–179

Influence of Alcohol Exposure on S-100b Serum Levels

P. Biberthaler[1], **T. Mussack**[1], **E. Wiedemann**[1], **K. G. Kanz**[1], **T. Gilg**[2], **C. Gippner-Steppert**[3], and **M. Jochum**[3]

[1] Chirurgische Klinik, Kliniken Innenstadt, Ludwig-Maximilians-Universität, München
[2] Institut für Rechtsmedizin, Ludwig-Maximilians-Universität, München
[3] Abteilung für Klinische Chemie und Klinische Biochemie/Kliniken Innenstadt, Ludwig-Maximilians-Universität, München

Summary

Recent assessment of the glia cell-derived neuroprotein S-100b in serum has been considered as a screening method for possibly occult brain injury in patients with minor head trauma (MHT). Since MHT is associated with alcohol intoxication in up to 50% of patients requiring emergency treatment, the blood-brain barrier (BBB) as well as neuronal cell integrity may be also affected by alcohol abuse. So far, however, no valid data are available on the release of S-100b after alcohol exposure. Thus, the aim of our study was to investigate S-100b serum levels in a controlled alcohol exposure paradigm. 22 healthy volunteers were included in the study, blood samples were drawn prior to and about 90 minutes after drinking. The amount of alcohol was adjusted to the body weight. A mean of 66.7 ± 14.81 g was consumed giving raise to a blood alcohol concentration of 0.827 ± 0.158‰. S-100b serum levels assayed by a luminescence immunoassay were compared with those of MHT patients. The still preliminary results suggest no increase of the serum S-100b levels (0.0509 ± 0.048 ng/ml versus 0.0422 ± 0.044 ng/ml) after moderate alcohol consumption. In contrast, MHT patients with alcohol intoxication (1.6 ± 0.77‰) revealed a significant up to 10fold elevation of S-100b serum levels. Because of the much higher blood alcohol concentration in the MHT patients compared to the control collective, a potential relationship between excessive alcohol consumption and the release of S-100b in minor head trauma can still not be excluded. Further investigations on this topic are in progress.

Keywords: Minor head trauma; S-100b; alcohol.

Introduction

Patients with minor head trauma (MHT) are causing 400.000–450.000 emergency room admissions per year in the U.S.A. [7]. The patients are characterized by a history of trauma, a Glasgow Coma Scale (GCS) of 13–15 points on admission, and various neurological symptoms, such as nausea, vomitus, headache and amnesia. The management of these patients continues to be debated in literature. In contrast to patients with severe (GCS < 8) or moderate (GCS 9–12) head trauma [9], the frequency of pathological findings (e.g. hemorrhage, edema) detected by cranial computed tomography (CT) is clearly lower (between 5.9% [1] and 21.6% [11]). The need for immediated surgical intervention (such as burr hole, craniotomy) in MHT ranges from 0.3% [4] up to 4.1% [11]. Due to the great number of MHT patients, however, identification of those at risk of intracerebral complications depends on safe and effective screening methods. Some authors [2, 12] are favoring a generous use of CT, since according to their experience the clinical judgement is not safe enough to identify patients requiring immediate surgery. Nevertheless, with regard to the above mentioned large number of patients with MHT, diagnosis by routine CT-scan in all of these cases constitutes logistic and pecuniary problems. Other authors assume [6, 8] a careful neurological examination as the best assessment procedure to discover serious complications in MHT. Yet, in these patients the suitability of the neurological examination of trauma-induced disorders is often adulterated in the presence of neurological symptoms which are caused by alcohol intoxications in at least 30 to 50% of patients with minor head injuries [5]. Thus, the proper assessment of the severity of head injury in those patients is still confronted with the open question about the most effective and safe screening procedure.

In order to improve identification of high-risk patients with MHT, the measurement of serum levels of the neuroprotein S-100b has recently been suggested [3]. Glial cells produce S-100b which may be released into the circulation during brain tissue injury evoked by trauma or hypoxia [10]. First results seem to indicate that the serum S-100b levels correlate with the outcome of patients suffering from severe head trauma

Table 1. *Distribution of Body Weight, Alcohol Consumption and Blood Alcohol Concentration (BAC) of Volunteers*

	Body weight [kg]	Alcohol consumption [g]	BAC [‰]
Whole group (n = 22)	75.7 ± 12.4	66.7 ± 14.8	0.827 ± 0.158
Male (n = 15)	81.3 ± 9.0	74.0 ± 15.0	0.825 ± 0.15
Female (n = 7)	63.67 ± 8.7	53.3 ± 8.2	0.86 ± 0.2

Table 2. *S-100b Serum Concentration in ng/ml of Volunteers Before and After Alcohol Exposure*

	Before exposure	After exposure
Whole group (n = 22)	0.0509 ± 0.048	0.0422 ± 0.044
Male (n = 15)	0.051 ± 0.055	0.037 ± 0.048
Female (n = 7)	0.045 ± 0.029	0.048 ± 0.039

[13]. Notwithstanding the prognostic value of S-100b in these patients, the diagnostic suitability of S-100b serum measurements remains unclear in patients with MHT. In particular, the high frequency of alcohol intoxication in MHT patients raises the question, whether release of S-100b into serum is influenced by this presumable blood brain barrier damaging substance. So far, no valid data are available on the release of S-100b by alcohol exposure. Therefore, the objective of the current study was to investigate S-100b serum levels following controlled alcohol exposure in healthy volunteers in comparison to MHT patients with alcohol intoxication.

Patients and Methods

22 healthy volunteers with a GCS of 15 points were included in the study group. They were informed in detail about the potentially negative consequences of alcohol consumption especially during pregnancy, running machines or participation in road traffic. Throughout the actual drinking period and the following three hours an experienced emergency physician was attending to provide medical assistance if necessary. All the study participants signed an informed consent.

The receiving alcohol dosis was adjusted to the body weight. A mean of 66.7 ± 14.81 g (mean ± SD) alcohol were administered (Table 1). Blood samples were drawn prior and about 90 minutes after drinking. Blood alcohol concentrations (BAC) were determined by routine head-space gas chromatography based on forensic criteria in duplicates. The levels are expressed in g/kg whole blood resp. ‰ S-100b serum levels (ng/ml) was assayed by a luminescence immunoassay (LIA: Byk-Sangtec Diagnostica, Dietzenbach, Germany).

The data were compared with those of a positive control group of patients (n = 18) with MHT and alcohol intoxication presenting with GCS 13–15 on admission.

Results

The 22 participants of the study group comprised 15 men and 7 woman with a mean body weight of 81.3 ± 9.0 kg and 63.6 ± 8.7 kg, respectively. Alcohol consumption within roughly 30 minutes amounted to a mean of 66.7 ± 14.81 g in the whole study group with 74.0 ± 15.0 g in male and 53.3 ± 8.2 g in female (Table 1). Blood samples taken prior to the drinking period revealed no alcohol in the circulation. The second blood samples drawn 86.4 ± 9.0 min after the start of the experiments showed alcohol concentrations of 0.83 ± 0.15‰ in all volunteers with 0.82 ± 0.15‰ in the males and 0.86 ± 0.20‰ in the females. The S-100b concentrations in serum prior to alcohol consumption were 0.0509 ± 0.048 ng/ml in all participants and 0.051 ± 0.055 ng/ml or 0.045 ± 0.029 ng/ml, respectively, in the two gender groups. Following the alcohol exposure an overall S-100b serum level of 0.0422 ± 0.044 ng/ml was measured which could be stratified into 0.037 ± 0.048 ng/ml in males and 0.048 ± 0.039 in females (Table 2). Statistical analysis did not reveal significant differences between serum concentrations before and after alcohol consumption either in the whole study collective ($p = 0.41$) or in both gender groups (male: $p = 0.31$; female: $p = 0.87$).

For comparison data were procured of 18 patients, who were admitted to our hospital from September 1998 until March 1999 with MHT (GCS of 13–15 points) and alcohol intoxication. This positive control group comprised 17 men and 1 woman. The alcohol blood level observed in the whole group was 1.6 ± 0.77‰ and the S-100b serum concentration amounted to 0.53 ± 0.80 ng/ml the latter being about 10 fold that of the voluntary study group. Statistical analysis revealed that blood alcohol and S-100b serum concentration were significantly ($p < 0.001$) different between the healthy volunteers with moderate alcohol consumption and MHT patients with alcohol intoxication.

Discussion

The proper treatment of patients with MHT continues to be debated, because the implementation of a clear management algorithm is hampered by various factors as stated in the introduction. In this context, neurological disorders due to excessive blood alcohol concentrations may confound trauma-related disturbances in MHT patients with a high frequency of alcohol intoxication.

Thus, the objective of the present study was to elucidate the influence of an increased blood alcohol level on the detection of the glial cell-derived neuroprotein S-100b in the circulation of healthy volunteers. The results indicate that a moderate consumption of alcohol (not exceeding a blood concentration of 1‰) does not influence normal S-100b concentrations in serum. The S-100b levels in this group of volunteers were significantly lower than those found in patients with MHT and alcohol intoxication.

Since, however, MHT patients showed blood alcohol concentrations almost twice as high as those found in the volunteers a potential influence of excessive alcohol consumption on the release of the neuroprotein S-100b can still not be excluded. Therefore, we are already in progress to perform further studies in individuals with and without MHT but comparable levels of blood alcohol concentrations to evaluate the suitability of S-100b serum measurements as a reliable indication of brain tissue injury in MHT.

Conclusions

The current results of our study reveal that moderate alcohol consumption does not increase the S-100b serum concentration. However, it remains to be clarified whether higher blood alcohol concentrations, as e.g. found in MHT patients, have an influence on the cerebral release of S-100b.

References

1. Borczuk P (1995) Predictors of intracranial injury in patients with mild head trauma. Ann Emerg Med 25: 731–736
2. Harad FT, Kerstein MD (1992) Inadequacy of bedside clinical indicators in identifying significant intracranial injury in trauma patients. J Trauma 32: 359–361
3. Ingebrigtsen T, Romner B (1996) Serial S-100 protein serum measurements related to early magnetic resonance imaging after minor head injury. Case report. J Neurosurg 5: 945–948
4. Jeret JS, Mandell M, Anziska B, Lipitz M, Vilceus AP, Ware JA, Zesiewicz TA (1993) Clinical predictors of abnormality disclosed by computed tomography after mild head trauma. Neurosurgery 32: 9–15
5. Kelly DF (1995) Alcohol and head injury: an issue revisited. J Neurotrauma 12: 883–890
6. Klauber MR, Marshall LF, Luerssen TG, Frankowski R, Tabaddor K, Eisenberg HM (1989) Determinants of head injury mortality: importance of the low risk patient. Neurosurgery 24: 31–36
7. Kraus JF (1987) Epidemiology of head injury. In: Cooper PR (ed) Head injury, 2nd eds. Wiliams & Wilkins, Baltimore, pp 1–19
8. Miller EC, Holmes JF, Derlet RW (1997) Utilizing clinical factors to reduce head CT scan ordering for minor head trauma patients. J Emerg Med 15: 453–457
9. Murray GD, Teasdale GM, Braakman R, Cohadon F, Dearden M, Iannotti F, Karimi A, Lapierre F, Maas A, Ohman J, Persson L, Servadei F, Stocchetti N, Trojanowski T, Unterberg A (1999) The European brain injury consortium survey of head injuries. Acta Neurochir (Wien) 141: 223–236
10. Rosen H, Rosengren L, Herlitz J, Blomstrand C (1998) Increased serum levels of the S-100 protein are associated with hypoxic brain damage after cardiac arrest. Stroke 29: 473–477
11. Shackford SR, Wald SL, Ross SE, Cogbill TH, Hoyt DB, Morris JA, Mucha PA, Pachter HL, Sugerman HJ, O'Malley K (1992) The clinical utility of computed tomographic scanning and neurologic examination in the management of patients with minor head injuries. J Trauma 33: 385–394
12. Stein SC, Ross SE (1990) The value of computed tomographic scans in patients with low-risk head injuries. Neurosurgery 26: 638–640
13. Woertgen C, Rothoerl RD, Holzschuh M, Metz C, Brawanski A (1997) Comparison of serial S-100 and NSE serum measurements after severe head injury. Acta Neurochir (Wien) 139: 1161–1164

Correspondence: Dr. P. Biberthaler, Chirurgische Klinik/Kliniken Innenstadt, Ludwig-Maximilians-Universität, München, Nussbaumstrasse 20, 80336 Munich, Germany.

Acta Neurochir (2000) [Suppl] 76: 181–184

Laser Doppler Scanning: How Many Measurements are Required to Assess Regional Cerebral Blood Flow?

M. Soehle, A. Heimann, and **O. Kempski**

Institute for Neurosurgical Pathophysiology, Johannes Gutenberg-University, Mainz, Germany

Summary

This study was initiated to determine the optimal number of measuring sites necessary to estimate regional cerebral blood flow (CBF) under pathophysiological conditions.

25 rats were exposed to 15 minutes of global cerebral ischemia. Local CBF was sequentially measured by laser Doppler (LD) at 32 locations during baseline conditions, ischemia and reperfusion using a computer-controlled scanning technique. A simulation study was performed based on 800 local measurements at each time point: random samples (size 1–100) were repeatedly drawn to estimate the variability of median flow. Accuracy was defined as probability that the simulated median differed less than ±5 LD-units from the true median of the 800 data.

Above a single location, CBF was measured with an accuracy of 21.6 ± 0.4% (baseline conditions, n = 100 simulations, mean ± SEM), 85.8 ± 0.4% (ischemia) and 11.1 ± 0.3% (30th min. reperfusion). Accuracy increases to 75.2 ± 0.5% (baseline conditions), 100 ± 0% (ischemia) and 41.8 ± 0.6% (30th min. reperfusion) if 24 locations are scanned.

Scanning, therefore, improves accuracy and reduces variability of CBF measurements. With enough local CBF measurements laser Doppler assessment of *regional* CBF is possible. Single location CBF assessment is sufficiently accurate only during ischemia. During reperfusion, when accuracy is half reduced compared to baseline conditions, larger sample sizes are required.

Keywords: Cerebral blood flow; laser Doppler scanning; global cerebral ischemia; rat.

Introduction

Laser Doppler flowmetry (LDF), commonly used to assess changes in microcirculatory blood flow [2, 5, 7], allows non-invasive, instantaneous and continuous measurements with a high spatial resolution of approximately 1 mm^3. Tissues show a substantial spatial variation of perfusion, and LDF measurements vary considerably even at adjacent sites [2]. Therefore it has been suggested that scanning over multiple locations would reflect tissue perfusion, i.e. regional flow, more precisely than local single point measurements. Scanning techniques have been introduced which permit to estimate regional blood flow from many local measurements [4, 9, 10].

How many locations must be scanned in an LDF study to obey a given precision standard is so far undetermined as to tissue, species or pathophysiological condition under investigation. Previous studies have shown that a minimum of four to six measurements is required for human skin, gastric mucosa and pig kidney for an acceptable precision estimate [6], whereas at least fifteen sites should be scanned in rat diaphragm [1]. In contrast, sample sizes above 25 are recommended in rabbit cerebral microcirculation [5]. These studies were performed under physiological conditions, and no information is available about the precision of LDF under pathological circumstances such as cerebral ischemia or reperfusion.

The current study was performed to determine the number of measurements required to achieve sufficient reliability during baseline conditions, cerebral ischemia and reperfusion. Samples from data pools collected during experiments in rats were randomly and repeatedly drawn applying a simulation technique [5]. The accuracy of LDF, defined as the probability that the simulated median differs less than ±5 laser Doppler units (LDU) from the true median cerebral cortical blood flow, was calculated for a given number of measuring sites ranging from 1 to 100 locations.

Materials and Methods

Twenty-five male Wistar rats (250 to 370 g body weight (bw), Charles River) were anesthetized with intraperitoneal chloral hydrate (360 mg/kg). Animals were orally intubated and ventilated during the entire experiment. Rectal temperature was controlled at 37 °C by means of a feedback-controlled homeothermic blanket

Table 1. *Accuracy (= Probability that the Median of the Sample Differs less than ±5 LDU from the true Median of the 800 CBF data) of Laser Doppler Scanning Depending on Different Sample Sizes. Values were Calculated for Time Points Before, During and after 15 min Global Cerebral Ischemia*

Sample size	Baseline	Ischemia	Reperfusion 15th min	30th min	60th min
1	21.6 ± 0.4	85.8 ± 0.4	7.8 ± 0.3	11.1 ± 0.3	16.6 ± 0.4
4	43.3 ± 0.4	95.7 ± 0.2	18.8 ± 0.4	17.3 ± 0.4	26.7 ± 0.5
8	52.9 ± 0.5	99.5 ± 0.1	20.2 ± 0.4	24.8 ± 0.5	37.2 ± 0.6
16	67.3 ± 0.6	100 ± 0	28.4 ± 0.6	34.2 ± 0.6	49.9 ± 0.5
24	75.2 ± 0.5	100 ± 0	32.7 ± 0.5	41.8 ± 0.6	59.4 ± 0.5
32	81.3 ± 0.4	100 ± 0	37.3 ± 0.5	47.4 ± 0.5	66.1 ± 0.5
40	85.7 ± 0.4	100 ± 0	42.3 ± 0.5	53.5 ± 0.6	72.1 ± 0.7
80	95.9 ± 0.2	100 ± 0	57.1 ± 0.6	70.5 ± 0.7	88.6 ± 0.4

Data are mean ± SEM, *n* 100 simulations.

control unit (Harvard, Edenbridge GB). A loose thread was looped around the left common carotid artery for temporary ligation during ischemia. A polyethylene catheter was inserted into the right common carotid artery for continuous monitoring of arterial blood pressure, and for blood gas analysis. The head was fixed in a stereotactic frame (Stoelting, Wood Dale, IL, USA) and the skull exposed by a 20 mm midline sagittal skin incision. Access to the brain surface was gained via a 5 × 3 mm large cranial window, centered 4 mm lateral and 4 mm caudal to the bregma. The dura was left intact. The lower body portion of the animals was placed in a sealable chamber, connected to an electronically controlled vacuum pump for later induction of hypobaric hypotension [3]. To do so, the barometric pressure within the chamber could be reduced down to −30 cm H_2O (−2.9 kPa), thereby causing a pooling of venous blood in the lower body portion of the rat.

Local cortical blood flow (lCBF) was measured using a laser flow blood perfusion monitor (model BPM 403a, Vasomedics, St. Paul, MN, USA) with a 0.8 mm needle probe. lCBF is expressed in 'LD units' since the calibration of laser Dopplers (LD) to absolute flow units remains controversial. The LD system has a reproducible low biological zero [4], and LD-units are valid for Vasomedics laser Dopplers only. lCBF was sequentially measured at 32 (8 × 4) cortical locations 300 μm apart in a computer-controlled micromanipulator scanning technique.

After a 15 min control phase, 15 min of global cerebral ischemia were initiated by bilateral occlusion of the common carotid arteries and MABP-reduction to 42 mmHg by hypobaric hypotension [8]. Reperfusion was monitored for one hour. LD-scanning was performed at baseline conditions, ischemia and reperfusion (15th, 30th, 60th min).

In order to assess the variability of regional CBF by determining the median flow from multiple local measurement sites, a simulation technique was applied [5]. Data from the 32 individual sites in 25 rats were pooled and considered as independent samples which represent the possible range of data to be encountered in the parietal cortex of ventilated rats in chloral hydrate anesthesia.

To determine the variability of the flow median with different observation numbers, a computer program was written in Visual Basic (Microsoft), that allowed to randomly draw samples from the total data pool. Repetitive drawings from the same location were prohibited during individual sample collections. Sample sizes between n = 1 and n = 100 were studied, representing between 1 and 100 measurement locations. For each sample the median was calculated. Sampling was repeated 100 times for each sample size, thus yielding 100 median values for each given sample size.

To express the variability of the median values thus found, the probability for the 100 medians to differ less than ±5 LD-units from the true median of the entire data pool was calculated and defined as accuracy. To achieve more reliable data, the described simulation procedure was repeated 100 times and accuracy expressed as mean ± SEM. The technique was used to calculate the mean accuracy for baseline conditions, ischemia, and 15th, 30th, 60th min of reperfusion.

Results

Mean arterial blood pressure (MABP) and arterial blood gases sampled at baseline were within physiological range.

The individual baseline CBF in the 800 locations of 25 rats varied considerably, and displayed a non-Gaussian distribution. The median CBF of the entire data pool dropped from 24.0 LD-units at baseline to 2.7 LD-units during global cerebral ischemia. A postischemic hyperperfusion occured during early reperfusion (15th min) with a median CBF of 63.1 LD-units. After one hour of reperfusion, median CBF reached preischemic values (24.8 LD-units) again.

Accuracy of laser Doppler scanning changed during baseline conditions, global cerebral ischemia and reperfusion, as shown in Table 1: Accuracy during baseline conditions was between 21.6 ± 0.4% (1 location measurement, n = 100 simulations) and 85.7 ± 0.4% (40 location measurement). It reached its maximum during ischemia with values between 85.8 ± 0.4% (1 location) and 100 ± 0% (40 locations). During reperfusion, accuracy increased with time, but never reached preischemic values: An accuracy between 7.8 ± 0.3% (1 location) and 42.3 ± 0.5% (40 locations) was found at 15th min. reperfusion and values between 16.6 ± 0.4% (1 location) and 72.1 ± 0.7% (40 locations) at 60th min of reperfusion.

Accuracy during reperfusion was approximately only half of that found during baseline conditions, no matter how many locations were scanned. In contrast, even with a single point measurement an accuracy of 85.8 ± 0.4% could be achieved during global cerebral ischemia that increases above 95% when scanning more than four locations or above 99% when measuring more than seven locations.

Discussion

In a normally distributed population, the error probability of a given sample size can be calculated using conventional statistics. With a non-normal distribution, simulation studies have to be applied, particularly if the mathematical transformation into a normal distribution is difficult or even impossible. We decided to apply a simulation technique previously used for the rabbit cerebral microcirculation [5]. This technique draws samples of a given size from a total data population and estimates the deviation of the sample median from the median of the entire population. We expressed the results as probability of the sample median to differ less than a certain amount from the median of the total population. We choose the difference of ±5 LD units from the true median to be acceptable. Had we chosen a larger or smaller difference, the results would have been similar, just shifted towards higher or lower accuracy values. Anyway, simulation studies can only answer questions on how many locations should be scanned to achieve a desired level of accuracy with a certain probability. Therefore we compared accuracy data at baseline conditions, during ischemia and reperfusion rather than trying to determine exactly how many measurements are required to describe regional CBF.

The larger the data pool from which the samples are drawn the more reliable will be the simulation. In practice, the data pool will always be finite (n = 800 in our study) resulting in errors when estimating the accuracy. It could be argued that by pooling data sets with varying distributions from 25 animals into one large data pool, the non-homogeneity of the data pool might be increased, resulting in an overestimation of the acceptable sampling numbers. Therefore Chang *et al.* [1] applied another statistical method, based on ANOVA, to obtain β values, defined as the length of a 95% confidence interval for the mean of repeated measurements [6]. The authors demonstrated a linear relationship between β values of the sampling and the ANOVA method. Furthermore, the β values of the sampling method were on average minimally larger than those of the ANOVA method. Therefore these authors excluded a vast overestimation of the required number of sample sizes using the same sampling method as in our study.

As described for the rabbit [5], we found a wide range of CBF readings during baseline conditions. As expected, the accuracy of LD scanning rises with an increasing number of measurement locations. During ischemia, CBF was found to be close to zero with only a small range of individual CBF readings. Therefore even a single point measurement revealed a high and sufficient accuracy of 86%. With 8 locations, an almost 100% accuracy can be achieved, therefore scanning more locations increases only measurement time but not accuracy. During reperfusion, accuracy of LD scanning increased little by time but was approximately only half as accurate as compared to baseline conditions. This is presumably caused by a much more heterogeneous and widespread microcirculatory blood flow during reperfusion than under resting conditions.

Therefore, if laser Doppler scanning is only used to assess ischemic rCBF, as little as 1 to 4 measuring sites are sufficient. In contrast, if reperfusion CBF is to be investigated, even more locations are necessary than during physiological conditions.

Previous studies recommend a sample size of 5–6 using statistical methods assuming a Gaussian distribution of LD readings [6]. In contrast, just as in the present study Kempski *et al.* [5] in rabbits found a non-Gaussian distribution and quite remarkable error probabilities of observed median flows as compared to a 'true' median flow. The error probability might be underestimated when assuming a Gaussian distribution, therefore the authors then recommended sample sizes above 25 to achieve reliable information on rCBF. In our study, we also found remarkable error probabilities, indicated by low accuracy values at low sample sizes.

Laser Dopplers provide noninvasive, instantaneous and continuous measurements of CBF with a high spatial resolution, and are hence commonly used. Their major disadvantage, the rather local than regional measurement can be overcome be the use of a scanning technique. Scanning is recommended especially in tissues with a heterogeneous microvasculature such as brain.

References

1. Chang HY, Chan CS, Chen JH, Tsai MC, Wu MH (1997) Evaluation of the number of laser Doppler measurements in assessing regional diaphragmatic microcirculation. Int J Microcirc 17: 123–129
2. Dirnagl U, Kaplan B, Jacewicz M, Pulsinelli W (1989) Continuous measurement of cerebral cortical blood flow by laser Doppler flowmetry in a rat stroke model. J Cereb Blood Flow Metab 9: 589–596
3. Dirnagl U, Thoren P, Villringer A, Sixt G, Them A, Einhäupl KM (1993) Global forebrain ischemia in the rat: controlled reduction of cerebral blood flow by hypobaric hypotension and two-vessel occlusion. Neurol Res 15: 128–130
4. Heimann A, Kroppenstedt S, Ulrich P, Kempski OS (1994) Cerebral blood flow autoregulation during hypobaric hypotension assessed by laser Doppler scanning. J Cereb Blood Flow Metab 14: 1100–1105
5. Kempski O, Heimann A, Strecker U (1995) On the number of measurements necessary to assess regional cerebral blood flow by local laser Doppler recordings: a simulation study with data from 45 rabbits. Int J Microcirc 15: 37–42
6. Line PD, Mowinckel P, Lien B, Kvernebo K (1992) Repeated measurement variation and precision of laser Doppler flowmetry measurements. Microvasc Res 43: 285–293
7. Öberg PA (1990) Laser Doppler flowmetry. Crit Rev Biomed Eng 18: 125–163
8. Soehle M, Heimann A, Kempski O (1998) Postischemic application of lipid peroxidation inhibitor U-101033E reduces neuronal damage after global cerebral ischemia in rats. Stroke 29: 1240–1247
9. Ungersböck K, Heimann A, Kempski O (1993) Cerebral blood flow alterations in a rat model of cerebral sinus thrombosis. Stroke 24: 563–570
10. Ungersböck K, Heimann A, Kempski O (1993) Mapping of cortical microcirculation by laser Doppler flowmetry. Microcirculatory stasis in the brain. In: Tomita M, Mchedlishvili G, Rosenblum WI, Heiss WD, Fukuuchi Y (eds) Elsevier Science Publishers, pp 405–414

Correspondence: Univ.-Prof. Dr. med. O. Kempski, Institute for Neurosurgical Pathophysiology, Johannes Gutenberg-University, Langenbeckstr. 1, 55101 Mainz, Germany.

Experimental Studies/Models

The wide range of experimental models described represents the remarkable ingenuity of the contributors to this section. All the models are relevant to clinical conditions in which brain oedema prevails.

Robertson *et al.* used magnetic resonance imaging (MRI) to measure tissue water and cerebral blood flow (CBF) in a cortical impact model. 2-chloroadenosine inhibited the oedema and ischaemia. Very early and frequent assessment of MRI with diffusion weighted Tensor (trace D) by Kuroiwa *et al.* was used to show that, following middle cerebral artery (MCA) occlusion, *cytotoxic* oedema can be detected within minutes of onset. Similarly, *vasogenic* oedema can be detected in the cryogenic injury model. This type of MRI should be able to differentiate the different oedema types clinically.

Using more conventional methodology (wet/dry) Ikeda *et al.* showed that L-Histidine inhibited vasogenic brain oedema following cryogenic injury.

Monitoring is being introduced into many clinical intensive therapy unit (ITU) environments and two new brain probes were evaluated experimentally: the tissue oxygen electrode was shown to correlate well with cerebral perfusion pressure (CPP) reduction in pigs. A new glutamate probe (directly sensitive to changes in tissue glutamate) was used to demonstrate the complex additive effect of traumatic brain injury (TBI) and hypoxia by Matsushita *et al.* This large measured increase in tissue glutamate holds great promise for its use as a simple clinical monitoring tool for the prevention of secondary insults in human head injury.

Traumatic subarachnoid haemorrhage (SAH) was studied and Thomas *et al.* described a new heparinised SAH model. The similarity between traumatic SAH and spontaneous SAH was highlighted by the Jackson (Mississippi) group who drew parallels between traumatic and spontaneous SAH. Therapeutic advances in traumatic SAH would seem to be just around the corner!

The interplay between traumatic SAH, Diffuse Axonal Injury (DAI), subdural haemorrhage and contusions in these experimental studies correlates well with the Marshall CT classification of head injury, which is now universally accepted in clinical TBI.

Ghabriel *et al.* describe an excellent new model of vasogenic oedema induced by the intraperitoneal injection of Clostridium perfringens type D epsilon protoxin.

There are now a wide variety of experimental models available to the researcher wanting to study the different types of brain oedema.

Acta Neurochir (2000) [Suppl] 76: 187–189

Assessment of 2-Chloroadenosine Treatment After Experimental Traumatic Brain Injury in the Rat Using Arterial Spin-Labeled MRI: A Preliminary Report

C. L. Robertson[1,6], **K. S. Hendrich**[7], **P. M. Kochanek**[1,2,6], **E. K. Jackson**[5], **J. A. Melick**[1,6], **S. H. Graham**[4], **D. W. Marion**[3], **D. S. Williams**[7], and **C. Ho**[7,8]

[1] Department of Anesthesiology and Critical Care Medicine, University of Pittsburgh, Pennsylvania
[2] Department of Pediatrics, University of Pittsburgh, Pennsylvania
[3] Department of Neurological Surgery, University of Pittsburgh, Pennsylvania
[4] Department of Neurology, Geriatric Research Educational and Clinical Center, VA Pittsburgh Health System, Pennsylvania
[5] Center for Clinical Pharmacology, University of Pittsburgh, Pennsylvania
[6] The Safar Center for Resuscitation Research, and the Brain Trauma Research Center, University of Pittsburgh, Pennsylvania
[7] Pittsburgh NMR Center for Biomedical Research, Carnegie Mellon University, Pennsylvania
[8] Department of Biological Sciences, Carnegie Mellon University, Pennsylvania

Summary

Adenosine is a putative endogenous neuroprotectant. Its action at A1 receptors mitigates excitotoxicity while action at A2 receptors increases cerebral blood flow (CBF). We hypothesized that cerebral injection of the adenosine analog, 2-chloroadenosine, would decrease swelling and increase CBF early after experimental traumatic brain injury (TBI). To test this hypothesis, rats were anesthetized and subjected to TBI using a controlled cortical impact (CCI) model (n = 5/group). Immediately after injury, 2-chloroadenosine (0.3 nmole in 2 μl) or an equal volume of vehicle were stereotactically injected lateral to the area of contusion. Using magnetic resonance imaging (MRI), *in vivo* spin-lattice relaxation time of tissue water (T_{1obs}) and CBF (arterial spin labeling) were measured in a 2-mm thick slice in the injured and non-injured hemispheres at 3–4 h after CCI. In a separate, preliminary experiment, the effect of 2-chloroadenosine injection in normal rat brain was studied. Rats (n = 2) were anesthetized and a burr hole was made for injection of 2-chloroadenosine into the same site as in the TBI model. One rat received the standard dose of 0.3 nmole and one rat received a 6 nmole injection. T_{1obs} and CBF studies were obtained 1.5–3.5 h after injection, using the same MRI methods as in the TBI study. In rats subjected to TBI, treatment with 2-chloroadenosine attenuated the increase in T_{1obs} after injury ($p < 0.05$ for treatment vs vehicle) in both hippocampus and cortex ipsilateral to injury. However, treatment with 2-chloroadenosine did not improve post-traumatic hypoperfusion. In normal rats, injection of 0.3 nmole of 2-chloroadenosine did not increase CBF, but the higher dosage of 6 nmole dramatically increased hemispheric CBF by 1.5–2.0-fold. The effect of local injection of 2-chloroadenosine at a dose of 0.3 nmole after experimental TBI on T_{1obs} presumably represents a reduction in post-traumatic edema. This reduction in edema, along with the augmentation of CBF seen in normal rats at higher dosage (6 nmole), supports a role for adenosine in neuroprotection following TBI.

Keywords: Adenosine; 2-chloroadenosine; traumatic brain injury; cerebral blood flow; post-traumatic cerebral edema.

Introduction

Adenosine is a putative endogenous neuroprotectant. Its biological activity is mediated by interaction with pre- and postsynaptic receptors. Adenosine action at A1 receptors mitigates excitotoxicity in the brain [12], while action at the A2 receptors increases cerebral blood flow (CBF) [8, 10]. Headrick *et al.* evaluated the effect of augmentation of adenosine following traumatic brain injury (TBI), using a fluid percussion injury model in rats [6]. Injection of the adenosine analog, 2-chloroadenosine, via the intracerebroventricular route produced improvement in metabolic energy disturbances and neurologic outcome following TBI in rats [6]. We hypothesized that cerebral injection of 2-chloroadenosine would attenuate the posttraumatic increase in the *in vivo* spin-lattice relaxation time of tissue water (T_{1obs}) and mitigate posttraumatic hypoperfusion early after experimental TBI in the rat. In separate studies, we also evaluated the effect of 2-chloroadenosine on both T_{1obs} and CBF studies in normal rats.

Materials and Methods

Mature, male Sprague-Dawley rats (n = 5/group) were studied. Animals were allowed free access to food and water before surgery. This study was approved by the University of Pittsburgh Animal Care and Use Committee. The care and handling of animals were in accord with National Institute of Health guidelines.

Rats were anesthetized, endotracheally intubated and mechanically ventilated. Rats underwent TBI using a controlled cortical impact (CCI) model as previously described [3]. Immediately after injury, 2-chloroadenosine (0.3 nmole in 2 μl) or vehicle was stereotactically injected lateral to the contusion in the left parietal cortex. The bone flap was replaced and sealed, and the scalp incision was closed. Anesthesia was discontinued, and rats were awakened, extubated and transported to the NMR center. CBF studies were performed at approximately 3 and 4 hours after TBI. T_{1obs} maps were obtained between perfusion studies.

In a separate, preliminary experiment, the effect of 2-chloroadenosine injection in normal rat was studied. Rats (n = 2) were anesthetized, intubated and mechanically ventilated. A burr hole was made and 2-chloroadenosine was injected into the same site as in the TBI model. One rat received the standard dose of 0.3 nmole and one rat received a 6 nmole injection. CBF studies and T_{1obs} maps were obtained 1.5–3.5 hours after injection.

MR images were acquired from a 2-mm thick coronal slice ~2.5 mm posterior to bregma. Spin-echo perfusion images (continuous arterial spin labeling) [2, 15] were acquired in duplicate using a single RF coil for both arterial spin labeling and for detection of the MR image. The spatial dependence for T_{1obs} was determined from a series of spin-echo maps acquired with variable TR.

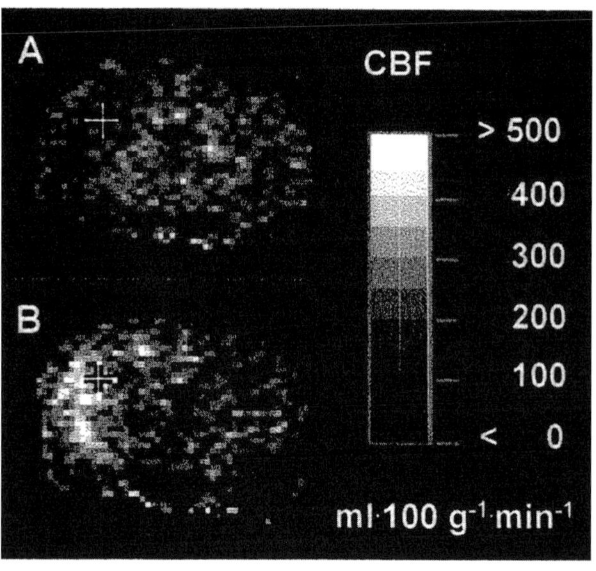

Fig. 1. MR perfusion maps in normal rat brain generated ~1.5 h after injection with 2-chloroadenosine (A) 0.3 nmole; (B) 6.0 nmole. The injection site is noted by the symbol (+)

Results

In rats subjected to TBI, injection of 2-chloroadenosine (0.3 nmole) dramatically attenuated the increase in T_{1obs} in both hippocampus and cortex ipsilateral to injury versus vehicle in the injured hemisphere (Table 1). In contrast, CBF was reduced in the injured hemisphere by TBI but not significantly different in any structure in the treatment vs vehicle groups (Table 1).

In the evaluation of normal rat brain, injection of 0.3 nmole of 2-chloroadenosine did not increase CBF. Interestingly, injection of 6 nmole dramatically increased CBF in a 2-mm slice through the ipsilateral hemisphere by 1.5–2.0-fold (Fig. 1).

Discussion

The effect of local injection of 2-chloroadenosine (0.3 nmole) on T_{1obs} after experimental TBI presumably represents a reduction in post-traumatic edema. This is consistent with the fact that 2-chloroadenosine demonstrates a five- to ten-fold selectivity for the A1 vs A2 receptor [7]. The therapeutic potential of augmenting adenosine after brain injury has been extensively reviewed [5, 14]. Evans *et al.* demonstrated protection against CA1 hippocampal cell death with local injection of 2-chloroadenosine following incomplete forebrain ischemia in the rat [4]. Similar neuroprotective effects have been demonstrated with other

Table 1. *Regional CBF (ml · 100 g^{-1} · min^{-1}) and $T_{1obs}(s)$ Measured at 4.7 Tesla in Rats at ~1.5 h After Experimental TBI*

Region	CBF(ml · 100 g^{-1} · min^{-1})				T_{1obs}(s)			
	2-chloroadenosine (n = 5)		Saline (n = 5)		2-chloroadenosine (n = 4)		Saline (n = 4)	
	Left	Right	Left	Right	Left	Right	Left	Right
Hippocampus	124 (39)	122 (34)	96 (20)	147 (20)	1.79 (0.09)[a]	1.74 (0.11)	2.08 (0.05)	1.86 (0.10)
Cortex	87 (28)	107 (28)	96 (29)	151 (44)	1.94 (0.05)[b]	1.84 (0.05)	2.13 (0.29)	1.81 (0.08)
Contusion enriched cortex	70 (34)	103 (31)	76 (24)	144 (34)	2.02 (0.13)[c]	1.88 (0.07)	2.29 (0.44)	1.82 (0.11)
Hemisphere	109 (26)	111 (27)	117 (40)	143 (54)	1.80 (0.04)	1.77 (0.02)	1.88 (0.14)	1.77 (0.08)

Values given are mean (standard deviation, SD). SD in CBF represents the intergroup variability in the perfusion %-change maps.
2-chloroadenosine dose for studies in TBI was 0.3 nmole (see text for details).
Contusion Enriched Cortex includes full cortical thickness within slice, but extends only to midpoint of arc defining maps.
[a] $p < 0.01$ for treatment vs saline vehicle in hippocampus.
[b] $p < 0.05$ for treatment vs saline vehicle in cortex.
[c] $p \leq 0.06$ overall ANOVA for treatment vs saline vehicle in contusion-enriched ROI.

A1-selective adenosine analogs after brain ischemia [11, 13]. Headrick *et al.* showed neuroprotective effects in a TBI model using 2-chloroadenosine [6]. The exact mechanism affording this neuroprotection is unknown, but it has been linked to an anti-excitotoxic action involving reduction of glutamate release and inhibition of calcium influx [1].

In this preliminary study of adenosine augmentation, injection of higher doses of 2-chloroadenosine (6 nmole) appears to have a significant effect on increasing CBF in normal rat brain. This likely reflects action at A2 receptors when a higher dose is applied. Interestingly, the effect on T_{1obs} was seen at 3–4 hours after TBI, and the effect on CBF in normal rats persisted at least 5 hours, although the plasma half-life of 2-chloroadenosine is only 5–10 minutes [9]. Future studies, using the higher 6 nmole 2-chloroadenosine dose are needed in rats subjected to TBI to determine if beneficial effects on both T_{1obs} and CBF can be obtained.

References

1. Arvin B, Neville LF, Pan J, Roberts PJ (1989) 2-Chloroadenosine attenuates kainic acid-induced toxicity within the rat striatum: relationship to release of glutamate and Ca^{2+} influx. Br J Pharmacol 98: 225–235
2. Detre JA, Leigh JS, Williams DS *et al* (1992) Perfusion imaging. Magn Reson Med 23: 37–45
3. Dixon CE, Clifton GL, Lighthall JW *et al* (1991) A controlled cortical impact model of traumatic brain injury in the rat. J Neurosci Meth 39: 253–262
4. Evans MC, Swan JH, Meldrum BS (1987) An adenosine analogue, 2-chloroadenosine, protects against long term development of ischaemic cell loss in the rat hippocampus. Neurosci Lett 83: 287–292
5. Fredholm BB (1997) Adenosine and neuroprotection. In: Neuroprotective agents and cerebral ischaemia. Academic Press Limited, New York
6. Headrick JP, Bendall MR, Faden AI, Vink R (1994) Dissociation of adenosine levels from bioenergetic state in experimental brain trauma: potential role in secondary injury. J Cereb Blood Flow Metab 14: 853–861
7. Ijzerman AP, vonFrijtag Drabbe Kunzel JK, Vittori S *et al* (1994) Purine-substituted adenosine derivatives with small N^6-substituents as adenosine receptor agonists. Nucleos Nucleot 13: 2267–2281
8. Kim YB, Gidday JM, Gonzales ER *et al* (1994) Effect of hypoglycemia on postischemic cortical blood flow, hypercapnic reactivity, and interstitial adenosine concentration. J Neurosurgery 81: 877–884
9. Mathot RAA, Soudijn W, Breimer DD *et al* (1996) Pharmacokinetic-haemodynamic relationships of 2-chloroadenosine at adenosine A1 and A2a receptors *in vivo*. Br J Pharmacol 118: 369–377
10. Park TS, Gidday JM, Gonzales E (1991) Local cerebral blood flow response to locally infused 2-chloroadenosine during hypotension in piglets. Brain Res Dev Brain 61: 73–77
11. Roucher P, Meric P, Correze JL *et al* (1991) Metabolic effects of R-phenylisopropyl-adenosine during reversible forebrain ischaemia studied by *in vivo* ^{31}P nuclear magnetic resonance spectroscopy. J Cereb Blood Flow Metab 11: 453–458
12. Rudolphi KA, Schubert P, Parkinson FE, Fredholm BB (1992) Adenosine and brain ischaemia. Cerebrovasc Brain Metab Rev 4: 346–369
13. von Lubitz DKJE, Dambrosia JM, Redmond DJ (1989) Protective effect of cyclohexyladenosine in treatment of cerebral ischaemia in gerbils. Neuroscience 30: 451–462
14. von Lubitz DKJE (1997) Adenosine and acute treatment of cerebral ischemia and stroke – "put out more flags". In: Jacobson KA, Jarvis MF (eds) Purinergic approaches in experimental theraputics. Wiley-Liss, Inc., New York
15. Williams DS, Detre JA, Leigh JS *et al* (1992) Magnetic resonance imaging of perfusion using spin inversion of arterial water. Proc Natl Acad Sci USA 89: 212–216

Correspondence: Patrick M. Kochanek, M.D., Safar Center for Resuscitation Research, 3434 Fifth Avenue, Pittsburgh, PA 15260.

Acta Neurochir (2000) [Suppl] 76: 191–194

Time Course of Trace of Diffusion Tensor [Trace(D)] and Histology in Brain Edema

T. Kuroiwa[1], **T. Nagaoka**[2], **N. Miyasaka**[1], **H. Akimoto**[3], **F. Zhao**[4], **I. Yamada**[4], **M. Ueki**[5], and **S. Ichinose**[6]

[1] Department of Neuropathology, Medical Research Institute, Tokyo Medical and Dental University, Tokyo, Japan
[2] Department of Neurosurgery, Tokyo Medical and Dental University, Tokyo, Japan
[3] Department of Gynecology and Obstetrics, Tokyo Medical and Dental University, Tokyo, Japan
[4] Department of Neurology, Tokyo Medical and Dental University, Tokyo, Japan
[5] Department of Radiology, Tokyo Medical and Dental University, Tokyo, Japan
[6] Department of Anesthesiology and Laboratory of Electronmicroscopy, Tokyo Medical and Dental University, Tokyo, Japan

Summary

We examined the correlation between changes in the trace of diffusion tensor [Trace(D)], regional water content and tissue ultrastructure relating to cellular (cytotoxic) and vasogenic brain edema. Cellular edema was induced by left middle cerebral artery occlusion in cats (Kuroiwa T *et al.*, 1998). Vasogenic edema was induced in the white matter of cats by a cold lesion (Kuroiwa T *et al.*, 1999). In cellular edema, the water content increase correlated linearly with the Trace(D) decrease in both the gray and white matter. However, both the slopes and intercepts of the correlation lines were significantly different. Hydropic astrocytic swelling was seen in both structures, and in the white matter, oligodendrocytic and myelinated axonal swelling were observed. In vasogenic edema, the increase in Trace(D) showed a significant linear correlation with the increase in tissue water content. Histologically, nerve fibers were dissociated and the extracellular space was markedly enlarged with protein-rich fluid. These result showed that the different slopes and intercepts of the water content – Trace(D) correlation lines for different subtype of brain edema, which reflect different ultrastructural localization of water, should be taken into account when evaluating brain edema using Trace(D) mapping.

Keywords: Trace of diffusion tensor; brain edema; ultrastructure; and water content.

Introduction

Brain edema has been classified as being either vasogenic or cellular (cytotoxic), according to whether the water accumulation is extracellular or intracellular, respectively [3]. It is clinically important to be able to differentiate between types of brain edema as early as possible after the onset of disease in order to start the appropriate treatment. It has been observed in in vitro experiment that changes in the ADC are linearly correlated with changes in the extracellular water fraction [1]. ADC mapping with MRI will therefore provide important information for quantitatively analyzing edematous brain tissue.

However, ADC varies with the orientation of structures within the tissue, such as the white matter, which has a regularly ordered microstructure (diffusion anisotropy). We therefore evaluated changes in the ADC by using the trace of diffusion tensor [Trace(D)] which is defined as the sum of diagonal elements of the diffusion tensor and unaffected by tissue orientation.

This paper is a summary of our recent studies on the Trace(D) mapping in cellular and vasogenic brain edema [5, 6].

Materials and Methods

The animal experiments were performed in accordance with institutional guidelines for animal care and experimentation. Twenty-one adult cats weighing 3.5 to 4.5 kg were used in the following experiments. The animal was intubated and artificially ventilated under isoflurane anesthesia. The body temperature was maintained at 37 °C by using a feed-back controlled water jacket.

1) For induction of early ischemic edema (cellular or cytotoxic edema), a middle cerebral artery (MCA) occlusion device was implanted in each cat via a transorbital approach. The animal was placed in an experimental MRI scanner (4.7-T experimental imager/spectrometer system) and T2-, diffusion weighted- and perfusion imaging was performed before and 15, 30, 60, 120 and 180 min after MCA occlusion. Trace(D) maps were generated as described previously [5, 6]. Shortly after obtaining the final MRI image, the animal was sacrificed under anesthesia. Tissue samples were cut from a coronal slice of the brain 10 mm anterior to the auditory meatus, and tissue water content was determined by gravimetry [7]. For morphological examination, each animal was perfused transcardially with fixative while under anesthesia.

2) For induction of cold lesion edema (vasogenic edema), a left parietal craniotomy was made on the left suprasylvian gyrus, the animal was placed into the MRI scanner and T2- and diffusion-weighted imaging was performed before and every 30 min during the initial 4.5 h after cold lesioning. A cortical cold lesion was made by applying a metal plate cooled to −40 °C with acetone dry ice to the dura for 90 s [10]. A 2% solution of Evans blue dye was injected intravenously shortly after the lesioning. Tissue water content was determined by the gravimetry. For morphological examination, each animal was perfused transcardially with fixative under anesthesia. The brain was cut into coronal sections and sampled from the sites corresponding to the regions of interest for Trace(D) measurement. The results are expressed as means ± standard deviation (S.D.). Differences at $p < 0.05$ were considered to be statistically significant.

Results

Cellular (Cytotoxic) Brain Edema

Perfusion imaging revealed perfusion deficits corresponding to the MCA territory in all animals. Trace(D) at 3 h after ischemia onset at the ectosylvian gyrus declined significantly to 424 ± 25.3 and $361 \pm 42.2 \times 10^{-6}$ mm^2/s in the moderate perfusion deficit group (perfusion index [5] between 0.6 and 0.2) and severe perfusion deficit group (perfusion index less than 0.2), respectively. The gray and white matter tissue water contents at the ectosylvian gyrus increased significantly from to 0.788 ± 0.0067 and 0.663 ± 0.0045 g. water/g. tissue to 0.814 ± 0.009 and 0.679 ± 0.007 g. water/g. tissue, respectively. The tissue water content increases paralleled the Trace(D) decreases in both the gray and white matter in these. However, both the slopes and intercepts of the correlation lines for the gray and white matter differed significantly (Table 1). Electron-microscopy revealed hydropic swelling of the astrocytes. Some neurons located in the ischemic center showed dark neuron change, whereas many others appeared normal. Cell membrane was not disrupted in the neurons showing either of the above changes. In the ischemic white matter, edematous rarefaction of the myelinated fibers was observed with light-microscopy. Electron-microscopy revealed marked cytoplasmic swelling of the oligodendrocytes as well as the astrocytes. Myelinated axonal swelling and periaxonal space enlargement was also observed.

Table 1. *Correlation Between Trace(D) and Tissue Water Content*

	Correlation line	Regression coefficient
Cellular brain edema		
Gray matter	$y = -10105x + 8533$	0.86
White matter	$y = -6174^*x + 4611^*$	0.67
Vasogenic brain edema		
Subcortical white matter	$y = 45.5x - 2367$	0.94
Deep white matter	$y = 37.0x - 1769$	0.93

x Water content (g water/g tissue), y Trace(D) ($\times 10^{-6}$ mm^2/s), * significantly different from the corresponding gray matter value ($p < 0.05$).

Vasogenic Brain Edema

Trace(D) map showed a high-intensity area in the subcortical white matter. Trace(D) gradually increased in the white matter, and the area also spread into the deep white matter during the observation period. At 4.5 h after cold lesioning, Trace(D) of the control side was measured $517 \pm 68 \times 10^{-6}$ mm^2/s and $581 \pm 46 \times 10^{-6}$ mm^2/s in the subcortical white matter and deep white matter, respectively. In the lesioned side, Trace(D) significantly increased to $1148 \pm 139 \times 10^{-6}$ mm^2/s $975 \pm 92 \times 10^{-6}$ mm^2/s, respectively. The water content of the subcortical and deep white matter of the control side was 0.638 ± 0.018 and 0.641 ± 0.022 g. water/g. tissue, respectively, and that the water content in the lesioned side significantly increased to 0.819 ± 0.0073 and

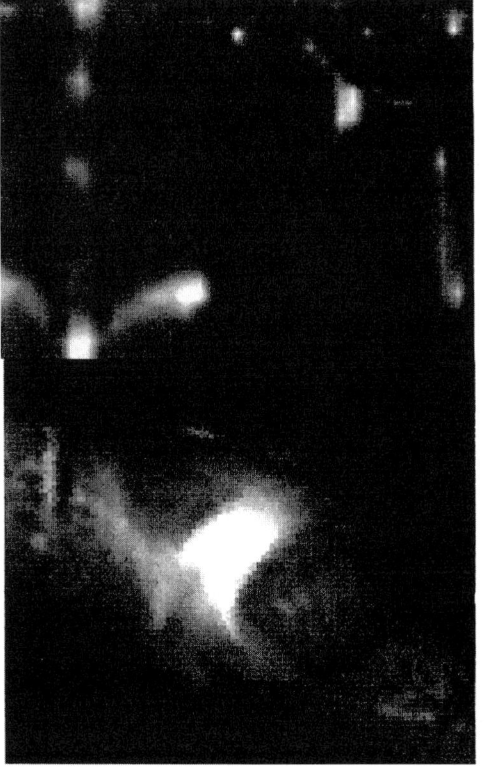

Fig. 1. Representative trace (D) maps after middle cerebral artery (*MCA*) occlusion (upper) and cortical cold lesioning (lower) in cats

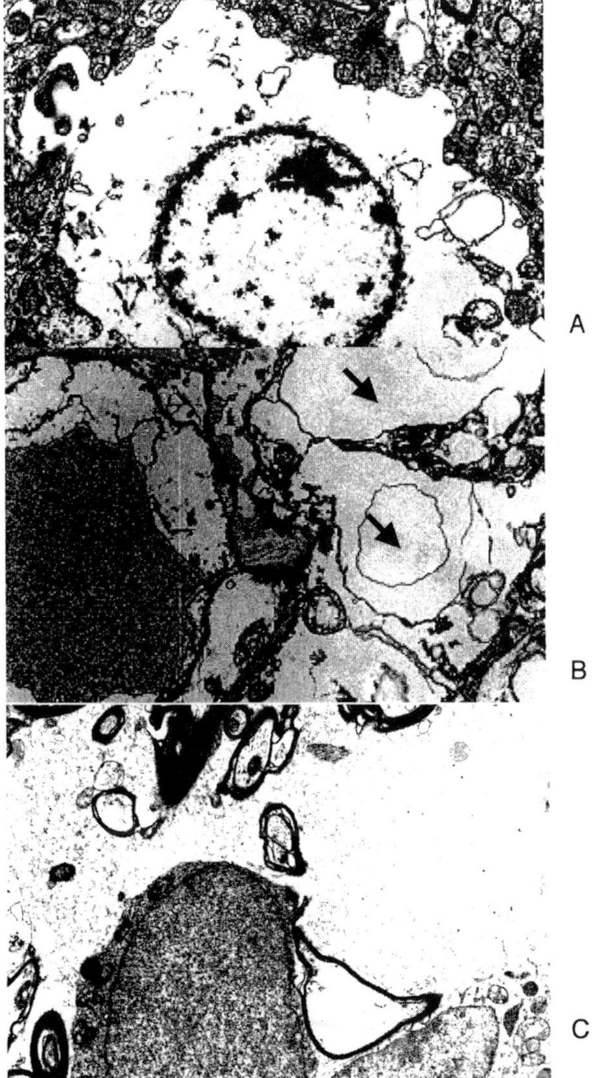

Fig. 2. Electron micrograms of ischemic white matter showing swelling of oligodendrocyte (A) and astrocytic perivascular endfeet (arrow) (B), and white matter after cold lesioning showing enlargement of extracellular space (C)

0.769 ± 0.025 g. water/g. tissue, respectively. The increase in Trace(D) and tissue water content showed a significant linear correlation both in the subcortical and deep white matter. The slopes and intercepts were not significantly different between the two correlation lines.

Light microscopically, most of the nerve fibers in the subcortical white matter run in parallel, whereas in the deep white matter the bundles of nerve fibers were often intermingled in the control side. In the lesioned side, the nerve fibers were dissociated and the interfiber space was enlarged both in the subcortical and the deep white matter. Electron microscopy revealed enlargement of the extracellular space with protein-rich fluid in the edematous white matter. No swelling of the cellular components was observed. Thus, enlargement of the extracellular space with protein-rich edema fluid corresponded to the occurrence of vasogenic edema in the white matter.

Discussion

A device designed for intramagnet MCA occlusion was used in cats to induce cellular cytotoxic edema (early ischemic edema), which enable us to record MR images keeping the animal in the magnet. We measured Trace(D) that is defined as the sum of diagonal elements of the diffusion tensor to avoid any influence of diffusion anisotropy of the edematous bran tissue.

In cellular edema, we observed that Trace(D) decreased in parallel to the increase in tissue water content. Electron microscopic examination showed cellular swelling in both the gray and white matter, which corresponded to the Trace(D) decreases in both structures. Cellular swelling in the gray matter takes place mainly in the astrocytes, whereas in the white matter, hydropic swelling of the oligodendrocytes as well as the astrocytes, intracellular water accumulation in the axon and periaxonal space enlargement was observed. The observed different localization of edema fluid in the ischemic gray and white matter probably accounts for the different slopes and intercepts of the Trace(D) and water content correlation lines.

To induce vasogenic brain edema, a cold lesion was made in the cat cerebral cortex. The advantage of the cold lesion model is that it results in predominantly vasogenic edema, which is different from many other lesions. Traumatic edema, for example, causes a mixture of both cellular and vasogenic edema [2]. In this model, the edema fluid spreads via the subcortical white matter to the deep white matter 3–6 h after lesioning. We observed a significant linear correlation between the increase in extracellular water content and Trace(D) in white matter manifesting vasogenic edema. The difference in the arrangement of nerve fibers in the subcortical and deep white matter (parallel vs. intermingled pattern) did not result in a significant difference in the correlation between extracellular water accumulation and Trace(D). The observed positive correlation is strikingly different from that which is observed following cellular edema.

The results described here show that Trace(D) is a suitable parameter for the differentiation of the brain edema subtype; this can not be done by CT [4] or conventional MRI. Since both types of edema are induced by most common disease processes in the brain such as ischemia, trauma and hypertension, the ability to differentiate between them using a non-invasive procedure is highly advantageous from the clinical point of view.

Acknowledgments

The authors wish to thank Dr. Shu Endo, Ms. Yoshie Furusawa, Ms. Tayoko Tajima, Ms. Hiromi Tanizawa, Mr. T Yoshizawa and Mr. N Shirato for their excellent technical assistance.

References

1. Andrasko J (1976) Water diffusion permeability of human erythrocytes studied by a pulsed gradient NMR technique. Biochemica et Biophysica Acta 428(2): 304–311
2. Ito J, Marmarou A, Barzo P, Faatouros P, Corwin F (1996) Characterization of edema by diffusion-weighted imaging in experimental traumatic brain injury J Neurosurg 84: 97–103
3. Klatzo I (1967) Presidential address, Neuropathological aspects of brain edema J Neuropathol Exp Neurol 26: 1–14
4. Kuroiwa T, Seida M, Tomida S, Hiratsuka H, Okeda R, Inaba Y (1986) Discrepancies among CT, histological, and blood brain barrier findings in early cerebral ischemia J Neurosurg 65: 517–524
5. Kuroiwa T, Nagaoka T, Ueki M, Yamada I, Miyasaka Akimoto H (1998) Different apparent diffusion coefficient – water content correlations of gray and white matter during early ischemia Stroke 29: 859–865
6. Kuroiwa T, Nagaoka T, Ueki M, Yamada I, Miyasaka N, Akimoto H, Ichinose S, Okeda R, Hirakawa K (1999) Correlation between the apparent diffusion coefficient, water content and ultrastructure relating to vasogenic brain edema. J Neurosurg 90: 499–503
7. Marmarou A, Tanaka K, Schulman K (1982) An improved gravimetric measure of cerebral edema. J Neurosurg 56: 246–253

Correspondence: Toshihiko Kuroiwa, M.D., Department of Neuropathology, Medical Research Institute, Tokyo Medical and Dental University, Yushima 1-5-45, Bunkyo-ku, Tokyo 113-8510, Japan.

Acta Neurochir (2000) [Suppl] 76: 195–197

L-Histidine but not D-Histidine Attenuates Brain Edema Following Cryogenic Injury in Rats

Y. Ikeda, Y. Mochizuki, H. Matsumoto, Y. Nakamura, K. Dohi, H. Jimbo, M. Shimazu, M. Hayashi, and **K. Matsumoto**

Department of Neurosurgery, Showa University School of Medicine, Tokyo, Japan

Summary

Oxygen free radicals have been implicated in the genesis of traumatic brain injury and brain edema (BE). Recent studies have suggested that hydroxyl radical can initiate lipid peroxidation, thus producing lipid-free radicals that may become important sources of singlet oxygen. L-histidine, a singlet oxygen scavenger, potentially can be used to treat BE. In this study we investigated the effects of L-histidine and D-histidine on BE following cryogenic injury in rats. Male Wistar rats were anaesthetized with chloral hydrate. Vasogenic BE was produced by a cortical freezing lesion. Generation of singlet oxygen from photoactivation of rose bengal was studied by electron spin resonance (ESR). Animals were separated into four groups: sham rats (n = 5), saline-treated rats (n = 10), L-histidine treated rats (n = 6) and D-histidine treated rats (n = 7). Each agent (100 mg/kg) was administered intravenously at 30 minutes before lesion production. Animals were sacrificed at 24 hours after lesion production and the brain water content was determined by the dry-wet weight method. L-histidine had no effect on rectal and brain temperature. Election Spin Resonance studies demonstrated that L-histidine is a singlet oxygen scavenger. L-histidine but not D-histidine significantly attenuated BE following cryogenic injury ($p < 0.05$). In conclusion, L-histidine is useful in the treatment of traumatic BE.

Keywords: Free radicals; L-histidine; brain injury; brain edema.

Introduction

Oxygen free radicals have been implicated in the genesis of traumatic brain injury and brain edema [2]. Among oxygen free radicals, the only species blamed for the tissue injury is hydroxyl radical. Recent reports [4] have suggested that in myocardial ischemia/reperfusion injury, the hydroxyl radical can initiate lipid peroxidation, thus producing lipid-free radicals that may become important sources of singlet oxygen (Fig. 1). No direct demonstration of singlet oxygen formation in vivo has been published to date. L-histidine, a singlet oxygen scavenger, potentially can be used to treat brain edema. In this study we investigated the effects of L-histidine and D-histidine on brain edema following cryogenic brain injury in rats.

Materials and Methods

Generation of Singlet Oxygen

Singlet oxygen was generated by photoexcitation of the light-sensitive dye rose bengal, which is one of the most effective sources of singlet oxygen generation. The spin trapping studies were performed by mixing rose bengal with spin trap 2,2,6,6-tetramethylpiperidine (TEMP) and illuminating for 10 minutes with light. Electron spin resonance detction of the spin adduct was performed at room temperature by a JES-RE3X, X-band, spectrometer (Joel, Tokyo) [5]. Inhibition of singlet oxygen by 25, 50 and 100 mM of L-histidine was also investigated.

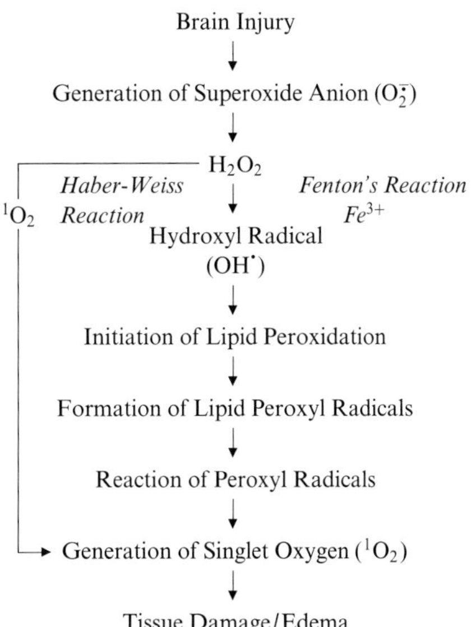

Fig. 1. Possible mechanisms of oxidant injury

Surgical Procedure and Experimental Protocols

Male Wistar rats, weighing 250 to 300 g each, were anesthetized intraperitoneally with chloral hydrate (360 mg/kg). A midline scalp incision and a craniectomy were made in the right parietal region. Cortical cryogenic injury was produced by application of a metal probe cooled by dry ice to the dura mater of the right parietal region. The dura was left intact. The skin was closed with sutures.

Animals were separated into four groups: sham rats ($n = 5$), saline-treated rats with lesion production ($n = 10$), L-histidine treated (100 mg/kg) rats with lesion production ($n = 6$) and D-histidine treated (100 mg/kg) rats with lesion production ($n = 7$). Each agent was administered intravenously at 30 minutes before lesion production. Animals were sacrificed at 24 hours after lesion production and the brain water content was determined by the dry-wet weight method. 24 hours after lesion production, animals were sacrificed by decapitation. The brain was removed immediately and divided into right injured hemisphere and left non-injured hemisphere. The tissue was then dried in a 100 °C oven for 24 hours and reweighted to obtain the dry weight. The water contents, expressed as a percentage of the wet weight, were calculated as (wet weight − dry weight)/wet weight × 100. Data are presented as mean ± standard deviation. Student t-test was used to assess significance, with $p < 0.05$ considered to indicate statistical significance.

Results

Electron spin resonance study showed that singlet oxygen was produced by photoactivation of rose bengal and was detected as singlet oxygen-TEMP product. The formation of TEMPO signal was strongly inhibited by L-histidine in a dose-dependent manner (Fig. 2).

The cortical cryogenic injury produced an increase in brain water contents at 24 hours (ipsilateral hemisphere: 80.43 ± 0.15% versus 79.06 ± 0.36%, contralateral hemisphere: 79.54 ± 0.27% versus 78.75 ± 0.24%, $P < 0.01$). At 24 hours after lesion production, L-histidine significantly attenuated an increase in brain water contents (ipsilateral hemisphere: 80.43 ± 0.15% versus 79.43 ± 0.52%, contralateral hemisphere: 79.54 ± 0.09 versus 78.76 ± 0.49%, $p < 0.01$) (Fig. 3). D-histidine did not attenuate an increase in water contents (ipsilateral hemishere: 80.43 ± 0.15% versus 80.53 ± 0.49%, contralateral hemisphere: 79.54 ± 0.09% versus 79.54 ± 0.32) (Fig. 4).

Discussion

L-histidine is an efficient scavenger of highly active singlet oxygen and a somewhat weaker scavenger of hydoxyl radicals. L-histidine is a naturally occurring amino acid that can be easily synthesized, stored and should have minimal toxicity. L-histidine has been shown to provide effective preservation of the canine heart and to protect against reperfusion injury in the

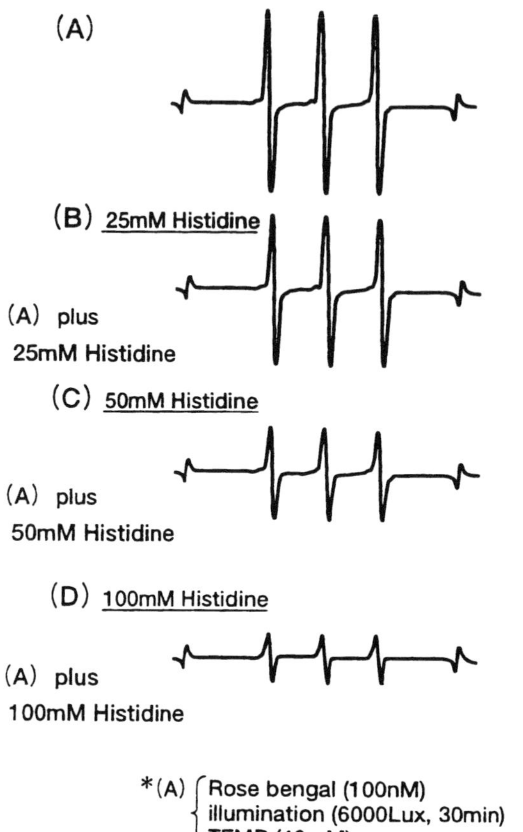

Fig. 2. ESR spectra of illuminated rose bengal in the presence of TEMP, TEMP: 2,2,6,6-tetramethylpiperidine

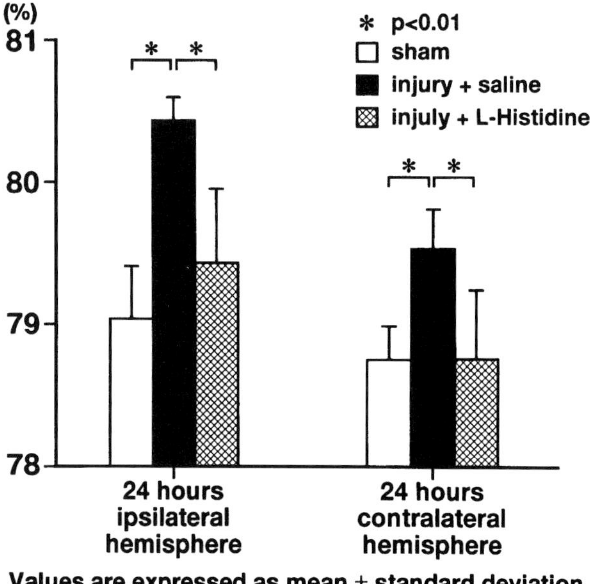

Fig. 3. Effects of L-histidine on brain water contents at 24 hours after cryogenic brain injury

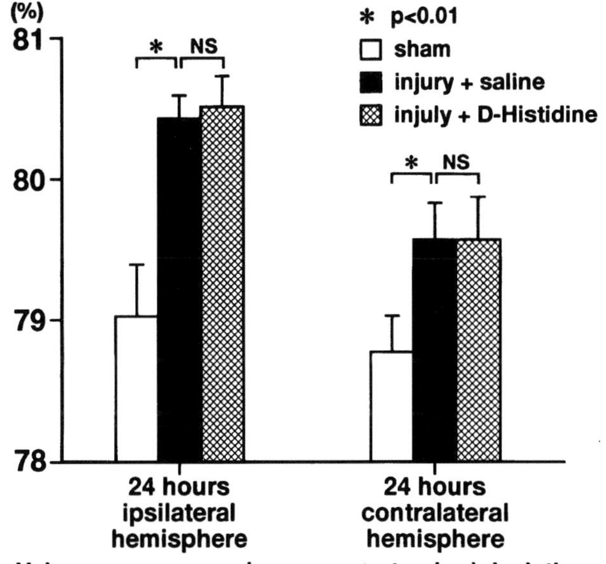

Fig. 4. Effects of D-histidine on brain water contents at 24 hours after cryogenic brain injury

heart, a pathogenic event in which free radical mechanisms paricipate. Kawamoto and Ikeda [3] demonstrated that L-histidine protected the elevation of extracellular glutamate concentrations and neuronal damage after reperfusion of cerebral ischemia in the rat hippocampus. Fadel *et al.* [1] showed that L-histidine reduces the amount of cerebral vasospasm occurring subsequent to experimental subarachnoid hemorrhage.

Oxygen free radicals have been implicated in the genesis of traumatic brain edema. The results of this study demonstrate that L-histidine reduced cryogenic induced brain edema at 24 hours after lesion production and singlet oxygen might be important in the genesis of traumatic brain edema.

We must clearly show by additional experiments that L-histidine is effective when applied after the injury and clinical application awaits expanded studies.

References

1. Fadel MM, Foley PL, Kassell NF *et al* (1995) Histidine attenuates cerebral vasospasm in a rabbit model of subarachnoid hemorrage. Surg Neurol 143: 52–58
2. Ikeda Y, Long DM (1990) The molecular basis of brain injury and brain edema: The role of oxygen free radicals. Neurosurgery 27: 1–11
3. Kawamoto T, Ikeda Y, Teramoto A (1997) Protective effect of L-histidine (singlet oxygen scavenger) on transient forebrain ischemia in the rat. No to sinnkei 49: 612–618
4. Kukreja RC, Jesse RL, Hess ML (1992) Singlet oxygen: a potential culprit in myocardial injury? Mol Cell Biochem 111: 17–24
5. Mizukawa H, Okabe E (1997) Inhibition by singlet molecular oxygen of the vascular reactivity in rabbit mesenteric artery. Br J Pharmacol 121: 63–70

Correspondence: Yukio Ikeda, M.D., D.M. Sc, Department of Neurosurgery, Showa University School of Medicine, 1-5-8 Hatanodai, Shinagawa-ku, Tokyo, Japan.

Acta Neurochir (2000) [Suppl] 76: 199–202

Oxygen Delivery and Oxygen Tension in Cerebral Tissue During Global Cerebral Ischaemia: A Swine Model

S. Rossi[1], **M. Balestreri**[2], **D. Spagnoli**[3], **G. Bellinzona**[2], **V. Valeriani**[1], **P. Bruzzone**[1], **M. Maestri**[1], and **N. Stocchetti**[1]

[1] Department of Anaesthesia and Intensive Care, Ospedale Maggiore, Policlinico IRCCS, Milano, Italy
[2] Institute of Neurosurgery, Ospedale Maggiore, Ospedale Maggiore, Policlinico IRCCS, Milano, Italy
[3] Department of Anaesthesia and Intensive Care and Experimental Surgery of Pavia University, Policlinico S. Matteo IRCCS, Pavia, Italy

Summary

Interest in tissue oxygen (PtiO2) monitoring is increasing. However the exact interactions between ptiO2, systemic and cerebral variables are a matter of debate. Particularly, the relationship between ptiO2, cerebral oxygen supply and consumption needs to be clarified. We designed a model to achieve progressive Cerebral Blood Flow (CBF) reduction through 3 steps: 1. baseline, 2. CBF between 50–60% of the baseline, 3. CBF < 30% of the baseline. In 7 pigs, under general anaesthesia, Cerebral Perfusion Pressure (CPP) and CBF were reduced through the infusion of saline in a lateral ventricle. PtiO2 and CBF were monitored respectively through a Clark electrode (Licox, GMS) and laser doppler (Peri-Flux). Blood from superior sagittal sinus and from an arterial line was simultaneously drawn to calculate the artero-venous difference of oxygen (AVDO2). Brain oxygen supply was calculated by multiplying relative CBF change and arterial oxygen content. PtiO2 reflected CBF reductions, as it was 27.95 (±10.15) mmHg during the first stage of intact CBF, declined to 14.77 (±3.58) mmHg during the first CBF reduction, declined to 3.45 (±2.89) mmHg during the second CBF reduction and finally fell to 0 mmHg when CBF was completely abolished. CBF changes were also followed by a decline in O2 supply and a parallel increase in AVDO2. Conclusion: this model allows stable and reproducible steps of progressive CBF reduction in which ptiO2 changes can be studied together with oxygen supply and consumption.

Keywords: Cerebral ischaemia; brain oxygenation; ICP; CBF.

Introduction

The primary goal in the management of acute cerebral damage is the minimisation of ischaemic/hypoxic secondary damage and possibly the preservation of adequate supply of oxygen and metabolites to the brain. In fact the maintenance of appropriate substrates delivery to the tissue is the premise for its viability and eventually for the restoration of its function.

Recently, techniques for local measurement of cerebral oxygenation are increasingly used in acute neurosurgical patients in order to assess cerebral blood flow (CBF) adequacy and metabolic substrates delivery [2, 9]. Particularly, the measurement of brain tissue oxygen pressure (ptiO2) using a polarographic Clark-type microcatheter is gaining increasing interest. However, many pathophysiological aspects of this technique still need to be clarified. Even though it is generally accepted that ptiO2 values are strictly dependent on cerebral blood flow (CBF), the levels of ptiO2 sufficient to maintain aerobic metabolism have not yet been identified. Furthermore the interrelations between oxygen delivery, consumption and brain oxygen tension are not fully understood. For these reasons the meaning of ptiO2 changes in response to clinical interventions is still uncertain.

Many experimental models have been developed to investigate the relationship between ptiO2, cerebral perfusion pressure (CPP), and CBF; however, as far as we know, none of the animal models currently used is suitable to achieve conditions of reduced CBF stable enough to allow the investigation of ptiO2, oxygen supply and consumption in a steady state [4, 8]. This study was designed to define a swine model of progressive cerebral ischaemia and to reach stable and reproducible steps of CBF decline in which ptiO2 responses to superimposed perturbations and interventions could be investigated.

Materials and Methods

In performing the experiments, the authors followed the guidelines for animal research published by the European Union and acknowledged by the Italian legislation in law n° 116/92.

Seven 8-week-old domestic pigs, weighing 18–22 kg were used. General anaesthesia was induced by propofol (2 mg/kg) and succinylcholine (1 mg/kg), and maintained by isofluorane 1.5% and 0.3 mg/kg/h pancuronium. The animals were ventilated by "controlled volume modality" to achieve paCO2 around 35 mmHg; inspiratory oxygen concentration was maintained at 30%. Internal temperature was continuously monitored by a rectal temperature probe and maintained between 37.5 and 38.5 °C. Saline infusions were administered at the rate of 3 ml/kg/h. Deep branches of the carotid artery and the jugular vein were surgically exposed and cannulated respectively for arterial pressure and blood gas monitoring and infusion of fluids.

The animal was placed in a prone position and a linear incision was performed in the midline from the inion to the nasion. The scalp was exposed and 3 burr holes were placed 1.5 cm from the midline on the right side through and across the coronal suture. Two more burr holes were made through the sagittal suture and through the left coronal suture (1.5 cm aside the midline). Through a dural incision in the cerebral parenchyma (from the front to the rear and on the right side) we placed the tip of the CBF probe, of the ptiO2 probe and of the ICP transducer. Through the burr hole on the left side a ventricular catheter was placed and connected to an infusion pump. The burr hole through the sagittal suture gave access to the superior sagittal sinus and was punctured for monitoring of blood gases and haemoglobin oxygen saturations.

ICP was measured by a parenchymal device (Camino). PtiO2 was measured by a polarographic Clark-type microcatheter (Licox, GMS). PtiO2 was allowed to stabilize for 2 hours after the insertion of the catheter and it was corrected for rectal temperature during the experiment. CBF estimation was obtained continuously by laser doppler flowmetry (Peri-flux, Perimed). CBF was calculated as the percentage change compared to the baseline value.

Intermittent samples were drawn simultaneously from superior sagittal sinus and from the artery in order to determine artero-venous oxygen difference (AVDO2). Cerebral electrical activity was monitored by a three point EEG.

The model was developed to obtain progressive CBF reduction through 3 stable steps: baseline (CBF = 100%), CBF between 50–60% of the baseline, CBF < 30% of the baseline. CBF reduction was obtained by inducing intracranial hypertension by means of the infusion of saline in the left lateral ventricle through a catheter connected with an infusion pump. ICP was raised in a stepwise fashion by a bolus of saline. After the end-point (in terms of reduction of CPP and CBF) was reached the velocity of fluid infusion into the ventricles was titrated to maintain stable values of ICP, CPP and CBF during each step. Cushing response, elicited by ICP increase, was inhibited by the infusion of β-blockers.

At the end of the experiment the animals were sacrificed by increasing isoflurane concentration up to 4% and by infusing 60 mEq of KCl.

Results

The course of intracranial variables during the steps of the experiment is shown in Fig. 1. CPP and CBF reduction were the result of both the increase in ICP and of the slight reduction of MAP as a consequence of the use of β-blockers to blunt the Cushing reflex. The end-points in terms of reduction in CPP and thus in CBF were reached. The 2 parameters were stable during the 3 steps. The mean duration of the 3 phases

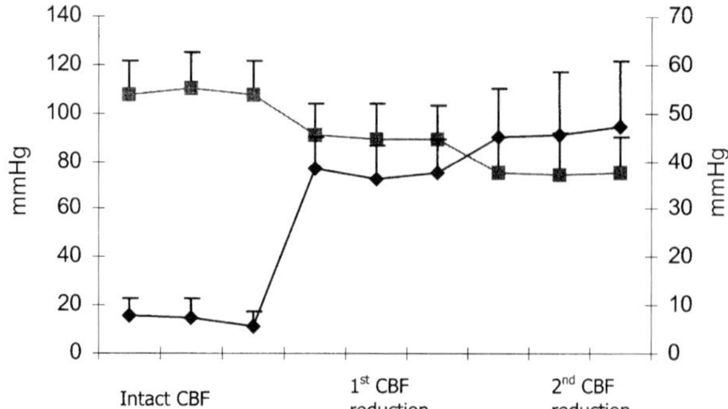

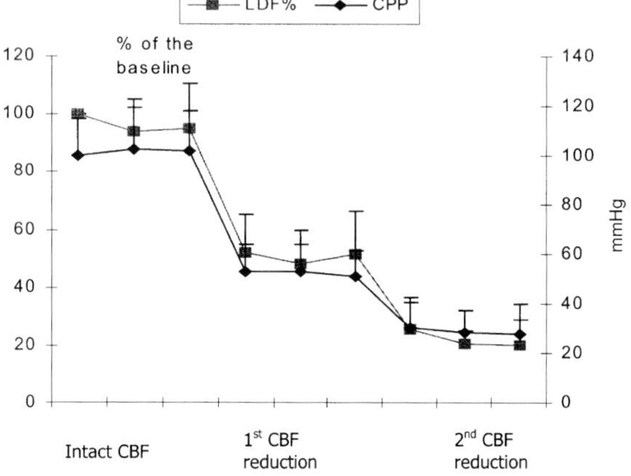

Fig. 1. MAP, ICP (upper part), CPP and CBF (lower part) course during the experiment. CBF reductions were calculated as the percentage change of laser doppler with respect to the baseline value. Error bars represent standard deviations. -■- MAP, -◆- ICP

was 49.8 (±10.49), 55.7 (±19.8) and 48.28 (±11.32) minutes, respectively.

During the baseline and the two phases of CBF reduction, the values of blood gases and internal temperatures remained constant; a mild decrease in hemoglobin concentration, probably due to frequent blood sampling, was observed (Table 1).

Progressive CBF impairment was accompanied by electroencephalographic (EEG) changes characterised by a reduction in EEG amplitude during the first phase (CBF = 50–60% of the baseline), which was more pronounced during the second (CBF = 20–30% of the baseline). PtiO2 changes reflected CBF reductions, since it was 27.95 (±10.15) mmHg during the first stage of intact CBF, declined to 14.77 (±3.85) mmHg during the first CBF reduction, declined to 3.45 (±2.89) mmHg during the second CBF reduction, and finally fell to 0 mmHg when CBF was completely abolished (Fig. 2).

CBF reduction was accompanied by a parallel decrease in O2 supply and increase in AVDO2. Fig. 3

Table 1. *Blood Gases, Temperature and Haemoglobin During the Three Phases of the Experiment*

	Hb (g/dl)	PaO2 (mmHg)	PaCO2 (mmHg)	SaO2%	pH	T °C
CBF 100%	9.0 (±1.25)	120 (±19.9)	38 (±2.58)	100	7.40 (±0.064)	37.8 (±0.30)
CBF 50–60%	8.3 (±1.43)	121 (±24.5)	37.1 (±3.07)	100	7.41 (±0.054)	37.5 (±0.45)
CBF 20–30%	7.9 (±1.13)	113 (±26.9)	37.7 (±1.97)	100	7.40 (±0.044)	37.9 (±0.29)
ANOVA	NS	NS	NS	NS	NS	NS

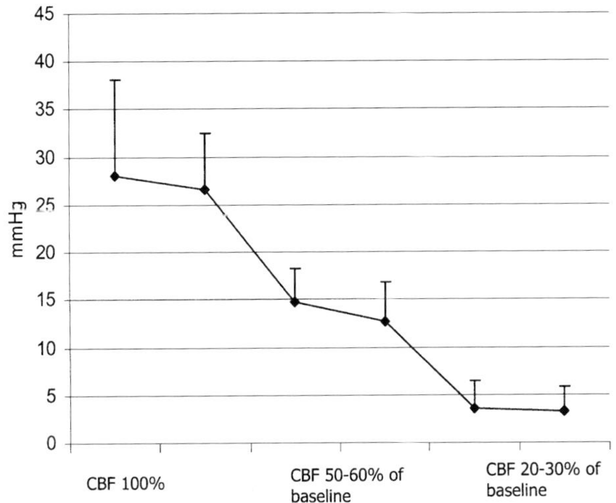

Fig. 2. PtiO2 changes in response to CBF decline. ◆ PtiO2

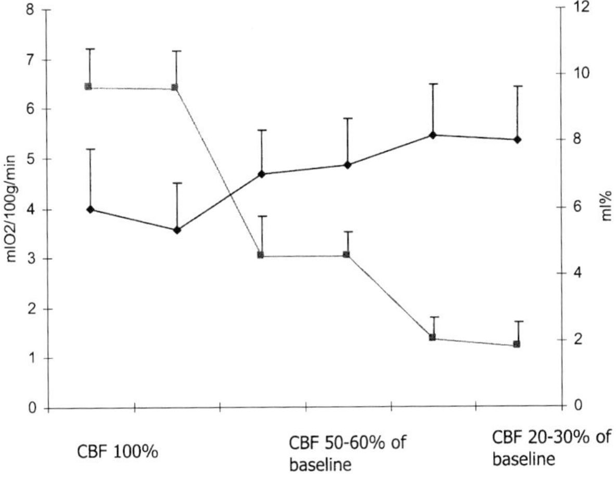

Fig. 3. AVDO2 and brain oxygen delivery. The latter was calculated by multiplying arterial oxygen content by the relative change of blood flow, assuming that the intact CBF corresponded to a value of 50 ml/100 g/min. ■ DO2, ◆ AVDO2

shows cerebral oxygen delivery and AVDO2 values during the baseline and the two phases of progressive and sustained CBF impairment.

Discussion

PtiO2 monitoring is gaining considerable interest and is widely used to study traumatic or vascular cerebral damage [2, 3, 7]. In particular, we have focused on the study of cerebral oxygenation in focal lesions. It is our policy to place the sensor in cerebral areas surrounding the core of the damage, therefore presumably in "penumbra" like areas [6]. These areas are in a "precarious" situation with respect to the energy supply: PtiO2 values recorded in such areas could provide guidance for a therapy aimed at preserving the portions of the brain more at risk of being permanently damaged.

From this standpoint we wanted to reproduce in the laboratory an animal model of progressive cerebral ischaemia and, particularly, a functional ischaemic penumbra, however simplified [1]. In the model the reduction of cerebral blood flow is achieved by injecting volume into the ventricular system, a technique that is amply reported in the literature [4]. The main purpose of the model was to obtain reproducible steps of CBF decline, stable enough to allow the study of PtiO2, oxygen delivery and AVDO2 in response to superimposed perturbations and interventions.

The end-points of CPP and CBF reduction were obtained in all the animals that were studied with only small variations. The continuous infusion of volume into the system enabled us to maintain the desired CBF reduction and, by administering β blockers, we were able to limit the Cushing response, which would tend to restore CBF closer to physiological levels by increasing the arterial pressure.

The PtiO2 decrease was parallel to the reduction of flow, as already described, and was stable during each phase. In such conditions it has been possible to estimate the brain oxygen delivery. Unfortunately, as we do not know the absolute value of CBF, the measurement has been extrapolated: however, with the stable conditions and a global reduction of flow, this extrapolation should give a good approximation of the variation of oxygen supply to the brain at different levels of CBF. The symmetrical variations of AVDO2 further confirm the existence of situations where CBF is progressively inadequate to meet the metabolic demand of the tissue [5].

The implementation of the model has some limits, both structural (over-simplification of a more complex situation, such as ischaemic penumbra) and instrumental (semi-quantitative measurement of CBF). Nevertheless, we believe it is a useful instrument to understand the interactions between parenchymal O2 tension and O2 content, especially when these latter are manipulated (arterial hyperoxia, haemotransfusion or infusion of O2 carrier) with important effects on the therapy.

References

1. Astrup J, Siesjo BK, Symon L (1981) Thresholds in cerebral ischemia – the ischemic penumbra. Stroke 12(6): 732–725
2. Doppenberg EMR, Watson JC, Broaddus WC, Holloway KL, Young HF, Bullock R (1997) Intraoperative monitoring of substrate delivery during aneurysm surgery and hematoma surgery: initial experience in 16 patients. J Neurosurg 87: 809–816
3. Kieneing KL, Unterberg AW, Bardt TF, Schneider GH, Lanksch W (1996) Monitoring of cerebral oxygenation in patients with severe head injuries: brain tissue PO2 versus jugular vein oxygen saturation. J Neurosurg 85: 751–757
4. Maas AIR, Fleckenstein W, deJong DA, vanSantbrink H (1993) Monitoring cerebral oxyenation: Experimantal studies and preliminary clinical results of continuous monitoring of cerebrospinal fluid and brain tissue oxygen tension. Acta Neurochir (Wien) 59: 50–57
5. Robertson CS, Narayan RK, Gokaslan ZL, Pahwa R, Grossman RG, Caram P, Allen E (1989) Cerebral arteriovenous oxygen difference as an estimate of cerebral blood flow in comatose patients. J Neurosurg 70: 222–230
6. Stocchetti N, Chieregato A, De Marchi M, Croci M, Benti R, Grimoldi N (1998) High cerebral perfusion pressure improves low values of local brain tissue O2 tension in focal lesion. Acta Neurochir (Wien) 71: 162–165
7. Valadka AB, Gopinath SP, Contant CF, Uzura M, Robertson CS (1998) Relationship of brain tissue pO2 to outcome after severe head injury. Crit Care Med 26: 1576–1581
8. Zauner A, Bullock R, Di X, Young HF (1995) Brain oxygen, CO2, pH, and temperature monitoring: evaluation in the feline brain. Neurosurgery 37: 1168–1177
9. Zauner A, Doppenberg EMR, Woodward JJ, Choi SC, Young HF, Bullock R (1997) Continuous monitoring of cerebral substrate delivery and clearance: initial experience in 24 patients with severe acute brain injuries. Neurosurgery 41: 1082–1093

Correspondence: Dr. Sandra Rossi, Neuro-ICU, Dept Anaesthesia and Intensive Care, Padiglione Beretta Neuro, Ospedale Maggiore Policlinico IRCCS, Via F. Sforza, 35 20122 Milano, Italy.

Acta Neurochir (2000) [Suppl] 76: 203–205

ICP and MABP Following Traumatic Subarachnoid Hemorrhage in the Rat

S. Thomas[1], **F. Tabibnia**[1], **M. U. Schuhmann**[2], **T. Brinker**[1], and **M. Samii**[1]

[1] Department of Neurosurgery, Nordstadt Hospital, Hannover, Germany
[2] Medical School, Hannover, Germany

Summary

Traumatic subarachnoidal hemorrhage (t-SAH) is a common finding in head-injured patients occurring with a frequency of 39% according to data of the Traumatic Coma Data Bank. The present study is the first description of a t-SAH-model with particular emphasis on patterns of intracranial pressure (ICP) changes and mean arterial blood pressure (MABP) response.

Diffuse brain injury was produced in intubated and ventilated adult Sprague-Dawley rats (N = 24) using a brass weight (500 gm) free falling from a predetermined height (1.5 m) on a steel disc glued to the skull of the rat. Before induction of the injury, heparin was administered intra-arterially (i.a.) and antagonised after injury by protamine. MABP-recordings and ICP-recordings were performed continuously. Histopathology was undertaken.

Following injury MABP decreased from 138 ± 14 mmHg to 89 ± 22 mmHg. During 5 to 15 min ICP increased up to 89.4 ± 50.4 mmHg, decreasing slowly within 60 min in surviving animals. The mortality rate was 41.6%. All brains showed a severe subarachnoid hemorrhage in the basal cisterns and cell-loss within the brainstem.

Experimental t-SAH is possible. Following t-SAH there is a subacute increase of ICP due to the actual bleeding. The model may provide deeper understanding in the basic physiological patterns of t-SAH.

Keywords: Traumatic subarachnoidal hemorrhage; rat; ICP; blood pressure.

Introduction

Traumatic subarachnoidal hemorrhage is common following traumatic brain injury. According to data of the American Traumatic Coma Data Bank based on 753 patients t-SAH was found in 39% cases [1]. In a Japanese series by Kobayashi *et al.* (1988) t.-SAH was detected in 23% of 414 severely head injured patients [7]. A European multicenter study known as the Head Injury Trial No.2 (HIT II) indicated t-SAH in 33% of 819 patients [6]. In addition the outcome of patients with t-SAH was unfavourable in 60% compared to 30% of noSAH patients. The mortality rate was 42% versus 14% with 40% of deaths occurring within the first 2 days after injury [5].

Traumatic subarachnoid hemorrhage became a particularly interesting topic because of an apparent positive effect of treatment with nimodipine. Whereas an overall treatment with Nimodipine in all trauma patients did not reveal any positive effect, Nimodipine significantly decreased the percentage of unfavourable outcomes in t-SAH patients. The occurrence of t-SAH in trauma patients appears to represent a particular pathophysiological subgroup rendering them suitable for specifc pharmaceutical treatment.

In previous experiments determining MABP changes in developing rats several pups exhibited t-SAH following administration of heparin to prevent the MABP-catheter from clotting [10]. Therefore, this subgroup of animals was examined more closely. By reviewing the relevant literature no experimental studies were detected dealing with t-SAH.

The aim of the present study was to develop a traumatic brain injury model to produce t-SAH in the rat. Utilizing that model continuous ICP-measurements and cardiovascular responses were determined before, during, and after the injury. In addition histological examinations were performed. In studies previously conducted in adult rats [8] no significant changes of ICP were measured following a single traumatic brain injury produced by the weight-drop-model. It was expected that t-SAH would result in a marked rise of ICP following early after injury.

Material and Methods

As approved by the Animal Research Committee of the Medical School of Hannover, 24 male Sprague-Dawley rats (350–400 g) were used for this study. They were initially anesthetized with isoflurane and then intubated and artificially ventilated with a gas mixture of N_2O (70%) and O_2 (30%) with isoflurane. Body temperature was maintained between 37° and 38 °C with a thermostatically controlled heating pad. Polyethylene catheters (PE-50) were placed into the femoral artery and connected to a Statham-transducer. Continuous blood pressure recordings were performed until one hour after injury.

The injury device first described by Marmarou *et al.* was used to produce trauma [3]. Following a midline scalp incision the skin and periosteum were reflected and the skull carefully dried. A stainless steel disc serving as a helmet was mounted on the skull using cyanoacrylate. A brass weight (500 g) fell free onto the helmet guided by a 2 m Plexiglas tube. The animal was placed in prone position on foam (20 × 20 × 50 cm; spring constant 30/50) held within a wooden frame. The lower end of the tube was placed directly above the helmet. Immediately following the initial impact the box was slid horizontally to prevent a second impact. Five minutes before trauma a high-dose heparin (10 I.E./g) was injected i.a.. Five minutes following trauma the equivalent dose of protamine (10 I.E./g) was administered and anesthesia reinstated.

Measurements of ICP were performed using a catheter (PE-50) placed subdurally through a lateral-frontal burr hole into the anterior fossa. The catheter was connected to a Statham-transducer and ICP was recorded up to one hour after injury.

All brains were processed for hematoxylin-eosin staining using 20 μm coronal sections. Surviving animals were perfused transcardially one day after injury and the brains were removed and postfixed in 4%-formalin. Sections were studied under light-microscopy for cell loss and hemorrhages.

All measurements were stored and analyzed using commercially available software (Dasy Lab V.3, Datalog, Mönchengladbach, Germany). Statistical analysis was performed using Wilcoxon signed rank test for paired data. Data are presented as mean ± SD.

Results

A traumatic subarachnoid hemorrhage was achieved in 12 (50%) of all injured animals as determined by histological evaluation. In addition, animals suffering a t-SAH exhibited a typical ICP-pattern (Fig. 1) which is presented now. All following results are dealing with the group of 12 rats with t-SAH.

Mortality rate for animals suffering a t-SAH was 41.6% (5/12). Death occurred usually within one hour after injury. The animals did not start breathing following termination of mechanical ventilation.

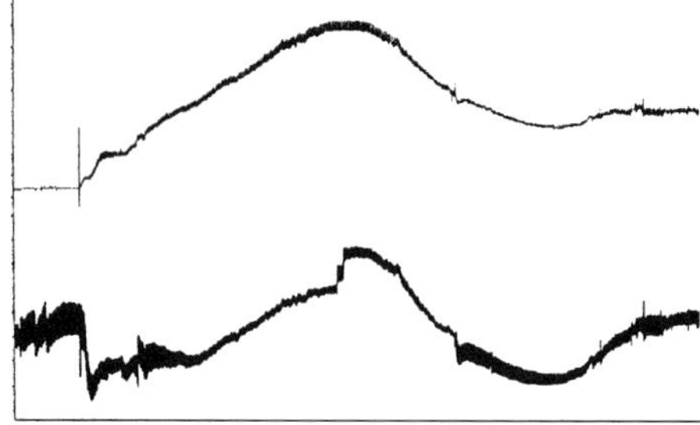

Fig. 1. Typical ICP (upper line) and MABP (lower line) pattern before and 60 min following t-SAH

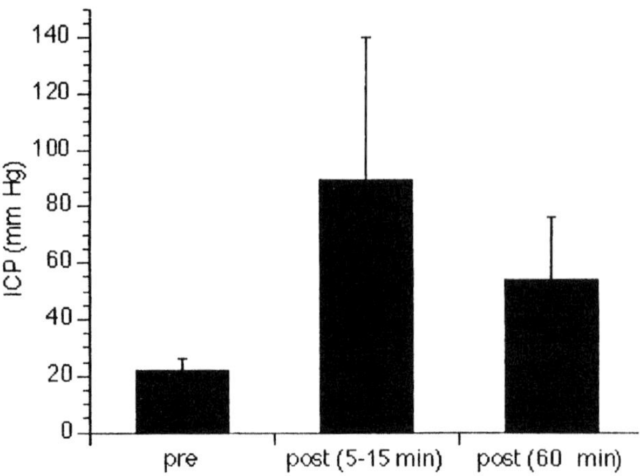

Fig. 2. Intracranial pressure (mean ± SD) before and after injury

Within 9.6 ± 5.4 min following injury all animals with t-SAH exhibited a significant rise of ICP from 21.9 ± 4.4 mmHg to 89.4 ± 50.4 mmHg ($p < 0.05$), gradually returning to lower levels. One hour after injury ICP was about 53.7 ± 22.5 mmHg. The ICP-pattern was quite heterogenous reaching the maximum between 5 and 15 min (Fig. 2).

In contrary to the ICP-increase, MABP decreased following injury from 138 ± 14 mmHg to 89 ± 22 mmHg at 30 to 180 sec. However, it then started to increase up to 178 ± 41.4 mmHg 5 to 15 min after trauma (Fig. 3). The blood pressure increased compared to base-line levels lasted as long as ICP was increased.

Gross pathological examination of the t-SAH animals did not reveal any skull fractures. Following removal of the brain, extensive subarachnoid hemor-

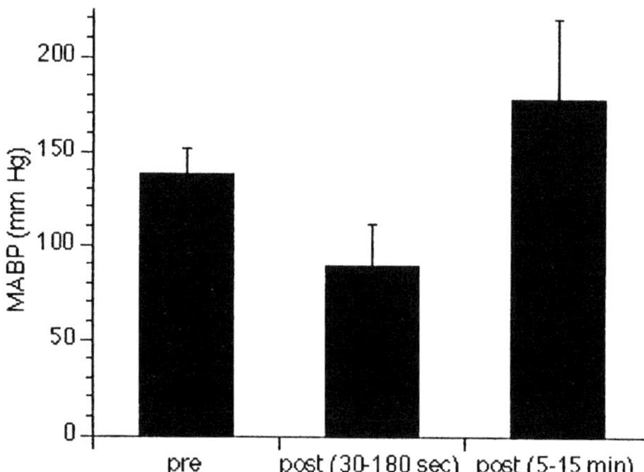

Fig. 3. Mean arterial blood pressure (mean ± SD) before and after injury

rhage was observed within the basal cisterns and in the whole subarachnoid space. Histological investigation confirmed the gross pathological inspection and showed in addition diffuse neuronal cell loss in all cortical areas, the hippocampus, and brain-stem. In addition minor perivascular bleeding was detected in the brainstem.

Discussion

The present study indicates that a modification of the weight-drop-model can be applied to produce a reproducible t-SAH. The incidence of 50% of t-SAH using the modified weight-drop injury model is higher compared to results from clinical series with severe brain injury. The mortality rate of 41.6% is in the range of mortalities reported in clinical studies and very close to the 42 % in the HIT II study.

The ICP and MABP-pattern can be explained in two different ways. The decrease of blood pressure immediately after injury is similar to results observed in studies previously [3, 9, 10] and attributable to a direct brainstem damage. The histological investigation revealed diffuse cell loss and minor perivascular bleedings within the brainstem. The increase of ICP is a result of the actual bleeding caused by the rupture of the subarachnoid vessels. The following increase of MABP is a compensatory response to preserve a sufficient cerebral perfusion pressure (CPP).

However, ICP and MABP-patterns may also be interpreted vice versa. The initial blood pressure decrease is a result from primary brainstem damage. Following this initial decrease MABP increases due to dysregulation within the brainstem. The ICP-increase would be secondary as a reaction due to impaired autoregulation.

The first explanation, indicating the ICP-increase to a direct bleeding from ruptured subarachnoid vessels is supported by our previous studies. Utilizing the weight-drop model in adult and developing rats without secondary injury or heparin no significant alteration of ICP was detected [8, 10]. The brainstem dysfunction caused by the initial impact should be comparable in both models. The impaired autoregulation would also be expected. Therefore, we believe that the ICP-increase is attributable to the subarachnoid bleeding with a secondary MABP-increase to preserve CPP.

In conclusion, the present model offers the opportunity to perform experimental studies on t-SAH. Several therapeutic strategies have been offered for SAH [2, 4, 11]. Utilizing the present model, pharmaceutical strategies can be evaluated also in t-SAH.

References

1. Eisenberg HM, Gary HE, Aldrich EF *et al* (1990) Initial CT findings in 753 patients with severe head injury. A report from the NIH Traumatic Coma Data Bank. J Neurosurg 73: 688–698
2. Hall ED, Travis MA (1988) Effects of nonglucocorticoid 21-aminosteroid U74006F on acute cerbral hypoperfusion following experimental subarachnoid hemorrhage. Exp Neurol 102: 244–248
3. Marmarou A, Foda MAA, Van den Brink W, Campbell J, Kita H, Demetriadou K (1994) A new model of diffuse brain injury in rats. Part I: pathophysiology and biomechanics. J Neurosurg 80: 291–300
4. Macdonald RL, Weir BKA, Runzer TD *et al* (1992) Effect of intrathecal superoxide dismutase and catalase on oxyhemoglobin-induced vasospasm in monkeys. Neurosurgery 30: 529–539
5. Kakarieka A, Braakman R, Schakel EH (1994) Clinical significance of the finding of subarachnoidal blood on CT scan after head injury. Acta Neurochir (Wien) 129: 1–5
6. Kakarieka A (1997) Traumatic subarachnoidal haemorrhage. Springer, Berlin Heidelberg New York Tokyo, p 21
7. Kobayashi S, Nakazawa S, Hiroyuki Y *et al* (1988) Traumatic subarachnoid hemorrhage in acute severe head injury. No To Shinkei 40: 1131–1135
8. Schuhmann MU, Thomas S, Hans VHJ, Beck H, Brinker T, Samii M (1998) CSF dynamics ina rodent model of closed head injury. Acta Neurochir [Suppl] (Wien) 71: 300–302
9. Shima K, Marmarou A (1991) Evaluation of brain-stem dysfunction following severe fluid-percussion head injury to the cat. J Neurosurg 74: 270–277
10. Thomas S, Tabibnia F, Schuhmann MU, Hans VHJ, Brinker T, Samii M (1998) Traumatic brain injury in the developing rat pup: Studies of ICP, PVI and neurological response. Acta Neurochir [Suppl] (Wien) 71: 135–137
11. Vollmer DG, Kassekk NF, Hongo K *et al* (1989) Effect of the nonglucocorticoid 21-aminosteroid U-74006F on experimental cerebral vasospasm. Surg Neurol 31: 190–194

Correspondence: Sebastian Thomas, M.D., Neurochirurgische Klinik, Nordstadt Hospital, Haltenhoffstrasse 41, D-30167 Hannover, Germany.

Acta Neurochir (2000) [Suppl] 76: 207–212

Real Time Monitoring of Glutamate Following Fluid Percussion Brain Injury with Hypoxia in the Rat

Y. Matsushita, K. Shima, H. Nawashiro, K. Wada, N. Tsuzuki, and **T. Miyazawa**

Department of Neurosurgery, National Defense Medical College, Tokorozawa, Saitama, Japan

Summary

In this study, extracellular glutamate (Glu) was monitored in real time using a biosensor following traumatic brain injury (TBI) either with or without inducing hypoxia in the rat Fluid-percussion model. We also measured the cortical contusion volume at 3 days after the insult. The animals were divided into 3 groups. Group 1 was subjected to TBI only, Group 2 to TBI followed by 20 min of moderate hypoxia (F_iO_2: 10%) and Group 3 to 20 min of moderate hypoxia without TBI. The surge increase in the extracellular Glu concentration occurred immediately after TBI in Groups 1 and 2. Group 2 showed a prolonged efflux of Glu during hypoxia. Group 3 Glu showed low continuous steady levels. The contusion volume in Group 2 was significantly larger than in Group 1. To test the possible involvement of apoptosis in Groups 1 and 2, rats were sacrificed at 1, 6, 24 and 72 h after TBI. Immunohistochemical studies showed an increased number of both CPP32 positive cells at 24 h and TUNEL cells at 72 h in Group 2. These results suggest that TBI with moderate hypoxia induced a prolonged efflux of Glu that resulted more cortical damage due to necrosis and apoptosis.

Keywords: Apoptosis; biosensor; glutamate; lateral fluid-percussion.

Introduction

Hypoxia and arterial hypotension are the most frequent causes of secondary brain damage in head-injured patients, and such insults after trauma may adversely affect the outcome of head-injured patients [2, 3, 13, 33]. Laboratory studies have demonstrated that early secondary hypoxia and hypotension aggravate brain damage following experimental traumatic brain injury (TBI). Our previous studies showed that secondary hypoxia also enhanced the vulnerability of the hippocampal CA3 pyramidal cells after mild closed head injury [26]. In addition, we previously reported that hypoxia caused a greater efflux of glutamate (Glu) in a concussion model [19]. In the present study, since Glu has been proposed to play a critical role in TBI pathophysiology in the brain, we monitored the extracellular Glu concentration in real time following TBI in a contusion model with and without hypoxia in the rat using an enzyme electrode biosensor. The successful application of the biosensor has been reported to be a real-time method for monitoring the Glu level in vivo in the extracellular space during epilepsy and ischemia [1, 23, 30]. We also determined the cortical contusion volume to investigate the effect of hypoxia following TBI histopathologically by staining with 2, 3, 5-triphenyltetrazolium chloride (TTC), which was reported to be useful for determining the lesion volume following TBI [27]. Furthermore, to clarify the effect of the increased extracellular Glu on apoptotic cell death in this double insult model, we immunohistochemically investigated the time course of CPP-32 expression which is a member of the interleukin-1ß converting enzyme (ICE) family that leads to apoptosis through the proteolytic cleavage of nuclear proteins [11, 29, 32], and also observed nuclear fragmentation using the terminal deoxynucleotidyl transferase-mediated biotin-dUTP nick-end labeling method (TUNEL).

Materials and Methods

Animals

Adult male Sprague-Dawley (SD) rats (300–400 g) were housed individually under controlled environmental conditions (12 / 12 h light / dark cycle) for at least one week, with food and water available *ad lib*, before being used in the experiments.

Dialysis Electrode (Biosensor)

The dialysis electrode was purchased from Sycopel International Ltd. (Boldon, Tyne and Wear, UK). The structure and principle of a dialysis electrode for measuring Glu were described by Walker *et al.* [30]. Before the beginning of this study, we had to set up the Biosensor. The response of the enzyme electrodes and their stability were tested in vitro.

Fluid Percussion Traumatic Brain Injury (TBI) Procedure

We used the Dragonfly fluid percussion device (MODEL #HPD-1700) to produce TBI in rats [6, 24]. To produce comparable injury severity, we determined that a higher pressure is required with this fluid percussion injury device than has been reported for the device commonly used in other laboratories [6, 8]. This is apparently due to a need for relatively greater pressure to yield a comparable fluid displacement through the smaller orifice and tubing diameter associated with this device design.

Surgery and Electrode Placement

On the day before we started this study, we conducted the surgery described below. A craniectomy, measuring 4.8 mm in diameter, was performed over the right parietal cortex (3.8 mm posterior to the bregma and 2.5 mm lateral to the midline), leaving the dura intact [7]. A plastic luer adapter (2.6-mm i.d., approx 4.8-mm o.d.) was positioned over the exposed dura, and a small hole was made in the ipsilateral temporal bone without penetrating the dura for insertion of the biosensor. The small hole was made obliquely at 5.0-mm posterior to the bregma and 6.0-mm lateral to the midline. A plastic luer adapter was cemented with cyanoacrylate to the skull surrounding the craniectomy site, and dental acryl was poured around the syringe hub avoiding the small hole. We thereafter returned the rats to their home cages and allowed them to recover overnight.

On the next day, the rats were intubated and ventilated with halothane (1–1.5%), 30% oxygen and 70% nitrous oxide under controlled respiration, fitted with femoral artery catheters for arterial blood sampling and pressure recording, and fixed in a stereotaxic frame. The blood pressure and blood gas levels were monitored throughout this study. The brain temperature was monitored indirectly via a thermocouple probe inserted into the temporal muscle [16] and maintained at 37.0 °C using an automatic heating lamp. The rectal temperature was also monitored and maintained at 38.0 °C using a heating pad.

After that, the cranial luer connector was exposed, filled with saline, and attached to the fluid percussion device, and then the electrode was inserted 2 mm into the cortex through a hole that had been previously made. Parasagittal fluid percussion TBI of moderate severity (3.5–4.0 atm, 16 ms duration) was induced.

We made 3 experimental groups of male SD rats. Group 1 ($n = 10$) was subjected to TBI only, Group 2 ($n = 10$) to TBI followed by 20 min of moderate hypoxia (F_iO_2: 10%) and Group 3 ($n = 4$) to moderate hypoxia only. The rats were ventilated with 0.5% halothane for 20 min after TBI, and then with 1.0-% halothane for 60 min. In Group 1, the rats were ventilated with 30% oxygen and 70% nitrous oxide under controlled respiration throughout the study. In Group 2, immediately after TBI, the rats were subjected to moderate hypoxia for 20 min, and then ventilated with 30% oxygen and 70% nitrous oxide after hypoxia for 60 min. In Group 3, the rats were subjected to hypoxia only for 20 min without TBI. These animals were subjected to all of the same procedures except for the actual insult, including preparatory anesthesia and placement of a plastic injury tube. After this study, we returned the rats to their home cages.

TTC Staining Procedure

Seventy-two hours after FP brain injury, the brains were then removed carefully after intracardiac perfusion with saline and refrigerated for 12 min. Each brain was cut into 1-mm coronal sections using a rat brain matrix (Muromachi Kikai, Co., Ltd., Tokyo). The tissue sections were immersed in 2% TTC (Sigma Chemical Co., St. Louis, MO), and then incubated at 37 °C for 30 min. After that, the brain sections were ranged and photographed. We determined the contusion volume using a computer-assisted image analyzer system (NIH Image 1.61). The total contusion volume was calculated by the summation of the contusion volumes measured in the component brain slices.

Immunohistochemistry and TUNEL Staining

To evaluate the possible involvement of apoptosis in Groups 1 and 2, separate rats were anesthetized and perfused via the aorta with 0.1 M phosphate buffered saline (PBS) and then with 4% formaldehyde / 0.1 M PBS after 1, 6, 24 and 72 hours after insult ($n = 2$ / group). Their brains were removed, and the paraffinembedded brains were sectioned at 6 μm, and processed for immunohistochemistry. The sections were reacted with rabbit polyclonal antibody against CPP32 at a dilution of 1:200 (CPP32 (h-277), Santa Cruz Biotechnology. Inc., U.S.A.). Immunohistochemistry was performed using the avidin-biotin technique, the DAKO LSAB2 kit, peroxidase for use on RAT Specimens (DAKO, Co., Ltd.).

To detect apoptotic cell death, the sections were subjected to the modified TUNEL procedure [9]. Apoptotic cells were detected using the Genzyme TACS^{TM} in situ apoptosis detection kit (Genzyme diagnostics Cambridge, MA), according to manufacturer's instruction.

Statistical Analysis

All data are expressed as means ± SEM. Data of physiological variable was analyzed by one way ANOVA. The concentration of Glu and the contusion volume in Groups 1 and 2 was analyzed by the unpaired t- test. A p value of less than 0.05 was considered to be statistically significant.

Results

Physiologic Findings

The physiological findings, including blood PCO_2, PO_2 and pH were all within the normal ranges before the insult in both groups. The mean arterial blood pressure (MABP) increased immediately after TBI(>200 mmHg) and normalized within 2 min in Groups 1 and 2. In Groups 2 and 3, PaO_2 was 32.1 ± 1.8 vs. 37.5 ± 1.7 mmHg and MABP decreased during hypoxia, but normalized after reoxygenation. The other physiological parameters, PCO_2 and pH, showed no significant differences after reoxygenation.

Real-Time Monitoring of Glutamate

Figure 1 shows a typical Glu change after trauma. Glu increased immediately (>200 μmol/l), but there was no significant concentration of Glu after 1 min following TBI. Group 2 showed that the Glu concen-

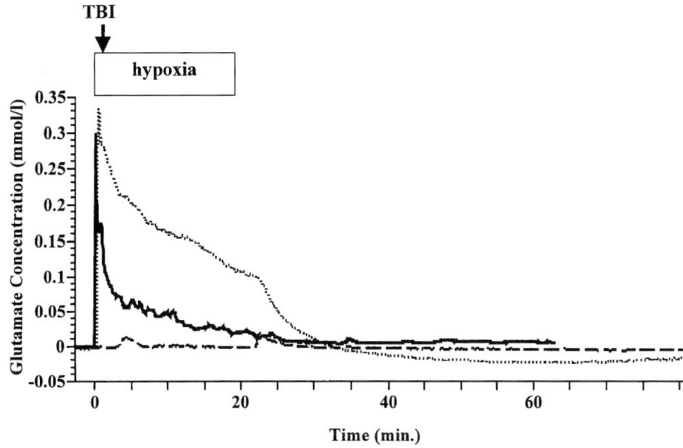

Fig. 1. Typical change of Glutamate in 3 groups. Group 2 showed that Glu increased immediately after TBI and kept high concentration during hypoxia in opposition to group 1, and thereafter that Glu fell to the same level of group 1 after reoxygenation. —— Group 1 (TBI only), ········ Group 2 (TBI + hypoxia), - - - Group 3 (hypoxia only)

tration increased immediately after TBI and thereafter remained high during hypoxia, in contrast to in Group 1, and thereafter Glu decreased to the same level as in Group 1 after reoxygenation. In Group 3, Glu continued to show a mild increase in spite of the hypotension (MABP = 50–60 mmHg) due to hypoxia.

TTC Staining

The cortical contusion volume in Group 2 was significantly greater than that in Group 1 (14.81 ± 1.99 vs. 23.71 ± 3.40 mm^3). A portion of the increased contusion volume observed in Group 2 appeared to be due to the increase in the relatively posterior extent of the cortical injury.

Immunohistochemistry and TUNEL Staining

CPP 32-positive neurons were seen at 24 h and TUNEL-positive neurons were seen at 72 h after insult in the cortex adjacent to the contusion area in Group 2. No CPP 32-positive neurons were seen in Group 1 and the opposite side of Group 2. The TUNNEL positive cells demonstrated nuclear condensation and fragmentation.

Discussion

In the present study, the use of the Dragonfly fluid percussion device (MODEL #HPD-1700) was the most important factor in producing TBI in the rats [6, 24] while a special biosensor was used to measure the extracellular concentration of Glu.

The Dragonfly fluid percussion device is more compact and sophisticated than previous deices and thus TBI can be induced from any direction. However, to produce a comparable severity of injury, we found that a higher pressure is required with this fluid percussion injury device than the devices commonly used in other laboratories [6, 8]. Because a craniectomy, measuring 4.8 mm in diameter, was performed over the right parietal cortex (3.8 mm posterior to the bregma and 2.5 mm lateral to the midline), leaving the dura intact, a contusion was made at relatively posterior from the impact portion. This procedure may thus have induced a significant degree of percussion-induced brain displacement and subsequent vascular damage [7], and may have also ensured the stable reproducibility of the extent of brain damage.

In the TTC study, the cortical contusion volume was found to significantly increase with TBI following hypoxia. The contusion area extended to posterior cortex from impact site. The cause of the posterior extension of the contusion area is not known, but it may be due to the fact that the contusion was made at a position relatively posterior from the impact portion in this fluid percussion model. Numerous studies have reported that transient arterial hypotension after cerebral trauma leads to vasodilatation, endothelial damage, impaired metabolism in the muscle wall of the cerebral blood vessel, and reduced vascular responsiveness to hypotension, hypoxia, or hypercapnia [14, 20, 21, 31]. In addition, less severe hypoxia has been shown to cause adverse effects on histopathology of the injured brain [15].

We introduce the principle of the biosensor as follows; the analyte being studied is measured using a specific enzyme or enzymes. Many oxidase enzymes produce hydrogen peroxide, which is detected amperometrically on the electrode at +550 mV. As the amperometric technique is used, oxidation is produced which is linearly proportional to the concentration of Glu, until the enzyme activity is saturated. Here we show a sample chemical reaction which is used to measure the Glu:

$$2\ \text{L-Glu} + O_2 + H_2O\text{–(L-Glu oxidase)} \rightarrow \text{2-oxoglutamate} + NH_4 + H_2O_2$$

$$H_2O_2\text{–(Platinum, +550 mV)} \rightarrow O_2 + 2H^+ + 2e^-$$

We obtained the raw data in amperes (A) and converted them into mole (M) by calibrating the data in vitro.

Our results demonstrated that Glu increased immediately (>200 μmol/l) following TBI and thereafter maintained a high level during hypoxia. In Group 3, MABP was reduced as well as in Group 2, but the Glu concentration was not significantly elevated during hypoxia alone. Therefore the reduction of MABP following hypoxia was not responsible for the prolonged efflux of Glu. It is conceivable that extracellular efflux of Glu is mediated by K^+, Glu transporter and Ca^{2+}. Katayama *et al.* reported that more severe traumatic brain injury produced a more pronounced, longer-lasting increase in the extracellular K^+ ($[K^+]_e$), and that an increase in the extracellular Glu concentration was concomitantly induced with the increase in $[K^+]_e$ [17]. The surge increase of Glu in the acute phase (within 1 min) may be due to impact depolarization [12], and the prolonged efflux of Glu during hypoxia may be caused by anoxic depolarization [18, 19]. Glu transporter also plays an important role in the increase of Glu after TBI. The postsynaptic released Glu is transported into cells via a Na^+/K^+ dependent Glu transporter, and thus ignoring both the ion and voltage gradients. The Glu transporter utilizes a Na^+/K^+ ion gradient, which acts as an energy-dependent pump. After changes in the Na^+/K^+ ion gradient, such as during anoxic depolarization, the Glu transporter loses its Glu transport activity when the concentration of extracellular K^+ increases to 10–12 mM. When the concentration of extracellular K^+ increases to 10–12 mM, the Glu transporter allows the release of Glu from the metabolic pool in the neurons and glial cells through reverse transport [10].

The increased extracellular Glu also influences the apoptotic process of the moribund neurons. The activation of CPP32 (caspase-3) – like proteolytic activity, a key mediator of apoptosis, precedes neuronal death. CPP32 was immunohistochemically expressed at 24 hours and TUNEL positive cells were observed at 72 h, respectively, in Group 2. In contrast, neither CPP32 protein nor TUNEL positive cells were observed in Group 1 (TBI alone). Since the caspase-3 mRNA levels were elevated approximately five-fold in the cortex of injured side at 4 h and two-fold in the hippocampus of injured side at 24 h after TBI [32], the increase in CPP-32 protein in the cortical cells was considered to be a reasonable finding. TUNEL staining is a marker of DNA fragmentation that supports apoptotic cell death [4, 22]. Conti *et al.* reported the temporal pattern of apoptosis in the rat after lateral fluid-percussion (FP) brain injury using TUNEL [5]. They thus demonstrated that, in the cortex, the average number of TUNEL-positive cells exhibiting apoptotic morphology peaked at 24 h and delayed peak at 1 week after lateral FP without hypoxia. In our data, we could not observe TUNEL-positive cells at any time in Group 1 (TBI alone), but we observed the nuclear condensation and fragmentation in the cortex adjacent to contusion area at 72 h after insults in Group 2. The cause of this difference might be due to some difference in the impact pressure or the device used.

Sengpiel *et al.* reported that *N*-methyl-D-aspartate (NMDA) was capable of inducing programmed cell death in cultured rat hippocampal neurons, which was sensitive to the irreversible caspase-1 inhibitor. Moreover, NMDA-induced programmed cell death was associated with a significant increase in the intracellular superoxide production, and sublethal NMDA exposure also stimulates intracellular superoxide production [28]. Mattson *et al.* reported evidence of synaptic apoptosis [25]. They observed that the caspase inhibitor zVAD-fmk prevented mitochondrial membrane depolarization, while glutamateinduced increases in the caspase activity were first observed in the dendrite and later in the cell body. In the case of TBI with secondary hypoxia, Glu released by TBI was not taken up but released from the metabolic pool because of energy failure. A large amount of Glu is not only neurotoxic, inducing necrosis, but may also induce apoptosis. In this model, it was difficult to induce apoptosis by an initial temporary increase of extracellular Glu following TBI but it was easy to induce apoptosis by a prolonged increase of extracellular Glu by loading hypoxia following TBI. Moreover, prolonged excessive Glu in the synaptic space is also considered to induce caspase activation and mitochondrial membrane depolarization of the dendrites at first and thereafter the apoptotic signal induces nuclear condensation and DNA fragmentation in the neuron body. In our data, the appearance of the apoptotic cells was adjacent to or remote from the contusion area.

We concluded that an excessive accumulation of Glu and prolonged burst-firing through excitatory pathways played an important role in the increased vulnerability of neurons by leading not only to necrosis but also to apoptosis. In addition, a reduction in the contusion volume may thus be possible by administering anti-apoptotic agents to TBI patients following hypoxia.

Acknowledgments

The authors gratefully thank Namiko Nomura and Akiko Yano for their excellent technical assistance. We carefully adhered to the animal welfare guidelines set forth in the *Guide for the Care and Use of Laboratory Animals* (US Dept. of Health and Human Services, Publ. No. 85–23, 1985).

References

1. Asai S, Iribe Y, Kohno T, Ishikawa K (1996) Real time monitoring of biphasic glutamate release using dialysis electrode in rat acute brain ischemia. NeuroReport 7: 1092–1096
2. Chesnut RM, Marshall LF, Klauber MR, Blunt BA, Baldwin N, Eisenberg HM, Jane JA, Marmarou A, Foulkes MA (1993) The role of secondary brain injury in determining outcome from severe head injury. J Trauma 34: 216–222
3. Chesnut RM, Marshall SB, Piek J, Blunt BA, Klauber MR, Marshall LF (1993) Early and late systemic hypotension as a frequent and fundamental source of cerebral ischemia following severe brain injury in the Traumatic Coma Data Bank. Acta Neurochir [Suppl] (Wien) 59: 121–125
4. Clark RS, Kochanek PM, Dixon CE, Chen M, Marion DW, Heineman S, DeKosky ST, Graham SH (1997) Early neuropathologic effects of mild or moderate hypoxemia after controlled cortical impact injury in rats. J Neurotrauma 14: 179–189
5. Conti AC, Raghupathi R, Trojanowski JQ, McInotosh TK (1998) Experimental brain injury induces regionally distinct apoptosis during the acute and delayed post-traumatic period. J Neurosci 18: 5664–5672
6. Dave JR, Bauman RA, Long JB (1997) Hypoxia potentiates traumatic brain injury-induced expression of c-fos in rats. Neuroreport 8: 395–398
7. Dietrich WD, Alonso O, Halley M (1994) Early microvascular and neuronal consequences of traumatic brain injury: a light electron microscopic study in rats. J Neurotrauma 11: 289–301
8. Dietrich WD, Alonso O, Halley M, Busto R (1996) Delayed posttraumatic brain hyperthermia worsens outcome after fluid percussion brain injury: a light and electron microscopic study in rats. Neurosurgery 38: 533–541
9. Gavrieli Y, Sherman Y, Ben-Sasson SA (1992) Identification of programmed cell death in situ via specific labeling of nuclear DNA fragmentation. J Cell Biol 119: 493–501
10. Graham DI, Ford I, Adams JH, Doyle D, Teasdale GM, Lawrence AE, McLellan DR (1989) Ischaemic brain damage is still common in fatal non-missile head injury. J Neurol Neurosurg Psychiatry 52: 346–350
11. Harada J, Sugimoto M (1997) Polyamines prevent apoptotic cell death in cultured cerebellar granule neurons. Brain Res 753: 251–259
12. Hayes RL, Jenkins LW, Lyeth BG (1992) Neurotransmitter-mediated mechanisms of traumatic brain injury: acetylcholine and excitatory amino acids. J Neurotrauma 9 [Suppl] 1: S173–187
13. Hovda DA, Becker DP, Katayama Y (1992) Secondary injury and acidosis. J Neurotrauma 9 [Suppl] 1: S47–60
14. Ishige N, Pitts LH, Berry I, Carlson SG, Nishimura MC, Moseley ME, Weinstein PR (1987) The effect of hypoxia on traumatic head injury in rats: alterations in neurologic function, brain edema, and cerebral blood flow. J Cereb Blood Flow Metab 7: 759–767
15. Ishige N, Pitts LH, Hashimoto T, Nishimura MC, Bartkowski HM (1987) Effect of hypoxia on traumatic brain injury in rats: part 1. Changes in neurological function, electroencephalograms, and histopathology. Neurosurgery 20: 848–853
16. Jiang JY, Lyeth BG, Clifton GL, Jenkins LW, Hamm RJ, Hayes RL (1991) Relationship between body and brain temperature in traumatically brain- injured rodents. J Neurosurg 74: 492–496
17. Katayama Y, Becker DP, Tamura T, Hovda DA (1990) Massive increases in extracellular potassium and the indiscriminate release of glutamate following concussive brain injury. J Neurosurg 73: 889–900
18. Katayama Y, Kawamata T, Tamura T, Hovda DA, Becker DP, Tsubokawa T (1991) Calcium-dependent glutamate release concomitant with massive potassium flux during cerebral ischemia in vivo. Brain Res 558: 136–140
19. Katoh H, Shima K, Nawashiro H, Wada K, Chigasaki H (1997) The effect of MK-801 on extracellular neuroactive amino acids in hippocampus after closed head injury followed by hypoxia in rats. Brain Res 758: 153–162
20. Lewelt W, Jenkins LW, Miller JD (1980) Autoregulation of cerebral blood flow after experimental fluid percussion injury of the brain. J Neurosurg 53: 500–511
21. Lewelt W, Jenkins LW, Miller JD (1982) Effects of experimental fluid-percussion injury of the brain on cerebrovascular reactivity of hypoxia and to hypercapnia. J Neurosurg 56: 332–338
22. Li Y, Chopp M, Jiang N, Yao F, Zaloga C (1995) Temporal profile of in situ DNA fragmentation after transient middle cerebral artery occlusion in the rat. J Cereb Blood Flow Metab 15: 389–397
23. Liu Z, Stafstrom CE, Sarkisian MR, Yang Y, Hori A, Tandon P, Holmes GL (1997) Seizure-induced glutamate release in mature and immature animals: an in vivo microdialysis study. NeuroReport 8: 2019–2023
24. Long JB, Gordon J, Bettencourt JA, Bolt SL (1996) Laser-Doppler flowmetry measurements of subcortical blood flow changes after fluid percussion brain injury in rats. J Neurotrauma 13: 149–162
25. Mattson MP, Keller JN, Begley JG (1998) Evidence for synaptic apoptosis. Exp Neurol 153: 35–48
26. Nawashiro H, Shima K, Chigasaki H (1995) Selective vulnerability of hippocampal CA3 neurons to hypoxia after mild concussion in the rat. Neurol Res 17: 455–460
27. Perri BR, Smith DH, Murai H, Sinson G, Saatman KE, Raghupathi R, Bartus RT, McIntosh TK (1997) Metabolic quantification of lesion volume following experimental traumatic brain injury in the rat. J Neurotrauma 14: 15–22
28. Sengpiel B, Preis E, Krieglstein J, Prehn JH (1998) NMDA-induced superoxide production and neurotoxicity in cultured rat hippocampal neurons: role of mitochondria. Eur J Neurosci 10: 1903–1910
29. Steller H (1995) Mechanisms and genes of cellular suicide. Science 267: 1445–1449

30. Walker MC, Galley PT, Errington ML, Shorvon SD, Jefferys JG (1995) Ascorbate and glutamate release in the rat hippocampus after perforant path stimulation: a "dialysis electrode" study. J Neurochem 65: 725–731
31. Wei EP, Dietrich WD, Povlishock JT, Navari RM, Kontos HA (1980) Functional, morphological, and metabolic abnormalities of the cerebral microcirculation after concussive brain injury in cats. Circ Res 46: 37–47
32. Yakovlev AG, Knoblach SM, Fan L, Fox GB, Goodnight R, Faden AI (1997) Activation of CPP32-like caspases contributes to neuronal apoptosis and neurological dysfunction after traumatic brain injury. J Neurosci 17: 7415–7424
33. Young W (1988) Secondary CNS injury. J Neurotrauma 5: 219–221

Correspondence: Dr. Y. Matsushita, Department of Neurosurgery, National Defense Medical College, 3-2 Namiki, Tokorozawa, Saitama 359-8513, Japan.

Acta Neurochir (2000) [Suppl] 76: 213–216

The Synergistic Effect of Acute Subdural Hematoma Combined with Diffuse Traumatic Brain Injury on Brain Edema

Y. Tomita, S. Sawauchi, A. Beaumont, and **A. Marmarou**

Division of Neurosurgery, Medical College of Virginia, Richmond, Virginia, U.S.A.

Summary

It is well-documented that acute subdural hematoma (ASDH) following diffuse traumatic brain injury (dTBI) contributes to severe disability and high mortality. The objective of this study was to characterize edema formation in a model of ASDH and ASDH following dTBI.

Eighteen Sprague-Dawley rats were separated into three groups: Sham operated ($n = 6$), ASDH ($n = 6$), ASDH following dTBI ($n = 6$). Diffuse TBI was produced via the Impact-Acceleration Model [10]. ASDH was induced in the left hemisphere using the well-described method [11]. Total tissue water content was determined 4 hours after TBI utilizing wet-weight/dry-weight assessment.

Our results show that ASDH causes a significant increase in tissue water content in the left hemisphere ($79.2 \pm 0.7\%$) compared with the contralateral hemisphere ($78.5 \pm 0.5\%$, $p = 0.009$). Animals exposed to ASDH following dTBI had significantly greater edema formation than those with ASDH (right: $80.9 \pm 0.4\%$, left: 80.5 ± 0.7, $p = 0.008$). There was no significant difference between the left and right hemisphere.

We conclude that edema formation in ASDH is worsened by the combination of dTBI and ASDH. Furthermore a diffuse and focal injury in combination retain the features of the diffuse injury, but with increased severity. Further studies are required to elucidate the synergistic mechanisms involved in these pathological processes.

Keywords: Cerebral edema; diffuse traumatic brain injury; acute subdural hematoma; intracranial pressure.

Introduction

Despite considerable advancements in understanding the pathological processes that contribute to traumatic brain injury, the pathophysiology of acute subdural hematoma (ASDH) remains elusive. This lack of understanding has resulted in little being done so far to reduce the mortality of patients with ASDH below 50%. The combination of subdural hematoma with traumatic brain injury may be particularly devastating [13]. Several elegant studies utilizing an established rodent model of ASDH have been published [2, 7, 11]. However little or no attention has been paid to the interaction between trauma and ASDH, and in particular, there is no model currently available to assess such interaction.

The aim of this study therefore was to develop and characterise a model of ASDH with traumatic brain injury, and to evaluate the extent and severity of edema formation associated with the model.

Material and Methods

Physiological Assessment

Adult Sprague-Dawley rats, weighing 350–400 g were divided into the following experimental groups: (1) Sham Control ($n = 6$), (2) Acute Subdural Hematoma (ASDH) ($n = 6$), (3) Diffuse Traumatic Brain Injury + Subdural Hematoma (TBI + ASDH) ($n = 6$). All animals used received humane care in compliance with the Guide for the Care and Use of Laboratory Animals" (NIH Publication No. 86–23, 1985).

The animals were intubated and mechanically ventilated with 66% N_2O, 33% O_2, and 1.0% Halothane. Cannulae were sited in the femoral artery and vein for measuring mABP, blood gases, withdrawal of autologous blood and delivery of fluid. Mean arterial blood pressure was maintained at 100 mmHg. Blood gases were maintained throughout the entire experiment with a pO_2 of 100–150 mmHg and a pCO_2 of 35–45 mmHg. The animals were hydrated with 10 cc/kg/hr saline and their temperature maintained at 36.5–37.5 °C using s rectal temperature probe and a heating lamp.

After stabilization of blood gases and blood pressure the animal was positioned in a stereotaxic frame (David Kopf Instruments) using ear bars to secure the head. A midline incision in the scalp was made with all overlying tissue reflected. Three burr holes were made with the following coordinates in relation to bregma: 1) 1 mm caudal and 2 mm right-lateral for the ICP sensor (Codman ICP Sensor), 2) 3 mm caudal and 2 mm right-lateral for the CBF probe, 3) 1 mm caudal and 2 mm left-lateral for the insertion of a needle for induction of ASDH. This latter burr-hole was enlarged to permit unrestricted visualization of the dura.

Diffuse Traumatic Brain Injury

The impact-acceleration model was used to induce diffuse traumatic brain injury [3, 10]. After burr holes were made and baseline data was collected for 15 minutes, a 10 mm round stainless steel disk was fixed to the calvarium in the midline lying between bregma and lambda, using rapid drying cyanoacrylic glue. Animals were then disconnected from the respirator and placed in a prone position on a foam bed of known spring constant under a hollow plexiglas tube. A sectioned brass weight of 450 g was dropped from a height of 2 m onto the center of the metal disk. After injury, the rat was rapidly reconnected to anesthesia and artificially ventilated.

Model of ASDH

The methodology of experimental acute subdural hematoma has been discribed by Miller *et al.* [11]. Immediately after reconnection to the ventilator, non-heparinized autologous venous blood was withdrawn. Then under an operating microscope, the dura underlying the third burr-hole was incised and a tangent curved blunt-tipped needle (23-gauge) was placed carefully into the subdural space. The needle was cemented into position using bone wax and cyanoacrylic glue. Ten minutes after diffuse brain injury, 400 μL of blood was injected into the subdural space at a rate of 50 μL/min with a microinfusion pump (CMA Instruments, North Chelmsford, MA). In the sham group, the same procedures were performed without diffuse brain injury and blood injection and in the ASDH alone group, the same procedures were completed without diffuse brain injury.

Cerebral Water Content

The water content of brain tissue was measured by the wet and dry weight method. Rats were sacrificed with air embolization and the brains were rapidly removed. Cerebral tissue was divided into right and left hemispheres, and placed on a piece of preweighed aluminum foil and then reweighed. Brain samples were dried to constant weight at 100 °C and weighed again. The percentage water content was calculated as follows: water (%) = (wet weight-dry weight)/wet weight × 100.

Statistical Analysis

All values reported are means ± standard deviation of the means. Statistical analysis was performed using paired and unpaired t-tests. A 95% confidence level was considered statistically significant.

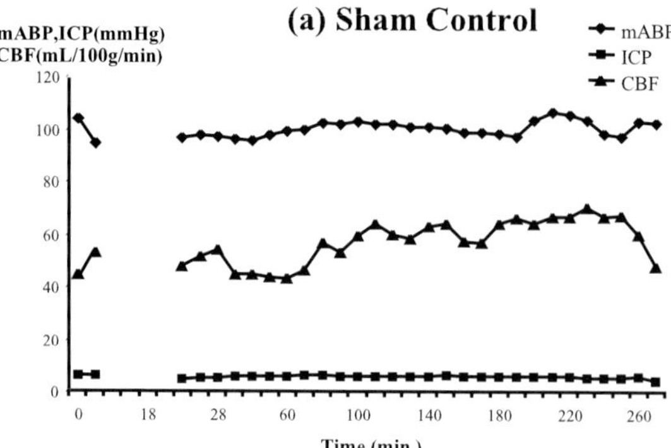

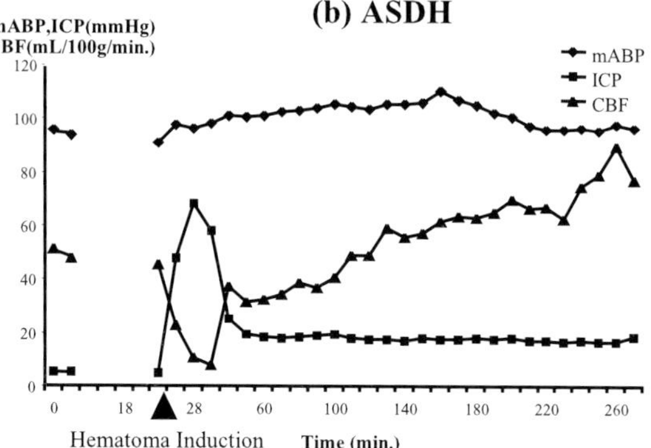

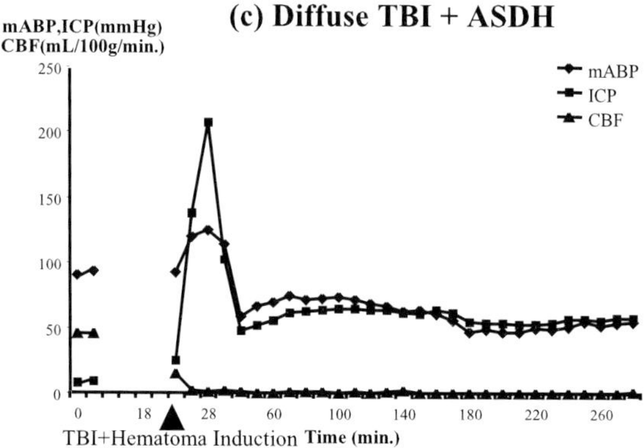

Fig. 1. Physiological variables in groups; mean ABP, ICP and CBF are shown. (a) Physiological parameters are stable throughout the experiment. (b) ICP reached highest value of 71.5 ± 18.3 mmHg. However, all parameters are restored. (c) Maximum ICP value was 207.6 ± 13.2 mmHg at the termination of injection. Cerebral autoregulation was destroyed and ICP became refractory

Results

Physiological Parameters

Acute Subdural Hematoma. ICP started to rise 30 seconds after induction of ASDH (Fig. 1. b). At the end of infusion, ICP reached a mean peak value of 71.5 ± 8.3 mmHg, and then immediately began to fall to 15.0 ± 3.4 mmHg at 4 hours following injury. These findings were in accordance with the results of Miller *et al.* [10]. During infusion a marked Cushing's response was apparent, which resolved immediately at the end of infusion. Baseline CBF was 47.7 ± 13.7 mL/100 g/min. that was reduced to 7.5 ± 5.9 mL/100 g/min. at the completion of infusion. Three minutes later CBF had increased to 25.8 ± 24.8 mL/100 g/min and continued to increase

Table 1. *Percentage of Brain Water*

	Sham control (n = 6)	ASDH (n = 6)	Diffuse TBI + ASDH (n = 6)
Right hemisphere (non-ASDH side)	78.3 ± 0.3	78.5 ± 0.5	80.7 ± 0.4*
Left hemisphere (ASDH side)	78.2 ± 0.2	79.2 ± 0.7*	80.5 ± 0.7*

Values are mean ± SD. *$p < 0.01$ compared with sham control (unpaired t-test).

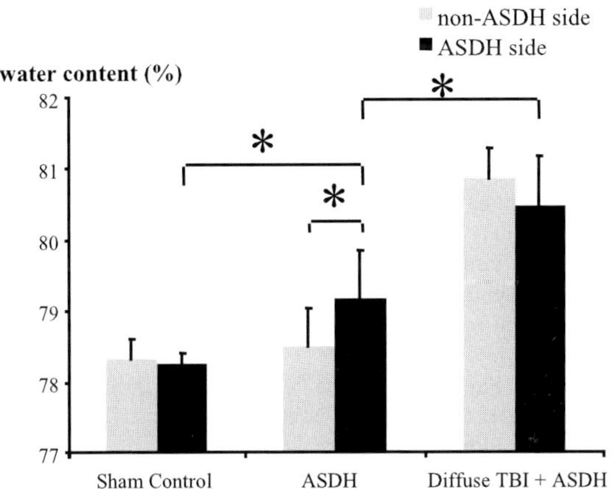

to 87.1 ± 39.8 mL/100 g/min. towards the end of experiment.

ASDH Following Diffuse TBI. Ten minutes after diffuse TBI, ICP was 24.9 ± 9.5 mmHg which rose immediately after induction of ASDH (Fig. 1. c). The mean peak value at the termination of injection was 207.6 ± 13.2 mmHg. A Cushing's response appeared transiently in this case, but within 4 minutes of blood infusion ICP greatly exceeded mABP. With increasing time ICP continued to rise, and mABP began to fall. At this point CBF as measured with Laser Doppler was reduced to 1.4 ± 2.7 mL/100 g/min. and this value did not vary for the remainder of the experiment.

Cerebral Edema Formation. In ASDH, the percentage water content of the infused hemisphere was significantly greater than the contralateral side ($p = 0.009$, Table 1, Fig. 2). Following TBI with ASDH, however tissue water was higher than that seen with ASDH alone (right: 80.9 ± 0.4%, left: 80.5 ± 0.7%, $p = 0.008$), and importantly edema formation occurred equally in both hemispheres.

Discussion

This study has for the first time described a model of acute subdural hematoma with traumatic brain injury. The model was generated by combining the Impact Acceleration model of diffuse TBI with the well-established infusion model of ASDH. Physiological parameters and tissue water were evaluated. With ASDH alone ICP showed a modest transient rise, and CBF showed a transient decline. With TBI and ASDH, however, ICP rose to very high levels, and exceeded mABP, therefore reducing the effective CPP to zero. CBF in this case fell to extremely low levels and did not return for the remainder of the experiment. With ASDH alone, tissue water increase is confined to the ipsilateral hemisphere, however with diffuse TBI + ASDH, edema formation is considerably greater, and it occurs equally in both hemispheres, irrespective of the hematoma site.

ASDH is an important clinical problem when combined with traumatic brain injury, in which estimates of mortality of between 50–90% have been made [4, 14, 15]. One factor partially responsible for the severity of this problem, is the rapidity with which the brain can swell under such conditions. The synergy between ASDH and traumatic brain injury is complicated which makes therapeutic decisions difficult. Even the optimal time for hematoma evacuation has not been fully defined. ASDH alone can cause swelling as a result of a mass effect with ischemia, and also through neurotoxic components [2, 11]. These factors in conjunction with cytotoxic injury arising from TBI [1], create an environment rich for edema formation. Furthermore blood in the subdural space, reduces compliance volume and therefore limits compensation for increases in tissue pressure.

In order to be able to understand the pathology of this problem better, a suitable experimental model is required. To date, no such model has been described in the literature. This study describes the physiological effects and degree of edema formation in a model of TBI with ASDH developed by combining an existing model of Impact Acceleration with a well-established model of ASDH.

ASDH alone caused a marked but transient drop in CBF as measured in the contralateral hemisphere, however CBF on the side of the lesion is known to be below ischemic levels [2], and this explains the asymmetry of edema formation. TBI with ASDH, caused a prolonged period of ischemia, as measured in the contralateral hemisphere, and this coupled with the knowledge of CBF in the ipsilateral hemisphere explains the symmetry of edema formation seen in this model.

TBI and ASDH clearly interact synergistically to enhance edema formation following injury. There are several possibilities which could explain this phenomenon. TBI causes a brief and rapid opening of the BBB, which is then followed by a phase of cytotoxic brain swelling [1]. TBI also triggers a cascade of events including neurotransmitter release and membrane depolarization [8] which leads to disruption of ionic homeostasis, calcium accumulation and increased energy demand [12]. ASDH is known to have both ischemic and neurotoxic effects on the brain [2, 11], and therefore the enhanced edema may represent an additive effect. Alternatively components of ASDH may add additional phases of vasogenic swelling, or limitation of energy production which prevent the response to an increased tissue energy demand. Of these, the effects on energy production are most likely.

Heath and Vink [5], utilizing the impact acceleration model, have demonstrated that mitochondrial oxidative capacity is actually elevated within one hour after trauma. Moreover, they report that the cytosolic phosphorylation ratio is reduced, representing an increased demand or hypermetabolic state of the injured brain. However, mitochondria are remarkably sensitive to ischemic injury [6]. Inglis *et al.* [7] show that in the ASDH model, energy demand outstrips the blood supply in tissue around the ischemic zone. The ability of the tissue to produce more energy may define the limits of the penumbra zone.

In combining TBI with ASDH, it is clear that both trauma and hematoma make considerable metabolic demands, which cannot be met by the injured tissue. It is this disparity, which is most likely the origin of the rapid and diffuse formation of cerebral edema.

We conclude that the model presented is a suitable model by which to study ASDH with TBI. Moreover we have observed that edema formation in TBI is worsened by a combination of diffuse TBI and ASDH. Further studies, which focus on tissue ion concentration, brain tissue osmolality, ion movement and mitochondrial function, are required to elucidate the synergistic mechanisms involved in this pathological process. However we feel that an increased energy demand, with limited resources to meet the demand is the most likely explanation for the synergistic effect.

Acknowledgments

The authors thank Ms. Christina Marmarou and Ms. Jana G Dunbar for their technical assistance.

References

1. Barzo P, Marmarou A, Fatouros P, Hayasaki K, Corwin F (1997) Contribution of vasogenic and cellular edema to traumatic brain swelling measured by diffusion-weighted imaging. J Neurosurg 87: 900–907
2. Bullock R, Butcher SP, Chen MH, Kendall L, McCulloch J (1991) Correlation of the extracellular glutamate concentration with extent of blood flow reduction after subdural hematoma in the rat. J Neurosurg 74: 794–802
3. Foda MAA, Marmarou A (1994) A new model of diffuse brain injury in rats. Part 2: morphological characterization. J Neurosurg 80: 301–313
4. Haselsberger K, Pucher R, Auer LM (1988) Prognosis after acute subdural or epidural haemorrhage. Acta Neurochir (Wien) 90: 111–116
5. Heath DL, Vink R (1995) Impact acceleration-induced severe diffuse axonal injury in rats: characterization of phosphate metabolism and neurologic outcome. J Neurotrauma 12: 1027–1034
6. Hillered L, Siesjo BK, Alfors K-E (1984) Mitochondrial response to transient forebrain ischemia and resuscitation in the rat. J Cereb Blood Flow Metab 4: 438–446
7. Inglis FM, Bullock R, Chen MH, Graham DI, Miller JD, McCulloch J (1990) Ischemic brain damage associated with tissue hypermetabolism in acute subdural hematoma: reduction by a glutamate antagonist. Acta Neurochir [Suppl] (Wien) 51: 277–279
8. Katayama Y, Becker DP, Tamura T, Hovda DA (1990) Massive increase in extracellular potassium and the indiscriminate release of glutamate following concussive brain injury. J Neurosurg 73: 889–900
9. Marmarou A (1994) Traumatic brain edema: an overview. Acta Neurochir [Suppl] (Wien) 60: 421–424
10. Marmarou A, Foda MA, Brink W, Campbell J, Kita H, Demetriadou K (1994) A new model of diffuse brain injury in rats, part 1. J Neurosurg 80: 291–300
11. Miller JD, Bullock R, Graham DI, Chen MH, Teasdale GM (1990) Ischemic brain damage in a model of acute subdural hematoma. Neurosurgery 27: 433–439
12. Muizelaar JP, Ward JD, Marmarou A, Newlon PG, Wachi A (1989) Cerebral blood flow and metabolism in severely head-injured children. J Neurosurg 71: 72–76
13. Sahuquillo-Barris J, Lamarca-Ciuro J, Vilalta-Castan J, Rubio-Garcia E, Rodriguez-Pazos M (1988) Acute subdural hematoma and diffuse axonal injury after severe head trauma. J Neurosurg 68: 894–900
14. Seelig JM, Becker DP, Miller JD, Greenberg RP, Ward JD, Choi SC (1981) Traumatic acute subdural hematoma. Major mortality reduction in comatose patients treated within four hours. N Engl J Med 304: 1511–1518
15. Stone JL, Rifai MHS, Sugar O, Lang RG, Oldershaw JB, Moody RA (1983) I. Acute subdural hematoma: progress in definition, clinical pathology, and therapy. Surg Neurol 19: 216–231

Correspondence: Anthony Marmarou, Division of Neurosurgery, P.O. Box, 508, MCV Station, Sanger Hall, Room 8004, 1101 E. Marshall Street, Richmond, Virginia 23298.

Acta Neurochir (2000) [Suppl] 76: 217–221

Mitogen-Activated Protein Kinase Plays an Important Role in Hemolysate-Induced Contraction in Rabbit Basilar Artery

A. Y. Zubkov, K. Ogihara, A. Patllola, A. D. Parent, and **J. Zhang**

Department of Neurosurgery, University of Mississippi Medical Center, Jackson, Mississippi

Summary

Object. Mitogen-activated protein kinase (MAPK) is an important signaling factor in the vascular proliferation and contraction, the two features of cerebral vasospasm following subarachnoid hemorrhage. We studied the possible involvement of MAPK in hemolysate-induced signal transduction and contraction in rabbit basilar artery.

Methods. Isometric tension was used to record the contractile response of rabbit basilar artery to hemolysate. Western blots using antibodies for MAPK were conducted. 1) Hemolysate produced a concentration-dependent contraction of rabbit basilar artery. Pre-incubation of arteries with MAPK kinase inhibitor PD-98059 markedly reduced the contraction induced by hemolysate. PD-98059 also relaxed, in a concentration-dependent fashion, the sustained contraction induced by hemolysate (10%). 2) Hemolysate produced a time-dependent elevation of MAPK immunoreactivity in Western blot in rabbit basilar artery. MAPK was enhanced 3 min after hemolysate exposure and the effect reached maximum at 5 min. The immunoreactivity of MAPK decayed slowly with time, but the level of MAPK was still higher than the basal level even at two hours after exposure to hemolysate. 3) Pre-incubation of arteries with MAPK kinase inhibitor PD-98059 abolished the effect of hemolysate on MAPK immunoreactivity.

Conclusion. Hemolysate produced contraction of rabbit basilar artery possibly by activation of MAPK. MAPK inhibitors may be useful in the treatment of cerebral vasospasm.

Keywords: MAP kinase; hemolysate; rabbit basilar artery; cerebral vasospasm.

Introduction

Cerebral vasospasm is featured by a prolonged contraction of cerebral arteries [8] and a proliferation in the vessel wall [23, 24]. The pathogenesis of cerebral vasospasm is not clear but probably relates to spasmogens released from blood clot such as hemolysate, oxyhemoglobin and adenosine triphosphate (ATP) or spasmogens, released from vascular tissues such as endothelin [14].

Mitogen-activated protein kinase (MAPK) is a family of serine/threonine protein kinases involved in cell growth, differentiation and transformation [20]. The mechanism of MAPK-regulated contraction is probably related to the phosphorylation of caldesmon which is involved in prolonged smooth muscle contraction [3]. However, the role of MAPK in the regulation of contraction in cerebral arteries has not been studied. We investigated the effect of hemolysate on MAPK phosphorylation and the effect of MAPK inhibitor on hemolysate-induced contraction in rabbit basilar artery. The possible involvement of some upstream protein tyrosine kinases in hemolysate-induced signaling was also studied.

Materials and Methods

Hemolysate Preparation

Hemolysate was prepared from dog arterial blood as described previously [19]. Concentration of oxyhemoglobin in the preparation of 100% hemolysate was 12.20 ± 0.93 mM (n = 5).

Isometric Tension

New Zealand white rabbits (n = 45) of either sex, 2–3 pounds weight, were anesthetized with an intravenous injection of thiopental (20 mg/kg) and euthanitized by exsanguination.

The basilar arteries were divided into 2 groups and the following studies were performed. The rings were incubated for 30 min with MAPK kinase inhibitor PD-98059 (30 μM). Concentration-dependent contractions were produced with hemolysate in the presence of this inhibitor. In the control group, concentration-dependent contractions were induced with hemolysate (0.01, 0.1, 1 and 10%) in the absence of inhibitor.

In another study, the rings were pre-contracted with hemolysate (10%) and, when a stable plateau contraction was maintained, PD-98059 was applied on the sustained contraction induced by hemolysate. Relaxation was calculated as a percentage of the maximum contraction to hemolysate.

Western Blot

The basilar arteries were removed from the brainstem and incubated with 10% hemolysate diluted in Krebs-Henseleit buffer. The arteries were treated for 1, 3, 5, 10, 30, 60 and 120 minutes, and then immediately frozen in the liquid nitrogen. The arteries were homogenized in (mM) 50 Tris-HCl pH 7.5, 100 NaCl, 5 EDTA, 1 PMSF and 100 μl of IGEPAL CA-630 for 20 minutes at 4 °C. The samples (20 μg protein) were applied to 12% SDS-PAGE. After electrophoretic transfer of the separated polypeptides to nitrocellulose membrane, the membranes were blocked using 5% non-fat milk in Tween-PBS for 1 hour. The membranes were washed with Tween-PBS and incubated at room temperature for 2 hours in a 1 : 5000 dilution of mouse anti-MAPK (Zymed Laboratories, San Francisco, CA). Nitrocellulose membranes were incubated with 1 : 5000 dilution of sheep anti-mouse IgG antibody, linked with horseradish peroxidase. The enhanced chemiluminescence (ECL) system (Amersham, Buckinghamshire, England) was used for visualization of protein bands. The results were quantified by laser (Molecular Dynamics, Image Quant^{TM}, Sunnyvale, CA, USA).

Results

Effects of Inhibitors on Hemolysate-Induced Contractions

Figure 1 shows the concentration-dependent contractions to hemolysate in the absence and presence of PD-98059 (Fig. 1A). PD-98059 pre-incubated with rings for 30 minutes almost abolished the contractions to hemolysate ($p < 0.05 - 0.001$, ANOVA).

In another study, the rings of rabbit basilar artery were contracted with hemolysate (10%) and once a stable contraction was obtained, cumulative concentrations of PD-98059 (1–100 μM) were applies on the sustained contraction induced by hemolysate. PD-98059 produced significant relaxation ($p < 0.05$, ANOVA, Fig. 2A) at high concentration (100 μM).

Phosphorylation of MAPK by Hemolysate

Hemolysate (10%) activates MAPK (ERK 1/2) in the first 3 minutes after exposure and induced peak MAPK enhancement at 5 minutes. The effect of hemolysate decayed with time but was still above the resting level even at 2 hours after exposure (Fig. 3).

In a separate study, rabbit basilar arteries were treated for 30 minutes with saline or PD-98059 (30 μM) and then exposed to hemolysate (10%) for 5 minutes. Figure 4 demonstrates that hemolysate enhanced significantly MAPK immunoreactivity and PD-98059 abolished the effect of hemolysate. PD-98059 did not markedly reduce the resting level of MAPK in rabbit basilar arteries.

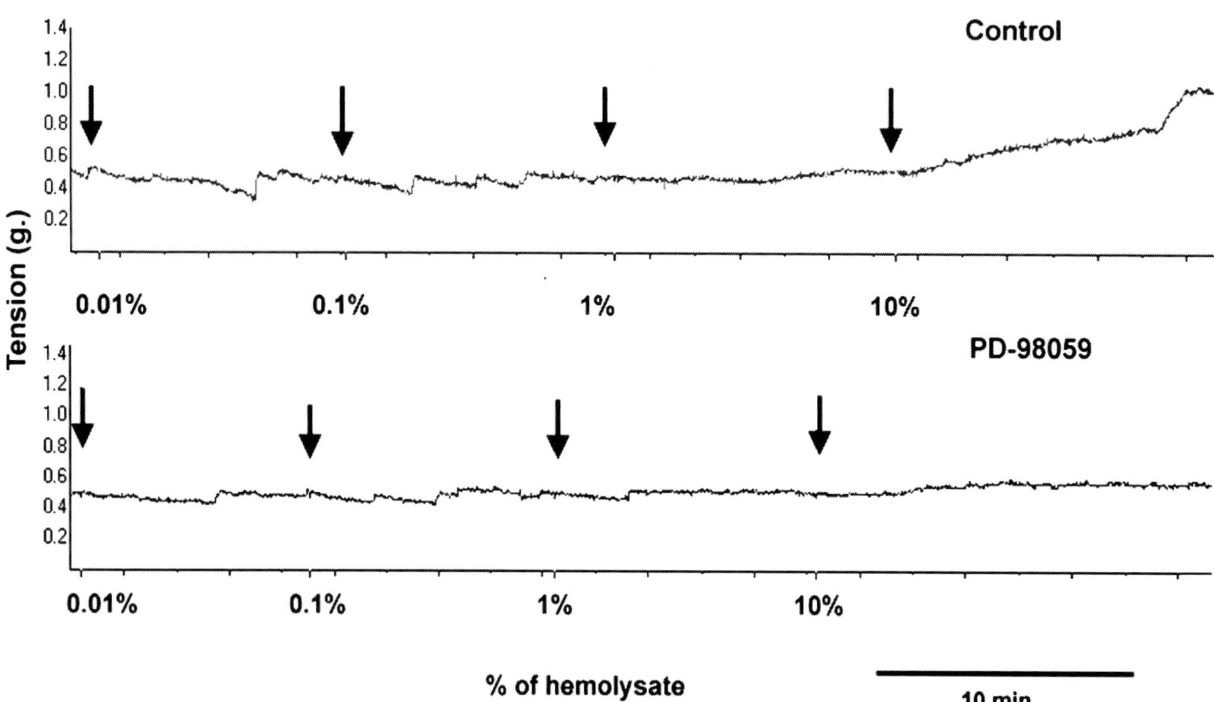

Fig. 1. Graphs displaying the inhihitory effects of the PD-98059. Real tracing of dose-dependent contraction of control arterial ring to hemolysate (upper tracing) is to the dose-dependent contraction after inhibition with PD-98059

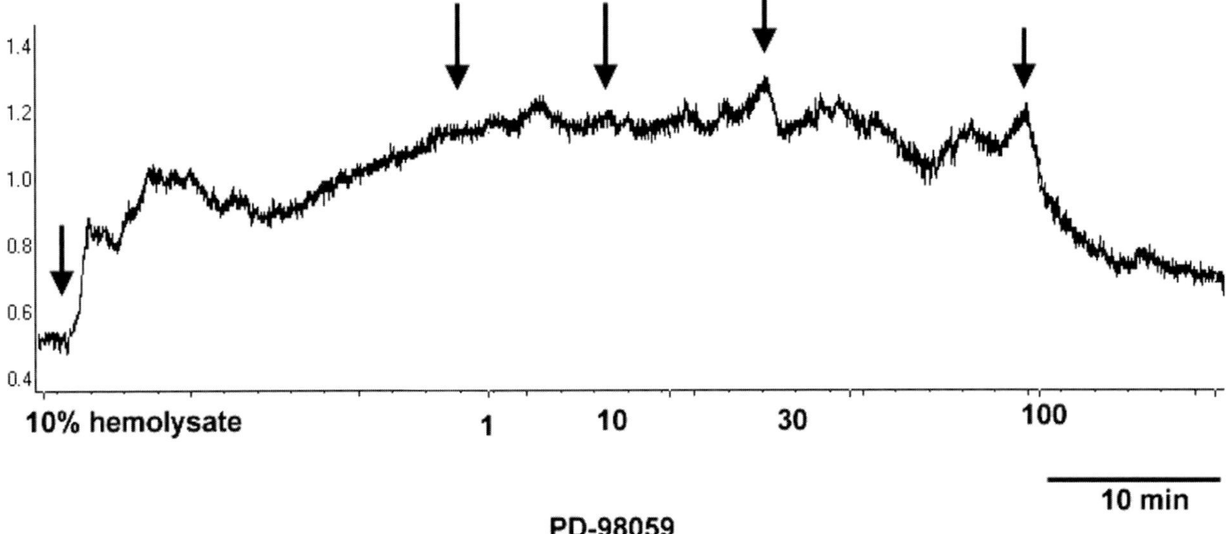

Fig. 2. Graphs displaying the relaxant effects of PD-98059 on sustained contraction induced by 10% hemolysate. PD-98059 significantly relaxed contracted artery in dose-dependent manner

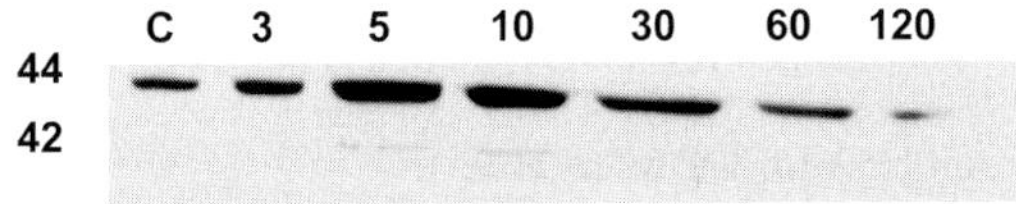

Fig. 3. Time course of activation of MAPK after stimulation with 10% hemolysate. A. MAPK was activated within 3 minutes, peaked by 5–10 minutes and maintained activity above baseline for at least 120 minutes. Abbreviations used: 42 – $p42^{ERK}$, 44 – $p44^{ERK}$.

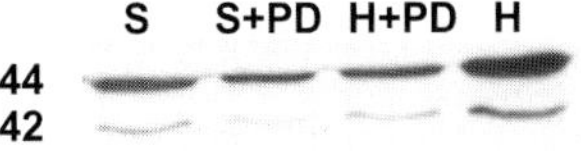

Fig. 4. Western blot picture demonstrating effect of PD-98059 on activation of MAPK after stimulation with hemolysate (10%). Incubation of control vessel with PD-98059 insignificantly decreased level of basal activity of MAPK. The effect of hemolysate (10%) on MAPK was abolished after the pre-incubation with PD-98059 for 30 minutes. Abbreviations used: S – saline treated group of arteries, S + PD – vessels were pre-incubated with PD-98059 for 30 minutes and, then, treated with saline for 5 minutes. H + PD – vessels were pre-incubated with PD-98059 for 30 minutes and, then, treated with hemolysate (10%) for 5 minutes. H – vessels treated with hemolysate (10%) for 5 minutes

Discussion

We have demonstrated 1) hemolysate produced concentration-dependent contractions in rabbit basilar artery and pre-incubation with MAPK kinase inhibitor PD-98059 abolished the contraction to hemolysate. 2) PD-98059 relaxed significantly sustained contraction of rabbit basilar arteries induced by hemolysate. 3) Hemolysate enhanced MAPK immunoreactivity in rabbit basilar artery. The initial effect on MAPK was observed at 1 minutes and the peak response obtained at 5 minutes after exposure to hemolysate. The effect of hemolysate on MAPK lasted up to 2 hours. 4) PD-98059 abolished the effect of hemolysate on MAPK immunoreactivity.

MAPK and Cerebral Vasospasm

Besides regulation of cell growth and differentiation, MAPK is involved in the regulation of smooth muscle contraction by phosphorylating thin filament associated proteins such as caldesmon [2]. Two isoforms 42 and 44 kDa (ERK 1/2) are the most well studied MAPK and they are activated by dual phosphorylations of the threonine and tyrosine residues [7]. Both 42 and 44 kDa were shown presented in vascular smooth-muscle cells [22]. Membrane depolarization and agonist activation increased MAPK activity in swine carotid artery [9] MAPK activity was enhanced within 0.5–1 minute, reached maximal level within 2 minutes and maintained high level of activity for at least 30 minutes [4]. We have observed similar results in rabbit basilar artery when MAPK activation was observed within 3 minutes and reached the peak level by 5 minutes. The prolonged activity of MAPK for up to 2 hours after exposure to hemolysate indicates that

MAPK may play an important role in cerebral vasospasm, a prolonged vasoconstriction.

PKC activation has been demonstrated to be involved in cerebral vasospasm [16, 21]. Activation of PKC may lead to the activation of MAPK [10, 18]. PKC inhibitor staurosporine abolished vasopressin-induced MAPK activity in rat aortic smooth muscle cells [12]. In addition, activation of MAPK may regulate smooth muscle contractility by phosphorylating thin filament associated proteins such as caldesmon. Caldesmon has been shown to be involved in prolonged vasoconstriction such as in cerebral vasospasm [5]. Activation of PKC and elevation of intracellular Ca^{2+} may activate protein tyrosine kinases Genistein and tyrphostin, two structurally different tyrosine kinase inhibitors, reduced hemolysate-induced Ca^{2+} elevation in cultured endothelial cells [15] and hemolysate-induced contraction of rabbit basilar artery [11]. Activation of tyrosine kinase may stimulate Ras and Raf-1 and lead to MAPK activation [6]. PD-98059 inhibits MEK activation by Raf-1 and thus inhibits MAPK [1]. Indeed, pre-incubation of tissues with PD-98059 in this study abolished MAPK immunoreactivity and the contractile response of rabbit basilar artery to hemolysate. However, when tissues were pre-contracted with hemolysate (or when MAPK was activated), PD-98059 produced only partial relaxation.

Conclusions

Cerebral vasospasm is probably a process of prolonged vascular contraction [13] and vascular wall proliferation [17]. Etiological factors and their signal transduction pathways may need to cover both contraction and proliferation of cerebral arteries. MAPK is involved in cell proliferation and in smooth muscle contraction. Hemolysate may produce contraction in rabbit basilar artery by activation of MAPK. This study raises a possibility that MAPK may be involved in the signal transduction in cerebral vasospasm and inhibition of MAPK may open a new avenue in the management of cerebral vasospasm. Probably the tyrosine kinase and PKC pathways are involved in the activation of MAP kinase.

Acknowledgment

This work was partially supported by a grant-in-aid to J. Z. from the American Heart Association.

References

1. Alessi DR, Cuenda A, Cohen P, Dudley DT, Jaltiel AR (1995) PD 098059 is a specific inhibitor of the activation of mitogen-activated protein kinase kinase in vitro and in vivo. J Biol Chem 270: 27489–27494
2. Childs TJ, Mak AS (1993) Smooth-muscle mitogen-activated protein (MAP) kinase: purification and characterization, and the phosphorylation of caldesmon. Biochem J 296: 745–751
3. Earley JJ, Su X, Moreland RS (1998) Caldesmon inhibits active crossbridges in unstimulated vascular smooth muscle: an antisense oligodeoxynucleotide approach. Circ Res 83: 661–667
4. Epstein AM, Throckmorton D, Brophy CM (1997) Mitogen-activated protein kinase activation: an alternate signaling pathway for sustained vascular smooth muscle contraction. J Vasc Surg 26: 327–332
5. Fukami M, Tani E, Takai A, Yamaura I, Minami N (1995) Activity of smooth muscle phosphatases 1 and 2A in rabbit basilar artery in vasospasm. Stroke 26: 2321–2327
6. Glenney JR, Jr. (1992) Tyrosine-phosphorylated proteins: mediators of signal transduction from the tyrosine kinases. Biochim Biophys Acta 1134: 113–127
7. Griendling KK, Ushio-Fukai M, Lassegue B, Alexander RW (1997) Angiotensin II signaling in vascular smooth muscle. New concepts. Hypertension 29: 366–373
8. Kassell NF, Helm G, Simmons N, Phillips CD, Cail WS (1992) Treatment of cerebral vasospasm with intra-arterial papaverine. J Neutosurg 77: 848–852
9. Katoch SS, Moreland RS (1995) Agonist and membrane depolarization induced activation of MAP kinase in the swine carotid artery. Am J Physiol 269: H222–H229
10. Khalil RA, Morgan KG (1993) PKC-mediated redistribution of mitogen-activated protein kinase during smooth muscle celll activation. Am J Physiol 265: C406–C411
11. Kim C-J, Kim K-W, Park J-W, Lee J-C, Zhang JH (1998) Role of tyrosine kinase in erithrocyte lysate-induced contraction in rabbit cerebral arteries. J Neurosurg 89: 289–296
12. Kribben A, Wieder ED, Li X, van PV, Granoty, Schrier RW, Nemenoff RA (1993) AVP-induced activation of MAP kinase in vascular smooth muscle cells is mediated through protein kinase C. Am J Physiol 265: C939–C945
13. Macdonald RL, Wang X, Zhang J, Marton LS (1996) Molecular changes with subarachnoid hemorrhage and vasospasm. The molecular biology of neurosurgical disease In: Raffel C, Harsh G (eds) Wikkiams & Wilkins, Baltimore, pp 278–293
14. Zuccarello M, Boccaletti R, Romano A, Rapoport RM (1998) Endothelin B receptor antagonists attenuate subarachnoid hemorrhage-induced cerebral vasospasm. Stroke 29: 1924–1929
15. Marton LS, Weir BK, Zhang H (1996) Tyrosine phosphorylation and $[Ca^{2+}]$i elevation induced by hemolysate in bovine endothelial cells: implications for cerebral vasospasm. Neurol Res 18: 349–353
16. Matsui T, Asano T (1996) Protein kinase C and vasospasm. J Neurosurg 85: 1197–1198
17. Mayberg MR, Okada T, Bark DH (1990) Morphologic changes in cerbral arteries after subarachnoid hemorrhage. Neurosurg Clin N Am 1: 417–432
18. Minami N, Tani E, Maeda Y, Yamaura I, Fukami M (1992) Effects of inhibitors of protein kinase C and calpain in experimental delayed cerebral vasospasm. J Neurosurg 76: 111–118
19. Onoda K, Ono S, Ogihara K, Shiota T Asari S, Ohmoto T, Ninomiya Y (1996) Inhibition of vascular contraction by intracisternal administration of preproendothelin-1 mRNA antisense oligoDNA in a rat experimental vasospasm model. J Neurosurg 85: 846–852

20. Pelech SL, Sanghera JS (1992) MAP kinases: charting the regulatory pathways. Science 257: 1355–1356
21. Sato M, Tani E, Matsumoto T, Fujikawa H, Jmajoh-Ohmi S (1997) Generation of the catalytic fragment of protein kinase C alpha in spastic canine basilar artery. J Neurosurg 87: 752–756
22. Watson MH, Venance SL, Pang SC, Mak AS (1993) Smooth muscle cell proliferation. Expression and kinase activities of p34cdc2 and mitogen-activated protein kinase homologues. Circ Res 73: 109–117
23. Zhang J, Lewis AI, Bernanke DH, Zubkov AY, Clower B (1998) Stroke: anatomy of a catastrophic event. The Anat Rec (New Anat) 253: 58–63
24. Zubkov AY, Lewis AI, Scalzo D, Bernanke DH, Harkey HL (1999) Morphological changes after percutaneous transluminal angioplasty. Surg Neurol 51: 399–403

Correspondence: John Zhang, M.D., Ph.D., Department of Neurosurgery of the University Mississippi Medical Center, 2500 North State Street, Jackson, MS.

Acta Neurochir (2000) [Suppl] 76: 223–226

Morphological Presentation of Posttraumatic Vasospasm

A. Y. Zubkov[1], **A. S. Pilkington**[2], **A. D. Parent**[1], and **J. Zhang**[1]

[1] Department of Neurosurgery, The University of Mississippi Medical Center, Jackson, Mississippi, USA
[2] Department of Surgical Intensive Care Unit, The University of Mississippi Medical Center, Jackson, Mississippi, USA

Summary

Posttraumatic vasospasm is a well-recognized sequela of head injury. The risk factors associated with posttraumatic vasospasm have not been well defined. We studied 119 consecutive patients with head injury to determine the risk factors for posttraumatic vasospasm.

Posttraumatic vasospasm was detected in 32 (35.6%) of 90 patients. Among these patients, 29 (90.6%) had severe head injury and 3 (9.4%) had moderate head injury. None of the patients with mild head injury suffered posttraumatic vasospasm. In most cases, the onset of posttraumatic vasospasm began on the fifth day and lasted 1 to 9 days. In 8 (25%) patients, posttraumatic vasospasm began within the first three days of the head injury. Clinical deterioration was documented in two (2.5%) patients.

Morphologically, posttraumatic vasospasm resembled features of aneurysmal vasospasm. We found increased corrugation of the internal elastic lamina and increased amounts of connective tissue in the subendothelial layer.

These findings showed that posttraumatic vasospasm, although clinically more mild, demonstrated the same morphological changes as did aneurysmal vasospasm.

Keywords: Head injury; cerebral vasospasm; morphology.

Introduction

Head injury is one of the leading causes of mortality and morbidity in young people. Most of the patients are males between 15 and 29 years old, and motor vehicle collisions are the leading cause of head injury [6]. The pathogenesis of head injury and the secondary factors affecting its outcome are still not completely understood. One of the suggested factors of secondary insult is posttraumatic vasospasm (PTV).

Following severe head injury, autoregulation is absent, diminished, or delayed in about 50% of patients [1]. In the absence of autoregulation, moderate or transient hypotension can cause ischemia. Ischemia after head injury may result from generalized increase in intracranial pressure (ICP), local brain compression secondary to hematomas, contusions, or cerebral vasospasm.

Morphological features of PTV are not defined. The purposes of this study were to investigate the morphology of PTV and to correlate morphological findings with clinical findings in the patients with PTV.

Materials and Methods

Clinical Studies

One hundred patients with head injury were admitted to the University Mississippi Medical Center from March 1996 to December 1997. In addition to standard management, transcranial Doppler (TCD) ultrasonographic measurements were performed daily, to obtain Doppler blood flow velocities in the arteries of the anterior circulation and in the extracranial internal carotid arteries. Transcranial Doppler ultrasonographic studies were performed by one operator (AYZ) using the TC2-64B Doppler ultrasound (EME, Germany) and 500M Doppler Ultrasound (Multigon Industries, Inc.). Posttraumatic cerebral vasospasm was detected when the Lindegaard index (ratio of middle cerebral artery (MCA) velocity to ipsilateral extracranial intracranial cerebral artery (ICA) velocity) was more than 3 [8]. The threshold for cerebral vasospasm was established as 100 cm/s because most patients had high intracranial pressure (ICP) and concomitant decreased cerebral blood flow [2, 12].

Morphological Studies

The arteries were fixed with 4% paraformaldehyde in 0.1 M sodium phosphate buffer, pH 7.3 for 7 days. Samples for light microscopy were embedded in paraffin or epoxy resin, and sections were stained with Gomori's trichrome stain or toluidine blue stain.

Samples for scanning electron microscopy were postfixed with osmium tetroxide, dehydrated in a graded series of acetone, dried using PelDri II®, mounted on aluminum studs, coated with 200 Å gold, and examined with a JOEL T300 scanning electron microscope.

Samples for transmission electron microscopy were postfixed with osmium tetroxide, dehydrated in a graded series of acetone, embedded in epon-araldite epoxy resin, sectioned at 60 Å, and examined with a LEO 906 transmission electron microscope.

Arteries obtained during autopsy of a patient who died immediately after head injury were used as a control.

Results

Cerebral vasospasm was detected in 32 (35.6%) of 90 patients. The onset of posttraumatic vasospasm ranged from 2 to 8 days (mean 5 days) after the injury and peaked at 5 to 7 days. In 8 (25%) of 32 patients posttraumatic vasospasm began within 3 days after head injury. This early onset is unique to posttraumatic vasospasm.

Autopsy was performed in three patients who died from severe head injury. Microscopic features of PTV closely resembled those of post-aneurysmal subarachnoid hemorrhage (SAH) cerebral vasospasm [14].

In the first case, a 39-year-old patient was admitted to the hospital with GCS 4. Computed tomography demonstrated acute subdural hematoma and multiple brain contusions. Despite emergent surgery, the patient's condition did not improve. Transcranial Doppler ultrasonography demonstrated diffuse severe PTV, which was confirmed with cerebral angiography. Posttraumatic vasospasm which peaked at day 8 with maximum velocity of 170 cm/sec and the Lindegaard index of 5, lasted for 13 days as measured by TCD. By day 19, TCD velocities had decreased to 100 cm/sec. On day 15, the patient developed pneumonia and multiorgan failure and died on day 20 after head injury.

Morphological studies revealed increased thickness of the tunica intima, increased corrugation of the internal elastic membrane (IEL), deposition of connective tissue under the IEL. (Fig. 1A,B)

In the second case, a 32-year-old patient presented with a GCS 3 and an acute subdural hematoma. The patient had high ICP (upper 20s), in spite of all the effort to decrease it. Transcranial Doppler ultrasonographic measurements revealed hyperemia during the first two days of the hospital stay ($V_{MCA} > 100$ cm/sec, Lindegaard index < 3). After the second day, the TCD velocities returned to normal values. But from day 5, TCD velocities rose again above 115 cm/sec and the Lindegaard index was more than 3 in the left MCA. Posttraumatic vasospasm peaked on day 7 with TCD velocities of 120 cm/sec and the Lindergaard index of 3.5; these values persisted for 3 days. The patient's neurological condition was unchanged GCS 3, despite normalization of TCD values. Having developed acute renal failure on day 4 after head injury, the patient died on day 10.

Morphologic studies revealed increased amounts of connective tissue under the IEL and in the subendothelial layer and fibrosis of the tunica media. Corrugation of IEL accompanied the arterial constriction. Desquamation of endothelial cells was also evident. Marked edema under the IEL was found in all samples. (Fig. 2A,B) These changes were demonstrated only in the MCA, affected by posttraumatic vasospasm. The opposite MCA, which did not have TCD signs of vasospasm, was normal morphologically. (Fig. 2C,D)

All these findings are quite characteristic for cerebral vasospasm. In the normal arteries, all endothelial cells were intact, and the cell-to-cell contacts and cell-

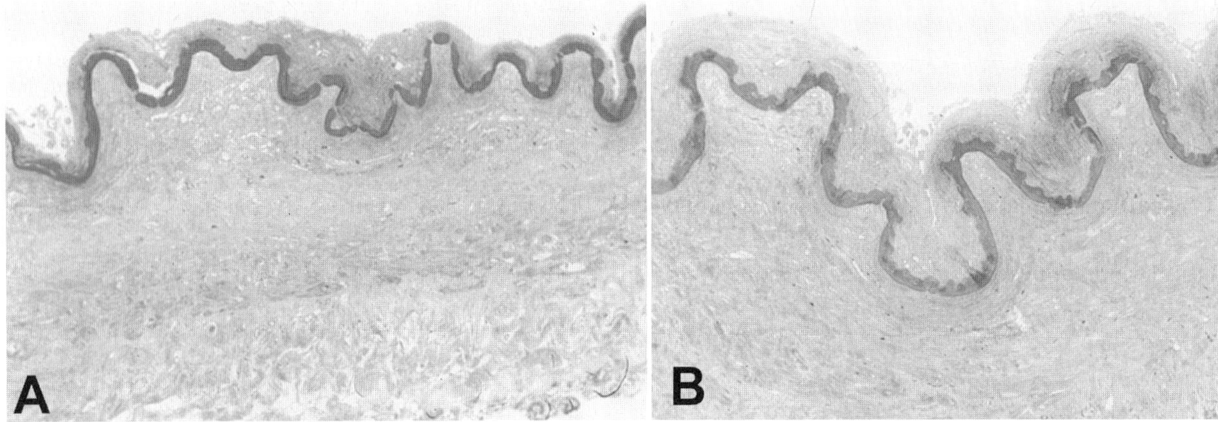

Fig. 1. Changes in middle cerebral arteries (*MCA*) from patient with diffuse posttraumatic vasospasm. (A) 200×; (B) 200×; toluidine blue stained epoxy resin embedded sections) Increases thickness of intima (small arrow), corrugation of internal elastic lamina (large arrow), edema of muscle layer and increased amount of connective tissue (opened arrow) are the characteristic changes in posttraumatic vasospasm

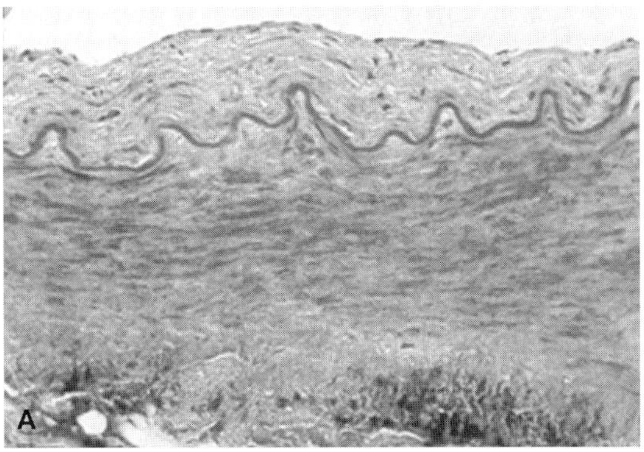

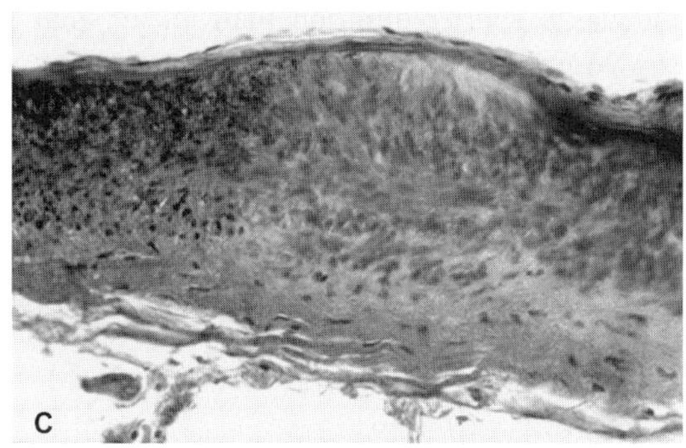

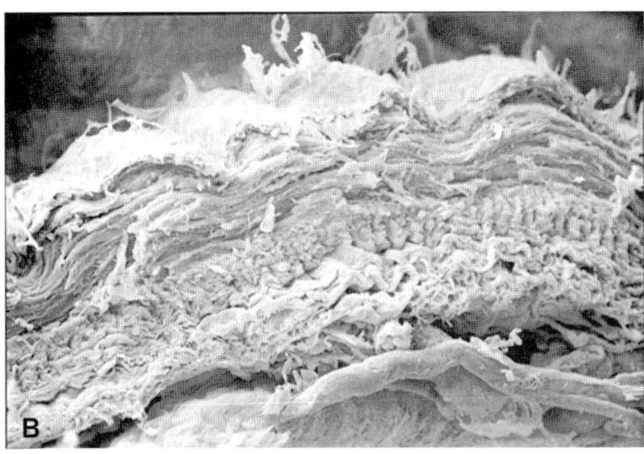

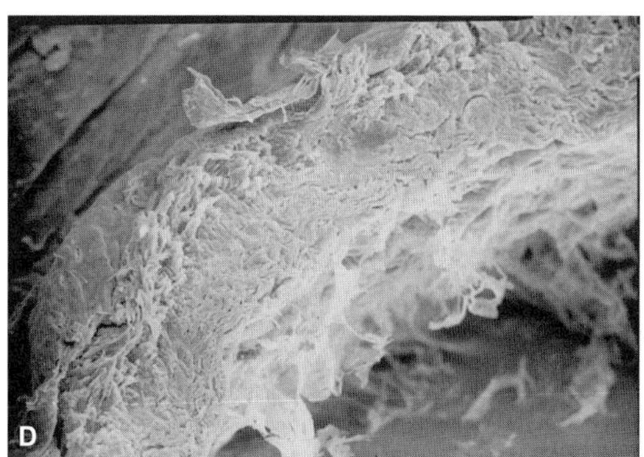

Fig. 2. Sections stained with Gomori trichrome stain (200×) (a) and scanning EM samples (350×) (b) from the patient with moderate vasospasm of left MCA demonstrating increased thickness of intimal layer (small arrows), corrugation of internal elastic lamina (large arrow). There is an increased amount of connective tissue which is demonstrated by light staining in muscle layer (double-headed arrow).

For comparison samples (c,d) of right MCA from the same patient that had not shown increased velocities did not have these changes, and resemble normal morphological findings in cerebral arteries. Arrows are pointing to the same areas as in (a) and (b)

basal membrane contacts were preserved. The IEL was not corrugated, smooth muscle cells appeared flat and no dystrophic changes were detected in these cells.

Discussion

We found a 35.6% incidence of PTV among the head injury patients in this study. The morphologic features of posttraumatic vasospasm resembled those of cerebral vasospasm after aneurysmal SAH. Posttraumatic vasospasm was presented with the changes in the intimal and muscle layers. Endothelial cells were dystrophic and desquamated, the IEL was corrugated and connective tissue in the tunica media increased markedly.

Many authors observed similarities between posttraumatic vasospasm and vasospasm occurring after aneurysm rupture, assuming similar pathogenesis [13]. This certainly is true for PTV accompanied by SAH, but in 10% of PTV cases there is no visible blood in the CSF [3, 5, 7, 11]. A cooperative study of the National Institute of health, based on CT examinations of 753 patients with severe head injury, reported that SAH appeared in only 40% of the patients [4].

Posttraumatic vasospasm certainly plays a role in patients' outcome. Macpherson and Graham found vasospasm in 41% of patients who died from head injury. They found ischemia of cerebral hemispheres in 51% of patients as compared to 32% with vasospasm without ischemia [9, 10]. Taneda *et al.* found that ischemic symptoms directly attributable to vasospasm occurred in 7.7% of the patients [11].

Conclusions

There are still a lot of controversies about posttraumatic vasospasm. It certainly plays a definite role in the pathogenesis of head injury. Clinically, posttraumatic vasospasm develops in about 1/3 of the patients, mainly with severe head injury. It starts earlier and has a shorter duration than aneurysmal vasospasm. Morphological features of posttraumatic vasospasm closely resemble aneurysmal vasospasm. That may mean that similar pathogenic factors are involved in both of these types of cerebral vasospasm and the approach to treatment has to be the same.

Acknowledgment

The authors thank Glenn Hoskins for assistance with transmission electron microscopy. This work was in part supported by NIH grand 1 S10 RR11321-01A1.

References

1. Bouma GJ, Muizelaar JP (1992) Cerebral blood flow, cerebral blood volume, and cerebrovascular reactivity after severe head injury. J Neurotrauma 9 [Suppl] 1: S333–S348
2. Chan KH, Miller JD, Dearden NM, Andrews PJ *et al* (1992) The effect of changes in cerebral perfusion pressure upon middle cerebral artery blood flow velocity and jugular bulb venous oxygen saturation after severe brain injury. J Neurosurg 77: 55–61
3. Echlin, Francis A (1980) Cerebral vasospasm due to local trauma. Cerebral arterial spasm: proceedings of 2nd International Workshop, Amsterdam, The Netherlands. Williams and Wilkins, Baltimore, pp 251–255
4. Eisenberg HM, Gary HE, Jr., Aldrich EF, Saydjari C *et al* (1990) Initial CT findings in 753 patients with severe had injury. A report from the NIH Traumatic Coma Data Bank. J Neurosurg 73: 688–698
5. Frenidenfelt H, Sundctrom R (1963) Local and general spasm in the internal carotid system following trauma. Acta Radiol 1: 278–283
6. Gardner D (1986) Acute management of the head-injured adult. Nurs Clin N Am 21: 555–562
7. Hamer J, Krastel A (1976) Cerebral vasospasm after brain injury. Neurochirurgia 19: 185–189
8. Lindegaard KF, Bakke SJ, Sorteberg W, Nakstad P *et al* (1986) A non-invasive Doppler ultrasound method for the evaluation of patients with subarachnoid hemorrhage. Acta Radiol [Suppl] 369: 96–98
9. Macpherson P, Graham DI (1973) Arterial spasm and slowing of the cerebral circulation in the ischaemia of head injury. J Neurol Neurosurg Psychiatry 36: 1069–1072
10. Macpherson P, Graham DI (1978) Correlatioon between angiographic findings and the ischaemia of head injury. J Neurol Neurosurg Psychiatry 41: 122–127
11. Taneda M, Kataoka K, Akai F, Asai T *et al* (1996) Traumatic subarachnoid hemorrhage as a predictable indicator of delayed ischemic symptoms. J Neurosurg 84: 762–768
12. Weber M, Grolimund P, Seiler RW (1990) Evaluation of posttraumatic cerebral blood flow velocities by transcranial Doppler ultrasonography. Neurosurgery 27:106–112
13. Wilkins RH, Odom GL (1970) Intracranial arterial spasm associated with craniocerebral trauma. J Neurosurg 32: 626–633
14. Zubkov AY, Lewis AI, Scalzo D, Bernanke DH *et al* (1999) Morphological changes after percutaneous transluminal angioplasty. Surg Neurol 51: 399–403

Correspondence: Alexander Y. Zubkov, M.D., Department of Neurosurgery of the University Mississippi Medical Center, 2500 North State Street, Jackson, MS, 39216-4505.

Acta Neurochir (2000) [Suppl] 76: 227–230

Role of Tyrosine Kinase in Fibroblast Compaction and Cerebral Vasospasm

A. Patlolla, K. Ogihara, A. Zubkov, K. Aoki, A. D. Parent, and **J. H. Zhang**

Departments of Neurosurgery, University of Mississippi Medical Center, Jackson, Mississippi

Summary

Hemolysate, a proposed causative agent for cerebral vasospasm following subarachnoid hemorrhage, produces contraction of cerebral arteries by activation of tyrosine kinases. In addition, hemolysate accelerates fibroblast collagen compaction that could play a role in cerebral vasospasm. We studied the effect of hemolysate on tyrosine phosphorylation and fibroblast collagen compaction in cultured dog cerebral and human dermal fibroblasts using tyrosine kinase inhibitors and tyrosine antibodies (Western blot).

1) Hemolysate was found to enhance tyrosine phosphorylation of two proteins approximately 64 and 120 kDa. The effect of hemolysate was time- and concentration-dependent. 2) Two main components in hemolysate, oxyhemoglobin and adenosine triphosphate (ATP), produced similar results to that of hemolysate. 3) Tyrosine kinase inhibitor genistein and tyrphostin A51 (30 μM) markedly reduced the effect of hemolysate on tyrosine phosphorylation. 4) In another study, hemolysate increased fibroblast collagen compaction and the effect of hemolysate was reduced by genistein and tyrphostin A51.

We conclude that hemolysate activates tyrosine kinase that may lead to acceleration of fibroblast compaction. This effect of hemolysate may contribute to cerebral vasospasm.

Keywords: Tyrosine phosphorylation; hemolysate; collagen-lattice compaction.

Introduction

Cerebral vasospasm, a persisted narrowing of major cerebral arteries, is a major cause of mortality and morbidity following subarachnoid hemorrhage (SAH) [4, 6]. The etiological factors for cerebral vasospasm are subarachnoid blood clots, especially the lysate of erythrocyte [6]. However, the pathogenesis of cerebral vasospasm and the signal transduction pathways responding to the spasmogens remain unclear. Besides smooth muscle contraction, vascular fibroblasts, non-muscle components can produce and maintain vascular constriction [8].

Thus, we studied the effect of hemolysate and its components on tyrosine phosphorylation and fibroblast collagen compaction in cultured canine basilar artery and human dermal fibroblasts.

Materials and Methods

Cell Culture

Neonatal normal human dermal fibroblast cells (NHDF-Neo) were purchased from Clonetics (San Diego, CA) and were cultured in FBM medium in a 5% CO_2 incubator. Canine basilar arterial fibroblast cells were obtained using explant methods and cultured in Dulbecco's modified Eagle's medium (Gibco Brl, Grand Island, NY) with 10% fetal bovine serum. These cells were stained negative to factor VIII and α-smooth muscle actin. Cells from the 3rd and 8th passages were used.

Western Blot

Western blot for tyrosine phosphorylation was described previously [3]. The results were quantified by laser densitometry of the films and integrated whole band analysis (Molecular Dynamics, Image Quant^{TM}, Sunnyvale, CA).

Fibroblast-Populated Collagen Lattices (FPCL) Compaction

Fibroblast-populated collagen lattices (FPCLs) were formed by mixing fibroblasts in DMEM (1.6 ml) with rat tail tendon collagen (Type I) with a vortex mixer. The mixture was immediately transferred to 16 mm wells (24-well Plates) and allowed to gel at 37 °C. The repolymerization process typically occurred within minutes, trapping the cells in the resulting lattice matrix. To assure even contraction, each FPCL was freed from the dish walls and surface with a fine needle after formation.

To test the effect of hemolysate and tyrosine kinase inhibitor on lattice compaction, 0.1 ml of hemolysate and tyrosine kinase inhibitors was added after the lattice was freed. During incubation, the fibroblasts were progressively compacted the collagen fibrils in all three dimensions in a process known as lattice contraction. At 24-hour intervals after the addition of hemolysate, lattice contraction was determined as a reduction in area. Lengths of the longer and shorter axes of each contracting lattice were measured using a scale of graph paper beneath the dish. The areas were then calculated, considering each lattice as an ellipse.

Data Analysis

Data are expressed as mean ± S. E. Statistical differences between the control and other groups were compared by analysis of variance (ANOVA), and a value of $P < 0.05$ was considered statistically significant.

Results

Hemolysate (10%) was found to enhance tyrosine phosphorylation of two proteins approximately 64 and 120 kDa in canine basilar artery (Fig. 1.) and human dermal (not shown). The effect of hemolysate was time-dependent and the phosphorylation lasted for more than 60 minutes.

Two major components in hemolysate, oxyhemoglobin and ATP were studied separately. Oxyhemoglobin (10 μmol/L) and ATP (10 μmol/L) were found to enhance tyrosine phosphorylation of two proteins approximately 64 and 120 kDa, similar to that of hemolsyate (not shown). The effect of oxyhemoglobin and ATP was time-dependent that the peak response was obtained at 3 min.

Pre-incubation with tyrosine kinase inhibitors, Genistein (30 μmol/L) and Tyrphostin A51 (30 μmol/L), for 60 minutes, markedly ($P < 0.05$) reduced the effect of hemolysate (10%, 5 min treatment) on tyrosine phosphorylation in cultured canine basilar artery fribroblast cells (Fig. 2).

In another study, Hemolysate increased FPCL compaction on day 1, 2 and 3 with statistical significance compared to the corresponding days with the control. Tyrosine kinase inhibitors genistein and tyrphostin A51 (30 μmol/L) reduced the effect of hemolysate (not shown).

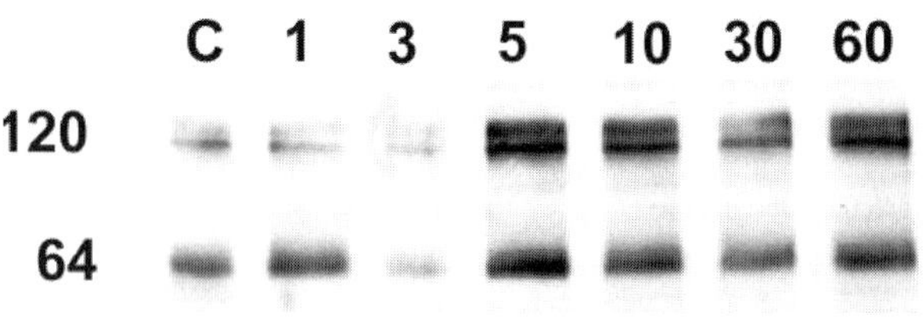

Fig. 1. Time course of hemolysate induced tyrosine phosphorylation in cultured canine basilar arterial fibroblasts. Western blot stained with monoclonal antibody to phosphotyrosine. Hemolysate (10%) was added to canine basilar arterial fibroblast cells for the indicated times. Equal amounts of protein were loaded into each lane. Hemolysate enhanced tyrosine phosphorylation of the 120 and 64 kDa proteins in a time-dependent fashion. The peak response to hemolysate was observed at 5 min and then the signal decayed slightly and maintained an elevated level above the resting level up to 60 min

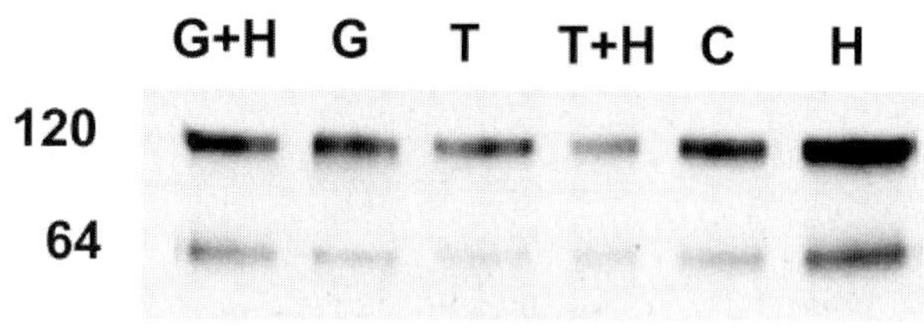

Fig. 2. Effect of tyrosine kinase inhibitors. A. Hemolysate (*H*, 10%) was added to canine basilar arterial fibroblasts for 5 min in the presence of tyrosine kinase inhibitors genistein ($G + H$, 30 μM) and tyrphostin A51 ($T + H$, 30 μM). Saline (*C*) was used in the control group. Genistein (*G*) and tyrphostin A51 (*T*) were used without hemolysate in two groups. Hemolysate enhanced tyrosine phosphorylation of the 120 and 64 kDa proteins and the effect of hemolysate was abolished by genistein and tyrphostin A51

Discussion

Yamamoto *et al.* [12] reported that myofibroblasts isolated from human cerebral arteries of vasospasm patients increased the collagen lattice compaction. This suggests that myofibroblasts in human cerebral arteries differ from medial smooth muscle cells and can generate a force rearranging the proliferated collagen matrix and this reorganization can contribute to, or be responsible for, sustained vasoconstriction. The possible role for fibroblasts in cerebral vasospasm was studied in vitro in both dermal and cerebral fibroblasts, and found to play an active role in collagen compaction induced bloody cerebrospinal fluid of vasospasm patients [8, 12]. Dermal and cerebral fibroblasts were used recently in the investigation of the possible role of protein kinase C in the fibroblasts-collagen compaction [9].

However, the mechanisms of spasmogen-induced compaction have not been clearly documented. Tyrosine kinases have shown to be involved in the contraction of peripheral smooth muscle either by activation of receptors or by opening of Ca^{2+} channels [1]. The role tyrosine kinases in endothelial [7] and smooth muscle cells [3, 5] have been described in our previous studies. This report demonstrated for the first time that hemolysate activated tyrosine kinases and increased collagen-lattice compaction in canine cerebral and human dermal fibroblasts. The participation of tyrosine kinases in the effect of hemolysate in fibroblasts was further supported by the effect of tyrosine kinase inhibitors genistein and tyrphostin A51. In this study, genistein and tyrphostin A51, two structurally different inhibitors, reduced the effect of hemolysate, indicating that the effect of genistein and tyrphostin A51 was probably not non-specific. The inhibitory effect of tyrphostin A51 in hemolysate induced tyrosine phosphorylation and lattice compaction was more pronounced when compared to genistein may indicate that different tyrosine kinases or isotypes were activated by hemolysate in the arteries. The differential effects between tyrphostin A51 and genistein are not unexpected since there are many forms of tyrosine kinases in cells and inhibitors such as tyrphostins have shown considerable differences in potency in their action against different tyrosine kinases or different isotypes [1].

It has been established that the etiology of cerebral vasospasm is subarachnoid blood clots. Spasmogenic substances released from subarachnoid blood clots include oxyhemoglobin and ATP [15]. Hemolysate has been shown to increase $[Ca^{2+}]_i$ in cerebral smooth muscle cells [13], and cerebral endothelial cells [14] and to produce contraction of cerebral arteries [10]. The effect of hemolysate on $[Ca^{2+}]_i$ mobilization has been suggested to be mediated, at least partly, by tyrosine kinase phosphorylation [3]. Hemolysate produced a dose-dependent increase in the level of tyrosine phosphorylation of two proteins approximately 70 and 110 kD in cultured smooth muscle cells [3] and in cultured bovine endothelial cells [7]. In this study, hemolysate produced a rapid and prolonged increase of tyrosine phosphorylation of two proteins, approximately 64 and 120 kD in canine basilar artery and human dermal fibroblast cells. Oxyhemoglobin and ATP each produced a smaller scaled but same bands of tyrosine phosphorylation in human dermal and canine basilar artery fibroblast cells.

The mechanism of hemolysate-induced tyrosine phosphorylation and lattice compaction is not clear. There are several possibilities. (a) Activation of G protein-coupled receptors either causes hydrolysis of inositol phospholipids by phospholipase C, or activation of tyrosine kinase, possibly by the $\beta\gamma$ subunits of heterotrimeric G proteins [1, 2]. Therefore, activation of G protein-coupled receptors may activate tyrosine kinases. (b) Oxyhemoglobin was suggested to activate tyrosine kinases [11] and may be involved in the effect of hemolysate since hemolysate contained oxyhemoglobin in this study. (c) In speculation, other molecules in hemolysate may contribute to tyrosine phosphorylation.

Conclusions

We conclude that hemolysate enhances tyrosine phosphorylation in canine cerebral and human dermal fibroblast cells. The effects of hemolysate were mediated by oxyhemoglobin, ATP and other unknown molecules. Elevated tyrosine phosphorylation may play a role in collagen compaction. The tyrosine kinase pathway may be involved not only in the contraction of smooth muscle cells but also in the compaction of fibroblasts. Thus, tyrosine kinases may be important in the pathogenesis of cerebral vasospasm and tyrosine kinase inhibitors may be useful in the management of cerebral vasospasm.

Acknowledgment

This work was partially supported by a grant-in-aid to J.H.Z. from the American Heart Association.

References

1. Di Salvo J, Kaplan N, Semenchuk LA (1996) Protein tyrosine phosphorylation and regulation of intracellular calcium in smooth muscle cells. In: Barany M(ed) Biochemistry of smooth muscle contraction. Academic Press, San Diego, pp 283–293
2. Hollenberg MD (1994) Tyrosine kinase pathways and the regulation of smooth muscle contractility. Trends Pharmacol Sci 15: 108–114
3. Iwabuchi S, Marton LS, Zhang J (1999) Tyrosine kinase mediated the effect of hemolysate on $[Ca^{2+}]_i$ in rat basilar smooth muscle cells. J Neurosurg 90: 127–135
4. Kassell NF, Sasaki T, Colohan AR, Nazar G (1985) Cerebral vasospasm following aneurysmal subarachnoid hemorrhage. Stroke 16: 562–572
5. Kim CJ, Kim KW, Park JW, Lee JC, Zhang J (1998) Role of tyrosine kinase in erythrocyte lysate-induced contraction of rabbit cerebral arteries. J Neurosurg 89: 289–296
6. MacDonald RL, Weir B (1994) Cerebral vasospasm and free radicals. Free Radical Biol Med 16: 633–643
7. Marton LS, Weir BKA, Zhang H (1996) Tyrosine phosphorylation and $[Ca^{2+}]_i$ elevation induced by hemolysate in bovine endothelial cells: Implications for cerebral vasospasm. Neurol Res 18: 349–353
8. Smith RR, Yamamoto Y, Bernanke DH, Clower BR (1990) Cerebrospinal fluid factors following SAH accelerate collagen lattice contraction by fibroblasts. Neurol Res 12: 41–44
9. Shiota T, Bernanke DH, Parent AD, Kouichi H (1996) Protein kinase C has two different major roles in lattice compaction enhanced by cerebrospinal fluid from patients with SAH. Stroke 27: 1889–1895
10. Sima B, MacDonald RL, Weir B, Marton LS, Zhang J (1996) Effect of P-purinoceptor antagonista on hemolysate and ATP induced contractions of dog basilar artery in vitro. Neurosurgery 39: 815–822
11. Vollrath B, Cook D, Megyesi J, Findlay JM, Ohkuma H (1998) Novel mechanism by which hemoglobin induces constriction of cerebral arteries. Eur J Pharmacol 361: 311–319
12. Yamamoto Y, Smith RR, Bernanke DH (1992) Accelerated

nonmuscle contraction after subarachnoid hemorrhage: culture and characterization of myofibroblasts from human cerebral arteries in vasospasm. Neurosurgery 3: 337–345

13. Zhang H, Weir B, Marton L, Macdonald, Bindokas V, Miller R & Brorson J (1995) Mechanisms of hemolysate induced calcium elevation in cerebral smooth muscle cells. Am J Physiol 269: H1874–1890
14. Zhang H, Weir B, MacDonald RL, Marton LS, Solenski N, Kwan A, Lee K (1996) Mechanisms of $[Ca^{2+}]_i$ elevation induced by erythrocyte components in endothelial cells. J Pharmacol Exp Ther 277: 1501–1509
15. Zhang H, Lewis A, Bernanke D, Zubkov A, Clower B (1998) Stroke – anatomy of a catastrophic event. Anat Rec (New Anat) 253: 58–63

Correspondence: John H. Zhang, M.D, Ph.D., Department of Neurosurgery, University of Mississippi Medical Center, 2500 North State Street, Jackson, Mississippi 39216-4505.

Acta Neurochir (2000) [Suppl] 76: 231–236

Toxin-Induced Vasogenic Cerebral Oedema in a Rat Model

M. N. Ghabriel[1], **C. Zhu**[1], **P. L. Reilly**[2], **P. C. Blumbergs**[3,4], **J. Manavis**[4], and **J. W. Finnie**[4]

[1] Department of Anatomical Sciences, University of Adelaide, Australia
[2] Department of Neurosurgery, University of Adelaide, Australia
[3] Department of Pathology, University of Adelaide, Australia
[4] Institute of Medical and Veterinary Science, Adelaide, Australia

Summary

Vasogenic cerebral oedema (VCO) was induced in Hooded Wistar rats by intraperitoneal injection of *Clostridium perfringens* type D epsilon prototoxin. Animals were killed, 1 h to 14 d postinjection, by perfusion fixation under general anaesthesia. VCO was detected by the presence of endogenous albumin in the brain, visualised by immunocytochemistry. As early as 1 h postinjection, albumin was detected in the walls of cerebral microvessels. Maximal diffuse leakage within the neural parenchyma was seen at 24 and 48 h and immunoreactivity was still present at 4 d. At 7 d only few foci were seen, and at 14 d albumin distribution was similar to that in controls. Ultrastructural assessment of the microvessels showed swelling of many astrocytic processes and abnormalities of the endothelial cells varying from swelling with loss of cytoplasmic organelles to cells showing increased electron density. Immunostaining for the endothelial barrier antigen (EBA) showed strongly immunoreactive vessels throughout normal brains. Experimental animals showed partial reduction in EBA expression, most evident at 24 and 48 h, with gradual recovery to normal by 14 d. The exact role that EBA plays in the intact BBB remains obscure.

Keywords: Blood-brain barrier; cerebral oedema; albumin; endothelial barrier antigen.

Introduction

Experimental evidence supports a causal relationship between blood-brain barrier (BBB) changes and the ensuing neuronal structural and functional perturbation in brain pathology. Human vasogenic cerebral oedema (VCO) secondary to breakdown of the BBB is believed to contribute to the morbidity and mortality resulting from head injury [10]. VCO may produce secondary insult in the brain by interfering with the microcirculation and by raising the intracranial pressure. The leakage of plasma proteins in the oedema fluid and the accumulation of neurotoxic substances such as glutamate may also contribute to the secondary insult [10].

The endothelial barrier antigen (EBA), a protein triplet of 30, 25 and 23.5 kDa, is specifically expressed by rat CNS endothelial cells (ECs) which possess barrier function [7, 11, 12]. A monoclonal antibody (anti-EBA) has been used to probe the distribution of the protein in the rat brain. In diseases associated with alteration in BBB permeability, the expression of EBA correlated with the state of the disease. In experimental allergic encephalomyelitis (EAE), anti-EBA labeling was abolished in brain vessels surrounded by inflammatory cells and in vessels located in residual lesions, but returned to normal levels after recovery from the acute phase [13]. In stab-wound of the brain, directly injured and adjacent vessels lacked EBA, but labelling with anti-EBA was restored after two weeks [11]. In oedema associated with spinal cord trauma, EBA expression was reduced, but returned to normal levels at 9 days [9]. Thus, the reduction in EBA expression as detected by immunocytochemistry appears to be a useful criterion for identifying sites of BBB disruption.

As part of a project to study the BBB we have been investigating a model for toxin-induced brain oedema in the rat. The *Clostridium Perfringens* (*Cl P*) type D epsilon toxin produces VCO in mice as detected by a significant increase in the water content of the brain [5]. The mechanism of action of the toxin is not fully understood. It has been shown that the toxin preferentially binds to the brain and that this binding is inhibited by prior injection of the prototoxin [8]. The prototoxin is an inactive form and is thought to compete with the toxin for certain presumed sites [8]. In the course of the investigation we employed the *Cl P* toxin and prototoxin. The prototoxin produced mild and reversible changes in the BBB and the expression of EBA, which are reported here.

Materials and Methods

Hooded Wistar rats (23 females and 20 males, 7–9 weeks old, 140–220 g) were studied. Experimental animals (n = 36) were injected intraperitoneally (i. p.) with a single dose of *Cl P* type D epsilon prototoxin (CSL Ltd, Victoria) diluted in distilled water (4 ml of 1:400, n = 9 or 1:500, n = 27). Control animals were either not injected (n = 5) or injected with an equal volume of the vehicle only (n = 2) with 24 h survival period. Animals were killed under pentobarbitone anaesthesia (Sagatal, 60 mg/kg) by cardiac perfusion with Dulbecco's phosphate buffered saline, followed by the fixative. Animals used for the ultrastructural study (n = 11) were fixed with 4% paraformaldehyde – 2% glutaraldehyde fixative in 0.1 M phosphate buffer. Tissue blocks from the brains were processed in Taab resin and ultrathin sections cut for electron microscopy. Animals used for the immunocytochemical study were fixed with 4% paraformaldehyde only, in 0.1 M phosphate buffer (n = 32). Brains were embedded in paraffin and 8 μm sections cut for light microscopy (LM). Experimental animals were killed at 1 h (n = 4), 6 h (n = 4), 9 h (n = 1), 12 h (n = 4), 18 h (n = 1), 24 h (n = 5), 48 h (n = 4), 4 d (n = 4), 7 d (n = 5), and 14 d (n = 4), postinjection.

Immunocytochemistry for endogenous albumin was used to investigate the development of VCO. LM sections were incubated overnight at 4 °C in a goat anti-rat albumin primary antibody (ICN Pharmaceuticals Inc., USA) at dilutions of 1:1000–1:3000 in 1% normal rabbit serum (NRS). A biotinylated rabbit anti-goat IgG secondary antibody (Vector Laboratories, USA) was used at a dilution of 1:500 in 1% NRS. For immunocytochemical detection of EBA in brain vessels, LM sections were incubated overnight at 4 °C in a monoclonal primary antibody to EBA (anti-EBA, SMI 71, Sternberger Monoclonals Inc., USA) diluted 1:3000 or 1:5000 in 1% normal horse serum (NHS). Sections were incubated in a biotinylated horse anti-mouse IgG secondary antibody (Vector Lab.) diluted 1:500 in 1% NHS. The secondary antibodies were detected using the avidin-biotin peroxidase method (ABC kit, Vector Lab.) and 3,3′-diaminobenzidine tetrahydrochloride with nickel enhancement. Negative controls included the omission of the primary antibody, or the primary and secondary antibodies.

Results

Positive immunoreactivity (IR) for endogenous albumin appeared as a black reaction product (Fig. 1). Immunostaining in controls generally showed faint IR in brain parenchyma (Fig. 1a), with the following observations. Firstly, certain brain regions showed small foci of weak IR for albumin. These foci were seen in the periventricular zone, hypothalamus, neurohypophysis, diencephalon, rostral midbrain, superior cerebellar peduncles and small areas in the floor of the fourth ventricle. Secondly, in the above regions, often some microvessels were highlighted by immunostaining of their walls. Thirdly, the white matter had a relatively higher IR compared to the grey matter.

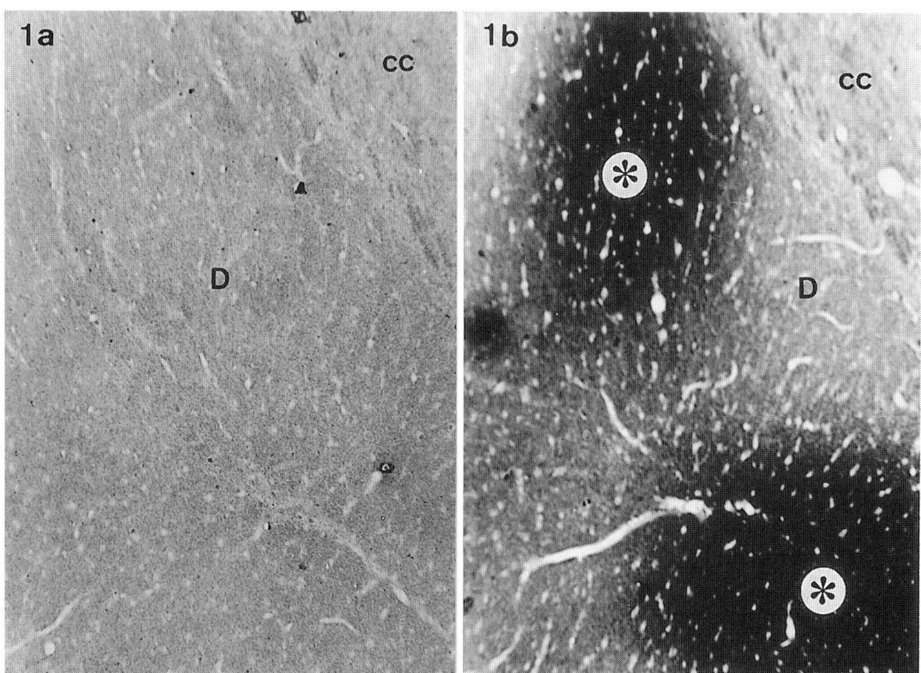

Fig. 1. (a, b) Light micrographs of brain sections from control (a) and experimental animal (b) injected with *Cl P* prototoxin 48 h previously, showing IR for albumin. In "b" increased IR is seen as black reaction product (asterisks) in the parenchyma. A faint IR is seen in "a" which was not seen in negative controls, not incubated with the primary antibody. *CC* Corpus callosum; *D* diencephalon. ×97

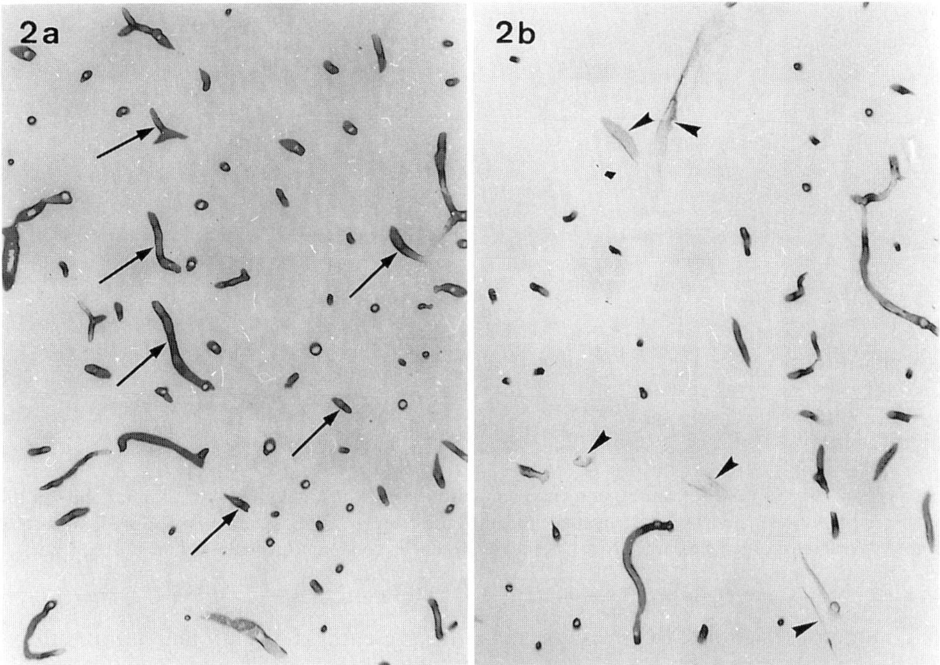

Fig. 2. (a, b) Light micrographs of brain sections from control (a) and experimental animal (b) injected with *Cl P* prototoxin 24 h previously, showing IR for EBA. Anti-EBA selectively stained brain vessels. In "a" microvessels are strongly IR (arrows). In "b" a general reduction in IR is seen in microvessels with many vessels showing pronounced loss of IR (arrowheads). ×195

Finally, the choroid plexus showed IR for albumin in the core of the plexus and in the cytoplasm of choroidal epithelium. Sections used as negative control by omission of the primary or the primary and secondary antibodies consistently showed complete absence of any reaction product.

Experimental animals showed dose- and time-dependent albumin leakage. However, at the 14 d time-interval, albumin distribution was similar to that seen in controls. As early as 1 h postinjection, in addition to the areas noted above in control material, blood vessel IR was seen in the frontal cortex, brainstem and cerebellar cortex at the depth of cerebellar fissures. Staining at 6, 9, 12 and 18 h was similar to 1 h, with the additional staining of the cytoplasm of many neurons and perivascular spaces and parenchyma. At 24 and 48 h, granular black reaction product was present throughout the brain (Fig. 1b). In addition, multiple foci of higher IR were apparent at low magnification. By 4 d there was a notable reduction in albumin IR and by 7 d only a small number of reactive foci was seen in the cerebrum and brainstem.

In control animals, immunostaining for EBA gave a dramatic demonstration of the extensive vascular bed of the brain (Fig. 2a). Microvessels in the grey and white matter were labelled and demonstrated the well known dense capillary network of the grey matter compared to the wider mesh of vessels in the white matter. Vessels were seen in longitudinal, transverse and oblique views with branching patterns. Medium-sized vessels in the parenchyma and pia mater showed strong labelling at the plane of the intima. Larger cerebral vessels in the subarachnoid space showed discontinuous intimal labelling. Some vessels in the choroid plexus and neurohypophysis were also labelled. Neurons and glia were unstained.

In experimental animals, none of the time intervals examined showed complete elimination of EBA expression in brain vessels. At 1–18 h, examination of the blood vessels revealed an increasing number of less reactive or non-reactive vessels. At 24 and 48 h sections showed a general reduction of labelling intensity throughout the brain (Fig. 2b). At 4 and 7 d although unstained vessels were not difficult to find, the majority of vessels were strongly IR. By 14 d post-injection, the staining pattern appeared similar to controls.

A continuum of ultrastructural changes was seen from 1 h to 14 d, with maximal changes seen at 48 h (Fig. 3). At each time interval a range of EC changes was seen among vessels in the same section and in the same vascular profile. Ultrastructural changes (Fig. 3)

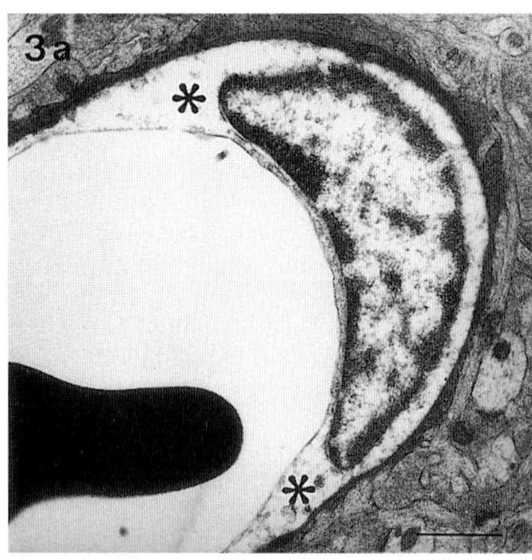

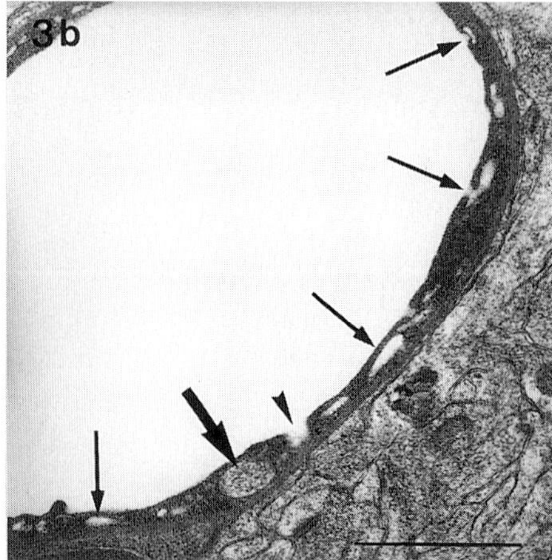

Fig. 3. (a, b) Electron micrographs of brain cortical vessels, from experimental animals injected with *Cl P* prototoxin 24 h (a) and 4 d (b) previously. ECs show swelling and loss of organelles (asterisks) or attenuated electron dense cytoplasm with several vesicles (small arrows), a deep crater (arrowhead), and presumed degenerated organelle (large arrow). Some of the vesicles communicate with the lumen. Bar, 1 μm

included: increased microvilli, numerous vacuoles, EC swelling, degenerated organelles, deep craters, thickened basal lamina, and subendothelial clefts detaching ECs from the basal lamina and pericytes. Intercellular junctions (ICJs) on the whole remained apposed, although some showed focal widening. Occasional EC channels were seen. Some ECs had electron dense attenuated cytoplasm. At 7 d many of the described changes were still apparent. At 14 d many ECs had not resumed the normal appearance and some retained a large number of vesicles. Pericytes showed large vacuoles.

Discussion

To our knowledge, there is no previous report in the literature of a study on the BBB in the rat using *Cl P* prototoxin. In the current study, animals injected i.p. with the prototoxin showed mild rapid opening of the BBB and demonstrated morphologically diffuse leakage of plasma proteins in brain parenchyma, ultrastructural changes in ECs and partial reduction in EBA expression in brain ECs. Recovery was noted by 14 d as indicated by reversal of the above changes. Thus the use of *Cl P* prototoxin as a sublethal agent appears to be a useful model for the induction of reversible generalised VCO in the rat.

Endogenous albumin is a naturally occurring macromolecule, and its distribution in CNS parenchyma may be used as an indicator of oedema [3]. One h after i.p. injection of *Cl P* prototoxin in rats, the walls of many blood vessels were IR for endogenous albumin, suggesting the presence of the protein intramurally. Such a rapid effect was also noted in a previous study of whole brains of mice injected with the active toxin, where 1.5% of injected ^{125}I-human serum albumin entered the brain within 3 min [16]. In mice, the toxin preferentially binds to the brain and the binding is inhibited by prior injection of prototoxin [8]. Using ^{125}I labelling, maximum binding of the toxin to the brain occurred 30 s after its i.v. injection. It was suggested that the *Cl P* toxin binds to presumed receptor sites in the brain and the same sites are competitively inhibited by the prototoxin [8]. The protective effect of the prototoxin was found to be only effective in the first 10 min after its injection, despite being detected in the whole brain by radiolabelling for at least 60 min. It was concluded that the prototoxin is internalised into cells in the brain, so that after 10 min the receptor sites become free to bind to the toxin [8].

EC ultrastructural features which are thought to contribute to extravasation of albumin, differ according to the aetiology of BBB breakdown [15]. Knowledge of ultrastructural changes in ECs, albumin permeability at the BBB and molecular anatomy of brain microvessels [2] is valuable to our understanding of BBB mechanisms. Previous studies on mice injected with a lethal dose of *Cl P* toxin, reported rapid ultrastructural changes indicating vascular endothelial damage [4, 5]. In the current study in the rat, at 1 h following *Cl P* prototoxin injection, as a sublethal dose, minimal ultrastructural changes in ECs were noted. At later time-intervals, some ECs showed swelling, reduced organelles and vacuoles, while others showed shrinkage and increased electron density of their cytoplasm and nuclei. These ultrastructural findings together with leakage of plasma proteins seen in this study of prototoxin, and the speed of toxin binding reported in previous studies [8] lead the authors to suggest that the effect of the toxin and prototoxin is primarily on EC and that the binding sites suggested by previous studies are located on ECs. The ultrastructural changes noted in perivascular astrocytic processes might indicated an additional effect of the prototoxin on astrocytes. Disturbance of astrocyte biology may further compromise BBB integrity [6].

EBA is a biochemical marker of the BBB [2, 12]. The exact function of EBA is not known. Its significance in the normal BBB is deduced from its strong expression by brain barrier vessels, but weak or no expression by non-barrier vessels (7, 12, 13, this study). Experimental evidence supports an inverse relationship between permeability and the level of expression of EBA. In EAE [13] and stab-wound injury of the brain [11], EBA expression is lost in vessels with compromised barrier function. However, some aspects of EBA expression hinder a conclusive account of its function. Firstly, we have found that some vessels in the choroid plexus and neurohypophysis, which are considered to lie outside the BBB, express EBA. Secondly, EBA is weakly expressed or absent in endoneurial vessels at the blood-nerve barrier [7]. Thirdly, EBA expression by brain vessels is a postnatal event [11], whereas the barrier properties of these vessels are established prenatally [14]. EBA is specific to the rat BBB [12]. We have found that anti-EBA does not stain blood vessels of sheep or human brains (unpublished observation). The BBB in species other than the rat may have a corresponding protein, with similar function to EBA, but different amino acid sequence and epitopes.

It is not known if the loss of EBA leads to a breakdown in the BBB or whether the reverse is true. At 1 h post-toxin injection, there was evidence of mild albumin leakage and a small degree of loss of EBA immunoreactivity. At 48 h time-interval, maximal leakage of albumin was seen and was associated with the lowest level of EBA expression. At 4, 7 and 14 d progressive reduction in albumin leakage accompanied progressive restitution of EBA expression. Since the alterations in EBA expression and albumin leakage seen in this study represent a continuum of changes, it was not possible to conclude which precedes the other.

The factors which lead to the disappearance and reexpression of EBA in this study are not known. Whether the loss of EBA expression is due to (a) a direct effect of *Cl P* prototoxin on ECs, (b) an indirect effect on ECs via perturbation of astrocytes [6], (c) a consequence of the development of vasogenic oedema or (d) a combination of the above is speculative. Other experimental models, such as EAE [13], angiogenesis following stab-wound injury of the brain [11] and spinal cord trauma [3, 9] also show reduction of EBA expression during the acute phase of the pathology followed by restoration of the expression to normal levels in a similar pattern to that noted in the current study. All the above models show cerebral oedema associated with the pathology. Thus, it is feasible to suggest that the changes in the expression of EBA are a consequence of the development of cerebral oedema. An alternative hypothesis is that all the above models lead to a certain EC dysfunction which is a 'final common pathway' leading to a reduction in EBA expression and secondary development of cerebral oedema.

Acknowledgment

We wish to thank Mrs. Gail Hermanis, Mrs. Nadia Gagliardi, Mr. Chris Leigh and Dr Damien Kent for advice and assistance. C Zhu is supported by a University of Adelaide grant and is a holder of an "Overseas Postgraduate Research Scholarship".

Abbreviations

BBB Blood-Brain Barrier
Cl P *Clostridium perfringens*
VCO Vasogenic Cerebral Oedema
EBA Endothelial Barrier Antigen
EC(s) Endothelial Cell(s)
ICJ(s) Intercellular Junction(s)
IR Immunoreactive, Immunoreactivity

References

1. Cassella JP, Lawrenson JG, Allt G, Firth JA (1996) Ontogeny of four blood-brain barrier markers: an immunocytochemical comparison of pial and cerebral cortical microvessels. J Anat 189: 407–415
2. Dermietzel R, Krause D (1991) Molecular anatomy of the blood-brain barrier as defined by immunocytochemistry. Int Rev Cytol 127: 57–109
3. Farooque M, Zhang Yi, Holtz A, Olsson Y (1992) Exudation of fibronectin and albumin after spinal cord injury in rats. Acta Neuropathol 84: 613–620
4. Finnie JW (1984) Ultrastructural changes in the brain of mice given *Clostridium perfringens* type D epsilon toxin. J Comp Path 94: 445–452
5. Gardner DE (1974) Brain oedema: an experimental model. Br J Exp Path 55: 453–457

6. Janzer RC (1993) The blood-brain barrier: cellular basis. J Inher Metab Dis 16: 639–647
7. Lawrenson JG, Ghabriel MN, Reid AR, Gajree TN, Allt G (1995) Differential expression of an endothelial barrier antigen between the CNS and the PNS. J Anat 186: 217–221
8. Nagahama M, Sakurai J (1991) Distribution of labeled *Clostridium perfringens* epsilon toxin in mice. Toxicon 29: 211–217
9. Perdiki M, Farooque M, Holtz A, Li GL and Olsson Y (1998) Expression of endothelial barrier antigen immunoreactivity in blood vessels following compression trauma to rat spinal cord. Temporal evolution and relation to the degree of the impact. Acta Neuropathol 96: 8–12
10. Povlishock JT and Dietrich WD (1992) The blood-brain barrier in brain injury: an overview. In: Globus M, Dietrich WD (eds) The role of neurotransmitters in brain injury. Plenum Press, New York
11. Rosenstein JM, Krum JM, Sternberger LA, Pulley MT, Sternberger NH (1992) Immunocytochemical expression of the endothelial barrier antigen (EBA) during brain angiogenesis. Dev Brain Res 66: 47–54
12. Sternberger NH, Sternberger LA (1987) Blood-brain barrier protein recognized by monoclonal antibody. Proc Natl Acad Sci USA 84: 8169–8173
13. Sternberger NH, Sternberger LA, Kies MW, Shear CR (1989) Cell surface endothelial proteins altered in experimental allergic encephalomyelitis. J Neuroimmunol 21: 241–248
14. Stewart PA, Hayakawa K (1994) Early ultrastructural changes in blood-brain barrier vessels of the rat embryo. Dev Brain Res 78: 25–34
15. Vorbrodt AW, Lossinsky AS, Dobrogowska DH, Wisniewski HM (1993) Cellular mechanisms of the blood-brain barrier (BBB) opening to albumin-gold complex. Histol Histopath 8: 51–61
16. Worthington RW, Mülders MSG (1975) The effect of *Clostridium perfringens* epsilon toxin on the blood brain barrier of mice. Onderstepoort J Vet Res 42: 25–28

Correspondence: Dr. M. N. Ghabriel, Department of Anatomical Sciences, The University of Adelaide, Frome Road, Adelaide, South Australia 5005.

Experimental Ischaemia

Sato *et al.* report the function of WATER CHANNELS of which there are 6 in mammalian cells. One of these, the AQ4 water channel, is affected by the expression of mRNA, which is decreased after ischaemia. The water content of tissues [modified by aquaporin inhibitors] may affect PtiO2 levels. Also, Rossi *et al.* showed that PtiO2 did not correspond to oxygen delivery in conditions of critical ischaemia in their swine model of CPP reduction. This interplay of factors was also reported by Matsushita *et al.* who showed that high potassium levels produced a larger increase in glutamate with ischaemia. Kempski *et al.* studied spreading depression in penumbra-like conditions and showed that it was associated with oedema and that the extent was time dependent. Friedrich *et al.* have shown that focal necrosis, induced with a cold lesion, reduces CBF which improves with infusion therapy. In a focal middle cerebral artery occlusion model Davis *et al.* have shown that proteolytic enzymes do not play a significant role in the ischaemic process.

Diffusion weighted MRI was used in experimental conditions to show that early cytotoxic oedema [measured by ADC] *does* play a role in TBI especially if associated with secondary insults. Park *et al.* have quantified the volume effect that occurs with ischaemic oedema.

The effect of reperfusion on oedema needs careful interpretation. In a cold lesion model of VASOGENIC OEDEMA there was an increase in CBF with infusion therapy but this did not prevent necrosis (Friederich *et al.*). In a Middle Cerebral Artery Occlusion (MCAO) model of CYTOTOXIC OEDEMA in the aging rat, Kattner *et al.* showed that intermittent reperfusion increased infarct volume. These models may not be representative of the clinical situation where early oligaemia can be reversed with early reperfusion.

Acta Neurochir (2000) [Suppl] 76: 239–241

Expression of Water Channel mRNA Following Cerebral Ischemia

S. Sato[1], **F. Umenishi**[2], **G. Inamasu**[1], **M. Sato**[1], **M. Ishikawa**[1], **M. Nishizawa**[1], and **T. Oizumi**[1]

[1] Center for Neurological Diseases, International University of Health and Welfare, Tochigi, Japan
[2] Department of Physiology, Cardiovascular Center, University of California San Francisco, USA

Summary

Water channel is a protein which regulates transcellular water permeability. Among mRNA expression of six principal mammalian water channels, AQ4 mRNA expression was highest in the brain. Water channels are supposed to regulate cerebral edema but the detailed physiological and pathological function is unknown. Brain edema has been analyzed as an aspect of ion channel injury or membrane injury. However the transportation of water molecule itself following cerebral ischemia is unknown. As water channels transport only water molecules, the functional changes of water channels following cerebral ischemia are of great interest. To evaluate the role of water channels in cerebral edema following cerebral ischemia, the changes of water channel mRNA expression were evaluated. Cerebral edema was induced by suture method. The extraction of water channel mRNA was performed according to Chomczynsli and Sacchi. RT-PCR was applied to extracted mRNA. Water channel mRNA electrophoresis was performed. For semi-quantified evaluation of water channel, mRNA intensities of the infarct hemisphere and normal hemisphere were compared. The expression of water channel mRNA was decreased following cerebral ischemia. This damage leads to loose physiological control of water permeability of the cell membrane in the neuron, glia and endothelial cells which leads to brain edema.

Keywords: Aquaporin 4; blood-brain barrier; brain edema; water channel.

Introduction

The homeostasis of water and electrolyte is important for cellular environment in the brain. Water metabolism plays a great role in the cerebral function in either physiological or pathological state. Various energy insufficiency induce neuronal and glial damages, as well as edema and BBB disruption [1] and this BBB disruption deteriorates clinical symptoms. In the acute stage of cerebral infarction, one of the main goals to treat the patient is to minimize the cerebral edema. Water metabolism in the brain has been studied for a long time, but the detailed molecular mechanism of water transportation is unknown.

Water molecules can pass through the cell membrane by simple diffusion, but it was found that human erythrocyte had a high water permeability which can not be explained by simple diffusion. It has been discussed that the water molecule passes through an aqueous pore transversing the membrane or passes through an active channel selectively. Water channel is found in erythrocytes and is cloned as Aquaporin 1 (CHIP28 or AQ1) [2, 3, 45].

Water channel is a protein which regulates transcellular water permeability and transports only the water molecule. Water channel family members have been cloned and six water channels (AQ 0 $\sim$ 6) have been reported [6, 7]. Fourth mammalian members of the aquaporin water channel family, AQ4. showed the highest expression in brain [8]. This water channel is supposed to regulate cerebral edema or cerebrospinal fluid metabolism [9, 10]. But the detailed physiological and pathological function is unknown. To elucidate the water channel function following cerebral ischemia, AQ4 water channel mRNA expression following cerebral ischemia was analyzed.

Methods and Materials

Male Sprague-Dawley rats (Bantin and Kingman, Fremont, CA) weighing 190–210 gm were anesthetized with xylazine (4 mg/kg) and chloral hydrate (350 mg/kg). Until the pedal and corneal reflexes were no longer responsive. If the pedal or corneal reflex returned prior to completion of the procedure, more intraperitoneal xylazine was administered at 1/2 the initial dose and the procedure stopped until the pedal and corneal reflexes were gone. To induce cerebral infarction, the suture method was employed. After the separation of common, internal and external carotid arteries, a 4-0 nylon suture was retrogradely inserted from the external carotid artery to the internal carotid artery about 22 mm. Brains were removed at 30 minutes, 6 hours and 24 hours after cerebral ischemia (n = 4), separated in the midline infarct and normal hemispheres were homogenized in 4 M guanidine thiocyanate, followed by phenol/chloroform extraction. After centrifugation(12000 G, 10 min., 4 °C), total RNA was collected in the aqueous phase and precipitated. The RNA was recovered by centrifugation, and the pellet was resuspended in guanidine thiocyanate solution and precipitated. The RNA pellet was resuspended in diethyl pyrocarbonate-treated water, and RNA content and purity were assessed by absorbance at 260 nm and 280 nm. RNA aliquots (30 μg) were stored at −80 °C for further assay [11]. One microgram of total RNA was reverse-transcribed using random hexamer primers and reverse transcriptase (GIBCO laboratory, Grand Island, NY). The reverse-transcribed cDNA was amplified by PCR using primers specific for AQ4, nucleotides 235–572. The PCR amplification was performed for 30 cycles under the following conditions: denaturation at 94 °C for 30 sec. PCR products, 5 μg/lane were loaded onto a 1.8% agarose gel containing ethidium bromide (0.3 g/ml) and electrophoresed at 90 V for 2 hours. The mRNA was visualized and photographed using ultraviolet transillumination (300 nm wavelength). Water channel mRNA expression in infarct and normal hemispheres were evaluated semi-quantitively by NIH image analysis.

Results

The water channel mRNA expression in the infarct area was slightly attenuated at 30 minutes and 6 hours after ischemia compared to normal hemisphere but remarkably decreased at 24 hours after ischemia (Fig. 1).

Discussion

Postischemic brain swelling is a common consequence of membrane dysfunction and damage [12]. It is also considered that BBB disruption plays a great role in the progression of cerebral ischemia. It is supposed that endothelial damage leads to vasogenic edema and glia and neuronal damage induce the cytotoxic edema. But the exact molecular mechanisms for sensing changes in extracellular osmolality and regulating water balance in the pathological state is unknown.

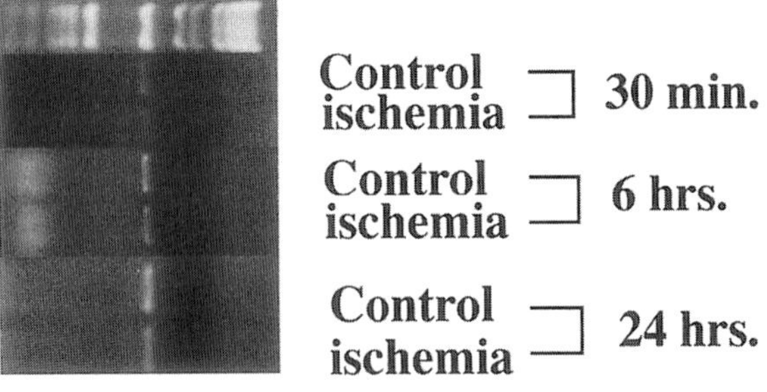

Fig. 1. The electrophoresis of water channel mRNA of infarct and normal hemisphere following 30 min., 6 and 24 hours after ischemia. The expression of water channel mRNA at 30 min., 6 and 24 hours after ischemia is decreased to compare the control hemisphere

The aquaporins transport only water molecules through membranes of numerous tissues [10]. The water channel monomers associate to form tetrameric structures around the 4-fold axes normal to the membrane [13, 14]. As AQ4 mRNA expression was highest in the brain [8, 15], AQ4 is supposed to regulate the osmoreceptor which regulates body water balance and mediates water flow within the central nervous system [9, 10]. The functional role of water channel expression in the neuromuscular system is uncertain but the tissue-specific expression of water channel suggests a role in fluid transport and/or cell volume in brain [8, 15]. Water channels, transporting only water molecules, are important to elucidate the mechanism of edema formation following cerebral ischemia.

In this experiment, water channel mRNA expression was reduced after cerebral ischemia. It is supposed that the active regulation of water molecule transports decreased. This result indicated that the physiological control of the water molecule by the water channel was disturbed progressively and water molecule passed through the damaged ion channel passively.

The factors leading to water channel suppression remain unclear but from our result some mechanism can be speculated. First, the direct energy failure reduces water channel in the endothelial cell. Second, water channel formation is disturbed as the result of general protein synthesis disturbances. It was shown that water channels are localized in basolateral membranes of the brain and it was strongly expressed in the ependymal layer lining the aqueductal system, endothelial cell, and in astrocytes [8, 15]. After ischemia, energy insufficiency in the endothelial cells induces BBB disruption(endothelial injury) and water channel distribution is high in the astrocyte and endothelial cells. It is suspected that BBB disruption is the result of releasing the foot of the astrocyte from BBB due to the suppression of water channel in endothelial astrocyte. Damaged endothelial water channel (BBB disruption) eventually induces vasogenic edema and direct energy failure to the water channel of neuron or glia induces cytotoxic edema.

Water channel suppression in 30 min. following ischemia is attributed to the effect of direct energy failure of the water channel in the endothelial cells. But a significant decrease of water channels following cerebral ischemia were observed 24 hours after ischemia. BBB breakdown may result in the extravasation of plasma components which either directly or indirectly injure cells via the induction of superoxide anion or releasing glutamate by damaged cell excitation. This delay may account for the mechanism of BBB disruption at 24 hours after ischemia and is due to secondary excitotoxicity of the superoxide anion or glutamate.

Brain edema is considered as a homeostatic response and seems to compensate the damaged energy support by enlarging the third space [16]. It is unknown whether the water channel suppression is the result of a compensative failure for damaged ion channels or some active response to regulate water balance following cerebral ischemia.

As the brain edema is related to the susceptibility of the brain region to BBB disruption [17, 18] and the water channels are expressed in glia more than in neuron, this may explain the greater contribution of glia to brain edema then by the neurons. It is thought that neurons are the most vulnerable to injury followed by glia and then endothelial cells.

Furthermore, an apoptotic process was detected in energy failure [19, 20, 21]. This indicates that the functional changes of water channel distorts apoptosis.

In conclusion, mild water channel mRNA suppression is an early event followed by profound water channel mRNA suppression after cerebral ischemia. We speculate that the water channel mRNA expression is damaged due to direct energy failure in the early stage and secondary excitotoxicity of the superoxide anion or glutamate in the late stage. This damage leads to loose physiological control of water permeability of the cell membrane in the neuron, glia and endothelial cells which induces brain edema.

References

1. Ito U, Go KG, Walker Jr, JT, Spatz M, Klatzo I (1976) Experimental cerebral ischemia in Mongolian gerbils III. Behaviour of the blood-brain barrier. Acta Neuropathol (Berl) 34: 1–6
2. Hasegawa H, Ma T, Skach W, Matthay MA, Verkman AS (1994) Molecular cloning of a mercurial-insensitive water channel expressed in selected water-transporting tissues. J Biol Chem 269: 5497–5500
3. Preston GM and Agre P (1991) Isolation of the cDNA for erythrocyte integral membrane protein of 28 kilodaltons: member of an ancient channel family. Proc Natl Acad Sci U S A 88: 11110–11114
4. Preston GM, Jung JS, Guggino WB, Agre P (1993) The mercury-sensitive residue at cysteine 189 in the CHIP28 water channel. J Biol Chem 268: 17–20
5. Smith BL, Baumgarten R, Nielsen S, Raben D, Zeidel ML, Agre P (1993) Concurrent expression of erythroid and renal aquaporin CHIP and appearance of water channel activity in perinatal rats [see comments]. J Clin Invest 92: 2035–2041
6. Agre P, Nielsen S (1996) The aquaporin family of water channels in kidney. Nephrologie 17: 409–415
7. King LS, Agre P (1996) Pathophysiology of the aquaporin water channels. Annu Rev Physiol 58: 619–648
8. Umenishi F, Verkman AS, Gropper MA (1996) Quantitative analysis of aquaporin mRNA expression in rat tissues by RNase protection assay. DNA Cell Biol 15: 475–480
9. Nielsen S, Arnulf Nagelhus E, Amiry-Moghaddam M, Bourque C, Agre P, Petter Ottersen O (1997) Specialized membrane domains for water transport in glial cells: high-resolution immunogold cytochemistry of aquaporin-4 in rat brain. J Neurosci 17: 171–180
10. Jung JS, Bhat RV, Preston GM, Guggino WB, Baraban JM, Agre P (1994) Molecular characterization of an aquaporin cDNA from brain: candidate osmoreceptor and regulator of water balance. Proc Natl Acad Sci USA 91: 13052–13056
11. Chomczynski P, Sacchi N (1987) Single-step method of RNA isolation by acid guanidinium thiocyanate-phenol-chloroform extraction. Anal Biochem 162: 156–159
12. Chan PH, Schmidley JW, Fishman RA, Longar SM (1984) Brain injury, edema, and vascular permeability changes induced by oxygen-derived free radicals. Neurology 34: 315–320
13. Mitra AK, Yeager M, van Hoek AN, Wiener MC, Verkman AS (1994) Projection structure of the CHIP28 water channel in lipid bilayer membranes at 12-A resolution. Biochemistry 33: 12735–12740
14. Mitra AK, van Hoek AN, Wiener MC, Verkman AS, Yeager M (1995) The CHIP28 water channel visualized in ice by electron crystallography [letter]. Nat Struct Biol 2: 726–729
15. Frigeri A, Gropper MA, Umenishi F, Kawashima M, Brown D, Verkman AS (1995) Localization of MIWC and GLIP water channel homologs in neuromuscular, epithelial and glandular tissues. J Cell Sci 108: 2993–3002
16. Suga S, Sato S, Yunoki K, Mihara B (1994) Sequential change of brain edema by semiquantitative measurement on MRI in patients with hypertensive intracerebral hemorrhage. Acta Neurochir [Suppl] (Wien) 60: 564–567
17. Sato S, Toya S, Ohtani M, Suga S, Harada S, Ikeda Y (1990) Effect of blood-brain barrier disruption on the permeability of peritumoral edema. Adv Neurol 52: 555
18. Sato S, Suga S, Yunoki K, Mihara B (1994) Effect of barrier opening on brain edema in human brain tumors. Acta Neurochir [Suppl] (Wien) 60: 116–118
19. Sato S, Gobbel GT, Li Y, Kondo T, Murakami K, Sato M, Hasegawa K, Copin JC, Honkaniemi J, Sharp FR, Chan PH (1997) Blood-brain barrier disruption, HSP70 expression and apoptosis due to 3-nitropropionic acid, a mitochondrial toxin. Acta Neurochir [Suppl] (Wien) 70: 237–239
20. Sato S, Gobbel GT, Honkaniemi J, Li Y, Kondo T, Murakami K, Sato M, Copin JC, Chan PH (1997) Apoptosis in the striatum of rats following intraperitoneal injection of 3-nitropropionic acid. Brain Res 745: 343–347
21. Sato S, Gobbel GT, Honkaniemi J, Li Y, Kondo T, Murakami K, Sato M, Copin JC, Sharp FR, Chan PH (1998) Decreased expression of bcl-2 and bcl-x mRNA coincides with apoptosis following intracerebral administration of 3-nitropropionic acid. Brain Res 808: 56–64

Correspondence: Shuzo Sato, M.D., Center for Neurological Diseases, International University of Health and Welfare, Iguchi 537-3, Nishinasunomachi, Nasugun, Tochigi, Japan 329-2763.

Acta Neurochir (2000) [Suppl] 76: 243–245

Brain Oxygen Tension During Hyperoxia in a Swine Model of Cerebral Ischaemia

S. Rossi[1], **L. Longhi**[1], **M. Balestreri**[2], **D. Spagnoli**[3], **A. deLeo**[2], and **N. Stocchetti**[1]

[1] Department of Anaesthesia and Intensive Care, Ospedale Maggiore Policlinico IRCCS, Milano, Italy
[2] Department of Anaesthesia and Intensive Care and Experimental Surgery of Pavia University, Policlinico S. Matteo IRCCS, Pavia, Italy
[3] Institute of Neurosurgery, Ospedale Maggiore Policlinico IRCCS, Milano, Italy

Summary

Arterial hyperoxia improves oxygen tension measured into the cerebral tissue (ptiO2). The extent of this improvement in ameliorating O2 delivery to the cerebral tissue, when cerebral blood flow (CBF) is reduced, is still unclear. The present experiment was developed to investigate the effect of arterial hyperoxia at normal or reduced CBF (baseline, CBF = 50–60%, and CBF = 20–30% of the baseline). CBF reduction was achieved in 7 pigs by saline infusion in a lateral ventricle. PtiO2 was measured by Licox equipment. Artero-venous oxygen difference (AVDO2) was calculated as the difference between arterial oxygen content and superior sagittal sinus oxygen content. Hyperoxia was induced by increasing inspired oxygen fraction to 100%. PtiO2 moved respectively from 27.95(±10.15) to 45.98 (±15.31), from 14.77 (±3.58) to 30.71 (±12.2), and from 3.45 (±2.89) to 11.1 (±12.6) mmHg at normal CBF, after the first reduction and after the second reduction. O2 supply showed only a negligible increase. AVDO2 decreased during the phases of intact and moderate CBF impairment, while it did not change during the phase of severe CBF impairment. In conclusion: an increase of ptiO2 does not necessarily correspond to an improvement of brain oxygen delivery. The small increase in oxygen delivery due to hyperoxia may cause a slight improvement in the balance between O2 delivery and consumption during mild CBF reduction, but such improvement is negligible when severe CBF reduction occurs.

Keywords: Brain oxygenation; ptiO2; ischaemia; hyperoxia.

Introduction

The ultimate purpose of clinical interventions in acute cerebral damage is the restoration of adequate cerebral oxygenation. Recently a great interest has arisen in the investigation of arterial hyperoxia to restore normal or supranormal values of brain oxygen tension (ptiO2) [3]. Our group developed a swine model of stepwise reduction of cerebral blood flow (CBF). The model was designed to achieve three steps of stable CBF values: the first with intact CBF, the second with a mild CBF reduction and the third with a severe CBF impairment; in each of these steps brain oxygen tension, oxygen delivery and artero-venous oxygen content difference (AVDO2) could be investigated. The goal of our investigation was to quantify whether the increase in paO2 and consequently in ptiO2, seen after ventilation with pure oxygen, represented an improvement in oxygen supply to the brain during phases of decreased CBF; thus whether the increase in O2 tension achieved by hyperoxia meant a real advantage for the brain in terms of volumes of O2 delivered to the brain itself.

Materials and Methods

In performing the experiments, the Authors followed the guidelines for animal research published by the European Union and acknowledged by the Italian legislation in law n° 116/92. Seven 8-week-old domestic pigs, weighing 18–22 Kg were used. The model has been previously extensively described. Briefly, it was developed to obtain progressive CBF reduction through 3 stable steps: baseline (CBF = 100%), CBF between 50–60% of the baseline, 3. CBF < 30% of the baseline. CBF reduction was accomplished by infusing saline in the left lateral ventricle through a 22 G catheter connected with an infusion pump. The velocity of infusion was titrated to maintain stable values of intracranial pressure (ICP), cerebral perfusion pressure (CPP) and CBF during each step. Cushing response, elicited by ICP increase, was inhibited by the infusion of β-blockers.

During each step of the experiment an hyperoxia test was performed by increasing inspired oxygen fraction from 30 to 100%. Hyperoxia was maintained until a steady state of ptiO2 was reached. Before, during and after hyperoxia, simultaneous blood samples were drawn from the arterial line and from the superior sagittal sinus in order to calculate AVDO2 and brain oxygen delivery. The latter was extrapolated by multiplying arterial oxygen content and the relative change of CBF measured by laser doppler flowmetry, assuming that the intact CBF corresponded to a value of 50 ml/100 g/min. AVDO2 was calculated as follow: arterial oxygen content–superior sagittal sinus oxygen content.

Table 1. *ICP, MAP and paCO2 Modifications During Hyperoxia in the Three Phases of the Experiment. Differences were not Statistically Significant*

	MAP mmHg		ICP mmHg		PaCO2 mmHg	
Hyperoxia	Normoxia	Hyperoxia		Normoxia	Hyperoxia	Normoxia
CBF 100%	107.8 (13.8)	110 (14.6)	8 (3.1)	7.3 (4.2)	38.2 (3.2)	36.4 (5.59)
CBF 50–60%	91.42 (12.7)	89.2 (14.6)	38.5 (6.5)	36.4 (6.77)	37.1 (3.07)	37.4 (4.11)
CBF 20–30%	75.28 (14.6)	74.1 (17.7)	45 (10)	45.5 (12.9)	37.7 (1.97)	39.8 (3.5)

Results

Due to the saline infusion in the ventricular system, cerebral perfusion pressure (CPP) decreased from 100 (±14.8) mmHg, to 53 (±11.2) mmHg and to 30 (±10.4) mmHg in the three phases of the experiment. CBF was parallel to the CPP reduction, as it was intact in the first stage, decreased to 50–60% of the baseline in the second and decreased to 20–30% during the third one. Intracranial and extracranial parameters, which may have influenced the response to hyperoxia, remained stable during the test. PaO2 increments caused by ventilation with pure oxygen, were not different during the three phases of the experiment, (intact, moderately reduced, and severely impaired CBF) (Table 1). PaO2 moved respectively from 120 (±19.9) to 485 (±55.3), from 121 (±24.55) to 466.6 (±83.2) and from 113 (±26.8) to 509 (±33.7) mmHg. Hyperoxia always caused a ptiO2 increase, as it moved respectively from 27.95 (±10.15) to 45.98 (±15.31), from 14.77 (±3.58) to 30.71 (±12.2), and from 3.45 (±2.89) to 11.1 (±12.6) mmHg. To clarify whether the increase of ptiO2 due to hyperoxia reflected an increase of oxygen supply, the latter was calculated by multiplying the arterial oxygen content by the relative value of the measured CBF. Compared with the huge increase in ptiO2, O2 supply showed only a negligible raise as shown in Fig. 1 (upper part).

In order to establish if the ptiO2 increase following hyperoxia had an impact on the coupling between oxygen supply and consumption, AVDO2 values were compared, respectively during normo and hyperoxia for the 3 CBF levels. AVDO2 changes are shown in Fig. 1 (lower part).

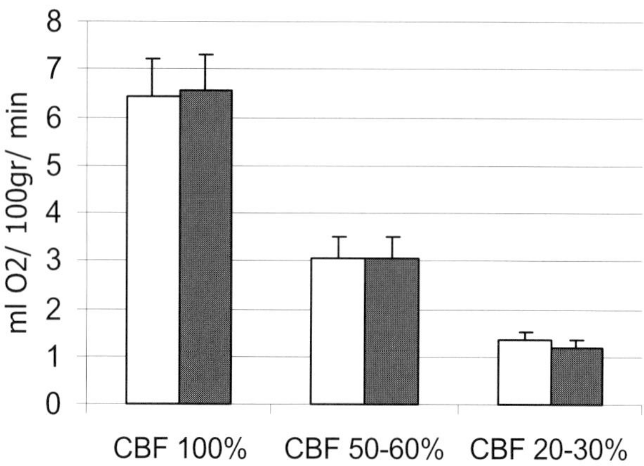

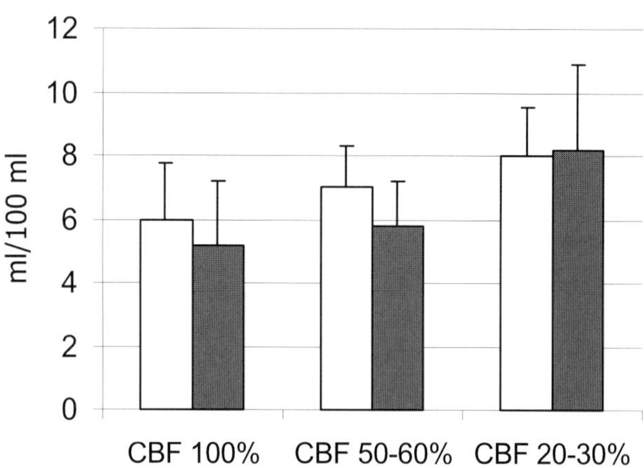

Fig. 1. O2 delivery (upper) and AVDO2 during normoxia and hyperoxia. ■ Normoxia, □ Hyperoxia

Discussion

The degree of increase in ptiO2 seen after ventilation with supranormal O2 concentrations has been used as an indirect method to explore the pathophysiology of ptiO2 [2]; besides ptiO2 reactivity to arterial oxygen tension seems to have a prognostic value, since it has been shown that an high reactivity during the first 24 hours after human head injury is associated with an higher rate of mortality [4]. Recently, it has been shown that arterial hyperoxia was able to produce not only the expected increase in ptiO2, but also a decrease in cerebral extracellular lactate (Zauner, personal communication). This finding suggests that the ptiO2 increase might correspond to an incrase of O2 "bioavailability" at the parenchymal level and, therefore, might substantially improve O2 delivery to the tissue. The extent of this improvement in ameliorating O2 delivery to the cerebral tissue, when cerebral blood flow is reduced, is still unclear. According to the physiology of O2 content and transport, an increase in the O2 dissolved fraction has a modest impact on O2 content, which is predominantely due to the fraction bound to the haemoglobin. That was confirmed in our experimental setting: O2 supply showed only a negligible increase, since the gain in O2 delivery was non significant in each phases. AVDO2 decreased during the phases of intact and moderately CBF reduction, while it did not change during the phase of severe CBF impairment. The AVDO2 reduction following hyperoxia during the phases of intact and moderately reduced CBF needs to be clarified: in fact it can be interpreted as an improvement of the balance between O2 delivery and consumption when CBF is moderately reduced, while its meaning during the phase of intact CBF is uncertain. The measurement of cerebral glucose, lactate and pyruvate might help to better elucidate this issue. In conclusion: the increase in paO2 and consequently in ptiO2, seen after ventilation with pure oxygen, does not correspond to an improvement in oxygen supply to the brain during phases of defective CBF.

References

1. Maas AIR, Fleckenstein W, deJong DA, vanSantbrink H (1993) Monitoring cerebral oxyenation: experimantal studies and preliminary clinical results of continuous monitoring of cerebrospinal fluid and brain tissue oxygen tension. Acta Neurochir (Wien) 59: 50–57
2. Meixenberger J, Dings J, Kuhnigh H, Roosen K (1993) Studies of tissue PO2 in normal and pathological human brain cortex. Acta Neurochir (Wien) 59: 58–63
3. Menzel M, Rieger A, Roth S, Soukup J, Peuse C, Hennig C, Molnar P, Furka I, Radke J (1998) Simultaneous continuous measurement of pO2, pCO2, pH and temperature in brain tissue and sagittal sinus in a porcine model. Acta Neurochir (Wien) 71: 183–185
4. van Santbrink H, Maas AIR, Avezaat CJJ (1996) Continuous monitoring of partial pressure of brain tissue oxygen in patients with severe head injury. Neurosurgery 38: 21–31

Correspondence: Dr. Sandra Rossi, Neuro-ICU, Dept Anaesthesia and Intensive Care, Padiglione Beretta Neuro, Ospedale Maggiore Policlinico IRCCS, Via F. Sforza, 35, 20122 Milano, Italy.

Acta Neurochir (2000) [Suppl] 76: 247–249

The Synergistic Effect of High K^+ and Hypoxia on Extracellular Concentrations of Neuroactive Amino Acid in Hippocampus

Y. Matsushita, K. Shima, H. Katoh, and **H. Nawashiro**

Department of Neurosurgery, National Defense Medical College, Tokorozawa, Saitama, Japan

Summary

In the present study, we examined extracellular concentrations of glutamate (Glu) in hypoxia using ringer solution with a high potassium (K^+) level using microdialysis. Based on our findings, we hypothesized that the concentration of extracellular K^+ caused a greater efflux of Glu. We used male SD rats and separated them into 3 groups based on the K^+ concentration of Ringer solution (RS), consisting of normal (4 mM), 40 mM and 150 mM groups. We stereotactically inserted the microdialysis probe into the hippocampus, and perfused the RS for 60 min before imposing hypoxia. Subsequently, while perfusing RS, hypoxia (7% O_2 + 93% N_2 gas) was induced in all 3 groups for 20 min. In the normal and 40 mM of K^+ concentration groups, the Glu level did not increase, but in the 150 mM of K^+ concentration group, the Glu level increased while being perfused with RS and a larger increase in Glu was observed after inducing hypoxia. This result suggests that the extracellular concentration of K^+ plays a role in the mechanism of increased neuronal vulnerability caused by hypoxia after TBI.

Keywords: Glutamate; potassium; traumatic brain injury; HPLC.

Introduction

The extracellular concentrations of potassium (K^+) and glutamate (Glu) are known to increase just after Traumatic Brain Injury (TBI) and this is assumed to play an important role in the pathophsiology of brain concussion. Our previous studies showed an increase in the neuronal vulnerability to hypoxia in hippocampal CA3 pyramidal cells after a mild closed head injury [7]. In addition, we already reported that TBI caused a greater efflux of Glu following hypoxia [5]. The present study was undertaken to determine the concentration of extracellular K^+, as a factor participating in the prolonged and extremely augmented accumulation of Glu in hippocampus after the combined insults of TBI and hypoxia, and we also examined the synergistic effects of a high extracellular K^+ concentration and hypoxia on Glu in hippocampus without TBI using microdialysis.

Materials and Methods

Animals

Fifteen adult male Sprague-Dawley rats (350–450 g) were divided into 3 groups according to the concentrations of K^+ which were perfused through the microdialysis probe. Group 1 (n = 5) was subjected to normal (4 mM) of K^+ concentration, Group 2 (n = 5) to 40 mM of K^+ concentration and Group 3 (n = 5) to 150 mM of K^+ concentration.

Preparation of Animals

At 72 hours before we started this experiment, the rats underwent surgery as described below. A midline scalp incision was made exposing the calvaria. A small right parietal craniectomy was made with its center positioned 4 mm caudal to the bregma and 3 mm lateral to the midline. A guide catheter was inserted 3 mm from the calvaria surface vertically. As the microdialysis probe was 3 mm longer than the guide catheter, the expected position of the microdialysis probe was the hippocampus. Subsequently, a concentric microdialysis probe (EICOM A-1) was inserted through the guide catheter. We returned the rats to their home cages. On the day of the experiment, the rats were intubated and ventilated with halothane (1–1.5%), oxygen (0.5 l/min.) and nitrous oxide (1.0 l/min.) under controlled respiration. Rectal temperature was maintained at 37.0 °C using a heat lamp.

In Vivo Microdialysis

The microdialysis probe was perfused with normal Ringer solution (RS) at a rate of 4 μl/min., and 60 min later, the sampling of microdialysis was started. The dialysate was collected every 10 min. In Group 1, the microdialysis probe was perfused with the normal K^+ concentration of RS throughout this experiment. In groups 2 and 3, the microdialysis probe was perfused with the normal K^+ concentration of RS from 0–60 min and with the high K^+ concentration of RS from 60–110 min, and again with the normal K^+ concentration of RS from 110–180 min. Hypoxia (7% O_2 + 93% N_2 gas) was induced in all 3 groups from 90–110 min, and then 100% oxygen was given from 110–180 min after hypoxia.

Analysis of Neuroactive Amino Acids

The dialysate from the hippocampus was analyzed for Glu concentrations using the EICOM high-performance liquid chromatography system with Eicompak MA-50DS column. The derivatives were detected by an electrochemical detector (EICOM ECD-100), and the peak areas were integrated and quantified based on the linear calibration with the known amino acid standards. The mean and SDs for the concentrations of each amino acid were analyzed by Fisher's protected least significant difference (PLSD) test with 5% significance levels.

Results

In Group 1, 20 min of hypoxia did not induce any significant increase in Glu concentration. In Group 2, 30 min of perfusion with the high K^+ concentration of RS did not induce any increase in the Glu concentration. Furthermore, additional hypoxia did not induce any significant increase in the Glu concentration. In Group 3, 30 min of perfusion with the high K^+ concentration of RS induced an increase in the Glu concentration while additional hypoxia also induced an increase in the Glu concentration (Table 1).

Discussion

In ischemia or anoxia, an initial slow increase in the extracellular K^+ concentration, presumably caused by impaired uptake, to a level ranging from 6 to 10 mM is followed by an increase to a level ranging from 50 to 60 mM. The intracellular influx of Na^+, Cl^- and Ca^{2+} occurs concomitantly. This drastic increase in the extracellular K^+ concentration, called an anoxic depolarization (AD) occurs during ischemia resulting in a massive release of Glu [2]. The surge increase in the extracellular Glu concentration occurs concomitantly with the increase in K^+ induced AD (the first phase) and a gradual increase subsequently persists (the second phase) [4]. On the other hand, the massive increase in extracellular K^+ concentration induced by AD results in the release of neurotransmitter after TBI [3]. Massive ion movement was found to occur effectively in neuronal cells, such as AD, and this phenomenon has also been observed in spreading depression (SD), which is known to occur in TBI [8]. However, Katoh *et al.* have observed the change of DC potential during hypoxia after TBI and was consistent with AD [6]. These results suggest that the increase in Glu induced by hypoxia can thus be attributed to AD as well as the change just after TBI. Takahashi *et al.* reported that TBI induced a significant increase in the extracellular K^+ concentration from the control level of about 4 mM to 20–50 mM [9]. The present study showed that an increase in the extracellular K^+ concentration promotes the efflux of Glu following hypoxia. Perfusion with the 40 mM K^+ concentration of RS did not induce the increase in Glu concentration, but perfusion with 150 mM K^+ concentration of RS induced the increase in Glu concentration while additional hypoxia induced the increase in Glu concentration. No efflux of Glu in the group of 40 mM K^+ concentration of RS under AD conditions suggest that the extracellular efflux of K^+ and the intracellular influx of Na^+, Cl^- and Ca^{2+} may thus not necessarily occur

Table 1.

Time(min)	Ringer + hypoxia	KCL(150) + hypoxia	KCL(40) + hypoxia
−20	0.389 ± 0.172	0.294 ± 0.119	0.531 ± 0.245
−10	0.375 ± 0.168	0.302 ± 0.074	0.548 ± 0.197
0	0.370 ± 0.172	0.268 ± 0.093	0.641 ± 0.212
10	0.370 ± 0.192*	1.439 ± 0.970*	0.559 ± 0.192
20	0.618 ± 0.345*	2.722 ± 1.418*,**	0.913 ± 0.740**
30	0.447 ± 0.180*	2.472 ± 1.355*,**	0.556 ± 0.324**
40	0.604 ± 0.507*	3.981 ± 2.334*,**	0.771 ± 0.527**
50	0.436 ± 0.276*	3.890 ± 2.176*,**	0.875 ± 0.513**
60	0.407 ± 0.323*	3.212 ± 1.700*,**	0.923 ± 0.554**
70	0.430 ± 0.377	2.695 ± 2.194	1.126 ± 0.912
80	0.361 ± 0.245	1.092 ± 0.777	1.044 ± 0.958
90	0.358 ± 0.233	1.188 ± 0.924	0.835 ± 0.547
100	0.545 ± 0.615	1.980 ± 1.552	0.832 ± 0.531
110	0.309 ± 0.198	0.411 ± 0.266	0.653 ± 0.329
120	0.296 ± 0.172	0.359 ± 0.146	0.443 ± 0.172

Temporal change in extracellular concentration of glutamate. Mean ± SD.
$P < 0.05$; *: KCL(150) + hypoxia vs. KCL(40) + hypoxia; **: KCL(150) + hypoxia vs. Ringer + hypoxia.

concomitantly. The postsynaptic release Glu is transported into the cell by the Na^+/K^+ dependent Glu transporter, regardless of the ion and voltage gradient. The Glu transporter utilizes the Na^+/K^+ ion gradient, which maintains an energy dependent pump. Changing of the Na^+/K^+ ion gradient such as under AD condition, the Glu transporter loses the capability of Glu transport when the concentration of extracellular K^+ is increased up to 10–12 mM. As a result, the Glu transporter allows the release Glu from metabolic pool in neurons and glial cells by reverse transport [1]. Energy demand increases to maintain the ion gradient under the high K^+ concentration. We thus consider that such additional hypoxia (1) exacerbated the energy insufficiency and (2) thus causes a reversal in the Glu transport and (3) also induces the Glu from the metabolic pool which is present in a large portion of the brain, and thereby causes an increase in the extracellular concentration of Glu under these circumstances.

References

1. Graham DI, Ford I, Adams JH, Doyle D, Teasdale GM, Lawrence AE, McLellan DR (1989) Ischaemic brain damage is still common in fatal non-missile head injury. J Neurol Neruosurg Psychiatry 52: 346–350
2. Ishige N, Pitts LH, Hashimoto T, Nishimura MC, Bartkowski HM (1987) Effect of hypoxia on traumatic brain injury in rats: part 1. Changes in neurological function, electroencephalograms, and histopathology. Neurosurgery 20: 848–853
3. Katayama Y, Becker DP, Tamura T, Hovda DA (1990) Massive increases in extracellular potassium and the indiscriminate release of glutamate following concussive brain injury. J Neurosurg 73: 889–900
4. Katayama Y, Tamura T, Becker DP, Tsubokawa T (1991) Calcium-dependent component of massive increase in extracellular potassium during cerebral ischemia as demonstrated by microdialysis in vivo. Brain Res 567: 57–63
5. Katoh H, Shima K, Nawashiro H, Wada K, Chigasaki H (1997) The effect of MK-801 on extracellular neuroactive amino acids in hippocampus after closed head injury followed by hypoxia in rats. Brain Res 758: 153–162
6. Katoh H, Shima K, Nawashiro H, Wada K, Chigasaki H (1997) The effect of hypoxia on extracellular neuroactive amino acids in traumatized rat hippocampus. Neurotraumatology 20: 7–13
7. Nawashiro H, Shima K, Chigasaki H (1995) Selective vulnerability of hippocampal CA3 neurons to hypoxia after mild concussion in the rat. Neurol Res 17: 455–460
8. Sunami K, Nakamura T, Kubota M, Ozawa Y, Namba H, Yamaura A, Makino H (1989) Spreading depression following experimental head injury in the rat. Neurol Med Chir (Tokyo) 29: 975–980
9. Takahashi H, Manaka S, Sano K (1981) Changes in extracellular potassium concentration in cortex and brain stem during the acute phase of experimental closed head injury. J Neurosurg 55: 708–717

Correspondence: Dr. Y. Matsushita, Department of Neurosurgery, National Defense Medical College 3-2 Namiki, Tokorozawa, Saitama 359-8513, Japan.

Acta Neurochir (2000) [Suppl] 76: 251–255

Spreading Depression Induces Permanent Cell Swelling Under Penumbra Conditions

O. Kempski, H. Otsuka, T. Seiwert, and **A. Heimann**

Institute for Neurosurgical Pathophysiology, Johannes Gutenberg-University, Mainz, Germany

Summary

Background. Spreading depression (SD) is known to go along with temporary breakdown of ion gradients and cell swelling which spontaneously normalizes. Here, the effects of SD at reduced flow conditions as encountered in the ischemic penumbra are examined.

Methods. In rats the right carotid artery was permanently occluded. MABP was lowered to 50 mmHg for 30 min. This is sufficient to reduce CBF to penumbra-like conditions in the right hemisphere. The following parameters were assessed: rCBF, DC potential, and tissue impedance. 5 or 15 min after onset of flow reduction one SD wave was initiated by microinjection of KCl. Histology was performed after 7 days.

Results. In animals with hypotension there was depolarization resembling anoxic depolarization after SD induction and an uncoupling of CBF and metabolism only in the right hemisphere. Impedance increased with SD but did not recover spontaneously as long as rCBF remained reduced. 15 min of SD-induced cell swelling was tolerated without permanent damage, whereas 25 min were followed by severe neuron loss in the affected cortex after 7 days.

Conclusions. The study demonstrates the induction of penumbra conditions in the cortex of one hemisphere. SD is followed by cell swelling which persists as long as flow is critically reduced. The experiments illustrate how peri-infarct depolarizations may detrimentally affect the penumbra.

Keywords: Penumbra; spreading depression; tissue impedance; cell swelling.

Introduction

Cell swelling occurrs regularly with a delay of 2–3 min after onset of cerebral ischemia. It is characterized by a complete breakdown of ion gradients and an uptake of extracellular fluid into the intracellular compartment. Extracellular K^+-concentrations rise to 50–70 mM. The only other known pathophysiologic condition with similar disturbances of electrolyte concentrations is cortical spreading depression (CSD). CSD goes along with a *temporary* (appr. 3 min) breakdown of ion gradients [11] and a massive increase of cerebral metabolic rate [7]. This increase of cortical metabolism is required to reestablish ion gradients. It has been reported that glucose consumption increased threefold by CSD [5], that oxygen consumption showed a 45% increase during CSD passage, and that these changes were coupled to augmentation of CBF and oxygen transport [4, 12]. Cortical ATP concentration is significantly reduced during CSD [10, 13]. CSD, hence, is an energy-requiring process that leads to substantial activation of energy metabolism [2]. In cerebral ischemia the energy required to normalize ion gradients is not available and cell swelling persists. Hence, ischemia has been compared to spreading depression under conditions of impaired energy supply. However it is undetermined so far, whether cell swelling contributes to neuronal damage or just constitutes an epiphenomenon.

Especially in the ischemic penumbra an onset of cell swelling may allow to identify regions which will soon be incorporated into the ischemic core. In their original description Astrup *et al.* [1] characterized the ischemic penumbra as tissue in the close neighborhood of an ischemic core where blood flow ranges between two thresholds, the upper threshold of electrical failure (18 $ml^{*}100\ g^{-1*}min^{-1}$) and the lower of energy and ion pump failure (10–12 $ml^{*}100\ g^{1*}min^{-1}$). The penumbra has been further characterized by electrical silence with normal or slightly elevated extracellular protassium concentrations [1]. Outcome from stroke is determined by the fate of the penumbra. In penumbra tissue flow reserves are not available. Therefore it is currently thought that additional energetic demands may contribute to the decay of penumbra tissue [3]. Such additional demands can arise from peri-infarct depolarization, i.e. CSD [7]. Nedergaard & Astrup [15] found periinfarct CSD characterized by longer duration and spontaneous generation as compared to normal tissue. More detailed analyses show that there is a correlation between the number of CSD waves and infarct volume [3, 14].

Hence it appeared of high interest to study the effect of CSD at conditions of critically reduced CBF. Therefore, a reproducible rat model was established with defined flow reduction restricted to the cortex of one hemisphere, i.e. with penumbra-like conditions. It was attempted to generate a large penumbra-like territory but without producing an infarct. In the current study we have used spreading depression also as a tool to identify penumbra-like conditions: penumbra conditions are to be accepted, if regional CBF (rCBF) does not increase during CSD, i.e. flow reserves are no longer available. Furthermore, the kinetics of cell swelling and the recovery of cell volume were evaluated using tissue impedance as a measure of the extra/intracellular fluid distribution.

Methods

The experiments were carried out in male Wistar rats (322 ± 47 g, range 280–410 g body weight, Charles River, Germany). Animals were anesthetized by intraperitoneal injection of chloral hydrate (36 mg/100 g body wt.). The trachea was intubated with silicon tube (OD 2.5 mm), and lungs were mechanically ventilated with 30% oxygen under respiration monitor control (Artema MM206C, Heyer, Sweden). The rectal temperature was kept close to 37.0 °C by a feedback-controlled heating pad. Polyethylene catheters were inserted into the right carotid artery. The arterial line served for continuous registration of mean arterial blood pressure (MABP), and arterial blood gas sampling. Rats were mounted in a stereotactic frame (Stoelting, Wood Dale, IL, U.S.A). After a 20-mm midline skin incision, a frontoparietal cranial window was made to access to the brain surface using a high-speed drill under an operating microscope. The dura was left intact, and the frontoparietal cortex was exposed.

Local CBF was measured by laser flow blood perfusion monitor (Model BPM 403a, Vasomedics, St. Paul, MN, U.S.A.) with a 0.8-mm needle probe and was expressed in LD-units. The LD probe was placed close to the brain surface avoiding visible vessels.

ADC potential electrode was made of glass tube using a micropipette puller and was inserted into the right occipital cortex (0.2–0.4 mm depth). The amplified DC potential between this electrode and a silver wire electrode placed in the neck muscle was recorded throughout the experiment.

The bipolar impedance electrode, which was made of two stainless steel wires (OD 0.5 mm) covered by polyvinyl chloride for electrical isolation except its 0.3 mm sharp-pointed tip, was also inserted into the cortex (0.4–0.5 mm depth). Impedance (1 kHz) was measured using a precision LCR monitor (4284A, Hewlett Packard, U.S.A.).

The lower body portion of the animals was placed in a sealable steel chamber, connected to tunable vacuum pump for later induction of hypobaric hypotension [6]. To do so, the barometric pressure within the steel chamber could be reduced down to −30 cm H2O, thereby causing a pooling of venous blood. After a 30 min control phase, 30 min of cerebral hypoperfusion were performed by MABP reduction to exactly 50 mmHg. Thereafter reperfusion was monitored for 15–30 minutes.

Ten minutes after impedance electrode insertion, a micropipette KCl injector (OD 15–20 μm), filled with 150 mmol/L KCl solution, was inserted into the right parietal cortex. It was connected to a microsyringe. In Group A (n = 8), all rats received a single injection of KCl solution (5.0 μl) into the parietal cortex 5 min after beginning of hypotension. In Group B (n = 8), all rats received a KCl injection into the parietal cortex at the fifth minute at normotension. Results were compared to previous experiments (n = 11) where CSD had been induced 10 min later, i.e. 15 min after onset of hypotension (Seiwert *et al.*, in preparation).

Seven days after the operation, the rats were subjected to perfusion fixation with 4% paraformaldehyde. Brains were embedded in paraffin to obtain coronal sections of the parietal region. Sections were stained with hematoxylin/eosin and luxol fast blue. The density of cortical neurons was counted at identical coordinates in all rats.

Results

There were no statistical differences in physiological parameters of MABP, arterial blood gases (PaO_2, $PaCO_2$, and pH), electrolytes (Na^+ and K^+), and blood glucose among the groups throughout the experiment.

In group A, tissue impedance more than doubled and remained significantly elevated for 30 minutes (6–35th min) immediately after KCl injection (Fig. 1 top) beginning 30–60 seconds after KCl injection. After normalization of systemic arterial pressure tissue impedance returned to baseline values. DC potential decreased significantly after KCl injection. In group B the impedance increase persisted only for five minutes (6–10th min) (Fig. 1 bottom). In previous experiments where KCl was injected after 15 min hypotension, a similar impedance increase had been recorded which also persisted as long as hypotension was maintained.

Local CBF decreased for 30 minutes (1–30th min) significantly in the right hemisphere (occluded carotid artery) as compared with baseline 1CBF during hypotension. No 1CBF increase was observed after CSD in group A (Fig. 2 top), whereas a significant three min CBF increase was seen in group B after KCl injection (Fig. 2 bottom).

Neuron density was significantly decreased to 31% of normal in the right hemisphere of group A animals. This is in sharp contrast to rats where the impedance increase lasted only 15 min, although penumbra-like conditions were also present for 30 min: in these animals no comparable loss of neurons had been found (Seiwert *et al.,* in preparation).

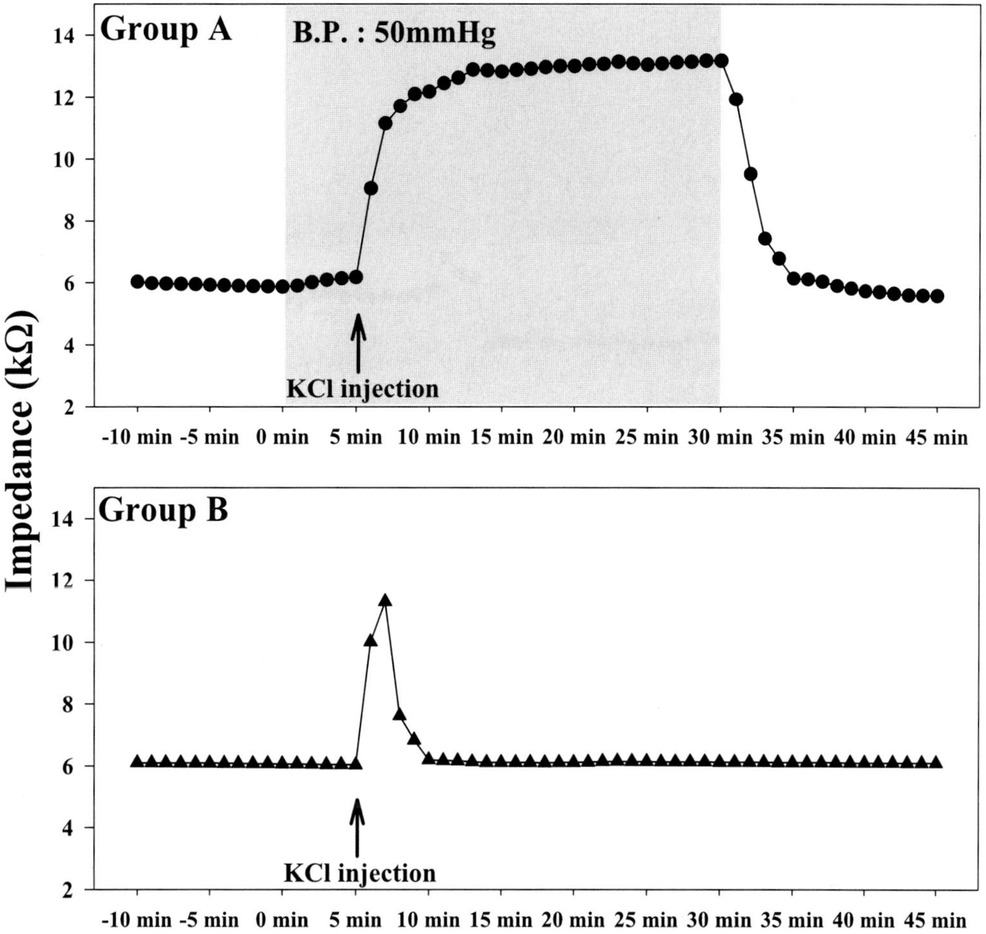

Fig. 1. Typical impedance changes in animals from group A (top) and group B (bottom). The shaded area marks the interval of hypotension in group A animals. A single microinjection of KCl into the parietal cortex was initiated 5 min after beginning of hypotension. (arrow). In the group B animal impedance increases temporarily, whereas in group A the impedance increase remained as long as systemic blood pressure remained reduced

Discussion

Cerebral tissue impedance is determined mainly by the size of the extracellular space, owing to the high electrical resistance of cell membranes [18], and is a suitable parameter to evaluate the degree of glial swelling. Impedance increases if the extracellular space shrinks. In our study it proved to be extremely reliable, easy to use, and was the most sensitive indicator of spreading depression. It is well established that during spreading depression the impedance increases temporarily as a consequence of the breakdown of ion gradients, and, hence, cell swelling [8, 17].

Impedance was still significantly elevated 15 or 25 min after CSD was induced by a single injection of isotonic KCl. In other words, the tissue suffered an insult very similar to the changes seen during anoxic 'terminal' depolarization, which in global cerebral ischemia determines whether ischemic brain injury occurs if it lasts longer than 15 min [9].

The current study suggests therefore, that a single CSD event was sufficient to cause a breakdown of ion gradients which could only be overcome after normalization of rCBF during recovery of systemic blood pressure 15 or 25 min later. Interestingly, widespread neuron loss was only encountered if the breakdown of ion gradients and cell swelling lasted 25 min but not 15 min.

The current data nicely illustrate how periinfarct depolarizations triggered by anoxic release of K^+ or glutamate in the core can accelerate or even initiate the transformation of penumbra tissue to infarct. The data indicate that this will happen in all those regions of the penumbra where flow is too low to cope with the dra-

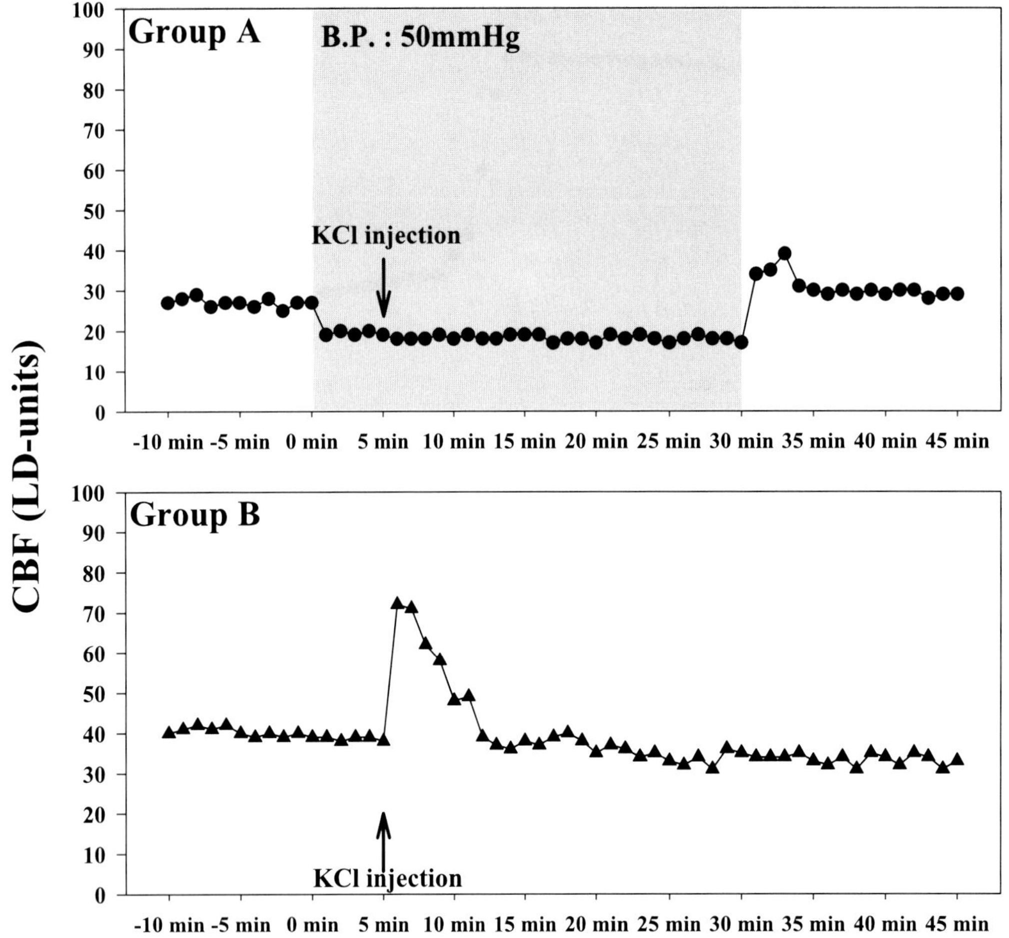

Fig. 2. Typical changes of local cortical blood flow in animals from group A (top) and group B (bottom). The shaded area marks the interval of hypotension in group A animals. A single microinjection of KCl into the parietal cortex was initiated 5 min after beginning of hypotension. (arrow). Note the decrease of CBF after blood pressure reduction and the absence of a flow response upon KCl injection. The typical temporary CBF stimulation during CSD is seen in the goup B animal

matic increase of the metabolic demands during CSD. In normal brain CSD in normal brain is not associated with neuronal injury [16].

If the flow reserves are exhausted, however, the energy supplies necessary to rebuild the ion gradients are not available, and tissue can only recover if flow is normalized within a critical time frame. The data available so far illustrate that 15 min can be tolerated without infarction or severe loss of cortical neurons. In global cerebral ischemia, 15 min of 'anoxic depolarization' are sufficient to cause neuronal death [9], suggesting that secondary mechanisms such as reperfusion damage contribute to nerve cell loss in global ischemia. It remains to be clarified which secondary mechanisms are turned on during the 25 min episode of 'terminal depolarization' in the current experiments which explain the delayed neuronal death observed after 7 days.

References

1. Astrup J, Siesjö, BK, Symon L (1981) Thresholds in cerebral ischemia – the ischemic penumbra. Stroke 12: 723–725
2. Back T, Kohno K, Hossmann KA (1994) Cortical negative DC deflections following middle cerebral artery occlusion and KCl-induced spreading depression: effect on blood flow, tissue oxygenation, and electroencephalogram. J Cereb Blood Flow Metab 14: 12–19
3. Back T, Ginsberg M, Dietrich WD, Watson BD (1996) Induction of spreading depression in the ischemic hemisphere following experimental middle cerebral artery occlusion: effect on infarct morphology. J Cereb Blood Flow Metab 16: 202–213
4. deCrespigny A, Röther J, van Bruggen N, Beaulieu C, Moseley M (1998) Magnetic resonance imaging assessment of cerebral hemodynamics during spreading depression in rats. J Cereb Blood Flow Metab 18: 1008–1017
5. Gjedde A, Hansen AJ, Quistorff B (1981) Blood-brain glucose transfer in spreading depression. J Neurochem 37: 807–812
6. Heimann A, Kroppenstedt S, Ulrich P, Kempski O (1994) Cerebral blood flow autoregulation during hypobaric hypo-

tension assessed by laser Doppler scanning. J Cereb Blood Flow Metab 14: 1100–1105
7. Hossmann K-A (1996) Periinfarct depolarizations. Cerebrovasc Brain Metabol Rev 8: 195–208
8. Jing J, Aitken PG, Somjen GG (1994) Interstitial volume changes during spreading depression (SD) and SD-like hypoxic depolarization in hippocampal tissue slices. J Neurophysiol 71: 2548–2551
9. Kaminogo M, Suyama K, Ichikura A, Onizuka M, Shibata S (1998) Anoxic depolarization determines ischemic brain injury. Neurol Res 20: 343–348
10. Lauritzen M, Hansen AJ, Wieloch T (1987) Metabolic changes with spreading depression in rat cortex. J Cereb Blood Flow Metab 7: S125
11. Leão AAP (1944) Spreading depression of activity in cerebral cortex. J Neurophysiol 7: 359–390
12. Mayevsky A, Weiss HR (1991) Cerebral blood flow and oxygen consumption in cortical spreading depression. J Cereb Blood Flow Metab 11: 829–836
13. Mies G, Paschen W (1984) Regional change of blood flow, glucose, and ATP content determined on brain sections during a single passage of spreading depression in rat brain cortex. Exp Neurol 84: 249–258
14. Mies G, Iijima T, Hossmann K-A (1993) Correlation between periinfarct DC shifts and ischemic neuronal damage in rat. Neuroreport 4: 709–711
15. Nedergaard M, Astrup J (1986) Infarct rim: Effect of hyperglycemia on direct current potential and [^{14}C] 2-deoxyglucose phosphorylation. J Cereb Blood Flow Metab 6: 607–615
16. Nedergaard M, Hansen AJ (1988) Spreading depression is not associated with neural injury in the normal brain. Brain Res 449: 395–398
17. Nicholson C, Kraig RP (1981) The behavior of extracellular ions during spreading depression. The application of ion-selective microelectrodes. Zeuthen (ed) Elsevier/North-Holland Biomedical Press, pp 217–238
18. Van Harreveld A, Ochs S (1956) Cerebral impedance changes after circulatory arrest. Am J Physiol 187: 180–192

Correspondence: Univ. -Prof. Dr. med. O. Kempski, Institute for Neurosurgical Pathophysiology, Johannes Gutenberg-University, Langenbeckstr. 1, 55101 Mainz, Germany.

Acta Neurochir (2000) [Suppl] 76: 257–259

Cerebral Blood Flow and the Secondary Growth of Brain Tissue Necrosis After Trauma

D. H. Friedrich, N. Plesnila, J. Eriskat, M. Stoffel, and **A. Baethmann**

Institute for Surgical Research, Klinikum Großhadern, Ludwig-Maximilians-Universität, München, Germany

Summary

A local brain tissue necrosis from trauma progresses during the following 24 hours or longer. A decrease in cerebral blood flow has been observed both in the necrotic as well as adjacent cortical region, which may influence expansion of the lesion into the perifocal brain tissue. Currently the regional cortical blood flow (rCBF) was assessed by using scanning laser Doppler fluxmetry. Brain tissue necrosis was induced by a highly standardised cold lesion. We attempted to inhibit the development of posttraumatic ischemia in and around the focal lesion by infusion of a hypertonic/hyperoncotic saline/starch solution. The infusion therapy resulted in a temporary improvement of posttraumatic blood flow in both necrotic and distant cortical regions. However, the expansion of the focal necrosis was not reduced. Additional investigations are in progress to determine whether further amelioration with a longer duration of rCBF increase is effective in combination with methods of neuroprotection to inhibit the secondary lesion growth after a traumatic insult.

Keywords: Posttraumatic hypoperfusion; focal necrosis; hypertonic/hyperoncotic saline/hydroxyethyl starch solution.

Introduction

A local brain tissue necrosis from trauma expands progressively during the following 24 hours [2]. The final increase of the necrosis ranges from 150% to 300% [4, 6, 7] dependent on the lesion model and species. A marked posttraumatic depression of rCBF has been observed, not only in the necrotic, but also in remote cortical regions, including the initially viable perifocal tissue [8]. In order to find out whether the acute cerebral hypoperfusion causes the spread of necrosis, we attempted to improve the regional cortical blood flow by infusing a hypertonic/hyperoncotic solution (HHS). The focal necrosis was induced by a highly standardised cold lesion. The regional cortical blood flow was measured by laser scanning Doppler fluxmetry of the exposed cerebral cortex, by means of a computerised positioning system [5]. The volume of the brain tissue necrosis was quantified by histomorphometry at 5 min and 24 h after trauma using Nissl stained coronal brain sections.

Material and Methods

17 male Sprague-Dawley rats (b.w. 280–320 g) were oro-tracheally intubated and mechanically ventilated using a combination of Halothane 0.8% in N_2O 70% and O_2 30%. The rectal temperature was kept constant at 37.5 °C to 38 °C using a heating pad. A catheter was introduced into the tail artery for continuous blood pressure monitoring and drawing arterial samples to control blood gases. The femoral vein was catheterised for administration of fluids and drugs. The skull was fixed in a stereotactic frame, and the right parietal squama was trephined forming a window of 4 mm × 7 mm by a liquid cooled dental drill, leaving the dura mater intact. A crown was placed on the skull enclosing the window and the scalp was stretched to form a reservoir, allowing continuous superfusion of the cortex by isotonic saline. The temperature of the superfusate was kept at 37.5 °C to 38 °C. The regional cortical blood flow (rCBF) was measured by using a laser Doppler monitor (Perimed 4001 Master). The tip of the laser Doppler probe was positioned to hover at minimal distance above the dura using an operating microscope. A computer controlled micromanipulator attached to the probe scanned over a grid of 6 × 10 points, at 500 µm steps. Thereby the necrotic area as well as the proximal and distant cortex was assessed. Each point was measured for 5 seconds. Following the baseline measurements, a focal lesion was induced by a stereotactically guided copper cylinder (∅ 3 mm) cooled to minus 68 °C by a mixture of dry ice and acetone. Animals were then randomly allocated to either (a) an acute, (b) a control, or (c) a therapy group. Animals of the acute group were perfusion fixed for histology immediately after trauma. Animals of the control and the therapy groups were infused at 10 minutes after trauma with 4 ml/kg b.w. of a 90 sec bolus of NaCl 0.9% or HyperHaes® (NaCl 7.2% + Hydroxyethylstarch MW 200,000 6%), respectively. Following a continuing observation period of 5 hours, the animals were extubated, allowed to wake up, and perfusion fixed at 24 hours after trauma during anaesthesia. Histology was carried out by using Nissl stained coronal brain sections and morphometric software (Optimate). Data are given as mean ± SEM.

Results

The laser Doppler flow (LDF) findings reached a stable baseline throughout the last 30 minutes before trauma over the entire brain surface. Following induction of the lesion, rCBF fell immediately and equally in all regions, attaining a minimum of 55% or 65% baseline after 20 minutes in the control and therapy groups, respectively. In the cortical regions distant from the lesion rCBF returned to baseline values at 60 minutes in both therapy and untreated animals, with only some more rapid recovery in the therapy group. In both groups, the necrotic as well as the perifocal region demonstrated improvement in blood flow during the subsequent observation period. The LDF-data showed a faster recovery in the necrotic region of animals with hypertonic/-oncotic fluid as compared to the control group until 120 minutes post trauma, when both groups reached 70% of baseline (non significant). In the penumbra, however, rCBF of treated animals was significantly improved during a period of 45 minutes ($p < 0.01$), commencing 15 minutes after trauma. The flow improvement continued to exceed rCBF of the untreated animals until the end of the observation period.

In animals sacrificed immediately after trauma, a lesion volume of 3.47 ± 0.51 mm^3 was obtained by histomorphometry. Untreated animals had an increase of the volume of necrosis to 4.68 ± 0.42 mm^3 at 24 hours, while animals infused with HHS had an increase to 4.84 ± 0.64 mm^3. The secondary growth of necrosis within 24 hours was significant for both groups with and without HHS, while there was no statistically significant difference in lesion growth between both groups.

Discussion

The current investigations confirm previous findings of a marked post traumatic decrease of rCBF in both the necrotic lesion and adjacent penumbral tissue. The various mechanisms for the decrease of the tissue perfusion include: release of vasoconstrictor mediator agents, such as PAF [3] or endothelin and depression of the neuronal function as well as lowering of energy metabolism, and hence blood flow. Irrespective of the nature of the underlying mechanisms, they were active for a brief period only, as widespread recovery of blood flow was noticeable during the subsequent 5 hours following trauma in both animals with and without treatment. Even though HHS significantly improved blood flow in the initially viable perifocal tissue, this did not prevent the penumbral tissue adjacent to the necrosis from perishing during the following 24 hours.

The failure of hypertonic/hyperoncotic solutions to protect perifocal brain parenchyma against secondary demise, in spite of marked improvement of penumbral flow, may have various reasons. One is insufficient recovery of the depressed blood flow on a quantitative and qualitative basis and of a duration less than would be necessary. A second reason may be spread of necrosis due to adverse factors and compounds accumulating in the perifocal brain from spill over of the necrotic tissue. A third reason may be tissue acidosis and vasoconstrictory prostanoids among others causing hypoperfusion. Obviously further studies are required to elucidate the complex pathophysiology underlying the secondary expansion of traumatic brain tissue necrosis. Nevertheless, administration of HHS may be beneficial for the treatment of patients with severe head injury, because CBF improves, and the systemic blood pressure stabilises, both of which are helpful, particularly in polytrauma cases suffering from additional multiple peripheral injuries. Moreover hypertonic/-oncotic solutions have been shown to lower intracranial pressure from traumatic brain oedema [1], which would also support recovery of an impaired post traumatic cerebral blood flow.

Acknowledgement

Supported by BMBF-Verbund "Neurotrauma" München FKZ 90 30 911.

References

1. Berger S, Schürer L, Härtl R, Messmer K, Baethmann A (1995) Reduction of post-traumatic intracranial hypertension by hypertonic/hyperoncotic saline/dextran and hypertonic mannitol. Neurosurgery 37: 98–108
2. Eriskat J, Schürer L, Kempski O, Baethmann A (1994) Growth kinetics of a primary brain tissue necrosis from a focal lesion. Acta Neurochir [Suppl] (Wien) 60: 425–427
3. Frerichs KU, Lindsberg PJ, Hallenbeck JM, Feuerstein GZ (1990) Platelet activating factor and progressive brain damage following focal brain injury. J Neurosurg 73: 223–233
4. Lindsberg PJ, Frerichs KU, Burris JA, Hallenbeck JM, Feuerstein G (1991) Cortical microcirculation in a new model of focal laser-induced secondary brain damage. J Cereb Blood Flow Metab 11 (1): 88–98
5. Ungersböck K, Heimann A, Strecker U, Kempski O (1993) Mapping of cerebral blood flow by laser-Doppler flowmetry. In: Tomita M, Mchedlishvili G, Rosenblum WI, Heiss WD, Fukuuchi Y (eds) Microcirculatory stasis in the brain. Elsevier, Amsterdam, pp 405–413

6. Vonhof S (1995) Die zerebrale Proteinsynthese nach Schädel-Hirn-Trauma: eine experimentelle Untersuchung zur Quantifizierung der sekundären Hirngewebsnekrose. Inauguraldissertation. Ludwig-Maximilians-Universität, München
7. Wyrwich W (1994) Die Entwicklung einer sekundären Hirngewebsnekrose nach primärem Trauma. Methodische Ansätze ihrer Quantifizierung. Inauguraldissertation. Ludwig-Maximilians-Universität, München
8. Yamakami I, McIntosh TK (1991) Alterations in regional cerebral blood flow following brain injury in the rat. J Cereb Blood Flow Metab 11 (4): 655–660

Correspondence: David Friedrich, Institute for Surgical Research, Klinikum Großhadern, Ludwig-Maximilians-Universität, Marchioninistr. 15, D-81366 München, FRG.

Acta Neurochir (2000) [Suppl] 76: 261–264

The Role of Proteolytic Enzymes in Focal Ischaemic Brain Damage

M. Davis[1], **D. Mantle**[1], and **A. D. Mendelow**[2]

[1] Departments of Medicine, The University of Newcastle upon Tyne, UK
[2] Department of Surgery (Neurosurgery), The University of Newcastle upon Tyne, UK

Summary

Although various neuroprotective and fibrinolytic drugs are currently under evaluation in the acute stages of ischaemic stroke, their therapeutic potential is likely to be limited by unwanted side effects and a narrow time window of opportunity for intervention. Proteolytic enzymes are involved in the catabolism of peptide neurotransmitters and structural cellular proteins in normal brain and have been implicated in the pathogenesis of neurodegenerative disorders. We hypothesised that activation of these enzymes might also play a crucial role in effecting ischaemic neuronal injury, thereby providing a potential site for therapeutic intervention in human stroke. Focal cerebral ischaemia was induced by thermocoagulation of the left middle cerebral artery in aged (30 month) male Wistar rats who were pre-treated with saline or the competitive N-methyl-D-Aspartate antagonist D-CPP-ene, which has been shown to be neuroprotective in young animal models of stroke. Major protease activities were analysed in the left (ischaemic) and right (non-ischaemic) hemispheres, following tissue homogenisation. Data have been analysed using Mann-Whitney tests and are presented as means $\pm$ standard errors. Enzyme activity decreased in ischaemic brain; for example, the mean activity of dipeptidyl aminopeptidase I was 23 ± 3 and 43 ± 6 nmol substrate/hour/ml brain extract in the left and right hemispheres respectively ($n = 10$, $p < 0.05$). Ischaemic neuronal injury is not effected by the early activation of proteolytic enzymes and protease inhibitors are therefore unlikely to be of benefit in human stroke.

Keywords: Proteases; focal; cerebral; ischaemia; aged.

Introduction

Stroke is the most common cause of severe neurological disability in adults worldwide and is also a common cause of death. Over the past few decades, experimental research has led to major advances in our understanding of the complex pathophysiological mechanisms that underlie ischaemic neuronal injury, leading to the development of numerous potential therapeutic strategies. However, for the mostpart, the interventions that have been shown to limit ischaemic brain damage in animal stroke models have not enjoyed similar therapeutic success in the aftermath of human stroke. There are many explanations for the apparent differential response in human and experimental stroke. These include the use of animal models of an inappropriate age, the moderation of dosing regimes in humans to accommodate for intolerable side effects, the added complexity of the collateral circulation, with the potential for spontaneous recanalisation in stroke patients, and the delays that are encountered in the administration of potential drug treatments in the face of narrow therapeutic time windows [3, 4, 9]. Thus, despite the recent emergence of neuroprotective drugs with fewer side effects, such pharmacological agents that target hyperacute events in the ischaemic cascade are unlikely ever to provide a therapeutic option for the majority of stroke victims. By contrast, loss of structural cellular protein from ischaemic cerebral cortex is a protracted process and continues over several days [13]. The mechanisms underlying disruption of the cytoskeletal architecture might therefore provide a timelier and potentially safer target for therapeutic intervention, possibly leading to the development of protease inhibitors as a more universally applicable treatment in human stroke.

Proteolytic enzymes are responsible for the catabolism of structural intracellular proteins and neurotransmitter peptides in normal brain tissue and have been implicated in tissue damage in neurodegenerative disorders [12, 15, 24]. We hypothesised that proteolytic enzymes would also be activated in the ischaemic penumbral zone of an evolving cerebral infarct.

As stroke is a disease of elderly humans, we tested our hypothesis by using an experimental model of a relevant age [5, 6]. Thus, we measured the activity of a comprehensive range of cytoplasmic and lysosomal proteases in ischaemic and non ischaemic brain tissue from aged male Wistar rats, following permanent occlusion of the left middle cerebral artery (LMCAO). To elucidate the effect of prior administration of a neuroprotective drug, animals were pre-treated intravenously with the competitive N-methyl D Aspartate antagonist D-CPP-ene, or 0.9% normal saline.

Materials and Methods

All experiments were conducted in accordance with the Animals (Scientific Procedures) Act 1986, in aged (30 month) male Wistar rats. Anaesthesia was induced by the inhalation of 4% halothane in nitrous oxide and oxygen (70%/30%). Ventilation was monitored continuously via pulse oximetry and a capnograph. Core temperature was maintained using a heating pad and a rectal thermistor probe. The femoral vessels were cannulated for the monitoring of arterial blood pressure, the measurement of arterial blood gases, glucose and haematocrit, and the administration of drugs and fluid. Animals were randomly allocated into treated and untreated groups. Treated rats received intravenous D-CPP-ene (15 mg/kg) 15 minutes prior to cerebral infarction, followed by an infusion (0.17 mg/kg/min) for the duration of the experiment. Untreated rats received a similar regime using the vehicle (0.9% normal saline). The left middle cerebral artery was exposed via a microcraniectomy and occluded by thermocoagulation using microbipolar diathermy, proximal to the origin of the lenticulostriate branch [21]. After 6 hours, the animals were decapitated, their brains were rapidly removed, the hemispheres were separated and divided into 4 coronal slices, corresponding (in the lesioned hemisphere) to histological sections depicting core, penumbral and non ischaemic tissue [17]. Specimens were snap frozen in liquid nitrogen and subsequently stored at $-70\,^{\circ}C$ for subsequent analysis. Tissue sections were homogenised 1:20 (w/v) in extraction buffer (50 mM Tris-acetate pH 7.5, 0.15 M NaCl, 1 mM dithiothreitol, 0.02% (w/v) NaN_3) using an Ultra-Turrax homogeniser (2×10 seconds at 5000 rpm). Following centrifugation at 2000 g for 15 minutes, tissue supernatants were assayed for the activities of the cytoplasmic proteases dipeptydyl aminopeptidase IV (DAP-4), proline endopeptidase (PRO-EP), alanyl, arginyl- and leucyl- aminopeptidases (ALA-AP, ARG-AP, and LEU-AP), and the lysosomal enzymes dipeptidyl aminopeptidases I and II, (DAP1, DAP2), as described previously [20]. Protein levels in tissue supernatants were determined by the method of Lowry *et al.* [14] with BSA as standard.

Data from coronal section one (representing penumbral tissue in the lesioned hemisphere and non ischaemic brain in the right hemisphere) are presented as means $\pm$ their standard errors (SEM) and comparisons have been made using Mann-Whitney tests.

Results

Overall in aged animals, cytoplasmic protease activity was significantly lower in the ischaemic section from the left hemisphere, in comparison with values from the corresponding coronal brain section in the right (non-ischaemic) hemisphere. Thus the mean activities of ALA-AP, ARG-AP, LEU-AP, DAP4, and PRO-EP from the ischaemic penumbral section in the left hemisphere were 433 ± 94, 995 ± 148, 21 ± 3, 47 ± 7 and 162 ± 3 nmol substrate/hour/ml soluble extract, compared with mean values in the corresponding section from the non ischaemic right hemisphere of 816 ± 122 ($p < 0.05$), 1835 ± 117 ($p < 0.001$), 38 ± 4 ($p < 0.01$), 99 ± 10 ($p = 0.001$) and 422 ± 44 ($p < 0.001$) nmol substrate/hour/ml brain extract.

In ischaemic aged brain, similar decreases were documented in the activities of the lysosomal enzymes DAP1 and DAP2, in comparison with brain tissue from the non-ischaemic hemisphere. Thus the mean activities of DAP1 and DAP2 in ischaemic brain were 23 ± 3 and 73 ± 16 nmol substrate/hour/ml brain extract respectively, compared with mean values from the corresponding section in the right hemisphere of 43 ± 6 ($p < 0.01$), and 230 ± 33 ($p < 0.001$) nmol substrate/hour/ml brain extract.

Pre-treatment with the neuroprotective drug D-CPP-ene moderated the decline in cytoplasmic and lysosomal protease activity in ischaemic aged brain. Thus the mean activities of LEU-AP in ischaemic and non ischaemic brain from treated aged rats were 24 ± 4 and 37 ± 7 nmol substrate/hour/ml brain extract respectively ($p = 0.21$ not significant), whilst corresponding activities of DAP1 were 30 ± 5 and 49 ± 10 nmol substrate/hour/ml brain extract respectively ($p = 0.09$ not significant).

Discussion

We have demonstrated that proteolytic enzyme activity declines significantly in ischaemic brain tissue from aged rats. Our findings contrast with the activation of caspases and matrix metalloproteinases that has been documented in the aftermath of transient global cerebral ischaemia followed by reperfusion [2, 7, 16, 23]. This might be in part due to the assay of different enzymes in the current study (i.e. those involved in generalised intracellular protein catabolism), but it might also reflect differences in the mechanisms which effect neuronal injury in permanent focal, as opposed to transient global cerebral ischaemia. In the latter experimental model, reperfusion may enhance free radical induced injury and the global ischaemic insult selectively targets hippocampal neurons, which undergo delayed apoptosis after several days. In contrast, proximal thermocoagulation of the middle cerebral artery produces permanent vascular occlusion without reperfusion, which initially induces early ischaemic necrosis of the cerebral cortex and basal ganglia within hours of the ischaemic insult [21].

An alternative explanation might lie in the time lapse between the induction of the focal ischaemic injury and the analysis of enzyme activity. As the analysis of protease activity was performed 6 hours after middle cerebral artery occlusion in our experiments, it is possible that either "delayed" or "hyperacute" enzyme activation has been missed. However, this is unlikely, because in the first instance, the depletion of cortical protein substrates is initiated within fifteen minutes of focal cerebral ischaemic injury [18] and in the second case, protein degradation has been reported to continue over several hours, maximising more than 24 hours after the onset of ischaemia [19].

The synthesis of structural proteins and neuropeptide transmitters is inhibited in ischaemic brain [10] and the reduction in enzyme activity might therefore reflect a decline in enzyme *production*, with subsequent depletion of cellular stores. Alternatively, changes in protease activity may result from modulation of neuronal genes [1, 8, 11]. This could lead to the induction of proteolytic enzyme inhibitors [22], or result in the modification of protease structure, with subsequent moderation of enzyme activity [2].

The neuroprotective drug D-CPP-ene has been shown to reduce cerebral infarct size in senescent animals subjected to permanent middle cerebral artery occlusion [5, 6]. Therefore, the relative preservation of enzyme activity seen in aged animals pretreated with this drug might merely reflect a reduction in the volume of infarcted tissue, with preservation of protein synthesis, rather than a specific effect on protein catabolic pathways.

Our experiments suggest that ischaemic neuronal injury in aged brains is not effected by early activation of proteolytic enzymes and therefore, such enzyme inhibitors are unlikely to be of benefit in human stroke.

References

1. Akins PT, Liu PK, Hsu CY (1996) Immediate early gene expression in response to cerebral ischaemia. Friend or foe? Stroke 27: 1682–1687
2. Chen J, Nagayama T, Jin K, Stetler RA, Zhu RL, Graham SH, Simon RP (1998) Induction of caspase-3-like protease may mediate delayed neuronal death in the hippocampus after transient cerebral ischaemia. J Neurosci 18: 4914–4928
3. Davis M, Barer DH (1995) Theoretical aspects of neuroprotection in acute ischaemic stroke. I: basic mechanisms. Vascular Medicine Review 6: 283–298
4. Davis M, Barer DH (1999) Neuroprotection in acute ischaemic stroke. II: clinical potential. Vascular Med 4: 149–163
5. Davis M, Mendelow AD, Perry RH, Chambers IR, James OFW (1995) Experimental stroke and neuroprotection in the aging rat brain stroke 26: 1072–1078
6. Davis M, Perry RH, Mendelow AD (1997) The effect of non-competitive N-Methyl-D-Aspartate receptor antagonism on cerebral oedema and cerebral infarct size in the aging ischaemic brain. Acta Neurochir (Wien) 70: 30–33
7. Gillardon F, Bottiger B, Schmitz B, Zimmermann M, Hossmann KA (1997) Activation of CPP-32 protease in hippocampal neurons following ischemia and epilepsy. Brain Res 50: 16–22
8. Giordano MJ, Mahadeo DK, He YY, Geist Rt, Hsu C, Gutmann DH (1996) Increased expression of the neurofibromatosis 1 (NF 1) gene product neurofibromin in astrocytes in response to cerebral ischemia. J Neurosci Res 43: 246–253
9. Grotta J (1995) Why do all drugs work in animals but none in stroke patients? 2. Neuroprotective therapy. J Intern Med 237: 89–94
10. Hossman KA (1993) Disturbances of cerebral protein synthesis and ishaemic cell death. Prog Brain Res 96: 161–177
11. Kim HS, Lee SH, Kim SS, Kim YK, Jeong SJ, Ma J, Han DH, Cho BK, Suh YH (1998) Post-ischaemic changes in the expression of Alzheimer's APP isoforms in rat cerebral cortex. Neuroreport 9: 533–537
12. Kuda T, Shoji M, Arai H, Kawashima S, Saido TC (1997) Reduction of plasma glutamyl aminopeptidase activity in sporadic Alzheimer's disease. Biochem Biophys Res Comm 231: 526–530
13. Kuwaki T, Satoh H, Takahuro O, Shibayama F, Yamashita T, Nishimura T (1989) Nilvadipine attenuates ischaemic degradation of gerbil brain cytoskeletal proteins. Stroke 20: 78–83
14. Lowry OH, Rosebrough NJ, Farr AL, Randall RJ (1951) Protein measurement with the Folin phenol reagent. J Biol Chem 193: 265–275
15. Mackay EA, Ehrhard A, Moniatte M, Guenet C, Tardif C, Tarnus C, Sorokine O, Heintzelmann B, Nay C, Remy JM, Higaki JVan Dorsselaer A, Wagner J, Danzin C, Mamomt P (1997) A possible role for Cathepsins D, E, and B in the processing of beta-amyloid precursor protein in Alzheimer's disease. Eur J Biochem 244: 414–425
16. Mun-Bryce S, Rosenberg GA (1998) Matrix metalloproteinases in cerebrovascular disease. J Cereb Blood Flow Metab 18: 1163–1172
17. Osborne KA, Shigeno T, Balarsky AM, Ford I, McCulloch J, Teasdale GM, Graham DI (1987) Quantitative assessment of early brain damage in a rat model of focal cerebral ischaemia. J Neurol Neurosurg Psychiatry 50: 402–410
18. Pettigrew LC, Holtz ML, Craddock SD, Minger SL, Hall N, Geddes JW (1996) Microtubular proteolysis in focal cerebral ischemia. J Cereb Blood Flow Metab 16: 1189–1202
19. Romanic AM, White RF, Arleth AJ, Ohlstein EH, Barone FC (1998) Matrix metalloproteinase expression increases after cerebral focal ischaemia in rats: inhibition of matrix metalloproteinase-9 reduces infarct size. Stroke 29: 1020–1030
20. Shaw PJ, Ince PG, Falkous G, Mantle D (1996) Cytoplasmic, lysosomal and matrix protease activities in spinal cord tissue from ALS and control patients. J Neurol Sci 139: 71–75
21. Tamura A, Graham DI, McCulloch J, Teasdale GM (1981) Focal cerebral ischaemia in the rat I. Description of technique and early neuropathological consequences following middle cerebral artery occlusion. J Cereb Blood Flow Metab 1: 53–60
22. Tsuda M, Kitagawa K, Imaizumi K, Wanaka A, Tohyama M, Takagi T (1996) Induction of SPI-3 mRNA, encoding a serine

protease inhibitor, in gerbil hippocampus after transient forebrain ischemia. Brain Res 35: 314–318

23. Yamashima T, Kohda Y, Tsuchiya K, Ueno T, Yamashita J, Yoshioka T, Kominami E (1998) Inhibition of ischaemic hippocampal neuronal death in primates with cathepsin B inhibitor CA-074: a novel strategy for neuroprotection based on "calpain-cathepsin hypothesis". Eur J Neurosci 10: 1723–1733
24. Saido TC, Yokota M (1997) Neurodegenerative diseases as proteolytic disorders: brain ischaemia and Alzheimer's disease. Tanpakushitsu Kakusan Koso – Protein, nucleic acid, enzyme 42: 2408–2417

Correspondence: Michelle Davis, Prof. A. D. Mendelow, Newcastle General Hospital, Westgate Road, Newcastle upon Tyne NE4 6BE, UK.

Acta Neurochir (2000) [Suppl] 76: 265–267

Effect of Intracerebral Lesions Detected in Early MRI on Outcome After Acute Brain Injury

B. M. Hoelper[1], **F. Soldner**[1], **L. Choné**[2], and **T. Wallenfang**[1]

[1] Department of Neurosurgery, City Hospital Fulda, Germany
[2] Institute of Radiology, City Hospital Fulda, Germany

Summary

In the present study we classified intracerebral lesions likely to influence the outcome of head injured patients according to localization, lesion type, lesion number and lesion volume. A score of intracerebral lesions based on findings in early MRI is presented.

Early MRI studies were performed in 30 patients (average 5–6 days after trauma) and outcome (GOS) was determined after 3 and 12 months. Lesions were classified and lesion volume V was calculated ($V = \pi abc/6$). The applied intracerebral lesion score included lesions in the frontal cortex, basal ganglia, corpus callosum and brainstem.

Patients in a persistent vegetative state (PVS) showed a higher number ($p = 0.018$) and volume ($p = 0.013$) of frontal lesions as compared to the non-vegetative group (NPVS). Lesion volume in basal ganglia differed significantly between PVS and NPVS ($p = 0.01$) and correlated to outcome ($r = -0.65$, $p < 0.005$). Volume difference in the corpus callosum between PVS and NPVS was significant ($p = 0.02$). The number ($r = -0.61$, $p < 0.005$) and volume ($r = -0.62$, $p < 0.005$) of brainstem lesions correlated to outcome and PVS differed in number ($p = 0.012$) and volume ($p = 0.006$). The intracerebral lesion score correlated to the GOS ($r = -0.57$, $p = 0.001$) and PVS and NPVS differed significantly.

A lesion volume exceeding 40 ml in the frontal cortex, 3.5 ml in the basal ganglia, 4 ml in the corpus callosum or 1.5 ml in the brainstem is likely to lead to an unfavorable outcome. More than 4 lesions in the frontal cortex or 3 lesions in the brainstem appeared more frequent in patients with unfavorable outcome. Treatment strategies in the early phase after brain injury could be modified by the knowledge of certain lesions only visible on MRI.

Keywords: Human traumatic brain injury; diffuse axonal injury; contusion; corpus callosum; brainstem; intracerebral lesion score; magnetic resonance imaging.

Introduction

Magnet resonance imaging (MRI) in ventilated patients is described as the preferred method compared to computed tomography (CT) in the observation of intracerebral lesions following traumatic brain injury, particularly in the brainstem and corpus callosum [2, 4, 5, 9, 10]. These lesions might affect the outcome of patients after brain injury [3, 7, 8] and thus MRI becomes more important in the diagnosis of traumatic brain injury. We report an analysis of the impact of intracerebral lesions, which were determined by volume and number of lesions in early MRI and/or CT, on the outcome of 30 patients after human traumatic brain injury. Based on anatomical and radiological classifications, we suggest an intracerebral lesion score that combines multiple lesions and enables correlation to the outcome.

Patients and Methods

In 30 patients early MRI studies were performed on the average of 5–6 days after trauma. Mass lesions were evacuated immediately and all patients received ICP directed management according to a standardized protocol. The clinical outcome (GOS) was determined 3 and 12 months after trauma [6]. Lesions were classified according to their anatomic localization. The lesion volume V (ml) was estimated according to an ellipsoid ($V = \pi abc/6$) determined by 3 orthogonal radius. The volume within one anatomical structure was summed for each patient to enable comparison of the lesion volume in further analysis. All data were entered into an SQL-database along with the clinical data of each patient. Unpaired groups were compared by the Mann-Whitney U test assuming that the data were not normally distributed. Contingency tables were performed by the Chi-square test and the Fisher's exact test. Correlation were computed with the Spearman and Kendall's rank correlation. An intracerebral lesion score (Table 1) was applied taking into account lesions in the frontal lobes, basal ganglia, corpus callosum and brainstem.

Results

A total of 288 intracranial lesions were classified as intracerebral hematoma, contusions and DAI. Patients in the persistent vegetative state (PVS) show a higher number ($p = 0.018$) and volume ($p = 0.013$) of

Table 1. *Intracerebral Lesions in the Frontal Lobe, Basal Ganglia, Corpus Callosum and Brainstem Classified for Lesion Number (N) and Volume (V). The Score is Shown in italic of each anatomic localization. One Score is Added if Frontal Lesions Exceed 40 ml in Volume or More than 3 Lesions were Found in the Brainstem. The Range of the Score is Minimally Zero and Maximally ten*

Frontal lobe		Basal ganglia		Corpus callosum		Brainstem	
1	$N \leq 4$	*1*	$V \leq 3.5$ ml	*1*	$V \leq 4$ ml	*1*	$V \leq 1.5$ ml
2	$N > 4$	*2*	$V > 3.5$ ml	*2*	$V > 4$ ml	*2*	$V > 1.5$ ml
+1	$V > 40$ ml					*+1*	$N > 3$

frontal lesions compared to the non-vegetative group (NPVS). Parietal (2.7%), insular (1.0%) and occipital (4.2%) lesions represented only a small number of the intracerebral lesions without a significant correlation to the outcome. Lesion volume in basal ganglia differed significantly between PVS and NPVS ($p = 0.01$). An increasing volume of basal ganglia lesions correlated significantly to worse outcome ($r = -0.65$, $p < 0.005$). The lesion volume of basal ganglia correlated significantly to the lesion volume of the brainstem ($r = 0.54$, $p < 0.05$). Volume difference in the corpus callosum between PVS and NPVS was significant ($p = 0.02$), but no significant correlation was found between increasing lesion volume and worse outcome for lesions in the corpus callosum. Number ($r = -0.61$, $p < 0.005$) and volume ($r = -0.62$, $p < 0.005$) of brainstem lesions correlated to outcome and PVS differed in number ($p = 0.012$) and volume ($p = 0.006$). The intracerebral lesion score correlated to the GOS ($r = -0.57$, $p = 0.001$) and PVS and NPVS differed significantly. The Analysis of the coincidence of intracerebral lesions in the frontal cortex, basal ganglia, corpus callosum and brainstem, showed only a slightly significant correlation for the lesion volume in the brainstem and in the basal ganglia ($r = 0.54$, $p < 0.05$, Fig 6). The intracerebral lesion score (table 1) correlated significantly to the outcome ($r = -0.59$, $p = 0.001$), and it is suggested that an increasing score indicated a significantly impaired outcome. Also the differences between the patients whom remained in the vegetative state 12 months after injury compared to the non-vegetative group (X^2 test ($p < 0.0001$) and Fisher exact test ($p < 0.001$)) were significant, based on the intracerebral lesion score of each patient.

Discussion

The differentiation of traumatic intracerebral lesions according to anatomical and morphological aspects is shown in this report to be crucial with regard to the outcome of patients. As our results suggest, the identification of lesion combinations in different anatomical regions, such as the corpus callosum, the brainstem, and the basal ganglia might have profound consequences on secondary brain injury, which determines clinical recovery. A lesion volume exceeding 40 ml in the frontal cortex, 3.5 ml in the basal ganglia, 4 ml in the corpus callosum or 1.5 ml in the brainstem is likely to lead to an unfavorable outcome. More than 4 lesions in the frontal cortex or 3 lesions in the brainstem appeared more frequent in patients with reduced outcome. Treatment strategies in the early phase after brain injury could be modified by the knowledge of certain lesions only visible on MRI. We suggest, that callosal and brainstem lesions, together with lesions in the basal ganglia, have potential effects on the clinical presentation and recovery. We observed that lesions in both the corpus callosum and the brainstem had also an important influence on the ability of the patient to recover after trauma. Even if small cortical contusions do not seem to influence the outcome of patients to a great extent, large cortical lesions can induce elevated intracranial pressure, increase of excitotoxic aminoacids [1] and extracellular potassium, all effects likely to be inversely correlated to outcome. However, alterations in the neuronal connective pattern and metabolic changes leading to cellular damage invisible on MRI might have a considerable effect on recovery. In the report of Kampfl *et al.*, 74% of the patients in a persistent vegetative state showed diffuse axonal injury in the posterolateral brainstem [7]. However, our approach in studying patients ranging from mild to severe traumatic brain injury indicates, that patients with a favorable outcome might also show brainstem or callosal lesions. In addition, we observed a rather linear relationship between the volume of brainstem lesions and the outcome. Therefore, we suggest that in addition to the incidence and anatomical structure of observed brainstem lesions, the lesion volume might also be an important predictor for the outcome of patients.

References

1. Bullock R, Zauner A, Woodward J, Young HF (1995) Massive persistent release of excitatory amino acids following human occlusive stroke. Stroke 26(11): 2187–2189
2. Cecil KM, Hills EC, Sandel ME, Smith DH, McIntosh TK, Mannon LJ, Sinson GP, Bagley LJ, Grossmann RI, Lenkinski RE (1998) Proton magnetic resonance spectroscopy for detection of axonal injury in the splenium of the corpus callosum of brain-injured patients. J Neurosurg 88: 795–801
3. Firsching R, Woischneck D, Dietrich M, Klein S, Rueckert A, Wittig H, Doehring W (1998) Early magnetic resonance imaging of brainstem lesions after severe head injury. J Neurosurg 89: 707–712
4. Gentry LR, Godersky JC, Thompson B (1988) MR imaging of head trauma: review of the distribution and radiopathologic features of traumatic lesions. AJR Am J Roentgenol 150(3): 663–672
5. Gentry LR, Thompson B, Godersky JC (1988) Trauma to the corpus callosum: MR features. AJNR Am J Neuroradiol 9(6): 1129–1138
6. Jennett B, Bond M (1975) Assessment of outcome after severe brain damage. Lancet 1: 480–484
7. Kampfl A, Franz G, Aichner F, Pfausler B, Haring HP, Felber S, Luz G, Schocke M, Schmutzhard E (1998) The persistent vegetative state after closed head injury: clinical and magnetic resonance imaging findings in 42 patients. J Neurosurg 88(5): 809–816
8. Kampfl A, Schmutzhard E, Franz G, Pfausler B, Haring HP, Ulmer H, Felber S, Golaszewski S, Aichner F (1998) Prediction of recovery from post-traumatic vegetative state with cerebral magnetic-resonance imaging [see comments]. Lancet 351(9118): 1763–1767
9. Teasdale E, Hadley DM (1997) Imaging the injury. In: Bullock Ra (ed) Head injury. Chapman & Hall, London, pp 167–207
10. Teasdale G, Teasdale E, Hadley D (1992) Computed tomographic and magnetic resonance imaging classification of head injury. J Neurotrauma 9 [Suppl] 1: S249–257

Correspondence: Bernd Hoelper, M.D., Department of Neurosurgery, City Hospital Fulda, Pacelliallee 4, 36043 Fulda, Germany.

Acta Neurochir (2000) [Suppl] 76: 269–271

Effects of Brain Oedema in the Measurement of Ischaemic Brain Damage in Focal Cerebral Infarction

C.-K. Park and **S.-G. Kang**

Department of Neurosurgery, College of Medicine, The Catholic University of Korea, Seoul, Korea

Summary

In a model of focal cerebral ischaemia, enlargement of ischaemic tissue by ischaemic brain oedema is one of the major problems in the measurement of infarction volume. To minimize an error of this overestimation, several methods have been proposed. However, there has been no attempt to compare these methods to elucidate their eligibility in the measurement of ischaemic area.

The authors used three different morphometric analyses in the measurement of infarction volume to assess the antiischaemic affects of a competitive NMDA antagonist, D-CPPene in MCA occlusion model of the rat: a direct measurement, the Swanson's method, and a measurement using a diagram.

Post-occlusion treatment of D-CPPene (4.5 mg/kg, i.v.+3 mg/kg/h, i.v.) produced reduction of infarction volume to about 40% compared to the control ($P < 0.05$). The volume of infarction determined by the direct measurement was much larger than that by Swanson's or diagram method ($P < 0.05$), about 70% larger in the control and by two times in the treated. However, there was no significant difference in the measured volume between the Swanson's and diagram methods. The protection rate, which was calculated as % = (infarct volume of the control – that of the treated/infarct volume of the control) ×100%, was larger in the Swanson's and diagram methods than in the direct measurement.

In conclusion, it is confirmed that the direct measurement at the peak time of ischaemic brain oedema brings about not only an overestimation of infarction volume but lower protection rate also, compared to the methods designed to minimize the overestimation. Our results also demonstrate the diagram method is useful in reducing overestimation of infarct volume that may be caused by ischaemic brain oedema, though this method was not designed for the purpose of avoiding oedema at first.

Keywords: Focal cerebral infarction; brain oedema; D-CPPene; neuroprotection.

Introduction

Morphometric analysis of infarct volume in animal models of focal cerebral ischaemia represents an objective and quantitative means to estimate the extent of ischaemic brain injury and is employed to determine the efficacy of neuroprotective agents in preclinical trials. Swelling of ischaemic tissue may result in enlargement of the infarcted zone, leading to overestimation of infarct volume and misinterpretation of experimental results [1]. To minimize the error that may be introduced by brain oedema, several methods have been proposed [4, 6, 11]. However, there were few reports to compare these methods in the same study and to assess which method would be more useful in minimizing the error.

The authors tried to compare three different methods, the direct measurement [2, 3, 5, 10], Swanson's method [11] and the diagram method [4, 7] in the left middle cerebral artery (MCA) infarction model of the rat, and to assess the effect of brain oedema on the measurements of infarct volume. The rat was administered a competitive N-methyl-D-aspartate (NMDA) antagonist, D-(E)-4-(3-phosphonoprop-2-enyl) piperazine-2-carboxylic acid (D-CPPene) to assess the effect of brain oedema upon the protection rate.

Materials and Methods

We studied twenty adult male Sprague-Dawley rats weighing 300 to 350 g. The animals were anesthetized using halothane and nitrous oxide-oxygen mixture (70:30%) during the surgical procedure. Spontaneous respiration was maintained by a face mask. Cannulation of the femoral artery and vein was first carried out, and the animals were maintained normothermic. The animals were divided into two groups: middle cerebral artery (MCA) occlusion control group ($n = 10$) and MCA occlusion treated group ($n = 10$). All animals underwent the occlusion of the left MCA via a subtemporal approach without removal of the zygomatic arch or temporal muscle. Under high power magnification, the left MCA was coagulated with a micro-bipolar coagulator from the olfactory tract to the most proximal portion of the MCA and divided. In the treated group, a competitive NMDA antagonist D-CPPene was administered i.v. 15 minutes after MCA occlusion (4.5 mg/kg of initial bolus and

3 mg/kg/h of maintenance), while in the control group, saline was administered in the same fashion.

Twenty-four hours following MCA occlusion, the rats were sacrificed. The brain was removed from the calvaria immediately after sacrifice. Coronal sections (20 μm thick) were cut with a cryostat and stained with haematoxyline-eosin. The infarcted area was readily delineated. Eight coronal sections, which corresponded to planes of the predetermined forebrain, were selected among stained slices, and the volumes of infarction and each hemisphere were computed from the areas of ischaemic damage and the hemisphere measured at the different coronal planes and their anteroposterior coordinates, as described previously.

For morphometric measurement of infarct volume, three different methods were employed: direct measurement, Swanson's method and the diagram method. Morphometric determination of in infarct volume by the direct and diagram methods has been described previously [8, 10]. Briefly, in the direct measurement, the coronal section area of infarction in the cerebral cortex of the left MCA territory of each brain slice was measured with a plannimeter after transcribing a real brain slice on a paper (×4.0 actual size) by a zoom stereoscope. In the diagram method, the area of infarction was also measured with a plannimeter after being drawn on a scale diagram (×4.0 actual size). Infarct volume was integrated with the area measured by each method. In Swanson's method [11], a formula using measured volume with the direct method was followed: LI = RT-LN, where LI = infarct volume in the left hemisphere measured by this method, RT = total cortex volume in the right hemisphere of the same brain, and LN = noninfarcted cortex volume in the left hemisphere of the same brain. To further determine if the effect of brain oedema on the protection rate of D-CPPene differed between three different methods, the protection rate was also calculated as % = (infarct volume of the control − that of the treated/infarct volume of the control) ×100%.

The neuroprotective effect of D-CPPene was assessed by Student's t-test, and significance of the difference between the methods were assessed by ANOVA for randomized block design & Dunnet's multiple comparison. P < 0.05 was required for significance.

Results

Post-occlusion treatment of D-CPPene significantly attenuated infarct volume to about 40% of the control, which was observed in all three different methods ($P < 0.05$) (Fig. 1).

In comparison of three methods employed in the current study, the mean volume of focal cerebral infarction in the control based on the direct measurement appeared to be larger than the results by the other two methods, Swanson's and the diagram methods (285.6 vs. 160.1 and 170.7 mm^3) (P < 0.05). The mean infarct volume in the treated based on the direct measurement appeared to be much larger than above two methods (182.2 vs. 92.1 and 96.7 mm^3) (P < 0.05). In the mean time, there was no difference between Swanson's and the diagram methods.

The protection rate of D-CPPene against ischaemic damage based on the direct measurement was the lowest. The protection rate based on Swanson's and the diagram methods appeared to be about 7% higher than that of the direct measurement (Table 1).

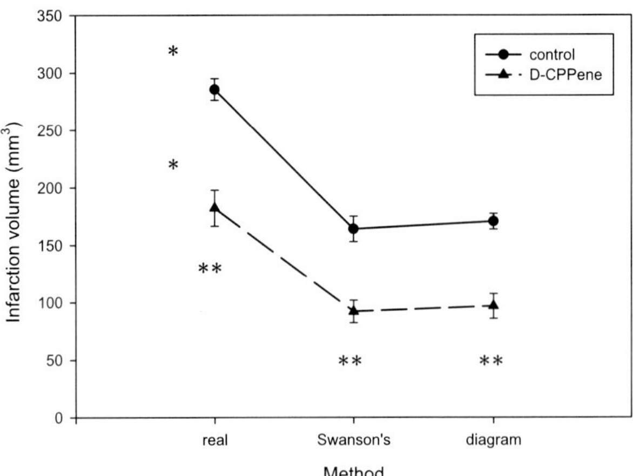

Fig. 1. Effect of D-CPPene on infarction volume (mm^3) of the cerebral hemisphere measured by different methods. The results are expressed as the means ± SE. *; $P < 0.05$, diagram compared to the other methods by ANOVA for randomized block design & Dunnett's multiple comparison. **; $P < 0.05$, compared to the control by Student's t-test. -●- control, –▲– D-CPPene

Table 1. *Protection Rate (%) of D-CPPene Against Ischaemic Brain Damage Based on Each Different Method*

Method	Direct measurement	Swanson's method	Diagram method
Protection rate (%)	36.5	43.9	43.5

Discussion

Brain swelling resulting from ischaemic oedema may play an important role in the pathogenesis of a focal cerebral infarction. Brain oedema reaches its maximal intensity 24–48 hours after initiation of ischaemia, and resulting increased regional tissue pressure exerts compressive effects on the surrounding vasculatures, and subsequently enhances ischaemic brain damage. D-CPPene has been known to attenuate ischaemic brain damage [9], as confirmed in the current study, but not to have specific protection effects upon ischaemic brain oedema [10].

Our results demonstrate that the effect of brain oedema at the early stage is significant enough to overestimate infarct volume. The mean volume of infarction based on the direct measurement appeared to be about 70% larger in the control and about 90%

larger in the treated, compared to the results of the Swanson's and the diagram methods. Considering that the effect of oedema is not avoided in the direct measurement, these results herald the effect of oedema is much more significant in the treated than in the control, indicating no effect of a competitive NMDA antagonist, D-CPPene on ischaemic brain oedema. Even in the protection rate, the direct measurement resulted in lower protection rate than the other methods. Recently, Lin and his colleagues [6] reported that infarct volume determined by direct measurement showed a wide fluctuation according to the evolution of brain oedema.

The indirect measurement proposed by Swanson and his colleagues [11] is based on the assumption that oedema does not occur outside the infarcted region in the hemisphere. The lack of significant difference in infarct volume between Swanson's and the diagram methods suggests that potential errors secondary to oedema-induced changes of noninfarcted cortex are minimal. Based on the original paper of diagram method written by Osborne and coworkers [7], this method was designed only to integrate consistent infarct volume. But in the current study, it was confirmed that measurement of infarct volume based on the diagram method is useful in reducing overestimation, which may be caused by oedema.

In conclusion, ischaemic brain oedema exerts a significant influence on the direct measurement at the acute stage to overestimate infarct volume and underestimate the protection rate of neuroprotective drugs in focal cerebral infarction. To eliminate overestimation of infarct volume during a period when brain oedema is prominent, indirect measurements such as Swanson's and the diagram methods offer desirable alternatives.

References

1. Avendano C, Roda JM, Carceller F, Dies-Tejedor E (1995) Morphometric study of focal cerebral ischemia in rats: a stereological evaluation. Brain Res 673: 83–92
2. Brint S, Jacewick M, Kiessling M, Tanabe J, Pulsinelli WA (1988) Focal brain ischemia in the rat: Method for reproducible neocortical infarction using tandem occlusion of the distal middle cerebral and ipsilateral common carotid arteries. J Cerebr Blood Flow Metab 8: 474–485
3. Hiramatsu K, Kassell NF, Goto Y, Soleau S, Lee KS (1993) A reproducible model of reversible, focal, neocortical ischemia in Sprague-Dawley rat. Acta Neurochir (Wien) 120: 66–71
4. Jacewicz M, Brint S, Tanabe J, Wang XJ, Pulsinelli WA (1990) Nimodipine pretreatment improves cerebral blood flow and reduces brain edema in conscious rats subjected to focal cerebral ischemia. J Cereb Blood Flow Metab 10: 903–913
5. Kondo T, Reaume AG, Huang TT, Carison E, Murakami K, Chen SF, Hoffman EK, Scott RW, Epstein CJ, Chan PH (1997) Reduction of CuZn-Superoxide dismutase activity exacerbates neuronal cell injury and edema formation after transient focal cerebral ischemia. J Neurosci 17: 4180–4189
6. Lin TN, He YY, Wu G, Kohan M, Hsu CY (1993) Effect of brain edema on infarct volume in a focal cerebral ischemia model in rats. Stroke 24: 117–121
7. Osborne KA, Shigeno T, Balarsky AM, Ford I, McCulloch J, Teasdale GM (1978) Quantitative assessment of early brain damage in a rat model of focal cerebral ischaemia. J Neurol Neurosurg Psychiatry 50: 402–410
8. Park CK, Nehls DG, Graham DI, Teasdale GM, McCulloch J (1988) The Glutamate antagonist MK-801 reduces focal ischemic brain damage in the rat. Ann Neurol 24: 543–551
9. Park CK, McCulloch J, Kang JK, Choi CR (1992) Efficacy of D-CPPene, a competitive N-methyl-D-aspartate antagonist in focal cerebral ischemia in the rat. Neurosci Lett 147: 41–44
10. Park CK, McCulloch J, Kang JK, Choi CR (1994) Pretreatment with competitive NMDA antagonist D-CPPene attenuate focal cerebral infarction and brain swelling in awake rats. Acta Neurochir (Wien) 127: 220–226
11. Swanson RA, Morton MT, Taso-Wu G, Salvalos RA, Davdson C, Sharp FR (1990) A semiautomated method for measuring brain infarct volume. J Cereb Blood Flow Metab 10: 290–293

Correspondence: Chun-Kun Park. M.D., Ph.D., Department of Neurosurgery, Kang Nam St. Mary's Hospital, Seoul, 137-040, Korea.

Acta Neurochir (2000) [Suppl] 76: 273–275

Characterizing Edema Associated with Cortical Contusion and Secondary Insult Using Magnetic Resonance Spectroscopy

G. Portella[1], **A. Beaumont**[2], **F. Corwin**[3], **P. Fatouros**[3], and **A. Marmarou**[2]

[1] Rianimazione, Ospedale S Gerardo, Monza, Milan, Italy
[2] Division of Neurosurgery, Medical College of Virginia, Richmond, VA, USA
[3] Division of Radiation Physics, Medical College of Virginia, Richmond, VA, USA

Summary

It is traditionally believed that edema associated with brain contusion is vasogenic. The objective of this study was to quantify and characterize the edema in cortical contusion coupled with early hypoxia and hypotension.

Sprague-Dawley rats were randomised into six groups: Sham, Trauma moderate (Tm), Trauma severe (Ts), Hypoxia and Hypotension (HH), Tm and Ts with HH (THHm; THHs). Trauma was induced with controlled cortical impact; associated secondary insults lasted 30 minutes. Water content was measured using tissue longitudinal relaxation time (T1). Apparent diffusion coefficient of water (ADC) was calculated from diffusion-weighted imaging and single voxel spectroscopy.

In the trauma groups ICP increased at 30 minutes post trauma ($p < 0.05$) and then gradually decreased. Only in the THH groups, ICP showed a trend to continually rise. No ICP variations were seen in the others groups. The increase in water content at 4 hours post trauma was inversely related to ADC variation ($p < 0.0001$). A significant increase in water content with low ADC, developed in the injured region in Ts, THHm ($p < 0.05$) and THHs ($p < 0.01$) compared to Sham. Intracellular water rose in the whole brain in THH groups although more severely in the THHs ($p < 0.01$). Immediately after trauma ADC fell in the THH groups, but gradually increased in the THHm, whereas there was no recovery in THHs.

The results indicate that the type of edema in the injured area, with and without superimposed secondary insult, is predominantly cytotoxic (cellular). Moreover, secondary insults act synergistically with focal injury to increase cellular water in both injured tissue and remote regions.

Keywords: Traumatic brain edema; secondary insult; water content; diffusion weighted imaging.

Introduction

The nature of edema, vasogenic versus cytotoxic, after traumatic head injury is still controversial and the role of secondary insults to eventually worsen edema is not clear.

Edema surrounding a contusional area has been classified as vasogenic, however recent studies in models of cortical contusion have demonstrated a predominant component of intracellular edema [7]. Secondary insults are common during the acute post-injury phase following a traumatic brain injury. They might increase brain damage and influence a worst outcome [1, 6, 8].

The aim of this study was to quantify and characterize the predominant type of brain edema (vasogenic versus cytotoxic), using MRI techniques, when early secondary insults were superimposed to a focal cortical contusion in rats.

Methods

A model of controlled cortical impact (CCI) [2] was used to induce a lateral cortical contusion in rats. Two different levels of severity of trauma were obtained using a depth of impact of 3 mm and 3.5 mm at a constant velocity of 2.3–2.7 m/sec. Immediately following head injury, 30 minutes of hypoxia (paO2 30–40 mmHg) and hypotension (mean arterial pressure of 30–40 mmHg) were superimposed. Animals were subsequently resuscitated.

We measured water content and ADC by experiments carried out in the MRI. The measurements were obtained in a region of interest (ROI) in the cortex directly under the site of impact, in the homotopic region within contralateral cortex and in the whole brain, at baseline and about 4 hours after trauma. To quantify the edema, precise estimate of longitudinal relaxation time (MRI T1 weighted imaging) of tissue was converted in percentage of water (water content grams of water / 100 grams of tissue) [3]. Intracellular increase of water was considered as cytotoxic edema whereas an extracellular rise of water was attributed to barrier compromise and vasogenic edema. The apparent diffusion coefficient of water (ADC) was calculated from MRI diffusion weighted imaging (DWI). From previous studies, ADC has been demonstrated to decrease in case of intracellular edema and increase with extracellular accumulation of

Table 1. *Water Content is Expressed in Grams of Water / 100 Grams of Tissue and ADC is 10^{-3} mm^2/sec*

Groups	ROI (injured region)		Whole brain	
	Water content %	ADC 10^{-3} mm^2:/sec	Water content %	ADC 10^{-3} mm^2:/sec
Sham	1.2 ± 1.03	0.64 ± 0.10	0.5 ± 0.9	0.71 ± 0.05
HH	4.2 ± 2.23	0.62 ± 0.04	1.9 ± 1.1	$0.62 \pm 0.06^*$
Tm	3.1 ± 1.00	0.56 ± 0.11	0.9 ± 1.0	0.74 ± 0.03
THHm	$4.5 \pm 3.42^*$	$0.42 \pm 0.08^{**}$	$2.3 \pm 1.2^*$	$0.57 \pm 0.02^{**}$
Ts	$6.3 \pm 1.89^{**}$	$0.39 \pm 0.06^{**}$	2.3 ± 2.4	$0.63 \pm 0.02^*$
THHs	$7.9 \pm 2.98^{**}$	$0.37 \pm 0.10^{**}$	$4.2 \pm 0.9^{**}$	$0.45 \pm 0.09^{**}$

* = $p < 0.05$; ** = $p < 0.01$ compared to Sham.

water [4, 5]. A fast acquisition (DWI single voxel spectroscopic technique) was used to follow the temporal course of ADC. Eighty-five adult Sprague-Dawley rats were randomized in six groups: Sham, Trauma moderate (Tm) and severe (Ts) Hypoxia Hypotension (HH), Tm and Ts with HH (THHm; THHs).

Technical problems made it impossible to record intracranial pressure (ICP) and cerebral perfusion pressure (CPP) inside of the magnet, so parallel bench studies were carried out to measure those parameters.

All data are shown as mean $\pm$ SD. Statistical analysis was performed by means of ANOVA and LSD post hoc test when multiple comparisons were made. Correlation between water map and ADC was analysed by Pearson Product-Moment correlation. Repeated measure analysis was used to follow the temporal course of the ADC and physiology data.

Results

In the trauma groups, ICP increased at 30 minutes post trauma (31 ± 10 mmHg Tm and 21 ± 6 mmHg Ts; $p < 0.05$), then gradually decreased. ICP showed a permanent trend to rise when trauma was associated with secondary insults (THH groups). No changes were seen in the sham groups.

The increase in water content in the whole brain was inversely related to the variation of ADC ($r = 0.70$, $p < 0.0001$) at four hours post trauma. This result suggested a predominant role of intracellular water in the developing edema. A significant increase in water content associated with low ADC was found in the injured region in THHm ($p < 0.05$) and Ts and THHs ($p < 0.01$) compared to Sham. In the THH groups the cytotoxic edema was not only confined to regions of trauma, but affected the entire brain. The rise in water content with low ADC was more severe in the THHs when compared to all others groups. ($p < 0.01$) (Table 1). The analysis of temporal course showed an immediate ADC drop after trauma in the THH groups. ADC was 0.44 ± 0.07 10^{-3} mm^2/sec in THHm and 0.32 ± 0.06 10^{-3} mm^2/sec in THHs by 30 minutes post-trauma. After this period, ADC recovered to 0.60 ± 0.11 10^{-3} mm^2/sec by the end of the study in THHm whereas there was no recovery of ADC values in THHs.

Conclusion

The inverse relation between water content and decreased ADC suggests a predominant role of intracellular water in the developing edema. Moreover, our results show that at 4 hours after a focal traumatic damage, there is an ipsilateral increase of water which is predominantly cellular proportional to the severity of trauma. Superimposed secondary insults increase the amount of edema associated with the mechanical insult. Trauma and secondary insults seem to act synergically to increase cellular edema in the entire brain and is not only restricted to the site of focal injury.

References

1. Chesnut RM, Marshall LF, Klauber MR *et al* (1993) The role of secondary brain injury in determining outcome from severe head injury. J Trauma 34: 216–222
2. Dixon CE, Clifton GL, Lighthall JW, Yaghnai AA, Hayes RL (1991) A controlled cortical impact model of traumatic brain injury in the rat. Neurosci Meth 39: 253–261
3. Fatouros PP, Marmarou A, Kraft KA, Inao S, Schwarz FP (1991) In vivo brain water determination by T1 measurements: effect of total water content, hydratation fraction and field strenght. Magnetic Resonance Med 17: 402–413
4. Ito J, Marmarou A, Barzo P, Fatouros P, Corwin F (1996) Characterization of edema by diffusion-weighted imaging in experimental traumatic brain injury. J Neurosurg 84: 97–103
5. Ebisu T, Naruse S, Horikawa *et al* (1993) Discrimination between different types of white matter edema with diffusion-weighted MR imaging. JMRI 3: 863–868

6. Miller JD, Butterworth JF, Gudeman SK *et al* (1981) Further experience in the management of severe head injury. J Neurosurg 54: 289–299
7. Stroop R, Thomale UW, Pauser S *et al* (1998) Magnetic resonance imaging studies with cluster algorithm for characterization of brain edema after Controlled Cortical Impact Injury (CCII). Acta Neurochir [Suppl] (Wien) 71: 303–305
8. Stocchetti N, Furlan A, Volta F (1996) Hypoxemia and arterial hypotension at the accident scene in head injury. J Trauma 40: 1–4

Correspondence: Anthony Marmarou, Ph.D., Division of Neurosurgery, Medical College of Virginia, Box 980508 Sanger Hall, 1101 E. Marshall St., Richmond Virginia 23298-0508.

Acta Neurochir (2000) [Suppl] 76: 277–278

Plasminogen Activator Inhibitor-1 in Patients with Ischemic Stroke

E. Haapaniemi[1], **T. Tatlisumak**[1], **L. Soinne**[1], **M. Syrjälä**[2], and **M. Kaste**[1]

[1] Department of Neurology, Helsinki University Central Hospital, Helsinki, Finland
[2] Department of Laboratory Medicine, Helsinki University Central Hospital, Helsinki, Finland

Summary

Low fibrinolytic activity may increase the risk of thrombosis. Plasminogen activator inhibitor-1 (PAI-1) is an inhibitor of the fibrinolytic system. We examined the PAI-1 levels in patients with ischemic stroke. Plasma levels of PAI-1 were measured using enzyme-linked immunosorbent assay (ELISA) in 55 consecutive patients (age 60.2 ± 11.4, 40 males and 15 females) with ischemic stroke. The PAI-1 assessments as well as neurological examinations using validated stroke scales were conducted at admission and 1 week, 1 month, and 3 months after stroke. Sex- and age-matched controls (± 4 years) underwent plasma PAI-1 measurement once. Etiology of the stroke was classified using the Trial of Org 10172 in Acute Stroke Treatment (TOAST) criteria. All pertinent stroke risk factors were recorded. All patients were contacted 3 years after stroke for recurrent vascular thrombotic disease. The plasma PAI-1 levels were 17.2 ± 7.8 IU at admission, 11.2 ± 9.2 IU at 1 week, 14.4 ± 7.9 IU at 1 month, and 17.8 ± 7.8 IU at 3 months among patients and 11.8 ± 9.5 IU among controls (p values are $<.002$, .7, .12, and $<.0005$, respectively). As a rule, the neurological scores did not show a correlation to the PAI-1 levels. Presence of diabetes, hypertension, obesity, smoking, anticoagulant treatment, and sleep apnea did not affect the PAI-1 levels at any time point. Females had slightly higher PAI-1 levels. Age was a strong determinant for PAI-1 levels being higher in younger patients at every sampling time point (p values .02, .02, .02, and .03 respectively). The etiology of the ischemic stroke did not have an impact on PAI-1 levels. In 16 patients recurrent thrombosis had occurred. The high PAI-1 levels at admittance may reflect either an acute phase response or a chronic state. Normalized levels at 1 week and 1 month may be due to hospital diet, antithrombotic medication, weight loss, active physical therapy, and better care for diabetes. PAI-1 levels at 3 months after stroke did not predict recurrent thrombosis.

Keywords: Plasminogen; stroke; fibrinolysis; thrombosis

Introduction

The fibrinolytic system counteracts thrombus formation in vessels. The proenzyme plasminogen is activated to plasmin by tissue-type plasminogen activator (t-PA). PAI-1 inhibits the activity of tPA and thereby the fibrinolytic process. Thus, PAI-1 has a critical role in the inhibition of fibrinolysis. A low level of fibrinolytic activity is a determinant of ischemic heart disease in younger men [1] and increased concentration of PAI-1 were found in patients with myocardial infarction [2]. Previously, both normal [3] and increased [4] levels of PAI-1 have been observed in the acute phase of stroke. A recent study with a design similar to ours reported high levels of PAI-1 in the patients with stroke [5]. High levels of PAI-1 may increase the risk of thrombosis by inhibiting fibrinolytic activity. This study was designed as a prospective, observational, descriptive, and clinical study aiming to describe PAI-1 levels in consecutive patients with ischemic stroke during the acute and chronic phases. Furthermore, a long follow-up study is planned to find if high PAI-1 levels 3 months after stroke predict stroke recurrence.

Materials and Methods

This study was approved by our local ethical committee (Department of Neurology, Helsinki University Central Hospital, Helsinki, Finland). All patients gave written informed consent. Fifty-five consecutive patients with clinically and radiologically proven brain infarction were included. Patients unable to give informed consent for various reasons and patients who refused to participate in the study were excluded. Fasting blood specimens were collected via the venous route at admittance (within 2 days), at one week (7 ± 1 days), at one month (30 ± 3 days), and at 3 months (90 ± 7 days). All specimens were taken at 8 to 10 am because of the diurnal variation of the PAI-1 activity [6, 7]. The blood was collected into vacuum tubes containing sodium citrate, centrifuged immediately, and plasma was frozen at $-70\,^{\circ}$C until analyzed. Plasma PAI-1 levels were then measured using enzyme-linked immunosorbent assay (ELISA). Sex- and age-matched (± 4 years) controls without any known thrombotic or hemorrhagic disease underwent blood sampling, sample handling, and PAI-1 measurement only once. All patients were examined neurologically at each blood sampling timepoint using several neurological scales (National Institute Health Stroke Scale, Scandinavian Stroke Scale, Glasgow Coma Scale,

Barthel Index, Modified Rankin Score, and Mini-Mental State Examination). All stroke risk factors, body mass index, and all medications were recorded. The etiology of brain infarction was determined according to TOAST criteria. All values are expressed as mean ± standard deviation. PAI-1 levels of the patients and of the controls were compared by paired *t*-test. Correlation between the PAI-1 levels and the neurological scores was calculated by linear regression. Patients with certain risk factors and patients without that particular risk factor were compared by the *t*-test. A *p*-value < .05 was considered significant.

Results

Of 55 patients (age 60.2 ± 11.4 years), 40 were males (61.5 ± 10.6) and 15 were females (56.9 ± 13.0). In the control group (age 60.0 ± 11.4 years), age distribution was 61.7 ± 10.3 for males and 56.7 ± 13.4 for females. PAI-1 levels among patients were 17.2 ± 7.8 IU at admittance (range 2.9–38.3), 11.2 ± 9.2 IU at one week (range 0.0–37.8), 14.4 ± 7.9 IU at one month (range 0.0–34.1), and 17.8 ± 7.8 IU at 3 months (range 2.9–37.8). In controls, PAI-1 level was 11.8 ± 9.5 IU (range 0.0–39.2). *P* values were <.002, 0.7, 0.12, and <.0004, respectively. Neurological scores (NIHSS, SSS, GCS, Barthel Index, Modified Rankin Scale, and MMSE) did not correlate with PAI-1 levels. Patients with diabetes (n = 7) had slightly, but insignificantly higher PAI-1 values measured compared to patients without diabetes (n = 48). Patients with hypertension (n = 27) showed a similar trend. Patients with BMI > 27 (n = 26) had slightly higher PAI-1 levels at all timepoints; cigarette smokers (n = 34) had a similar pattern. None of these measurements reached statistical significance. Patients with sleep apnea (n = 21) surprisingly had consistently lower PAI-1 values. Patients receiving either heparin or warfarin had lower PAI-1 levels at admittance ($p = .02$), but at later measurements, no difference was observed. Females (n = 15) had slightly higher PAI-1 levels at every timepoint compared to males (n = 40). The etiology of brain infarction did not disclose a significant relationship to the PAI-1 levels at any measurement timepoint. These data are not shown. Age appeared to be a significant determinant of plasma PAI-1 concentrations. The PAI-1 levels of the patients younger than 60 years (n = 29) were compared to the PAI-1 levels of the patients over 60 years (n = 26). The *p* values were .02, .02, .02, and .025 for the respective timepoints. At all timepoints, PAI-1 levels were significantly higher in the younger patients group (data not shown).

Discussion

High PAI-1 levels among the patients at admittance may suggest either an acute phase response or a chronic state. High PAI-1 levels at 3 months suggest chronically high concentrations with a probable increased risk for thrombosis among the patients (a 3-year follow-up study is under way). Normalized PAI-1 levels at one week and at one month timepoints may suggest an improvement in the fibrinolytic activity among the patients, probably due to the use of anticoagulants and antithrombotic agents, better care for diabetes and hypertension in the hospital, hospital diet, cessation of smoking, vigorous physical rehabilitation, and possibly due to other less well-known factors. PAI-1 levels showed a wide range and large standard deviation both among the patients and the controls suggesting a highly variable fibrinolytic activity among individuals. In most patients, the first blood sampling time after the index stroke was close to 2 days which may not necessarily have a rapid increase and decrease of the PAI-1 levels acutely in less than 2 days.

References

1. Meade TW, Ruddock V, Stirling Y, Chakrabarti R, Miller GJ (1993) Fibrinolytic activity, clotting factors, and long-term incidence of ischemic heart disease in the Northwick Park Heart Study. Lancet 342: 1076–1079
2. Hamsten A, Wiman B, de Faire U, Blombäck M (1985) Increased plasma levels of a rapid inhibitor of tissue plasminogen activator in young survivors of myocardial infarction. N Engl J Med 313: 1557–1563
3. Fisher M, Francis R (1990) Altered coagulation in cerebral ischemia: platelet, thrombin, and plasmin activity. Arch Neurol 47: 1075–1079
4. Feinberg WM, Bruck DC, Jeter MA, Corrigan JJ Jr (1991) Fibrinolysis after acute ischemic stroke. Thromb Res 64: 117–127
5. Lindgren A, Lindoff C, Norrving B, Åstedt B, Johansson BB (1996) Tissue plasminogen activator and plasminogen activator inhibitor-1 in stroke patients. Stroke 27: 1066–1071
6. Angleton P, Chandler WL, Schmer G (1989) Diurnal variation of tissue-type plasminogen-activator and its rapid inhibitor (PAI-1). Circulation 79: 101–106
7. Eliasson M, Evrin P-E, Lundblad D, Asplund K, Rånby M (1993) Influence of gender, age and sampling time on plasma fibrinolytic variables and fibrinogen: a population study. Fibrinolysis 7: 316–323

Correspondence: Dr. Turgut Tatlisumak, Department of Neurology, Helsinki University Central Hospital, Helsinki, Finland.

Acta Neurochir (2000) [Suppl] 76: 279–281

Experimental Study on Brain Oxygenation in Relation to Tissue Water Redistribution and Brain Oedema

E. Titovets, N. Nechipurenko, T. Griboedova, and **P. Vlasyuk**

Basic Research Department, Research Institute of Neurology and Neurosurgery, Minsk, Belarus

Summary

The aim of the present experimental research was to study brain oxygenation parameters in relation to tissue water movement and brain cortex oedema caused by focal brain ischemia. It has been demonstrated that local osmotic dehydration of the parietal brain cortex, mercury compounds (aquaporin inhibitors) and brain cortex oedema resulting from focal brain ischemia all influence extra-capillary oxygen transport lowering tissue respiration rates and oxygen transfer coefficients. The changes of brain oxygenation parameters in case of cortex ischemic oedema are reflected in the gas composition (oxygen and carbon dioxide partial pressure) of the blood in *v. jugularis.* A short course of hyperbaric treatment results in normalization of water content in the brain. The results are interpreted in terms of the functioning of tissue microcirculation that might participate, at the extra-capillary level, in brain oxygenation.

Keywords: Oxygen; water; brain oedema.

Introduction

Brain oedema presents a complex pathological manifestation. It results from malfunctioning of the mechanisms maintaining brain homeostasis and the disparity between the inflow and the outflow of tissue water. Microcirculation of water in brain tissue might be influenced by the oxygen transport system which has wide implications to brain respiration, energy metabolism and hypoxia. The present study investigates the problem of brain cortex oxygenation in its relation to tissue water and oedema. We have concentrated onthe investigation of brain respiration and extra-capillary oxygen transport and the effects of various agents and conditions influencing tissue water distribution.

Materials and Methods

The experiments were carried out on Chinchilla rabbits of both sexes weighing 3.1–3.5 kg kept under intravenous *Hexenal* (50–70 mg/kg) anesthesia. Access to the parietal brain cortex was achieved by drilling two burr holes, 8 mm diameter lateral to the sagittal sinus and removing the dura mater. Local tissue oxygenation parameters were measured either on the dural aspect of the arachnoidea or on the cortex parenchyma after extirpation of the leptopmeningies. Focal brain-cortex ischemia (FBCI) in rabbits was induced by clipping for three hours both *a carotis communis.*

Water content in the parietal brain cortex was determined by the gravimetric method as described elsewhere in the literature [6]. Oxygen and carbon dioxide partial pressure determinations in the blood were carried our using Model ABL50 Radiometer, Copenhagen. The brain oxygenation parameters k (oxygen transfer coefficient) and V (tissue respiration rate at 150 mm Hg oxygen partial pressure) were both derived from the oxygen consumption curves obtained by surface application of Clark-type oxygen sensors with 15 μm diameter platinum cathodes [9].

The mercury compounds used in our experiments to study aquaporin participation in water transfer were: mercury acetate, mercury sulfate, and mercury cyanide – all of analytical grade. In the experiments on local effects of these compounds their solutions were applied on a 6 mm diameter filter paper on the tissue surface for five minutes.

Results

Oxygen consumption by the brain tissue when measured by the surface contact technique closely follows first-order kinetics. The oxygen consumption curves are thus characterized by oxygen transfer coefficients, k, having the reversed time dimension. It should be observed here that it is the extra-capillary oxygen mass-transfer that has been monitored by the above approach.

In the experiments presented in Fig. 1 the measurements have been carried out using two oxygen sensors placed over symmetrical areas of the parietal cortex. Such an approach, along with the simultaneous oxygen monitoring, makes it possible to compare accurately the oxygenation parameters of the arachnoidea and the cortex parenchyma in the right and the left hemispheres.

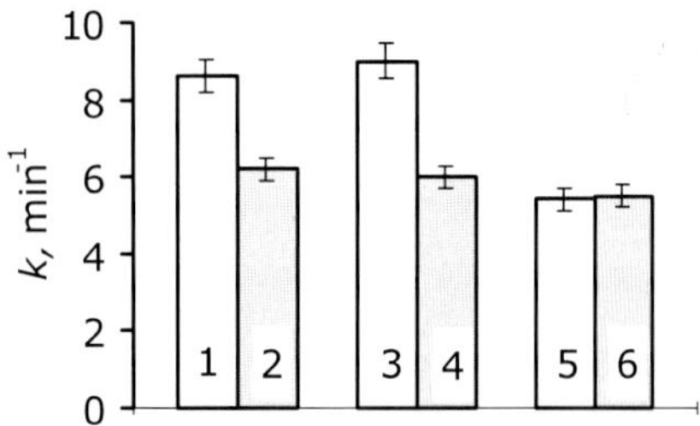

Fig. 1. Oxygen transfer coefficients in the arachnoidea (1,2) and cortex parenchyma (3–6) of the right (even numbers) and the left (odd numbers) hemispheres. Explanations in text

A statistically significant difference in the k values for the symmetrical brain structures was revealed with higher values in the left hemisphere. Such a pattern has been observed in 80% of the animals while the rest demonstrated a reversed picture – higher values for the right hemisphere. With any asymmetry pattern k values for the cortex parenchyma have been higher than those for the arachnoid. Brain ischemia brought about by cardiac arrest results in lowering and leveling off the k values (cf. columns 5 and 6).

The apparent first-order rate constants for oxygen reduction by cytochrome oxidase *in situ* are orders of magnitude higher than those for oxygen mass-transfer observed in our experiments, cf. [1, 2]. This fact indicates that under our experimental conditions extra-capillary oxygen-mass transfer controls the rate of mitochondrial respiration and, consequently, brain energy production. This allows the measurement of the effect of various factors influencing upon the brain water distribution, the effect of the latter on tissue respiration and extra-capillary oxygen transport.

Application on the arachnoid of 0.6 M sodium chloride solution resulted in a reduced oxygen transfer coefficient by 33% (3.6 $\pm$ 0.3 min^{-1} (n = 29) in control and 2.4 $\pm$ 0.3 min^{-1} (n = 22) after the sodium chloride exposure). The respiration rate followed the above pattern with 510 $\pm$ 36 O_2 mm Hg/min (n = 28) before and 372 $\pm$ 42 O_2 mm Hg/min (n = 26) after the hypertonic solution exposure thus resulting in a 27% decrease of tissue respiration rate.

Mercury compounds inhibit some aquaporins [7] and might serve a powerful tool for assessing the effect of control of water movements on cortex oxygenation. Of the three chosen compounds – mercury acetate, mercury sulfate and mercury cyanide – neither mercury acetate nor mercury sulfate applied on the cortex surface at the concentration of 3 mM produced any significant effect on cortex oxygenation. This might have been expected in view of the fact that brain AQP4 is insensitive to mercury inhibition [8]. Mercury acetate at an enhanced concentration of 16 mM resulted in a 64% lowering of k. This might implicate indirect involvement of aquaporins other then AQP4 in the oxygen tissue transport via a water micro-flow mechanism.

Mercury cyanide at 3 mM caused 79% reduction in both the respiration rate and the oxygen transfer coefficients. A possible explanation might have been that the cyanide anion is a well-known inhibitor of cytochrome oxidase [10] hence lowering of the tissue respiration rate. But it is hardly a satisfactory explanation in view of the fact that cyanide also interferes with the oxygen mass-transfer resulting in a 79% decrease of k. As has been shown above tissue respiration under our experimental conditions is controlled by oxygen mass-transfer. Thus the inhibition of the respiration rate might have been primarily due to cyanide interference with the oxygen transfer to cytochrome oxidase. It poses a new question regarding mechanism and we find it difficult to supply an answer at this stage.

As seen from Table 1 focal ischemia results in the expected parietal cortex oedema and the increase was statistically significant. At the same time there was a lowering by 27% of both the respiration rate and oxy-

Table 1. *Parameters of Brain Cortex Oxygenation in Control and Brain Oedema. Parietal Lobe. Focal Ischemia as Described Under Materials and Methods*

Experimental step	K, min^{-1}	V, O_2 mmHg/min	H_2O, % wet weight
Control	5.1 $\pm$ 0.24 (32)	750 $\pm$ 35 (32)	77.5 $\pm$ 0.49 (36)
Focal 3-hour ischemia	3.7 $\pm$ 0.18* (32)	545 $\pm$ 31* (32)	81.2 $\pm$ 0.35* (25)
5 days after the ischemia	6.6 $\pm$ 0.36* (32)	997 $\pm$ 52* (32)	80.5 $\pm$ 0.27* (23)

Figures in brackets indicate the number of observations. * Statistically significant changes in respect to control.

gen transfer coefficient. Thus cortex oedema reflects negatively upon oxygen transport which might further maintain tissue hypoxia. After five days we observed a 30–33% increase of the oxygenation parameters over the control values although the oedema was still present.

Measurements in the above experiments of oxygen partial pressure in the *v. jagularis* showed values of 41.5 ± 3.1 mm Hg (n = 14) and 25.6 ± 2.3 mm Hg (n = 6) for the control and the focal-ischemia animals, respectively. Carbon dioxide partial pressure equaled 42.2 ± 0.7 mm Hg (n = 14) in control animals and 44.9 ± 0.5 mm Hg (n = 6) after focal hypoxia. Lower oxygen partial pressure in the outflow blood accompanied by hypercapnia, when considered together with the brain oxygenation parameters, might be interpreted as indication of an increased oxygen consumption by the cortex at this stage due to enhanced oxygen extra-capillary transport.

A short course of hyperbaric-oxygen therapy (three daily exposures for 40 min. at 2 ata) conducted after 5 days of brain ischemia produced a positive effect on the brain oxygenation parameters and the venous blood gas composition.

Discussion

Brain oedema presents a complex pathological manifestation that includes many aspects important for elucidation of its pathogenic mechanisms [3–6]. In our present research we have considered a rather narrow tentative aspect of the issue – tissue water as a vehicle for the extra-capillary transport of oxygen to cytochrome oxidase while extracellular and intracellular swelling might interfere with this process. Within this framework brain oedema might be viewed as an extreme condition of tissue water accumulation impairing the oxygen transport mechanism with important implication to tissue oxygenation.

We hypothesize that extra-capillary oxygen-mass transfer is related to vector micro-flows of water that occur laterally along the cell membranes as well as in the trans-membrane fashion via catalytic action of aquaporins. Together they form a system that might be involved into the mechanism of extra-capillary oxygen transfer. The above experimental results with the hypertonic exposure, mercury compounds, and brain cortex oedema demonstrate the characteristic lability of tissue oxygenation parameters.

References

1. Chance B, Quistorff A (1978) Study of tissue oxygen gradients by single and multiple indicators. Oxygen transport to tissue. In: Silver TA (ed) Plenum Press, New York London, pp 331–338
2. Clark J B, Niclkas WJ, Degn H (1976) The apparent K_m for oxygen of rat brain mitochondrial respiration. J Neurochem 26: 409–411
3. Go KG (1997) The normal and pathological physiology of brain water. Adv Tech Stand Neurosurg 23: 47–142
4. Kimelberg HK (1995) Current concepts of brain edema. J Neurosurg 83: 1051–1059
5. Kimelberg HK, Norenberg MD (1994) The neurobiology of central nervous system trauma. Oxford University Press, New York. 193–208
6. Klatzo I, (1967) Presidential address: neuropathological aspects of brain edema. J Neuropathol Exp Neurol 26: 1–13
7. Kuwahara M, Gu Y, Ishibashi K, Marumo F, Sasaki S (1997) Mercury-sensitive residues and pore site in AQP3 water channel. Biochemistry 36(46): 13973–13978
8. Lee MD, King LS, Agre P (1997) The aquaporin family of water channel proteins in clinical medicine. Medicine 76(3): 141–156
9. Titovets E, Parkhach L (1998) Method for monitoring oxygen mass-transfer in the biological tussues. Patent N^0 2813, Belarus
10. Yoshikawa S, and Orii Y, (1973) The inhibition mechanism of cytochrome oxidase reaction. IV. The nature of kinetically inactive complex of cytochrome oxidase with cyanide. J Biochem 73: 637–645

Correspondence: Prof. Ernst Titovets, MD, Ph.D, Basic Research Department, Research Institute of Neurology and Neurosurgery, Filatova, 9, 220026, Minsk, Belarus.

Pharmacology/Therapy

The only clinical paper in this group is presented by Hartmann and co-workers yielding practical important results i.e. Furosemide has very limited usefulness in brain oedema therapy. The authors found a decrease in global CBF following Furosemide treatment. The best effect was observed after Sorbitol and Mannitol administration.

The possible usefulness of pretreatment with hyperbaric oxygenation (HBO) in order to enhance ischemia tolerance was studied by Wada and co-workers. The authors report positive effects of pretreatment with HBO sessions on the apoptosis regulating protein and free radical scavenging system (Mn-SOD).

Two papers presented by the Uppsala group concern therapy for spinal cord injury. The authors provide results of the effects of neurotrophic pre-treatment which provide a new way forward in pharmacotherapy.

In both cold-induced (vasogenic) and ischaemia (cytotoxic) oedema models Mima *et al.* showed that Lipocortin – I and dexamethasone were ineffective at reducing oedema. By contrast, hepatocyte growth factor (Tsuzuki *et al.*) and Lidocaine (Hirayama *et al.*) did reduce oedema. The understanding and interpretation of these findings must be restricted to the very specific conditions which applied during the studies.

A number of agents were shown to have neuroprotective potential in experimental focal ischaemia:

- Takahashi *et al.* showed that Niraboline reduced vasogenic oedema in a tumour model.
- Tatlisumak *et al.* showed that glycine site antagonists reduced infarct volume.
- Takemori *et al.* showed that nitric oxide synthase inhibition reduced brain weight in spontaneously hypertensive stroke prone rats.
- Kubota *et al.* showed that sphingolipids improved cortical function.
- Ikeda *et al.* showed that vitamin E derivatives reduced vasogenic brain oedema.
- Tatlisumak *et al.* described a new calcium channel inhibitor.

Whether such Neuroprotective potential can be translated into clinical effectiveness or not remains to be seen.

Acta Neurochir (2000) [Suppl] 76: 285–290

Mn-SOD and Bcl-2 Expression After Repeated Hyperbaric Oxygenation

K. Wada[1,2], **T. Miyazawa**[1], **N. Nomura**[1], **A. Yano**[1], **N. Tsuzuki**[1], **H. Nawashiro**[1], and **K. Shima**[1]

[1] Department of Neurosurgery, National Defense Medical College, Saitama, Japan
[2] Undersea Medical Center, Japan Maritime Self Defense Force, Kanagawa, Japan

Summary

To clarify the mechanism of ischemic tolerance induced by HBO, we investigated the effect of HBO on immunoreactivity to Bcl-2 and Bax, apoptosis-regulating protein, or Mn-SOD, a radical scavenging system, in the CA1 sector of the gerbil hippocampus.

Pretreatment comprising, five sessions at 2 ATA (atmosphere absolute) every other day, but not that comprising, ten sessions at 3 ATA every day, caused significant increases in Bcl-2 and Mn-SOD immunoreactivity in the CA1 sector compared with in the sham pretreatment group. No significant differences in Bax immunoreactivity and neuronal density in the CA1 hippocampal neurons was observed between the groups.

These results suggest that protection against mitochondrial alterations after ischemia through Mn-SOD and/or Bcl-2 expression is related to the ischemic tolerance induced by repeated HBO pretreatment.

Keywords: Ischemic tolerance; hyperbaric oxygen; Bcl-2, Bax; Mn-SOD; gerbil.

Introduction

Even brief global cerebral ischemia causes irreversible damage to hippocampal CA1 neurons in rodents. The selective vulnerability of CA1 neurons results in delayed neuronal death [16]. This delayed neuronal death can be reduced by some pretreatments or diverse environmental changes, such as non-lethal hyperthermic stress [5], non-lethal ischemic stress [17, 18], oxidative stress [26], and TNF-α [24]. This phenomenon has been designated as "ischemic tolerance". If ischemic tolerance could be applied clinically to humans, it would be helpful in patients undergoing ischemia-producing procedures, such as temporary clipping of major intracranial vessels during aneurysmal or bypass surgery. We have already reported that repeated hyperbaric oxygenation, which is used in humans in the treatment of stroke, CO poisoning, air embolism and decompression sickness, induces ischemic tolerance in gerbil hippocampal CA1 pyramidal neurons [35].

Recently, a disturbance of mitochondria was reported to be a cause of ischemic delayed neuronal death [1]. In this regard, to clarify the mechanism of ischemic tolerance induced by HBO, we investigated whether or not HBO induced protective mechanisms against mitochondrial dysfunction. Firstly, since recent studies suggested that activation of the apoptotic process is involved in the delayed neuronal death of the hippocampal CA1 sector [15, 25, 30], we investigated immunohistochemically the influence of HBO on the expression of apoptosis-regulating proteins, Bcl-2 (suppressor of apoptosis) and Bax (promotor of apoptosis). Secondly, mitochondrial manganese superoxide dismutase has been reported to reduce ischemic brain injury [14]. Therefore, we investigated the influence of HBO on Mn-SOD expression, by means of immunohistochemical staining.

Materials and Methods

A total of 15 male Mongolian gerbils, weighing 60–80 g, were used. They were allowed free access to food and water prior to and following the treatment. The animals were divided into the following three groups: sham-HBO (n = 5), five-session HBO (2-ATA (atmospheres absolute)) pretreatment (n = 5), and ten-session HBO (3-ATA) pretreatment (n = 5) groups.

For HBO treatment, pure oxygen was supplied continuously at a pressure of either 2-ATA for 1 hour once every other day five times or 3-ATA for 1 hour every day ten times. Compression was performed at 1 $kg/cm^2/min$, and decompression was carried out at 0.2 $kg/cm^2/min$. No seizure was observed in any animals during the procedure. The animals in the sham-HBO group were placed in the chamber, which was not pressurized for sham-treatment, with the same schedule as for the five-time HBO pretreatment group.

Two days following sham-pretreatment, 5-session HBO at 2-ATA pretreatment or 10-session HBO pretreatment at 3-ATA, the gerbils were anesthetized and their brains were briefly washed by transcardiac perfusion with heparinized saline, followed by perfusion-fixation with 4% paraformaldehyde in 0.1 *M* phosphate buffer for 20 min. The brains were removed 1 h later, immersed in the same fixative for 1 day, and then embedded in paraffin. Paraffin sections, 5 μm in thickness, were prepared at the level of the dorsal hippocampus. The paraffin sections of the gerbil brains were immunohistochemically stained with a human polyclonal antibody raised against Bcl-2 (Santa Cruz, CA, USA), a mouse polyclonal antibody raised against Bax (Bcl-associated X protein) (Santa Cruz, CA, USA), or a human polyclonal antibody against manganese superoxide dismutase (Mn-SOD) (Biogenesis, NH, USA) to examine the mitochondrial response following HBO pretreatment. The sections were stained using antibodies against Mn-SOD, Bcl-2 or Bax. Briefly, the sections were deparaffinized, and then heated and boiled for 1 min by microwaving in 10 mM citrate buffer, pH 6.0. Then, these were preincubated with 10% normal serum in PBS for 1 h at room temperature, followed by 1-hour incubation with a antibody against Mn-SOD diluted 1:200 at room temperature, followed by overnight incubation with an antibody against Bcl-2 or Bax diluted 1:500 at room temperature. The sections were then incubated with a biotinylated anti-mouse IgG + IgA + IgM antibody for 1 h and then placed in streptavidin-horseradish peroxidase conjugate for 30 min. The final reaction product was visualized using 0.05% 3,3i-diaminobenzidine as the chromogen in the presence of 0.02% hydrogen peroxide for 5 min. The sections for Bcl-2 and Bax staining were counterstained using Mayer's hematoxylin. Sections were then washed in water for 5 min, mounted on silicon-coated slides, dehydrated in a graded alcohol series and coverslipped. For the controls for nonspecific staining, the primary antibody was omitted. The immunoreactivity of the medial and lateral parts of both sides, totally four parts of the CA1 sector of the hippocampus, was graded semi-quantitatively using a scale of 0 (only faintly visible), 1 (weak), 2 (moderate) to 3 (definite) by the examinor (A. Y.) in a blind fashion, and the scores were summed.

Other paraffin sections, 5 μm in thickness, were prepared, stained with hematoxylin and eosin, and then examined under a light microscope. The neuronal density of the hippocampal CA1 subfield, i.e., the number of intact pyramidal cells per 1 mm length of CA1, was determined in a blind fashion (K.W.) according to the method of Kirino [16].

Statistical comparisons were made by means of one-way ANOVA and the post-hoc Fisher test. Values of $p < 0.05$ were considered to be significant, and the results were expressed as means ± SD.

Results

The immunohistochemical results for Mn-SOD (Fig. 1), Bcl-2 (Fig. 2), and BAX (Fig. 3) at 2 days after pretreatment are illustrated.

Immunohistochemistry using an antibody against Bcl-2 revealed only faint immunoreactivity in the sham-pretreatment group. Increased staining of the cytoplasm of pyramidal cells of the hippocampus was observed in the five-session HBO (2-ATA) pretreatment group. However, immunoreactivity in the ten-session HBO (3-ATA) group did not increase. Five-session HBO pretreatment, but not ten-session HBO pretreatment, significantly increased Bcl-2 expression compared with sham pretreatment (1.0 ± 1.2, $p < 0.05$).

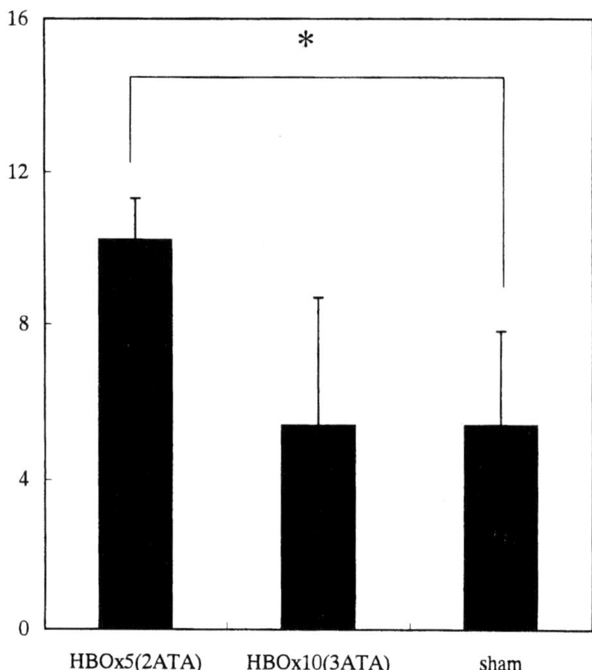

Fig. 1.

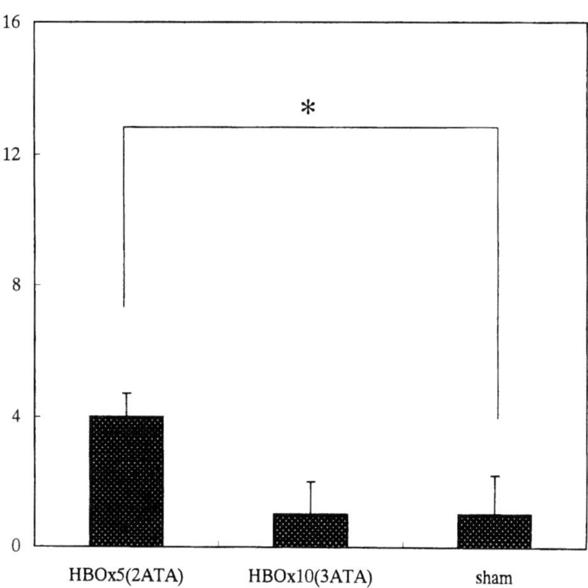

Fig. 2.

Immunoreactivity to Bax revealed cytoplasmic granular immunostaining in the sham-pretreatment group, but no differences in immunoreactivity were observed in the three groups. The immunoreactivity to

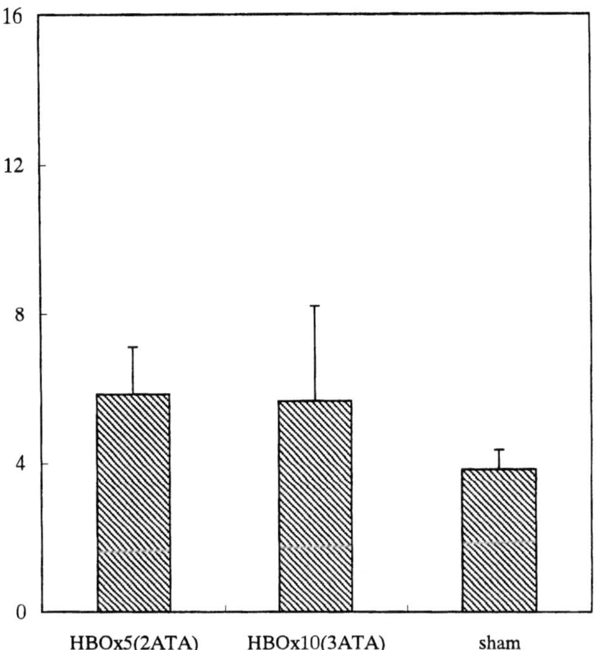

Fig. 3.

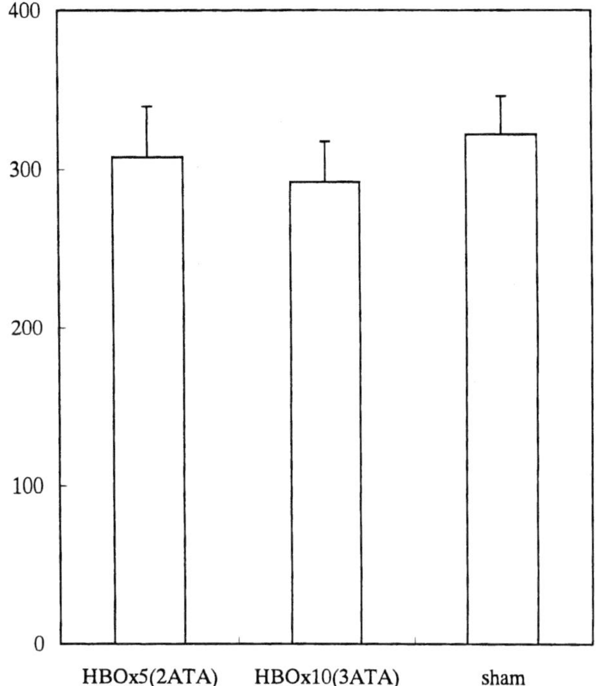

Fig. 4.

Bax was 3.8 ± 0.5 in the sham-pretreatment group, 5.8 ± 1.3 in the 5-session HBO pretreatment group, and 5.6 ± 2.6 10-session HBO pretreatment group.

Immunohistochemistry with an antibody against Mn-SOD revealed only faint immunoreactivity in the sham-pretreatment group. Increased staining of the cytoplasm of many CA1 pyramidal cells in the hippocampus was observed in the five-session HBO (2-ATA) pretreatment group. However, the immunoreactivity in the ten-session HBO (3-ATA) group did not increase. The Mn-SOD immunoreactivity was significantly increased in the five-session HBO pretreatment group (10.2 ± 1.1) compared with in the ischemic control group (5.4 ± 2.4, $p < 0.05$), but it was not observed in the ten-session HBO pretreatment group (5.4 ± 3.3, $p < 0.05$).

The results of histologic examination of CA1 sectors at 2 days following pretreatment are illustrated in Fig. 4. HBO pretreatment caused no neuronal death. The neuronal density in the CA1 sector at 2 days after pretreatment was not significantly different in the sham-pretreatment group (321.4 ± 23.8/mm), the five-session HBO pretreatment group (307.2 ± 31.9/mm), or the ten-session HBO pretreatment group (291.6 ± 25.4/mm).

Discussion

Activation of the apoptotic process involved in the delayed neuronal death (DND) of the hippocampal CA1 sector is controversial. However, recent studies have suggested that apoptosis might play an important role in DND, based on the detection of DNA fragmentation [15, 25] and protection against apoptosis through inhibition of protein synthesis [30].

Bcl-2 and a related protein, Bcl-associated X (Bax), have been identified as apoptosis-regulating molecules, influencing mitochondrial alterations associated with apoptosis. It is known that overexpression of the Bax protein induces apoptotic cell death [19]. Bax has been reported to be localized in the cytosol under physiological conditions. Bax is thought to move to mitochondria from the cytosol during apoptosis [36], to anchor the mitochondrial membrane, and to release cytochrome c, which is an apoptosis-inducing factor in mitochondria, with or without the formation of pores within the mitochondrial membrane [10]. Once cytochrome c is released into the cytosol from mitochondria, it promotes the assembly of a multiprotein complex that induces proteolytic processing and activation of cell death proteases known as caspases [20].

On the other hand, Bcl-2 has been shown to inhibit apoptosis and to promote cell survival (Hockenbery *et al.*, 1991). Overexpression of Bcl-2 has been shown to protect neurons from ischemia [21]. Bcl-2 is localized to the endonuclear membrane, endoplasmic reticulum, and outer mitochondrial membranes [22]. The mechanism by which Bcl-2 protects cells from apoptotic cell death is unknown. But, one possibility is that Bcl-2 forms a heterodimer with the Bax protein, and thus the apoptosis-inducing function of Bax is blocked [38]. Secondly, Bcl-2 protects cells from the damaging effects of reactive oxygen species (ROS). Because, Bcl-2 have been shown to inhibit ROS-inducing necrosis [12] as well as apoptotic cell death [11]. Third, Bcl-2 prevent apoptotic cell death through maintenance of mitochondrial membrane potential [32] and prevention of the release of cytochrome c [37].

Shimazaki *et al.* [31] reported that 2 min sublethal ischemia induced tolerance to subsequent lethal ischemia and prevented delayed neuronal death. Under these conditions, increased expression of the Bcl-2 protein was observed in the CA1 sector of the gerbil hippocampus. Furthermore, increasing Bax immunoreactivity, that peaks before DNA fragmentation, has been reported in the pyramidal cells in the hippocampal CA1 sector which destined to undergo delayed neuronal death [8]. In this study, we clearly demonstrated that immunoreactivity to Bcl-2, but not to Bax, increased in the 5-session HBO pretreatment group, these conditions having been reported to induce ischemic tolerance [35]. Therefore, it is conceivable that HBO administration induced an apoptotic-suppressing protein, which prevented apoptosis, leading to reduced delayed neuronal death. However, some studies have indicated that DND is different typical apoptosis, judging from inhibition of protein synthesis as well as RNA synthesis, or morphological findings [17]. Therefore, further study is necessary to prove the tolerance induced by HBO through the apoptotic process.

Hara *et al.* [8] have been reported that Bax immunoreactivity peaked at 72 h following 5-min ischemia and that no Bcl-2 immunoreactivity was detected in the CA-1 sector. On the contrary, our data indicated that an increase in Bcl-2 and no significant difference in Bax immunoreactivity were observed following HBO pretreatment. But, following HBO pretreatment, the mean value of Bax immunoreactivity was slightly higher than in the sham-pretreatment group. The induction mechanism for Bcl-2 is not clear, but tumor necrosis factor-α, which is one of the pro-inflammatory cytokines and is expressed in the ischemic brain, pretreatment has been reported to induce ischemic tolerance [24]. Therefore, this slightly increased expression of Bax might be related to the induction of Bcl-2.

Reactive oxygen species (ROS) are generated during and after cerebral ischemia, and have been suggested to play an important role in ischemia-induced neuronal damage, and have been considered to be common mediators of necrosis as well as apoptosis (reviewed by Buttke and Sandstrom [4]). ROS have been shown to react with nitric oxide to form highly cytotoxic peroxynitrite [3]. ROS also cause increased output of excitatory amino acids and trigger delayed neuronal death following transient ischemia [28]. Mitochondria are considered to be a major subcellular source of ROS (Piantadosi and Zhang., 1996). SODs are the most effective endogenous scavenging enzymes implicated in the regulation of cellular defense against ROS [23]. Two types of SODs are known, cytosolic copper-zinc SOD and mitochondrial Mn-SOD [7]. Akai *et al.* [1] have shown, by the localization of Mn-SOD in the hippocampus, that CA1 pyramidal cells were weakly immunostained under physiological conditions, whereas CA3 pyramidal cells were strongly reactive. Therefore, they concluded that the differences in the density of Mn-SOD immunostaining might be related to the vulnerability of CA1. In fact, the protective effect of SOD administration on DND has been reported [34]. Furthermore, increased immunoreactivity to Mn-SOD of tolerance-acquired CA1 following sublethal pretreatment has been shown [13, 27]. Under hyperbaric oxygen conditions, increased Mn-SOD activity has been reported [9]. In the lung, increased tolerance to oxygen toxicity has been reported after a preconditioning with non-toxic level of hyperbaric oxygen [6]. We also demonstrated in this study increased immunoreactivity to Mn-SOD (manganese superoxide dismutase) in the 5-session HBO pretreatment group. In this regard, Mn-SOD induced by repeated hyperbaric oxygenation may play an important role in ischemic tolerance.

However, animals treated with hyperbaric oxygenation at 3 ATA every day ten times did not show increased immunoreactivity to Bcl-2 or Mn-SOD. This might indicate that there are preferential conditions of hyperbaric oxygenation for the induction of ischemic tolerance. Further study is neccessary to determine the most preferential HBO conditions for inducing ischemic tolerance.

Acknowledgments

The authors would like to thank Ms. T. Hayashi, Ms. O. J. Natsume, Dr. M. Sato, and Mr. K. Murata for their excellent technical assistance.

References

1. Abe K, Aoki M, Kawagoe J, Yoshida T, Hattori A, Kogure K, Itoyama Y (1995) Ischemic delayed neuronal death. A mitochondrial hypothesis. Stroke 26: 1478–1489
2. Akai F, Maeda M, Suzuki K, Inagaki S, Takagi H, Taniguchi N (1990) Immunocytochemical localization of manganese superoxide dismutase (Mn- SOD) in the hippocampus of the rat. Neurosci Lett 115: 19–23
3. Beckman JS, Koppenol WH (1996) Nitric oxide, superoxide, and peroxynitrite: the good, the bad, and ugly. Am J Physiol 271: C1424–1437
4. Buttke TM, Sandstrom PA (1994) Oxidative stress as a mediator of apoptosis. Immunol Today 15: 7–10
5. Chopp M, Chen H, Ho KL, Dereski MO, Brown E, Hetzel FW, Welch KM (1989) Transient hyperthermia protects against subsequent forebrain ischemic cell damage in the rat. Neurology 39: 1396–1398
6. Crapo JD, Tierney DF (1974) Superoxide dismutase and pulmonary oxygen toxicity. Am J Physiol 226: 1401–1407
7. Fridovich I (1975) Superoxide dismutases. Annu Rev Biochem 44: 147–159
8. Hara A, Iwai T, Niwa M, Uematsu T, Yoshimi N, Tanaka T, Mori H (1996) Immunohistochemical detection of Bax and Bcl-2 proteins in gerbil hippocampus following transient forebrain ischeia. Brain Res 711: 249–253
9. Ito T, Yufu K, Mori A, Packer L (1996) Oxidative stress alters arginine metabolism in rat brain: effect of sub- convulsive hyperbaric oxygen exposure. Neurochem Int 29: 187–195
10. Jürgensmeier JM, Xie Z, Deveraux Q, Ellerby L, Bredesen D, Reed JC (1998) Bax directly induces release of cytochrome c from isolated mitochondria. Proc Natl Acad Sci USA 95: 4997–5002
11. Kane DJ, Sarafian TA, Anton R, Hahn H, Gralla EB, Valentine JS, Ord T, Bredesen DE (1993) Bcl-2 inhibition of neural death: decreased generation of reactive oxygen species. Science 262: 1274–1277
12. Kane DJ, Ord T, Anton R, Bredesen DE (1995) Expression of bcl-2 inhibits necrotic neural cell death. J Neurosci Res 40: 269–275
13. Kato H, Kogure K, Araki T, Liu XH, Kato K, Itoyama Y (1995) Immunohistochemical localization of superoxide dismutase in the hippocampus following ischemia in a gerbil model of ischemic tolerance. J Cereb Blood Flow Metab 15: 60–70
14. Keller JN, Kindy MS, Holtsberg FW, St Clair DK, Yen HC, Germeyer A, Steiner SM, Bruce-Keller AJ, Hutchins JB, Mattson MP (1998) Mitochondrial manganese superoxide dismutase prevents neural apoptosis and reduces ischemic brain injury: suppression of peroxynitrite production, lipid peroxidation, and mitochondrial dysfunction. J Neurosci 18: 687–697
15. Kihara S, Shiraishi T, Nakagawa S, Toda K, Tabuchi K (1994) Visualization of DNA double strand breaks in the gerbil hippocampal CA1 following transient ischemia. Neurosci Lett 175: 133–136
16. Kirino T (1982) Delayed neuronal death in the gerbil hippocampus following ischemia. Brain Res 239: 57–69
17. Kirino T, Tsujita Y, Tamura A (1991) Induced tolerance to ischemia in gerbil hippocampal neurons. J Cereb Blood Flow Metab 11: 299–307
18. Kitagawa K, Matsumoto M, Tagaya M, Hata R, Ueda H, Niinobe M, Handa N, Fukunaga R, Kimura K, Mikoshiba K, Kamada T (1990) 'Ischemic tolerance' phenomenon found in the brain. Brain Res 528: 21–24
19. Krajewski S, Mai JK, Krajewska M, Sikorska M, Mossakowski MJ, Reed JC (1995) Upregulation of bax protein levels in neurons following cerebral ischemia. J Neurosci 15: 6364–6376
20. Liu X, Kim CN, Yang J, Jemmerson R, Wang X (1996) Induction of apoptotic program in cell-free extracts: requirement for dATP and cytochrome c. Cell 86: 147–157
21. Martinou JC, Dubois-Dauphin M, Staple JK, Rodriguez I, Frankowski H, Missotten M, Albertini P, Talabot D, Catsicas S, Pietra C, Huarte J (1994) Overexpression of BCL-2 in transgenic mice protects neurons from naturally occurring cell death and experimental ischemia. Neuron 13: 1017–1030
22. Merry DE, Korsmeyer SJ (1997) Bcl-2 gene family in the nervous system. Annu Rev Neurosci 20: 245–267
23. Nakazawa H, Genka C, Fujishima M (1996) Pathological aspects of active oxygens/free radicals. Jpn J Physiol 46: 15–32
24. Nawashiro H, Tasaki K, Ruetzler CA, Hallenbeck JM (1997) TNF-alpha pretreatment induces protective effects against focal cerebral ischemia in mice. J Cereb Blood Flow Metab 17: 483–490
25. Nitatori T, Sato N, Waguri S, Karasawa Y, Araki H, Shibanai K, Kominami E, Uchiyama Y (1995) Delayed neuronal death in the CA1 pyramidal cell layer of the gerbil hippocampus following transient ischemia is apoptosis. J Neurosci 15: 1001–1011
26. Ohtsuki T, Matsumoto M, Kuwabara K, Kitagawa K, Suzuki K, Taniguchi N, Kamada T (1992) Influence of oxidative stress on induced tolerance to ischemia in gerbil hippocampal neurons. Brain Res 599: 246–252
27. Ohtsuki T, Matsumoto M, Suzuki K, Taniguchi N, Kamada T (1993) Effect of transient forebrain ischemia on superoxide dismutases in gerbil hippocampus. Brain Res 620: 305–309
28. Pellegrini-Giampietro DE, Cherici G, Alesiani M, Carla V, Moroni F (1990) Excitatory amino acid release and free radical formation may cooperate in the genesis of ischemia-induced neuronal damage. J Neurosci 10: 1035–1041
29. Piantadosi CA, Zhang J (1996) Mitochondrial generation of reactive oxygen species after brain ischemia in the rat. Stroke 27: 327–331
30. Shigeno T, Yamasaki Y, Kato G, Kusaka K, Mima T, Takakura K, Graham DI, Furukawa S (1990) Reduction of delayed neuronal death by inhibition of protein synthesis. Neurosci Lett 120: 117–119
31. Shimazaki K, Ishida A, Kawai N (1994) Increase in bcl-2 oncoprotein and the tolerance to ischemia-induced neuronal death in the gerbil hippocampus. Neurosci Res 20: 95–99
32. Shimizu S, Eguchi Y, Kamiike W, Waguri S, Uchiyama Y, Matsuda H, Tsujimoto Y (1996) Bcl-2 blocks loss of mitochondrial membrane potential while ICE inhibitors act at a different step during inhibition of death induced by respiratory chain inhibitors. Oncogene 13: 21–29
33. Siesjo BK, Agardh CD, Bengtsson F (1989) Free radicals and brain damage. Cerebrovasc Brain Metab Rev 1: 165–211
34. Uyama O, Matsuyama T, Michishita H, Nakamura H, Sugita M (1992) Protective effects of human recombinant superoxide dismutase on transient ischemic injury of CA1 neurons in gerbils. Stroke 23: 75–81
35. Wada K, Ito M, Miyazawa T, Katoh H, Nawashiro H, Shima K, Chigasaki H (1996) Repeated hyperbaric oxygen induces ischemic tolerance in gerbil hippocampus. Brain Res 740: 15–20

36. Wolter KG, Hsu YT, Smith CL, Nechushtan A, Xi XG, Youle RJ (1997) Movement of Bax from the cytosol to mitochondria during apoptosis. J Cell Biol 139: 1281–1292
37. Yang J, Liu X, Bhalla K, Kim CN, Ibrado AM, Cai J, Peng TI, Jones DP, Wang X (1997) Prevention of apoptosis by Bcl-2: release of cytochrome c from mitochondria blocked. Science 275: 1129–1132
38. Yin XM, Oltvai ZN, Korsmeyer SJ (1994) BH1 and BH2 domains of Bcl-2 are required for inhibition of apoptosis and heterodimerization with Bax. Nature 369: 321–323

Correspondence: Dr. Takahito Miyazawa, Department of Neurosurgery, National Defense Medical College, 3-2 Namiki, Tokorozawa, Saitama 359, Japan.

Acta Neurochir (2000) [Suppl] 76: 291–296

Neurotrophic Factors Attenuate Alterations in Spinal Cord Evoked Potentials and Edema Formation Following Trauma to the Rat Spinal Cord

T. Winkler[1], **H. S. Sharma**[2], **E. Stålberg**[1], and **R. D. Badgaiyan**[2,3]

[1] Department of Clinical Neurophysiology, University Hospital, Uppsala, Sweden
[2] Laboratory of Neuroanatomy, Department of Anatomy, Biomedical Centre, Uppsala University, Sweden
[3] Department of Psychiatry, Harvard University, Harvard Medical School and Massachusetts General Hospital, Cambridge, MA, USA

Summary

Influence of brain derived neurotrophic factor (BDNF) and insulin like growth factor-1 (IGF-1) on spinal cord injury induced disturbances in spinal cord conduction, edema formation and cellular stress response was examined in a rat model. Pretreatment with BDNF or IGF-1 significantly attenuated the loss of SCEP negative amplitude seen immediately after spinal cord injury. In these neurotrophins treated rats, upregulation of heat shock protein (HSP 72 kD) immunoreactivity, a measure of cellular stress response and spinal cord edema formation were considerably reduced 5 h after injury. These results suggest that neurotrophic factors improve spinal cord conduction after trauma and this beneficial effect of growth factors may be related with their ability to attenuate trauma induced cellular stress response, not reported earlier.

Keywords: Neurotrophic factors; spinal cord conduction; heat shock protein response; spinal cord edema.

Introduction

Spinal cord injury is a serious problem to clinicians because this situation is associated with severe neurological deficit and a long-term rehabilitation problem [7, 16]. Until now no suitable drug therapy has been worked out which can minimise the neurological outcome and tissue damage in spinal cord trauma victims [7, 16, 21]. Thus, further studies using new therapeutic principles are highly needed to improve spinal cord function following trauma. One important approach to enhance functional recovery after spinal cord injury is to reduce secondary tissue damage [7]. In addition, preservation of tissues and fiber tracts responsible for restoration of bioelectrical conduction through remaining fiber tracts is also necessary [9, 17, 21]. The secondary inflammatory reaction occurring around the lesion site will determine the final consequences of the cell injury and influence spinal cord bioelectrical activity [14, 16]. Although the cascade of tissue reactions and cell injury develop within days or weeks, the most extensive cell death in spinal cord injury occurs within hours after trauma [7, 16, 21]. This suggests that an early intervention by therapeutic agents would be the most promising approach to rescue the cord from further and irreversible cell damage. Thus influencing these early secondary injury processes around the lesion by pharmacological and/or neurotrophic agents seems to be highly relevant for therapy and to minimise cord dysfunction following trauma [1, 3, 4]. The early consequences of cell injury following trauma is still a neglected subject which require detailed investigations in order to develop suitable therapeutic strategy.

Experiments carried out in our laboratory during the last decade suggest that recording of spinal cord evoked potentials (SCEP) from the epidural electrodes placed around the lesion site after peripheral stimulation of tibial and sural nerves reliably predict the disturbances in the cord function following trauma [14, 21]. There is a strong correlation between decrease in SCEP amplitude with later development of spinal cord edema and cell injury [9, 10, 12–14]. Thus, changes in SCEP response within 0 to 10 minutes following trauma are well correlated with the development of spinal cord pathology seen 5 h after injury [9, 10]. Spinal cord trauma may induce profound cellular "shock" or "stress" response resulting in blockade of spinal cord conduction. Thus, it seems likely that attenuation of these early shock or stress response by neuroprotective agents may improve spinal cord recovery and function.

Recent reports suggest that several neurotrophic factors are neuroprotective in ischemia and brain injury [7, 17, 18]. Thus a possibility exists that neurotrophic factors may also induce some beneficial effects in the spinal cord following injury. Neurotrophic factors may provide trophic support to injured neurons and thus improve their metabolism and function after injury [1]. Neurotrophic factors influence neurochemical transmission and improve cell to cell communication [4]. An improved neuronal communication may thwart neuronal "shock" or "stress" phase [19]. Thus a possibility exists that neurotrophins in spinal trauma will influence cord conduction and cellular stress response. The present investigation was carried out to find out whether topical application of brain derived neurotrophic factor (BDNF) or insulin like growth factor-1 (IGF-1) will influence the trauma induced cellular stress response and if so, whether the beneficial effects of these growth factors will be reflected in early SCEP recordings.

Materials and Methods

Animals

Experiments were carried out on 30 male Sprague Dawley rats (body weight 300–350 g) housed at controlled room temperature with 12 h light and 12 h dark schedule. Rat food pellets and tap water were provided ad libitum.

Spinal Cord Injury

Under Equithesin anaesthesia (3 ml/kg, i.p.), one segment laminectomy (T10–11) was made. The spinal cord injury was inflicted by making a longitudinal incision into the right dorsal horn [14]. The wound was covered with cotton soaked saline in order to prevent a direct exposure of the cord to air. Normal animals served as controls. This experimental condition is approved by the Ethical Committee of Uppsala University, Uppsala, Sweden and the Banaras Hindu university, Varanasi, India.

Recording of SCEP

Spinal cord evoked potentials were recorded from the epidural electrodes placed over the right dorsal surface of the spinal cord of the T9 (rostral) and the T12 (caudal) segments following stimulation of right tibial and sural nerves as described earlier [14]. The reference electrodes were placed in corresponding paravertebral muscles of the active exploratory epidural electrodes. The ground electrode was placed over the proximal end of the tail [20, 21].

Treatment with Neurotrophins

Two potent neurotrophic factors, BDNF and IGF-1 were used for topical application over the exposed surface of the spinal cord repeatedly [9, 12]. Thus, repeated topical application of BDNF or IGF-1 (20 μg/kg for 30 sec) applied 30 min before followed by 0 min (at the time of injury), 10 min, 30 min, 60 min after and thereafter every 1 h, i.e. 120 min, 180 min, 240 min and 300 min [20] and the SCEP was recorded using standard protocol [14, 20, 21]. In controls, the treatment schedule was exactly followed except that the animals were not injured.

Spinal Cord Edema

At 5 h, spinal cord tissue pieces from the injured (T10–11) and the caudal (T12) segments were taken out to determine edema formation by measuring water content [9].

Heat Shock Protein Immunoreactivity

In order to determine traumatic stress response and its modification with neurotrophins, heat shock protein (HSP-72) expression in the T9 segment of the spinal cord was examined on free floating Vibratome sections (40 μm thick) using commercial antiserum (StressGene, Canada; Affiniti, UK) as described earlier [15, 19]. The immunostaining was developed using peroxides-antiperoxidase technique and the control, spinal cord injured and neurotrophins treated control or spinal cord injured were processed for HSP immunostaining in parallel.

Statistical Analysis

ANOVA followed by Dunnet test or unpaired Student's t-test were applied to determine the statistical significance of the data obtained. A p-value less than 0.05 was considered to be significant.

Results

Effects of Neurotrophins on SCEP Changes

A focal trauma to the rat spinal cord produced by incision of the right dorsal horn at T10–11 segment resulted in an immediate depression of SCEP amplitude (mean depression 60%) which lasted for about 1 h. At the end of 5 h there was some recovery in SCEP amplitude whereas the latency of SCEP continued to increase (Fig. 1).

Repeated topical application of BDNF or IGF-1 (20 μl of a 1 μg/ml solution for 30 sec) applied 30 min before followed by 0 min (at the time of injury), 10 min, 30 min, 60 min after and thereafter every 1 h [3, 5], resulted in a marked protection of SCEP amplitude seen after injury (Fig. 1). Thus in the neurotrophins treated rats, the SCEP amplitude did not diminish after trauma. In fact there was a significant increase in SCEP amplitude (mean 20%) from the pre-injury level.

Effects of Neurotrophins on Spinal Cord Edema

Water content at 5 h spinal cord traumatised rats treated with neurotrophins showed a significantly less

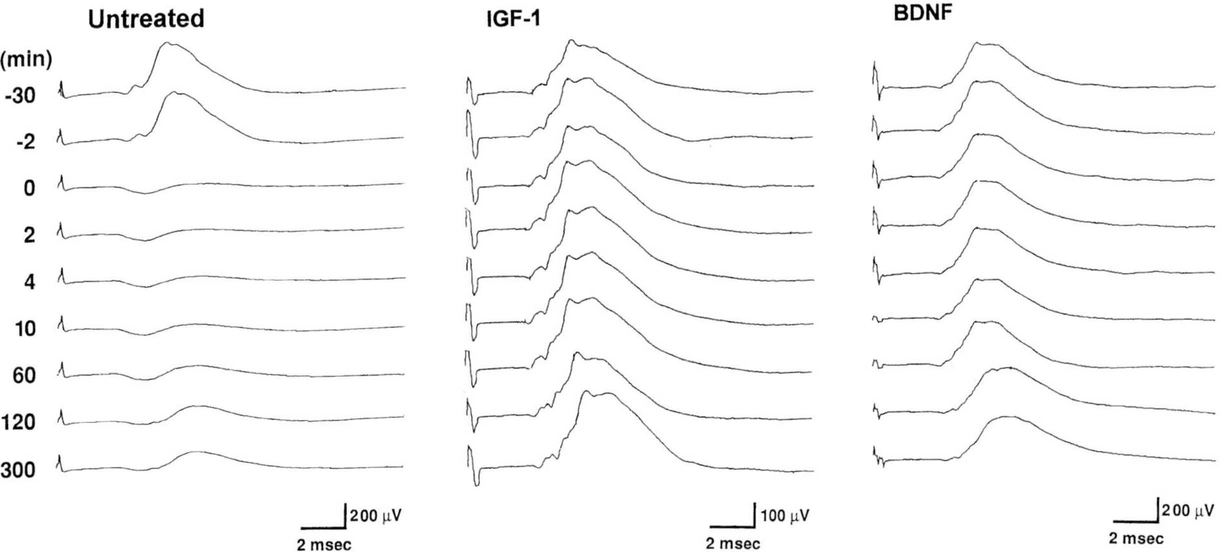

Fig. 1. A representative SCEP recordings obtained from the epidural electrode placed over the T9 segment of the cord following stimulation of the right tibial and sural nerves in one spinal cord traumatised rat and its modification with BDNF and IGF-1 pretreatment. In neurotrophins treated rats, depression of SCEP amplitude seen immediately after injury (0 min) in untreated rat is not evident

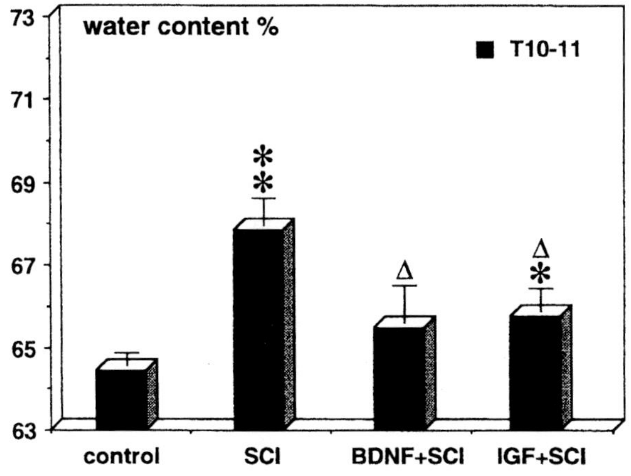

Fig. 2. Spinal cord edema formation in the T10–11 segments after 5 h injury in untreated rats and its modification with BDNF or IGF-1 pretreatment. * = $P < 0.05$; ** = $P < 0.01$ compared to control; Δ = $P < 0.05$, Compared to spinal cord injury *(SCI)*. Values are mean ± SD

edema formation compared to the untreated traumatised group (Fig. 2).

Effects of Neurotrophins on HSP Immunoreactivity

Expression of heat shock protein (HSP 72 kD), a measure of cellular stress, was quite pronounced in the perifocal T9 and T12 segments. This upregulation of HSP response was much less evident in neurotrophins treated rats (Fig. 3).

Discussion

The present results for the first time provide evidence that neurotrophic factors attenuate the cellular stress response and improve spinal cord conduction following trauma. These observations further confirm that SCEP can be used as a reliable indicator of edema formation and spinal cord pathology.

The mechanism behind improved spinal cord conduction following injury by neurotrophic factors is not clear from this investigation. However, our observations suggest that growth factors have the capacity to attenuate cellular stress response following trauma. This hypothesis is in line with our findings that BDNF and IGF-1 treatment significantly attenuated HSP-72 response following injury.

The HSP response is mainly related to the cellular stress [8, 19]. Thus signals emanating from the damaged or distorted cells will explicitly express HSP response. However, there are certain reports in ischemia that upregulation of HSP is neuroprotective in nature [19]. Although, this assumption is still controversial, our data further suggest that HSP response could simply serve as an indication of cellular stress signals. This

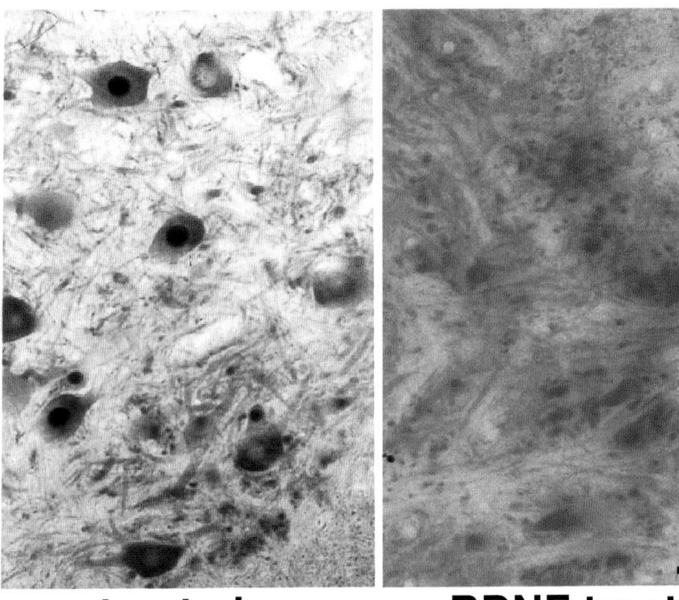

Fig. 3. Heat shock protein (HSP 72 kD) immunoreactivity in the T9 segment of its spinal cord in one untreated rat (left) and its modification with BDNF (right) pretreatment. Pretreatment with BDNF markedly reduced the expression of HSP immunoreactivity indicating a profound reduction in the cellular stress response following trauma (bar = 50 μm) [15]

idea is well supported by our previous observations in hyperthermic brain injury or spinal cord injury [8, 19, 21]. Thus drugs which are able to achieve neuroprotection in either spinal cord trauma or hyperthermia induced brain injury were able to reduce the expression of HSP response [19, 21]. This indicates that HSP expression is somehow related to the cell injury factors. To our knowledge, this observation is the first report which demonstrates a reduction in HSP response following trauma by neurotrophic factors.

Since in vivo situation, no single chemical compound or factor is responsible for all the pathological changes seen in any traumatic, ischemic or metabolic diseases of the CNS [8, 9, 11], it seems quite likely that a balance between endogenous neuroprotective and neurodestructive agents determine the final outcome. Based on these principles, it sounds reasonable to assume that growth factors may have shifted the sequences of events towards neuroprotection by either inhibiting the release of endogenous neurodestructive agents or augmenting the role of endogenous neuroprotective agents. To that end, attenuating stress response could be one important signal for enhancing endogenous neuroprotection seen in our model of spinal cord trauma. This idea is in agreement with the observation that pretreatment with neurotrophic factors reduces the cell injury, edema formation and disturbances in the blood-spinal cord barrier (BSCB) permeability [8, 21]. Thus, it may be that disturbances in the fluid microenvironment of the cord plays an important role in cellular stress mechanisms and consequently injury. These observations clearly demonstrate that BDNF and IGF-1 are capable of providing neuroprotection by attenuating endogenous cellular stress as one neurodestructive agent.

The mechanisms by which BDNF and IGF-1 attenuate SCEP disturbances following spinal cord trauma is not clearly known. Neurotrophic factors are released following membrane depolarisation and application of neurotrophic factors in cell culture attenuates such disturbances in membrane electrical activity [5, 6]. However, it seems likely that reduction in the early events around lesion following BNDF or IGF treatment plays a major role. Trauma induced secondary injury factors are involved in SCEP disturbances following spinal cord injury. Thus, serotonin, prostaglandins, histamine or opioids influence SCEP changes following trauma [21]. Prevention of release of serotonin and prostaglandins following trauma attenuates SCEP disturbances [8, 21]. The present study further suggests that presence of BDNF or IGF around the lesion site is also beneficial on SCEP activity. One possibility would be that a focal trauma may cause a loss of growth factors needed to maintain cell survival. Exogenous supplement of growth factors will induce sufficient trophic support to the cells around lesion resulting in their survival. Obviously maintenance of normal cell survival will improve electrical conduction.

The possibility of BDNF or IGF-1 induced preservation of SCEP response following trauma may be due to the fact that these growth factors may attenuate the spinal "shock" or cellular "stress" phenomena, commonly seen following trauma [2, 17]. When cells following trauma enter into the shock phase they lost their normal conduction properties resulting in a loss of SCEP activity. Exogenous growth factors may attenuate this "shock" phase response after trauma resulting in less SCEP disturbances. This idea is in line with the findings of a reduced HSP expression in growth factor treated injured animals.

This study further confirms our hypothesis that SCEP changes are reliable in predicting later edema formation and cell pathology of the spinal cord. Thus edema formation and cell injury were considerably reduced in animals which received BDNF or IGF-1 treatment. In these rats, the disturbances in SCEP changes were mainly absent. These observations suggest that early SCEP changes are mainly due to release of several secondary injury factors at the time of initial insult. If these secondary injury factors are modified with neurotrophic factors given before the injury, a possibility exists that the SCEP disturbances will be minimal. Obviously, a minor disturbance in the fluid microenvironment of the cord following injury, or modification of secondary injury factors by growth factors treatment is directly responsible for the later outcome of the edema formation and cord pathology.

In conclusion, our observations using BDNF and IGF-1 provide new insights in exploring therapeutic strategies in the spinal cord injury research to preserve spinal cord conduction and to reduce the final outcome of edema and cell injury. It would be interesting to explore whether repeated application of BDNF or IGF-1 treatment at various time intervals after the primary injury is still neuroprotective and can restore spinal cord conduction, a feature which is currently under investigation in our laboratory.

Acknowledgments

This investigation is supported by grants from Swedish Medical Research Council nrs. 135 (ES), 02710 (JW, HSS), Göran Gustafsson Stiftelse (HSS), Sweden and The University Grants Commission (HSS), New Delhi, India. The technical assistance of Kärstin Flink and Ingamarie Olsson is highly appreciated.

References

1. Apfel SC (1999) Neurotrophic factors in peripheral neuropathies: therapeutic implications. Brain Pathol 9: 393–413
2. Badgaiyan RD, Schacter DL, Alpert NM (1999) Auditory priming within and across modalities: evidence from positron emission tomography. J Cog Neuroscience 11: 337–348
3. Ibanez CF (1998) Emerging themes in structural biology of neurotrophic factors. TiNS 21: 438–444
4. Liu Y, Kim DH, Himes BT, Chow SY, Schallert T, Murray M, Tessler A, Fischer I (1999) Transplants of fibroblasts genetically modified to express BDNF promote regeneration of adult rat rubrospinal axons and recovery of forelimb function. J Neurosci 19: 4370–4387
5. Rodriguez-Capote K, Cespedes E, Arencibia R, Gonzalez-Hoyuela M (1998) Indicators of oxidative stress in rat brain during ageing. The effect of nerve growth factor. Rev Neurol 27: 494–500
6. Sashihara S, Tsuji S, Matsui T (1998) Oncogene and signal transduction pathways in the regulation of Na+ channel expression. Crit Rev Oncogen 9: 19–34
7. Schwab ME, Bartholdi D (1996) Degeneration and regeneration of axons in the lesioned spinal cord. Physiol Rev 76: 319–370
8. Sharma HS (1999) Pathophysiology of blood-brain barrier, brain edema and cell injury following hyperthermia: New role of heat shock protein, nitric oxide and carbon monoxide. an experimental study in the rat using light and electron microscopy. Acta Universitatis Upsaliensis 830: 1–94
9. Sharma HS, Nyberg F, Gordh T, Alm P, Westman J (1998) Neurotrophic factors attenuate neuronal nitric oxide synthase upregulation, microvascular permeability disturbances, edema formation and cell injury in the spinal cord following trauma. Spinal cord monitoring. Basic principles, regeneration, pathophysiology and clinical aspects. In: E Stålberg, HS Sharma, Y Olsson (eds) Springer, Wien New York, pp 181–210
10. Sharma HS, Nyberg F, Westman J, Gordh T, Alm P, Lindholm D (1998) Brain derived neurotrophic factor and insulin like growth factor-1 attenuate upregulation of nitric oxide synthase and cell injury following trauma to the spinal cord. Amino Acids 14: 121–129
11. Sharma HS, Alm P, Westman J (1998) Nitric oxide and carbon monoxide in the pathophysiology of brain functions in heat stress. Prog Brain Res 115: 297–333
12. Sharma HS, Nyberg F, Gordh T, Alm P, Westman J (1997) Topical application of insulin like growth factor-1 reduces edema and upregulation of neuronal nitric oxide synthase following trauma to the rat spinal cord. Acta Neurochir [Suppl] (Wien) 70: 130–133
13. Sharma HS, Westman J, Olsson Y, Alm P (1996) Involvement of nitric oxide in acute spinal cord injury: an immunohistochemical study using light and electron microscopy in the rat. Neurosci Res 24: 373–384
14. Sharma HS, Winkler T, Stålberg E, Olsson Y, Dey PK (1991) Evaluation of traumatic spinal cord edema using evoked potentials recorded from the spinal epidural space. An experimental study in the rat. J Neurol Sci 102: 150–162
15. Sharma HS, Nyberg F, Gordh T, Alm P, Westman J (2000) Neurotrophic factors influence upregulation of constitutive isoform of heme oxygenase and cellular stress response in the spinal cord following trauma. Amino Acids 19: 351–361
16. Stålberg E, Sharma HS, Olsson Y (1998) Spinal cord monitoring. Basic principles, regeneration, pathophysiology and clinical aspects. Springer, Wien New York, pp 1–527
17. Tonra JR (1999) Classical and novel directions in neurotrophin transport and research: Anterograde transport of brain-derived neurotrophic factor by sensory neurons. Micros Res Tech 45: 225–232

18. van Ooyen A, Willshaw DJ (1999) Competition for neurotrophic factor in the development of nerve connections. Proc Royal Soc Lond 266: B883–B892
19. Westman J, Sharma HS (1998) Heat shock protein response in the CNS following heat stress. In: Brain functions in hot environment. In: Sharma HS, Westman J (eds) Prog Brain Res 115: 207–239
20. Winkler T, Sharma HS, Stålberg E, Badgaiyan RD, Alm P, Westman J (1998) Spinal cord evoked potentials and edema in the pathophysiology of rat spinal cord injury. Involvement of nitric oxide. Amino Acids 14: 131–139
21. Winkler T, Sharma HS, Stålberg E, Westman J (1998) Spinal cord monitoring. Basic principles, regeneration, pathophysiology and clinical aspects. In: E Stålberg, HS Sharma, Y Olsson (eds) Springer, Wien New York, pp 283–364

Correspondence: Hari Shanker Sharma, Ph.D., Laboratory of Neuroanatomy, Department of Medical Cell Biology, Box 571, Biomedical Centre, Uppsala University, S-75123 Uppsala, Sweden.

Acta Neurochir (2000) [Suppl] 76: 297–301

Spinal Cord Injury Induced *c-fos* Expression is Reduced by p-CPA, a Serotonin Synthesis Inhibitor. An Experimental Study Using Immunohistochemistry in the Rat

H. S. Sharma[1], **J. Westman**[1], **T. Gordh**[3], and **F. Nyberg**[2]

[1] Laboratory of Neuroanatomy, Department of Medical Cell Biology, Department of Pharmaceutical, Uppsala, Sweden
[2] Department of Pharmacentical Biosciences, Biomedical Centre Uppsala University, Uppsala, Sweden
[3] Department of Anaesthesiology, University Hospital, Uppsala University, Uppsala, Sweden

Summary

Influence of serotonin on upregulation of cellular-*fos* (c-*fos*) following a focal spinal cord injury was examined using immunohistochemistry in a rat model. Spinal cord injury was produced by making a unilateral longitudinal incision of the dorsal horn of the T10–11 segments. A focal lesion to the cord markedly upregulated c-*fos* immunohistochemistry at 5 h which was mainly located in the edematous regions of the cord in the injured as well as in the perifocal T9 and T12 segments. Pretreatment with p-CPA, a serotonin synthesis inhibitor, significantly attenuated the c-*fos* upregulation along with the edematous expansion of the cord. These results for the first time suggest that trauma induced release of serotonin and edema formation are important biological signals inducing c-*fos* expression.

Keywords: Spinal cord injury; c-*fos* immunohistochemistry; p-CPA; spinal cord edema.

Introduction

Spinal cord injury is a serious clinical problem. Depending upon the magnitude and severity of the initial impact, spinal trauma will lead to life time disability of the victims involving huge amount of financial burden on the society [9, 15, 16]. Thus every efforts should be made to minimise the consequences of spinal injury in order to preserve the integrity and function of the spinal cord. One way to understand this problem is to identify series of events that are taking place in early phase of spinal cord trauma. This would expand our knowledge regarding the mechanisms of spinal cord dysfunction following trauma.

There are reports indicating that events occurring within 8 h periods following primary insult will set the stage for the later spinal cord dysfunction leading to permanent disability [3, 9, 16]. Thus suitable pharmacological therapy if introduced within 8 h time window after insult will have some beneficial effects on the recovery of spinal cord function in patients. Any therapy given after 8 h primary insult is simply ineffective [9, 16]. Thus, further studies should be carried out in greater details to understand the basic early events following trauma. This would help to explore probable therapeutic measures to minimise spinal cord dysfunction leading to permanent disability.

Our laboratory is engaged since the last 13 years to understand the basic mechanisms of early cell reactions following trauma in a rat model [10, 11, 16]. Our observations show that trauma to the spinal cord upregulates several cellular proteins and enzymes such as heat shock protein (HSP 72 kD), glial fibrillary acidic protein (GFAP), nitric oxide synthase (NOS), heme oxygenase (HO-2), cyclooxygenase-1 (COX-1) and COX-2 enzymes in the spinal cord following trauma at 5 h [10–15]. Most of these proteins and enzymes participate in the pathophysiological reactions of spinal cord cell injury. This is evident from the fact that drugs or compounds which offer significant neuroprotection in the spinal cord following trauma are also able to attenuat expression of these proteins or enzymes [10–12, 15, 16]. These observations suggest that trauma induced pathophysiology of spinal cord injury is a complex phenomenon and several injury factors, proteins and enzymes are involved which, however, require further investigation.

One possible mechanisms for altered protein or enzyme expression is the disturbances of the fluid microenvironment of the cord following trauma which may influence gene expression [4, 8, 9, 16]. However, it is not certain whether early spinal trauma is associated with gene expression, and if so, whether these molecular events are related with the cell survival or cell death. The cellular *fos (c-fos)* is a primary response gene which can be detected within the neurons in vivo by immunohistochemical techniques 20–90 min after neuronal excitation and prolonged *c-fos* expression precedes programmed cell death in vitro [5, 6]. This indicates that *c-fos* can be used as a neuronal marker for cell injury. However, the expression of *c-fos* and its functional significance in CNS trauma is not well known.

In present investigation, c-*fos* immunoreactivity was examined in the spinal cord segments in order to find out whether activation of c-*fos* occurs following trauma induced cellular stress, injury or activation of spinal cord neurons. Furthermore, to understand the contribution of serotonin following trauma, c-*fos* immunostaining was examined in p-CPA treated rats which results in less cellular stress and injury compared to untreated animals.

Materials and Methods

Animals

Experiments were carried out on 20 male Sprague Dawley rats (200–250 g) housed at controlled room temperature at 21 ± 1 °C with 12 h light and 12 h dark schedule. Food and tap water were supplied ad libitum before the experiment.

Spinal Cord Injury

Under Equithesin anaesthesia (0.3 ml/100 g, i.p.) one segment laminectomy over T10–11 segments was done and a longitudinal incision (about 5 mm) over the right dorsal horn was made using a sterile scalpel. The deepest part of the lesion was mainly located 1.5 to 2 mm deep around the Rexed's laminae VIII to X [11, 12]. The haemorrhage, if any, over the dorsal surface of the cord was removed and surface of the lesion was covered with cotton soaked in saline in order to avoid the direct exposure of air [11]. Animals (n = 5) were allowed to survive 5 h after the insult. Normal intact rats (n = 5) served as controls. This experimental condition is approved by the Ethical Committee of Uppsala University, Uppsala, Sweden and Banaras Hindu University, Varanasi, India.

p-chlorophenylalanine Treatment

In separate group of 10 rats, a serotonin synthesis inhibitor drug, p-chlorophenylalanine (p-CPA, Sigma Chemical Co., USA) was administered intraperitoneally (100 mg/kg/day) for 3 consecutive days [12]. On the fourth day, these animals were divided into the two groups. One group was subjected to 5 h spinal cord injury and the remaining 5 animals were used as drug treated controls.

c-fos Immunohistochemistry

The *c-fos*-immunohistochemistry was examined on free floating vibratome sections obtained from the T9 segment of the cord using monoclonal *c-fos* antiserum (Calbiochem, USA) according to the commercial protocol [13].

Perfusion and Fixation

Immediately after 5 h spinal cord injury, rats were perfused with about 50 to 80 ml with 0.1 M phosphate buffer (pH 7.0) at room temperature via heart in order to washout the remaining blood from the blood vessels followed by about 150 ml of 4 % paraformaldehyde in 0.1 M phosphate buffer. The perfusion pressure was constantly maintained at 90 torr throughout the process of perfusion [12].

Spinal Cord Edema

In separate groups of rats, spinal cord edema formation was examined in the T9 segment of the cord using measurement of the spinal cord water content [10, 11]. In another group of rats, edematous expansion of the spinal cord was examined using standard light microscopy technique to conform the water content measurements [11].

Statistical Evaluation

The quantitative or semi-quantitative data obtained were analysed using Student's unpaired t-test for their statistical significance according to the standard procedures using a personal computer. A p-value less than 0.05 was considered to be significant.

Results

Effect of p-CPA on c-fos Immunohistochemistry

Normal rats did not express *c-fos* immunostaining in the spinal cord. A focal spinal cord injury markedly upregulated c-*fos* immunoreactivity in neurons of the injured as well as the adjacent rostral T9 and caudal T12 segments of the spinal cord (Fig. 1). The magnitude of *c-fos* upregulation was most marked in the ipsilateral side. Interestingly, p-CPA pretreatment significantly attenuated the c-*fos* immunostaining caused by trauma (Figs. 1 and 2).

A representative example of c-*fos* immunoreactivity in the ipsilateral ventral gray matter is shown in Fig. 2. Marked upregulation of c-*fos* immunostaining is seen in the neurons located into the ventral grey matter of the traumatised cord. Expansion of the ventral horn of the spinal cord and general sponginess and edema is quite apparent along with the c-*fos* immunostained nerve cells (Fig. 2). On the other hand p-CPA pretreated and injured spinal cord, did not show much c-*fos*-immunolabelled nerve cells (Fig. 2). In general, the sponginess, edema and general expansion of the ventral horn are mainly absent (Fig. 2).

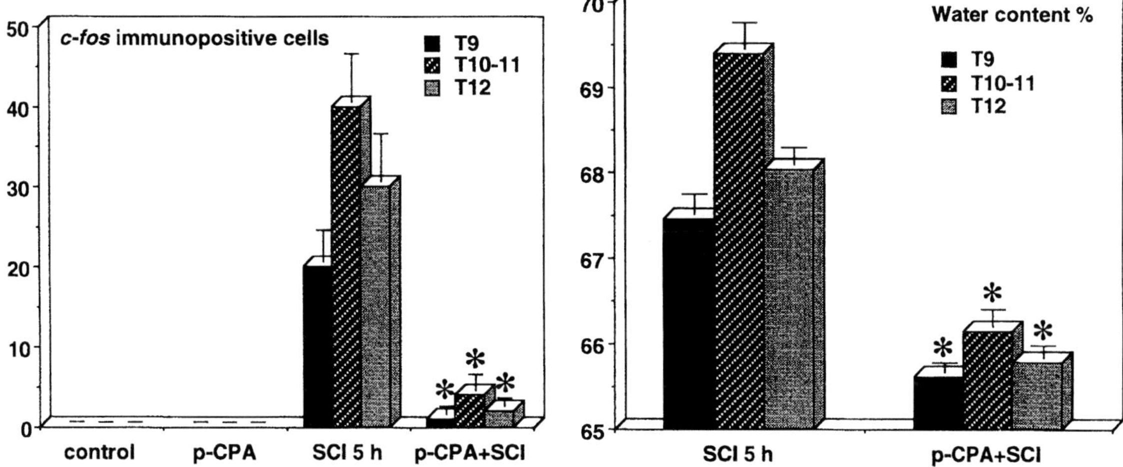

Fig. 1. *c-fos* immunohistochemistry (left) and spinal cord water content (right) in 5 h spinal cord traumatised rats and their modification with p-CPA pretreatment. p-CPA, a serotonin synthesis inhibitor was given (100 mg/kg/day, i.p.) for 3 days and the animals were traumatised on the 4th day (for details see text). Marked increase in c-fos immunohistochemistry and spinal cord edema is evident in untreated spinal cord traumatised rats. Pretreatment with p-CPA significantly attenuated upregulation of *c-fos* expression and spinal cord edema following injury. *** = $P < 0.001$ compared with spinal cord injured (*SCI*) group, Student's unpaired t-test

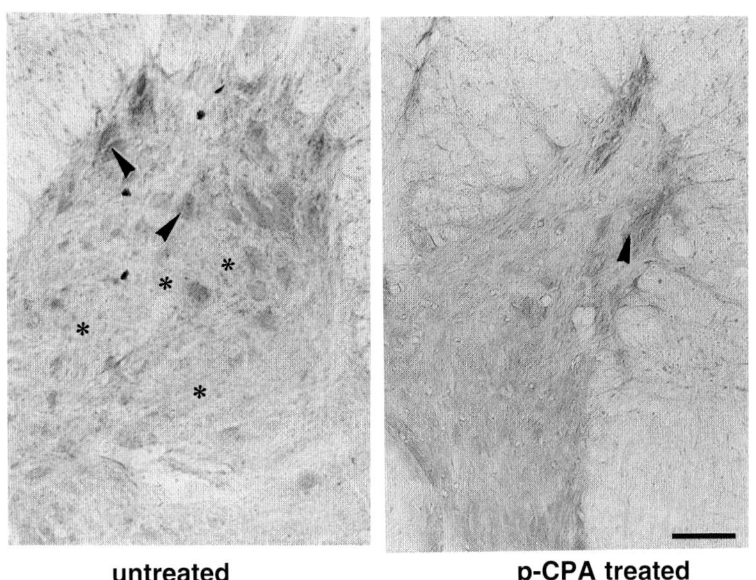

Fig. 2. *c-fos* immunolabelled neurons in the ventral horn of one 5 h spinal cord traumatised rat (a) and its modification with p-CPA pretreatment (b). Many *c-fos* immunolabelled cells can be seen in the traumatised rat (arrow heads). Spinal cord edema and expansion (*) is clearly visible in the untreated rat. Pretreatment with p-CPA markedly reduced the expression of *c-fos* and the edematous swelling and expansion of the cord in this drug-treated rat is mainly absent (bar = 100 μm)

Effect of p-CPA on Spinal Cord Water Content

Measurement of the water content showed profound increase in edema formation in the T9, T10–11 and T12 segments of the cord following 5 h injury (Fig. 1). This increase in the water content was significantly attenuated by pretreatment with p-CPA (Fig. 1).

Discussion

The salient new finding of the present investigation is a marked upregulation of the c-*fos* immunoreactivity following trauma to the spinal cord. This upregulation of *c-fos* was located within the edematous expansion of the spinal cord. The *c-fos* immunoreactivity and edema are no longer evident in the serotonin depleted traumatised rats. This observation indicates that edema formation and serotonin release following trauma are important biological factors in the *c-fos* upregulation, not reported earlier.

Upregulation of c-*fos* is reported in different parts of the CNS following stress, ischemia, chemical infusion, bacterial endotoxins or under influence of several neurochemicals and hormones [2, 4–8]. It seems quite likely that nerve cells showing an upregulation of c-*fos* may represent an increased excitation or activation of their cellular activity [5]. Increased c-*fos* immunoreactivity in the non traumatised regions of the cord and pronounced expression of the immunoreaction in vicinity of the lesion are in good agreement with this idea.

The present results further suggest that trauma induced cellular stress can be one important signal in inducing c-*fos* expression. This is supported by the observation that c-*fos* immunoreactivity is observed in present study in far remote areas of the spinal cord which are not directly influenced by the incision. A focal trauma to the cord can induce severe cellular stress response in the vicinity of the lesion as well as in remote regions probably by altering the spinal cord fluid microenvironment [11]. Increased permeability of the blood-spinal cord barrier (BSCB) as well as expression of heat shock protein (HSP 72 kD) in the remote T9 and T12 regions in this model [11, 12, 16] are in good agreement with this idea.

Serotonin is a well known mediator of stress reaction [1, 16] and has the capacity to induce brain edema formation [1, 3] and breakdown of the blood-brain barrier (BBB) or the BSCB permeability [11, 14]. Release of serotonin in the CNS and in periphery occurs in a wide variety of emotional, physical and psychological stressful conditions [1, 16]. Blockade of serotonin release following p-CPA pretreatment attenuates stress response and prevents the BBB or BSCB breakdown following traumatic, emotional or psychological stressors [1, 9, 11, 15, 16]. Thus an increased release of the amine is associated with edema formation probably via opening of the BBB permeability [11]. Obviously, breakdown of the BBB permeability will allow serum proteins to enter into the extracellular compartment of the brain leading to vasogenic edema formation. Increased release of serotonin is also associated with the trauma induced cellular stress response [1, 12, 16].

How serotonin can influence c-*fos* gene expression? This is not clear from this study. It may be that the traumatic stress is less severe in animals in which serotonin synthesis is inhibited with p-CPA prior to trauma [1]. p-CPA given in the present dose can inhibit long lasting decrease in the serotonin synthesis in the CNS as well as in the periphery [10, 12, 16]. Thus, the levels of serotonin in the CNS, blood plasma and all its stores are considerably reduced [1]. Trauma in serotonin depleted rats will not increase the serotonin levels in the plasma or in the cord. Thus, the actions of serotonin on the microvessels leading to disruption of the BSCB permeability and edema formation will be considerably reduced or prevented [12, 16].

Alternatively, the cellular stress phenomenon is also inhibited following trauma in serotonin depleted animals [12]. Previous studies showing inhibition of HSP response in perifocal regions in serotonin depleted animals following trauma is in line with the above idea [12]. However, a direct effect of serotonin on c-*fos* expression cannot be ruled out. There are some evidences that serotonin can upregulate c-*fos* expression [5]. Thus, in absence of serotonin release c-*fos* expression may not be upregulated. To further confirm this point, specific serotonergic receptor blockers are needed which require further investigation.

In conclusion, our results show that c-*fos* is markedly upregulated following trauma to the spinal cord and this upregulation of c-*fos* can be attenuated by prior depletion of serotonin in the spinal cord. These observations suggest that depletion of serotonin has an inhibitory influence on c-*fos* upregulation caused by trauma, not reported earlier.

Acknowledgments

This investigation is supported by grants from Swedish Medical Research Council nrs. 2710 (JW, HSS), 9077 (TG, HSS) Göran Gustafsson Stiftelse (HSS), Sweden and The University Grants Commission (HSS), New Delhi, India. The technical assistance of Kärstin Flink and Kerstin Rystedt is highly appreciated.

References

1. Chaouloff F (1993) Physiopharmacological interactions between stress hormones and central serotonergic systems. Brain Res Rev 18: 1–32
2. Chapman V, Buritova J, Honoré P, Besson J-M (1995) 7-Nitroindazole, a selective inhibitor of neuronal nitric oxide synthase, reduces formalin evoked *c-fos* expression in dorsal horn neurons of the rat spinal cord. Brain Res 697: 258–261
3. Faden AI (1993a) Experimental neurobiology of central nervous system trauma. Crit Rev Neurobiol 7: 175–186
4. Huang W, Simpson RK (1999) Antisense of c-fos gene attenuates Fos expression in the spinal cord induced by unilateral constriction of the sciatic nerve in the rat. Neurosci Lett 263: 61–64
5. Hughes P, Dragunow M (1995) Induction of immediate-early genes and the control of neurotransmitter-regulated gene expression within the nervous system. Pharmacol Rev 47: 133–178
6. Hunt SP, Pini A, Evan G (1987) induction of c-fos-like protein in spinal cord neurons following sensory stimulation. Nature (Lond) 328: 632–634

7. Lima D, Avelino A (1994) Spinal c-*fos* expression is differentially induced by brief or persistent noxious stimulation. Neuro Report 5: 1853–1856
8. Manabe YK, Shiro Y, Shomori T, Abe K (1999) Enhanced Fos expression in rat lumbar spinal cord cultured with cerebrospinal fluid from patients with amyotrophic lateral sclerosis. Neurol Res 21: 309–312
9. Schwab ME, Bartholdi D (1996) Degeneration and regeneration of axons in the lesioned spinal cord. Phys Rev 76: 319–370
10. Sharma HS, Dey PK (1982) Correlation of spinal cord tissue 5-HT with edema development following surgical spinal cord trauma in rats. Indian J Physiol Pharmacol 26 [Suppl] I: 8–9
11. Sharma HS, Olsson Y, Dey PK (1990) Early accumulation of serotonin in rat spinal cord subjected to traumatic injury. Relation to edema and blood flow changes. Neuroscience 36: 725–730
12. Sharma HS, Olsson Y, Westman J (1995) A serotonin synthesis inhibitor, p-chlorophenylalanine reduces the heat shock protein response following trauma to the spinal cord. An immunohistochemical and ultrastructural study in the rat. Neuroscience Res 21: 241–249
13. Sharma HS, Westman J, Olsson Y (1996) Spinal cord injury induced *c*-fos expression is reduced by p-CPA, a serotonin synthesis inhibitor. Neuropathol Appl Neurobiol 22: 15–16
14. Sharma HS, Westman J, Nyberg F (1997) Topical application of 5-HT antibodies reduces edema and cell changes following trauma to the rat spinal cord. Acta Neurochir [Suppl] (Wien) 70: 155–158
15. Stålberg E, Sharma HS, Olsson Y (1998) Spinal cord monitoring. Basic principles, regeneration, pathophysiology and clinical aspects. Springer, Wien New York, pp 1–527
16. Winkler T, Sharma HS, Stålberg E, Westman (1998) Spinal cord bioelectrical activity, edema and cell injury following a focal trauma to the spinal cord. An experimental study using pharmacological and morphological approach. Spinal cord monitoring. In: Stålberg E, Sharma HS, Olsson Y (eds) Springer, Wien New York, pp 281–348

Correspondence: Hari Shanker Sharma, Ph.D., Laboratory of Neuroanatomy, Department of Medical Cell Biology, Box 571, Biomedical Centre, Uppsala University, S-75123 Uppsala, Sweden.

Acta Neurochir (2000) [Suppl] 76: 303–306

Lipocortin-1 Fails to Ameliorate Ischemic Brain Edema in the Cat

T. Mima[1] and **T. Shigeno**[2]

[1] Department of Neurosurgery, Kochi Medical School, Japan
[2] Department of Neurosurgery, Kanto Rosai Hospital, Japan

Summary

It has been reported that corticosteroids exert their anti-inflammatory action through de novo synthesis of phospholipase-inhibitory proteins called lipocortins (annexins). We postulated that the following may lessen the effectiveness of corticosteroids on acute ischemic brain edema: 1) lipocortins are induced several hours after administration of steroids; 2) de novo synthesis of lipocortins is suppressed in the ischemic brain; and 3) lipocortins induced systemically do not pass through the blood-brain barrier (BBB) to reach the sites of ischemic edema. To test this hypothesis, we examined whether dexamethasone, given long before ischemia or direct administration of recombinant lipocortin-1, combined with or without BBB opening, ameliorate ischemic brain edema. Three hours before occlusion of the middle cerebral artery (MCA) in the cat, 4 mg/kg of dexamethasone was injected intravenously. The animals were subjected to 4 hours of ischemia. Alternatively, 2 ug/ml (total volume 10 ml) of recombinant human lipocortin-1 (annexin-I) was perfused intermittently into the ischemic focus by catheterization into the MCA. Artificial opening of the BBB was performed by intra-arterial mannitol infusion. None of these strategies demonstrated amelioration of ischemic edema. We conclude that: Dexamethasone and recombinant lipocortin-1 seem unlikely to have robust effects on amelioration of acute ischemic edema.

Keywords: Lipocortin 1; dexamethasone; cerebral ischemia; cytotoxic edema.

Introduction

In the early period of ischemia, the major compartment in which water accumulates is the astrocyte (cytotoxic edema). The blood-brain barrier (BBB) is not disrupted until 4–6 hours after ischemia [20, 26]. Release of arachidonic acid by phospholipase A2 constitutes one of the trigger mechanisms of edema formation of ischemic brain [1]. Corticosteroids, which are inhibitors of phospholipase A2, have been tried to prevent edema formation, but no satisfactory effect has been demonstrated on ischemic brain edema [11]. In the past, some evidence suggested that glucocorticoids exert their anti-inflammatory activity through de novo synthesis of proteins that inhibit phospholipase A2, later designated as lipocortins or annexins [5].

It is important to note that it takes several hours for lipocortins to be induced after administration of corticosteroids [5] and that protein synthesis is severely suppressed in the ischemic brain [33]. Even though lipocortins are induced in normal brain tissue outside the ischemic region, or systemically elsewhere, the BBB in the early periods of brain ischemia prevents these proteins from reaching the site of cytotoxic edema, the astrocyte. We hypothesized that corticosteroids, given long enough before ischemia, induce more lipocortins prior to the onset of ischemia, and artificial opening of the BBB helps transfer lipocortins to the astrocytes.

To test the hypothesis, we administered high doses of dexamethasone 3 hours before middle cerebral artery (MCA) occlusion in cats, combining this with BBB opening, and compared the severity of ischemic edema to controls. We also employed the direct administration of recombinant human lipocortin-1 (annexin-I) into the ischemic focus by direct catheterization of the MCA.

Material and Methods

Adults mongrel cats (2–3 kg) were anesthetized with 2–4% halothane/N_2O/O_2 under controlled ventilation. In each cat, a femoral artery and a femoral vein were cannulated for monitoring arterial blood pressure and arterial gas, and for administration of fluids. Physiological parameters were kept within the normal range (blood pressure > 100 mmHg, PaO_2 > 100 mmHg, $PaCO_2$ 30–40 mmHg, pH 7.3–7.5). Focal cerebral ischemia was produced by permanent occlusion of the MCA via the transorbital approach [19]. For direct intra-arterial perfusion into the ischemic area, we employed a technique of catheterization into the MCA distal to the occlusion site, as previously described [28, 29]. Immediately after occlusion, a polyethylene catheter (o.d. 1.2 mm, i.d. 0.8 mm) with a tapered tip was inserted through an arteriotomy in the MCA just distal to the occlusion site. The drug in solution, aerated with 95% O_2/5% CO_2, was perfused intermittently (15 seconds every 5 minutes), with a hydrostatic loading pressure of 20 mmHg. This ensured that the drug would perfuse the entire MCA territory [28, 29]. Otherwise a sufficient supply would not have reached the ischemic focus because of low cerebral blood flow. Cortical regional cerebral blood flow (rCBF) was measured by the hydrogen clearance technique at six sites in the lateral ischemic hemisphere. After 4 hours of ischemia, halothane-anesthetized animals were sacrificed with intravenous saturated KCl, and the specific gravity of the brain tissue samples was measured with an automated microgravimetric apparatus, as previously reported [27].

Experiment-1: Protocol for dexamethasone treatment. To open the BBB in the ischemic brain, hypertonic mannitol (total volume 10 ml) was perfused intermittently through the MCA catheter, starting 30 minutes after ischemia and extending for 3 hours. As Koenig and colleagues [16] have reported that the BBB opens with intra-arterial mannitol injection, we also confirmed the BBB opening in the specific region with evidence of Evans blue staining. Four groups were subjected to 4 hours of permanent MCA occlusion: 1) no treatment (n = 9), 2) BBB opening by mannitol (n = 5), 3) dexamethasone 4 mg/kg given intravenously 3 hours before MCA occlusion (n = 5), and 4) a combination of group 2 and 3, i.e., pretreatment with dexamethasone combined with BBB opening by mannitol (n = 5).

Experiment-2: Protocol for lipocortin-1 treatment. Recombinant human lipocortin-1 (35 kD) diluted with Krebs-Ringer solution (10-7 M; total volume 10 ml), was perfused intermittently through the MCA catheter, starting 30 minutes after ischemia and extending for 3 hours. Since the MCA catheter was used for lipocortin-1 administration, a bolus injection of mannitol (total volume 3 ml) was conducted through the intracarotid artery 30 minutes before ischemia for the purpose of BBB opening. This method of mannitol injection also provided BBB opening evidenced by Evans blue staining. Four groups were subjected to 4 hours of permanent MCA occlusion: 1) no treatment (n = 9), 2) BBB opening only (n = 4), 3) lipocortin-1 (n = 6), and 4) a combination of 2) and 3), i.e., lipocortin-1 and BBB opening (n = 5).

For statistical purposes, we used the analysis of variance (ANOVA) for comparison of multiple groups, and compared two groups by PLSD. P values of less than 0.05 were considered statistically significant.

Results

As we reported previously [14, 29], edema formation appeared only when rCBF fell below 30 ml/100 g/min, and there was an apparent dissociation of the severity of edema at an rCBF threshold of 15 ml/100 g/min (Figure 1 and 2). Furthermore, the rCBF stayed almost constant during the MCA occlusion. Therefore, the drug effect on ischemic edema in relation to specific gravity changes was compared in two separate ischemic windows, i.e., 0 to 15 ml/100 g/min (severe ischemia) and 15 to 30 ml/100 g/min (moderate ischemia).

Experiment-1: As compared to no treatment, pretreatment with 4 mg/kg dexamethasone failed to attenuate edema formation in either ischemic flow range

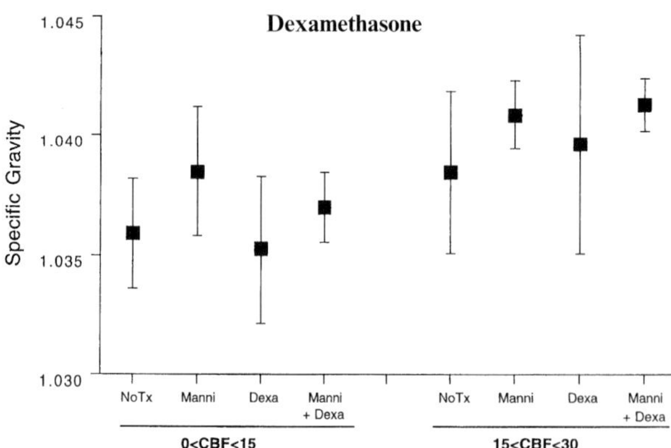

Fig. 1. Graphs comparing edema formation with severe ($0 < CBF < 15$) and moderately severe ischemia ($15 < CBF < 30$) caused by 4 hours of middle cerebral artery occlusion in cats. Severity of edema formation was indicated by specific gravity, and the values are given as mean with standard deviations shown by error bars. In moderate ischemia (the right side of the graphs), dexamethasone combined with BBB opening by mannitol (*Manni + Dexa*) ameliorated edema formation significantly ($p < 0.05$ by PLSD) as compared to the no treatment group (*NoTx*), however, this difference was not significant when compared to the mannitol alone group (*Manni*). Dexamethasone alone (*Dexa*) did not show any beneficial effect in either degree of ischemia

(Fig. 1). Mannitol perfusion into the ischemic focus showed slight reduction of edema formation compared to no treatment in the moderate ischemic range ($p < 0.05$ by PLSD). Dexamethasone combined with BBB opening also showed slight but significant amelioration in the moderate ischemic range compared to no treatment ($p < 0.05$ by PLSD). However, taking account of the edema-reducing effect of mannitol itself, no statistical effect of dexamethasone given 3 hours before ischemia was found.

Experiment-2: Recombinant human lipocortin-1 perfused into the MCA did not show any attenuation of edema formation (Fig. 2). Even the combined therapy of lipocortin-1 and BBB opening showed no beneficial effect. A bolus intra-carotid injection of mannitol 30 minutes before ischemia did not ameliorate brain edema (Fig. 2), although mannitol intermittently perfused into the brain focus during ischemia significantly reduced brain edema (Fig. 1).

Discussion

We hypothesized that the ineffectiveness of corticosteroids on ischemic edema [11, 21] is due to three factors: 1) Several hours' delay of lipocortins induction after administration of steroids weakens their effects, 2) de novo synthesis of lipocortins is suppressed in the

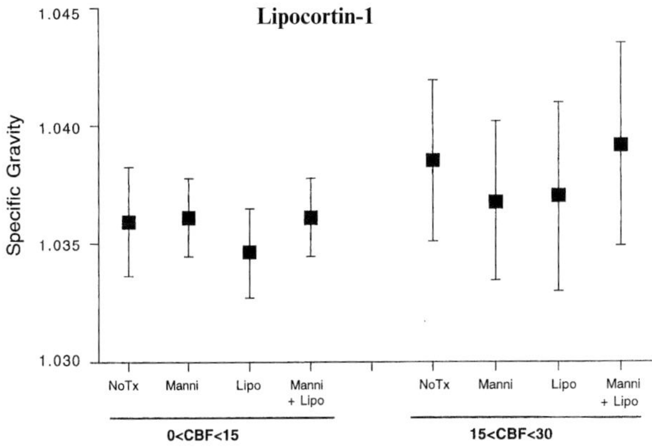

Fig. 2. The effect of recombinant lipocortin-1 on ischemic edema shown by graphs similar to those in Fig. 1. Neither lipocortin-1 alone (*Lipo*) nor lipocortin-1 combined with BBB opening by mannitol (*Manni* + *Lipo*) showed amelioration. BBB opening by mannitol injection through the intracarotid artery (*Manni*) did not ameliorate brain edema

ischemic brain [33], and 3) lipocortins, which are produced in non-ischemic brain and/or systemically elsewhere, cannot reach the ischemic site because of the intact BBB in the early period of ischemia.

In the present study, we aimed to solve these three problems in three ways: 1) dexamethasone was injected 3 hours before ischemia, 2) recombinant human lipocortin-1 was administered to the ischemic focus by catheterization of the MCA, and 3) the BBB in the ischemic brain was opened by mannitol infusion. However, none of these strategies demonstrated direct evidence of attenuating ischemic edema.

Lipocortin-1 is widely detected in neurons and glia in normal rat and human brain [15, 30, 31], and highly expressed in ependymal cells and tancytes lining the cerebral ventricles [31]. Marked increases of lipocortins in reactive astrocytes and macrophages were observed in pathological conditions such as infarcts (24 hours to 7 days after ischemia) [24, 25], tumor [15], and encephalomyelitis [10]. Outside of the central nervous system, lipocortins are also expressed in monocytes, macrophages, lymphocytes, and neutrophils [4, 10, 13, 22] as well as in organs such as lung, kidney, spleen, liver, skin, and placenta [2, 15, 32]. However, it still remains controversial whether the protein level of lipocortins is elevated by dexamethasone and whether lipocortins are secreted and/or taken up by relevant cells [3, 8, 9, 12, 18, 23].

Recently, it was reported that intracerebroventricular injection of lipocortin-1 fragment (1-188 amino acids) caused marked inhibition of infarct size and cerebral edema after MCA occlusion in the rat and its neutralizing antiserum aggravated the results [24, 25]. The authors stated that the lipocortin-1 fragment had greater activity and stability than the full molecule when administered intraventricularly. We used full length of recombinant lipocortin-1 and administered it intraarterially, but not intraventricularly. This difference may have caused negative data in the present study. However, there have been only a few in vivo studies supporting the anti-inflammatory effect of lipocortin-1 [7], and its efficacy in carrageenin-induced paw edema [7] is controversial [18]. As far as we have tested effects of lipocortin-1 on various types of edema such as carrageenin-induced paw edema (unpublished data), peri-tumoral edema in the rat [6], and cold-injured brain edema in the rat [17], we have not found any ameliorating effects.

In the present study, dexamethasone given 3 hours before ischemia or direct administration of lipocortin-1 did not ameliorate acute ischemic brain edema in the cat. It seems unlikely that full length of lipocortin-1 has a robust effect on reducing ischemic brain edema.

Acknowledgments

We thank Drs. T. Matsumoto and S. Ito (Kyowa Hakko Co. Ltd., Tokyo, Japan) for their generous gift of recombinant human lipocortin-1. We also thank Ms. R. Tokiwa for technical support in the experiments, Ms. Y. Muto for animal care, and Ms. Y. Tsuzuku for secretarial help in preparation of this manuscript.

References

1. Abe K, Kogure K, Yamamoto H, Imazawa M, Miyamoto K (1987) Mechanism of arachidonic acid liberation during ischemia in gerbil cerebral cortex. J Neurochem 48: 503–509
2. Ambrose M, Hunninghake G (1990) Corticosteroids increase lipocortin 1 in alveolar epithelial cells. Am J Resp Cell Mol Biol 3: 349–353
3. Beyaert R, Suffys P, Van Roy F, Fiers W (1990) Inhibition by glucocorticoids of tumor necrosis factor-mediated cytotoxicity. Evidence against lipocortin involvement. FEBS Lett 262: 93–96
4. Browning JL, Ward MP, Wallner BP, Pepinsky RB (1990) Studies on the structural properties of lipocortin-1 and the regulation of its synthesis by steroids. Prog Clin Biol Res 349: 27–45
5. Buckingham JC, Flower RJ (1997) Lipocortin 1: a second messenger of glucocorticoid action in the hypothalamo-pituitary-adrenocortical axis. Mol Med Today 3: 296–302
6. Chang CC, Shinonaga M, Kuwabara T, Mima T, Shigeno T (1990) Effect of recombinant human lipocortin I on brain oedema in a rat glioma model. Acta Neurochir [Suppl] (Wien) 51: 145–147
7. Cirino G, Peers SH, Flower RJ, Browning JL, Pepinsky RB (1989) Human recombinant lipocortin 1 has acute local anti-inflammatory properties in the rat paw edema test. Proc Natl Acad Sci USA 86: 3428–3432

8. Crompton MT, Moss SE, Crumpton MJ (1988) Diversity in the lipocortin/calpactin family. Cell 55: 1–3
9. Dennis DA, Davidson FF (1990) Phospholipase A2 and lipocortin effects. Prog Clin Biol Res 349: 47–54
10. Elderfield AJ, Bolton C, Flower R (1993) lipocortin 1 (annexin 1) immunoreactivity in the cervical spinal cord of Lewis rats with acute experimental allergic encephalomyelitis. J Neurol Sci 119: 146–153
11. Fenske M, Fisher M, Regli F, Hase U (1979) The response of focal ischemic cerebral edema to dexamethasone. Neurology 220: 199–209
12. Go KG, Zuiderveen F, De Ley L, Ter Haar JG, Parente L, Solito E, Molenaar WM (1994) Effect of steroids on brain lipocortin immunoreactivity. Acta Neurochir [Suppl] (Wien) 60: 101–103
13. Goulding N, Godolphin J, Sharland P, Peers S, Sampson M, Maddison P, Flower R (1990) Anti-inflammatory lipocortin 1 production by peripheral blood leukocytes in response to hydrocortisone. Lancet. 335: 1416–1418
14. Hanamura T, Shigeno T, Asano T, Mima T, Takakura K (1989) Prostaglandin profiles in relation to local circulatory changes following focal cerebral ischemia in cats. Stroke 20: 803–808
15. Johnson M, Kamso-Pratt J, Pepinski R, Whetsell W (1989) Lipocortin 1 immunoreactivity in the normal human central nervous system and lesions with astrocytes. Am J Clin Pathol 92: 424–429
16. Koenig H, Goldstone AD, Lu CY (1989) Polyamines mediate the reversible opening of the blood-brain barrier by the intracarotid infusion of hyperosmolar mannitol. Brain Res 483: 110–116
17. Mima T, Shigeno T (2000) Lipocortin-1 failed to ameliorate cold-injured brain edema in the rat. Acta Neurochir [Suppl] (Wien) 76: 309–312
18. Northup JK, Valentine-Braun KA, Johnson LK, Severson DL, Hollenberg MD (1988) Evaluation of the antiinflammatory and phospholipase-inhibitory activity of calpactin II/lipocortin I. J Clin Invest 82: 1347–1352
19. O'Brien M, Waltz A (1973) Transorbital approach for occluding the middle cerebral artery without craniotomy. Stroke 4: 201–206
20. O'Brien MD, Jordan MM, Waltz AG (1974) Ischemic cerebral edema and the blood-brain barrier. Arch Neurol 30: 461–465
21. Okamoto S, Peck RC, Lefer AM (1982) Protective actions of dexamethasone in acute cerebral ischemia. Circ Shock 9: 445–456
22. Peers S, Smillie F, Elderfield A, Flower R (1993) Glucocorticoid- and non-glucocorticoid induction of lipocortins (annexins) 1 and 2 in rat peritoneal leukocytes in vivo. Br J Phamacol 108: 66–72
23. Piltch A, Sun L, Fava RA, Hayashi J (1989) Lipocortin-independent effect of dexamethasone on phospholipase activity in a thymic epithelial cell line. Biochem J 261: 395–400
24. Relton J, Strijbos P, O'Shaughnessy C, Carey F, Forder R, Tilders F, Rothwell N (1991) Lipocortin-1 is an endogenous inhibitor of ischemic damage in the rat brain. J Exp Med 174: 305–310
25. Rothwell N, Relton J (1993) Involvement and lipocortin-1 in ischemic brain damage. Cereb Brain Metab Rev 5: 178–198
26. Schuier FJ, Hossmann KA (1980) Experimental brain infarcts in cats. II. Ischemic brain edema. Stroke 11: 593–601
27. Shigeno T, Brock M, Shigeno S Fritschka E, Cervós-Navarro J (1982) The determination of brain water content. Microgravimetry versus drying-weighing method. J Neurosurg 57: 99–107
28. Shigeno T, Asano T, Watanabe E, Johshita H, Takakura K (1985) Does capillary Na, K-ATPase plays a role in the development of ischemic brain edema? Brain edema. In: Inaba Y, Klatzo I, Spatz M (eds) Springer, Berlin Heiderberg New York Tokyo, pp 461–464
29. Shigeno T, Asano T, Mima T, Takakura K (1989) Effect of enhanced capillary activity on the blood-brain barrier during focal cerebral ischemia in cats. Stroke 20: 1260–1266
30. Strijbos P, Tilders F, Carey F, Forder R, Rothwell N (1990) Localization of lipocortin-1 in normal rat brain. Biochem Soc Trans (Engl) 18: 1234–1235
31. Strijbos PJLM, Tilders FJH, Carey F, Forder R, Rothwell NJ (1991) Localization of immunoreactive lipocortin-1 in the brain and pituitary gland of the rat. Effect of adrenalectomy, dexamethasone and colchicine treatment. Brain Res 553: 249–260
32. Vishwanath B, Frey F, Bradbury M, Dallman M, Frey B (1992) Adrenolectomy decreases lipocortin-1 messenger ribonucleic acid and tissue protein content in rats. Endocrinology 130: 585–591
33. Xie Y, Mies G, Hossmann KA (1989) Ischemic threshold of brain protein synthesis after unilateral carotid artery occlusion in gerbils. Stroke 20: 620–626

Correspondence: Tatsuo Mima, M.D., Ph.D., Department of Neurosurgery, Kochi Medical School, Nankoku City, Kochi 783-8505, Japan.

Acta Neurochir (2000) [Suppl] 76: 307–310

Lipocortin-1 Fails to Ameliorate Cold-Injury Brain Edema in the Rat

T. Mima[1] and **T. Shigeno**[2]

[1] Department of Neurosurgery, Kochi Medical School, Japan
[2] Department of Neurosurgery, Kanto Rosai Hospital, Japan

Summary

Based on evidence that corticosteroids exert their anti-inflammatory action via de novo synthesis of phospholipase A2 inhibitory proteins called lipocortins, we examined effects of high dose dexamethasone and recombinant human lipocortin-1 (annexin-I) on cold-injury brain edema in the rat. Since it takes several hours for lipocortins to be induced, dexamethasone (10 mg/kg) was injected intraperitoneally 3 hours before cold injury. Recombinant lipocortin-1 was administered intraventricularly at three different doses (0.01 mg/kg, 0.05 mg/kg, or 0.1 mg/kg: total volume 20 μl), or via the internal carotid artery at a dose of 10^{-7} M (2 ml). To induce cold injury, a liquid-nitrogen-cooled probe was placed on the exposed dura of male Wistar rats (330–370 kg) for 1 minute. Specific gravimetry and/or a wet-dry weighing method were used for measurement of brain edema at 24 or 48 hours after lesion production. In the present study, dexamethasone and recombinant lipocortin-1 failed to attenuate edema formation. The anti-inflammatory effects of dexamethasone or exogenous lipocortin-1 seemed unlikely to affect cold-injury brain edema.

Keywords: Lipocortin-1; annexin-I; dexamethasone; vasogenic brain edema.

Introduction

Clinically vasogenic edema associated with brain abscess or brain tumor (particularly meningioma and metastatic brain tumor) can be dramatically improved by corticosteroids, but vasogenic edema caused by trauma responds poorly to corticosteroids.

The anti-inflammatory effects of corticosteroids have been reported to derive from antiphospholipase A2 inhibitory proteins called lipocortins [7, 8]. Lipocortins have been collectively characterized as the lipocortin/calpactin family of Ca^{2+} dependent membranebinding proteins [5, 11]. According to the homology of sequences including other proteins, a consensus has been reached to name all the members of this supergene family "annexin" [1, 6, 10].

We hypothesized that the effectiveness of corticosteroids on brain edema depends on the amount of lipocortins induced. Importantly, it takes several hours for lipocortins to be synthesized after administration of corticosteroids [8]. In cold-injury brain edema, if a high does of dexamethasone is injected several hours before cold-injury or if exogenous lipocortin-1 is directly administered, more lipocortins at the acute stage may attenuate edema formation. To test the hypothesis, we examined effects of dexamethasone (injected 3 hours before cold injury) and recombinant human lipocortin-1 on cold-injury brain edema in the rat.

Materials and Methods

Adult male Wistar rats weighing 330 to 370 g were anesthetized with intraperitoneally injected pentobarbital (50 mg/kg). Upon sedation the parietal bone was craniectomized and a cold lesion was induced by applying a liquid-nitrogen-cooled cylinder for 60 seconds to the surface of the exposed dura matter (Fig. 1). Anesthetized animals were decapitated at 2 hours, 24 hours or 48 hours after the onset of cold-injury.

Two different methods for measuring edema formation were used in the separate experimental animals. The specific gravimetry technique was used for measuring brain edema in the specified small region in Experiments 1 and 2 (Fig. 1), with the aid of an automated apparatus as previously described [20]. The wet-dry weighing method was used in Experiments 3, 4, and 5, to measure more global edema in the edematous parietal cortex which contained the cold-injury cortex ("core") and its adjacent cortex ("periphery") (Fig. 1). Since edema was negligible in remote regions such as the frontal cortex, temporal cortex, and thalamus, the area of parietal cortex including "core" and "periphery" was excised (Fig. 1) and their tissue water content was determined by desiccation at 105 °C for 5 days. The cold-injury "core" was identified by staining with Evans blue injected 30 minutes before decapitation.

Recombinant human lipocortin-1 (35 kD), LC-10 (1.9 kD), and LC-24 (1.9 kD) were generous gifts from Drs. Matsumoto and Ito (Kyowa Hakko Co. Ltd., Tokyo). LC-10 and LC-24 are the peptides, which compose part of recombinant lipocortin-1 and possess

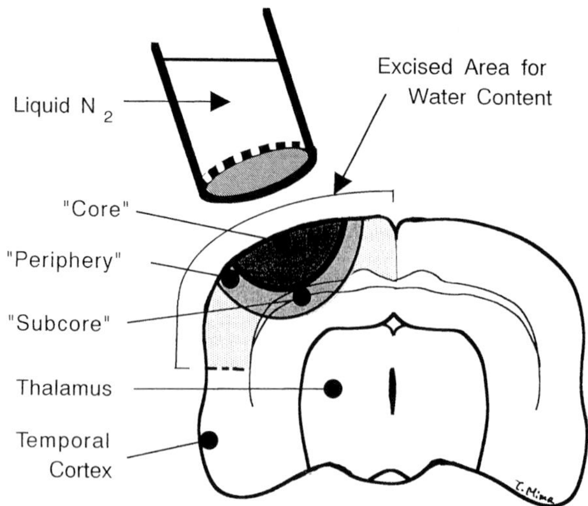

Fig. 1. Diagram for cold injury and the region of brain measured for edema formation. A liquid-nitrogen-cooled cylinder was attached to the exposed dura for 60 seconds. Water content of small tissue fragments (10 mg) in each site was determined by the specific gravimetry technique, as an indicator of region-specified edema such as the cold-injury "core" (severe edema) and "periphery" (moderate edema)

phospholipase A2 inhibitory activity. With regard to the inhibitory potency, LC-10 and LC-24 is 1/10 and 1/3 as potent as lipocortin-1, respectively. Those peptides were dissolved in 20 μl of mock cerebrospinal fluid (CSF) and infused into the right lateral ventricle (i.c.v.) 3 hours before cold-injury. Infusion took 5 minutes. In some experimental groups (Experiment 3 and 4), lipocortin-1 was injected intra-arterially (i.a.) via the right carotid artery. Dexamethasone was injected intra-peritoneally (i.p.) either 3 hours or immediately before cold-injury, combined with an intraventricular injection of mock CSF 3 hours before cold-injury.

Experiment 1: 24 hours after cold-injury. Seven groups were subjected to cold-injury. Albumin was injected as control to make the same osmolarity as 0.1 mg/kg of lipocortin-1. (1) no treatment (n = 5), (2) mock CSF i.c.v. (n = 8), (3) albumin 0.18 mg/kg i.c.v. (n = 4), (4) dexamethasone 10 mg/kg i.p. immediately before cold-injury with mock CSF i.c.v. (n = 6), (5) dexamethasone 10 mg/kg i.p. 3 hours before cold-injury with mock CSF i.c.v. (n = 6), (6) lipocortin-1 0.1 mg/kg i.c.v. (n = 5), and (7) lipocortin-1 0.01 mg/kg i.c.v. (n = 8).

Experiment 2: 48 hours after cold-injury. This experiment was designed to see longer-term effects of dexamethasone and lipocortin-1. (1) mock CSF i.c.v. (n = 5), (2) dexamethasone 10 mg/kg i.p. twice, 3 hours before and 24 hours after cold-injury, combined wit mock CSF i.c.v. 3 hours before cold-injury, (n = 9), (3) lipocortin-1 0.1 mg/kg i.c.v. once, 3 hours before cold injury (n = 8), (4) lipocortin-1 0.1 mg/kg i.c.v. twice, 3 hours before and 24 hours after cold-injury (n = 6), and (5) lipocortin-1 0.01 mg/kg i.c.v. twice, same schedule as (4) (n = 5).

Experiment 3: 24 hours after cold-injury. (1) sham operation (n = 6), (2) mock CSF i.c.v. (n = 8), (3) dexamethasone 10 mg/kg i.p. 3 hours before cold-injury with mock CSF i.c.v., (n = 10), (4) lipocortin-1 0.1 mg/kg i.c.v. (n = 6), (5) lipocortin-1 0.01 mg/kg i.c.v. (n = 8), (6) lipocortin-1 2 mL of 10^{-7} M i.a. 10 minutes before cold-injury (n = 8), (7) LC-10 0.01 mg/kg i.c.v. (n = 8), and (8) LC-24 0.01 mg/kg i.c.v. (n = 6).

Experiment 4: 48 hours after cold-injury. This experiment aimed to see the effects of dexamethasone and lipocortin-1 at the later stage (24–48 hours) of brain edema. (1) no treatment (n = 8), (2) dexamethasone 10 mg/kg i.p. 24 hours after cold-injury (n = 6), and (3) lipocortin-1 2 ml of 10^{-7} M i.a. same schedule as (2) (n = 5).

Experiment 5: 2 hours after cold-injury. This experiment focused on the effects at the earlier stage (0–2 hours) of brain edema. (1) mock CSF i.c.v. (n = 6), (2) dexamethasone 10 mg/kg i.p. 3 hours before cold-injury wit mock CSF i.c.v. (n = 6), and (3) lipocortin-1 0.05 mg/kg i.c.v. (n = 8).

For statistical purposes, we used the analysis of variance (ANOVA) for comparing multiple groups, and used Student's test for comparing two groups. P value of less than 0.05 was considered statistically significant.

Results

Experiment 1: At 24 hours after cold injury, brain edema in the no treatment group, indicated as specific gravity (mean +/– SD), was only prominent in the regions labeled as "core" (1.0254 +/– 0.0009), "periphery" (1.0407 +/– 0.0023) and "subcore" (1.0415 +/– 0.0011). Specific gravity of tissue in the remote regions such as the frontal cortex (1.0454 +/– 0.0009), the temporal cortex (1.0441 +/– 0.0006) and the thalamus (1.0450 +/– 0.0010) was the same as that in the contralateral cerebral cortex (1.0454 +/– 0.0004) and thalamus (1.0454 +/– 0.0004).

At the "periphery" and "core", none of the treatments showed significant edema reduction. High- and low-dose lipocortin-1 at "core" tended to ameliorate edema slightly, but the effect was not statistically significant (Fig. 2). Dexamethasone given 3 hours before cold injury, which aimed to induce more lipocortins at the acute stage of edema formation, was as ineffective as dexamethasone given immediately before the insult

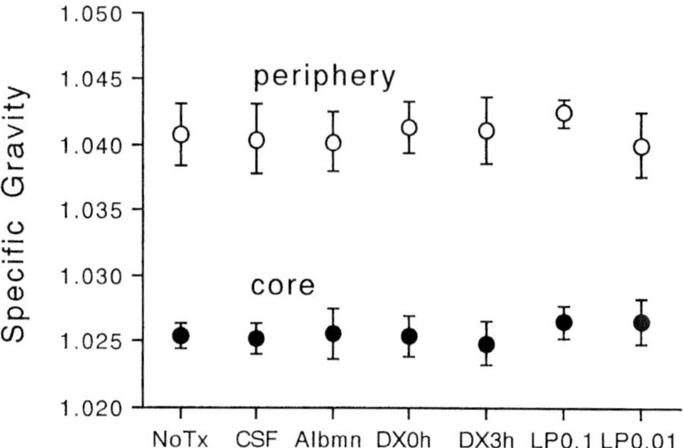

Fig. 2. Experiment 1: Specific gravity at 24 hours after cold injury (mean +/– SD). 10 mg/kg of dexamethasone injected immediately before cold-injury (DX0h), same dose of dexamethasone injected 3 hours before cold-injury (DX3h), 0.1 mg/kg of lipocortin-1 (LP0.1) or 0.01 mg/kg of lipocortin-1 (LP0.01) did not show any amelioration in either "core" or "periphery", compared with no treatment group (NoTx). Intraventricular injection of mock CSF (*CSF*) or albumin (Albmn) did not influence the results

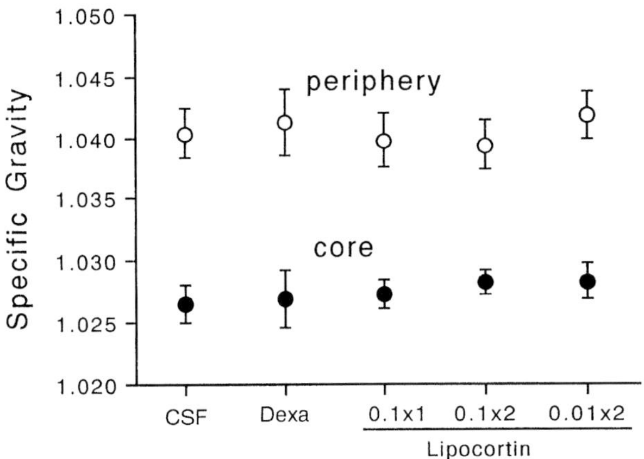

Fig. 3. Experiment 2: Specific gravity at 48 hours after cold injury (mean +/− SD). Dexamethasone *(Dexa)*, single injection of 0.1 mg/kg of lipocortin-1 (0.1 × 1), double injection of 0.1 mg/kg (0.1 × 2), or 0.01 mg/kg of lipocortin-1 (0.01 × 2) showed no beneficial effects compared with mock CSF injection *(CSF)*

(Fig. 2). Although the values at the "subcore" (mostly composed of corpus callosum, Fig. 1) showed large standard deviations in some groups, 0.1 mg/kg of lipocortin-1 aggravated edema formation as compared with no treatment or albumin ($p < 0.05$): (1) no treatment (1.0415 +/− 0.0011), (2) mock CSF (1.0401 +/− 0.0035), (3) albumin (1.0416 +/− 0.0020), (4) dexamethasone pre-0hr (1.0398 +/− 0.0048), (5) dexamethasone pre-3hr (1.0415 +/− 0.0009), (6) lipocortin-1 0.1 mg/kg (1.0378 +/− 0.0029), and (7) lipocortin-1 0.01 mg/kg (1.0418 +/− 0.0017).

Experiment 2: At 48 hours after cold injury, no treatments showed significant effects at the "core" and "periphery" (Fig. 3). Even double injection of dexamethasone or lipocortin-1 did not attenuate edema.

Experiment 3: When a larger area of edematous tissue was sampled to see the effects on more global edema at 24 hours after cold injury, no treatments ameliorated edema statistically. All of the lipocortin-1 treatments had a tendency to aggravate edema, but they were not statistically significant from control. The values of water content (mean +/− SD) were as follows: (1) sham (78.46 +/− 0.30%), (2) mock CSF (83.07 +/− 0.69%), (3) dexamethasone (82.89 +/− 1.10%), (4) 0.1 mg/kg of lipocortin-1 (83.80 +/− 0.73%), (5) 0.01 mg/kg of lipocortin-1 (83.61 +/− 0.42%), (6) intraarterial injection of lipocortin-1 (83.83 +/− 0.78%), (7) LC-10 (82.72 +/− 0.95%), and (8) LC-24 (83.18 +/− 0.37%).

Experiment 4: When the effects of drug were tested at the subacute stage of edema (24–48 hours after cold injury), dexamethasone or lipocortin-1 did not attenuate edema. Intraarterial infusion of lipocortin-1 significantly aggravated edema compared with no treatment or dexamethasone ($p < 0.05$). The values of water content (mean +/− SD) were as follows: (1) no treatment (83.31 +/− 1.06%), (2) dexamethasone (83.38 +/− 0.99%), and (3) lipocortin-1 (84.86 +/− 0.46%).

Experiment 5: At the earlier stage of edema formation (0–2 hours after cold injury), neither dexamethasone nor lipocortin-1 showed amelioration. The values of water content (mean +/− SD) were as follows: (1) no treatment (81.59 +/− 0.27%), (2) dexamethasone (82.19 +/− 0.91%), and (3) lipocortin-1 (82.18 +/− 0.51%).

Discussion

High dose dexamethasone did not attenuate edema formation even though pretreatment was designed to induce more lipocortins prior to the onset of injury. The effectiveness of corticosteroids on reducing cold-injury edema is still controversial. Although some groups reported positive data [12, 13, 21], others claimed that the effects are not robust [9, 16, 23, 24]. Reduction of water content with dexamethasone was not statistically significant [23]. Dexamethasone improved neurological outcome, but did not reduce water content [24]. The beneficial effect of corticosteroids was only detected by radioiodinated serum albumin (RISA) distribution [16] and by magnetic resonance imaging (MRI) [9], but was not found by the water content method in either study [9, 16].

Sugiura *et al.* [21] reviewed 25 experimental studies of steroid treatment, and concluded that "steroids given before or at the time of producing edema tend to bear more positive data than negative ones, while there have been no positive reports when steroids were given some time after the production of the lesions." Meinig and Diesenroth reported that much stronger effects were obtained with dexamethasone pretreatment, however the effect became minimal when the drug was given more than 30 minutes after injury [13]. The dissociation of steroid effectiveness between pretreatment and posttreatment suggests that the anti-edema mechanisms depend on de novo synthesis of anti-inflammatory proteins.

Protein synthesis is suppressed when ischemic cerebral blood flow falls to 55 ml/100 g/min [14], and even in the cortex adjacent to the cryogenic lesion, the cerebral blood flow is below that threshold [22]. After cold-injury, therefore, the core and periphery of cold-injury brain may be unable to synthesize anti-inflammatory proteins in response to steroids. This speculation may also explain why steroids have a greater effect on edema caused by tumor or abscess compared with that caused by ischemia, trauma, or cold-injury, because cerebral blood flow is preserved in the former edema but decreased in the latter.

In an ex vivo study such as an isolated perfusion lung model, recombinant lipocortin-1 was shown to be active and rapid in its onset of action when infused in small amounts 1 μg/ml [3]. However, only a few in vivo studies have been reported to support the anti-inflammatory effect of lipocortin-1 [4, 18, 19], and its efficacy in carrageenin-induced paw edema [4] was not duplicated [17]. Although we also tested the effects of lipocortin-1 in peritumoral edema in the rat [2] and in ischemic edema in the cat [15], both studies failed to ameliorate edema. Recently, Relton and Rothwell reported that a lipocortin-1 fragment (1–188 amino acids) attenuated infarct size and cerebral edema after MCA occlusion in the rat, and stated that the lipocortin-1 fragment had greater activity and stability than the full molecule they did not show from treatment data with the full molecule of lipocortin-1 [18, 19]

In the present study, dexamethasone and recombinant human lipocortin-1 failed to ameliorate cold-injury brain edema in the rat. The anti-inflammatory effects of dexamethasone or exogenous lipocortin-1 on cold-injury brain edema are minimal.

Acknowledgments

We thank Drs. T. Matsumoto and S. Ito (Kyowa Hakko Co. Ltd., Tokyo) for a generous gift of recombinant human lipocortin-1. We also thank Ms. R. Matsuura for technical assistance in the experiment, and Ms. Y. Muto for animal cares.

References

1. Browning JL, Ward MP, Wallner BP, Pepinsky RB (1990) Studies on the structural properties of lipocortin-1 and the regulation of its synthesis by steroids. Prog Clin Biol Res 349: 27–45
2. Chang CC, Shinonaga M, Kuwabara T, Mima T, Shigeno T (1990) Effect of recombinant human lipocortin I on brain oedema in a rat glioma model. Acta Neurochir [Suppl] (Wien) 51: 145–147
3. Cirino G, Flower RJ, Browning JL, Sinclair LK, Pepinsky RB (1987) Recombinant human lipocortin 1 inhibits thromboxane release from ginea-pig isolated perfused lung. Nature 328: 270–272
4. Cirino G, Peers SH, Flower RJ, Browning JL, Pepinsky RB (1989) Human recombinant lipocortin 1 has acute local anti-inflammatory properties in the rat paw edema test. Proc Natl Acad Sci USA 86: 3428–3432
5. Crompton MT, Moss SE, Crumpton MJ (1988) Diversity in the lipocortin/calpactin family. Cell 55: 1–3
6. Crumpton M, Dedman J (1990) Protein terminology tanglew. Nature 345: 212
7. Di Rosa M, Flower RJ, Hirata F, Parente L, Russo-Marie F (1984) Anti-phospholipase proteins. Prostaglandins 28: 441–442
8. Flower R (1990) Lipocortin. Prog Clin Biol Res 349: 11–25
9. Handa Y, Kobayashi H, Kawano H, Ishii H, Naguchi Y, Hayashi M (1990) Steroid and hyperosmotic diuretic effects on the early phase of experimental vasogenic oedema. Acta Neurochir [Suppl] (Wien) 51: 107–109
10. Johnson MD, Gray ME, Carpenter G, Pepinsky RB, Sundell H, Stahlman MT (1989) Ontogeny of epidermal growth factor receptor/kinase and of lipocortin-1 in the ovine lung. Pediatric Res 25: 535–541
11. Klee CB (1988) Ca2+-dependent phospholipid- (and membrane-) binding proteins. Biochemistry 27: 6645–6653
12. Maxwell RE, Long DM, French LA (1971) The effects of glucosteroids on experimental cold-induced brain edema. J Neurosurg 34: 477–487
13. Meinig G, Deisenroth K (1990) Dose- and Time-dependent Effects of Dexamethasone on Rat Brain Following Cold-injury Oedema. Acta Neurochir [Suppl] (Wien) 51: 100–103
14. Mies G, Ishimaru S, Xie Y, Seo K, Hossmann KA (1991) Ischemic thresholds of cerebral protein synthesis and energy state following middle cerebral artery occlusion in rat. J Cereb Blood Flow Metab 11: 753–761
15. Mima T, Shigeno T (2000) Lipocortin-1 failed to ameliorate ischemic brain edema in the cat. Acta Neurochir [Suppl] (Wien) 76: 305–308
16. Nakata H, Yen MH, Tajima A, Lin SZ, Pettigrew K, Blasberg R, Fenstermacher J (1990) Dexamethasone effects on the distribution of water and albumin in cold-injury cerebral edema. Adv Neurol 52: 335–342
17. Northup JK, Valentine-Braun KA, Johnson LK, Severson DL, Hollenberg MD (1988) Evaluation of the antiinflammatory and phospholipase-inhibitory activity of calpactin II/lipocortin I. J Clin Invest 82: 1347–1352
18. Relton J, Strijbos P, O'Shaughnessy C, Carey F, Forder R, Tilders F, Rothwell N (1991) Lipocortin-1 is an endogenous inhibitor of ischemic damage in the rat brain. J Exp Med 174: 305–310
19. Rothwell N, Relton J (1993) Involvement and lipocortin-1 in ischemic brain damage. Cereb Brain Metab Rev 5: 178–198
20. Shigeno T, Brock M, Shigeno S, Fritschka E, Cervós-Navarro J (1982) The determination of brain water content. Microgravimetry versus drying- weighing method. J Neurosurg 57: 99–107
21. Sugiura K, Kanazawa C, Muraoka K, Yoshino Y (1980) Effect of steroid therapy on cerebral cold injury oedema in the rat. Surg Neurol 13: 301–305
22. Tajima A, Yen MH, Nakata H, Lin SZ, Patlak C, Blasberg R, Fenstermacher J (1990) Effect of dexamethasone on blood flow and volume of perfused microvessels in traumatic brain edema. Adv Neurol 52: 343–350
23. Unterberg A, Schmidt W, Dautermann C, Baethmann A (1990) The effect of various steroid treatment regimens on cold-induced brain swelling. Acta Neurochir [Suppl] (Wien) 51: 104–106
24. Yoshida S, Alksne JF, Seelig JM, Bailey MD, Moore SS, Kitamura K (1989) Effect of uridine 5′-diphosphate on cryogenic brain edema in rabbits. Stroke 20: 1694–1699

Correspondence: Tatsuo Mima, M.D., Ph.D., Department of Neurosurgery, Kochi Medical School, Nankoku City, Kochi 783-8505, Japan.

Acta Neurochir (2000) [Suppl] 76: 311–316

Hepatocyte Growth Factor Reduces Infarct Volume After Transient Focal Cerebral Ischemia in Rats

N. Tsuzuki[1], **T. Miyazawa**[1], **K. Matsumoto**[2], **T. Nakamura**[2], **K. Shima**[1], and **H. Chigasaki**[1]

[1] Department of Neurosurgery, National Defense Medical College, Tokorozawa, Japan
[2] Division of Biochemistry, Biomedical Research Center, Osaka University Medical School, Suita, Osaka, Japan

Summary

Hepatocyte growth factor (HGF) was originally discovered as a powerful mitogen for hepatocytes. HGF functions both as a neurotrophic factor as well as an angiogenetic factor. Furthermore, HGF has an anti-apoptotic effect on vascular endothelial cells. The present study examined the neuroprotective effect of HGF after transient focal cerebral ischemia in rats, in which an anti-apoptotic and an angiogenetic effect of HGF was assumed to contribute to the reduction of the infarct volume. The intraventricular administration of human recombinant HGF (90 μg) significantly reduced the infarct volume after 120 minutes occlusion of both the right middle cerebral artery (MCA) and the bilateral common carotid arteries (CCAs). In a separate series of experiments, we investigated both the anti-apoptotic effect on neurons and the angiogenetic effect of HGF histopathologically. The number of survival neurons and vascular lumina in the HGF group were significantly higher than those in the vehicle group. A large number of TUNEL positive neurons were observed in the inner boundary of the infarct area in the vehicle group, whereas only a few TUNEL positive neurons were observed in a corresponding area in the HGF group. In the HGF group, Bcl-2 protein was obviously represented in survival neurons as well as in vascular endothelial cells and in glial cells subjected to ischemia. These data suggest that HGF prevents apoptotic neuronal cell death by upregulating the production of Bcl-2 protein and by an angiogenetic effect in the central nervous system which affected transient focal cerebral ischemia.

Keywords: Hepatocyte growth factor; cerebral ischemia; apoptosis; Bcl-2 protein.

Introduction

Hepatocyte growth factor (HGF) is a multifunctional cytokine originally identified and purified as a potent mitogen for hepatocytes [20, 21]. HGF specifically binds and activates a tyrosine kinase receptor encoded by the c-met proto-oncogene [1]. The activation of the c-Met/HGF receptor following HGF binding evokes diverse cellular responses, including mitogenesis, motogenesis, morphogenesis, and anti-apoptosis [13, 17].

Previous studies showed that HGF and c-Met/HGF receptor are expressed in various regions in the brain [12] and HGF enhances the survival of hippocampal and cerebral cortex neurons in vitro [11, 12]. Recently Miyazawa [19] demonstrated that HGF protected hippocampal neurons from delayed neuronal death after transient forebrain ischemia in gerbils. Based on the findings of these studies, we addressed whether or not the administration of HGF elicits any neuroprotective activity against transient focal cerebral ischemia in rats.

Increasing evidence suggests that apoptosis may contribute to the death of neurons subjected to focal cerebral ischemia [4, 6, 7, 14–16] and that apoptosis thus contributes to the expansion of the lesion [8]. Therefore, we next investigated whether or not HGF has an anti-apoptotic effect against focal cerebral ischemia. In addition, HGF has an angiogenetic activity in vitro as well as in vivo [2, 10]. We therefore investigated an angiogenetic effect of HGF after transient focal cerebral ischemia. As a result, we obtained evidence that HGF suppressed apoptotic neuronal cell death and had an angiogenetic effect. HGF is therefore considered to have a definite neuroprotective effect against transient focal cerebral ischemia in rats.

Materials and Methods

Animal Preparation

Adult male S-D rats (270–320 g) were divided into three groups consisting of: a control group, animals given transient focal ischemia only; a physiological saline solution (vehicle) group, animals given ischemic treatment and intraventricular administration of vehicle; the HGF group, animals given ischemic treatment and intraventricular administration of 90 μg hrHGF in 200 μl of vehicle (n = 9, for each group). HrHGF or vehicle was continuously infused stereotaxically into the right lateral ventricle during 24 hours using a mini-osmotic pump. Eleven hours after starting administration of hrHGF or vehicle, both CCAs and the right MCA were occluded by snares and mini-clip, respectively. Two hours later, the blood was reperfused by removing the artery snares and mini-clip.

The rectal temperature and the brain temperature (epidural space) were continuously monitored. Mean arterial blood pressure, PaO_2, $PaCO_2$ and pH were monitored via a polyethylene-50 tube introduced into the left femoral artery. The cerebral blood flow (CBF) was also monitored throughout the experiment using laser Doppler flowmeter.

Measurement of Infarct Volume

Seventy-two hours after reperfusion, the animal brain was removed and sliced into 2-mm coronal sections. Infarct areas were visualized by 2% TTC staining and were determined using a computer-assisted image analyzing system (NIH image 1.57). The total infarct volume was then calculated [22].

Histological Procedures

Other rats were treated with hrHGF or vehicle for histological examination (n = 5, for each group). Seventy-two hours after reperfusion, the brain was removed and embedded in paraffin. Several coronal brain sections were obtained at the level of the hippocampus. The sections were stained with hematoxylin-eosin to evaluate the neuroprotective and angiogenetic effect of hrHGF. We counted the viable neurons and vascular lumina in 24 non-overlapping microscopic fields covering the entire right MCA territory at a magnification of ×200.

Other sections were subjected to the modified TUNEL procedure [9]. TUNEL-stained cells were considered to undergo apoptosis only when cell shrinkage was observed and their nuclei were densely labeled with apoptotic bodies [3, 14, 15].

The other sections were immunohistochemically treated with anti-Bcl-2 antibody. Immunoreactive complex was detected with peroxidase-labeled streptavidin-biotin complex.

Statistical Analysis

All the values represent the mean ± standard deviation (SD). To evaluate any changes in the infarct volume, a one-way analysis of variance (ANOVA) with the Bonferroni/Dunn correction was used. To evaluate the neuroprotective effect and angiogenetic effect of hrHGF, the changes in the number of neurons and vascular lumina in infarct area were statistically analyzed using the unpaired t-test.

Results

Neuroprotective Effect of hrHGF

There were no significant differences in the physiological variables and CBFs among the three groups (data not shown).

In the vehicle group, the infarct regions were widespread in the territory of the right MCA. In the HGF group, the infarct regions were seen heterogeneously and peripherally in the cerebral cortex (Fig. 1, upper left). Infarct volume in the vehicle group was 114 ± 6.3 mm^3, and the volume was almost the same as that in the control group. In contrast, infarct volume in the HGF group decreased to 65.4 ± 6.5 mm^3. There was a significant reduction of infarct volume in the HGF group (Fig. 1, upper right).

Histological analysis showed that in the vehicle group, the infarct regions accurately corresponded to the right MCA territory. (Fig. 1, lower left, A). There were numerous dead neurons all over the infarct area (Fig. 1, lower left, C). In contrast, in the HGF group, the infarct regions were definitely reduced and some rescued regions were noticed in the right MCA territory (Fig. 1, lower left, B). The neurons is this region were apparently viable (Fig. 1, lower left, D). A statistically significant difference was seen in the number of viable neurons in the right MCA territory between the vehicle group and HGF group ($P < 0.01$) (Fig. 1, lower right).

Anti-Apoptotic Effect of hrHGF

In the vehicle group, the majority of apoptotic cells were located along the inner boundary of the infarct area (Fig. 2A). Apoptotic cells were densely labeled in their nuclei accompanied by small particles around the nuclei, which resembled apoptotic bodies (Fig. 2A, inset). In the HGF group, several neurons undergoing apoptosis were also distributed in the inner boundary of the infarct area (Fig. 2B), whereas the number of apoptotic neurons was much less than that of the vehicle group. Interestingly, in the infarct core in HGF group (Fig. 2D), there were a large number of cells in which nuclei were slightly diffuse TUNEL positive (Fig. 2D, inset). The staining pattern of these cells was consistent with necrotic ones [3, 14, 15]. In contrast, a vast majority of cells had already fallen off and disappeared in the infarct core in the vehicle group (Fig. 2C). These results indicate that hrHGF suppresses apoptotic neuronal death in the inner boundary of the infarct area, and in addition, hrHGF delays necrotic neuronal death in the infarct core.

Expression of Bcl-2 Protein

Few Bcl-2-positive neurons were seen in the infarct core in the vehicle group (Fig. 2E). On the other hand, an abundant expression of Bcl-2 protein was observed in survival neurons in the rescued region in the corre-

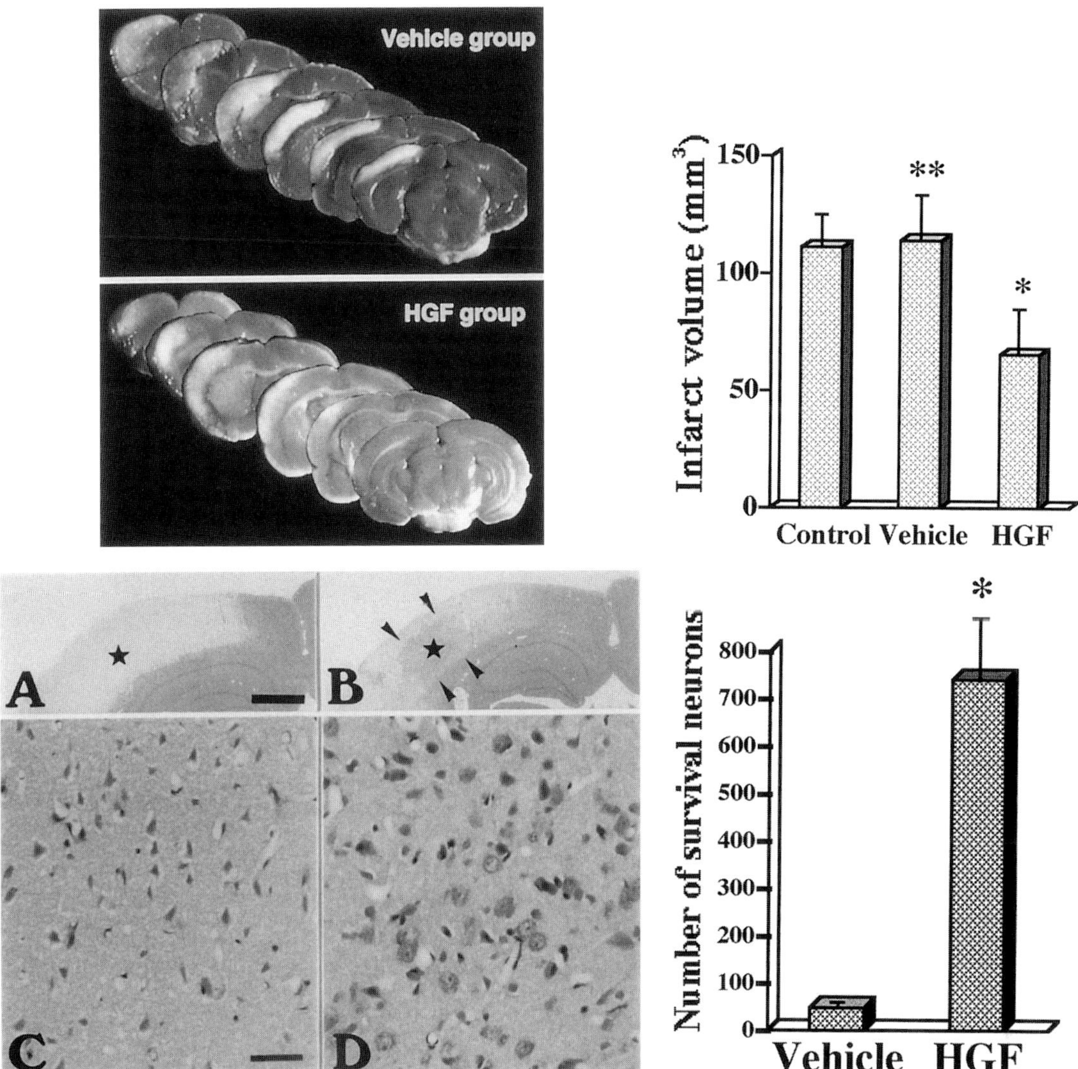

Fig. 1. (Upper left) 2% TTC staining of the brain slices. Note the marked reduction of the infarct area in the HGF group. (Upper right) A bar graph showing a significant reduction of infarct volume in the HGF group. $*P < 0.05$ compared with the control and vehicle group. ** Not significant compared with the control group. (Lower left) Histological appearances of the infarct regions in the rat brains. Note the significant infarction in the MCA territory in the vehicle group (A). Dead neurons were observed all over the MCA territory (C). In the HGF group, the infarct regions were not clearly indistinguishable from the surrounding brain and some rescued regions (arrowheads) were noticed in the corresponding area (B). Neurons in this region were apparently viable (D). Asterisks in A and B indicate the magnified areas shown in C and D, respectively. Scale bars = 1 mm for A and B, 100 μm for C and D. H&E stain. (Lower right) A bar graph showing statistical significance between the number of viable neurons in the vehicle and HGF group ($*P < 0.01$)

sponding area of the HGF group (Fig. 2F). A weak, diffuse expression of Bcl-2 protein was seen in the cells of the contralateral cerebral hemisphere of both the vehicle- and the HGF-treated rat brain (Fig. 2E, F, insets).

Protective Effect of hrHGF on Blood Vessels

In the HGF group, an increased number of vascular lumina was noticed in the rescued region in the right MCA territory, whereas a vast majority of vascular lumina had vanished in the vehicle group (Fig. 3, left, A and B). The number of vascular lumina in the right MCA territory of the HGF group was significantly larger than that in the corresponding area of the vehicle group ($P < 0.01$, Fig. 3). Furthermore, in the HGF group, the regional concentration of the number of vascular lumina in the rescued region was definitely larger than that in the contralateral brain cortex (Fig. 3, left, B, inset).

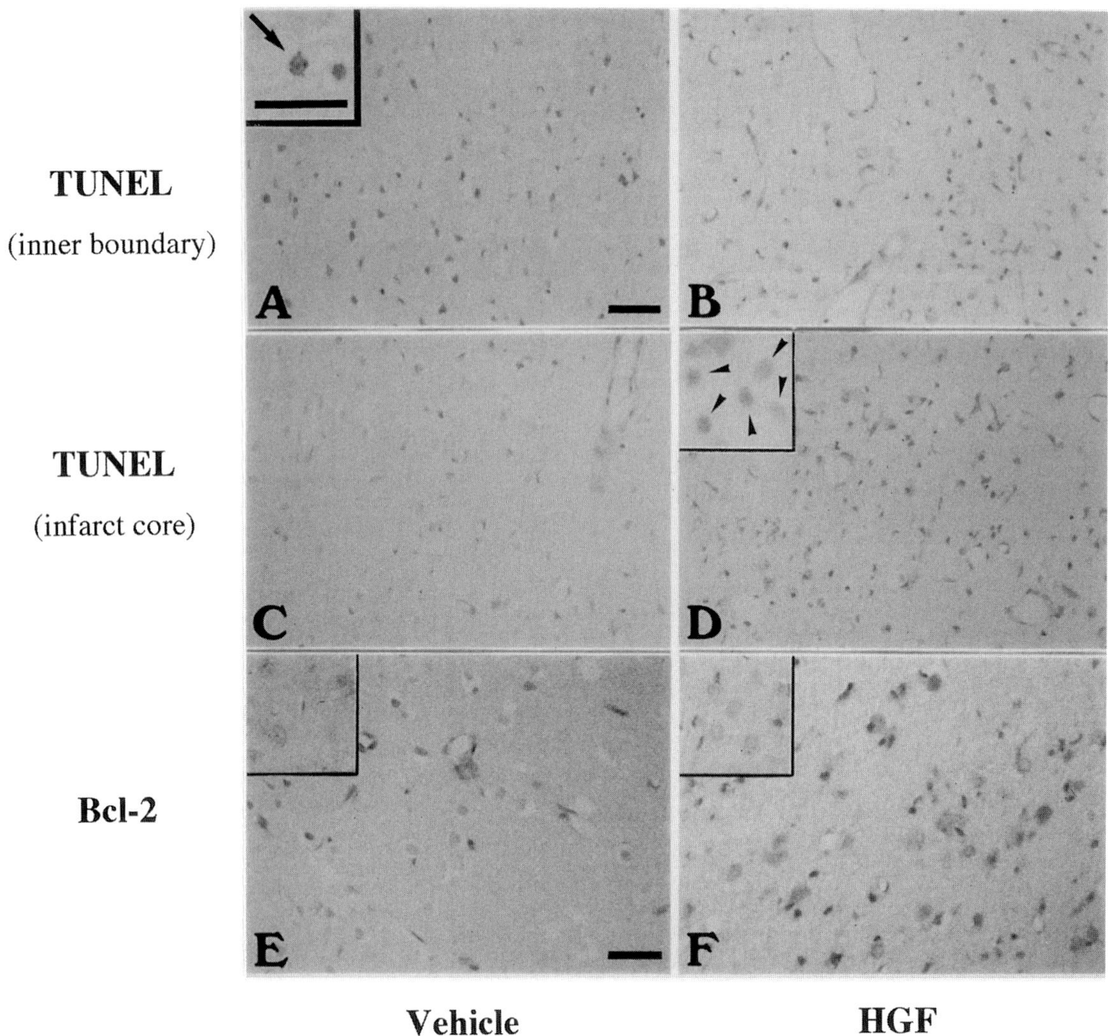

Fig. 2. TUNEL and Bcl-2 immunohistochemical staining in rat brains. Numerous apoptotic neurons are observed in the inner boundary of the infarct area of the vehicle group (A). A typical apoptotic neuron with small apoptoic bodies is presented in inset in A (arrow). In contrast, a smaller number of apoptotic neurons are observed in the corresponding area in the HGF group (B). A larger number of cells had fallen off and disappeared in the infarct core in vehicle group (C) whereas neurons which are undergoing to necrosis, with diffuse light labeling of DNA fragmentation (inset in D, arrowheads) are markedly observed in the infarct core in the HGF group (D). A few Bcl-2-positive cells are seen in infarct area in the vehicle group (E), while a marked expression of Bcl-2 protein is observed in the survival neurons, glial cells and vascular endothelial cells in the HGF group (F). A weak expression of Bcl-2 protein is seen in the contralateral cerebral cortex of both the vehicle and HGF group (insets in E and F). Scale bars = 500 μm for A through D, 100 μm for E, F and insets in A, D

Discussion

HGF functions as a survival factor for rat pheochromocytoma PC12 cells [17] and hippocampal neurons from fetal rat brains [12]. Likewise, HGF enhances the neurite outgrowth in neocortical explants of embryonic rat and promotes the survival of mesencephalic dopaminergic neurons [11].

We herein showed a marked neuroprotective effect of hrHGF against transient focal cerebral ischemia, by infusing hrHGF into the lateral ventricle of rat brain. The apoptotic neurons were much less detected in the HGF group compared with those in the vehicle group and a significant reduction of infarct volume in the HGF group was thus observed.

The present study also showed that hrHGF upregulated the expression of Bcl-2 protein on neurons after transient focal ischemia in rats' brain. Chen [5] reported that under the severe ischemic conditions induced by 120 minutes of MCA occlusion, the expression of Bcl-2 protein was only observed in a few scattered neurons in the border zone of the infarct

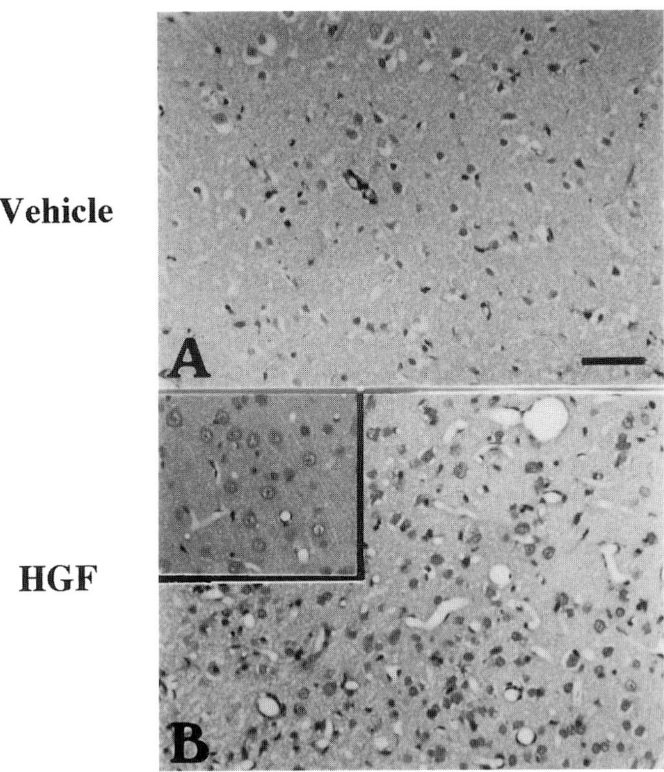

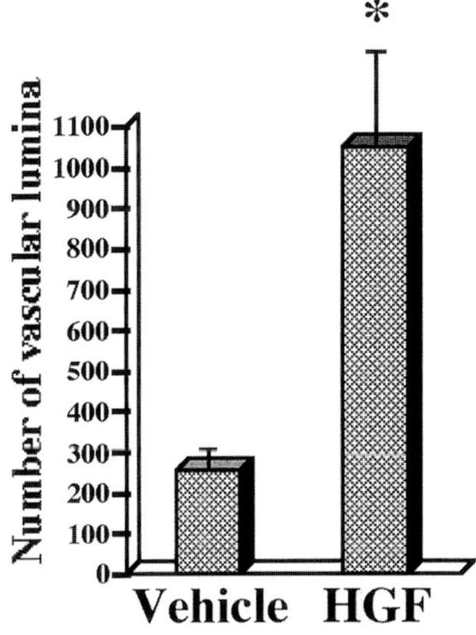

Fig. 3. (Left) Histological appearances of the infarct regions in the rat brains. In the HGF group, an increased number of vascular lumina is noticed in the rescued region in the right MCA territory (B) whereas a vast majority of vascular lumina have vanished in the vehicle group (A). Furthermore, the regional concentration of the number of vascular lumina in the rescued region is much higher than that in contralateral brain cortex in the HGF group (inset in B). Scale bar = 50 μm. H&E stain. (Right) A bar graph showing a statistical significance between the number of vascular lumina in the vehicle and the HGF group ($*P < 0.01$)

area. These patterns of neuronal Bcl-2 expression are comparable to those observed in our vehicle group. An important findings is that in the HGF group, the abundant expression of Bcl-2 protein in MCA territory was observed, in spite of the severe ischemic insult induced by occluding MCA and CCAs for 120 minutes. Chen [5] also reported that Bcl-2 protein could be an endogenous neuroprotectant in cerebral ischemia. Taken together, both these data and our results suggest that hrHGF might greatly increase the neuronal expression of endogenous Bcl-2 protein, which might be responsible for the anti-apoptotic effect of hrHGF on neurons subjected to focal cerebral ischemia, and thus hrHGF might contribute to a reduced infarct volume.

In addition to an anti-apoptotic effect, an angiogenetic effect of HGF in vivo has also been reported [2, 10]. In this study, we also demonstrated an angiogenetic effect of hrHGF in the rat brains subjected to ischemia. Unfortunately, we could not evaluate the cerebral blood flow during the reperfusion period, however, an improvement of microcirculation following angiogenesis might also contribute to a reduction of the infarct volume.

In conclusion, hrHGF has a definite neuroprotective effect after transient focal cerebral ischemia in rats' brain. An anti-apoptotic effect by upregulating the expression of Bcl-2 protein and an angiogenetic effect may be responsible for the neuroprotective effect of hrHGF.

References

1. Bottaro DP, Rubin JS, Faletto DL, Chan AM, Kmiecik TE, Vande Woude GF, Aaronson SA (1991) Identification of the hepatocyte growth factor receptor as the c-met proto-oncogene product. Science 251: 802–804
2. Bussolino F, Di Renzo MF, Ziche M, Bocchietto E, Olivero M, Naldini L, Gaudino G, Tamagnone L, Coffer A, Comoglio PM (1992) Hepatocyte growth factor is a potent angiogenic factor which stimulates endothelial cell motility and growth. J Cell Biol 119: 629–641
3. Charriaut-Marlangue C, Ben-Ari Y (1995) A cautionary note on the use of the TUNEL stain to determine apoptosis. Neuroreport 7: 61–64

4. Charriaut-Marlangue C, Margaill I, Represa A, Popovici T, Plotkine M, Ben-Ari Y (1996) Apoptosis and necrosis after reversible focal ischemia: an in situ DNA fragmentation analysis. J Cereb Blood Flow Metab 16: 186–194
5. Chen J, Graham SH, Chan PH, Lan J, Zhou RL, Simon RP (1995) bcl-2 is expressed in neurons that survive focal ischemia in the rat. Neuroreport 6: 394–398
6. Choi DW (1996) Ischemia-induced neuronal apoptosis. Curr Opin Neurobiol 6: 667–672
7. Chopp M, Li Y (1996) Apoptosis in focal cerebral ischemia. Acta Neurochir Suppl 66: 21–26
8. Du C, Hu R, Csernansky CA, Hsu CY, Choi DW (1996) Very delayed infarction after mild focal cerebral ischemia: a role for apoptosis? J Cereb Blood Flow Metab 16: 195–201
9. Gavrieli Y, Sherman Y, Ben-Sasson SA (1992) Identification of programmed cell death in situ via specific labeling of nuclear DNA fragmentation. J Cell Biol 119: 493–501
10. Grant DS, Kleinman HK, Goldberg ID, Bhargava MM, Nickoloff BJ, Kinsella JL, Polverini P, Rosen EM (1993) Scatter factor induces blood vessel formation in vivo. Proc Natl Acad Sci U S A 90: 1937–1941
11. Hamanoue M, Takemoto N, Matsumoto K, Nakamura T, Nakajima K, Kohsaka S (1996) Neurotrophic effect of hepatocyte growth factor on central nervous system neurons in vitro. J Neurosci Res 43: 554–564
12. Honda S, Kagoshima M, Wanaka A, Tohyama M, Matsumoto K, Nakamura T (1995) Localization and functional coupling of HGF and c-Met/HGF receptor in rat brain: implication as neurotrophic factor. Brain Res Mol Brain Res 32: 197–210
13. Kosai K, Matsumoto K, Nagata S, Tsujimoto Y, Nakamura T (1998) Abrogation of Fasinduced fulminant hepatic failure in mice by hepatocyte growth factor. Biochem Biophys Res Commun 244: 683–690
14. Li Y, Chopp M, Jiang N, Yao F, Zaloga C (1995a) Temporal profile of in situ DNA fragmentation after transient middle cerebral artery occlusion in the rat. J Cereb Blood Flow Metab 15: 389–397
15. Li Y, Chopp M, Jiang N, Zaloga C (1995b) In situ detection of DNA fragmentation after focal cerebral ischemia in mice. Brain Res Mol Brain Res 28: 164–168
16. Linnik MD, Zobrist RH, Hatfield MD (1993) Evidence supporting a role for programmed cell death in focal cerebral ischemia in rats. Stroke 24: 2002–2008; discussion 2008–2009
17. Matsumoto K, Kagoshima M, Nakamura T (1995) Hepatocyte growth factor as a potent survial factor for rat pheochromocytoma PC12 cells. Exp Cell Res 220: 71–78
18. Matsumoto K, Nakamura T (1997) Hepatocyte growth factor (HGF) as a tissue organizer for organogenesis and regeneration. Biochem Biophys Res Commun 239: 639–644
19. Miyazawa T, Matsumoto K, Ohmichi H, Katoh H, Yamashima T, Nakamura T (1998) Protection of hippocampal neurons from ischemia-induced delayed neuronal death by hepatocyte growth factor: a novel neurotrophic factor. J Cereb Blood Flow Metab 18: 345–348
20. Nakamura T, Nawa K, Ichihara A (1984) Partial purification and characterization of hepatocyte growth factor from serum of hepatectomized rats. Biochem Biophys Res Commun 122: 1450–1459
21. Nakamura T, Nawa K, Ichihara A, Kaise N, Nishino T (1987) Purification and subunit structure of hepatocyte growth factor from rat platelets. FEBS Lett 224: 311–316
22. Swanson RA, Morton MT, Tsao-Wu G, Savalos RA, Davidson C, Sharp FR (1990) A semiautomated method for measuring brain infarct volume [see comments]. J Cereb Blood Flow Metab 10: 290–293

Correspondence: Nobusuke Tsuzuki, Department of Neurosurgery, National Defense Medical College, 3-2 Namiki-cho, Tokorozawa, Saitama, 359-8513, Japan.

Acta Neurochir (2000) [Suppl] 76: 317–321

Clinical Use of Lidocaine for Control of Stroke Oedema in the Posterior Cranial Fossa Accompanied by Acute Hydrocephalus

A. Hirayama, S. Yamasaki, and **M. Miyata**

Division of Surgical Neurology, Chifune General Hospital, Osaka, Japan

Summary

Intravenous Lidocaine, in combination with steroid and Mannitol was used in 17 critical cases to control posterior fossa stroke oedema with jeopardised upward or downward herniation. Lidocaine successfully provided time for observation to select 5 correct candidates out of 17, indicated for aggressive decompression surgery in addition to ventricular drainage for acute hydrocephalus. There is no 'Golden-Rule' for this situation but the use of Lidocaine has a place in the management of it.

Keywords: Lidocaine; brain oedema; stroke; brain herniation.

Introduction

Contrary to expectations, that advanced neuroscientific technology in the study of brain oedema would ease the neurosurgeon's decision making, the reverse has been the case. This is due to conflicting parameters other than clinical signs being introduced.

Acute obstructive hydrocephalus, created by sudden hemorrhagic or ischemic stroke oedema in the posterior fossa, is one of the difficult situations encountered. There is no immediate solution to this problem.

From experiences using Lidocaine for controlling arrythmia, which accompanies the mass lesion, the authors recommend its use, in order to gain time of observation. The condition of either upward or downward herniation necessitates an immediate decision as to whether surgery is appropriate or not. The use of Lidocaine provides the vital time for decision making.

Materials and Methods

The 17 patients involved in this study were first diagnosed by CT or MR scan to assertain that they were suffering from posterior fossa stroke mass (either hemorrhagic or ischemic), large enough to induce brain oedema, obliteration of the IVth ventricle and create acute hydrocephalus.

If necessary tracheal intubation was carried out. Lidocaine 10% solution was administered by infusion pump syringe at a rate of 1.5–3 mg per minute, but less than 300 mg per hour. In addition to Lidocaine, 300 mls of manitol 20% and 4 mg of Dexamethasone were combined as an initial dosage. External ventricular drainage and ventricular pressure monitoring were instituted. The ventricular pressure was kept between 200 and 300 mm CSF by fractional removal of the CSF. Oxygen saturation was monitored by a skin probe. Blood pressure was controlled between 140 and 200 mm Hg systolic. Selective catheter angiography was made during the first 72 hours. Auditory brain stem evoked potentials were monitored every 6 hours.

Decompression surgery was done for clinical deterioration such as:

- Irregular respiration and failure to respond to arterial oxygen saturation, despite increasing the oxygen inhalation concentration up to 90% using a saturation monitor.
- In the case of tracheal intubation, where verbal response is difficult, failure to respond to a command to open the eyes was considered adequate.

Patients who were on respirators were not involved in this study, nor were cases of aneurysm and arteriovenous malformation.

Results

During a three month post operative period there were no surgical mortalities among the five patients who underwent decompression surgery.

Clinical profiles of the surgical cases are summarised in the accompanying Table 1 and Figs. 1–4. Of the seventeen patients involved in the study, twelve cases were hemorrhagic, including two surgically verified hemorrhagic infarctions. The remaining five cases were diagnosed as ischemic by selective catheter angiography study. (Two cases of occlusion at the origin of the vertebral artery from the subclavian arteries were diagnosed, accompanied by hypoplastic arteries on the opposite side. Also revealed was one spastic thin right superior cerebellar artery accompanied by a

Table 1. *5 Cases of Delayed Decompression Surgery*

Case	Age	Sex	Location of mass	Nature	Time of surgery after CT/MRI diagnosis (time after onset)	Outcome in 3 mo. time
1	62	male	Rt. hemisphere	ischemic	5 hr. (28 hr.)	independent
2	61	female	Vermis	hemorrhagic	5 hr. (9 hr.)	hydrocephalus
3	73	female	Rt. hemisphere	hemorrhagic	3 hr. (11 hr.)	independent
4	78	female	Lt. hemisphere	hemorrhagic	7 hr. (20 hr.)	hydrocephalus
5	65	male	Lt. hemisphere	hemorrhagic	15 hr. (17 hr.)	independent

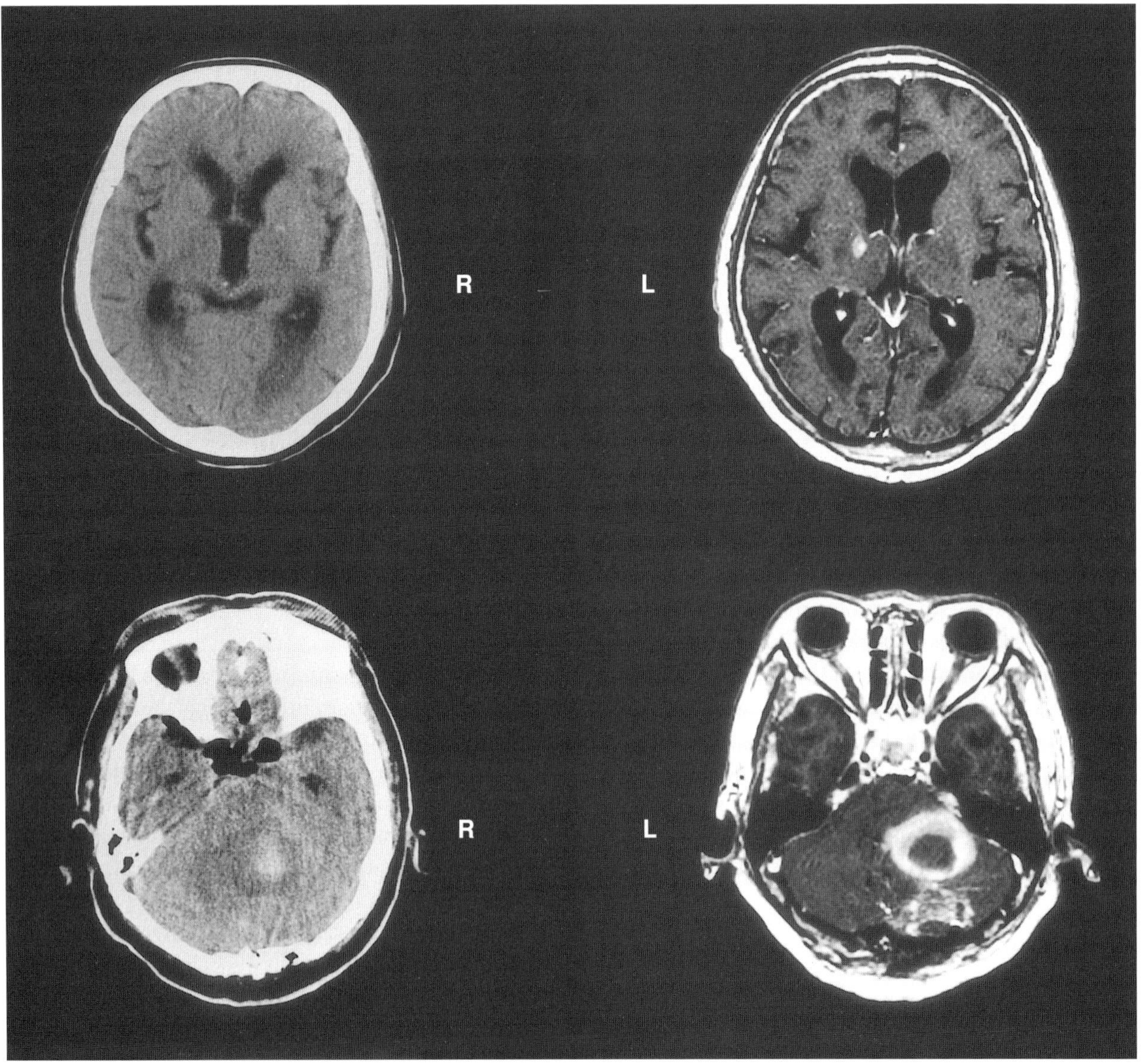

Fig. 1. Case 5 (Right) 2 pictures are preoperative MRI with contrast enhancement. (Left) 2 pictures are immediate postoperative X-CT

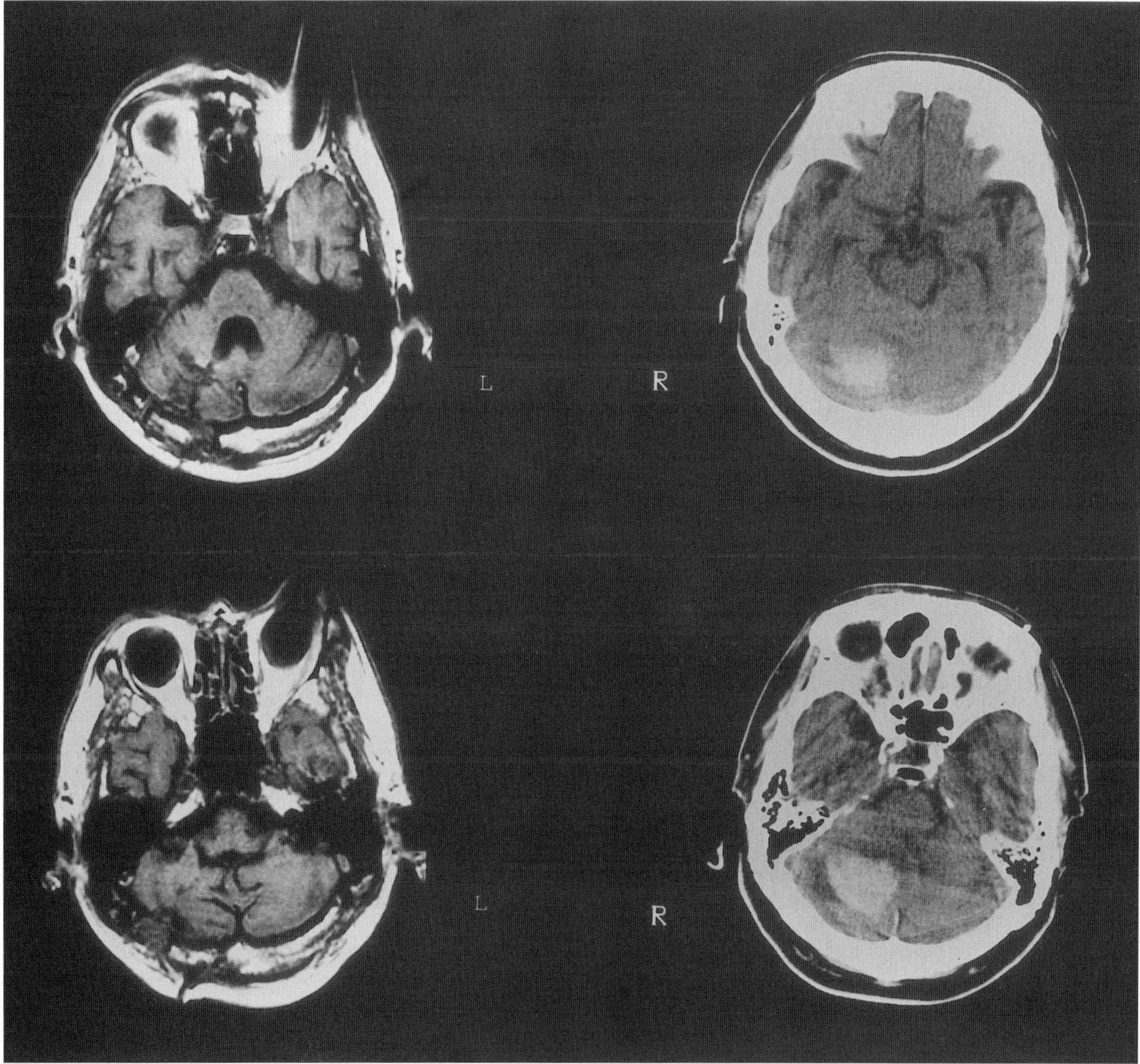

Fig. 2. Case 3 (Right) 2 pictures are preoperative X-CT. (Left) 2 pictures are postoperative MRI

hyproplastic right posterior communicating artery and one, possibly recanalized vertebral artery).

Although, intensive monitoring was maintained for 72 hours after diagnosis, surgical decisions were made, within 24 hours of the introduction of Lidocaine. Sustained improvement was noted 14 hours after ictus and 9 hours after institution of treatment in the earliest cases. On the other hand, in the latest cases improvement was noted 37 hours and 33 hours after.

Auditory brain-stem evoked potential studies disclosed delayed conduction time and even irregular amplitude, but no significant change during the observation period.

Discussion

In over 15 years in local community hospitals, unlike industrialised large institutions, members of neurosurgical teams spend more time in observation. The authors believe that time for neurological observation is most important.

Two patients with the same condition but not included in this study, died as a result of delayed decompression surgery. Immediate surgery could not only have saved their lives but also enabled them to return to independent status.

Stroke mass, either ischemic or hemorrhagic, in the

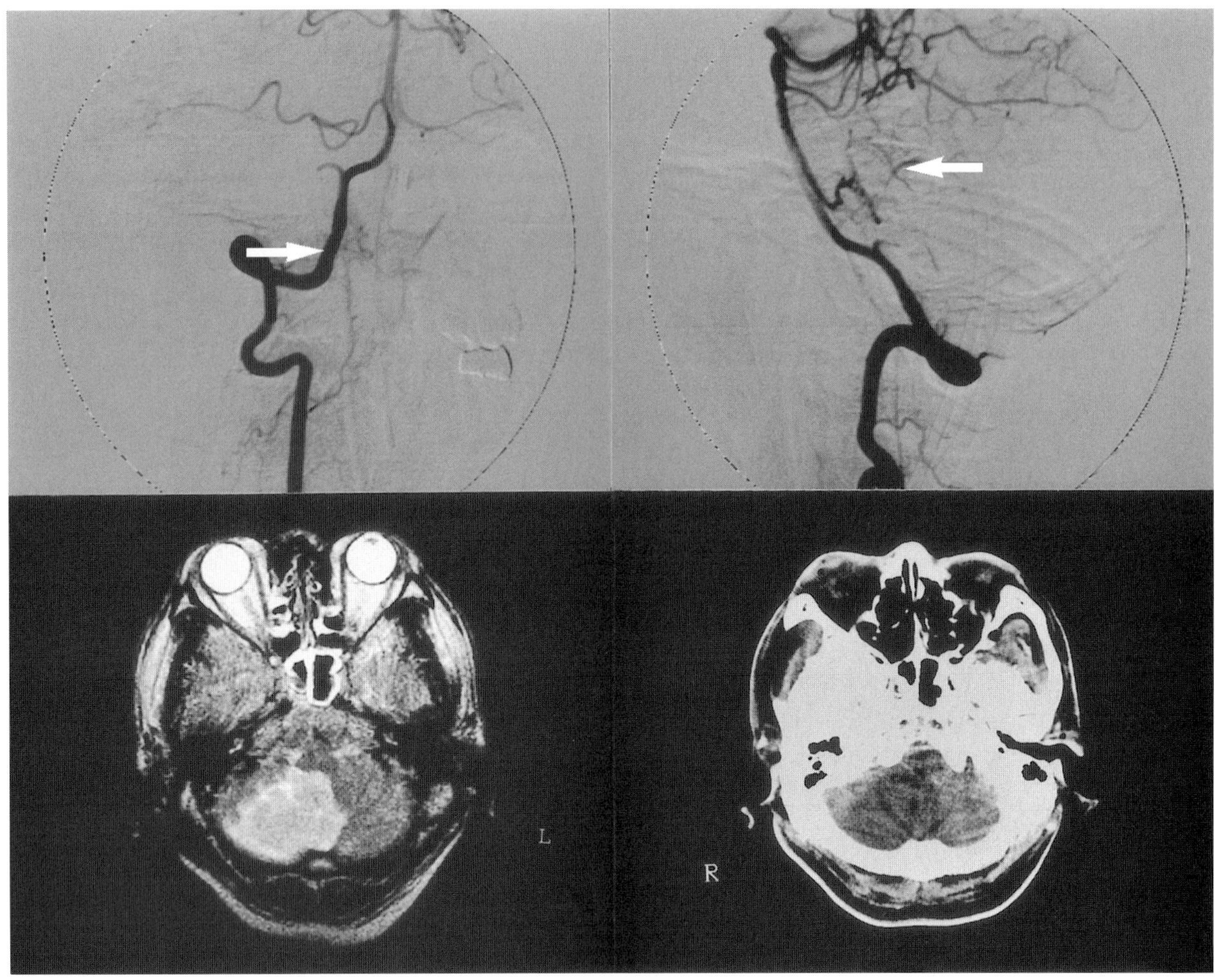

Fig. 3. Case 1 (Upper) 2 pictures indicate right posterior inferior cerebellar artery occlusion. (Lower) 2 pictures are preoperative MRI (left) and X-CT (right)

posterior cranial fossa is accompanied by significant oedema, which if large enough, can obliterate the IVth ventricle. In the case of subarachnoid hemorrhage, sudden deterioration can occur within the first 24 hours. Patients who require respirator control at this stage of diagnosis are unlikely to benefit from further treatment of any kind.

Likewise, patients who only suffer [4] small lesions are not subjects for further treatment but still require management. There is, however, a place for neurosurgical treatment for the patients between these two categories.

Intravenously applied Lidocaine at a relatively [9] high dosage can benefit those requiring control for cardiac arrythmia or lower intracranial pressure [1, 8]. Lidocaine is a depressant of the central nervous system [2] but does not affect consciousness in general [9]. The mechanism for action has been found to be receptor and acceptor based [2]. Animal experiments have suggested its protective effect on neural conditions such as, lack of glucose as in ischemia [7], accomplished by inhibiting the leak of cations across the cell membrane.

This hypothesis appears to be compatible with rapid reaction in the CSF pressure response. In this study, Lidocaine slowed down the rapid rise of local oedema, although, not the height of its peak, thus providing time for observation.

There is no 'golden rule' in this situation, but the use of Lidocaine can provide opportunities for neurosurgeons to treat this difficult problem more precisely from observed evidence than without it.

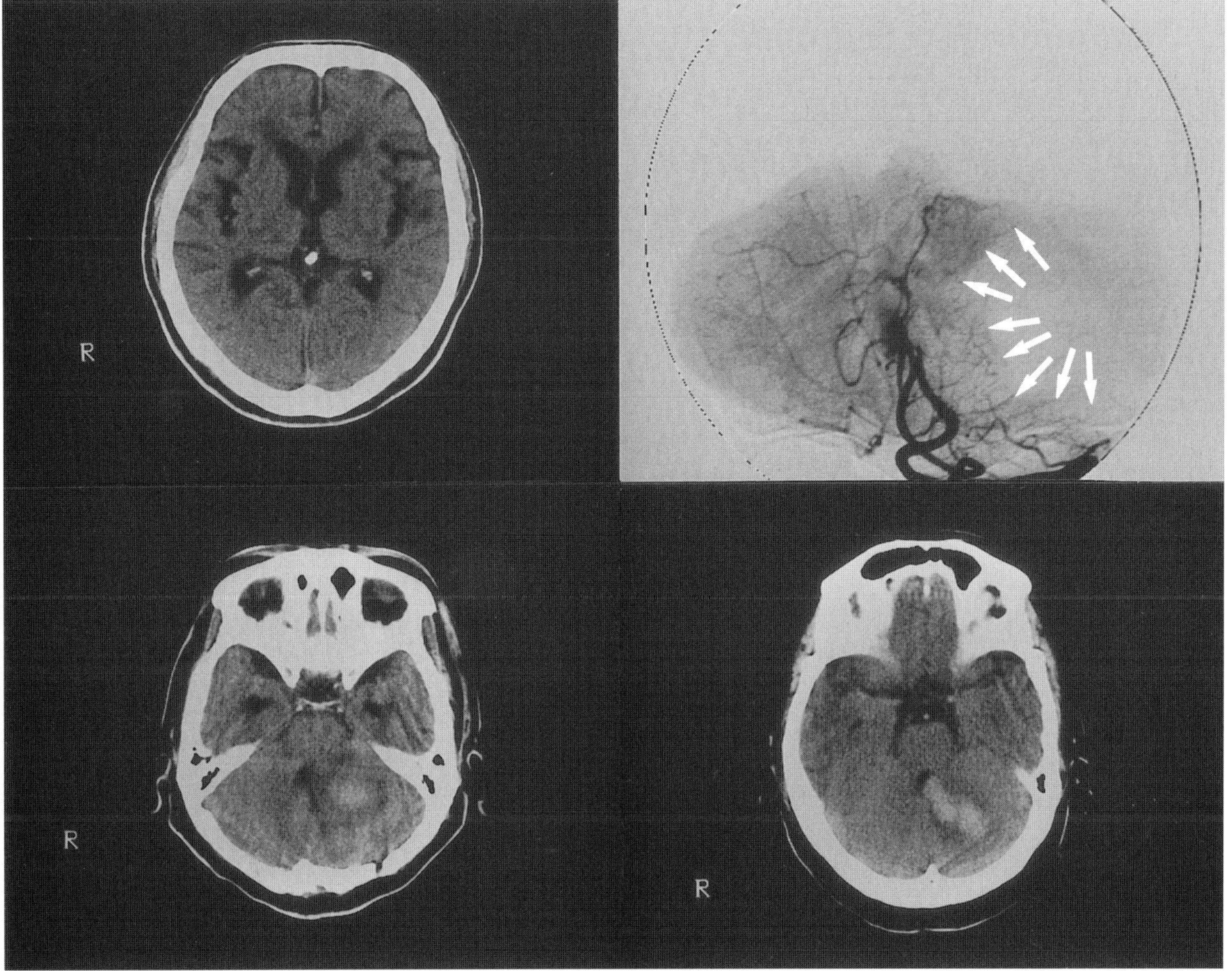

Fig. 4. Case 5 (Upper right) is preoperative angiography, (lower right) is preoperative X-CT. (Left) pictures are postoperative (4Wks) X-CT

References

1. Bedford RF, Persing JA, Pobereskin L, Butler A (1980) Lidocaine or thiopental for rapid control of intracranial hypertension. Anesth Analg 59: 435–437
2. Bradley PB (1989) Introduction to neuropharmacology, 1st edn. Butterworth, London, pp 119–120
3. Evans DE, Kobrine AI, LeGrys DC, Bradley ME (1984) Protective effect of lidocaine in acute cerebral ischemia induced by air embolism. J Neurosurg 60: 257–263
4. Hirayama A, Yamasaki S (1989) Therapeutic hydrocephalus for postoperative delayed coma patients. In: Bhatia R, Bhatia S (eds) Book of abstract, 9th International Congress of Neurological Surgery. New Delhi, pp 370
5. Hirayama A, Yamasaki S, Miyata M (1993) A pilot study on postoperative ICP control by glycerin combined with lidocaine or nitroglycerin. In: Avezaat CJ, Van Eijnhaven JM, Maas AR and Tanc JJ (eds) Intracranial pressure VIII. Springer, Berlin Heidelberg New York Tokyo, pp 609–611
6. Khayata M, Arbit E DiResta GR, Lau N, Galicich JH (1989) ICP Reduction by Lidocaine: Dose response curve and effect on CBF and EEG. In: Hoff JT, Betz AL (eds) Intracranial Pressure VII. Springer, Berlin Heidelberg New York Tokyo, pp 490–496
7. Nagao S, Murota T, Momma F, Kuyama H, Nishimoto A (1988) The effect of intravenous lidocaine on experimental brain edema and neural activities. J Trauma 28: 1650–1655
8. Rout A, Padmanabhan V, Rout D (1987) Role of lignocaine anesthesia in neurosurgery. In: Merry G (ed) Proceedings of the seventh Asian Australian congress of neurological surgery. Brisbane, pp 184
9. Salzer LB, Weinrib AB, Marina RJ, Lima JJ (1981) A comparison of methods of lidocaine administration in patients. Clin Pharmacol Ther 29: 617–624

Correspondence: A Hirayama, Division of Surgical Neurology, Chifune General Hospitals, Tsukuda, Nishiyodogawa, Osaka, Japan.

Acta Neurochir (2000) [Suppl] 76: 323–327

Usefulness of Niravoline, an Arginine Vasopressin Inhibitor, on Tumour-Origin Brain Oedema

H. Takahashi[1], **H. Hamada**[1], and **A. Teramoto**[2]

[1] Department of Neurosurgery, Nippon Medical School Dai-ni Hospital, Japan
[2] Department of Neurosurgery, Nippon Medical School, Japan

Summary

Niravoline is a selective agonist of κ-opioid receptors having potent aquaretic activity which may peripherally be mediated in animals. This effect of niravoline is thought to be due to inhibition of arginine vasopressin secretion. Niravoline does not cause an overt excretion of electrolytes that is seen with conventional diuretics, and it is anticipated that niravoline may prove useful in the treatment of oedema. In this study, effect of niravoline on tumour-origin brain oedema was investigated in a brain tumour model created by implantation of C6 glioma cells into the brains of Wistar rats.

Five weeks after the tumour cell implantation, niravoline was administered iv at 1 mg/kg a total of four times at one-hour intervals. In the control group (i.e., saline or vehicle-treated rats), this brain tumour model was found to result in a statistically significant increase in the water content in selected brain regions remote from the tumour. Administration of niravoline inhibited the increase in the water content in such selected brain regions.

Niravoline might be useful on tumour-origin brain oedema clinically.

Keywords: Niravoline; arginine vasopressin inhibitor; tumour-origin brain oedema; C6 glioma.

Introduction

Opioid receptors are currently classified into five subtypes, α, κ, δ, ε and σ, on the basis of their pharmacological action. Of these, the κ-opioid receptor is thought to act via dynorphins to express various physiological effects, such as inhibition of the secretion of antidiuretic hormone (arginine vasopressin; AVP), an analgesic effect, and a sedating effect [7, 8, 10, 11].

AVP is a peptide comprised of 9 amino acids, and it is synthesized in the hypothalamus and secreted from the posterior lobe of the hypophysis. AVP maintains the homeostasis of the body fluids through its antidiuretic activity [6].

Niravoline (RU599) is a selective agonist of κ-opioid receptors having potent aquaretic activity which may peripherally be mediated in animals. This effect of niravoline is thought to be due to inhibition of AVP secretion. Niravoline does not cause an overt excretion of electrolytes that is seen with conventional diuretics, and it is anticipated that niravoline may prove useful in the treatment of oedema [3]. Niravoline was found to show an aquaretic effect in cirrhotic rats with water retention [1], and research results indicate that it is effective in the treatment of hyponatremia or water retention accompanying cirrhosis. Niravoline has been found to reduce, in laboratory animals, the water content in the brain with experimental oedema induced by cryogenic injury [5], by middle cerebral artery occlusion [2] and by ischemia-reperfusion [4]. It is reported that niravoline reduced intracranial hypertension induced by balloon inflation due to the reduction in the brain water content [9].

The oedema which forms around a developing brain tumour often becomes extensive and this tumour-origin brain oedema has been treated with steroids, mannitol or glycerol preparations. However, these drugs can cause undesirable adverse effects, such as peptic ulcer or abnormalities of blood electrolytes. In view of this, the purpose of the present study was to investigate the effect of niravoline which expresses aquaretic activity by means of a new mechanism on oedema caused by brain tumours established in rats.

Materials and Methods

Experimental Animals and Groups

The experimental animals were 3-week-old female Wistar rats (body weight range: 100 ~ 200 g). These animals were allocated to three experimental groups: Group 1, a sham group; Group 2, a control group; and Group 3, a niravoline administration group. Niravoline was synthesized and supplied by Hoechst Marion Roussel (Romainville, France).

Preparation of Brain Tumour Model

The rats were anesthetized and immobilized in a stereotactic headholder (Kopf Instruments; CA, USA). The skull was exposed and a drill was used to create a burr hole in the skull at a point 3-mm right lateral and 0.5-mm posterior to the bregma. And a 0.5-mm microsyringe needle was slowly inserted perpendicularly to the brain surface to a depth of 5 mm, thus reaching exactly into the right caudoputamen. This needle was then used to infuse a 10^7 cells/20 μl suspension of C6 glioma cells in phosphate buffer solution (PBS) into the right candoputamen of the animals in the control group (Group 2) and the niravoline administration group (Group 3), while 20 μl of PBS was infused into the sham group animals (Group 1). The needle was gently removed 3 min after completion of the infusion. Finally, the burr hole was plugged with bone wax, and the scalp was sutured.

Measurement of Brain Water Content and Electrolytes

Five weeks after the implantation of the tumour cells, niravoline was intravenously administered to the animals in Group 3 by injection into the tail vein in a dosage of 1 mg/kg a total of four times at 1 hour intervals. The sham group (Group 1) and the control group (Group 2) were administered saline at 1 ml/kg. At one hour after the final administration, each rat was decapitated, a blood sample was collected, and the brain was removed.

The water content of the brain was measured by the wet-dry weight method for the seven regions of the brain diagrammed in Fig. 1. Measurement of the electrolytes (Na^+ and K^+) in the brain and serum was performed by high-performance liquid chromatography (HPLC) for regions 3 and 4 of the brain (Fig. 1).

Histopathological Studies

For the histopathological studies, sections of the bilateral cerebral hemispheres including the site of tumour cell implantation were prepared and evaluated using hematoxylin-eosin (HE) and Luxol fast blue (LFB) stains by light microscopy. In addition, for the purpose of investigating expansion of the area of cerebral ischemia, triphenyltetrazolium chloride (TTC) staining was also performed. Finally, the boundary of the tumour and normal tissues was observed by electron microscopy (EM). The results of these studies were presented as the mean ± S.E., and Dunnett's multiple comparison test was applied to determine the presence or absence of statistically significant differences.

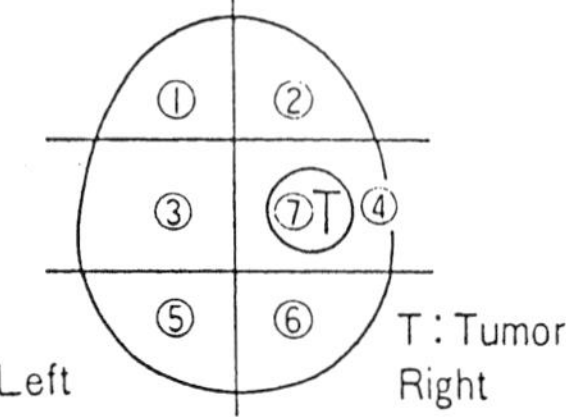

Fig. 1. Diagram of examined regions of the brain. The water content was determined for seven regions of the brain: region *7*, the tumour site; and regions *1*, *2*, *3*, *4*, *5* and *6*, separate from the tumour

Results

Brain Water Content

Figures 2 and 3 show the results of determination of the water content in the 7 analyzed regions of the brain in the three animal groups. At 5 weeks after the implantation of the tumour cells into the brains of the Group 2 (control) animals, the water content was significantly increased in all regions of the brain except for the frontal regions (i.e., regions 1 and 2) in comparison with the Group 1 (sham) animals which did not receive tumour cells. Treatment with niravoline (Group 3) reduced tumour-origin oedema in regions 3, 5 and 6 of the brain, but not in the regions most affected by the tumour (region 7, containing the tumour, and the adjacent region 4).

Electrolytes

Tables 1 and 2 show the results of measurement of the concentrations of Na^+ and K^+ in the brain tissue and serum specimens. The K^+ concentration in the brain was unchanged in the sham, control and niravoline groups. In contrast, Na^+ concentration in region 4 of the brains of the control animals was significantly increased compared with the sham group as a result of the implantation of tumour cells. Administration of niravoline (Group 3) did not alter the level of Na^+ in region 4 due to the presence of the tumour. The K^+ concentration in the serum showed – like its concentration in the brain tissue – no significant differences among the three animal groups. However, the serum Na^+ concentration was significantly higher in the niravoline administration group compared with the control group.

Histopathological Findings

In the histopathological studies, typical images of brain oedema and surrounding ischemic lesions were not observed in any of the animal groups.

Discussion

When niravoline was administered intravenously in the present study, the increase in the water content in the brain region remote from the implanted tumour was significantly suppressed. However, the increase in the water content in the tumour and the brain tissue

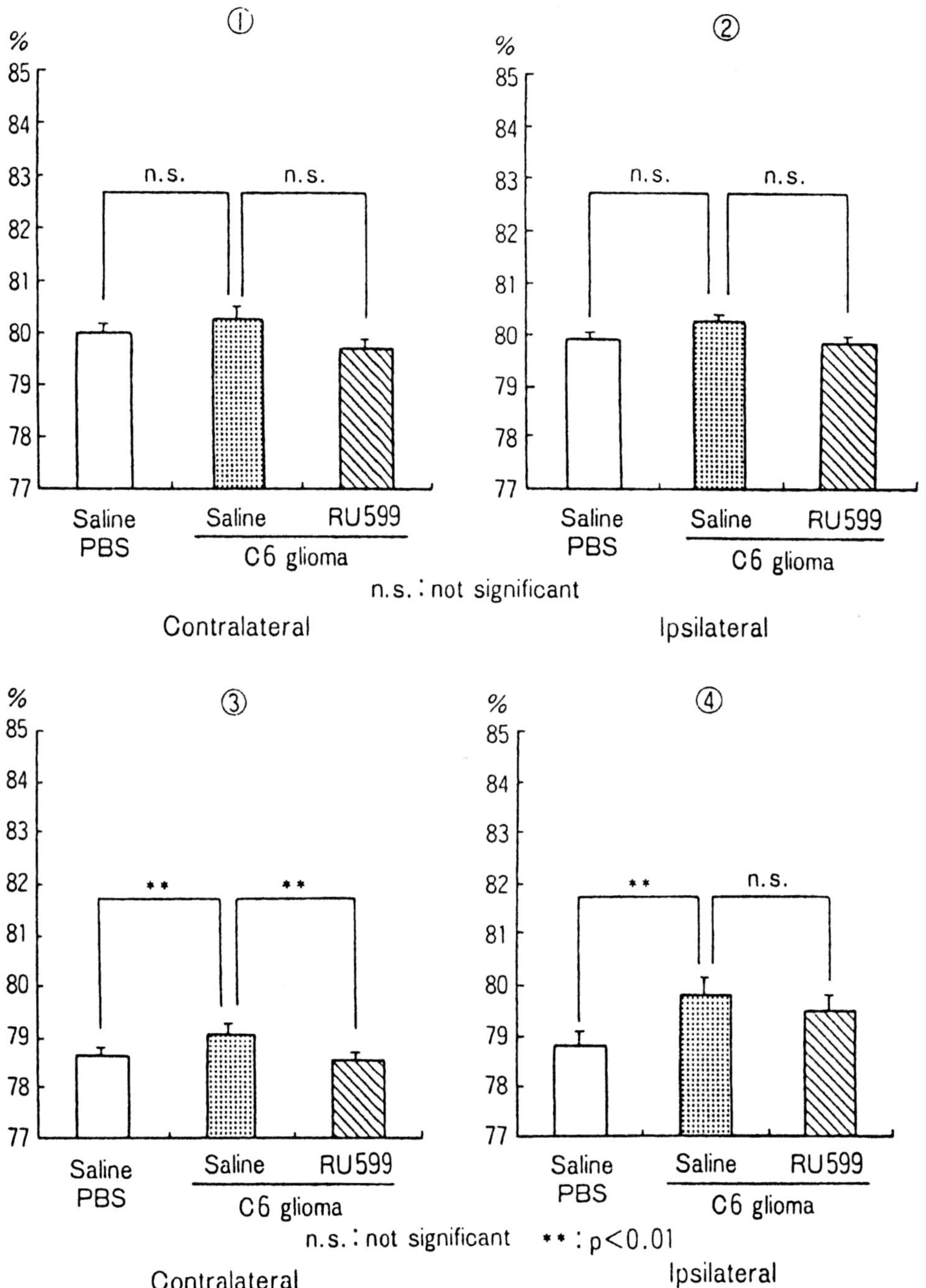

Fig. 2. Comparison of water contents of the frontal and middle brain regions in the three animal treatment groups. Sham group (n = 10), Control group (n = 9) and niravoline administration group (n = 8)

surrounding the tumour was not suppressed by niravoline. The decrease in the water content in the brain regions remote from the tumour can be explained on the concept that the increase in the brain water content is a result of inhibition of the AVP activity in the brain. On the other hand, it can be surmised that our inability to detect any decrease in the water content of the tumour and the surrounding brain tissue was due to an insufficient effect of niravoline, which is attributable to the marked increase in the water content inside the tumour and the various oedema-developing mechanisms in the tissues surrounding the tumour.

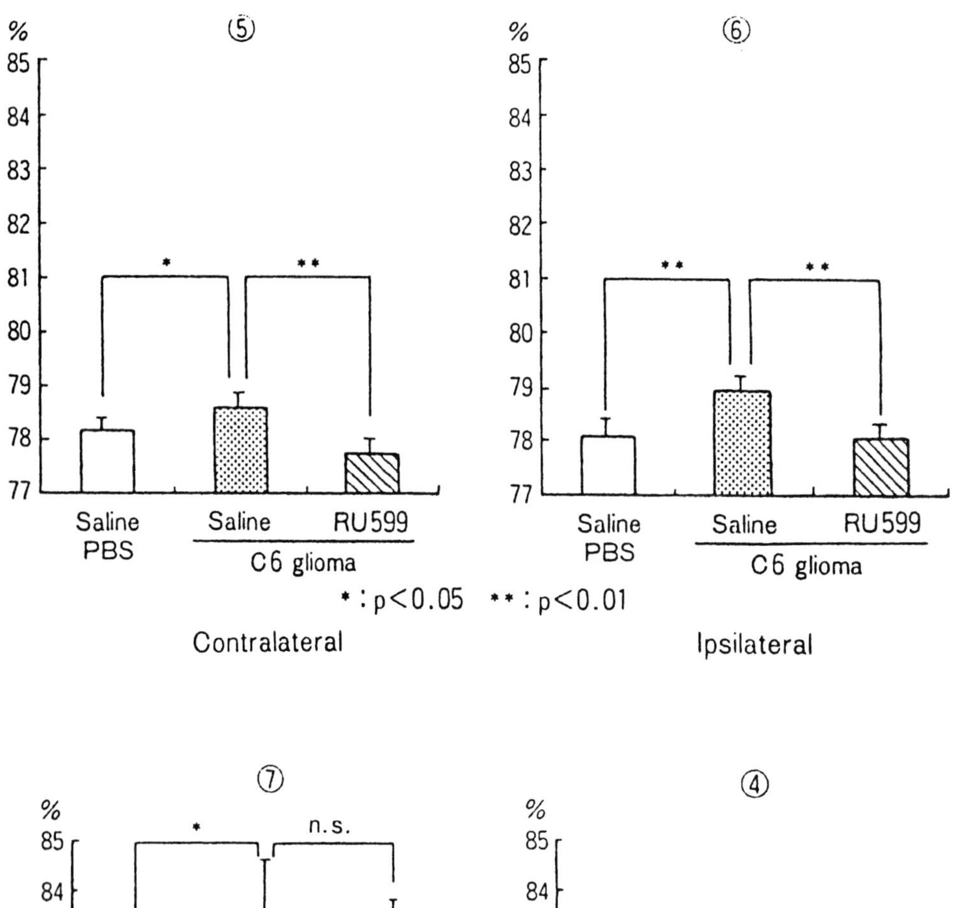

Fig. 3. Comparison of water contents of the occipital brain and tumor regions in the three animal treatment groups. Sham group (n = 10), Control group (n = 9) and niravoline administration group (n = 8)

We also found that niravoline increased the serum Na^+ concentration in this study. This increase is supposed to have been caused by dehydration of animals resulting from inhibition of AVP secretion. Simultaneously, niravoline might induce the release of diuretic factors of adrenomedullary origin and it could dehydrate animals.

On the basis of the results of our experiments, we surmise that niravoline, by means of its inhibition of AVP secretion through its agonist action on κ-opioid

Table 1. *Concentrations of Na^+ and K^+ in Brain Tissue Specimens (Regions 3 & 4)*

Experimental group	Brain tissue (region 3)		Brain tissue (region 4)	
	Na^+ (mM/kg)	K^+ (mM/kg)	Na^+ (mM/kg)	K^+ (mM/kg)
Sham	208.39 ± 3.53	474.53 ± 7.31	215.48 ± 2.31	479.59 ± 8.20
Control	210.92 ± 3.76	480.77 ± 3.71	236.80 ± 6.16*	478.18 ± 4.95
Niravoline	219.07 ± 2.38	490.99 ± 5.38	246.09 ± 8.78	492.54 ± 5.70

Mean ± SE, *: $p < 0.05$ vs. Sham group (Dunnett's test).

Table 2. *Concentrations of Na^+ and K^+ in Serum Specimens*

Experimental group	Na^+ (mEq/l)	K^+ (mEq/l)
Sham	141.40 ± 0.87	10.94 ± 0.35
Control	139.89 ± 1.09	10.51 ± 0.25
Niravoline	150.88 ± 0.81**	10.30 ± 0.25

Mean ± SE, **: $p < 0.01$ vs. Control group (Dunnett's test).

receptors, suppresses the increase in vascular permeability to water, thereby inhibiting the increase in accumulation of water in the brain and resulting in attenuation of brain oedema. However, in our present rat brain oedema model, niravoline was not able to suppress the accumulation of water in the brain region containing the implanted tumour or in the region periphery to the tumour. For this reason, we may not be able to expect this κ-opioid receptor agonist to show suppressive activity against brain tumours themselves. Nevertheless, niravoline may have potential for extensive future use in clinical medicine as a anti-oedema agent having a new action mechanism.

References

1. Bosch-MarcÈ M, JimÈnez W, Angeli P *et al* (1995) Aquaretic effect of the κ-opioid agonist RU51599 in cirrhotic rats with ascites, water retention. Gastroenterol 109: 217–223
2. Gueniau C, Berteleau L, Oberlander C (1995) Protection from ischemic focal cerebral oedema in mice by two kappa opioid receptor agonists, Niravoline and U50488H. J Cereb Flow Metab 15 [Suppl] 1: S383
3. Hamon G, Fortin M, Le Martret O *et al* (1994) Pharmacological profile of niravoline, a new aquaretic compound. J Amer Soc Nephrol 5: 272
4. Ikeda Y, Toda S, Kawamoto T, Teramoto A (1997) Arginine vasopressin release inhibitor RU51599 attenuates brain oedema following transient forebrain ischemia in rats. Acta Neurochir (Wien) 139: 1166–1172
5. Ikeda Y, Teramoto A, Nakagawa Y, Ishibashi Y, Yoshii T (1997) Attenuation of cryogenic induced brain oedema by arginine vasopressin release inhibitor RU51599. Acta Neurochir (Wien) 139: 1173–1180
6. Kimura T (1991) Vasopressin: recent advances. Med Today (Tokyo) 46(1): 76–82
7. Lord JH, Waterfield AA, Hughes J, Kosterlitz HW (1977) Endogenous opioid peptides: multiple agonists and receptors. Nature 267: 495–499
8. Martin WR, Eades CG, Thompson JA, Huppler RE, Gilbert PE (1976) The effects of morphine and nalorphine-like drugs in the nondependent and morphine-dependent chronic spinal dog. J Pharmacol Exp Ther 197: 517–531
9. Nagao S, Bemana I, Takahashi E, Nakamura T, Kuyama H (1997) Treatment of acute intracranial hypertension with RU 51599 a selective kappa opioid agonist. Acta Neurochir [Suppl] (Wien) 70: 198–201
10. Ueda H (1989) Molecular pharmacology of opioid receptor mechanisms. Folia Pharmacol Jap 94: 339–349
11. Ueda H (1994) Signal transduction of cloned opioid receptors. Folia Pharmacol Jap 104: 229–239

Correspondence: Hiroshi Takahashi, M.D., Department of Neurosurgery, Nippon Medical School Dai-ni Hospital, 1-396 Kosugicho, Nakahara-ku, Kawasaki City, Kanagawa 211-8533, Japan.

Acta Neurochir (2000) [Suppl] 76: 329–330

Broad-Spectrum Cation Channel Inhibition by LOE 908 MS Reduces Infarct Volume in Vivo and Postmortem in Focal Cerebral Ischemia in the Rat

T. Tatlisumak[1,2], **R. A. D. Carano**[3], **K. Takano**[2], **M. R. Meiler**[3], **F. Li**[2], **C. H. Sotak**[3], **U. Pschorn**, and **M. Fisher**[2]

[1] Department of Neurology, Helsinki University Central Hospital, Helsinki, Finland
[2] Department of Neurology, University of Massachusetts-Memorial Health Care, Worcester, MA
[3] Department of Biomedical Engineering, Worcester Polytechnic Institute, Worcester, MA
[4] Department of CNS Research, Boehringer Ingelheim Pharma KG, Ingelheim am Rhein, Germany

Summary

Cation channels conduct calcium, sodium, and potassium, cations that are likely deleterious in the evolution of focal ischemic injury. Diffusion-weighted magnetic resonance imaging (DWI) is a powerful tool for evaluation of acute cerebral ischemia. We studied the effects of a novel, broad-spectrum inhibitor of several cation channels, LOE 908 MS, on acute ischemic lesion development with DWI and on cerebral infarct size using 2,3,5-triphenyltetrazolium chloride (TTC) staining postmortem. Eighteen male Sprague-Dawley rats underwent middle cerebral artery occlusion (MCAO) and were randomly and blindly assigned to either LOE 908 MS (1 mg/kg bolus 30 min after MCAO and continuous iv infusion of 10 mg/kg for 4 h thereafter) or vehicle. Whole-brain DWI was done before initiation of treatment and repeated every 30 min for the next 3.5 h. The animals were reperfused in the magnetic resonance imaging (MRI) scanner 90 min after MCAO. At 24 h, the animals were killed, and the brains were cut into six 2-mm-thick slices and stained with 2% TTC. Percent hemispheric lesion volume (%HLV) was calculated for each animal. Physiological parameters, body weight, and premature mortality (3 in the placebo group and 1 in the treated group) did not differ between the groups. No hypotension, abnormal behavior, or other adverse effects were seen. Pretreatment, the DWI-derived %HLV did not differ between the groups (19.8 ± 6.2 in the control group and 17.9 ± 7.9 in the treated group), whereas at 4 h after MCAO, it was significantly smaller in the treated group (21.8 ± 15.4 vs 40.4 ± 15.5, $p = 0.03$). Postmortem, TTC-derived %HLV was significantly attenuated in the LOE 908 MS group (21.3 ± 11.9 vs 50.1 ± 10.7, $p = 0.0001$) and the neurological scores at 24 h were significantly better among the treated rats (2.1 ± 1.5 vs 4.0 ± 1.0, $p < 0.02$). LOE 908 MS significantly improved neurological outcome and reduced infarct size without observable effects in rats as demonstrated in vivo by DWI and confirmed postmortem by TTC staining. Blocking several distinct cation channels by LOE 908 MS showed significant neuroprotection.

Keywords: Stroke; ischemia; magnetic resonance imaging; calcium; rats.

Introduction

Focal brain ischemia is associated with a massive influx of calcium (Ca^{2+}), into the neurons, a process involving several distinct membrane channels and leading to neuronal death [1, 2]. LOE 908 MS is a novel and potent broad-spectrum inhibitor of several cation channels including the store- and voltage-operated Ca^{2+} channels, AMPA, NMDA, and Na^+ and K^+ channels and may prevent the ionic changes in the neuronal cytosol during ischemia. Diffusion-weighted MRI is based on the translational movement of water molecules in biological media and is sensitive for the early detection of focal brain ischemia [3]. We evaluated the effect of delayed application of LOE 908 MS on focal cerebral ischemia in vivo with diffusion-weighted magnetic resonance imaging (DWI) and postmortem with TTC staining in rats undergoing 90 minutes of temporary middle cerebral artery occlusion (MCAO).

Materials and Methods

This study was approved by the Animal Research Committee of the University of Massachusetts Medical School. Eighteen male Sprague-Dawley rats (300–350 g) underwent MCAO [4] under continuous monitoring of physiological parameters. The animals were then placed into the bore of the magnet where anesthesia was maintained with 1.0% of isoflurane. The animals were reperfused in the magnet 90 minutes after MCAO. Eight contiguous, 2-mm-thick coronal slices encompassing the whole brain were acquired by trace

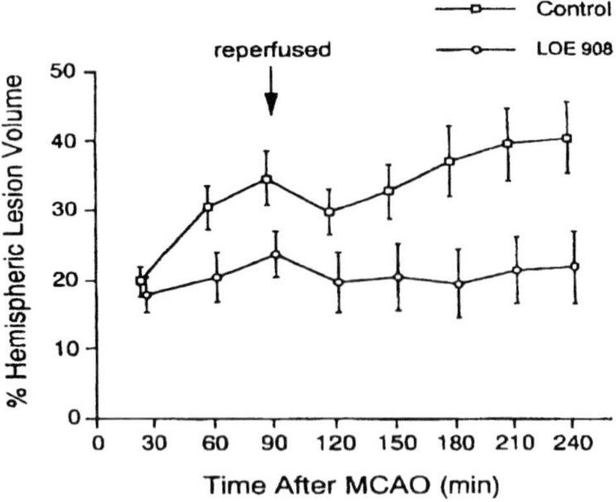

Fig. 1. The changes of %HLV in the control and LOE 908 MS treated groups over time assessed by DWI. Pretreatment the lesion volumes were similar. At 4 h, the %HLV in the treated group was significantly smaller (p = 0.03 by ANOVA)

DWI on a 2-Tesla MRI scanner at 25, 60, 85, 120, 150, 180, 210, and 240 minutes after MCAO. The average apparent diffusion coefficient (ADC_{av}) were used to calculate the percent hemispheric lesion volume (%HLV) at each imaging time point. Thirty min after MCAO, the rats received an i.v. bolus of LOE 908 MS at 1 mg/kg dose or vehicle (dextrose water) which was followed by a 10 mg/ml continuous i.v. infusion of LOE 908 MS or vehicle for 4 h, all in a randomized and blinded manner. 24 h after MCAO, the animals were scored neurologically [5], reanesthetized, and killed. The brains were coronally sectioned into six 2-mm-thick slices and stained with TTC [6]. The unstained area was defined as infarction. The areas of the infarcted tissue and the areas of both hemispheres were calculated for each brain slice. The %HLV, uncorrected and corrected infarct volumes were calculated for each animal [7].

Results

There were no significant differences in body weight, rectal (core) temperature, arterial blood pressure, or arterial blood gases (data not shown). We did not observe any adverse effects. Three animals among the controls and 1 animal in the treated group died prematurely and were graded 5 (= dead) on the neurological scale [5]. These animals underwent immediate craniectomy and TTC staining.

The TTC-derived %HLV, uncorrected and corrected infarct volumes, and neurological scores are presented in Table. The DWI-derived lesion volumes are presented in Fig. 1 and Table 1. In TTC derived infarct volumes, neurological scores, and DWI-derived lesion volumes, there was a significant benefit of the treatment (Table 1).

Table 1. *Major Results of the Study*

	Control (n = 9)	Treated (n = 9)	*P* value
%HLV	50.1 ± 10.7	21.3 ± 11.9	0.0001
Uncorrected infarct volume	354.5 ± 90.7	150.4 ± 90.7	< 0.0005
Corrected infarct volume	286.8 ± 76.9	85.6 ± 49.8	< 0.00001
Neurological scores	4.0 ± 1.0	2.1 ± 1.5	< 0.02
DWI %HLV at 25 min	19.8 ± 6.2	17.9 ± 7.9	N.S.
DWI %HLV at 4 h	40.4 ± 15.5	21.8 ± 15.4	0.03

Discussion

LOE 908 MS showed a robust anti-ischemic effect both in vivo and at postmortem without observable adverse effects. DWI excluded a possible pretreatment lesion size bias and disclosed an in vivo anti-ischemic effect as "lesion freezing" in the treated animals. LOE 908 MS showed significant neuroprotection in rats with temporary ischemia probably by inhibiting several kinds of cation channels.

References

1. Siesjö BK (1992) Pathophysiology and treatment of focal brain ischemia, part I: pathophysiology. J Neurosurg 21: 1445–1451
2. Kristian T, Siesjö BK (1998) Calcium in ischemic cell death. Stroke 29: 705–718
3. Baird AE, Warach S (1998) Magnetic resonance imaging of acute stroke. J Cereb Blood Flow Metab 18: 583–609
4. Takano K, Tatlisumak T, Bergmann AG, Gibson DG (III), Fisher M (1997) Reproducibility and reliability of middle cerebral artery occlusion using a silicon-coated suture (Koizumi) in rats. J Neur Sci 153: 8–11
5. Zea Longa E, Weinstein PR, Carlson S, Cummins R (1989) Reversible middle cerebral artery occlusion without craniectomy in rats. Stroke 20: 84–91
6. Bederson JB, Pitts LH, Germano SM; Nishimura MC, Davis RL, Bratkowski HM (1986) Evaluation of 2,3,5-triphenyltetrazolium chloride as a stain for detection and quantification of experimental cerebral infarction in rats. Stroke 17: 1304–1308
7. Tatlisumak T, Takano K, Carano RAD, Miller LP, Foster AC, Fisher M (1998) Delayed treatment with an adenosine kinase antagonist, GP683, attenuates infarct size in rats with temporary middle cerebral artery occlusion. Stroke 29: 1952–1958

Correspondence: Dr. Turgut Tatlisumak, Department of Neurology, Helsinki University Central Hospital, Helsinki, Finland.

Acta Neurochir (2000) [Suppl] 76: 331–333

A Glycine Site Antagonist ZD9379 Reduces Number of Spreading Depressions and Infarct Size in Rats with Permanent Middle Cerebral Artery Occlusion

T. Tatlisumak[1,2], **K. Takano**[2], **M. R. Meiler**[3], and **M. Fisher**[2]

[1] Department of Neurology, Helsinki University Central Hospital, Helsinki, Finland
[2] Department of Neurology, University of Massachusetts-Memorial Health Care, Worcester, MA
[3] Department of Biomedical Engineering, Worcester Polytechnic Institute, Worcester, MA

Summary

Spreading depressions (SDs) occur in experimental focal ischemia and contribute to lesion evolution. *N*-methyl-D-aspartate (NMDA) antagonists inhibit SDs and reduce infarct size. The glycine site on the NMDA receptor complex offers a therapeutic target for acute focal ischemia, potentially devoid of many side effects associated with competitive and non-competitive NMDA antagonists. We evaluated the effect of the glycine antagonist, ZD9379, on SDs and brain infarction. Male Sprague-Dawley rats (n = 18) weighing 290 to 340 g undergoing permanent middle cerebral artery occlusion (MCAO) were randomly and blindly assigned to receive drug or placebo: Group 1 (pre-MCAO treatment group, n = 5) a 5 mg/kg bolus of ZD9379 over 5 minutes followed by 5 mg/kg/hour drug infusion for 4 hours beginning 30 minutes before MCAO; Group 2 (post-MCAO treatment group, n = 7) a 5 mg/kg bolus of ZD9379 30 minutes after MCAO followed by 5 mg/kg/hour drug infusion for 4 hours; and Group 3 (control group, n = 6) vehicle for 5 hours beginning 30 minutes before MCAO. SDs were monitored electrophysiologically for 4.5 hours following MCAO by continuous recording of cortical direct current (DC) potentials and electrocorticogram (ECoG). Infarct volume was measured 24 hours after MCAO by 2,3,5 triphenyltetrazolium chloride (TTC) staining. Corrected infarct volume was 90 ± 72 mm^3 (mean ± standard deviation) in Group 1, 105 ± 46 mm^3 in Group 2, and 226 ± 41 mm^3 in Group 3 ($P < .001$). The corresponding numbers of SDs in the 3 groups were 8.2 ± 5.8, 8.1 ± 2.5, and 16.0 ± 5.1, respectively ($P < .01$). When all animals (n = 18) were analyzed, infarct volumes and the number of SDs were significantly correlated ($r = .68$, $P = .002$). This study demonstrated that ZD9379 initiated before or after MCAO significantly reduced the number of SDs and infarct volume in a permanent focal ischemia model, implying that ZD9379 is neuroprotective and its neuroprotective effect may be related to inhibiting ischemia-related SDs.

Keywords: Glycine; spreading depression; stroke; cerebral infarction.

Introduction

Leão's spreading depression (SD) is a generalized and stereotyped response of the cerebral cortex to a variety of noxious stimuli and characterized by a slowly moving, transient, and reversible depression of cortical electrical activity that spreads like ripples in a pond from the site of onset usually to the whole cortex of the ipsilateral brain hemisphere with a speed of 2 to 5 mm per minute [1]. Several studies have demonstrated the contribution of repetitive pathologic SDs in the periinfarct border zone to the expansion of ischemic brain injury [2–5]. SD is an energy-consuming process and repetitive SDs play an important role in the evolution of ischemic injury into infarction by exhausting the energy reserves of ischemic penumbra [6, 7]. Glycine is a co-agonist of the NMDA receptor channel-complex. The glycine site on the NMDA receptor complex may offer a therapeutic target for acute focal ischemia, potentially devoid of many side effects associated with competitive and non-competitive NMDA antagonists [8]. Recent studies concluded that glycine antagonists are neuroprotective in focal brain ischemia [9]. ZD9379 is a soluble, potent, bioavailable full antagonist at the glycine site penetrating highly into brain tissue and reduced infarct volume in rats up to 51,4% when started 30 minutes after induction of MCAO [10]. In the present study, we extended our observation to the effect of this drug on SDs.

Materials and Methods

This study was approved by the Animal Research Committee (ARC) of the University of Massachusetts Medical School (ARC protocol A-773). Eighteen male Sprague-Dawley rats (290 to 340 g) were anesthetized by chloral hydrate and continued with isoflurane. Rectal temperature was maintained at 37 °C. Mean arterial blood pressure arterial blood gas values were monitored. Two Ag/AgCl

Table 1. *Major Results of the Study*

	Group 1	Group 2	Group 3	*P* Value
Infarct volume (all animals included)	90.2 ± 72.3	104.7 ± 46.4	225.7 ± 40.1	.00092
Infarct volume (premature deaths excluded)	68.9 ± 62.7	100.7 ± 49.6	216.8 ± 35.1	.0035
Number of SDs (all animals included)	8.2 ± 5.8	8.1 ± 2.5	16.0 ± 5.1	.0084
Number of SDs (premature deaths excluded)	6.0 ± 3.5	7.3 ± 1.5	15.3 ± 3.5	.0011
Neurological Score (all animals included)	2.6 ± 1.3	1.9 ± 1.5	3.7 ± 1.1	.022

electrodes were placed into two burr holes in the right frontoparietal area allowing continuous recording of ECoG and DC potential. Focal cerebral ischemia was induced by the suture occlusion model of the MCA. The experiment was conducted in a blinded and randomized fashion: Group 1 received a 5 mg/kg bolus of ZD9379 over 5 minutes 30 minutes before MCAO, followed by 5 mg/kg/hour continuous drug infusion for 4 hours. Group 2 received a 5 mg/kg bolus of ZD9379 over 5 minutes 30 minutes after MCAO followed by a continuous infusion of a drug for 4 hours. Group 3 received vehicle only. Twenty-four hours later, the animals were examined neurologically and killed. The brains were sectioned coronally into six 2-mm-thick slices and stained with TTC. The unstained area was defined as infarcted tissue. Corrected infarct volume was calculated {lesion volume (total volume of the right hemisphere-total volume of the left hemisphere)}. Values are presented as mean ± standard deviation. One-factor analysis of variance (ANOVA) and subsequent post hoc Scheffe's test were used for continuous variables. Repeated measures ANOVA was applied for serial changes in physiological variables. Kruskal-Wallis *H* test followed by Mann-Whitney *U* test was applied for neurological scores. Linear regression analysis was used to correlate the number of SDs, infarct volumes, and neurological scores. A two-tailed *P* value $< .05$ was considered significant.

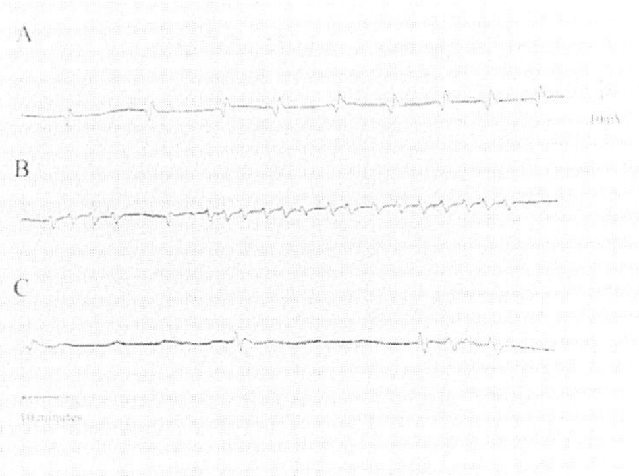

Fig. 1. DC recordings from 3 different animals. *A* The amplitude, shape, and duration of SDs were mostly identical in each animal over time. *B* A series of 15 SDs in 65 minutes in a control animal. *C* Occasionally, SDs changed in amplitude, shape, and duration in the same rat

Results

There were no significant differences in body weight, body temperature, mean arterial blood pressure, or arterial gases among the 3 groups. We did not observe any side effects or abnormal behavior. Two animals in the control group, and 1 animal from each treated group died prematurely. As shown in Table 1, neurological scores, infarct volumes, and number of SDs showed a significant difference in favor of the treated groups, analyzed either including the prematurely died animals or not. Infarct volume and the number of SDs showed a significant, positive correlation ($n = 18$, $r = .68$, $P = .002$). Similarly, infarct volume and neurological score were well-correlated ($r = .59$, $P = .01$). Number of SDs also correlated with the neurological scores ($r = .7$, $P = .001$).

Discussion

The glycine site antagonist, ZD9379, led to a substantial decrease in infarct size and in the number of SDs (Fig. 1), and improved the neurological outcome in rats with permanent MCAO without causing any observable adverse effects or any significant changes in physiological parameters. The mechanism whereby NMDA receptor antagonists prevent the elicitation of SD, most probably resides in their prevention of the glutamate binding to the receptor protein or to the blockade of the receptor-coupled ionophore. NMDA receptor has a binding site for glycine and glycine is required for NMDA receptor activation [12] suggesting that glycine antagonist might inhibit SD by a similar mechanism as NMDA antagonists. This presented study is the first to report simultaneous inhibition of SDs and attenuation of infarct size with a glycine site antagonist.

References

1. Marshall WH (1959) Spreading cortical depression of Leão. Physiol Rev 39: 239–279
2. Marrannes R, Willems R, De-Prins E, Wauquier A (1988) Evidence for a role of the N-Methyl1-D-Aspartate (NMDA) receptor in cortical spreading depression in the rat. Brain Res 457: 226–240

3. Gill R, Andiné P, Hillered L, Persson L, Hagberg H (1992) The effect of MK-801 on cortical spreading depression in the penumbral zone following focal ischemia in the rat. J Cereb Blood Flow Metab 12: 371–379
4. Iijima T, Mies G, Hossmann K-A (1992) Repeated negative DC deflections in rat cortex following middle cerebral artery occlusion are abolished by MK-801: effect on volume of ischemic injury. J Cereb Blood Flow Metab 12: 727–733
5. Chen Q, Chopp M, Bodzin G, Chen H (1993) Temperature modulation of cerebral depolarization during focal cerebral ischemia in rats: correlation with ischemic injury. J Cereb Blood Flow Metab 13: 389–394
6. Takano K, Latour LL, Formato JE, Carano RAD, Helmer KG, Hasegawa Y, Sotak CH, Fisher M (1996) The role of spreading depression in focal ischemia evaluated by diffusion mapping. Ann Neurol 39: 308–318
7. Hossmann K-A (1994) Viability thresholds and the penumbra of focal ischemia. Ann Neurol 36: 557–565
8. Kemp JA and Leeson PD (1993) The glycine site of the NMDA receptor-five years on. Trends Pharmacol Sci 14: 20–25
9. Gill R, Hargreaves RJ, Kemp JA (1995) The neuroprotective effect of the glycine site antagonist 3R-(+)-cis-4-methyl-HA966 (L-687,414) in a rat model of focal ischemia. J Cereb Blood Flow Metab 15: 197–204
10. Takano K, Tatlisumak T, Formato JE, Carano RAD, Bergmann AG, Pullan LM, Bare TM, Sotak CH, Fisher M (1997) A glycine site antagonist, ZD9379, attenuates infarct size in experimental focal ischemia: postmortem and diffusion mapping studies. Stroke 28: 1255–1263
11. Nellgård B and Wieloch T (1992) NMDA-receptor but not NBQX, an AMPA-receptor antagonist, inhibit spreading depression in the rat brain. Acta Physiol Scand 146: 497–503
12. Dalkara T, Erdemli G, Barun S, Onur R (1992) Glycine is required for NMDA receptor activation: electrophysiological evidence from intact rat hippocampus. Brain Res 576: 197–202

Correspondence: Dr. Turgut Tatlisumak, Department of Neurology, Helsinki University Central Hospital, Helsinki, Finland.

Acta Neurochir (2000) [Suppl] 76: 335–338

Effects of Inducible Nitric Oxide Synthase Inhibition on Cerebral Edema in Severe Hypertension

K. Takemori, H. Ito, and **T. Suzuki**

Department of Pathology, Kinki university School of Medicine, Osaka, Japan

Summary

In order to clarify the causative role of cytotoxic nitric oxide (NO) in hypertensive cerebral injury, the effects of inducible nitric oxide synthase (iNOS) inhibition on leukocytes and endothelial function were examined using stroke-prone spontaneously hypertensive rats (SHRSP).

For the iNOS inhibition, S-methylisothiourea (SMT) was administered to 12-week-old male SHRSP for 3 weeks. Immunohistochemical examination were carried out for the expression of intercellular adehesion molecule-1 (ICAM-1), glucose transporter-1 (GLUT-1), fibrinogen and grial fibrillary acidic protein (GFAP) in cerebral cortex. The effects of iNOS inhibition was also examined for Mac-1 expression by flow cytometric analysis.

Plasma NO metabolites level was significantly lower in the SMT group than in the control group. Mac-1 expression was inhibited by SMT. In the SMT group, brain weight was significantly lower than in the control. By SMT administration, ICAM-1 expression was suppressed, GLUT-1 was enhanced, fibrinogen was decreased and GFAP was decreased as compared to those in control group.

In hypertensive cerebral injury in SHRSP, iNOS-derived NO, mainly in activated leukocytes, could be an important causative factor for endothelial injury.

Keywords: Cerebral edema; hypertension; nitric oxide; leukocyte.

Introduction

Stroke-prone SHR (SHRSP) is the suitable animal model of human essential hypertension and almost all of them suffered from cerebral edema and softening. We had already revealed that lipid peroxidation in the cerebral cortex was much more intense in SHRSP after establishment of severe hypertension, but not before the occurrence of stroke lesions, as compared to that in normotensive WKY [7]. Furthermore, we had reported the important role of free radicals in the pathogenesis of cerebral injury in SHRSP, but the xanthine-xanthine oxidase system was not a major source of free radical generation in the SHRSP cerebral cortex [9]. In SHRSP cerebral cortex, many leukocytes are frequently seen within and/or around microvessels, suggesting the possible involvement of leukocytes in hypertensive cerebral injury. In ischemia-reperfusion injury, it has been well documented that leukocytes may play an important role in vascular changes via enhanced adhesion to endothelial cells [8]. Since leukocytes contain inducible nitric oxide synthase (iNOS) and produce cytotoxic NO by various stimuli [10], NO derived from activated leukocytes may be a key factor in inducing endothelial injury in the SHRSP cerebral cortex. Thus, it was hypothesized that increased adhesion of leukocytes to endothelial cells of brain microvessels and generation of NO-related radical(s) may play an important role in the endothelial injury and subsequent cerebral tissue damage. In the present study, to elucidate the mechanisms of microvascular changes in severe hypertension, effects of iNOS inhibition on expression of intercellular adhesion molecule-1 (ICAM-1, an adhesion molecule of endothelial cells), glucose transporter-1 (GLUT-1, a marker of blood-brain barrier), fibrinogen (marker of vascular permeability) and glial fibrillary acidic protein (GFAP, marker of neural damage) were examined in cerebral cortex of SHRSP.

Materials and Methods

Expression of ICAM-1, GLUT-1, Fibrinogen and GFAP in Cerebral Cortex of SHRSP and WKY

In order to elucidate the pathophysiological changes in cerebral cortex of SHRSP, expression of ICAM-1, GLUT-1, fibrinogen and GFAP were examined immunohistochemically using 23-week-old SHRSP in comparison with those in WKY. After sacrificing rats, brains were isolated under light ether anesthesia and 10 μm slices were stained by ABC methods using the specific antibody for rat ICAM-1, GLUT-1, fibrinogen and GFAP. Positive cells in cerebral cortex were counted by three different pathologists under microscope at magnification of ×400. Furthermore, ICAM-1 expression was examined by Reverse-transcription and a polymerase chain reaction (RT-PCR). Sense and antisense for ICAM-1 and β-actin were as follows: ICAM-1, 5′-CTGGAGAGCACAAACAGCAGAG-3′ and 5′-AAGGCCGCAGAGCAAAAGAAGC-3′, β-actin, 5′-TGTTTGAGACCTTCAACACC-3′ and 5′-TCAGGCAGCTCATAGCTCTT-3′, respectively. Base pair positions are those given in the published cDNA sequences for rat ICAM-1 and rat β-actin. RT-PCR was performed using the mRNA selective PCR Kit (Ver. 1.1, TaKaRa BIOCHEMICALS Co.) according to the Manufacturer's instructions.

Effects of iNOS Inhibition on Expression of ICAM-1, GLUT-1, Fibrinogen and GFAP

Male SHRSP were and at 12 weeks of age. For the iNOS inhibition, S-methylisothiourea (SMT, 10 mg/kg, i.p.) was administered to rats every other day for 3 weeks. Plasma NO metabolites, mainly NO_3^-, were measured using HPLC (TCI-NOX 1000; Tokyo Kasei Kogyo Co., Ltd., Tokyo), according to the methods of Green *et al.* [4]. Immunohistochemical examination of ICAM-1, GLUT-1, fibrinogen and GFAP expression was carried out as described above.

Effects of iNOS Inhibition on Expression of Mac-1 in Leukocytes

Polymorphoneutrophils (PMN) were obtained from 16-week-old SHRSP. Flow-cytometric analysis was carried out using FITC-conjugated mouse anti-rat Mac-1 antibody. Prior to incubation with antibody, PMN were incubated with S-methylisothiourea (SMT, final conc. 2.78 μg/ml) 37 °C for 30 min. for iNOS inhibition. Flow cytometric analysis was performed using Flow cytometer (FACS Calibur, Becton-Dickinson).

Results

In the baseline condition at 23 weeks of age, brain weight was significantly heavier in SHRSP than in WKY and some of SHRSP brains showed edematous changes in cerebral cortex. Immunohistochemical expression in SHRSP cerebral cortex was much more intense for ICAM-1, fibrinogen and GFAP, whereas much less for GLUT-1. In RT-PCR analysis, ratio of ICAM-1/β-actin was significantly higher in SHRSP than in WKY, being 0.18 ± 0.02 in the former and 0.27 ± 0.02 in the latter ($p < 0.01$).

Table 1. *Effects of iNOS Inhibition on Blood Pressure, Brain Weight and Plasma NO Metabolites Content in SHRSP*

	Control	SMT
Blood pressure (mmHg)	252 ± 8	250 ± 3
Brain weight (g)	2.302 ± 0.102	1.983 ± 0.053*
NO metabolits (μM)	39.5 ± 4.5	28.0 ± 3.5*

n = 7 in each group.
Mean ± SE, * $p < 0.01$ vs control.

Table 1 shows the effects of SMT on blood pressure, brain weight and plasma NO metabolites content in SHRSP. Although no difference was found in blood pressure between two groups, brain weight in SMT group was significantly lighter than in control. The effects of iNOS inhibition was confirmed by plasma NO metabolites content, i.e. it was significantly lower in SMT group. Furthermore, some of control group showed edematous change microscopically whereas no pathological changes were found in the cerebral cortex of SMT group. Figure 1 shows the immunohistochemically positive cells for ICAM-1, GLUT-1, GFAP and positive vessels for fibrinogen in both groups. In the SMT group, expression of ICAM-1 was

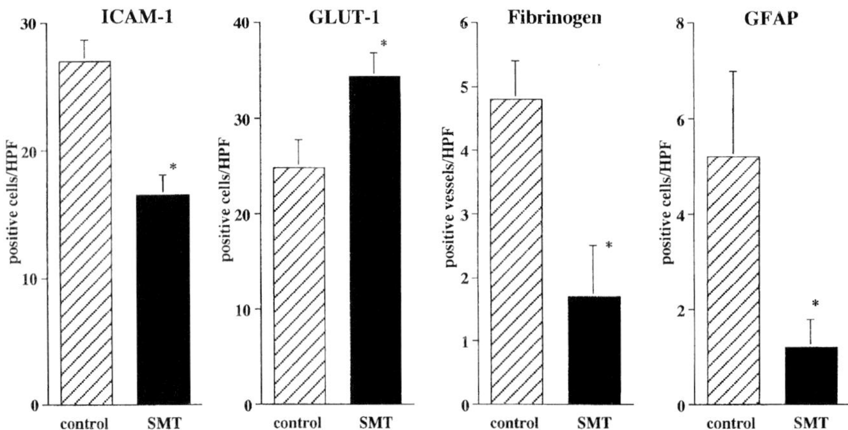

Fig. 1. Immunohistochemical analysis of ICAM-1, GLUT-1, fibrinogen and GFAP expression in cerebral cortex. *HFP* High power field (×400). Mean ± SE, * $p < 0.05$ or more

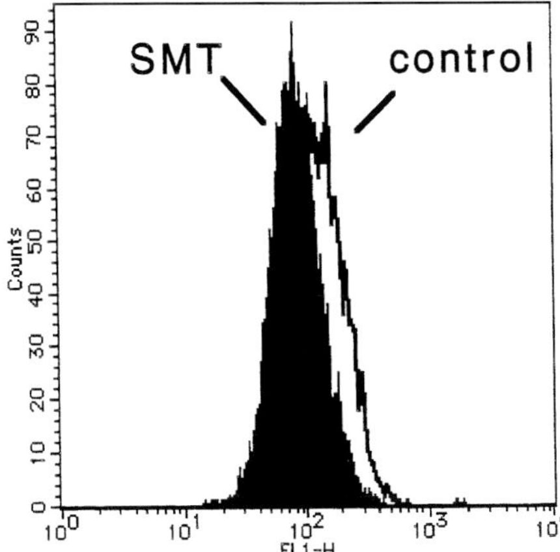

Fig. 2. Flow cytometric analysis of Mac-1 expression in leukocytes

less, GLUT-1 was much more intense, but fibrinogen and GFAP were much less than compared to those in control group. Furthermore, in vitro expression of Mac-1 in leukocytes was prohibited by addition of SMT, as shown in Fig. 2.

Discussion

Although it has been reported that leukocytes may be involved in the pathogenesis of hypertensive cardiovascular changes in SHR [11], the role of leukocyte-derived NO radicals in hypertensive cerebral injury remains unclear. It is well established that NO plays important roles in both the vascular function and pathophysiology of cardiovascular disorders (see reviews by Dusting [3]). NO is synthesized from arginine by nitric oxide synthase (NOS), and three types of isoforms of NOS have been identified; endothelial NOS (eNOS), neuronal NOS (nNOS), and inducible NOS (iNOS). Among these, the pathophysiological roles of NO derived from eNOS have been well documented, but little information is available on the role of iNOS-derived NO in cardiovascular pathology. Although eNOS-derived NO has protective effects against endothelial injury [1], the cytotoxicity of iNOS-derived NO would suggest that this isoform plays a causative role in endothelial injury (see review by Bredt and Snyder [2].

In the present study, although no difference in blood pressure was found between the control and SMT groups, brain weight was significantly lower in the SMT group than in the control group. In these lighter SMT group brains, immunohistochemical expression of ICAM-1 was greatly reduced, whereas GLUT-1 expression was well preserved. Such changes were parallel to those in fibrinogen expression, i.e., fibrinogen content was remarkably reduced in the cerebral cortex of the SMT group. These results indicate a number of protective effects of iNOS inhibition, such as inhibition of leukocyte-endothelial cells adhesion, prohibition of blood brain barrier dysfunction, and subsequent enhancement of vascular permeability. Since iNOS has been detected in the cells of several tissues, including PMN, monocyts, astrocyts, and vascular smooth muscle cells, the decrease in NO metabolites found here may not be exclusively related to PMN-derived NO. However, the changes in NO metabolites content and Mac-1 expression were parallel to iNOS inhibition under the present experimental condition, so that the major portion of NO metabolites changes can be considered the result of PMN activity. However, Ideacola *et al.* [5, 6] performed extensive studies on a rat model with transient, focal cerebral ischemia, and found that iNOS was induced earlier and predominantly conditions were in vascular cells rather than in neutrophils. Although no direct evidences on NO production (or content) were obtained in the present study, the results indicate the important role of leukocytes in hypertensive cerebral injury and suggest the beneficial effects of iNOS inhibition for the therapy of hypertensive cerebral edema.

References

1. Biffl WL, Moore EE, Moore FA, Barnett CC (1996) Nitric oxide reduces endothelial expression on intercellular adhesion molecule (ICAM)-1. J Surg Res 63: 328–332
2. Bredt D, Snyder SA (1994) Nitric oxide: a physiologic messenger molecule. Annu Rev Biochem 63: 175–195
3. Dusting GJ (1995) Nitric oxide in cardiovascular disorders. J Vasc Res 32: 143–161
4. Green LC, Wanger DA, Glogowski J, Skipper PL, Wishnok JS, Tannenbaum SR (1982) Analysis of nitrate, nitrite, and [15N] nitrate in biological fluids. Analy Biochem 126: 131–138
5. Iadecola C, Zheng F, Xu S, Casey R, Ross E (1995) Inducible nitric oxide synthase gene expression in brain following cerebral ischemia. J Cereb Blood Flow Metab 15: 378–384
6. Ideacola C, Zhang F, Casey R, Clark HB, Ross ME (1996) Inducible nitric oxide synthase gene expression in vasular cells after transient focal cerebral ischemia. Stroke 27: 1373–1380
7. Ito H, Torii M, Suzuki T (1993) A comparative study on lipid peroxidation in cerebral cortex of stroke-prone spontaneously hypertensive and normotensive rats. Int J Biochem 25: 1801–1805
8. Kochanek PM, Hallenbeck JM (1992) Polymorphonuclear leukocytes and monocytes/macrophages in the pathogenesis of cerebral ischemia and stroke. Stroke 23: 1367–1379

9. Maenishi O, Ito H, Suzuki T (1997) Acceleration of hypertensive cerebral injury by the inhibition of xanthine-xanthine oxidase system in stroke-prone spontaneously hypertensive rats. Clin Exp Hypertension 19: 461–477
10. Monchada S (1992) The L-arginine: nitric oxide pathway. Acta Physiol Scand 145: 201–227
11. Schmid-Schonbein GW, Seiffge D, DeLano FA, Shen K, Zweifach BW (1991) Leukocyte counts and activation in spontaneously hypertensive and normotensive rats. Hypertension 17: 323–330

Correspondence: H. Ito, Department of Pathology, Kinki University, School of Medicine, Osaka, Japan.

Acta Neurochir (2000) [Suppl] 76: 339–341

Sphingolipid Biosynthesis by L-PDMP After Rat MCA Occlusion

M. Kubota[1], **M. Nakane**[1], **T. Nakagomi**[1], **A. Tamura**[1], **H. Hisaki**[1], **N. Ueta**[1], **J. Inokuchi**[2], and **A. Hirayama**[3]

[1] Department of Neurosurgery & Biochemistry, Teikyo University School of Medicine, Tokyo, Japan
[2] Graduate School of Pharmaceutical Science, Hokkaido University, Sapporo, Japan
[3] Chifune Hospital, Osaka, Japan

Summary

L-PDMP (L-threo-1-phenyl-2-decanoylamino-3-morpholino-1-propanol) exhibits stimulatory effects on glycosphingolipid biosynthesis and its neurotrophic actions in cultured neuron. The effects of intraperitoneal administration of L-PDMP on sphingolipid metabolism and behavioral changes in the rat following permanent occlusion of the left middle cerebral artery (MCA) were investigated. The L-PDMP treatment induced increases in glucosylceramide (ganglioside precursor) and sphingomyelin (SM) levels in the ischemic cerebral cortex, and improved acquisition of memory and learning in the Morris water maze task. The pharmacological effects of L-PDMP have been proposed to have a significant activity on promoting cell survival and improving neural functions.

Keywords: Sphingolipid; focal ischemia; L-PDMP; memory.

Introduction

Focal cerebral ischemia was induced by occluding the proximal portion of the middle cerebral artery (MCA) [3, 4]. In this type of focal ischemia, there is an ischemic core (basal ganglia) confined in the territory of the MCA, and a perifocal penumbra (cerebral cortex) which receives collateral arterial supply, results in brain edema at 2–3 days after the arterial occlusion histologically. It is important for the pathophysiologic studies and development of drug therapies for stroke to establish convenient methods, and to evaluate impairment of neurological functions in rodent models. Supplementation of gangliosides and glucosylceramide facilitates neurite outgrowth following suppression of neuronal activity in vitro [2]. L-PDMP (L-threo-1-phenyl-2-decanoylamino-3-morpholino-1-propanol) enhanced the activities of glycosyltransferase, resulting in elevated cellular levels of glycosphingolipids including glucosylceramide and gangliosides in cultured cortical neuron, and exhibited stimulatory effects on neurite growth [1, 5]. To evaluate the role of sphingolipids on behavioral changes, we examined ceramide, sphingomyelin and cerebroside levels in the rat cerebral cortex during permanent focal ischemia. This paper presents our recent findings on the neurotrophic actions and effects of L-PDMP on sphingolipid metabolism in vivo.

Materials and Methods

Surgical Procedure

Twelve male Sprague-Dawley rats (Japan Slc Inc., Shizuoka, Japan), weighing 250–310 g, were trained in administered acquisition trials of the Morris water-maze task for 5 days. The rats were then anesthetized with 2% halothane and the left MCA was permanently occluded at a proximal site using a microbipolar coagulator [3, 4]. After operation, the rats were allowed free access to food and water. One week after MCA occlusion, L-PDMP (40 mg/kg) or vehicle (5% Tween 80) was injected i.p. twice a day for 14 days. From the 18th day to the 20th day following the MCA occlusion, postoperative acquisition trials were carried out at a same procedure (Fig. 1). After a 24 hr rest period, the rats were exposed to microwaves (Toshiba microwave applicator 4 kW, 1.5 seconds, Japan) under halothane inhalation, and the left frontal cortex was dissected from the cerebral hemisphere for lipid analysis. The Animal Research Committee of Teikyo University School of Medicine approved of all the experimental protocols.

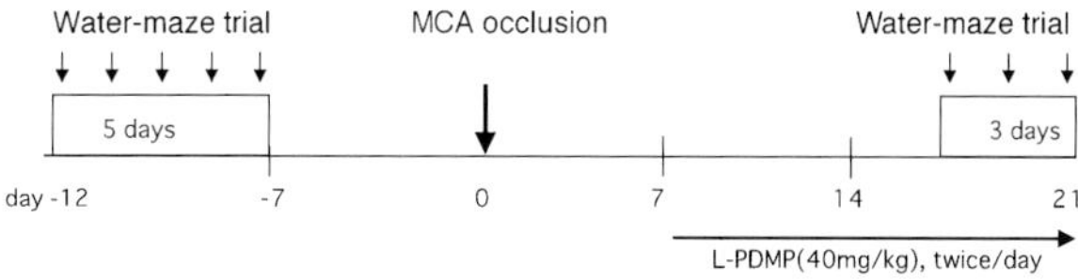

Fig. 1. Experimental Protocol: Twelve rats were trained in administered acquisition trials of the Morris water-maze task for 5 days. One week after MCA occlusion, L-PDMP (40 mg/kg) or vehicle (5% Tween 80) was injected i.p. twice a day for 14 days. From the 18th day to the 20th day following the MCA occlusion, postoperative acquisition trials were carried out at the same procedure

Lipid Analysis

Total lipids were extracted from the cortex (100–110 mg) with 20 volumes of chloroform-methanol (2:1, by volume) according to the Folch's method. The total lipids (5.0–6.0 mg) thus obtained were applied to HPTLC (Merck & Co,, Inc.) plate, using chloroform-methanol-acetic acid-formic acid (20:5:3:1, by volume) as a solvent system for the separation of cerebrosides and sphingomyelin. The spots of cerebrosides and sphingomyelin were identified after spraying the plate with Primuline and comparison with a corresponding authentic standard. The spot corresponding to sphingolipids on the plate was scraped directly into a test tube and methanolyzed with 5% anhydrous HCl at 85 °C for 6 hours. These amino-linked fatty acyl residues were then analyzed by gas liquid chromatography (GLC). To determine the sugar components of the cerebrosides the total lipids were subjected to Florisil (1 g) (Kanto Chemical Co. Inc. Japan) column chromatography (activated at 120 °C for 3 hours prior to use) and then eluted with chloroform-methanol (2:1, by volume) for the removal of glycerophospholipids. The solvent was evaporated under a stream of nitrogen gas and the lipid moiety was subjected to HPTLC. The plate was developed and the spot corresponding to cerebrosides was scraped into a test tube in the same manner as described above. The mixture containing silicic acid and cerebrosides was added chloroform-methanol (2:1, by volume) and filtrated. The filtrate was evaporated and subjected to Bond Elut column (NH2) using chloroform-methanol (2:1, by volume) as the elution solvent for the removal of silicic acids. After methanolysis of the cerebroside fraction, 2 ml of n-hexane was added to the reaction mixture, and fatty acid methylesters were removed. This procedure was repeated twice. The remaining methanolic phase was neutralized with 0.15 ml of pyridine (KANTO Chemical CO., Inc. Japan) and evaporated to dryness under a stream of nitrogen gas. The methylglycosides were trimethylsilylated with TMS-PZ (trimethylsilylating reagent) (Tokyo Kasei, Japan) and their TMS-derivatives were subjected to GLC.

For the quantification and identification of ceramides, the total lipids extracted using the above procedure were applied to HPTLC plate, using chloroform-methanol-acetic acid-formic acid (20:50:3:1, by volume) and then hexane-diethylether-acetic acid (50:50:1, by volume) as the solvent systems. The spots of ceramides on the plate were methanolyzed as described above and their amino-linked fatty acids were analyzed by GLC. On the other hand, ceramides containing silicic acids were dissolved in chloroform-methanol (2:1, by volume) and filtrated. The filtrate was evaporated to dryness, trimethylsilylated with TMS-PZ and the TMS-derivatives were subjected to GC-MS (Shimadzu QP 5000).

Gas Liquid Chromatography (GLC): GLC was carried out with a Shimadzu 14A Gas Chromatograph (Shimadzu Corp, Japan) equipped with a flame ionization detector using a capillary column of NEUTRA BOND-1 (30 m × 0.25 mm ID; GL Sciences Inc. Japan). The column temperatures were kept at 230–250 °C for the analysis of fatty acid methylesters and at 180 °C for that of glycoside-derivatives. The amounts of fatty acids were calculated by comparison with each internal standard.

Morris Water Maze Task

Spatial memory retention was examined using the Morris water maze task. The apparatus used was a 150 cm diameter cylindrical tank, filled with water to a depth of 28 or 32 cm, with a transparent 10 cm diameter platform placed at a constant position at the center of one of the four quadrants of the tank. Before surgery, acquisition trials were carried out twice a day for 5 days. The platform was set 2 cm below the water level where the rats could not see it directly. In each trial, the rats were placed into the water at a fixed starting position, and the time taken to escape to the hidden platform and the swimming path length were measured using a Video Image Motion Analyzer (MZ-30; MATYS, Toyama, Japan). The rats were given 120 sec to find the hidden platform during each acquisition trial and allowed to rest on the platform for 30 sec after finding it. Retention trials were carried out at same procedure as described above but were not placed onto the platform by the experimenter.

Results

Morris Water Maze Test

Two rats subjected to MCA occlusion died before the administration of L-PDMP and were excluded from the study. The body weights of the MCA-occluded rats in both the L-PDMP and vehicle groups decreased significantly comparing with those of pre-operative rats. Before surgery, there was no significant difference in the mean times taken to reach the criterion of success during the acquisition trial between L-PDMP and vehicle groups. The mean acquisition time of the first postoperative trial (18th day after surgery) was 69.9 sec in the L-PDMP group, and 72.6 sec in the vehicle group. The mean acquisition time in third postoperative trial, on the 20th day after surgery, was 37 sec in the L-PDMP, and 51.9 sec in the vehicle group (Fig. 2). This acquisition time on the 20th day after surgery was significantly shorter in the L-PDMP group than the vehicle group. Thus L-PDMP induced the improvement of re-acquisition time.

Lipid Analysis

In the rat brain, cerebrosides consisted of large amounts of galactosylceramide and smaller amounts

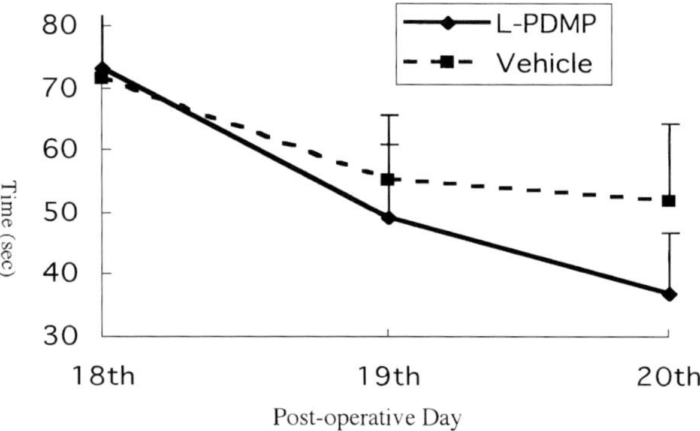

Fig. 2. Re-acquisition and memory retention of water-maze trial after MCA occlusion. The mean acquisition time of the first postoperative trial (18th day after surgery) was 69.9 sec in the L-PDMP group, and 72.6 sec in the vehicle group. The mean acquisition time in the third postoperative trial, on the 20th day after surgery, was 37 sec in the L-PDMP, and 51.9 sec in the vehicle group

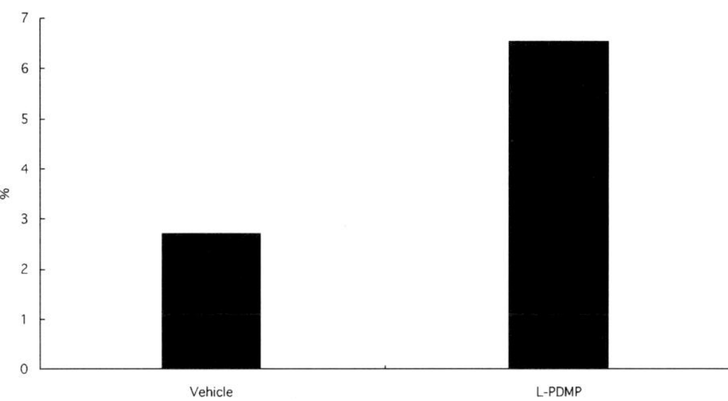

Fig. 3. GLC of sugar components of cerebroside (galactosyl- and glucosyl-ceramides) in rat ischemic cortex after L-PDMP treatment. The glucose/total sugar (galactose + glucose) ratio in the ischemic cortex of L-PDMP rats was 6.5% (vehicle; 2.7%)

Table 1. *Sphingomyelin and Ceramide Levels in Ischemic Cerebral Cortex with the Treatment of L-PDMP*

	Sphingomyclin (mmol/kg)	Ccramidc (μmol/kg)
Vehicle	3.92 ± 0.23	765.8 ± 324.6
L-PDMP	4.60 ± 0.41*	562.1 ± 235.3

*; < 0.05 significant vs. Vehicle.

of glucosylceramide, which is the precursor of ganglioside synthesis. We examined the sugar components of galactose and glucose by GLC analysis. As shown in Figure 3, the glucose/total sugar (galactose + glucose) ratio in the ischemic cortex of L-PDMP rats was 6.5% (vehicle; 2.7%), which was 2.4-fold that in the vehicle group. Sphingomyelin (SM) levels in the L-PDMP rats increased by 4.6 ± 0.4 mmol/kg (vehicle; 3.9 ± 0.2 mmol/kg) and its amino-linked fatty acids were mainly composed of stearic and palmitic acids, while the very long chain fatty acids (C24:0 C24:1) were only minor components. There was no significant difference in ceramide levels between the L-PDMP and vehicle rats.

Discussion

L-PDMP induced improvement in the re-acquisition time in the Morris water-maze task. It has been reported that L-PDMP increases the incorporation of serine into the sphingosine base and other sphingolipids in cultured cortex [5]. In our experiment, the glucosylceramide and SM levels in the ischemic cortex increased significantly following L-PDMP treatment. This suggests that serine palmitoyltransferase and sphingosine N-acyltransferase, and glucosylceramide synthetase in the ischemic cortex are activated by L-PDMP. The neurotrophic actions of L-PDMP may be associated with its stimulatory effects on the biosynthesis of sphingolipids.

References

1. Inokuchi J, Kuroda Y, Kosaka S, Fujiwara M (1998) L-threo-1-phenyl-2-decanoylamino-3-morpholino-1-propanol stimulates ganglioside biosynthesis, neurite outgrowth and synapse formation in culture cortical neurons, and ameliorates memory deficits in ischemic rats. Acta Biochim Pol 45: 479–492
2. Schwarz A, Rapaport E, Hirschberg K, Futerman HA (1995) A regulatory role for sphingolipids in neuronal growth. Inhibition of sphingolipid synthesis and degradation have opposite effects on axonal branching. J Biol Chem 270: 10990–10998
3. Tamura A, Graham DI, McCulloch J, Teasdale G (1981) Focal cerebral ischaemia in the rat: 1. Description of technique and early neuropathological consequences following middle cerebral artery occlusion. J Cereb Blood Flow Metabol 1: 53–60
4. Tamura A, Graham DI, McCulloch J, Teasdale G (1981) Focal cerebral ischemia in the rat: 2. Regional cerebral blood flow determined by [14C] iodoantipyrine autoradiography following middle cerebral artery occlusion. J Cereb Blood Flow Metabol 1: 61–69
5. Usuki S, Hamanoue M, Kohsaka S, Inokuchi J (1996) Induction of ganglioside biosynthesis and neurite outgrowth of primary cultured neuron by L-threo-1-phenyl-2-decanoylamino-3-morpholino-1-propanol. J Neurochem 67: 1821–1830

Correspondence: Masaru Kubota, Department of Neurosurgery, Teikyo University School of Medicine, 2-11-1, Kaga, Itabashi-ku, Tokyo 173-8605, Japan.

Acta Neurochir (2000) [Suppl] 76: 343–345

Protective Effect of a Novel Vitamin E Derivative on Experimental Traumatic Brain Edema in Rats – Preliminary Study

Y. Ikeda[1], **Y. Mochizuki**[1], **Y. Nakamura**[1], **K. Dohi**[1], **H. Matsumoto**[1], **H. Jimbo**[1], **M. Hayashi**[1], **K. Matsumoto**[1], **T. Yoshikawa**[2], **H. Murase**[3], and **K. Sato**[4]

[1] Department of Neurosurgery, Showa University School of Medicine, Tokyo
[2] Department of Medicine, Kyoto Prefectual University of Medicine, Kyoto, Japan
[3] CCI Co., Gifu, Japan
[4] Analysis Center, School of Pharmaceutical Sciences, Showa University, Tokyo, Japan

Summary

Oxygen free radicals have been proposed to be one of the major mechanisms of secondary brain damage in traumatic brain injury. Protective effect by vitamin E against oxidative damage has attracted much attention. Recent studies have demonstrated a novel vitamin E derivative, 2-(alpha-D-glucopyranosyl)methyl-2,5,7,8-tetramethylchroman-6-ol (TMG), has excellent water-solubility and antioxidant activity. The purpose of this study was to investigate protective effects of TMG on experimental traumatic brain edema (BE). Male Wistar rats were anaesthetized with chloral hydrate. Traumatic BE was produced by a cortical freezing lesion. Animals were separated into three groups: saline-treated rats ($n = 4$), TMG-treated (4 mg/kg) rats ($n = 7$) and TMG-treated (40 mg/kg) rats ($n = 8$). Saline or TMG was administered intravenously before lesion production. Animals were sacrificed at 6 hours after lesion production and the brain water content was determined by the dry-wet weight method. Half-life of TMG after intravenous administration of TMG was also investigated. The half life of TMG was approximately 5 minutes. TMG (40 mg/kg) significantly attenuated BE following cryogenic brain injury ($p < 0.01$). In conclusion, this preliminary study has demonstrated that a novel vitamin E derivative might be promising in the treatment of traumatic BE.

Keywords: Brain edema; brain injury; vitamin E; free radicals.

Introduction

Oxygen free radicals have been proposed to be one of the major mechanisms of secondary brain damage in traumatic brain injury [1]. Lipid peroxidation through oxygen free radicals is recognized as an important pathological process. Protective effect by vitamin E against oxidative damage has attracted much attention [2, 3]. It has been reported that vitamin E scavenges not only peroxyl radicals but also singlet oxygen and the superoxide radical [4–6]. Since the mobility of vitamin E in the biological membranes is restricted due to its long phytyl side chain, it seems unlikely to scavenge active oxygens which might be generated in the aqueous phase. Recent studies [7, 8] have demonstrated that a novel vitamin E derivative, 2-(alpha-D-glucopyranosyl)methyl-2,5,7,8-tetramethylchroman-6-ol(TMG), has excellent water-solubility and antioxidant activity (Fig. 1).

The purpose of this study was to investigate protective effects of TMG on experimental traumatic brain edema (BE).

Materials and Methods

Measurement of Superoxide Scavenging Activity of TMG

Determination of superoxide scavenging activity of TMG was performed by electron spin resonance spectrometry using 5,5-dimethyl-1-pyrroline-1-oxide (DMPO) as a spin trap. Fifty microliters of 2 mM hypoxanthine, 20 μl of 0.5 mM diethylenetriamine-pentaacetic acid (DETAPAC), 50 μl of TMG, 50 μl of DMPO and 30 μl of xanthine oxidase were put into a test tube and mixed by an automatic mixer. Then the solution was placed in a special flat cell and DMPO-O_2^-, spin adduct was analyzed by electron spin resonance spectrometry.

Surgical Procedure and Experimental Protocols

Male Wistar rats, weighing 250 to 300 g each, were anesthetized intraperitoneally with chloral hydrate (360 mg/kg). A midline scalp incision and a craniectomy were made in the right parietal region. Cortical cryogenic injury was produced by application of a metal probe cooled by dry ice to the dura of the right parietal region. The dura was left intact. The skin was closed with sutures. Animals were separated into three groups: saline-treated rats with lesion production ($n = 4$), TMG-treated (4 mg/kg) rats with lesion production ($n = 7$) and TMG-treated (40 mg/kg) rats with lesion production

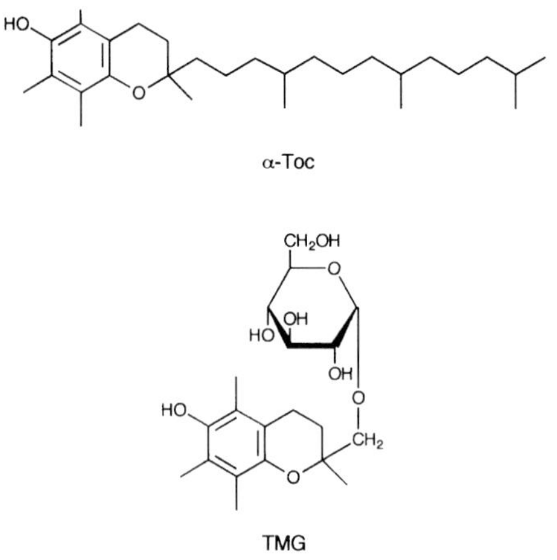

Fig. 1. Structure of TMG

($n = 8$). Saline or TMG was administered intravenously before lesion production. Animals were sacrificed at 6 hours after lesion production and the brain water content was determined by the dry-wet weight method. The brain was removed immediately and divided into right injured hemisphere and left non-injured hemisphere. The tissue was then dried in a 100 °C oven for 24 hours and reweighted to obtain the dry weight. The water contents, expressed as a percentage of the wet weight, were calculated as (wet weight − dry weight)/wet weight × 100. Half-life of TMG after intravenous administration of TMG was also investigated.

Data are presented as mean ± standard deviation. Student's t-test was used to assess significance, with $p < 0.05$ considered to indicate statistical significance.

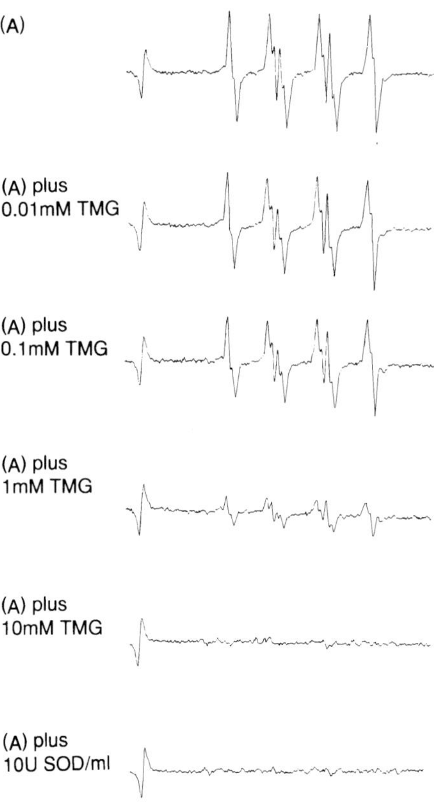

Fig. 2. Determination of superoxide scavenging activity of TMG by electron spin resonance (*ESR*). ESR spectra of DMPO-O_2^- spin adduct produced by xanthine oxidase

Results

The half-life of TMG was approximately 5 minutes after intravenous injection of TMG. Electron spin resonance study showed that the formation of superoxide-DMPO spin adduct was strongly inhibited by TMG in a dose-dependent manner (Fig. 2). TMG (4 mg/kg) did not reduce BE following cryogenic brain injury, however TMG (40 mg/kg) significantly attenuated BE (Fig. 3).

Discussion

Vitamin E is a major lipophilic antioxidant in cellular membranes and its excellent antioxidant activity is well recognized. Since the mobility of vitamin E in the biological membranes is restricted due to its long phytyl side chain, it seems unlikely to scavenge active oxygen which might be generated in the aqueous phase. Recently the efficiency of several water-soluble vitamin E analogs as biological antioxidants has been reported. Murase *et al.* [7, 8] succeeded in the synthesis of a novel water soluble vitamin E derivative, TMG, and demonstrated its excellent water solubility and the ability of superoxide scavenging activity.

We demonstrated that oxygen free radicals, which cause lipid peroxidation, play a role in traumatic brain edema and proposed that oxygen free radical scavengers could be used in the treatment of brain edema following head injury. For this purpose, several therapeutic methods were considered. Superoxide dismutase (SOD) was expected and was studied. However, we showed that free SOD does not reduce traumatic brain edema, because the molecular weight of SOD is 31000 and SOD cannot pass through the blood-brain barrier under normal conditions and half-life is very short [1]. Young *et al.* [9] reported that no statistical differences in neurological outcomes and mortality rates were observed between patients treated with polyethylene glycol-SOD, whose biological half-life was extended to 5 days, and those receiving placebo in their clinical study of 463 patients with severe head injuries. Yushida [3] reported the degree of traumatic brain edema resulting from focal brain compression in rats raised with vitamin E deficient diets. The degree of edema

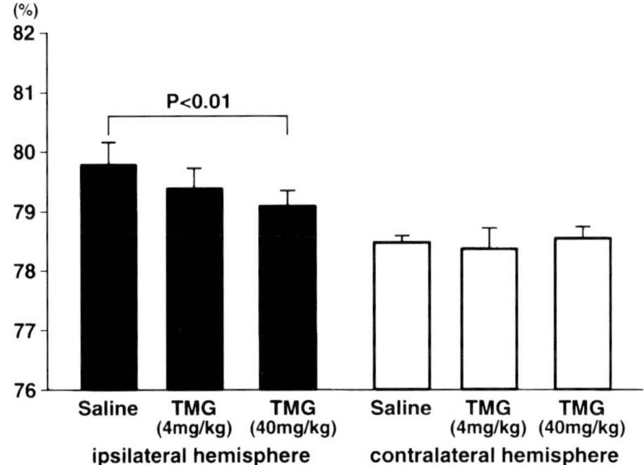

Fig. 3. Effects of TMG on brain water contents at 6 hours after cryogenic brain injury

was most pronounced in the vitamin E-deficient group. Tagami *et al.* [10] reported that vitamin E prevents apoptosis in cortical neurons during hypoxia and oxygen reperfusion in rats. Experimental studies have suggested the effectiveness of oxygen free radical scavengers such as vitamin E, SOD, catalase and iron chelating agent, but clinical application of oxygen free radical scavengers remains immature [11]. This TMG, vitamin E derivative, seems to be promising, especially for the purpose of clinical application.

References

1. Ikeda Y, Long DM (1990) The molecular basis of brain injury and brain edema. role of oxygen free radicals. Neurosurgery 27: 1–11
2. Busto R, Yoshida S, Ginsberg MD, Alonso O, Smith DW, Goldberg WJ (1984) Regional blood flow in compression-induced brain edema in rats. Ann Neurol 15: 441–444
3. Yoshida S, Busto R, Ginsberg MD, Abe K, Martinez E, Watson BD, Scheinberg P (1983) Compression induced brain edema: modification by prior depletion and supplementation of vitamin E. Neurology 33: 166–172
4. Grams GW (1971) Oxidation of alpha-tocopherol by singlet oxygen. Tetrahedron Lett 50: 4823–4825
5. Nishikimi M, Yamada H, Yagi K (1980) Oxidation by superoxide of tocopherols dispersed in aqueous media with deoxycholate. Biochem Biophys Acta 627: 101–108
6. Fukuzawa K, Gebicki JM (1983) Oxidation of alpha-tocopherol in micelles and liposomes by the hydroxy, perhydroxy and superoxide free radicals. Arch Biochem Biophys 226: 242–251
7. Murase H, Yamauchi, Kato K, Kunieda T, Terao J (1997) Synthesis of a novel E derivative, 2-(alpha-D-glucopyranosyl) methyl-2,5,7,8-tetramethylchroman-6-ol, by alpha-glucosidase-catalyzed transglycosylation. Lipids 32: 73–78
8. Murase H, Moon JH, Yamauchi R, Kato K, Kunieda T, Yoshikawa T, Terao J (1998) Antioxidant activity of a novel vitamin E derivative, 2-(alpha-D-glucopyranosyl)mrthyl-2,3,7,8-tetramethylchroman-6-ol. Free Radical Biol Med 24: 217–225
9. Young B, Runge JW, Waxman KS, Harrington T, Wilberger J, Muizelaar JP, Boddy A, Kupiec JW (1996) Effects of pegorgotein on neurologic outcome of patients with severe head injury: a multicenter, randomized controlled trial. JAMA 276: 538–543
10. Tagami M, Yamagata K, Ikeda K, Nara Y, Fujino H, Kubota A, Numano F, Yamori Y (1998) Vitamin E prevents apoptosis in cortical neurons during hypoxia and oxygen reperfusion. Lab Invest 78: 1415–1429
11. Shohami E, Yannai EB, Horowitz M, Kohen R (1997) Oxidative stress in closed-head injury: brain antioxidant capacity as an indicator of functional outcome. J Cereb Blood Flow Metab 17: 1007–1019

Correspondence: Yukio Ikeda, M.D., D.M.Sc, Department of Neurosurgery, Showa University School of Medicine, 1-5-8 Hatanodai, Shinagawa-ku, Tokyo 142-8666, Japan.

Head Injury

This was one of the largest sections and begins with mechanisms of increased ICP and secondary brain damage in head injury.

In the head injured patient, a rise in ICP is the most frequent cause of death, and is not caused by vascular engorgement, but is mainly caused by brain oedema. Traumatic brain oedema has always been considered to be of vasogenic origin as a result of BBB breakdown in the contusion. Dr. Marmarou *et al.* measured brain water and Apparent Diffusion Coefficients (ADC), in severely head injured patients, using MRI methods, and simultaneously measured cerebral blood flow using the stable Xenon method. This excellent study found that the main cause of oedema (increase in water content) was cytotoxic and factors other than ischaemia were responsible for the edema formation.

Recently, cellular compartmentation of brain metabolism has been considered. Astrocytes are thought to be processing plants of energy metabolism, locating at a key position between the capillaries on one side and the neurons and oligodendrocytes on the other. They convey all nutrients required for energy production such as glucose, oxygen and amino acids. Lactate and alanine are thought to be generated in the astrocytes and are transferred to neurons as fuels. Chen T. *et al.* measured cerebral dialysate lactate and glucose, and arterial lactate and glucose, before and after rat fluid percussion injury with and without i.v. infusion of lactate. They found that, after percussion injury, arterial lactate augmentation increases brain dialysate lactate and results in less reduction of glucose dialysate. Infused lactate accumulated at the injury site, where metabolism was probably the greatest. Eriskat J. *et al.* found, using the rat cold injury model, that interstitial lactate did not cause severe tissue acidosis which could be liable for the secondary growth of the area of traumatic tissue, necrosis.

Di X. *et al.*, to test the mechanism of astrocytic swelling after traumatic brain injury, measured volume regulatory ion currents using whole cell patch clamp electrophysiology, after stretch injury to the co-cultured astrocytes and neurons on a deformable, silastic membrane applying a timed pulse of pressurized air to the membrane. They found that activation of stretch-activated cation currents exacerbated cell swelling in the injured astrocyte.

Stoffel M. *et al.*, using the rat cold lesion model, histometrically measured the spread of the primary necrotic lesion and found that aminoguanidine, an iNOS inhibitor, led to significant attenuation of the expansion of the necrotic lesion.

Stover *et al.* found that prolonged isoflurane anaesthesia induced a significant increase in arterial plasma glutamate level and brain oedema. Woertgen *et al.* found that the highest Neuron Specific Enolase (NSE) serum level was detected six hours after experimental cortical impact injury to rats, reflecting neuronal damage after the injury. Sharma *et al.* found that repeated topical application of BDNF, over the exposed surface of the longitudinally incised traumatic spinal cord, attenuated the oedematous expansion and BBB break down of the injured cord. Tenedieva *et al.* found a marked decrease of thyroid function recorded by serum FT3 and T3 levels in head injured patients with a GCS of less than 8. They recommended adequate T3 therapy in the early period after head injury.

Markers of the severity of head injury have been identified and include S100b (Mussock *et al.*) and adrenomedullin (Robertson *et al.*). The role of secondary insults has been further clarified using elegant experimental models by Thomas *et al.* who showed that hypoxia exacerbated brain damage when added to trauma in young and adult rats. Ke *et al.* likewise showed that hyponatraemia does a similar thing.

The importance of Diffuse Axonal Injury (DAI) is outlined by Lubillo *et al.* and explored experimentally by De Mulder *et al.*

Decompressive craniectomy is reported by De Luca *et al.* and this paper should be read together with Meier *et al.*'s paper which appears earlier in this volume.

Clinical trials are required to confirm these and other observational studies, which purport to substantiate that Decompressive craniectomy is effective when elevated ICP becomes refractory to medical treatment.

Acta Neurochir (2000) [Suppl] 76: 349–351

Distinguishing Between Cellular and Vasogenic Edema in Head Injured Patients with Focal Lesions Using Magnetic Resonance Imaging

A. Marmarou[1], **G. Portella**[1], **P. Barzo**[1], **S. Signoretti**[1], **P. Fatouros**[2], **A. Beaumont**[1], **T. Jiang**[2], and **R. Bullock**[1]

[1] Division of Neurosurgery, Medical College of Virginia, Virginia Commonwealth University Richmond, Virginia
[2] Division of Radiation Physics, Medical College of Virginia, Virginia Commonwealth University

Summary

Having determined that edema and not vascular engorgement is the major factor leading to traumatic brain swelling, the objective of this study was to determine which type of edema, cellular or vasogenic, is responsible for increased tissue water in patients with focal lesions. Severely head injured patients (GCS 8 or less) were transported to imaging suites for measurement of brain water and apparent diffusion coefficient (ADC) using magnetic resonance technique. Cerebral blood flow by stable Xenon method was also measured in the regions of interest. Brain water was increased significantly in the hemisphere with lesion. The increase in water was associated with reduced ADC signifying a predominant cellular edema. The ADC in the contralateral hemisphere was near normal value. Cerebral blood flow values in the regions of interest were above ischemic levels suggesting that factors other than ischemia are responsible for the cytotoxic swelling in patients with focal injury.

Keywords: Brain edema; cellular; vasogenic; cytotoxic; brain swelling; MRI; water map.

Introduction

In head injured patients, the rise in intracranial pressure concomitant with uncontrolled brain swelling is the most frequent cause of death. Heretofore, the compartment responsible for the increase in brain volume remained unknown. Although edema was thought to play a role, the generally held view was that vascular engorgement secondary to vasoparalysis was responsible for increased brain bulk and subsequent rise in ICP. It has now been established, both in the laboratory [4] and clinical setting [5], that edema is responsible for the increased brain volume and that in patients, blood volume is actually reduced during the first five days post injury.

Our attention has now focused on describing the type of edema that is formed following injury. Traumatic brain edema has always been considered to be of vasogenic origin as a result of the breach in the blood brain barrier and particularly with contusion where edema is more easily visualized by computerize tomography. However, experimental studies in diffuse injury have shown that the breach of the blood brain barrier is short lived and is closed by 30 minutes post injury [1]. This would suggest that subsequent increase in brain water would be caused by cellular swelling or cytotoxic edema. This hypothesis was tested in the present study where the amount and type of edema in focal injury was characterized by MRI technique. A second objective was to measure the CBF in the same regions of interest to determine if ischemia was implicated in the pathogenesis of the swollen tissue.

Methods

All patients in this study group ($n = 16$) were either comatose upon admission or deteriorated to GCS 8 or less prior to imaging studies which took place during the acute management period. Patients were entered into the study only when they were considered stable and both ICP and CPP were under control. Patients were transported to the imaging suite for measurement of the apparent diffusion coefficient (ADC) obtained from diffusion weighted images. The DWI was performed on a 1.5 Tesla whole body clinical imager. (Siemens Vision MR system) with diffusion echo planar spin echo sequences. These pulses generated an ADC trace image using a single shot technique with 3b values: 0, 500, 1000 s/mm^2. Regions of interest (ROI's) were identified based on the location of the lesion (ipsilateral) and the identical region of the contralateral hemisphere was evaluated for comparison. Thus, the ADC of the lesion site and the similar site of the contralateral hemisphere was available for analysis. Brain water of the respective ROI's was measured using techniques described elsewhere [2]. Cerebral blood flow was also measured using the stable Xenon CT technique using a Siemens CT/plus scanner immediately following or immediately before measurement of brain water and DWI sequences. The order of studies was dictated by scanner availability. Scans were performed at three axial

Table 1. *Brain Water Content and ADC in Focal Injury*

		Ipsilateral hemisphere (lesion side)	Contralateral hemisphere
Brain water content	mean	81.4	77.4
	S.D.	2.9	3.09
ADC	mean	0.72	0.98
	S.D.	0.32	0.29
Number of patients		16	16

planes with a thickness of 5 mm each 20 mm apart. Two baseline scans were performed at each level followed by inhalation of 30% xenon and 70% oxygen. From measurements of the CT enhancement and the end-tidal curve, CBF images were calculated by means of the Kety-Schmidt equation.

Results

All studies were completed without complication and the patients returned safely to the ICU.

The ADC of the ipsilateral hemisphere averaged 0.72 ± 0.32 S.D. s/mm^2. (Table 1) In contrast, the ADC of the comparable site of the opposite hemisphere averaged 0.98 ± 0.29 and the difference were statistically significant. ($p = 0.017$). The reduction of ADC was associated with an increase in brain water averaging $81.4 \pm 2.9\%$ whereas the water in the contralateral hemisphere was within normal range. (77.4 ± 0.29). Interestingly, the increased water andreduced ADC associated with the site of lesion had CBF values above ischemic thresholds (Fig. 1). This also was the case in a larger study group of patients in whom both CBF and brain edema were measured (Fig. 2).

Discussion

The reductions in ADC values associated with focal lesion indicate that the type of edema in patients with focal injury is predominantly cellular. Moreover, the

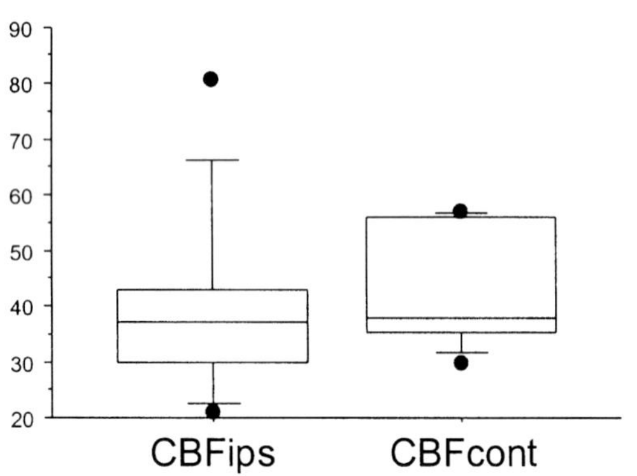

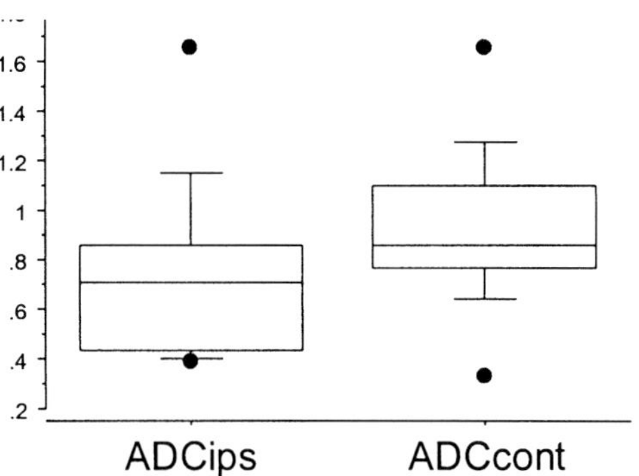

Fig. 1. ADC is reduced in the region adjacent to the lesion (*ips*) compared to the contralateral site (ADCcont). CBF (ml/min/100 gmt) in the lesion ROI (*CBFips*) is above ischemic thresholds

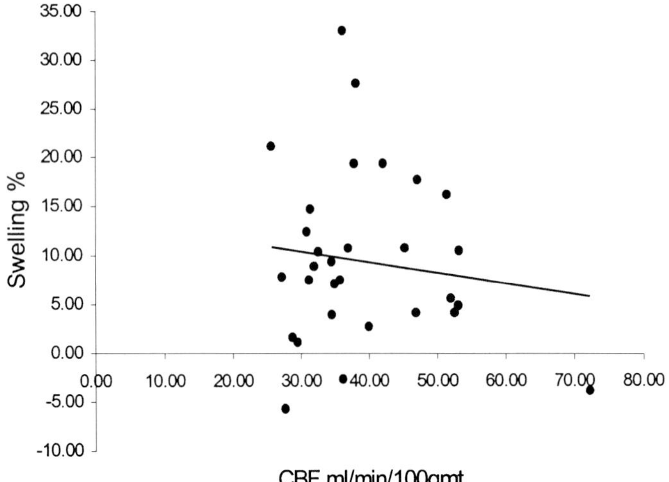

Fig. 2. CBF vs Brain Swelling in severely head injured patients. CBF remains above critical thresholds

cellular edema is associated with CBF levels that are above ischemic thresholds suggesting that factors other than blood flow play a role in the development of cytotoxic edema. This is illustrated in Fig. 2 which shows the relationship of traumatic brain swelling expressed in percent swelling vs CBF. The swelling percentage of the brain slice under study reached levels of 30% increase in the presence of CBF levels above 20 ml/100 gt/min. The observation that the edema occurs in the presence of adequate CBF at time of measurement does not exclude the possibility that an early ischemic event was responsible for the reduced ADC observed later in the patient's course. It will be necessary to measure CBF ultra-early (less than 4 hours) to identify those patients and those studies are currently underway.

It has been shown previously that ADC shifts positive for an extracellular edema and is reduced in the presence of cellular edema [3]. In application of diffusion weighted imaging, the ADC represents the algebraic sum of both increased (vasogenic) and decreased (cytotoxic) ADC components. Thus, a contribution of vasogenic edema to the water increase shown in these studies cannot be excluded. However, for vasogenic edema to play a role in the gradual swelling process, a sustained barrier opening is required. Preliminary studies by our group (unpublished) using Gadolinium as a tracer, suggest that the barrier rapidly closes and with exception of a mild halo surrounding a contusion, no indication of barrier opening has been observed during the first four days post injury when ICP is most apt to rise. Thus, there is little supportive evidence at this juncture to suggest that vasogenic edema plays a major role in the swelling process and in view of the reduction in ADC, one must conclude that the type of edema is predominantly cellular, most probably due to swelling of the astrocytes.

This work was supported by National Institutes of Health Grant No. NS19235-11 and the Lind Lawrence Foundation.

References

1. Barzo P, Marmarou A, Fatouros P, Corwin F, Dunbar J (1997) Magnetic Resonance Imaging-monitored acute blood brain barrier changes in experimental traumatic brain injury. J Neurosurg 87: 900–907
2. Fatouros PP, Marmarou A (1999) In vivo measurements of brain water in humans using magnetic resonance imaging: method and normal values. J Neurosurg 90: 109–115
3. Ito J, Marmarou A, Barzo P, Fatouros P, Corwin F (1996) Characterization of edema by diffusion weighted imaging in experimental brain injury J Neurosurg 84: 97–103
4. Kita H, Marmarou A (1994) The cause of acute brain swelling after closed head injury in rats. Acta Neurochir [Suppl] (Wien) 60: 425–455
5. Marmarou A, Barzo P, Fatouros P, Yamamoto T, Bullock R, Young H (1997) Traumatic brain swelling in head injured patients: brain edema or vascular engorgement? Brain edema X. In James HE, Marshall LF *et al* (eds) Acta Neurochir [Suppl] (Wien) 70: 68–70

Correspondence: Anthony Marmarou Ph.D., Division of Neurosurgery, PO Box 508, MCV Station, Sanger Hall Room 8004, 1101 East Marshall Street, Richmond Virginia, 23298.

8. Hovda DA, Lee SM, Smith ML, von Stuck S, Bergsneider M, Kelly D, Shalmon E, Martin N, Caron M, Mazziotta J, Phelps M, Becker DP (1995) The neurochemical and metabolic cascade following brain injury: moving from animal models to man. J Neurotrauma 12: 903–906
9. Maughan RJ (1982) A simple, rapid method for the determination of glucose, lactate, pyruvate, alanine, 3-hydroxybutyrate and acetoacetate on a single 20-μl blood sample. Clin Chim Acta 122: 231–240
10. Nilsson P, Hillered L, Ponten U, Ungerstedt U (1990) Changes in cortical extracellular levels of energy-related metabolites and amino acids following concussive brain injury in rats. J Cereb Blood Flow Metab 10: 631–637
11. Robertson CS, Grossman RG, Goodman JC, Narayan RK (1987) The predictive value of cerebral anaerobic metabolism with cerebral infarction after head injury. J Neurosurg 67: 361–368
12. Rosner MJ, Becker DP (1984) Experimental brain injury: successful therapy with the weak base, thromethamine. With an overview of CNS acidosis. J Neurosurg 60: 961–971
13. Siesjö BK, Katsura K-I, Zhao Q, Folbergrová J, Pahlmark K, Siesjö P, Smith M-L (1995) Mechanisms of secondary brain damage in global and focal ischemia: a speculative synthesis. J Neurotrauma 12: 943–956
14. Staub F, Baethmann A, Peters J, Weigt H, Kempski O (1990) Effects of lactacidosis on glial cell volume and viability. J Cereb Blood Flow Metab 10: 866–876
15. Stoffel M, Eriskat J, Plesnila N, Aggarwal N, Baethmann A (1997) The penumbra zone of a traumatic cortical lesion: a microdialysis study of excitatory amino acid release. Acta Neurochir [Suppl] (Wien) 70: 91–93
16. Wyrwich W (1994) Die Entwicklung einer sekundären Hirngewebsnekrose nach primärem Trauma. Methodische Ansätze ihrer Quantifizierung. Inauguraldissertation. Ludwig-Maximilians-Universität, München

Correspondence: Jörg Eriskat, Institute for Surgical Research, Klinikum Großhadern, Ludwig-Maximilians-Universität, Marchioninistr. 15, D-81366 München, FRG.

Acta Neurochir (2000) [Suppl] 76: 357–358

Attenuation of Secondary Lesion Growth in the Brain After Trauma by Selective Inhibition of the Inducible No-Synthase

M. Stoffel[2], **M. Rinecker**[1], **N. Plesnila**[1], **J. Eriskat**[1], and **A. Baethmann**[1]

[1] Institute for Surgical Research, Klinikum Großhadern, Ludwig-Maximilians-University, Munich, Germany
[2] Department of Neurosurgery, Rheinische Friedrich-Wilhelms-University, Bonn, Germany

Summary

In previous studies we have demonstrate that aminoguanidine *pretreatment* attenuates the secondary necrosis growth after focal brain trauma. Purpose of the present investigation was to elucidate the therapeutic potential of this iNOS-inhibitor when administered *post lesion*. Sprague-Dawley rats were subjected to a highly standardized cortical freezing lesion and administered with aminoguanidine (100 mg/kg i.p.) 15 min and 8 hrs *after* trauma or with isotonic saline, respectively. Animals were assigned to one of three experimental groups. The animals of group I – which served as reference for the histomorphometric determination of the spread of the primary lesion – were sacrificed 5 min after trauma. Group II, receiving isotonic saline and group III with aminoguanidine were subjected to perfusion fixation 24 hrs after trauma for evaluation of the necrosis growth. In controls with saline, the volume of the cortical necrosis increased from 6.07 ± 1.04 mm^3 (5 min) to 8.39 ± 1.57 mm^3 at 24 hrs (group II) after trauma. Treatment with aminoguanidine (group III) led to significant attenuation of the expansion of the necrosis to 6.77 ± 0.87 mm^3 at 24 hrs. Thus, the pathological role of activation of the inducible NO-synthase in the phenomenon of secondary lesion growth is confirmed by the present data on iNOS-inhibition. Attenuation of expansion of the lesion is achieved even when initiating therapy after trauma.

Keywords: Brain trauma; necrosis growth; nitric oxide; aminoguanidine.

Introduction

In brain trauma, the final parenchymal damage can be viewed as the result of the interplay of the primary lesion and the secondary damage mechanisms. While the primary damage produced by the initial insult can be influenced only by prophylactic procedures, the evolving secondary damage is responsive to therapeutic intervention. Among the various manifestations of secondary brain damage, the secondary growth of a focal contusion deserves special attention [1]. Previous experiments of our laboratory have demonstrated an impressive attenuation of the posttraumatic lesion growth by the selective iNOS-inhibitor aminoguanidine when administered *prior to trauma* [4]. These findings support strongly that expansion of the traumatic lesion must be considered as a manifestation of *secondary brain damage* which is amenable to therapeutic inhibition. Purpose of the current investigation was to elucidate, whether inhibition of the inducible NO-synthase by aminoguanidine is also affording protection when administered *post lesion*.

Material and Methods

Male Sprague-Dawley rats (n = 30) of 250 to 350 g b.w. were anaesthetized by halothane/O_2/N_2O, intubated and mechanically ventilated. The rectal and temporal muscle temperatures were kept constant at 37.0 °C by a feedback controlled heating pad and lamp, respectively. Systemic blood pressure, blood gases, and serum osmolarity were monitored via a catheter in the tail artery. A highly standardized cortical lesion was induced by focal freezing of the brain utilizing attachment of a metal cylinder (−68 °C) for 6 sec [2]. Animals were randomly assigned to one of three experimental groups. Animals of group I were sacrificed 5 min after trauma as reference to determine the spread of the primary brain tissue necrosis. Group II (sham treatment) received isotonic saline, group III aminoguanidine (100 mg/kg), at 15 min and 8 hrs post lesion intraperitoneally. 24 hrs later, animals of group II and III were sacrificed by perfusion fixation, and the brain was removed for histological investigation. The brain specimen were cut in 5 μm serial coronal sections at 150 μm intervals throughout the lesion proper and stained with cresyl violet according to NISSL. The area of necrosis was planimetrically assessed in all sections with lesion. The volume of necrosis was calculated by utilizing all sections with lesioned parenchyma by employment of the *Basic volume estimator* [5]. Expansion of the secondary lesion at 24 hrs was compared with the spread of the focal brain tissue necrosis of animals surviving trauma for only 5 min.

Results

Important physiological variables, such as the systemic blood pressure, paO_2, $paCO_2$, blood glucose, or serum osmolarity did not significantly differ between the experimental groups. The focal freezing lesion resulted in a cortical necrosis with a volume of 6.07 ± 1.04 mm^3 at 5 min after trauma in group I. Under sham treatment (group II), the lesion expanded to a volume of 8.39 ± 1.57 mm^3, corresponding to 138% at 24 hrs after the insult ($p < 0.01$, ANOVA on ranks). In animals with aminoguanidine treatment (group III) starting *post trauma*, the volume of necrosis was increased to only 6.77 ± 0.87 mm^3, indicating a lesion growth to only 112%. Thus, the selective iNOS-antagonist aminoguanidine was inhibiting the secondary growth of a traumatic brain lesion also when administered after trauma, i.e. from 138% (sham treatment) to 112% ($p < 0.05$ ANOVA on ranks) by more than two third.

Discussion

The high level of standardization and reproducibility of the presently used cold lesion model made it possible to produce a sharply defined, circumscribed area of necrosis, which is limited to cortical gray matter. Under this precaution, the growth kinetics of the traumatic cortical tissue necrosis has been analyzed in subtle details by our laboratory [1]. Thereby, a biphasic growth dynamics became recognizable, with a first growth phase during 6 hrs after insult and a second – more pronounced – between 12 and 24 hrs after trauma.

Administration of the iNOS-inhibitor aminoguanidine 15 min and 8 hrs *post injury* resulted again in significant attenuation of the growth of necrosis by more than two third. Thus, aminoguanidine may become known as the first pharmacological agent affording a marked therapeutical potency in this important manifestation of secondary brain damage. The current findings of a therapeutical efficacy of iNOS-inhibition by aminoguanidine – even when treatment commences only *post insult* may be explained by the recent data of Knerlich *et al.* [3]. The authors have obtained evidence from experiments using the same lesion model that iNOS mRNA is expressed at 6 hrs after trauma at the earliest, rendering plausible that inhibition of the NO-producing enzyme *after trauma* is not too late. On the other side, a mediator role of NO during the first phase of lesion growth (up to 6 hrs) is less likely according to results of Rinecker *et al.*, who could not antagonize or enhance, respectively, expansion of the necrosis, neither by cNOS-inhibition nor augmentation of the NO-production by L-NNA or l-arginine [4]. For the early post insult phase, other factors and mechanisms, such as excitatory amino acids, free radicals, arachidonic acid, bradykinin, and a posttraumatic tissue hypoperfusion must be considered.

References

1. Eriskat J, Schürer L, Kempski O, Baethmann A (1994) Growth kinetics of a primary brain tissue necrosis from a focal lesion. Acta Neurochir [Suppl] (Wien) 60: 425–427
2. Klatzo I, Piraux A, Laskowski EJ (1958) The relationship between edema, blood-brain barrier and tissue elements in a local brain injury. J Neuropathol Exp Neurol 17: 548–564
3. Knerlich F, Schilling L, Görlach C, Wahl M, Ehrenreich H, Siren AH (1999) Temporal profile of expression and cellular localization of inducible nitric oxide synthase, interleukin-1 beta and interleukin converting enzyme after cryogenic lesion of the rat parietal cortex. Mol Brain Res 68 (1–2): 73–87
4. Rinecker M, Stoffel M, Plesnila N, Eriskat J, Baethmann A (1999) Effect of NO on secondary growth of a brain tissue necrosis from focal injury. Restorat Neurol Neurosci 14: 226
5. Uylings HB, Van Eden CG, Hofman MA (1986) Morphometry of size/volume variables and comparison of their bivariate relations in the nervous system under different conditions. J Neurosci Methods 18: 19–37

Correspondence: Michael Stoffel, M.D., Department of Neurosurgery, Rheinische Friedrich-Wilhelms-University, Sigmund-Freud-Str. 25, 53105 Bonn, Germany.

Acta Neurochir (2000) [Suppl] 76: 359–364

Evidence for Lactate Uptake After Rat Fluid Percussion Brain Injury

T. Chen, Y. Z. Qian, X. Di, J. P. Zhu, and **R. Bullock**

Division of Neurosurgery Medical College of Virginia, Virginia Commonwealth University, Richmond, VA

Summary

Traumatic brain injury (TBI) places enormous early energy demand on brain tissue to reinstate normal ionic balance. Glucose declines and lactate increases after TBI as demonstrated in clinical and lab studies, suggesting increased glycolysis. This led us to hypothesize that high extracellular fluid (ECF) lactate may be beneficial after TBI. We measured cerebral dialysate lactate and glucose, and arterial lactate and glucose, before & after rat Fluid Percussion Injury (FPI) (2.06 ± 0.13 atm) with and without IV lactate infusion (100 mM $\times$ 4.5 hours) to test the hypotheses that arterial lactate determines ECF lactate. ^{14}C-lactate autoradiography was also performed, to demonstrate whether lactate is taken up by traumatized brain. **RESULTS:** Dialysate lactate was always significantly higher than arterial. After lactate infusion, both the dialysate and the arterial lactate were significantly increased ($P < 0.0001$). Dialysate lactate increased within 10 min. following FPI, with significantly higher values in the lactate infusion group (82% higher with lactate infusion after FPI). Dialysate glucose fell following FPI, with a more severe decline in the saline group (129% lower), suggesting lactate infusion preserves or "spares" glucose in ECF. In our autoradiographic study, IV ^{14}C-lactate accumulated at the injury site, with levels 2–4 times higher than in contralateral cortex. In conclusion, arterial lactate augmentation thus increases brain dialysate lactate and results in less reduction in ECF glucose, after FPI. Infused lactate accumulates at the injury site, where metabolism is probably the greatest.

Keywords: Traumatic brain injury; microdialysate; lactate; glucose; autoradiography.

Introduction

Over the last two decades, studies have repeatedly demonstrated extracellular lactate accumulation during cerebral ischemia and injury, in which a high degree of tissue lactic acidosis during brain ischemia impairs postischemic recovery [13, 14, 22]. In addition, different degrees of tissue lactic acidosis may explain why severe incomplete ischemia, in certain experimental models, is more deleterious than complete brain ischemia [13, 14, 22]. Moreover, head-injured patients have demonstrated increased brain lactate levels both locally in the cerebral spinal fluid (CSF) and in the regular venous blood, which has been regarded as a marker for poor clinical outcome [8, 25]. Andersen and Marmarou have demonstrated that whole brain lactate, as well as CSF lactate increased after fluid percussion TBI, even though simultaneously measured cerebral blood flow was unchanged, suggesting that TBI itself, rather than secondary ischemia, causes this lactate increase [2]. Increased glycolysis supports restoration of ionic homeostasis, and generates extracellular fluid (ECF) lactate [1, 21].

Recently, Pellerin and Magistretti showed, in a tissue culture model, that increased ECF glutamate causes lactate production into the ECF space, by astrocytes [21]. They hypothesize that lactate was thus made available for preferential uptake by neurons, and could directly enter oxidative metabolism, at the level of pyruvate, by the enzymatic action of lactate dehydrogenase [21]. After TBI, increased glutamate has been demonstrated, together with disturbed ionic homeostasis, both in humans, and animal models [3, 4, 10, 19, 29]. Moreover, a close relationship has been shown, between lactate and glutamate, in humen TBI [27].

More recently, several reports also indicate that lactate can serve as an energy substrate, for damaged and premature neonatal brain [9, 21, 23, 24]. Schurr also demonstrated that lactate, not glucose, fuels the recovery of synaptic function after hypoxia upon reoxygenation in hippocampal slices [23]. Thus we chose to investigate the role of lactate in the changes in metabolism that occur following traumatic brain injury. We tested the hypothesis that systemic lactate might be taken up by the brain, after TBI.

Materials and Methods

Exprimental Groups

All studies were approved by the Institutional Animal Care and Use Committee, of the Medical College of Virginia. Twenty-five adult male Sprague-Dawley rats, weighting 297 to 405 gm, were randomly allocated among three groups as follow: 1. Control group, sham operation with lactate iv infusion (n = 5), 2. Fluid percussion injury with saline infusion, saline-FPI (n = 7). 3. Fluid Percussion injury with lactate iv infusion, lactate-FPI (n = 7). Infusion of lactate (100 mM) or saline iv were at 0.6 ml/hr for 1 hour before, and 4 hours after the injury. 4. Fluid Percussion injury with ^{14}C-lactate iv injection(bolus) (n = 5). 5. Sham injury with ^{14}C-lactate iv injection(bolus) (n = 4).

Surgical Preparation

Animals were anesthetized with a nitrous oxide/oxygen mixture (70% : 30%) containing 2% halothane. Tracheal intubation was performed and positive-pressure ventilation was initiated. Both femoral artery and vein were canulated with PE50 Polyethylene tubing for monitoring blood pressure, blood gas analysis and infusion of lactate or saline. After cannulation, the wounds were sutured, and the animals were turned to the prone position. The animals were then placed in a stereotactic frame and the scalp was sagittally incised, after 0.5% lidocaine infiltration. A 4.8 mm diameter skull trephine opening was prepared, 2 mm to the left side of the midline between bregma and lambda. Two fixation screws were then placed 1 mm rostral to the bregma and 1 mm caudal to lambda. A Leur-Loc needle hub was placed into the skull hole and cemented in position with cyano acrylate glue. Dental acrylic was then poured around the needle hub, and the two screws for rigidity. A 1.5 mm burr hole was then drilled in the middle of the left occipital bone and a CMA/20 flexible microdialysis probe (active membrane 4 mm), was placed horizontally so that the active membrane lay under the subcortical region at the injury site. Dental acrylic was used to immobilize the probe. In the autoradiography study, instead of infusion of lactate or saline iv, 50 μCi ^{14}C-lactate was injected iv immediately after the FPI. 30 mins after the injury, the rat was sacrificed and brain was taken out instantly and frozen in isopentane in dry ice.

During the entire experiment, the mean arterial blood pressure (MABP) was continuously monitored and blood gases were measured every hour. A heating blanket maintained body temperature at 37 ± 2 °C, and physiological homeostasis was maintained.

Fluid Percussion

A fluid percussion device was used to produce TBI and has been described in detail previously [7]. Animals were injured at a moderate magnitude of injury (2.06 ± 0.13 atm), sham-injury animals received identical surgery and anesthesia but did not have the fluid percussion pulse delivered to the brain.

Microdialysis Procedure

Before the surgery, precalibration of the probe was performed to test the recovery rate from a standard solution of lactate and glucose. Following precalibration, the CMA/20 flexible probe was axially positioned in the subcortex just below the injection window for fluid percussion, via an occipital burr hole, as described above. Dialysate perfusion was performed using saline at a flow rate of 2.0 ul/min. Five 10 min samples were collected for baseline of extracellular lactate and glucose during 1 hr stabilization period. Then the lactate or saline infusion were started intravenously. Approximately 60 mins after beginning infusion of lactate or saline, the rat brains were injured by subjecting them to the fluid percussion pulse, which was used to produce experimental TBI, while the flexible microdialysis probe remained in the cortex to collect dialysate as early as possible posttrauma. The length of the outlet tube was shortened to 4 mm to keep the void volume small. The dialysate samples and the blood samples from the arterial line were collected every ten minutes for quantitation of lactate and glucose using the YSI 2700 Select Biochemistry Analyzer. Calibration of the probe after the experiment was also performed, and the microdialysate values were corrected according to the recovery rate of the probe.

Autoradiography Study

The frozen brain was cut into 20 μm thick sections on crystat at −20 °C, mounted on precoat slide, dried on a 60 °C hot plate and then exposed to Kodak Scientific Imaging Film for 14 days. The films were analyzed by a computer image system.

Statistical Analysis

Physiological data and microdialysate data, were analyzed using repeated measures analysis of variance (ANOVA). Significance was $p < 0.05$.

Results

Physiological Data and Injury Level

The mean physiological variables for the three experimental groups are shown in Table 1. There were no significant differences in any of these parameters between the two groups tested. The fluid percussion

Table 1. *Mean Arterial Blood Pressure (MABP), Arterial Blood Gases, and Rectal Temperature Before and After Fluid Percussion Injury in Both Control and Injury Groups*

Parameter	Lactate infusion		Lactate infus. + FPI		Saline infus. + FPI	
	Before infusion	After infusion	Before injury	After injury	Before injury	After injury
MABP (mmHg)	101.5 + 2.1	102.1 + 2.5	103.5 + 1.4	104.6 + 2.2	100.5 + 2.5	104.2 + 1.6
Rec. Temp. (°C)	36.3 + 0.2	36.5 + 0.1	36.5 + 0.1	36.5 + 0.1	36.6 + 0.1	36.5 + 0.0
PO2 (mmHg)	134.8 + 9.1	142 + 10.7	144.6 + 5.8	134.7 + 4.7	133.1 + 7.8	131.5 + 4.9
PCO2 (mmHg)	35 + 3.0	32.7 + 1.5	37.6 + 1.5	39.2 + 0.6	37.2 + 1.8	34.7 + 0.8
PH	7.4 + 0.1	7.41 + 0.0	7.41 + 0.0	7.41 + 0.0	7.41 + 0.0	7.4 + 0.0

* Values shown in table are mean ± SE.

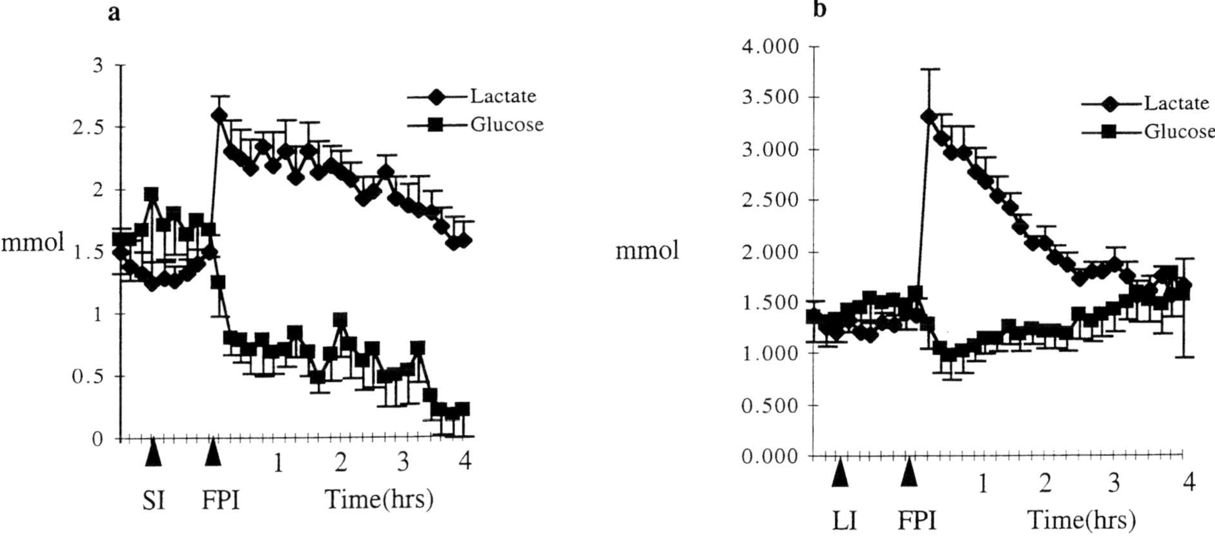

Fig. 1. (a, b) Corrected cerebral microdialysate lactate and glucose after fluid percussion, without lactate infusion. *SI* Saline infusion, *LI* Lactate infusion, *FPI* fluid percussion injury

injury level was between 1.85 to 2.28 atm (Mean $\pm$ SEM: 2.1 $\pm$ 0.14 atm). There were no significant differences between the two injury groups ($p = 0.36$).

Microdialysate Results

Lactate. In the saline-FPI group, the microdialysis lactate rose to 2.2 $\pm$ 0.08 mmol from 1.43 $\pm$ 0.15 mmol during the first half hour after the fluid percussion injury (54%) and remained around 2 mmol for the duration of the experiment (Fig. 1). In the lactate-FPI group, the dialysate lactate rose to 3.28 $\pm$ 0.07 mmol from 1.14 $\pm$ 0.1 mmol during the first half hour after the fluid percussion injury (100% increase) (Fig. 1). At the end of the first hour after injury, lactate increased 178% in the saline-FPI group, but increased 237% in the lactate-FPI group. These 1 hour increases were significantly different from baseline lactate ($p < 0.0001$). The dialysate lactate difference between the lactate infusion + FP group and the saline infusion + FP group at the end of the first hour after injury was also significantly different ($p < 0.022$).

Glucose: In contrast, the dialysate glucose level decreased from 1.96 $\pm$ 0.04 mmol to 1.36 $\pm$ 0.27 mmol during the first half hour after FPI in the lactate-FPI group, and from 1.72 $\pm$ 0.53 mmol to 0.77 $\pm$ 0.04 mmol in the saline-FPI group (Fig. 1). The most interesting observation was that the dialysate glucose increased back to the pre-injury level, by the 4th hour after the injury, while the lactate decreased in the lactate-FPI group. In contrast, in the saline FPI group, instead of increasing, the dialysate glucose remained significantly decreased at the 4th hour compared to the first hour after injury (Fig. 1). The dialysate glucose levels in both injury groups were significantly decreased during the first hour after the fluid percussion injury, compared to the baseline ($p < 0.001$) (Fig. 1). Only in the lactate FP group, the microdialysate glucose was seen to increase significantly from the nadir during the first hour after the FP injury ($p < 0.0001$) (Fig. 1). In the lactate sham group, the ECF lactate showed strong correlation with arterial lactate (Fig. 2).

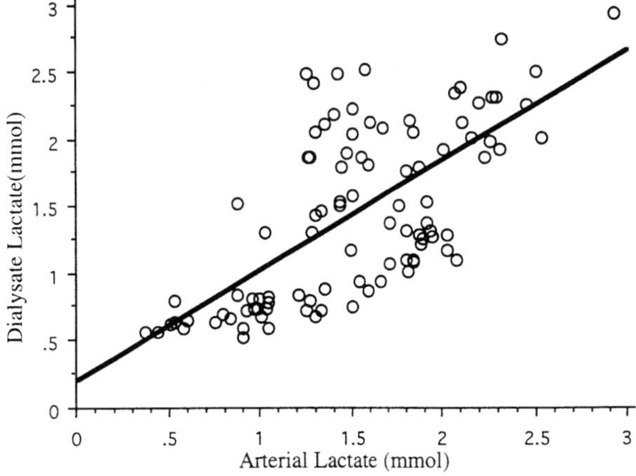

Fig. 2. Relationship between cerebral dialysate lactate and arterial lactate after lactate infusion, without fluid percussion injury ($R^2 = 0.455$, $p < 0.0001$)

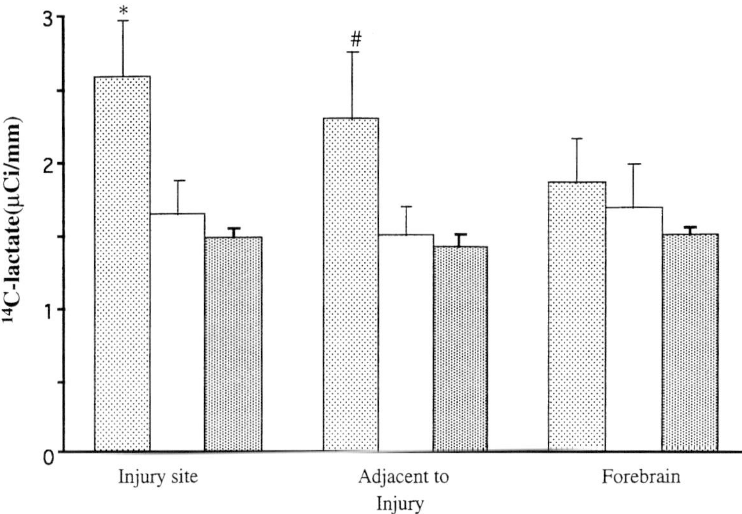

Fig. 3. Uptake of ^{14}C-lactate in different brain regions after TBI
* different from contralateral side at $p < 0.0008$, from sham at $p < 0.0003$
# different trom contralateral side at $p < 0.007$, from sham at $p < 0.001$
Injury side; Opposite side; Forebrain

In the ^{14}C autoradiography study, the sham injury animals show that the ^{14}C-lactate can cross the blood brain barrier into normal brain. In the injury animals, the uptake of ^{14}C-lactate was increased 4 times around the injury site. The injury site uptake was significantly different from the contralateral side (Fig. 3).

Discussion

Many studies have now described elevation of microdialysate lactate in head injury patients [5, 11, 12, 16] and in animal brain injury models [13, 14, 24]. In the present study, the dialysate glucose decreased while lactate level increased 10 mins after the fluid percussion injury, in both lactate and saline infusion groups. Moreover, in the lactate infusion group, the increase in microdialysate lactate after the fluid percussion TBI injury was much greater than in the saline infusion group. This indicates that the injured brain takes up lactate from the circulating blood. In addition, several studies report that the BBB in rats is readily penetrable to lactate by means of facilitated diffusion [20]. In humans, the BBB permeability to lactate is about one half that of glucose, by means of facilitated diffusion, and hypercapnia enhances the brain uptake of lactate [18]. Our data shows that after fluid percussion injury the microdialysate lactate was highly significantly increased from the pre-injury level (about 178% increase in the saline-FPI group, and 237% in the lactate-FPI group). Thus, lactate infusion clearly enhances the elevation of ECF lactate after brain injury. During the first hour after injury, the significant difference in dialysate lactate, between the saline and lactate infusion injury groups suggests that lactate in the blood can cross the BBB and be taken up by injured brain in rats. After the injury, the increase in dialysate lactate in the lactate infusion group is almost 2.5 fold larger compared to the saline infusion group.

There was a strong correlation between the blood lactate and the dialysate lactate in the lactate infusion group. These results, indicate that arterial lactate augmentation increases the brain ECF lactate, after TBI. More importantly, the decrease of the dialysate glucose in the lactate infusion group is only 63% of that seen in the saline infusion group.

The brain lactate level has been regarded as an indicator of poor prognosis following brain trauma in patients. Several early studies demonstrated a relationship between poor prognosis and high CSF lactate levels acutely following brain injury [6, 17, 25, 30]. Our study shows no significant increase in blood lactate level after injury in both injury groups, as showed also by Yuan and Wade [29]. However, the brain lactate level does increase after brain injury both in clinical and experimental studies [5, 11, 12, 13, 14, 16, 22]. Our data concur with these findings. But does this mean that the elevation of lactate in brain tissue plays a role in the secondary damage to the injured brain, after TBI? Pellerin and Magistretti have shown the ability of the excitatory neurotransmitter glutamate to stimulate aerobic glycolytic lactate production by astrocytes and its utilization by neurons [22]. Lactate has been reported to provide an energy source to support neuronal synaptic function in the hippocampal slice [15, 23, 26]. Schurr also reported that lactate can be utilized by brain tissue for energy metabolism during recovery from hypoxia and that lactate conversion to pyruvate does not require investment of ATP [23]. Our study shows that the lactate-FPI rats have a high brain lactate level shortly after the injury. As the lactate level decreases, the brain glucose level increases. More importantly, the decrease of dialysate glucose in the lactate infusion group is only 63% of that seen in the saline infusion group. In the saline injury group, the glucose levels stay low. Although the brain lactate levels have the same trend as seen in the lactate infusion injury group, the glucose levels in these rat brains decrease significantly instead of increasing as the lactate levels decrease.

In our autoradiographic study, radioactive lactate is seen to cross the blood barrier in sham rats and shows increased uptake in the injured brain. Thus we conclude that the injured brain can take up peripheral lactate and ultimately this correlates with an elevation of the ECF glucose. Both lactate and glucose can be used as an energy source to facilitate the recovery of ionic homeostasis in the injured brain tissue. In other words, infusing lactate seems not only to increase ECF lactate after TBI, but also to maintain ECF glucose, and prevent its prolonged reduction to low levels.

According to Schurr's study, following a hypoxic period long enough to deplete tissue ATP, lactate could be a preferred or even an obligatory energy substrate over glucose because of the lactate conversion to pyruvate without investment of ATP [24].

We conclude from our study that the infusion of lactate to the circulation can reduce the decrease in brain glucose. Thus, we speculate that lactate may serve as an energy source, to spare glucose acutely, and allow restoration of ionic homeostasis. Further studies in patients are needed.

References

1. Andersen BJ, Marmarou A (1992) Post-traumatic selective stimulation of glycolysis. Brain Res 585: 184–189
2. Andersen BJ, Unterberg AW, Clarke GD, Marmarou A (1988) Effect of posttraumatic hypoventilation on cerebral energy metabolism. J Neurosurg 68: 601–607
3. Brown JI, Baker AJ, Konasiewicz SJ, Moulton RJ (1998) Clinical significance of CSF glutamate concentrations following severe traumatic brain injury in humans. J Neurotrauma 15: 253–263
4. Bullock R, Zauner A, Woodward JJ, Myseros J, Choi SC, Ward JD, Marmarou A, Young HF (1998) Factors affecting excitatory amino acid release following severe human head injury. J Neurosurgery 89: 507–518
5. Bullock R, Zauner A, Myseros JS, Marmarou A, Woodward JJ, Young, HF (1995) Evidence for prolonged release of excitatory amino acids in severe human head trauma. Relationship to clinical events. Ann NY Acad Sci 765: 290–297; discussion 298
6. Crockard HA, Taylor AR (1972) Serial CSF lactate-pyruvate values as a guide to prognosis in head injury coma. Eur Neurol 8: 151–157
7. Dixon CE, Lyeth BG, Povlishock JT, Findling RL, Hamm RJ, Marmarou A, Young HF, Hayes RL (1987) A fluid percussion model of experimental brain injury in the rat. J Neurosurg 67: 110–119
8. Enevoldsen EM, Jensen FT (1977) Cerebrospinal fluid lactate and pH in patients with acute severe head injury. Clin Neurol Neurosurg 80: 213–225
9. Fernandes J, Berger R, Smit GP (1982) Lactate as energy source for brain in glucose-6-phosphatase deficient child [letter]. Lancet 1: 113
10. Globus MY, Alonso O, Dietrich WD, Busto R, Ginsberg MD (1995) Glutamate release and free radical production following brain injury: effects of posttraumatic hypothermia. J Neurochem 65: 1704–1711
11. Goodman JC, Valadka AB, Gopinath SP, Cormio M, Robertson CS (1996) Lactate and excitatory amino acids measured by microdialysis are decreased by pentobarbital coma in head-injured patients. J Neurotrauma 13: 549–556
12. Hamberger A, Runnerstam M, Nystrom B, Starmark JE, Von Essen C (1995) The neuronal environment after subarachnoid haemorrhage–correlation of amino acid and nucleoside levels with post-operative recovery. Neurol Res 17: 97–105
13. Hossmann KA, Kleihues P (1973) Reversibility of ischemic brain damage. Arch Neurol 29: 375–384
14. Inao S, Marmarou A, Clarke GD, Andersen BJ, Fatouros PP, Young HF (1988) Production and clearance of lactate from brain tissue, cerebrospinal fluid, and serum following experimental brain injury. J Neurosurg 69: 736–744
15. Izumi Y, Benz AM, Zorumski CF, Olney JW (1994) Effects of lactate and pyruvate on glucose deprivation in rat hippocampal slices. Neuroreport 5: 617–620
16. Kawamata T, Katayama Y, Hovda DA, Yoshino A, Becker DP (1995) Lactate accumulation following concussive brain injury: the role of ionic fluxes induced by excitatory amino acids. Brain Res 674: 196–204
17. King LR, McLaurin RL, Knowles HC Jr (1974) Acid-base balance and arterial and CSF lactate levels following human head injury. J Neurosurg 40: 617–625
18. Knudsen GM, Paulson OB, Hertz MM (1991) Kinetic analysis of the human blood-brain barrier transport of lactate and its influence by hypercapnia. J Cereb Blood Flow Metab 11: 581–586
19. Koizumi H, Fujisawa H, Ito H, Maekawa T, Di X, Bullock R (1997) Effects of mild hypothermia on cerebral blood flow-independent changes in cortical extracellular levels of amino acids following contusion trauma in the rat. Brain Res 747: 304–312
20. Oldendorf WH (1971) Blood brain barrier permeability to lactate. Eur Neurol 6: 49–55
21. Pellerin L, Magistretti PJ (1994) Glutamate uptake into astrocytes stimulates aerobic glycolysis: a mechanism coupling neuronal activity to glucose utilization. Proc Natl Acad Sci U S A 91: 10625–10629
22. Rehncrona S, Rosen I, Siesjo BK (1981) Brain lactic acidosis and ischemic cell damage: 1. Biochemistry and neurophysiology. J Cereb Blood Flow Metab 1: 297–311
23. Schurr A, Payne RS, Miller JJ, Rigor BM (1997) Brain lactate, not glucose, fuels the recovery of synaptic function from hypoxia upon reoxygenation: an in vitro study. Brain Res 744: 105–111
24. Schurr A, West CA, Rigor BM (1988) Lactate-supported syn-

aptic function in the rat hippocampal slice preparation. Science 240: 1326–1328
25. Siegel JH, Rivkind AI, Dalal S, Goodarzi S (1990) Early physiologic predictors of injury severity and death in blunt multiple trauma. Arch Surg 125: 498–508
26. Stittsworth JD, Jr, Lanthorn TH (1993) Lactate mimics only some effects of D-glucose on epileptic depolarization and long-term synaptic failure. Brain Res 630: 21–27
27. Valadka AB, Goodman JC, Gopinath SP, Uzura M, Robertson CS (1998) Comparison of brain tissue oxygen tension to microdialysis-based measures of cerebral ischemia in fatally head-injured humans. J Neurotrauma 15: 509–519
28. Vespa P, Prins M, Ronne-Engstrom E, Caron M, Shalmon E, Hovda DA, Martin NA, Becker DP (1998) Increase in extracellular glutamate caused by reduced cerebral perfusion pressure and seizures after human traumatic brain injury: a microdialysis study. J Neurosurg 89: 971–982
29. Yuan XQ, Wade CE (1993) Lactated Ringer's solution alleviates brain trauma-precipitated lactic acidosis in hemorrhagic shock. J Neurotrauma 10: 307–313
30. Zupping R (1970) Cerebral acid-base and gas metabolism in brain injury. J Neurosurg 33: 498–505

Correspondence: Ross Bullock, M.D., Ph.D., Division of Neurosurgery, Medical College of Virginia, Virginia Commonwealth University, Richmond, VA 23298.

Acta Neurochir (2000) [Suppl] 76: 365–369

Topical Application of Brain Derived Neurotrophic Factor Influences Upregulation of Constitutive Isoform of Heme Oxygenase in the Spinal Cord Following Trauma An Experimental Study Using Immunohistochemistry in the Rat

H. S. Sharma[1], **J. Westman**[1], **T. Gordh**[2], and **P. Alm**[3]

[1] Laboratory of Neuroanatomy, Department of Medical cell Biology; Biomedical Centre, Uppsala University
[2] Department of Anaesthesiology, University Hospital, Uppsala, Sweden
[3] Department of Pathology, University Hospital, Lund, Sweden

Summary

Influence of brain derived neurotrophic factor (BDNF) on carbon monoxide (CO) production following spinal cord injury was examined using expression of the constitutive isoform of the enzyme hemeoxygenase-2 (HO-2) in a rat model. A longitudinal incision of the right dorsal horn on the T10–11 segment markedly increased the HO-2 immunostaining in the cord at 5 h. At this time period, breakdown of the blood-spinal cord barrier (BSCB) and edema formation were quite prominent. Repeated topical application of BDNF (20 μl of a 1 μg/ml solution) over the exposed surface of the cord significantly attenuated the edematous expansion of the cord and the disturbances in the BSCB permeability. In BDNF-treated rats, expression of HO-2 immunoreactivity was considerably reduced. These results strongly suggest that BDNF is neuroprotective in spinal trauma and this growth factor has the capacity to attenuate CO production by downregulating HO-2 expression.

Keywords: Spinal cord injury; hemeoxygenase-2; brain derived neurotrophic factor; blood-spinal cord barrier.

Introduction

Brain derived neurotrophic factor (BDNF) is a well known neuroprotective agent in ischemia and trauma [2, 3, 4, 7, 10]. Long-term pretreatment with growth factors using slow release capsules implanted in the skin for several weeks is known to attenuate cell damage following ischemia or brain trauma indicating that neurotrophic factors may provide neuroprotection following ischemic or traumatic insults to the brain [8, 9, 11]. Spinal cord injury induces an upregulation of neurotrophic factor receptors [11, 13, 20] indicating that growth factors play some role in the pathophysiology of spinal cord trauma. Previous experiments from our laboratory suggest that BDNF is neuroprotective in spinal cord injury [18]. However, the detailed mechanisms of BDNF induced neuroprotection are not well characterised [18].

One of the main problems in neurotrophins induced neuroprotection is to deliver the adequate quantity of the growth factor within the central nervous system (CNS) in order to have an optimal effect [2, 19]. Since transport of the several growth factors across the blood-brain barrier (BBB) is limited, therefore, delivery of the growth factors in high quantity at the site of the CNS injury is an important factor in achieving neuroprotection [12, 13, 19]. A direct delivery of growth factors to the lesion site by topical application, tissue implants or intrathecal application in order to by pass the BBB are few desirable steps needed to achieve growth factor induced neuroprotection, which, however, require further investigation.

The mechanisms of neurotrophic factors induced neuroprotection is not completely understood [18]. Improved neuronal communication by modifying neurochemical transmission and enhanced cell metabolism are considered to be important in neurotrophins induced neuroprotection [4, 10]. Trauma induces a series of events including release of many endogenous neuroprotective and neurodestructive substances which finally determine the cell injury or cell survival [14, 21]. It seems probable that exogenous supplement of growth factors may tilt the balance toward neuroprotection either by neutralising the influence of neurodestructive agents or by enhancing the influence of neuroprotective substances. Alternatively, neurotrophic factors may have some inhibitory control over neurodestructive elements, a feature which require further study.

Previously, our laboratory showed that BDNF pretreatment attenuates nitric oxide (NO) production by inhibiting constitutive isoform of nitric oxide synthase (cNOS) enzyme in the spinal cord following trauma. This indicates that neurotrophic factors may have some inhibitory influence on NOS upregulation. Since, carbon monoxide (CO), is also a gaseous molecule like NO and plays important role in cell injury [18], the present investigation was undertaken to find out whether an upregulation of the hemeoxygenase-2 (HO-2) enzyme following spinal cord trauma is associated with cell injury and whether pretreatment with BDNF has any influence on CO production by influencing HO-2 expression.

Materials and Methods

Animals

Experiments were carried out on 30 male Sprague-Dawley rats (200–230 g) kept at controlled room temperature 21 ± 1 °C with 12 h light and 12 h dark schedule. The rat food pellets and tap water were supplied ad libitum.

Spinal Cord Injury

Under Equithesin anaesthesia (3 ml/kg, i.p.) one segment laminectomy was done over the T10–11 segment. Spinal cord injury was made by making a longitudinal incision of the right dorsal horn at the T10–11 (about 2 mm deep and 5 mm long) [13, 20]. Bleeding from the spinal cord was cleaned with cotton soaked saline and the surface of the exposed cord was covered with the same in order to avoid a direct exposure of the cord to air. This experimental condition is approved by the Ethical Committee of Banaras Hindu University, Varanasi, India and Uppsala University, Uppsala, Sweden.

Treatment with the BDNF

Separate groups of animals were treated with BDNF (n = 5) topically by applying the growth factor in a concentration of 1 μg/ml (20 μl) starting from 30 min before injury, immediately after injury followed by 30 min, 60 min, 120 min, 180 min and 240 min following trauma as described earlier [13, 14, 16, 18].

HO-2 Immunohistochemistry

Five h after injury, both treated (n = 10) and untreated rats (n = 10) were perfusion fixed and the spinal cord segments comprising T9 to T12 were removed and analysed for HO-2 immunostaining according to the standard protocol [12, 15, 17]. In brief, monoclonal HO-2 antibodies (1 : 500, StressGene, Canada) were applied on the free floating 40 μm thick vibratome sections obtained from the T9 and the T12 segments with constant agitation at the room temperature. The immunoreaction was developed using peroxidase-antiperoxidase reaction [12, 15]. The HO-2 positive cells if any were visualised and analysed by two independent observers and photographed using light microscopy at ×80 to 120.

Spinal Cord Edema

Edema of the spinal cord was analysed using water content of the cord from the differences in the wet and dry weight of the sample as described earlier [13, 20].

Blood-Spinal Cord Barrier Permeability

The BSCB permeability was examined using Evans blue albumin and ^{131}I-sodium as described earlier [12, 15, 21]. In brief, both tracers were administered into the right femoral vein through needle puncture. The intravascular tracer was washed-out by perfusion through heart 5 min after its initial administration. Immediately before perfusion, one ml of whole blood was collected from the left ventricle through needle puncture for determination of the blood radioactivity at the time of sacrifice [12].

Statistical Analysis

Student's unpaired t-test was used to analyse the statistical significance of the data obtained. A p-value less than 0.05 was considered to be significant.

Results

Effect of BDNF on HO-2 Immunohistochemistry

Subjection of rats to 5 h spinal trauma induced by an incision of the right dorsal horn at T10–11 segments markedly increased the expression of HO-2 immunostaining in the traumatised as well as the adjacent perifocal spinal cord segments (T9 and T12). Pretreatment with BDNF significantly attenuated the upregulation of trauma induced HO-2 expression in the cord. A representative example of increased HO-2 expression in the T12 segment following trauma is shown in Fig. 1. Pretreatment with BDNF significantly attenuated the upregulation of HO-2 expression in the cord (Fig. 1).

Effect of BDNF on Spinal Cord Edema

Subjection of animals to a 5 h spinal cord trauma significantly increased the edematous swelling of the spinal cord compared with the control group (Fig. 2). This increase in edema formation was significantly attenuated by pretreatment with BDNF (Fig. 2).

Effect of BDNF on BSCB Permeability

Pretreatment with BDNF has considerably reduced the extravasation of radioactive iodine in the spinal cord segments following trauma (Fig. 2). This effect was most pronounced in perifocal spinal cord segment. Pretreatment with the BDNF alone however, did not

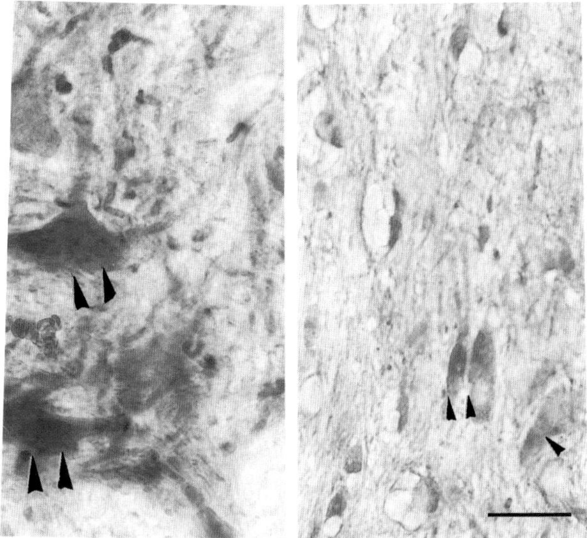

Fig. 1. Upregulation of HO-2 expression in the T12 segment of one spinal cord traumatised rat (left) and its modification with BDNF pretreatment (right). The upregulation of HO-2 is clearly seen in nerve cells (large arrow heads) and dendrites in spinal cord traumatised rat. Pretreatment with BDNF resulted in considerably reduced HO-2 immunoreactivity (small arrow heads) in the cord. In BDNF treated rat, general expansion of spinal cord and distortion of nerve cell is less apparent than the untreated traumatised rat (bar, left- = 50 μm, right = 80 μm)

influence the BSCB permeability to radioactive iodine (results not shown).

Discussion

The salient new findings of the present investigation show that BDNF pretreatment attenuated HO-2 immunoreactivity following a focal trauma to the cord. This indicates that the neurotrophic factor may have some inhibitory influence on CO metabolism, not reported earlier. Our results further show that BDNF treatment also attenuated the development of spinal cord edema and breakdown of the BSCB permeability indicating that alteration in the fluid microenvironment of the cord following trauma plays important role in HO-2 expression and cell injury. Previous observations from our laboratory show that BDNF treatment attenuates NO production following trauma (14). This indicates that like NO, CO production in spinal cord following trauma is also associated with cell injury.

Increased expression of HO is associated with increased production of CO [5]. Like NO, CO is also a gaseous molecule which influences neuronal transmission within the CNS by diffusing from one cell to the other after its production far away from its action site [1, 5]. Due to this rapid diffusion, and a very short half life of CO once formed within the CNS, it is very difficult to study its function in the CNS. Thus most of the studies of CO functions are confined to examine its synthesising enzymes HO-1 or HO-2 expression [1, 5, 15].

Few previous observations suggest that upregulation of HO-1 occurs following brain trauma in glial cells 1 day to several weeks after the initial insult [6]. This upregulation of HO-1 is interpreted by the authors as one form of protective mechanism because glial scar formation is helping in regeneration [1, 5, 6]. However, the role of CO or HO-2 expression in neurodegeneration or repair mechanisms are still unclear. We have used HO-2 immunostaining to study the

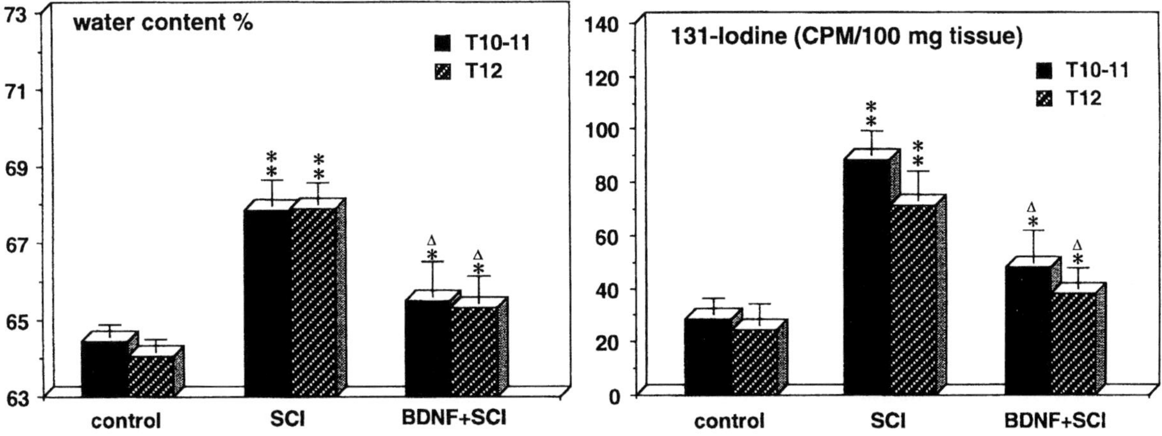

Fig. 2. Spinal cord water content (left) and blood-spinal cord barrier (*BSCB*) permeability (right) in spinal cord traumatised rats and their modification with BDNF pretreatment. ** = $P < 0.01$ compared from control; Δ = $P < 0.05$, compared from spinal cord injury (*SCI*)

function of CO. There are reasons to believe that upregulation of HO-2 is also associated with increased production of CO. However, an increased production of CO doesn't necessarily mean that the molecule is inducing damage to the CNS. Increased production of CO may be beneficial also because of its vasodilating action in several vascular beds.

In order to understand beneficial or harmful effects of HO-2 induced CO release in spinal cord trauma, we examined the influence of BDNF, a known neuroprotective agent on trauma induced HO-2 expression. Our results suggest that upregulation of HO-2 expression is injurious to the cord following trauma. This idea is supported by the fact that BDNF pretreatment significantly reduced HO-2 expression in the cord following injury. This observation is in good agreement with the previous study which clearly demonstrated a neuroprotective effect of HO inhibitors on trauma induced edema formation in cortical slices using ex-vivo techniques [6, 12]. Since drugs interfering with HO synthesis do not normally recognise different isoforms, it is not certain whether HO-2 or HO-1 blockade was related with the observed beneficial effect in this experiment. That upregulation of HO-2 is associated with cell injury is further supported by our observations in hyperthermic brain injury [15]. Thus, hyperthermia upregulated HO-2 expression in several brain regions associated with cell injury and pretreatment with drugs other than HO inhibitors, induced marked neuroprotection and also attenuated the HO-2 expression. This observation clearly suggests that HO-2 expression is injurious to the cell.

The mechanisms by which BDNF influences HO-2 expression is not clear from this study. Growth factors in general offer neuroprotection by either influencing neurochemical transmission or by exerting powerful trophic effects on the cell following injury [2, 7, 8, 18]. Cells do not cope with the magnitude and severity of trauma and thus, supply of their basic nutrients or energy metabolism deteriorates rapidly [11, 19]. In addition, release of secondary injury factors will directly influence cellular stress following trauma resulting in a "shock phase" response [21]. There are reason to believe that neurotrophic factors may interfere in all these mechanisms by enhancing trophic support, attenuating cellular "shock" or "stress" response by improving cell to cell communication, and/or by modifying sensory injury mechanisms probably via neuropeptides or other neurochemical receptors [7, 10, 19].

The essential biological signal responsible for BDNF induced attenuation of CO production is not known in all its details. CO production is influenced by neurochemicals, cytokines, hormones and many other events occurring during trauma or ischemia (5). BDNF can modify early cellular events by influencing the magnitude and severity of cellular "shock phase", secondary injury cascade and/or neuronal communication. Thus, it seems plausible that in BDNF treated animals, the endogenous neurodestructive signals are not sufficient enough to induce an upregulation of HO expression. Obviously, a less expression of HO-2 will not generate sufficient CO production responsible for cell injury.

In conclusion, our observations suggest that spinal cord trauma is associated with CO production as indicated by upregulation of HO-2 expression which contributes to the cellular injury process. BDNF treatment significantly attenuated HO-2 expression and cell injury. This indicates that BDNF may have some inhibitory influence on CO metabolism, a feature which requires further investigation.

Acknowledgments

This investigation is supported by grants from Swedish Medical Research Council nrs. 02710 (JW, HSS), 9077 (TG, HSS), 11205 (PA); Göran Gustafsson Stiftelse (HSS), Sweden; and The University Grants Commission (HSS), New Delhi, India. The technical assistance of Kärstin Flink, Ingamarie Olsson, Inga Hörte and Ulla Johansson is highly appreciated.

References

1. Applegate L, Luscher P, Tyrell R (1991) Inhibition of heme oxygenase: a general response to oxidant stress in cultured mammalian cells. Cancer Res 51: 974–978
2. Conner JM, Tuszynski MH (1998) Growth factor therapy. Ment Retard Develop Disab Res Rev 4: 212–222
3. Cotman CW, Berchtold NC (1998) Plasticity and growth factors in injury response. Ment Retard Develop Disab Res Rev 4: 223–230
4. Dijkhuizen PA, Verhaagen J (1999) The use of neurotrophic factors to treat spinal cord injury: Advantages and disadvantages of different delivery methods. Neurosci Res Commun 24: 1–10
5. Ewing JF, Maines MD (1992) In situ hybridisation and immunohistochemical localization of heme oxygenase-2 mRNA and protein in normal brain: Differential distribution of isozyme 1 and 2. Mol Cell Neurosci 3: 559–570
6. Fukuda K, Richmon JD, Sato M, Sharp FR, Panter SC, Noble LJ (1996) Induction of heme oxygenase-1 (HO-1) in glia after traumatic brain injury. Brain Res 736: 68–75
7. Oudega M, Hagg T (1999) Neurotrophins promote regeneration of sensory axons in the adult rat spinal cord. Brain Res 818: 431–438
8. Lee TT, Green BA, Dietrich WD, Yezierski RP (1999) Neuro-

trophic effects of basic fibroblast growth factor following spinal cord contusion injury in the rat. J Neurotrauma 16: 347–356
9. Liu Y, Kim DH, Himes BT, Chow SY, Schallert T, Murray M, Tessler A, Fischer I (1999) Transplants of fibroblasts genetically modified to express BDNF promote regeneration of adult rat rubrospinal axons and recovery of forelimb function. J Neurosci 19: 4370–4387
10. Lu J, Waite P (1999) Advances in spinal cord regeneration. Spine 24: 926–930
11. Schwab ME, Bartholdi D (1996) Degeneration and regeneration of axons in the lesioned spinal cord. Physiol Rev 76: 319–370
12. Sharma HS (1999) Pathophysiology of blood-brain barrier, brain edema and cell injury following hyperthermia: New role of heat shock protein, nitric oxide and carbon monoxide. an experimental study in the rat using light and electron microscopy, Acta Universitatis Upsaliensis 830: 1–94
13. Sharma HS, Nyberg F, Gordh T, Alm P, Westman J (1998) Neurotrophic factors attenuate neuronal nitric oxide synthase upregulation, microvascular permeability disturbances, edema formation and cell injury in the spinal cord following trauma. Spinal cord monitoring. Basic principles, regeneration, pathophysiology and clinical aspects. In: Stålberg E, Sharma HS, Olsson Y (eds) Springer, Wien New York, pp 181–210
14. Sharma HS, Nyberg F, Westman J, Gordh T, Alm P, Lindholm D (1998) Brain derived neurotrophic factor and insulin like growth factor-1 attenuate upregulation of nitric oxide synthase and cell injury following trauma to the spinal cord. Amino Acids 14: 121–129
15. Sharma HS, Alm P, Westman J (1998) Nitric oxide and carbon monoxide in the pathophysiology of brain functions in heat stress. Prog Brain Res 115: 297–333
16. Sharma HS, Nyberg F, Gordh T, Alm P, Westman J (1997) Topical application of insulin like growth factor-1 reduces edema and upregulation of neuronal nitric oxide synthase following trauma to the rat spinal cord. Acta Neurochir [Suppl] (Wien) 70: 130–133
17. Sharma HS, Alm P, Westman J (1997) Upregulation of hemeoxygenase-II in the rat spinal cord following heat stress. Thermal physiology. In: Nielsen-Johanssen B, Nielsen R (eds) The August Krogh Institute, Copenhagen, pp 135–138
18. Sharma HS, Nyberg F, Gordh T, Alm P, Westman J (2000) Neurotrophic factors influence upregulation of constitutive isoform of heme oxygenase and cellular stress response in the spinal cord following trauma. Amino Acids 19: 351–361
19. Skaper SD, Walsh FS (1998) Neurotrophic molecules: Strategies for designing effective therapeutic molecules in neurodegeneration. Mol Cell Neurosci 12: 179–193
20. Stålberg E, Sharma HS, Olsson Y (1998) Spinal cord monitoring. Basic principles, regeneration, pathophysiology and clinical aspects. Springer, Wien New York, pp 1–527
21. Winkler T, Sharma HS, Stålberg E, Westman J (1998) Spinal cord monitoring. Basic principles, regeneration, pathophysiology and clinical aspects. In: Stålberg E, Sharma HS, Olsson Y (eds) Springer, Wien New York, pp 283–364

Correspondence: Hari Shanker Sharma, Ph.D., Laboratory of Neuroanatomy, Department of Medical Cell Biology, Box 571, Biomedical Centre, Uppsala University, S-75123 Uppsala, Sweden.

Acta Neurochir (2000) [Suppl] 76: 371–373

Time Profile of Neuron Specific Enolase Serum Levels After Experimental Brain Injury in Rat

C. Woertgen, R. D. Rothoerl, and **A. Brawanski**

Department of Neurosurgery, University of Regensburg, Germany

Summary

The aim of this study was to investigate the time course of NSE serum levels after traumatic brain injury in rats.

65 male Wistar rats were subjected to severe cortical impact injury (100 PSI, 2 mm deformation). Blood samples were drawn directly after trauma, after 1 h, 6 h, 12 h, 24 h, and 48 h in the trauma group as well as in sham operated animals directly after craniotomy, after 6 h and after 48 h. NSE serum levels were estimated with a commercially available enzyme immuno assay (LIA-mat Sangtec®). The control animals showed a NSE serum level of 8.82 μg/l (mean, n = 10). We demonstrated a time dependent release of NSE into the serum after trauma. The highest NSE serum values were detected six hours after trauma (31.5 μg/l, mean, n = 10). NSE serum level seems to reflect neuronal damage after cortical contusion in the rat in a time dependent manner.

Keywords: NSE; traumatic brain injury.

Introduction

There is an increasing interest in serum markers after nervous system damage. Serum markers like Neuron Specific Enolase, CKBB, Myelin Basic Protein and S-100B are known to give useful additional information for outcome prediction after severe head injury, stroke and subarachnoid hemorrhage [2–9, 11–19]. The results concerning the serum levels of the Neuron specific enolase (NSE) after traumatic brain injury are contradictory. Skogseid found in 60 patients NSE serum levels correlating to the severity of trauma and correlating to the contusion volume seen on the CT scan [15]. Ross studied 51 patients with severe head injury, but he did not find a correlation of NSE serum levels to the Glasgow Coma Score after trauma [13]. These results could be confirmed in further studies [12, 19]. Experimental investigations concerning this issue are sparse [5, 16]. Uzan studied serum levels of NSE three hours after traumatic brain injury in rat. He found no correlation to the severity of trauma and no difference between the trauma and the sham group [16]. But he found an elevated NSE level in thc liquor 7.5 hours after severe traumatic brain injury. Hardemark saw an early peak (7.5 hours after trauma) and a peak after 1.5 days of NSE liquor levels after traumatic brain injury in 5 rats [5]. The aim of this study was to investigate the time course of NSE serum levels after traumatic brain injury in rat.

Materials and Methods

The experimental protocol was approved by the local animal protocol review commitee. All surgery was carried out under aseptic conditions. Male Wistar rats (150 g–200 g, n = 65) were anesthetized with 5% isoflurane in an anesthetic chamber. Anesthesia was maintained with 2,5% isoflurane and 100% oxygene until wound closure. The head of the animals was secured in a stereotaxic frame (Kopf, Heidelberg, Germany) and a 10 mm diameter craniotomy was performed using a dental drill. Rats were randomly assigned into one of the following groups: 1.) 100 PSI Trauma blood sample drawn directly after trauma (n = 10), 2.) 100 PSI Trauma blood sample drawn after 1 h (n = 10) 3.) 100 PSI Trauma blood sample drawn after 6 h (n = 10), 4.) 100 PSI Trauma blood sample drawn after 12 h (n = 10) 5.) 100 PSI Trauma blood sample drawn after 24 h (n = 10), 6.) 100 PSI Trauma blood sample drawn after 48 h (n = 5) 7.) Sham operated blood samples drawn directly after craniotomy (n = 4), 8.) Sham operated blood sample drawn after 6 h (n = 4) and 9.) Sham operated blood sample drawn after 48 h (n = 2). Traumatic brain injury was induced using a controlled cortical impact (Cci) device as described in detail by Dixon *et al.* 1991. The Cci device was adjusted so that the piston velocity was 7 m/s with a PSI of 100 and 2 mm deformation thereby inducing a severe level of injury. Sham operated animals underwent the same surgical manipulations as the animals in the traumatic brain injury group with the exception of inflicting cortical injury.

Blood samples were drawn under anesthetic conditions as described above by direct puncture of the left ventricel of the heart. The blood sample was allowed to clot for 20 minutes at room temperature and centrifugated at 4000 rounds per minute for 10 minutes. Serum was frozen until analyzation at a temperature of −40 °C. The animals were sacrifized after the blood samples were drawn.

Table 1. *NSE Mean Serum Levels and Range at the Different Studied Time Points in µg/l*

Blood sample	Direct	1 h Post trauma	6 h Post trauma	12 h Post trauma	24 h Post trauma	48 h Post trauma	Sham group
Mean	10.6[1]	28.45	31.5[2]	23.47	22.1	17.56	8.82[3]
Std. Dev.	2.66	13.5	7.2	10.98	9.77	13.4	2.96
Std. Error	0.84	4.27	2.28	3.47	3.1	5.99	0.94
Min.	6.5	14.5	20.6	11.95	9.82	7.61	3.3
Max.	13.8	53.87	41.15	41.51	40.89	40.51	13.7
Count	10	10	10	10	10	5	10

[1] $p < 0.005$ compared to NSE values after 1 h, 12 h, 24 h; $p < 0.0001$ compared to NSE values after 6 h.
[2] $p < 0.05$ compared to NSE values after 24 h.
[3] $p < 0.0005$ compared to NSE values after 1 h; $p < 0.0001$ compared to NSE values after 6 h. [3] $p < 0.005$ compared to NSE values after 12 h and 24 h.

Serum samples were analyzed with a commercial available light immuno assay (LIA-mat® NSE Prohifigen®, Byk-Sangtec Diagnostica GmbH & Co. KG, Dietzenbach, Germany).

Statistical analysis was performed using the StatView® computer programme version 4.5 including the t-test. The statistical significance was determined at a level of $p < 0.05$.

Results

The control animals showed a NSE serum level of 8.82 µg/l (mean, n = 10). Directly after trauma the NSE serum level had increased to 10.6 µg/l, 1 hour later the concentration had risen to 28.45 µg/l, 6 hours after trauma to 31.5 µg/l. After 12 and 24 hours the concentration decreased to 23.47 µg/l and 22.1 µg/l (mean, each group n = 10). After 2 days the NSE concentration dropped to 17.56 µg/l (mean, n = 5). The NSE levels of the control and direct group differed significantly from the 1, 6, 12 and 24 hour groups (t-test, see also Table 1).

Discussion

Uzan studied NSE serum levels in spraque dawley rats three hours after traumatic brain injury induced with a weight drop model [16]. He found no correlation of NSE serumlevels to the severity of trauma and no difference between the trauma and the sham group [16]. But he did find an elevated NSE level in the liquor 7.5 hours after severe traumatic brain injury. Uzan states that NSE serum levels are not useful to monitor traumatic brain injury.

We used the cortical impact model to induce traumatic brain injury. We demonstrated a time dependent release of NSE into the serum after trauma. The highest NSE serum values were found six hours after trauma. There was no second increase of the serum levels up to 48 hours after trauma.

Our results are in accordance with the immunohistochemical findings of Li *et al.*. They found a reduced immunoreactivity of NSE 1 to 2 hours after trauma at the impact side, and 4 to 6 hours after trauma almost all neurons had lost their NSE immunoreactivity [10]. Directly after trauma we could not detect a significantly elevated NSE serum level. Six hours after trauma we found the highest NSE serum levels reflecting neuronal cell death found by Li *et al.* (10). Because Uzan investigated the NSE serum level only at three hours after trauma, where he found no elevation, he probably failed to detect the highest serum level after trauma [16]. Furthermore he employed the use of a weight drop model producing a more diffuse trauma without a direct trauma to the cortex as is produced in the cortical impact model [16].

In different clinical studies the NSE serum level did not correlate to clinical assessment and outcome after traumatic brain injury. According to the literature and our experimental results it can be concluded that the NSE serum level seems to reflect only the direct neuronal damage after traumatic brain injury in a time dependent manner. However clinical outcome after traumatic brain injury is dependent on glial and neuronal damage. This fact could explain the clinical failure of the NSE serum level to be of prognostic value, because this marker seems not reflect the overall brain damage in the clinical setting.

Conclusions

NSE serum level seems to reflect neuronal damage after cortical contusion in the rat in a time dependent manner.

References

1. Dixon CE, Clifton GL, Lightball JW, Yaghami AA, Hyes RL (1991) A controlled cortical impact model of traumatic brain injury in the rat. J Neurosci Meth 39: 253–262
2. Fagnart OC, Sindic ChJM, Laterre Ch (1988) Practical counting immunassay of S100 protein in serum. Possible relevance in tumors and ischemic disorders of the central nervous system. Clin Chem 34/7: 1387–1391
3. Fassbender K, Schmidt R, Schreiner A, Fatar M, Mühlhauser F, Daffertshofer M, Hennerici M (1997) Leakage of brain-originated proteins in peripheral blood: temporal profile and diagnostic value in early ischemic stroke. J Neurol Sci 148: 101–105
4. Hardemark HG, Almquist O, Johansson T, Pahlmann S, Persson L (1989) S-100B protein in cerebrospinal fluid after aneurysmal subarachnoid hemorrhage. Acta Neurochir (Wien) 99: 135–144
5. Hardemark, HG, Ericsson, N, Kotwica, Z, Rundstrom, G, Mendel, HI, Olsson, Y, Pahlman, S, Persson, L (1989) S-100B protein and neuron-specific enolase in CSF after experimental traumatic or focal ischemic brain damage. J Neurosurg 71: 727–731
6. Ingebrigsten T, Romner B, Kongstad P, Langbrakk B (1995) Increased serum concentrations of protein S-100B after minor head injury: a biochemical serum marker with prognostic value? J Neurol Psychiatry 59: 103–104
7. Ingebrigsten T, Romner B, Trumpy JH (1997) Management of minor head injury: the value of early computed tomography and serum protein S-100B measurements. J Clin Neurosci 4: 29–33
8. Ingebrigtsen T, Rommer B (1996) Serial S-100B protein measurements related to early magnetic resonance imaging after minor head injury. J Neurosurg 85: 945–948
9. Johnson P, Lundqvist Ch, Lindgren A, Ferencz I, Alling Ch, Ståhl E (1995) Cerebral complications after cardiac surgery assessed by S-100B and NSE levels in blood. J Cardiothor Vasc Anesth 9: 694–699
10. Li R, Fujitani N, Jia JT, Kimuta H (1998) Immunihistochemical indicators of early brain injury: an experimental study using the fluid-percussion model in cats. Rhe Am J Forensic Med Pathol 19: 129–136
11. Missler U, Wiesmann M, Friedrich Ch, Kaps M (1997) S-100B protein and neuron-specific enolase concentrations in blood as indicators of infarction volume and prognosis in acute ischemic stroke. Stroke 28: 1956–1960
12. Raabe A, Grolms C, Keller M, Döhnert J, Sorge O, Seifert V (1998) Corelation of computed tomography findings and serum brain damage markers following severe head injury. Acta Neurochir (Wien) 140: 787–792
13. Ross SA, Cunningham RT, Johnston CF, Rowlands BJ (1996) Neuron-specific enolase as an aid to outcome prediction in head injury. Brit J Neurosurg 10: 471–476
14. Rothoerl RD, Woertgen C, Holzschuh M, Metz C, Brawanski A (1998) S-100B serum levels after minor and severe head injury. J Trauma 45: 765–767
15. Skogseid LM, Nordby HK, Urdal P, Paus E, Lilleaas F (1992) Increased Sserum creatine kinase BB ans neuron specific enolase following head injury indicates brain damage. Acta Neurochir (Wien) 115: 106–111
16. Uzan M, Hanci M, Güzel Ö, Sarioglu AC, Kuday C, Özlen F, Kaynar MY (1995) The significance of neuron specific enolase levels in cerebrospinal fluid and serum after experimental brain damage. Acta Neurochir (Wien) 135: 141–143
17. Westaby St, Johnson P, Parry AJ, Blomqvist St, Solem JO, Alling Ch, Pillai R, Taggart DP, Grebenik C, Ståhl E (1996) Serum S100 protein: a potential marker for cerebral events during cardiopulmonary bypass. Ann Thorac Surg 61: 88–92
18. Wiesmann M, Missler U, Hagenström H, Gottmann D (1997) S-100B Protein Plasma Levels after Aneurysmal Subarachnoidal Haemorrhage, Acta Neurochir (Wien) 139: 1155–1160
19. Woertgen C, Rothoerl RD, Holzschuh M, Metz C, Brawanski A (1997) Comparison of serial S-100B and NSE serum measurements after severe head injury. Acta Neurochir (Wien) 139: 1161–1165

Correspondence: Chris Woertgen M.D., Department of Neurosurgery, University of Regensburg, Franz-Josef-Strauss Allee 11, 93053 Regensburg, Germany.

Acta Neurochir (2000) [Suppl] 76: 375–378

Isoflurane Doubles Plasma Glutamate and Increases Posttraumatic Brain Edema

J. F. Stover[1], **S. N. Kroppenstedt**[1], **U. W. Thomale**[1], **O. S. Kempski**[2], and **A. W. Unterberg**[1]

[1] Department of Neurosurgery, Berlin, Germany
[2] Institute for Neurosurgical Pathophysiology, Mainz, Germany

Summary

Increased plasma and cerebral glutamate levels may contribute to posttraumatic edema formation. Since volatile anesthetics elevate plasma amino acid concentrations, the influence of isoflurane on arterial plasma glutamate levels and brain edema formation was investigated in brain-injured rats. Rats were anesthetized with chloral hydrate (380 mg/kg i.p.) or isoflurane (1.2–2.0 vol%) for four hours following controlled cortical impact injury. Isoflurane significantly increased arterial glutamate levels compared to chloral hydrate (124 ± 12 vs. 60 ± 5 μM; $p < 0.005$). At eight hours after trauma, water content was significantly increased in the traumatized hemisphere compared to the non-traumatized side ($p < 0.005$). In addition, four hours of isoflurane anesthesia caused a significant increase in brain water content of both hemispheres compared to chloral hydrate (80.1 ± 0.1 vs. 79.6 ± 0.1%; $p < 0.005$). Prolonged isoflurane anesthesia is associated with a significant increase in arterial plasma glutamate levels and brain water content. This increase in brain water content must be considered when performing prolonged isoflurane anesthesia.

Keywords: Brain edema; controlled cortical impact injury; glutamate; isoflurane.

Introduction

Apart from its physiological role in neuronal excitation, glutamate may induce glial and neuronal damage. Tightly regulated energy-dependent uptake mechanisms are required to maintain low cerebral extracellular glutamate levels and to prevent cellular damage and possibly cell death [14]. Under physiological conditions free access of plasma glutamate to the central nervous system is controlled by the blood-brain barrier [14].

Under pathological conditions, however, plasma glutamate levels have been shown to cross the damaged blood-brain barrier [9] and increase brain edema [7]. Selective glutamate-receptor antagonists could prevent evolving tissue damage [21] which underlines the importance of plasma glutamate within the pathophysiology of brain edema formation.

Volatile anesthetics as applied in clinical routine have been shown to reversibly increase plasma concentrations of essential and non-essential amino acids [6]. In a previous study we were able to show a significant doubling in plasma and cerebrospinal fluid glutamate levels in electively craniotomized neurosurgical patients during isoflurane anesthesia [18].

Based on these findings we investigated the influence of isoflurane on arterial plasma glutamate levels and brain edema formation in rats following traumatic brain injury mimicking the clinical situation in which anesthesia is performed approximately four hours after injury and maintained as long as four hours.

Materials and Methods

Anesthesia

All spontaneously breathing rats were first anesthetized with chloral hydrate for 30 minutes (360 mg/kg body weight i.p.) to cannulate the right femoral artery and assess basal blood values. Thereafter, anesthesia was switched to 1.2–2.0 vol% isoflurane in a 2:1 gas mixture of N_2O/O_2 under which trephination and induction of trauma were performed. Immediately after trauma scalp incision was closed, arterial lines were removed, isoflurane anesthesia was stopped, and rats were returned to their cages.

Four hours after trauma, animals were randomly assigned to receive either isoflurane (group 1) (1.2–2.0 vol%) or chloral hydrate (group 2) (360 mg/kg i.p.) for a period of four hours. All rats received new arterial lines. Thereafter, rats were positioned in a stereotaxic holder and a Codman ICP microsensor (Johnson & Johnson Medical Ltd. Berkshire, United Kingdom) was inserted with a micromanipulator to a depth of 6 mm in the contralateral parietal region. Rectal temperature was kept between 37° and 38 °C using a heating pad. Mean arterial blood pressure (MABP), intracranial pressure (ICP), cerebral perfusion pressure (CPP) and rectal temperature were recorded continuously during the entire study.

Arterial blood samples were drawn 30 minutes after administration of chloral hydrate, and 30 minutes after induction of isoflurane anesthesia. During four hours of anesthesia arterial samples were drawn at 30, 120, and 240 minutes.

Trauma

In 20 male Sprague-Dawley rats (250–350 g) a controlled cortical contusion to the left temporoparietal cortex was induced as described previously [10]. In brief, after positioning the head of the rat in a stereotaxic frame a 10-mm-diameter craniotomy was performed on the left side of the skull within the anatomical boundaries as outlined by the lambdoid, sagittal, coronal sutures and the cygomatic arch. The impactor tip (diameter of 8 mm) was centered in the craniotomy at an angle of 30 degrees to the vertical. The tip was lowered until it touched the dura. Thereafter, the impactor rod was retracted and the tip was advanced an additional 2 mm to produce a brain penetration of 2 mm. Velocity and impact duration were set at 7 m/sec (100 p.s.i) and 300 msec, respectively.

Determination of Brain Swelling and Hemispheric Water Content

Immediately after four hours of anesthesia rats were sacrificed by exsanguination. Upon removal of the brains the hemispheres were dissected along the interhemispherical line under a microscope. Both hemispheres were weighted to assess wet weight (WW) and to determine brain swelling (brain swelling [%]: $WW_{traumatized\ hemisphere} - WW_{non\text{-}traumatized\ hemsiphere}/WW_{non\text{-}traumatized} \times 100$). Thereafter, the hemispheres were dried for 24 hours at 104 °C to determine dry weight (DW). Based on wet and dry weight water contents of both, the traumatized and non-traumatized hemispheres were calculated: water content [%] = (WW-DW) WW × 100.

Analysis of Plasma Amino Acids

Amino acids were analyzed by high performance liquid chromatography (HPLC) using ortho-phthaldialdehyd pre-column derivatisation and fluorescence detection [19].

Statistical analysis

Results are presented as mean ± SEM. Parameters were compared for significant differences within the groups using one-way analysis of variances (ANOVA), and between the two groups using Student's *t*-test. Differences were rated significant at $p < 0.05$.

Results

Arterial Plasma Amino Acid Levels

Arterial plasma glutamate levels were significantly and reversibly increased during isoflurane anesthesia compared to chloral hydrate (Table 1). By four hours after stopping isoflurane anesthesia glutamate decreased, reaching basal glutamate levels as measured during initial administration of chloral hydrate (Table 1). Second administration of isoflurane resulted in a further significant increase in plasma glutamate levels exceeding those of the initial isoflurane anesthesia.

In addition, arterial plasma taurine, asparagine, and serine concentrations were also significantly increased while glutamine, aspartate, methionine, alanine, and lysine remained unchanged (Table 1).

Hemispheric Water Content and Brain Swelling

Following traumatic brain injury water content of the traumatized (left) hemisphere was significantly increased compared to the non-traumatized hemisphere in all rats. In addition, four hours of isoflurane anesthesia resulted in a further significant increase in water content of both hemispheres compared to rats receiving chloral hydrate (Table 2). Brain swelling tended to be increased after four hours of isoflurane anesthesia compared to chloral hydrate (Table 2).

MABP, ICP, CPP

MABP and CPP were maintained at stable values during the entire study period in all rats (Table 1). MABP remained between 78 and 90 mmHg. ICP was significantly increased during isoflurane anesthesia compared to chloral hydrate (mean: 6.5 ± 0.5 vs. $4.4 \pm 0.4\%$; $p < 0.05$). CPP was identical during isoflurane and chloral hydrate anesthesia, ranging from 74 to 86 mmHg (Table 1).

Discussion

Arterial plasma glutamate levels were significantly and reversibly increased during isoflurane anesthesia. After traumatic brain injury, four hours of isoflurane anesthesia was associated with significantly increased water content of the traumatized and non-traumatized hemisphere. Similar doubling in plasma glutamate levels were found to significantly increase brain edema formation in a focal cryogenic lesion [7].

Increases in plasma amino acid levels seems to be an unspecific effect related to diminished organ perfusion [5], sustained release [6] or attenuated renal elimination [13]. Under normal conditions, plasma glutamate concentrations exceed those within the cerebral extracellular space by a ten-fold [14]. This passive gradient directed from plasma towards the extracellular space is balanced by an anatomically and physiologically intact blood-brain barrier. Under pathological conditions with a damaged blood-brain barrier plasma glutamate levels will flood the extracelluar space [9], compromising brain homeostasis and putting neuronal

Table 1. *Changes in Arterial Plasma Glutamate, Lactate, and Hypoxanthine Levels, ICP and CPP Values Determined at Different Time Points During Isoflurane and Chloral Hydrate Anesthesia. Differences Within (#) and Between the Groups (§) are Rated Significant at $p < 0.05$*

	Trephination, trauma				Anesthesia, four hours after trauma					
	Chloral hydrate (n = 20) (360 mg/kg i.p.)		Isoflurane (n = 20) (mean: 1.4 ± 0.05 vol%)		Isoflurane (n = 10) (mean: 1.7 ± 0.1 vol%) group 1			Chloral hydrate (n = 10) (360 mg/kg i.p.) group 2		
	Group 1	Group 2	Group 1	Group 2	30 Minutes	120 Minutes	240 Minutes	30 Minutes	120 Minutes	240 Minutes
Glutamate [µM]	63 ± 5	68 ± 4	87 ± 4 #	79 ± 5 #	124 ± 12§	122 ± 8§	121 ± 8§	68 ± 8	61 ± 6	71 ± 6
Asparagine [µM]	100 ± 6	101 ± 5	114 ± 5	112 ± 6	127 ± 9 #§	152 ± 8 #§	156 ± 9 #§	93 ± 7	104 ± 12	112 ± 13
Serine [µM]	240 ± 20	220 ± 10	320 ± 10 #	270 ± 12 #	330 ± 20 #§	360 ± 10 #§	380 ± 15 #§	230 ± 20	240 ± 20	280 ± 20
Taurine [µM]	350 ± 40	340 ± 60	510 ± 30 #	500 ± 40	510 ± 40 #§	600 ± 50 #§	510 ± 30 #§	350 ± 20	370 ± 40	410 ± 40
Glutamine [µM]	550 ± 50	551 ± 8	540 ± 10	580 ± 12	550 ± 30	600 ± 50	600 ± 20	560 ± 10	580 ± 20	550 ± 30
Aspartate [µM]	11 ± 0.7	12 ± 0.5	12 ± 0.6	12 ± 0.4	13.3 ± 1.3	14.3 ± 1.8	14.7 ± 2.0	11.4 ± 1.0	12.6 ± 0.7	12.7 ± 0.8
Methionine [µM]	42 ± 2	40 ± 4	42 ± 1	43 ± 2	38 ± 4	39 ± 5	46 ± 4	40 ± 2	44 ± 3	48 ± 3
Alanine [µM]	558 ± 39	560 ± 40	662 ± 45	612 ± 30	409 ± 51	547 ± 75	641 ± 64	436 ± 34	613 ± 47	651 ± 52
Lysine [µM]	190 ± 14	194 ± 12	214 ± 11	212 ± 10	195 ± 11	186 ± 14	203 ± 19	174 ± 23	154 ± 18	187 ± 19
MABP [mm Hg]	88 ± 2	83 ± 1	85 ± 1	84 ± 1	87 ± 2	84 ± 2	80 ± 2	82 ± 2	83 ± 2	85 ± 2
ICP [mm Hg]	not determined		not determined		7.5 ± 0.6§	6.3 ± 0.4§	5.6 ± 0.5§	5.3 ± 0.6	4.4 ± 0.4	3.6 ± 0.3
CPP [mm Hg]	not determined		not determined		80 ± 1.3	78 ± 1.5	79 ± 1.4	77 ± 2.0	79 ± 2.1	81 ± 2.0

Table 2. *Changes in Hemispheric Water Content and Brain Swelling in Rats After Four Hours of Isoflurane and Chloral Hydrate Anesthesia. Differences in Hemispheric Water Contents Between Traumatized and Non-Traumatized Hemispheres (#) and Between Rats Anesthetized with Isoflurane and Chloral Hydrate (§) are Significant at $p < 0.05$*

	Hemispheric water content [%]		Brain swelling [%]
	Traumatized hemisphere	Non-traumatized hemisphere	
Isoflurane (n = 10)	80.1 ± 0.1 #,§	79.5 ± 0.1§	7.9 ± 1.1
Chloral hydrate (n = 10)	79.6 ± 0.1 #	79.2 ± 0.2	6.8 ± 0.9

and glial viability at stake [14]. In addition to its neurotoxic effects glutamate is known to also induce glial swelling [14], resulting in cytotoxic edema formation which, in turn, aggravates vasogenic edema.

As shown in several studies the brain is highly susceptible to secondary insults within the first eight hours following focal traumatic brain injury [4]. Evolving vasogenic [1, 20] and cytotoxic [20] brain edema is among other causes related to reduced pericontusional perfusion [3], increased formation of microthrombosis [12], sustained release of glutamate [15], and energetic perturbation as reflected by mitochondrial dysfunction [22] and increased extracelluar hypoxanthine levels [2]. Taken together possible damaging effects associated with prolonged isoflurane-induced increases in arterial plasma glutamate levels appear to confront a highly susceptible brain in this early vulnerable posttraumatic phase.

Increased hemispherical water content is accepted to reflect brain edema formation. The present findings are highly suggestive that increased arterial plasma glutamate levels could mediate, at least in part, some of the adverse effects leading to the significant increase in hemispherical water content during the four hour period of isoflurane anesthesia. Significantly increased water content of the non-traumatized hemisphere compared to chloral hydrate anesthesia cannot be explained by the present study design. These increases are not related to hemodynamic instability, hypoxia or contralateral blood-brain barrier damage since CPP was kept between 75 and 85 mm Hg, arterial blood gases remained within physiological limits, and extravasation of Evans Blue is only seen in the ipsilateral hemisphere [1, 20]. The hypothesis that sustained glutamate-mediated neuronal excitation persists during isoflurane anesthesia is strengthened by the facts that isoflurane (1–1.5 vol%) fails to influence brain metabolism despite depressed electroencephalographic activity [8] and that blocking of glutamate receptors significantly decreases cerebral oxygen consumption during isoflurane anesthesia [11]. Furthermore, volatile anesthetics are believed to cause conformational changes within the lipid bi-layer, consequently influencing receptor function and causing ionic derangement [17]. This, in turn, could result in cellular swelling and brain edema formation as shown by others [16, 17] and as described in the present study.

Apart from glutamate-mediated brain edema formation the observed elevated ICP during isoflurane anesthesia could be influenced by isoflurane-induced vasodilation which is suggested to contribute to posttraumatic edema formation [17].

Based on these results, the anesthetic regimen needs to be chosen carefully when investigating brain edema formation in experimental studies. It appears as if prolonged isoflurane anesthesia could negatively influence anticipated investigations. When transferred to the clinical situation, these data suggest that prolonged anesthesia with isoflurane should be avoided in the early phase following traumatic brain injury. Whether the increased plasma glutamate levels mediate the increased brain edema formation warrants further investigation.

References

1. Baskaya MK, Rao AM, Dogan A, Donaldson D, Dempsey RJ (1997) The biphasic opening of the blood-brain barrier in the cortex and hippocampus after traumatic brain injury in rats. Neurosci Lett 226: 33–36
2. Bell MJ, Kochanek PK, Carcillo JA, Mi Z, Schiding JK, Wisniewski SR, Clark RSB, Dixon CE, Marion DW, Jackson E (1998) Interstitial adenosine, inosine, and hypoxanthine are increased after experimental traumatic brain injury in the rat. J Neurotrauma 15: 163–170
3. Bryan RM, Cherian L, Roberston C (1995) Regional cerebral blood flow after controlled cortical impact injury in rats. Anesth Analg 80: 687–695
4. Cherian L, Robertson CS, Goodman JC (1996) Secondary insults increase injury after controlled cortical impact in rats. J Neurotrauma 13: 371–383
5. Gelman S, Fowler K, Smith L (1983) Cardiac output distribution and regional blood flow during isoflurane anesthesia. Anesthesiology 59: A68 (abstract)
6. Horber FF, Krayer S, Haymond MW (1988) Anesthesia with halothane and nitrous oxide alters protein and amino acid metabolism in dogs. Anesthesiology 69: 319–326
7. Kempski O, van Adrian U, Schürer L, Baethmann A (1990) Intravenous glutamate enhances edema formation after a freezing lesion. Adv Neurol 52: 219–222
8. Kochs E, Hoffman WE, Werner C, Albrecht RF, Schulte am Esch J (1993) Cerebral blood flow velocity in relation to cerebral blood flow, cerebral metabolic rate for oxygen, and electroencephalographam activity during isoflurane anesthesia. Anesth Analg 76: 1222–1226
9. Koizumi H, Fujisawa H, Ito H, Maekawa T, Di X, Bullock R (1997) Effects of mild hypothermia on cerebral blood flow-independent changes in cortical extracellular levels of amino acids following contusion trauma in the rat. Brain Res 747: 304–312
10. Kroppenstedt SN, Schneider G-H, Thomale U-W, Unterberg A.W (1998) Protective effects of Aptiganel Hcl (Cerestat®) following controlled cortical impact injury in the rat. J Neurotrauma 15: 191–197
11. Lu X, Sinha AK, Weiss HR (1997) Effects of excitatory amino acids on cerebral oxygen consumption and blood flow in rat. Neurochem Res 22: 705–711
12. Maeda T, Katayama Y, Kawamata T, Aoyamma N, Mori T (1997) Hemodynamic depression and microthrombosis in the peripheral areas of cortical contusion in the rat: role of platelet activating factor. Acta Neurochir [Suppl] (Wien) 70: 102–105
13. Mazze RI, Cousins MJ, Barr GA (1972) Renal effects and metabolism of isoflurane in man. Anesthesiology 40: 536–542
14. Obrenovitch TP, Urenjak J (1997) Altered glutamatergic transmission in neurological disorders: from high extracellular glutamate to excessive synaptic efficacy. Prog Neurobiol 51: 39–87
15. Palmer AM, Marion DW, Botscheller ML, Swedlow PE, Styren SD, DeKosky ST (1993) Traumatic brain injury-induced excitotoxicity assessed in a controlled cortical impact model. J Neurochem 61: 2015–2024
16. Schettini A, Furniss WW (1977) Brain water and electrolyte distribution during the inhalation of halothane. Br J Anaesth 51: 1117–1124
17. Smith AL, Marque JJ (1976) Anesthetics and cerebral edema. Anesthesiology 45: 64–72
18. Stover JF, Kempski OS (1996) Glutamate levels in CSF and plasma are elevated during neuroanesthesia. J Neurosurg Anesthesiol 9: 96
19. Stover JF, Morganti-Kossmann MC, Lenzlinger PM, Stocker R, Kempski OS, Kossmann T (1999) Glutamate and taurine are increased in ventricular cerebrospinal fluid of severely brain-injured patients. J Neurotrauma 16: 135–142
20. Unterberg AW, Stroop R, Thomale U-W, Kiening KL, Päuser S, Vollmann W (1997) Characterization of brain edema following "controlled cortical impact injury" in rats. Acta Neurochir [Suppl] (Wien) 70: 106–108
21. Westergren I, Johansson BB (1983) Blockade of AMPA receptors reduces brain edema after opening of the blood-brain barrier. J Cereb Blood Flow Metab 33: 603–608
22. Xiong Y, Gu Q, Peterson PL, Muizelaar JP, Lee CP (1997) Mitochondrial dysfunction and calcium perturbation induced by traumatic brain injury. J Neurotrauma 14: 23–34

Correspondence: John F. Stover, M.D., Department of Neurosurgery, Charité-Virchow Medical Center, Augstenburger Platz 01, D-13353 Berlin.

Acta Neurochir (2000) [Suppl] 76: 379–383

Mechanical Injury Alters Volume Activated Ion Channels in Cortical Astrocytes

X. Di, P. B. Goforth, R. Bullock, E. Ellis, and **L. Satin**

Division of Neurosurgery, Medical College of Virginia, Virginia Commonwealth University, Virginia, USA

Summary

Although astrocytic swelling is likely to mediate brain edema and high ICP after traumatic brain injury, the mechanism is not understood. We employed whole cell patch clamp electrophysiology and a stretch injury model to understand whether volume regulating ion currents are altered following cell injury. Mixed rat astrocytes and neurons were co-cultured on deformable silastic membranes. Mild-moderate cell injury was produced using a timed pulse of pressurized air to deform the silastic substrates by 6.5 mm. Then, ion currents were recorded with patch clamp methods. Cells were held at −65 mV and were stepped to +10 mV to monitor current changes.

Results: In unstretched astrocytes, small amplitude currents were obtained under isotonic conditions. Hypotonic solution activated an outwardly-rectifying current which reversed near −40 mV. This current resembled a previously reported anion current whose activation may restore cell volume by mediating a net solute efflux. In contrast, stretch injured cells exhibited a large amplitude, non-rectifying current. This current was not due to non-specific ionic leakage, since it was fully suppressed by the cation channel blocker gadolinium. Activation of novel stretch-activated cation currents may exacerbate cell swelling in injured astrocytes. Stretch injured astrocytes thus express a dysfunctional cation current as opposed to an osmoregulatory anion current. This mechanism, if present in vivo, may contribute to the cytotoxic swelling seen after traumatic brain injury.

Keywords: Whole cell patch clamp; ion channel; astrocyte; brain edema.

Introduction

Up to eighty percent (80%) of patients who die while under medical care following traumatic brain injury will do so due to raised intracranial pressure, (ICP) secondary to brain swelling within the first few days. Swelling of brain astrocytes probably plays the major role in overall brain swelling, since they play the major role in buffering ionic shifts. Astrocyte swelling, and concomitantly an inability to compensate for osmotic stresses, may contribute to overall brain edema and elevated ICP, as observed after trauma. This is supported by our recent observation that cytotoxic, not vasogenic edema is the major determinant of brain swelling in TBI.

Head injury, as studied both clinically and using in vivo animal models, is associated with widespread cortical depolarization and rapid increase in extracellular glutamate, other neurotransmitters, and potassium [2, 7]. These early post impact ionic shifts may be an important factor, to determine raised ICP and subsequent outcome [3]. Chloride ion channels exist in virtually all mammalian cells [6, 13]. Their relationship with astrocytic swelling have never been reported even though numerous studies of Cl- fluxes have shown permeability changes for Cl- in response to changes in other ions. Consequently, astrocytes have acquired an important role in "buffering" these ion shifts especially K^+, and they do so by volume change [8]

In the present study, we have studied the response of single astrocytes to quantifiable mechanical perturbation, especially with regards to the electrophysiology of astrocyte ion channels. We employed patch clamp techniques in control and stretched cells to test the hypotheses that membrane stretch injury alters the swelling-activated ion currents of astrocytes, and that injury thus modifies cell volume regulation in the face of osmotic stress.

Methods and Materials

Cell Culture

Primary cultures were prepared from 1- 2-day-old Zivic-Miller rats. Neocortices were minced in saline and then trypsinized (0.125%) for 10 min at 37C. Tissue then was transferred to culture medium containing Dulbecco's modified essential medium (DMEM) containing 4.5 g/l glucose supplemented with 10% fetal bovine serum, 100 U/ml penicillin and 100 ug/ml streptomycin (P/S), and 2 mM 1-glutamine. Tissue was washed and dispersed by trituration through Pasteur pipettes of successively smaller diameters. The resulting suspension was centrifuged for 10 min. The pellet was resuspended in culture medium and washed. The final suspension was filtered through a hylon Nitex sieve with a pore size of 88 μm. Cells were counted and plated at a density of 106 cells per well in six-well Flex plates (Flexcell International, McKeesport, PA). The bottom of each well consisted of a 25-mm diameter and 2-mm thick silastic membrane. Silastic membranes were collagen-coated before plating cells. Plates were incubated at 37C in a 95%–5% mixture of air/carbon dioxide, with 95% humidity. Culture medium was replaced with growth medium (DMEM, 30 mM glucose, P/S, and 5% horse serum) 2–3 days after plating and cultures were fed twice weekly. And then subsequently twice each week, the medium was changed to fresh growth medium that contained only 10% newborn calf serum. Cultures were confluent after 2 weeks and were examined electrophysiologically between 2 and 3 weeks, in vitro. More than 90% of the cells stain positively for GFAP using an immunoperoxidase procedure.

Delivery of Injury

Injury was delivered by use of a model 94A cell injury controller (Commonwealth Biotechnology, Richmond, VA) as previously reported [5]. This controller allowed pressure pulses of varying amplitude and duration to be applied to individual wells of the Flex Plates. A single 50-ms pressure pulse was used in all experiments. The stretched silastic membrane returned to its resting position within 250 ms of its initial movement toward maximum deformation. The amplitude was set to deform the silastic membrane 6.3 mm (corresponding to 38% stretch). Cells were stretched in culture medium or normal external solution. After injury, cells were washed 3 times with standard external solution and ready for the patch clamp. Drugs were made up as a concentrated stock solution and were diluted as required in external solution.

Electrophysiology

Whole cell patch clamps technique was used to measure Cl- current. Electrodes were made from borosilicate capillaries using a two-stage puller. Pipette and seal resistances ranged from 5 to 20 MΩ and 2 to 20 MΩ, respectively, capacitance and series resistance were compensated. A flowing KCl junction (FlexRef, World Precision Instruments, Sarasota, FL) was used as a reference electrode. Cells were voltage clamped at −65 mV. I_{cl} was isolated from other current using an external solution containing 115 mmol/l NaCl 3 mmol/l CaCl2, 5 mmol/l CsCl, 1 mmol/l MgCl2, 10 mmol/l tetraethylammonium (TEA)-Cl, 10 mmol/l HEPES, 5 × 10 −4 mmol/l tetrodotoxin (TTX, and 11.1 mmol/l glucose, pH 7.2 (274 ± 5 mOsm). Patch pipettes contained 114 mmol/l Cs-aspartate, 10 mmol/l CsCl, 2 Mg2ATP, 20 mmol/l HEPES, 10 mmol/l 4-aminopyridine (4-AP), and 1 mmol/l EGTA, pH 7.2 (269 ± 5 mOsm; isotonic with external solution). In all experiments, 0.2 mmol/l CdCl was added to the external solution to block Ca2+ current. Na+ currents were blocked by TTX, and K+ current were blocked by internal ATP, 4-AP, Cs+, and external TEA+. Thus, the remaining current should be mainly carried by anions. Hypotonic solution (223 ± 3 mOsm) was identical to the control solution, except NaCl was reduced 25% from 115 to 86.3 mmol/l. Hypertonic solution 305 mOsm) was made by adding 75 mmol/l sucrose to the hypotonic solution. The low Cl- hypotonic solution (210 mOsm) had the following composition: 91.3 mmol/l Na-aspartate, 3 mmol/l CaCl2, 1 mmol/l MgCl2, 10 mmol/l TEA-Cl, 10 mmol/l HEPES, 5 × 10 −4 mmol/l TTX, and 11.1 mmol/l glucose, pH 7.2. The liquid junction potential between the low Cl-CsAsp internal solution and high Cl- external solution was +8 mV. All chemicals were obtained from Sigma.

A 16-bit hardware interface (Instrutech, Elmont, NY) and Igor-Pro software (Wavemetrics, Lake Oswego, OR) were used with a Macintosh Quadra *00 computer to generate current-voltage (I–V) and monitoring test pulses and to digitize membrane currents at 5 kHz. Currents were filtered at 2 kHz before sampling. Software was provided by R. Bookman and J. Herrington of the University of Miami, Miami, FL. Pulse-evoked currents were analyzed as in Satin and Cook [14, 15].

Results

Control cortical astrocyte current was recorded using whole cell patch clamp methods and held at −65 mV. In isotonic external solution, a background outwardly-rectifying current was observed with basal current at near −150 pA at −120 mV, and +500 pA at +50 mV (Fig. 1). In marked contrast to control cells, astrocytes stretch-injured with a 6.5 mm deformation pulse showed markedly different responses to hypotonic solution within 15 minutes of injury. The application of hypotonic solution activated an outward current at +10 mV but the current-voltage characteristics of this current revealed not the outwardly-rectifying current seen in the control cells but rather a linear current which reversed near −15 mV instead of near −40 mV. This current was also much larger, e.g. −400 pA at −120 mV, and >+2000 pA at +50 mV in the hypotonic solution (Fig. 2). In addition, the application of the stretch-activated channel blocker gadolinium (30 uM) in hypotonic solution after the linear current was activated, *fully blocked* all, inward current (Fig. 3). The effect of stretch injury on hypotonically activated I_{cl} amplitude at +50 mV was thus significantly increased when compared with that of control astrocytes. A significant difference in peak amplitude was seen as determined using Student's *t* test (*p < 0.001) (Fig. 4).

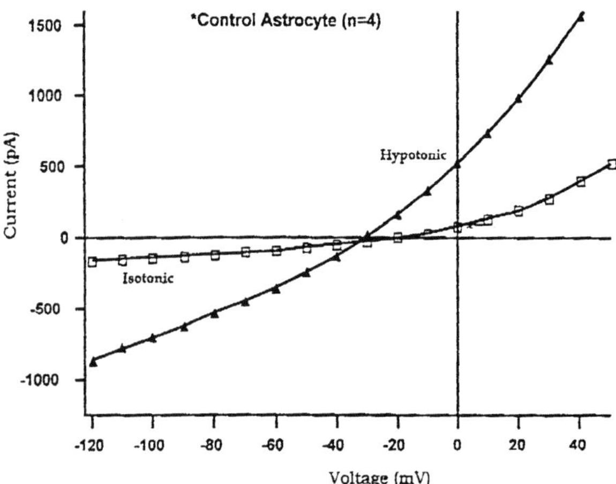

Fig. 1. Effect of hypotonic and isotonil external solutions upon current/voltage relationship, in control astrocytes.

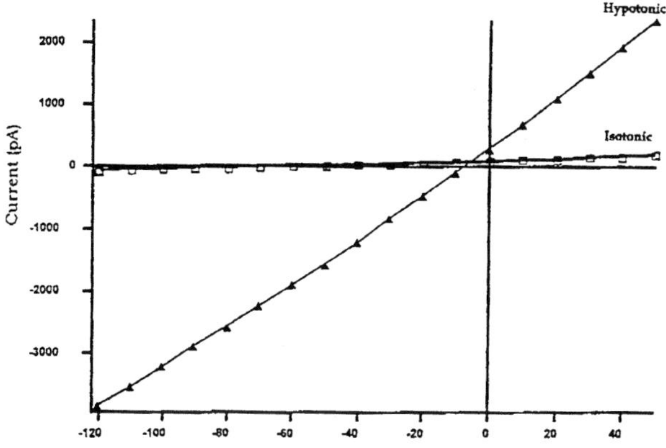

Fig. 2.

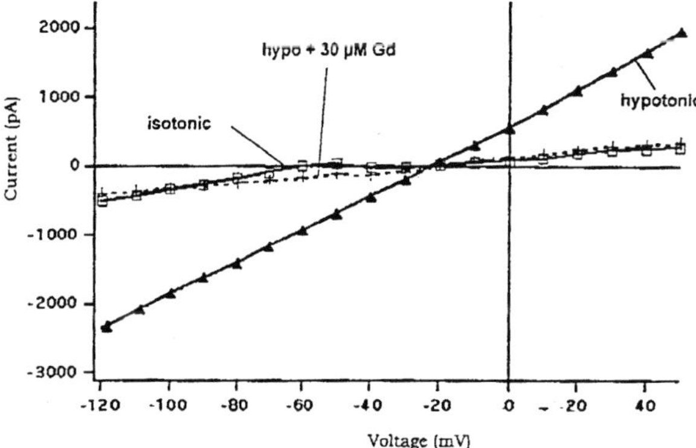

Fig. 3. Effect of hypotonic and isotonic external solutions upon current/voltage relationship, in stretch injured astrocytes with and without gadolinium

Hypotonic solution thus seems to activate a novel outwardly rectifying current in cortical astrocytes. Since hypotonic solutions are known to activate swelling-induced Cl- currents in other cell types [12], we tested whether lowering extracellular osmolarity (by 20%) activated a Cl- current in both control and injured cortical astrocytes. After establishment of baseline conditions, application of hypotonic solution increased cell volume within 0.5 min, followed by a 1.2 min delayed increase in inward (at-65 mV) and outward (at 10 mV) current. Cell volume increase induced maximal flow which then decreased again after application of isotonic solution, with the decrease in cell volume preceding the decrease in inward and outward current.

Discussion

Astrocytes are the major determinants of cytotoxic brain swelling after TBI. In the present study, our

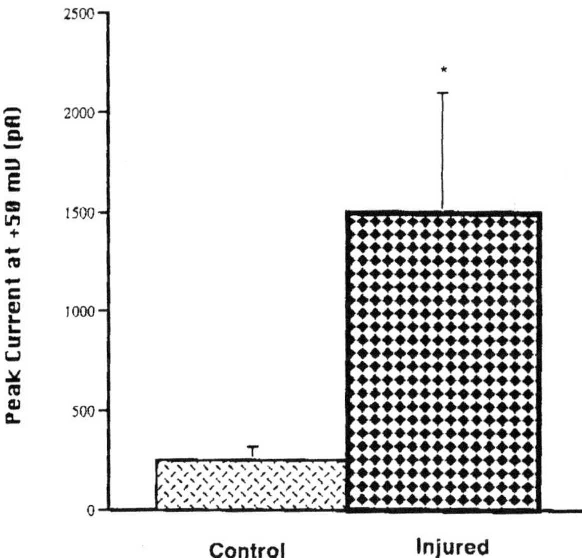

Fig. 4. Effect of Stretched-injury on Hypotonically Activated I_{cl} Amplitude at +50 mV

attention has, therefore, focused on the response of single astrocytes to quantifiable mechanical injury, since this is not well understood, especially with regards to the electrophysiology of astrocytes. However, much progress has been made in understanding and characterizing volume regulation, as well as volume-regulated ion channels in these cells [1, 9, 11]. Part of the gap in our knowledge of astrocyte swelling mechanisms in trauma and the role of ion channels stem from the lack of a suitable in vitro model for testing whether mechanical stress, alterations in brain energy metabolism and/or changes in second messengers, lead to cell swelling and abnormal cell volume regulation, in cortical astrocytes.

In this study, the properties of the current which activated at this time, showed an increased membrane slope conductance below ca. −60 mV and strong outward rectification above 0 mV. The current increased to −850 pA at −120 mV, and +1500 pA at +50 mV in the hypotonic solution. E_{rev} was ca. −40 mV, after correction for liquid junction potentials. This current was strikingly similar to swelling-induced Cl currents in astrocytes, previously reported in the literature [1, 11]. The slow time course of activation is intriguing, as in insulin secretary cells for instance the response to hypotonic solutions is much faster, ca. 3–5 minutes [10] vs. the 10–20 minute lag seen here. The signal transduction mechanism in both cell types is unknown. The pipette solution contained 6 mM [Cl], while the hypotonic bath solution contained 114 mM [Cl]. This yielded a calculated Nernst Erev for Cl of −74 mV. For a pure Cl current, this would mean that there would be net Cl efflux, mediating a net inward membrane current below Erev, and a net outward current above Erev due to net Cl influx, assuming all current flow was purely due to Cl. Alternatively, some small cation flux in hypotonic conditions could produce a similar shift. In any case, the current observed in control astrocytes in hypotonic conditions is similar to those reported previously, and would likely activate in a hypotonic solution in order to mediate a net anion efflux, to help promote cell shrinking as part of the cell regulatory volume decrease (RVC). In marked contrast to control cells, astrocytes stretch-injured with a 6.5 mm deformation pulse showed markedly different responses to hypotonic solution within 15 minutes of injury. Thus, the application of hypotonic solution in this case again activated an outward current at +10 mV but the current-voltage characteristics of this current revealed not the outwardly-rectifying current seen in the control cells but rather a linear or weakly inwardly-rectifying current which reversed near −15 mV instead of near −40 mV. This current was also much larger, e.g. −4000 pA at −120 mV, and >+2000 pA at +50 in hypotonic solution (Figure 2), unlike the outwardly rectifying current of control cells which appeared gradually after applying hypotonic solution. The current was not due to cell death or seal breakdown, because it deactivated after replacing hypotonic solution with isotonic control. In addition, the application of the stretch-activated channel blocker gadolinium, fully blocked all inward current in hypotonic solution, after the linear current activated. At 30 uM, Gd is relatively selective for *stretch-activated cation* channels and does not block outwardly rectifying anion channels [4, 16]. This strongly suggests that the hypotonic-induced current is not due to cell death or deterioration of the pipette seal but rather reflects a massive activation of stretch-activated cation channels primed by injury. Thus, the linearity of the current-voltage relation, its more positive Erev and its sensitivity to the blocker Gd suggest that stretch injury may have switched the astrocyte membrane conductance from one which was dominated by a Cl channel to one dominated by a cation channel. While the mechanism mediating this injury-induced alteration remains to be determined, the possible consequences of this shift in ion selective mechanosensitive channels are likely to be deleterious to the astrocyte and may have important ramifications for understanding of astrocytes and brain swelling.

In future studies, we will determine whether pharmacological agents such as tarantula spider venom, which block stretch-activated cation channels in other systems, will block pathophysiological cell volume regulation in astrocytes. This might open the door to new approaches for treating the component of raised ICP mediated by astrocytic ionic dysfunction and concomitant cell swelling.

Acknowledgments

Lind Lawrence Foundation and NIH Grant No. NS12587.

References

1. Bowman CL, Ding JP, Sachs F, Sokabe M (1992) Mechanotransducing ion channels in astrocytes. Brain Res 584: 272–286
2. Bullock R, Butcher SP, Chen MH, Kendall L, McCulloch J (1991) Correlation of the extracellular glutamate concentration with extent of blood flow reduction after subdural hematoma in the rat. J Neurosurg 74: 794–802
3. Bullock R, Zauner A, Woodward JJ, Myseros J, Choi SC, Ward JD, Marmarou A, Young HF (1998) Factors affecting excitatory amino acid release following severe human head injury. J Neurosurg 89: 507–518
4. Caldwell RA, Clemo HF, Baumgarten CM (1998) Using gadolinium to identify stretch-activated channels: technical considerations. Am J Physiol 275: C619–621
5. Ellis EF, McKinney JS, Willoughby KA, Liang S, Povlishock JT (1995) A new model for rapid stretch-induced injury of cells in culture: characterization of the model using astrocytes. J Neurotrauma 12: 325–339
6. Fahlke C, Rudel R (1995) Chloride currents across the membrane of mammalian skeletal muscle fibres. J Physiol (Lond) 484: 355–368
7. Katayama Y, Becker DP, Tamura T, Hovda DA (1990) Massive increases in extracellular potassium and the indiscriminate release of glutamate following concussive brain injury. J Neurosurg 73: 889–900
8. Kimelberg HK (1992) Astrocytic edema in CNS trauma. J Neurotrauma 9 [Suppl] 1: S71–81
9. Kimelberg HK, Goderie SK, Higman S, Pang S, Waniewski RA (1990) Swelling-induced release of glutamate, aspartate, and taurine from astrocyte cultures. J Neurosci 10: 1583–1591
10. Kinard TA, Satin LS (1996) Temperature modulates the Ca2+ current of HIT-T15 and mouse pancreatic beta-cells. Cell Calcium 20: 475–482
11. Lascola CD, Kraig RP (1996) Whole-cell chloride currents in rat astrocytes accompany changes in cell morphology. J Neurosci 16: 2532–2545
12. Leaney JL, Marsh SJ, Brown DA (1997) A swelling-activated chloride current in rat sympathetic neurones. J Physiol (Lond) 501: 555–564
13. Park K, Arreola J, Begenisich T, Melvin JE (1998) Comparison of voltage-activated Cl- channels in rat parotid acinar cells with ClC-2 in a mammalian expression system. J Membr Biol 163: 87–95

14. Satin LS, Cook DL (1985) Voltage-gated Ca2+ current in pancreatic B-cells. Pflugers Arch 404: 385–387
15. Satin LS, Cook DL (1988) Evidence for two calcium currents in insulin-secreting cells. Pflugers Arch 411: 401–409
16. Satin LS, Tavalin SJ, Kinard TA, Teague J (1995) Contribution of L- and non-L-type calcium channels to voltage-gated calcium current and glucose-dependent insulin secretion in HIT-T15 cells. Endocrinology 136: 4589–4601

Correspondence: Ross Bullock, M.D., Ph.D., Division of Neurosurgery, Medical College of Virginia, Virginia Commonwealth University, Box 980631, Richmond, VA 23298-0631, USA.

Acta Neurochir (2000) [Suppl] 76: 385–391

Thyroid Hormones in Comatose Patients with Traumatic Brain Injury

V. D. Tenedieva, A. A. Potapov, E. I. Gaitur, V. G. Amcheslavski, L. V. Micrikova, N. D. Tenedieva, and **V. G. Voronov**

Burdenko Neurosurgical Institute RAMS, Moscow, Russia

Summary

The objective was to study if thyroid hormones, cortisol, prolactin and brain injury marker levels were changed in traumatic brain injury (TBI) patients with changing levels of consciousness. We estimated the above named parameters in 32 patients (27 men and 5 women aged 11–55). Admission Glasgow Coma Score was <8. Follow-up period – 30 days. The length of coma was 3 to 25 days. There were significant decreases in TSH, TBG, FT3 and F_levels ($p < 0.05$, for each) and a T3 increase (as compared to very low preceding values) on day 1 before emergence from coma and considerable post-coma increase in TBG, FT3, TSH and F levels ($p < 0.001$ each) on days 1–3 in patients with diffuse axonal injury (DAI). In patients with contusions and epidural and subdural hematomas (CH) T3 and T4 levels continued to fall until 4–6 postcoma days. TSH values significantly increased up to average normal ranges ($p < 0.05$) on days "–" 2 and "–" 1 before emergence from coma and remained so. Significantly lower levels of TSH, F and PRL were found in patients with CH in the mostly remote period (on days "–" 12–"–" 8) before emergence from coma in comparison with DAI patients. In blood the following correlations of examined parameters were established: between NSE and T3 ($r = -0.39$), NSE and FT3 ($r = -0.59$), TNFα and TBG ($r = -0.64$), TNFα and T3 ($r = -0.3$) and S-100 and T3 ($r = -0.3$) ($p < 0.05$, for each). The results obtained confirmed a low T3 syndrome in comatose TBI patients. We demonstrated an objective and informative interdependence: the turning-point moment of the emergence from coma was accompanied by significant changes of examined hormone levels and brain injury marker levels. The results may serve as a base for recommending monitoring FT3 and T3 levels simultaneously with that of other injury markers and adequate T3 replacement therapy in the early posttraumatic period.

Keywords: Triiodothyronine; traumatic brain injury; coma.

Introduction

The brain thyronergic system as well as the influences of thyroid hormones on astroglial and immune responses, calcium homeostasis, axonal transport mechanisms and morphology are very important in functioning of the brain [4, 5, 8, 9, 11, 14]. Coma is the most severe level of consciousness depression with life threatening metabolic and neurotransmission disturbances. Emergence from coma as a principal important moment obviously must be characterised by significant brain biochemical changes. So the cornerstone of the study was a comparison of the data obtained in patients with traumatic brain injury (TBI) in coma versus post-coma. Beside hormones, markers of brain injury for control of brain tissue and metabolic changes during the examined period were investigated. Among them the marker of acute brain inflammatory response – tumour necrosis factorα (TNFα), metabolic disturbances and tissue destruction – neurone specific enolase (NSE) and protein S-100, respectively, were studied. The goals of the study were: 1) To evaluate thyroid hormone tests, cortisol and prolactin levels along with brain injury marker levels in comatose patients with TBI. 2) To analyse coma and post-coma hormone levels and to correlate them with clinical and radiography features – contusions with epidural and subdural hematomas (CH) and diffuse axonal injury (DAI).

Material and Methods

32 patients (27 men and 5 women aged 11–55, average age – 32.9) with TBI and with admission Glasgow Coma Score < 8 were enrolled in our study. Follow-up period – 30 days. The length of coma was 3 to 25 days. Fifteen patients had contusions with epidural and subdural hematomas, 14 had I–III type DAI, 3 patients were with missile trauma. The patient outcomes were estimated by Glasgow

outcome Scale (GOS). Four patients died. The serum thyroxine (T4), triiodothyronine (T3), free FT4 and FT3, thyroxine binding globulin (TBG), thyrotropin (TSH), cortisol (F) and prolactin (PRL); TNFα, NSE and protein S-100 were measured by RIA (Immunotech, Czech Republic) and ELISA (Innogenetics, Belgium).

Results

Figures 1 and 2 demonstrate the hormones and injury marker levels in TBI patients who survived. The investigated parameters are plotted against the "+" days which are related to post-coma days, while "–" days are related to coma days (the results are plotted in the reverse direction from the out-of-coma moment). As is seen on the diagrams, the results are as follows:

Coma – Post-Coma Days

Diffuse Axonal Injury (DAI). There were significant decreases in TSH, TBG, FT3 and F levels ($p < 0.05$, for each) and a T3 increase (as compared to very low preceding values) on day 1 before emergence from coma (day "–" 1) and considerable post-coma increase in TBG, FT3, TSH and F levels ($p < 0.001$ each) on days 1–3 (Fig. 1).

Contusion and Epidural and Subdural Hematomas (CH). T3 and T4 levels continued to fall until 4–6 postcoma days. The TSH values significantly increased up to average normal ranges ($p < 0.05$) on days "–" 2 and "–" 1 before emergence from coma and remained so (Fig. 2).

Hormone Levels in the Mostly Remote Period from Our-of-Coma ("–" Days) (Figs. 1–2)

Significantly lower levels of TSH, F and PRL were found in patients with CH in the mostly remote period (on days "–" 12–"–" 8) before emergence from coma in comparison with DAI patients.

Markers of Injury

All comatose patients had increased NSE, S-100 and TNFa levels with some value fluctuations. NSE level decreased on days 1–2 out of coma with a subsequent increase on days 17–20. The TNFα level normalization was noted 3 days before emergence from coma, while S-100 levels – on day 17 after it (Fig. 3). The following correlations of examined parameters in blood were established: between NSE-T3 ($r = -0.39$), NSE-FT3 ($r = -0.59$), TNFα-TBG ($r = -0.64$), TNFα-T3 ($r = -0.3$) and S-100 and T3 ($r = -0.3$), $p < 0.05$, for each.

The main hormonal pattern distinction in dead patients compared to survivors was as follows: there were more significant and monotonous decreased levels of cortisol, Prl, T3, FT3 and TBG, while T4 and FT4 levels had a tendency to some increased values which remained near the below normal range at the same time but abruptly diminished before death (day-"–" 1).

Discussion

The results obtained demonstrate that in TBI there is an interdependence of the patients condition clinical and examined hormone levels. There is a critical or turning-point moment at the emergence from coma which is accompanied by significant changes in biologically active molecule levels.

First of all, TNFα and NSE levels fall at this critical moment and most likely serve as a real reflection of an impending improvement in brain function.

Second, the significant increase of cortisol levels and Prl levels is probably indicative of stress ceasing and host immune defense mechanisms improving. Moreover, the increase in cortisol levels simultaneously with a decrease of TNFα levels on out-of-coma days can possibly be considered as a favorable prognostic sign.

It is interesting that the above-mentioned changes of Prl, F and TSH levels (i.e. an absence of F and Prl stress reactions, undetected TSH levels) were more expressed in patients with CH compared with DAI patients. This suggests more brain injury severity in CH than in DAI in the initial period of traumatic brain injury.

A low T3 syndrome was characterized for both groups of patients but it was more significant in patients with CH. Nevertheless, the early removal of hematomas had a tendency to result in an earlier "reverse" of low T3 syndrome. Thus, in CH T3 levels reached the normal range on days 7–9 after emergence from coma whereas in DAI they became normal only 11–20 days after emergence.

Many factors may cause the low T3 syndrome as part of the sick euthyroid syndrome (SES) in TBI. For example, low brain noradrenaline (NE) levels which

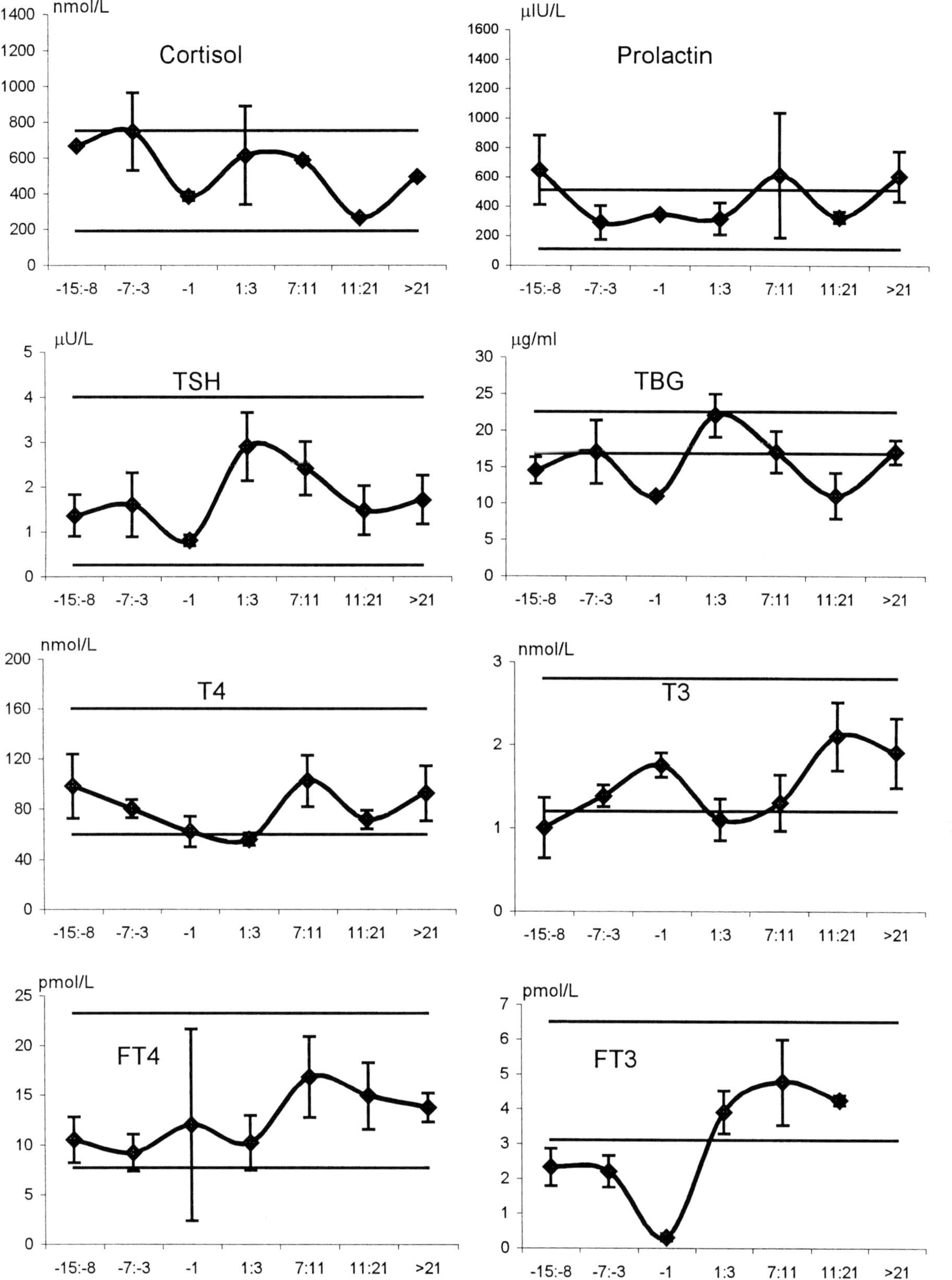

Fig. 1. Coma – post-coma plasma levels of examined hormones in traumatic brain injury (*TBI*) patients with diffuse axonal injuries (*arrows* show the turning-point moment of emergence from coma, *horizontal lines* mark the normal range, *days* "–" refer to coma period, *days* "+" refer to post-coma period)

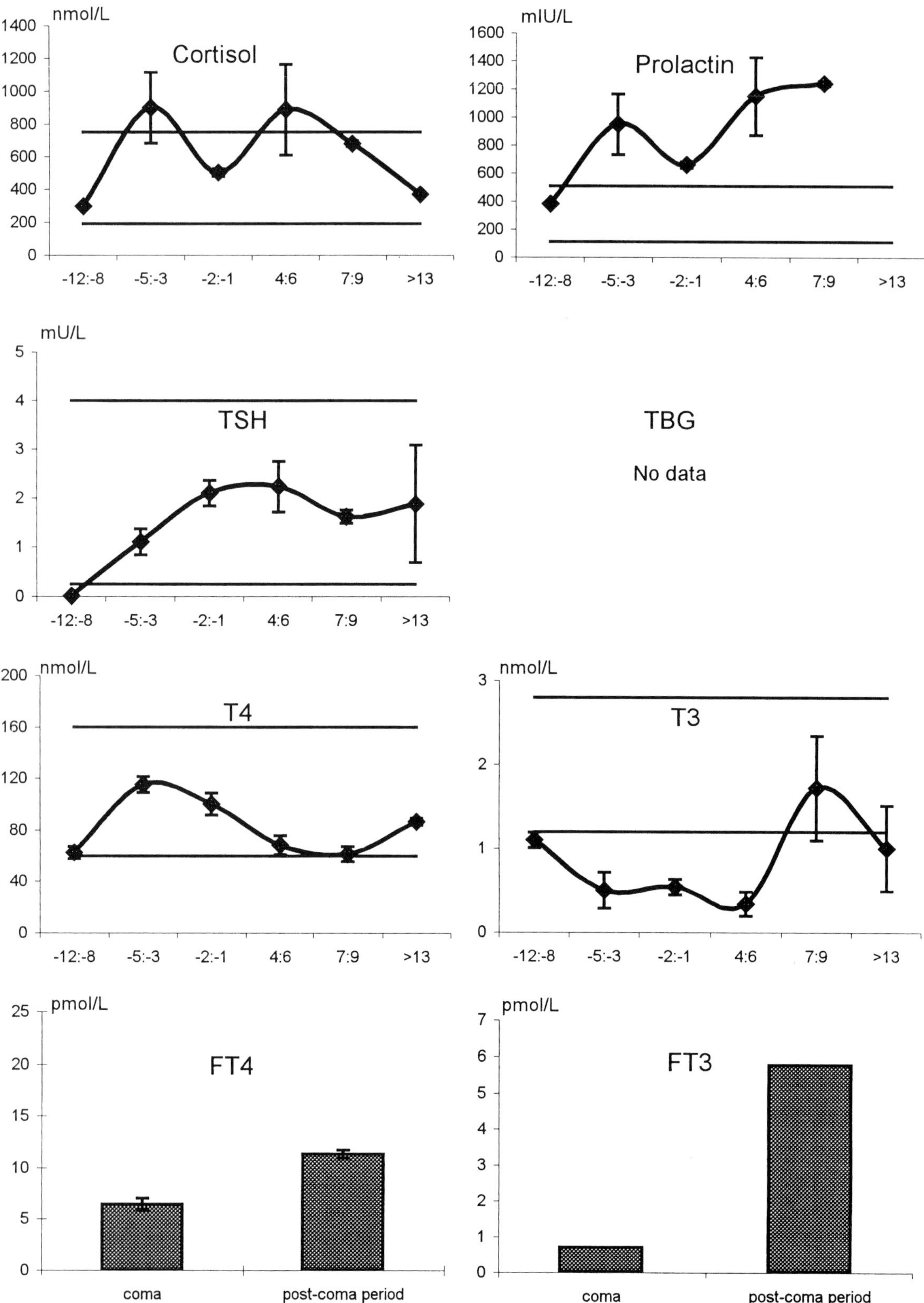

Fig. 2. Coma – post-coma plasma levels of examined hormones in traumatic brain injury (*TBI*) patients with contusion and epidural and subdural hematomas (*arrows* show the turning-point moment of emergence from coma, *horizontal lines* mark the normal range, *days* "–" refer to coma period, *days* "+" refer to post-coma period)

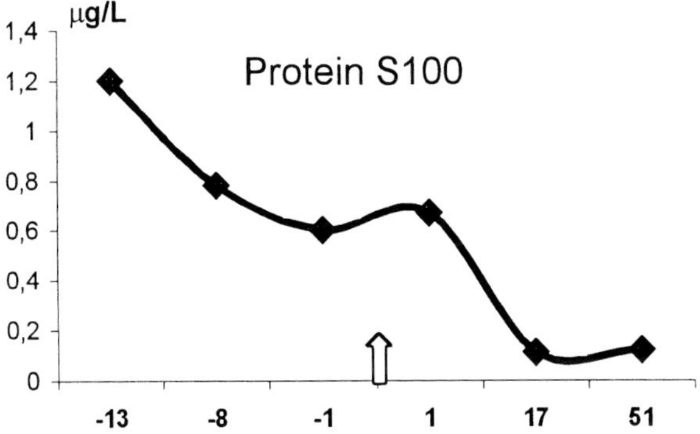

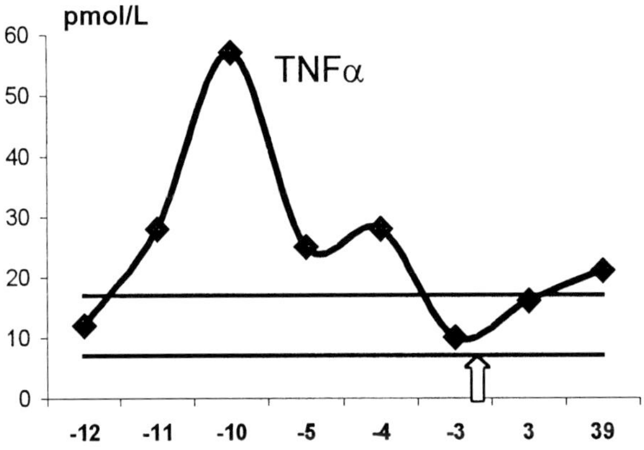

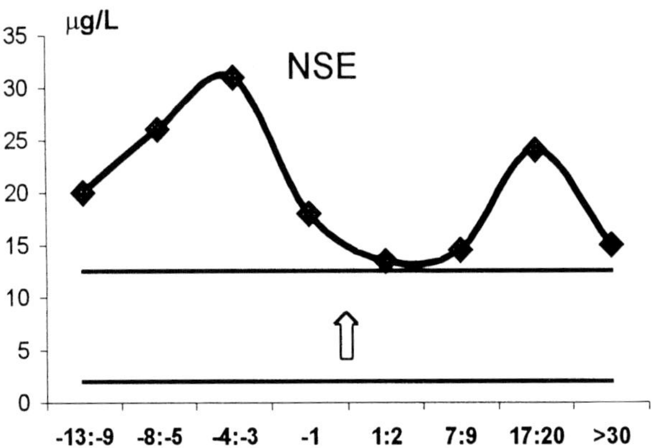

Fig. 3. Coma – post-coma serum levels of protein S-100, neuron specific enolase (*NSE*) and tumor necrosis factor α (*TNFα*) in traumatic brain injury patients (*arrows* show the turning-point moment of emergence from coma, *horizontal lines* mark the normal range, *days* "–" refer to coma period, *days* "+" refer to post-coma period)

normally promote brain T4 transformation to T3, disturbed T3 and NE axonal transport and internalisation; hormone delivery systems to the brain, dopamine infusion and glutamate which introduce or aggravate SES [2, 6, 13, 15]. We do not exclude a disturbance of activity of brain type II and III 5′-deiodinases in severe brain injury, because that can result in significant impairment of thyroid metabolism [2].

The increase of TBG levels on days 1–3 after emergence from coma accompanied by augmentation of FT3 and TSH levels possibly indirectly reflects an interconnection of consciousness clearing and heightening thyronergic system activity. The negative correlations between thyroid test values and brain injury marker levels confirm this interconnection at the molecular level.

These results suggest that the decreased level of T3 during the coma period and the increased T3 levels after emergence from coma (clearing consciousness level) may make T3 monitoring necessary for intensive care patients with TBI. Other investigators have shown early T3 (or TRH, T4) replacement to positively influence brain recovery [1, 3, 7, 10, 16].

Conclusion

Correlations between changes in T3 levels and brain injury marker levels and comparison with the consciousness level suggest a crucial T3 role in brain functioning after traumatic injury. Our results may serve as a basis for recommending FT3 and T3 level monitoring with possible replacement therapy in early posttraumatic brain injury.

References

1. Borromei A, Cavrini G, Guerra L, Lozito A, Parmeggiani A, Reggiani L, d'Orsi U, Vargiu B (1997) Elective neurotraumatology and therapeutic strategies in early post-trauma. Funct Neurol 2: 89–99
2. Cheng LY, Outterbridge LV, Covatta ND, Martens DA, Gordon JT, Dratman MB (1994) Film autoradiography identified unique features of [123I] 3,3′5′-(reverse) triiodothyronine transport from blood to brain. J Neurophysiol 72: 380–391
3. D' Alecy LG (1997) Thyroid hormone in neural rescue. Thyroid 7: 115–124
4. Dratman MB, Gordon JT (1996) Thyroid hormones as neurotransmitters Thyroid 6: 639–647
5. Garcia-Segura LM, Chowen JA, Naftolin F (1996) Endorcine glia: roles of glial cells in the brain actions of steroid and thyroid hormones and in the regulation of hormone secretion. Front Neuroendocrinol 2: 180–211
6. Hoyt KR, Reynolds IJ, Hastings TG (1997) Mechanisms of dopamine-induced cell death in cultured rat forebrain neurones: interactions with and differences from glutamate-induced cell death. Exp Neurol 143: 269–281
7. Hsu RB, Huang TS, Chen YS, Chu SH (1995) Effect of triiodothyronine administration in experimental myocardial injury. J Endocrinol Invest 18: 702–709

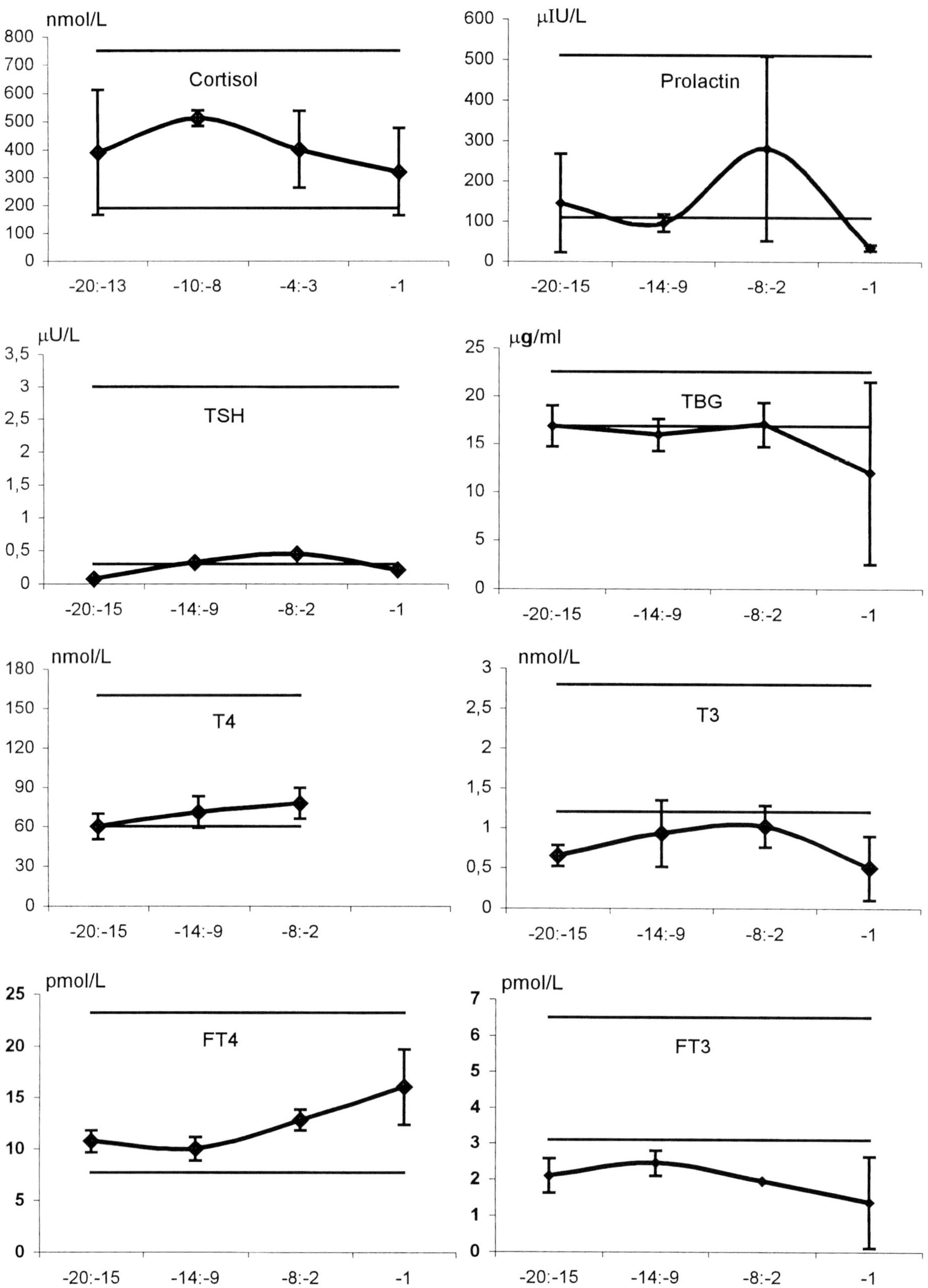

Fig. 4. Plasma levels of examined hormones in dead traumatic brain injury (*TBI*) patients in coma period (*horizontal lines* mark the normal range, *days* "–" refer to coma period up to lethal outcome)

8. Iniguez MA, De Lecea L, Guadano-Ferraz A, Morte B, Gerendasy D, Sutcliffe JG, Bernal J (1996) Cell-specific effects of thyroid hormone on RC3/neurogranin expression in rat brain. Endocrinology 3: 1032–1041
9. Knoblach SM, Kubek MJ (1997) Changes in thyrotropin-releasing hormone levels in hippocampal subregions induced by a model of human temporal lobe epilepsy: effect of partial and complete kindling. Neuroscience 1: 97–104
10. Köhrle J (1996) Thyroid hormone deiodinases – a selenoenzyme family acting as gate keeper to thyroid hormone action. Acta Med Austriaca 23: 17–30
11. Martin JV, Williams DB, Fitzgerald RM, Im HK, Vonvoigtlander PF (1996) Thyroid hormonal modulation of the binding and activity of the GABAA receptor complex of brain. Neuroscience 3: 705–713
12. Novitzky D (1996) Novel actions of thyroid hormone: the role of triiodothyronine in cardiac transplantation. Thyroid 6: 531–536
13. Schreiber G, Southwell BR, Richardson SJ (1995) Hormone delivery systems to the brain-transthyretin. Exp Clin Endocrinol Diabetes 2: 75–80
14. Sinha AK, Pickard MR, Kim KD, Ahmed MT, al Yatama F, Evans IM, Elkins RP (1994) Perturbation of thyroid homeostasis in the adult and brain function. Acta Med Austriaca 2: 35–43
15. Van den Berghe G, Zegher F, Lauwers P (1994) Dopamine and the sick euthyroid syndrome in critical illness. Clin Endocrinol 6: 731–737
16. Van den Berghe G, de Zegher F, Vlasselaers D, Schetz M, Verwaest C, Ferdinande P, Lauwers P (1996) Thyrotropin-releasing hormone in critical illness: from a dopamine-dependent test to strategy for increasing low serum triiodothyronine, prolactin, and growth hormone concentrations. Crit Care Med 24: 590–595

Correspondence: Dr. V. D. Tenedieva, Burdenko Neurosurgical Institute, Fadeev Street, 5, Moscow 125047, Russia.

Acta Neurochir (2000) [Suppl] 76: 393–396

S-100b as a Screening Marker of the Severity of Minor Head Trauma (MHT) – a Pilot Study

T. Mussack[1], **P. Biberthaler**[1], **E. Wiedemann**[1], **K. G. Kanz**[1], **A. Englert**[1], **C. Gippner-Steppert**[2], and **M. Jochum**[2]

[1] Chirurgische Klinik, Kliniken Innenstadt, Ludwig-Maximilians-Universität, München, Germany
[2] Abteilung für Klinische Chemie und Klinische Biochemie, Chirurgische Klinik, Kliniken Innenstadt, Ludwig-Maximilians-Universität, München, Germany

Summary

Due to its neural tissue specificity S-100b is considered as a screening marker of cerebral injury in head trauma patients. However, the occurrence and relevance of an increased S-100b serum level in minor head trauma (MHT) is still debated. Therefore, the purpose of our study was to evaluate the diagnostic utility of S-100b measurements in a level I trauma center emergency room (ER). Eighty patients presenting with clinical symptoms of MHT (GCS score of 13–15, transitory loss of consciousness, amnesia, nausea) were prospectively recruited. Blood samples were drawn at 0 h, 6 h and 24 h after admission, and a cerebral computed tomography (CT) was performed. The reference group consisted of 10 patients with severe head injury (GCS score < 8), the control group of 20 healthy volunteers. Concentrations of S-100b in serum were determined by an immunoluminometric assay. The results were compared with the plasma levels of polymorphonuclear (PMN) elastase as an established general trauma marker.

In the MHT group, the S-100b serum level revealed 1.26 ± 0.57 ng/ml at study entry (73.46 ± 47.53 min after trauma). In comparison, the S-100b concentration was significantly elevated in patients with severe head trauma (5.26 ± 1.65 ng/ml, $p = 0.009$), but no significant difference became evident in relation to the control group (0.05 ± 0.01 ng/ml). Starting values of PMN elastase in plasma amounted to 66.40 ± 14.92 ng/ml in severe trauma, and to 60.52 ± 10.75 ng/ml in MHT showing significant differences only in relation to the control group (23.36 ± 1.53 ng/ml). When correlated with the severity of the later clinical course, the first S-100b measurements exhibited steadily increasing values as demonstrated in MHT outpatients (0.29 ± 0.11 ng/ml), MHT in-hospital patients (0.70 ± 0.19 ng/ml) and MHT intensive care unit patients (5.03 ± 3.18 ng/ml). PMN elastase levels revealed no significant differences concerning the three MHT subgroups.

Thus, in contrast to the general trauma marker PMN elastase, assessment of the specific neuroprotein S-100b early after traumatic insult appears to be a promising laboratory marker for the prognosis of the severity of brain injury in MHT patients. Nevertheless, further investigations are required to better understand its predictive value.

Keywords: Minor head trauma; S-100b; PMN elastase; diagnostics.

Introduction

Minor head trauma (MHT) patients with a GCS score of 13–15 and clinical symptoms like transitory loss of consciousness, nausea, vomiting, amnesia and vertigo, represent an increasing number of patients in emergency rooms (ER) of level 1 urban trauma centers [8, 10]. The management of these patients is still under debate. Although head pathology, i.e. hemorrhage, skull fracture or brain oedema, detectable by computed tomography (CT) with a range between 5.9 and 21.6%, are less frequent than in cases of moderate (GCS score of 9–12) or severe head trauma (GCS score ≤ 8), emergency operations are still required in 0.3 to 4.1% of patients [2, 10]. Thus, in order to evaluate effectively MHT patients at risk routine CT scans may be applied as a screening tool at time of diagnosis. However, evidence of CT abnormalities is only one of many definitions of brain injury, and may therefore often not predict neurologic sequelae. Clinical examination also turned out as a good predictor of serious complications, but might be impaired by subjective symptoms after MHT [7]. For the identification of high-risk patients with subacute neurological impairments measurements of the neuroprotein S-100b released into the circulation have been considered as a reliable screening marker of isolated brain injury [5]. S-100b is normally present in the cytosol or bound to the membranes of glial cells, astrocytes and Schwann cells [3]. An early concentration peak of S-100b in serum 20 minutes after severe head trauma reflects both cellular damage and increased permeability of the blood-brain-barrier (BBB) [8, 9, 15].

The purpose of this study was to evaluate the diagnostic value of S-100b serum levels in relation to the general trauma marker PMN elastase [13] in patients attending a level I trauma center ER because of isolated MHT. The results were correlated with the clinical course and the severity of brain injury. Comparison with data of patients with severe head trauma (reference group) and of healthy control individuals was also performed.

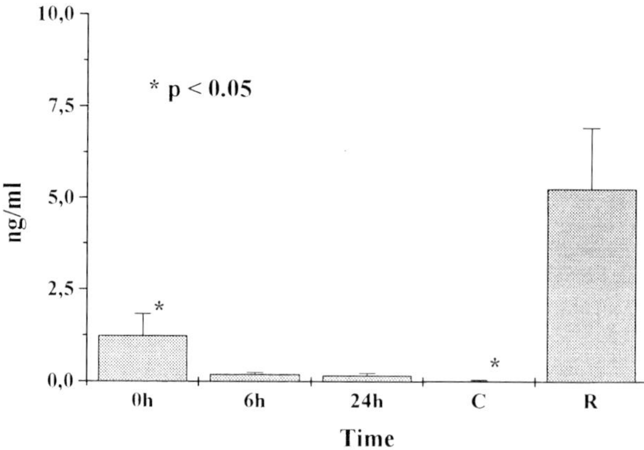

Fig. 1. S-100b serum levels of MHT patients at 0 h, 6 h and 24 h after admission to the emergency room in comparison to those of healthy controls (*C*) and a reference group (*R*) with severe isolated head trauma

Patients and Methods

Between October and December 1998 80 patients (51 male, 29 female) with isolated MHT and clinical symptoms of brain injury were prospectively enclosed in this study of our level I trauma center ER. The study was approved by the local research ethics committee. Informed consent was given by all patients, or, in case of unconscious patients, by their relatives. The trauma-ER admission interval was 73.46 ± 47.53 min on average. At time of diagnosis all patients had a GCS score of 13–15, transitory loss of consciousness and symptoms like amnesia, nausea, vomiting or vertigo. Blood samples were drawn at admission, and 6 h and 24 h afterwards. Spiral CT-scans (2 mm) of the skull base and sequential CT scans (8 mm) of the cerebrum were performed within the first 6 hours. According to their clinical course all patients were divided into an outpatient group (n = 57, discharge ≤ 6 h), an in-hospital group (n = 14, discharge ≥ 24 h) and an intensive care unit group (n = 9, discharge ≥ 72 h). The reference group consisted of 10 patients with isolated severe head injuries (GCS score ≤ 8), who had undergone an emergency operation due to acute brain oedema or intracerebral hemorrhage. A control group was established of 20 healthy volunteers.

Concentrations of S-100b in serum were determined by an immunoluminometric assay (LIA-mat® Sangtec® 100, Byk-Sangtec, Dietzenbach, Germany) with a minimum sensitivity of 0.02 ng/ml. Serum concentrations of S-100b were compared with polymorphonuclear (PMN) elastase in citrated plasma, an established general trauma marker, which was determined with a two-side sandwich ELISA (DPC Biermann, Bad Nauheim, Germany).

Statistical analysis was performed using the t-test for independent blood samples and the Chi-square-test or correlation rank test of Pearson and Spearman for clinical data. Significance was accepted at $p < 0.05$. All values are given as mean and standard error of the mean (mean ± sem).

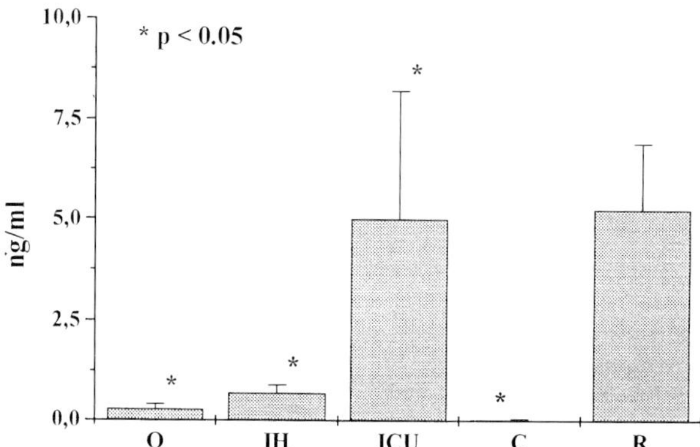

Fig. 2. S-100b serum levels of MHT patients stratified into outpatients (*O*), in-hospital patients (*IH*) and intensive care unit patients (*ICU*) versus healthy controls (*C*) and the reference group (*R*) with severe head trauma

Results

S-100b serum levels of the 80 MHT patients revealed 1.26 ± 0.57 ng/ml at 0 h, 0.21 ± 0.04 ng/ml at 6 h and 0.18 ± 0.06 ng/ml at 24 h after entry into the study (Fig. 1). The reference group with severe head trauma showed S-100b serum concentrations of 5.26 ±1.65 ng/ml at admission to our ER. Thus, the first measurements were significantly different ($p = 0.009$) in both head trauma collectives. In the control group S-100b serum levels of 0.05 ± 0.01 ng/ml were detected, the differences to the MHT group at 0 h were not significant ($p = 0.181$). Analysis of clinical courses revealed a significant correlation between elevated S-100b levels and neurological impairments leading to prolonged in-hospital stay (Fig. 2). First S-100b measurements in the MHT outpatient group (n = 57) showed 0.29 ± 0.11 ng/ml, in the MHT in-hospital group (n = 14) 0.70 ± 0.19 ng/ml and in the MHT intensive care unit group (n = 9) 5.03 ± 3.18 ng/ml. The values of this latter group were not significantly different to those of the reference group with severe isolated head trauma.

PMN elastase levels reached 60.52 ± 10.75 ng/ml at 0 h, 51.44 ± 4.84 ng/ml at 6 h and 45.33 ± 3.60 ng/ml at 24 h in MHT patients. Significant differences were determined in comparison to the control group

Table 1. *Correlation Between S-100b Serum Levels in MHT Patients at Admisssion and GCS Score, Mode of Accident, CT Scan or PMN Elastase*

	Parameter	p-value
S-100b (0 h)	GCS (severity of brain disorders)	0.001
	car accident	0.030
	bicycle accident	0.004
	CT scan (skull fracture)	0.016
	PMN elastase (0 h)	0.027

(23.36 ± 1.53 ng/ml, $p = 0.038$), but not to the reference group (66.40 ± 14.92 ng/ml, $p = 0.826$). Moreover, PMN elastase plasma levels determined at study entry also did not reveal significant differences in severity.

As depicted in Table 1 at time of admission, strong correlations of S-100b serum levels in MHT patients were shown with the severity of brain disorders according to the GCS score ($p = 0.001$), the mode of accident, the appearance of a skull fracture in CT scan ($p = 0.016$) and the PMN elastase level ($p = 0.027$).

Discussion

The measurement of the neuroprotein S-100b concentration in serum has been proposed as a reliable marker to determine brain damage from stroke or subarachnoid hemorrhage, and may be appropiate for the diagnosis of cerebral damage after severe head trauma [8]. Brain-specific S-100b protein is released into the blood circulation after neuronal cell damage [1]. Because of the rapid posttraumatic increase, followed by a probably even faster decrease, S-100b levels in serum must be determined as soon as possible after head trauma. Since the time between the onset of traumatic insult and the admission of the MHT patients to our level 1 trauma center ER was on average 73.46 ± 47.53 min, S-100b serum levels in individual patients might have already declined before the first blood sample has been drawn.

Nevertheless, the results of our prospective study seem to support previously published data [5] showing a predictive value of S-100b in the clinical course and severity of central nervous system (CNS) damage after MHT. Serum concentrations in patients of the MHT group were significantly lower than those of the reference group with severe head trauma. S-100b serum levels obtained early after brain injury were proposed as an accurate predictor of late neurological deficits [14]. Some authors decribed specific cognitive dysfunction, i.e. measures of reaction time, attention span and speed of information processing, in patients with elevated S-100b levels [12]. Repeated measurements may be used to monitor the effects of treatment in patients with CNS injury. These measurements may also permit early diagnosis of secondary insults such as vasospastic infarction or brain oedema. However, increases in serum concentrations of S-100b protein have been found after various modes of CNS injury indicating that elevations of circulating S-100b protein are not specific for types of CNS tissue or mechanisms of injury [14]. As claimed by some authors, S-100b serum concentrations may not serve as a sole prognostic determinant, but as a helpful tool in combination with radiological or clinical data for predicting neurological outcome after MHT [9]. Yet, some patients with elevated S-100b serum levels showed normal CT results, but magnetic resonance imaging (MRI) verified cerebral contusion [6].

At admission, we found highly significantly different S-100b serum levels in MHT patients with deviating clinical courses indicated by increasing times of discharge from the hospital (Fig. 2). This may be taken as a further suggestion of the predictive value of the circulating neuroprotein as an index of severity of brain damage due to MHT. S-100b serum levels at 0 h showed also a strong correlation to the severity of traumatic brain disorders according to the GCS score, the mode of accident, the appearance of a skull fracture in CT scan and to the PMN elastase level at 0 h (Tab. 1).

PMN elastase at 0 h, 6 h and 24 h after admission exhibited significantly higher plasma levels compared to the control group, but no differences to the reference group. As an established general trauma marker [13] PMN elastase is elevated in every kind of trauma, but it clearly does not specifically identify brain damage of various degrees in MHT patients.

Conclusions

Proper treatment of MHT patients is hampered by a diagnostic dilemma especially because of insufficient neurological and radiological findings. Measurement of the brain tissue derived S-100b in serum seems to be a helpful tool for identifying those patients at higher risk. Nevertheless further investigations are required to better understand its predictive value in MHT.

References

1. Blomquist S, Johnsson P, Luhrs C, Malmkvist G, Solem JO, Alling C, Stahl E (1997) The appearance of S-100 protein in serum during and immediately after cardiopulmonary bypass surgery: a possible marker for cerebral injury. J Cardiovasc Vasc Anesth 11: 699–703
2. Borczuk P (1995) Predictors of intracranial injury in patients with mild head trauma. Ann Emerg Med 25: 731–736
3. Haimoto H, Hosoda S, Kato K (1987) Differential distribution of immunoreactive S100-α and S100-β proteins in normal nonnervous human tissues. Lab Invest 57: 489–498
4. Harad FT, Kerstein MD (1992) Inadequacy of bedside clinical indicators in identifying significant intracranial injury in trauma patients. J Trauma 32: 359–361, discussion 361–363
5. Ingebrigtsen T, Romner B, Kongstad P, Langbakk B (1995) Increased serum concentrations of protein S-100 after minor head injury: a biochemical serum marker with prognostic value? J Neurol Neurosurg Psychiatry 59: 103–104
6. Ingebrigtsen T, Romner B (1996) Serial S-100 protein measurements related to early magnetic resonance imaging after minor head injury. J Neurosurg 85: 945–948
7. Miller EC, Holmes JF, Derlet RW (1997) Utilizing clinical factors to reduce head CT scan ordering for minor head trauma patients. J Emer Med 15: 453–457
8. Persson L, Haardemark HG, Gustafsson J, Rundstrom G, Mendel-Hartvig I, Esscher T, Pahlman S (1987) S-100 protein and neuron-specific enolase in cerebrospinal fluid and serum: Markers of cell damage in human central nervous system. Stroke 18: 911–918
9. Rothoerl RD, Woertgen C, Holzschuh M, Metz C, Brawanski A (1998) S-100 serum levels after minor and major head injury. J Trauma 45: 765–767
10. Shackford SR, Wald SL, Ross SE, Cogbill TH, Hoyt DB, Morris JA, Mucha PA, Pachter HL, Sugerman HJ, O'Malley K (1992) The clinical utility of computed tomographic scanning and neurologic examination in the management of patients with minor head injuries. J Trauma 33: 385–394
11. Stein SC, Ross SE (1992) Mild head injury: a plea for routine early CT scanning. J Trauma 33: 11–13
12. Waterloo K, Ingebrigtsen T, Romner B (1997) Neuropsychological function in patients with increased serum levels of protein S-100 after minor head injury. Acta Neurochir (Wien) 139: 26–31, discussion 31–32
13. Waydhas C, Nast-Kolb D, Trupka A, Zettl R, Kick M, Wiesholler J, Schweiberer L, Jochum M (1996) Posttraumatic inflammatory response, secondary operations, and late multiple organ failure. J Trauma 40: 624–630
14. Wiesmann M, Missler U, Hagenstroem H, Gottmann D (1997) S-100 protein plasma levels after aneurysmal subarachnoid haemorrhage. Acta Neurochir (Wien) 139: 1155–1160
15. Woertgen C, Rothoerl RD, Holzschuh M, Metz C, Brawanski A (1997) Comparison of serial S-100 and NSE serum measurements after severe head injury. Acta Neurochir (Wien) 139: 1161–1165

Correspondence: Dr. Thomas Mussack, Chirurgische Klinik, Kliniken Innenstadt, Ludwig-Maximilians-Universität, Nussbaumstrasse 20, D-80336 München, Germany.

Acta Neurochir (2000) [Suppl] 76: 397–399

Influences of Secondary Injury Following Traumatic Brain Injury in Developing Versus Adult Rats

S. Thomas[1], **F. Tabibnia**[1], **M. U. Schuhmann**[2], **T. Brinker**[1], and **M. Samii**[1,2]

[1] Departments of Neurosurgery, Nordstadt Hospital, Hannover, Germany
[2] Medical School, Hannover, Germany

Summary

Hypoxia and hypotension are both common findings following traumatic brain injury occuring with a frequency of up to 46% according to data of the Traumatic Coma Data Bank. In the present study the influence of secondary injury on intracranial pressure and the cardiovascular response is investigated in developing rats. Differences from adult rats are determined.

Diffuse brain injury was produced in intubated and ventilated 17–20 days old Sprague-Dawley rats (N = 16) using a modification of the Marmarou-model. Hypoxia was induced by reducing O_2-concentration to 8% lasting for 15/30 min. Mean arterial blood pressure recordings and intracranial pressure recordings were performed continuously. Animals were divided into two groups, sustaining hypoxia alone (N = 9) and trauma/hypoxia (N = 7). The results were compared to readings in adult animals subjected to hypoxia (N = 5) and trauma/hypoxia(N = 5) (450 gm/150 cm).

Immediately following the onset of hypoxia in the developing rat, MABP decreased from 76.5 ± 13 mm Hg to 35.8 ± 7 mm Hg. In the adult rat the decrease was more marked (from 93.3 ± 8 mm Hg to 33.5 ± 5.7 mm Hg) ($p < 0.05$). Mortality rate in developing rats with trauma/hypoxia was 43% with no significant change of ICP (from 13 ± 5.2 to 22.3 ± 11). All adult animals recovered following trauma/hypoxia with no relevant ICP-increase within one hour post-trauma.

Hypoxia induces hypotension in adult and developing rats. However, developing rats appear to be more vulnerable to hypoxia associated with trauma.

Keywords: Rat pup; traumatic brain injury; secondary injury; hypoxia.

Introduction

Hypoxia and hypotension are both common findings following traumatic brain injury. According to data of the Traumatic Coma Data Bank hypoxia occured in 46% of severely head injured patients and hypotension occured in 35% [2].

It is a clinical well known that the juvenile brain responds differently to traumatic brain injury compared to adults [8]. However, the pathophysiological causes still remain unclear. Experimental traumatic brain injury in the developing rat was first produced using the fluid percussion device [10, 13]. Recently, the weight-drop model, first established by A. Marmarou *et al.* [9], was introduced for traumatic brain injury in the developing rat [1, 14]. The aim of the present study was to determine ICP-changes and cardiovascular responses following traumatic brain injury in 17–20 days old rats compared to adults with emphasis on secondary injury.

Material and Methods

As approved by the Animal Research Committee of the Medical School of Hannover 17 to 20 days old Sprague-Dawley rats were obtained from the in-house breeding colony. The pups were nursed by their mother and weaned the day before the experiment. All animals were intubated using a 20 G venflon and artificially ventilated with a gas mixture of N_2O (70%) and O_2 (30%) with isoflurane. Polyethylene catheters (PE-10) were placed into the femoral artery and connected to a Statham-transducer. Mean arterial blood pressure was recorded continuously.

A diffuse brain injury was produced by using a modification of the injury device first described by A. Marmarou *et al.* [9, 14]. A brass weight fell free onto a brass helmet glued to the skull of the rat by cyanoacrylate. The weight was guided by a 1 m Plexiglass tube. The animal was placed in a prone position on foam (20 × 20 × 50 cm; spring constant 30/50) held within a wooden frame. The lower end of the tube was placed directly above the helmet. Immediately following the initial impact the box was slid horizontally to prevent a second impact.

Hypoxia was induced by reducing the O_2-concentration to 8% and reducing the respiratory rate from 80 to 35.

Measurement of ICP was performed using a catheter (PE-50) placed subdurally through a lateral-frontal burr hole into the anterior fossa. The catheter was connected to a Statham-transducer and ICP was recorded up to one hour after injury.

Animals were perfused transcardially 3 days after injury and the brains were removed and post-fixed in 4%-formalin. All brains were processed for hematoxylin-eosin staining using 20 μm coronal sections. Sections were studied under light-microscopy for cell loss and hemorrhages.

Animals were divided into two groups, sustaining hypoxia alone (N = 9) and trauma/hyoxia (N = 7). The results were compared to readings in adult animals subjected to hypoxia (N = 5) and trauma/hypoxia (N = 5). In adult animals a 450 g/1.5 m injury was performed.

All measurements were stored and analyzed using commercially available software (Dasy Lab V.3, Datalog, Mönchengladbach, Germany). Statistical analysis was performed using Wilcoxon signed rank test for paired data. Data are presented as mean ± SD.

Results

In the first series MABP was determined before, during, and 30 min. after hypoxia. The blood gas levels during hypoxia indicated a lower pO_2 in adult rats compared to pups (35.2 ± 2.33/49 ± 8.28). All other parameters were unremarkable (pups: pCO_2 46.2 ± 6.6, pH 7.236 ± 0.006, BE −6.5 ± 1.1; adults: pCO_2 50.13 ± 3.1, pH 7.228 ± 0.029, BE −7.5 ± 1.539). Immediately following the onset of hypoxia MABP decreased from 76.5 ± 13 mm Hg to 35.8 ± 7 mm Hg. The decrease was more marked (from 93.3 ± 8 mm Hg to 33.5 ± 5.7 mm Hg) ($p < 0.05$) in the adult animals (Fig. 1). The mortality rate for rat pups following 30 min hypoxia was 78%. However, all adult animals survived that duration of hypoxia.

Therefore, the duration of hypoxia following traumatic brain injury was reduced to 15 min. resulting in a mortality rate of 43% in pups. All adult animals survived trauma/15 min. hypoxia and regained consciousness. The MABP-pattern observed was similar to the one without trauma with a more marked decrease in adult rats (88 ± 18 mm Hg to 40 ± 13.2 mm Hg) compared to pups (72.4 ± 13 mm Hg to 43.75 ± 11 mm Hg). However, no statistically significant difference was achieved. In all animals no relevant ICP-changes were determined within one hour post-trauma (Figs. 2, 3).

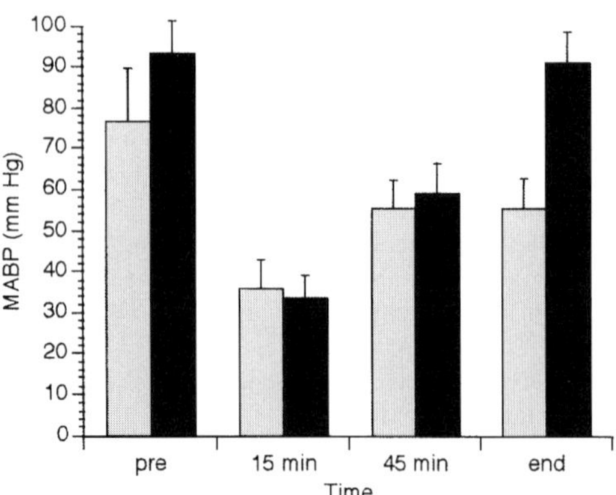

Fig. 1. Mean arterial blood pressure (mean ± SD) in developing and adult rats before, during and after hypoxia, ▢ pup, ■ adult

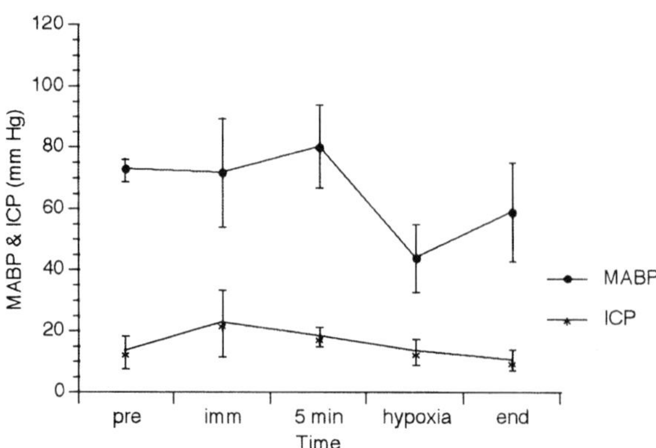

Fig. 2. Mean arterial blood pressure and intracranial pressure (mean ± SD) before, during, and after injury and hypotension in developing rats

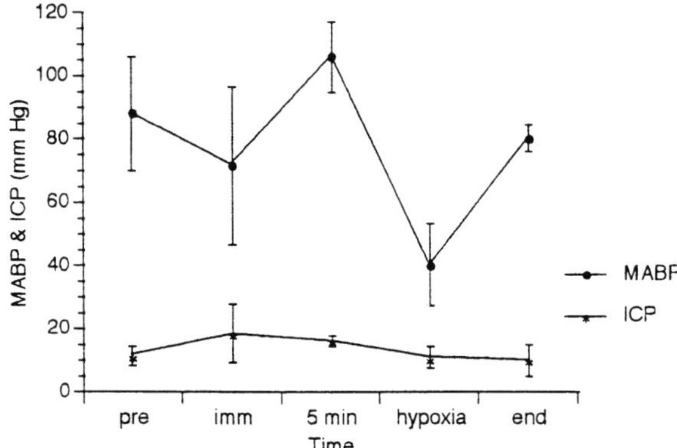

Fig. 3. Mean arterial blood pressure and intracranial pressure (mean ± SD) before, during, and after injury and hypotension in adult rats

Gross pathological examination of the surviving animals did not reveal any skull fractures. Histological investigation showed diffuse neuronal cell loss in all cortical areas and in the hippocampus.

Discussion

The decrease of blood pressure following hypoxia is a well known feature and has been described previously [4, 6, 11, 12, 15]. It has been attributed to an activation of central adenosine receptors [12, 15]. Following brief inhalation of an oxygen-deficient (5%) gas mixture caffeine was able to attenuate the hypoxia-evoked hypotension. 8-p-Sulphophenyltheophylline and xanthine amine congener, which did not penetrate the blood-brain barrier, had little effect on the magnitude of hypotension [12]. In addition to adenosine atrial natriuretic factor may play a role in mediating the physiologic response to hypoxia in the rat [6].

The present study indicates that immediately following onset of hypoxia a marked decrease of MABP occurs, resulting in a higher mortality in pups versus adult rats with no change of ICP. It was expected that hypoxia and hypotension would cause a rise of ICP as reported previously by utilization of the same model [3, 7]. In both studies, in addition to reduction of O_2, hypotension was induced by withdrawing arterial blood. In both reports an increase of ICP was observed reaching 35 mm Hg at 90 min post-injury. In the present study no blood withdrawal was performed because MABP was already reduced by hypoxia.

The difference in mortality rate between pups and adult rats was striking. The higher decrease of MABP in adult rats may be attributable to the higher base-line levels.

In conclusion the results of the present study indicate that adult rats appear to be less vulnerable to hypoxia. Therefore, children may be more sensitive to secondary injury and even greater care has to be taken to prevent secondary injury in pediatric brain trauma.

References

1. Adelson PD, Robichaud P, Hamilton RL, Kochanek PM (1996) A model of diffuse traumatic brain injury in the immature rat. J Neurosurg 85: 877–884
2. Aldrich EF, Eisenberg HM, Saydjari C, Luerssen TG, Foulkes MA, Jane JA, Marshall LF, Young H (1992) Diffuse brain swelling in severely head-injured children. A report from the NIH Traumatic Coma Data Bank. J Neurosurg 76: 450–454
3. Barzo P, Marmarou A, Fatouros P, Corwin F, Dunbar J (1996) Magnetic resonance imaging-monitored acute blood-brain barrier changes in experimental traumatic brain injury 85: 1113–1121
4. Bunt JE, Gavilanes AW, Reulen JP, Blanco CE, Vles JS (1996) The influence of acute hypoxemia and hypovolemic hypotension of neuronal brain activity measured by the cerebral function monitor in newborn piglets. Neuropediatrics 25: 260–264
5. Chesnut RM, Marshall LF, Klauber MR, Bennt BA, Baldwin N, Eisenberg HM, Jane JA, Marmarou A, Foulkes MA (1993) The role of secondary injury in determining outcome from severe head injury. J Trauma 34: 216–222
6. Colice G, Yen S, Ramirez G, Dietz J, Ou LC (1991) Acute hypoxia-induced diuresis in rats. Aviat Space Environ Med 62: 551–554
7. Ito J, Marmarou A, Barzo P, Fatouros P, Corwin F (1996) Characterization of edema by diffusion-weighted imaging in experimental traumatic brain injury. J Neurosurg 84: 97–103
8. Kraus JF, Rock A, Hemyari P (1990) Brain injuries among infants, children, adolescents, and young adults. AJDC 144: 684–691
9. Marmarou A, Foda MAA, Van den Brink W, Campbell J, Kita H, Demetriadou K (1994) A new model of diffuse brain injury in rats. Part I: pathophysiology and biomechanics. J Neurosurg 80. 291–300
10. Prins ML, Lee SM, Cheng CLY, Becker DP, Hovda DA (1991) Fluid percussion brain injury in the developing and adult rat: a comparative study of mortality, morphology, intracranial pressure and mean arterial blood pressure. Dev Brain Res 95: 272–282
11. Saiki C, Mortola JP (1997) Effect of 2,4-dinitrophenol on the hypometabolic response to hypoxia of conscious adult rats. J Appl Physiol 83: 537–542
12. Simpson L, Barraco RA, Phillis JW (1989) A central role for adenosine in the hypotension elicited by hypoxia in anesthetized rats. Brain Res Bull 23: 37–40
13. Thomas S, Hovda DA, Samii M, Becker DP (1991) Fluid percussion injury in the developing rat pup: Studies of cerebral metabolism. J Neurotrauma 9: 71
14. Thomas S, Tabibnia F, Schuhmann MU, Hans VHJ, Brinker T, Samii M (1998) Traumatic brain injury in the developing rat pup: Studies of ICP, PVI and neurological response. Acta Neurochir [Suppl] (Wien) 71: 135–137
15. Waaben J, Husum B, Hansen AJ, Gjedde A (1989) Regional cerebral blood flow and glucose utilization during hypocapnia and adenosine-induced hypotension in the rat. Anesthesiology 70: 299–304

Correspondence: Sebastian Thomas, M.D., Neurochirurgische Klinik, Nordstadt Hospital, Haltenhoffstrasse 41, 30167 Hannover, Germany.

Acta Neurochir (2000) [Suppl] 76: 401–404

The Role of Decompressive Craniectomy in the Treatment of Uncontrollable Post-Traumatic Intracranial Hypertension

G. P. De Luca, L. Volpin, U. Fornezza, P. Cervellini, M. Zanusso, L. Casentini, D. Curri, M. Piacentino, G. Bozzato, and **F. Colombo**

Division of Neurosurgery, Vicenza City Hospital, Italy

Summary

The benefit of decompressive craniectomy for the treatment of uncontrolled post-traumatic intracranial hypertension seems to be encouraging if medical management fails. We present our experience in 22 cases of cerebral edema due to head trauma. The edema alone was rarely the direct consequence of head trauma. Frequently it was associated with an acute subdural or extradural hematoma and contusion (with or without mass effect). First of all we treated the mass effect of the hematoma and contusion when the diameter was more than 3 cm. Intracranial pressure was monitored in the majority of patients. Bone decompression was performed in the operating theatre depending on the values of intracranial pressure. In our series 41% of patients had a good recovery, 18% a severe disability, 23% a vegetative state and 18% died. The findings showed that the bony decompression must be performed early before the situation becomes irreversible. We suggest that if intracranial pressure values remain greater than 30 mmHg with cerebral perfusion pressure below 70 mmHg, despite vigorous anti-edema therapy, decompressive craniectomy should be considered.

Keywords: Acute subdural hematoma; brain edema; cerebral contusion; decompressive craniectomy.

Introduction

It has been reported in numerous clinical studies on head injury that elevated intracranial pressure is related to increased death. The single most frequent cause of death is uncontrollable intracranial pressure. An intracranial pressure of 30–40 mmHg has been considered to be dangerous. Thus, reduction of ICP is one of the major goals when treating severely head injured patients. When the intracranial pressure value remains greater than 30 mmHg, with failure of anti-edema therapy, decompressive craniectomy should be considered.

Materials and Methods

In our Hospital all severe head injuries with a Glasgow Coma Score (GCS) of 8 or less are admitted to the intensive care unit (ICU): immediately we perform a computed tomographic (CT) scan, chest and spinal column x-ray, ICP monitoring and monitoring of jugular bulb oximetry. Generally for increased ICP we elevate the head by 30 degrees, insert an intraventricular catheter, and use hyperosmolar therapy with mannitol and mild hyperventilation (PCO2 of 30–35 torr). When these measures fail to maintain the ICP below 20 torr with cerebral perfusion pressure above 70 torr we use mild hypothermia to 35 degrees Celsius [13]. Pre and post-operative barbiturate therapy is used in selected patients with a worsening trend and increase of ICP above 20 torr. Ventriculostomy was performed in one patient [8].

Results

Between October 1996 and December 1998 we treated 22 patients with decompressive craniectomy. The patients were peaced in the supine position with a mild degree of reverse Trendelenburg positioning. The surgical procedure involved a bicoronal, horseshoe or reverse question mark-shaped skin flap based on the ear. A wide hemicraniectomy was performed with the removal of frontal, temporal and parietal bone. The dura was opened to the extent of the bone decompression. A large dural graft was used to augment the dura before closure. The temporalis musculature and skin were reapproximated. The results are reported in Tables 1 and 2. In our series 41% of patients had a good recovery, 18% a severe disability, 23% a vegetative state and 18% died [3, 10, 15].

Discussion

A decompressive craniectomy was performed when the intracranial pressure (ICP) remained steady above

Table 1. *Patients Undergoing Craniectomy for Uncontrollable Post-Traumatic Intracranial Pressure. Patient Characteristics and Treatment Information**

Pat. no	Age (Yr)	Diagnosis	Time craniec.	Bone flap
1	17	R AEH R O C	URG	R O
2	26	BIL F C	10	BIL F
3	29	L ASH	2	BIL FTP
4	22	R FTP C	2	R FTP TOILET
5	18	L F C R ASH	5	BIL F TOILET
6	12	R ASH R FT C L AEH	URG	R FT TOILET
7	52	L ASH R ASH R T C	URG	L FTP R TOILET
8	30	L ASH L FT C	URG	L FT TOILET
9	16	L ASH L TP C	URG	L FTP TOILET
10	62	L ASH L FT C	URG + 10	L FTP TOILET
11	9	L ASH L FT C	URG	L FTP
12	60	BIL ASH BIL F C	URG + 1	BIL F TOILET
13	27	L ASH	URG	BIL F
14	20	R ASH BIL F C	URG	R FTP
15	36	L FP AEH R P AEH BIL F C	URG 12 HRS	L FTP R P
16	30	L F C	URG + 4	L FTP TOILET
17	16	R F C L FP AEH	URG + 1	R F TOILET L FP
18	56	R FTP C	1	R FTP
19	24	L P AEH L P ASH	1	L FTP
20	44	R ASH R FTPO C	URG	R TP
21	52	L P ASH L PT C R TPO C	URG	R TP TOILET
22	31	L ASH L F C	5	L FTP TOILET

* *R* Right; *L* left; *ASH* acute subdural hematoma; *AEH* acute extradural hematoma; *C* contusion; *F* frontal; *T* temporal; *P* parietal; *O* occipital.

30 mmHg (the ICP was monitored with an intraparenchymal Codman transducer). Other criteria were the cerebral perfusion pressure (CPP) below 70 mmHg and failure of antiedema therapy [1, 2, 4, 5, 6, 7, 9, 12]. In our experience if we are not able to maintain the ICP below 30 mmHg and CPP above 30–60 mmHg, patients die or remain vegetative. Patient number 4 became midriatic for a few minutes with ICP of 33 and CPP of 50 mmHg. This is not valid for all the patients but it represents a border-line value. Sometimes the bony decompression was done without ICP monitoring when there was an imminent herniation during evacuation of a hematoma and/or the removal of cerebral contusions (Fig. 1). We always perform a wide bony decompression on the side of the edema (Figs. 2, 3) except when the edema is seen bilaterally [11, 14]. The intraoperative observations suggest that the target of bony decompression is to obtain a wide herniation of the cerebral parenchyma. In this way we avoid steps between cerebral parenchyma and bone. The dural graft must be wide and redundant. We suggest particular attention to soft tissue and the skin flap because frequently these patients undergo surgery more than once. We cut the bone so that the edges will not be sharp. In this way we reduce the possibility of infection (two cases) and improve wound healing. When the dura is opened, there is a 50% decrease in ICP but after the soft tissues are reapproximated we noticed an increase of 20%. To avoid increasing ICP by 20% we widely separated the soft tissues from bone. In this way we obtained more space to allow the brain to expand.

Conclusions

In our series the patients were young and most of them were treated as emergencies for acute subdural hematoma and brain contusions. Sometimes the decision is very hard but must be made early before the situation becomes irreversible. Early surgery seems to optimise the outcome. We believe that the decompression in a selected group of patients justifies the mor-

Table 2. *Patient Characteristics and Treatment Information**

Pat. no.	GCS	Preop. ICP (mmHg)	Preop. CPP	Postop. ICP	Postop. CPP	OS
1	12	N/A	N/A	15–33	60–90	1
2	6	40–50	60	30–70	20	5
3	3	70	60	30	30	5
4	12	33	50	20	70	1
5	11	70	10	15–22	60	1
6	7	N/A	N/A	15	70	1
7	5	N/A	N/A	N/A	N/A	4
8	3	N/A	N/A	15–20	70	3
9	8	N/A	N/A	N/A	N/A	1
10	4	37–50	60	14–36	70–80	3
11	4	N/A	N/A	7–30	60–70	1
12	3	N/A	N/A	N/A	N/A	5
13	3	70–80	30	30	30	5
14	3	N/A	N/A	10–15	85–90	1
15	6	30–39	40–50	20	50–60	4
16	5	27–60	60	8–15	70–80	1
17	4	41	44	16–26	70	3
18	4	70	45	20–50	50–70	4
19	10	NA	NA	18–20	60–80	3
20	3	NA	NA	16–32	60–70	4
21	3	NA	NA	12–29	60–80	4
22	3	51	40–60	10–15	70–90	1

* *Preop.* preoperative; *Postop.* postoperative; *GCS* Glasgow Coma Scale; *GOS* Glasgow Outcome Score (5 = death); *ICP* intracranial pressure; *CPP* cerebral perfusion pressure, *N/A* not available.

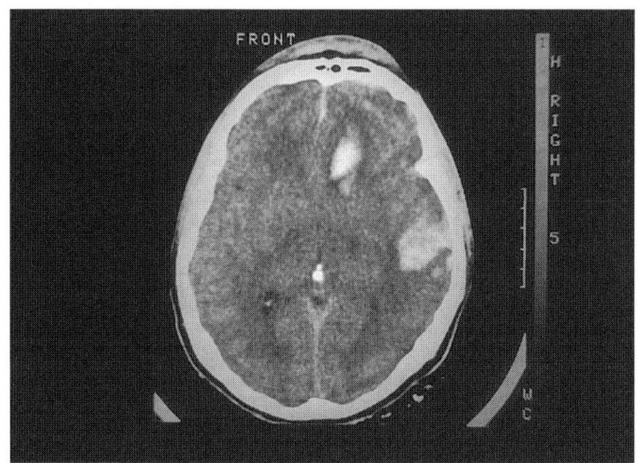

Fig. 1. CT scan obtained 2 days after admission in a 22 year old man (GCS 12). There is evidence of right frontal and temporal contusion. There was a sudden midriasis, ICP raised to 33 mmHg and CPP decreased to 50 mmHg. We performed a right fronto-tempor parietal bony decompression and toilette of frontal and temporal contusion

bidity, the added time and cost, the cosmetic disfigurement and the subsequent operation for replacement of the flap. We are aware that we need more cases to better understand the utility of this treatment and the comparison with other neurosurgical teams.

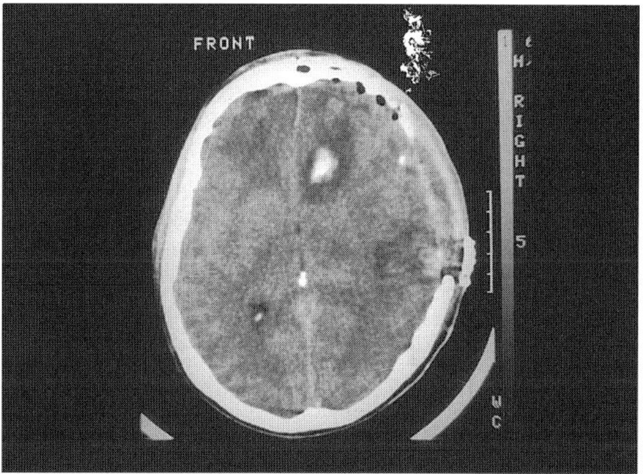

Fig. 2. CT scan obtained after the surgical treatment. We can see the edema around the contusions and the wide right bony decompression. The ICP decreased to 20 mmHg and CPP raised to 70 mmHg

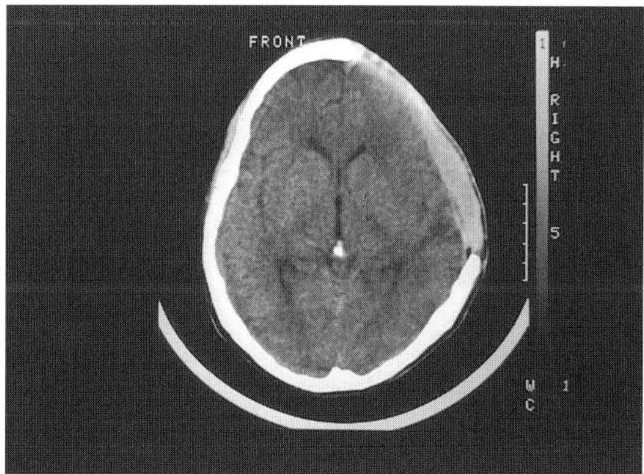

Fig. 3. In the last CT scan there is a complete reabsorption of right frontal and temporal contusion. The GOS at 6 months was good and the patient returned to his previous work after flap replacement

Acknowledgments

The authors wish to thank Mrs. Roberta Dalla Fontana for her assistance in preparing the manuscript and Mr. Piercarlo Facchin for preparing pictures.

References

1. Cooper PR, Rovit R, Ransohoff J (1975) Hemicraniectomy in the treatment of acute subdural hematoma: a re-appraisal. Surg Neurol 5: 25–28
2. Dam Hieu P, Sizun J, Person H, Besson G (1996) The place of decompressive surgery in the treatment of uncontrollable post-traumatic intracranial hypertension in children. Childs Nerv Syst 12: 270–275
3. Dent DL, Croce MA, Menke PG (1995) Prognostic factors after acute subdural hematoma. J Trauma 39: 36–43
4. Gaab MR, Rittierodt M, Lorenz M, Heissler HE (1990) Traumatic brain swelling and operative decompression: a prospective investigation. Acta Neurochir [Suppl] (Wien) 51: 326–328

5. Katayama Y, Tsubokawa T, Miyazaki S, Kawamata T, Yoshino A (1990) Oedema fluid formation within contused brain tissue as a cause of medically uncontrollable elevation of intracranial pressure: the role of surgical therapy. Acta Neurochir [Suppl] (Wien) 51: 308–310
6. Kjellberg RN, Prieto Jr A (1971) Bifrontal decompressive craniotomy for massive cerebral edema. J Neurosurg 34: 488–493
7. Jourdan CH, Convert J, Mottolese C, Bachour E, Gharbi S, Artru F (1993) Evaluation du benefice clinique de l'hemicraniectomie decompressive dans l'hypertension intracranienne non controlee par le traitement medical. Neurochirurgie 39: 304–310
8. Marmarou A, Maset AL, Ward JD, Choi S, Brooks D, Luts H, Moulton RJ, Muizalaar JP, DeSalles A, Young HF (1987) Contribution of CSF and vascular factors to elevation of ICP in severe head-injured patients. J Neurosurg 66: 883–890
9. Miller JD, Becker DP, Ward JD, Sullivan HG, Adams WE, Rosner MJ (1997) Significance of intracerebral hypertension in severe head injury. J Neurosurg 47: 503–516
10. Phuenpathom N, Choomuang M, Ratanalert S (1993) Outcome and outcome prediction in acute subdural hematoma. Surg Neurol 4: 22–25
11. Polin RS, Shaffrey ME, Bogaev CA, Tisdale N, Germanson T, Bocchicchio B, Jane JA (1997) Decompressive bifrontal craniectomy in the treatment of severe refractory posttraumatic cerebral edema. Neurosurgery 41: 84–94
12. Ransohoff J, Benjamin MV, Gage Jr EL, Epstein F (1971) Hemicraniectomy in the management of acute subdural hematoma. J Neurosurg 34: 70–76
13. Rinaldi A, Mangiola A, Anile C, Maira G, Amante P, Ferraresi A (1990) Hemodynamic effects of decompressive craniectomy in cold-induced brain edema. Acta Neurochir [Suppl] (Wien) 51: 394–396
14. Venes JL, Collins WF (1975) Bifrontal decompressive craniectomy in the management of head trauma. J Neurosurg 42: 429–433
15. Zumkeller M, Behrmann R, Heissler HE, Dietz H (1996) Computed tomographic criteria and survival rate for patients with acute subdural hematoma. Neurosurgery 39: 708–713

Correspondence: Dr. Gianpaolo De Luca, Divisione di Neurochirurgia, Ospedale Civile di Vicenza, V.le Rodolfi 37, 36100 Vicenza, Italy.

Acta Neurochir (2000) [Suppl] 76: 405–408

The Impact of Acute Hyponatraemia on Severe Traumatic Brain Injury in Rats

C. Ke[1], **W. S. Poon**[1], **H. K. Ng**[2], **N. L. S. Tang**[3], **Y. Chan**[1], **J. Y. Wang**[1], and **J. N. K. Hsiang**[1]

[1] Neurosurgical Unit, Department of Surgery, Prince of Wales Hospital, The Chinese University of Hong Kong, Hong Kong
[2] Department of Anatomical and Cellular Pathology, Prince of Wales Hospital, The Chinese University of Hong Kong, Hong Kong
[3] Department of Chemical Pathology, Prince of Wales Hospital, The Chinese University of Hong Kong, Hong Kong

Summary

The effect of experimental acute hyponatraemia on severe traumatic brain injury (TBI) was studied in a modified impact-acceleration model. The cortical contusional volume was quantified by image analysis on serial sections, injured axons were visualized and quantified by β-Amyloid Precursor Protein (β-APP) immunohistochemical staining. Regional brain water content was estimated by the wet-dry weight method. The experiment was conducted in Group I (injury only) and Group II (injury followed by acute hyponatraemia). Comparison between the two groups showed that acute hyponatraemia significantly increased contusional volume (3.24 ± 0.70 mm^3 *vs.* 1.80 ± 0.65 mm^3, $P = 0.009$) and the number of injured axons (128.7 ± 44.3 *vs.* 41.7 ± 50.1, $P = 0.04$) in the right thalamus & basal ganglia region. Water content of the brain stem region was also significantly increased by acute hyponatraemia (73.71 ± 0.14% *vs.* 72.28 ± 0.93%, $P = 0.004$). These results suggest that acute hyponatraemia potentiates secondary brain damage in severe TBI by augmentation of both focal contusion and diffuse axonal injury. The injured brain stem region is more susceptible to edema formation induced by experimental acute hyponatraemia.

Keywords: Head injury; hyponatraemia; rat.

Introduction

Acute hyponatraemia, a common event following traumatic brain injury (TBI), is associated with unfavourable clinical outcome [2, 5]. In this study, the effects of acute hyponatraemia on experimental TBI were examined to answer the classical question of whether hyponatraemia potentiates further brain damage or is simply an epiphenomenon.

Materials and Methods

Adult male Sprague-Dawley rats (360–410 g) were used. Physiological parameters were monitored through catheterization of the right femoral artery as shown in Table 1. Body temperature was controlled within 37.5 ± 0.5 °C. The injury was produced in a modified impact-acceleration model [7]. A small cylindrical peg-shaped projection was added to the peripheral aspect of the inferior surface of the original stainless metal disc and was inserted into a 2 mm burr hole at the right parietal cranium located 3.5 mm lateral to the middle point of the sagittal suture. The projection contacted the dura mater whilst the disc was glued on the cranium as previously reported. Both contact and inertial effects were employed to produce focal cortical contusion and widespread diffuse axonal injury in this model. Severe level (450 g–2 m) was used exclusively. After the impact, mechanical ventilation was required for 15–20 minutes.

Immediately after the injury, experimental acute hyponatraemia was induced by subcutaneous injection of 0.5 μg ddAVP (Ferring, Sweden) followed by intraperitoneal infusion of 30 ml 2.5% glucose solution (three injections of 10 ml at two-hourly intervals) [4, 9]. The temporal change of serum sodium concentration is shown in Fig. 1. Animal groups are shown in Table 2. The injury only group was defined as Group I, the injury followed by experimental acute hyponatraemia group was defined as Group II. 16 animals were used in the pilot study, 58 in the experiment-proper.

For histopathological observation, after perfusion fixation, a 1.5-mm thick coronal cerebral section with cortical contusion and another from brain stem at the level of 3 mm posterior to the pineal gland were taken, routinely processed and paraffin-embedded. In the cerebral section, ten 10 μm-thick serial sections were performed with 100 μm increments, and histochemically stained with 0.5% cresyl violet +1% acid fuchsin to identify the irreversible neuronal damage [3]. The contusional area (mm^2) of each cerebral section was calculated by CAS^{TM} 200 image analyzer (Becton-Dickinson). The contusion volume (mm^3) was equal to the sum of all the contusion areas in these serial sections.

For axonal injury quantification, one cerebral section and one of brain stem were stained with monoclonal antibody against β-Amyloid Precursor Protein (β-APP) (Boehringer, clone 22C11) and Histomouse SP Kit (Zymed). The number of positive-stained injured axons (axonal swellings and the retraction balls) within the following three areas, was counted under 100× magnification: 1) in coronal section of the corpus callosum, 2) in a single 100× field of area with the most dense positive axonal profiles of thalamus & basal ganglia region, 3) in the pyramidal tracts of the brain stem.

Measurement of brain water content was based on wet-dry weight method [10]. A 2 mm-thick cerebral coronal section with contusion was taken, as was one from the brain stem at the above-mentioned level. Then the cerebral section was dissected along the plane of corpus callosum and the midline. 5 samples were collected from

Table 1. *The Blood Gas Physiological Parameters Between the Control and Head Injury Groups*

Groups	pH	P_{CO2} (kPa)	P_{O2} (kPa)	O_2SAT	MABP (mmHg)
Control	7.435 ± 0.064	3.806 ± 1.472	19.883 ± 0.516	0.990 ± 0.002	91.100 ± 2.247
Head injury	7.476 ± 0.074	3.073 ± 0.494	21.228 ± 2.228	0.992 ± 0.001	87.735 ± 1.887
P value	0.283	0.268	0.121	0.081	0.033

* Student-t test was used for comparison. After 1 hr recovery, the MABP (Mean Arterial Blood Pressure) of head injury group returned back to normal range of 99.3 ± 6.658 mmHg (Mean $\pm$ SD).

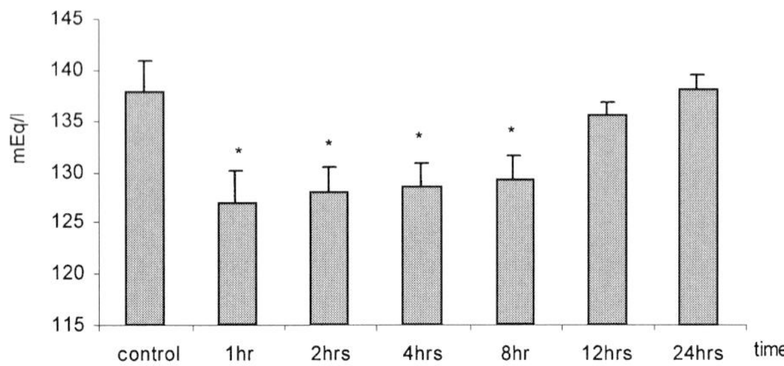

Fig. 1. Temporal curve of serum sodium concentration in normal rats with induced experimental acute hyponatremia. *The serum sodium concentration at 1 hr, 2 hrs, 4 hrs and 8 hrs post-induction groups were lower than that of the control group (Student's t test, $P < 0.05$)

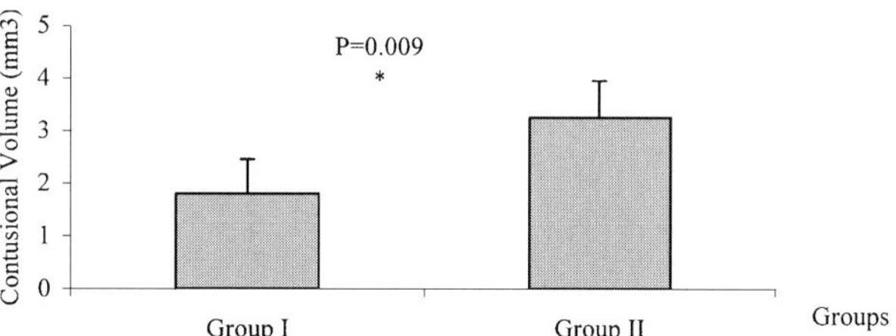

Fig. 2. Comparison of contusional volume at four hours post-injury. Group I was for injury only group, Group II was for the group with injury followed by acute hyponatraemia. (Mann-Whitney U Test)

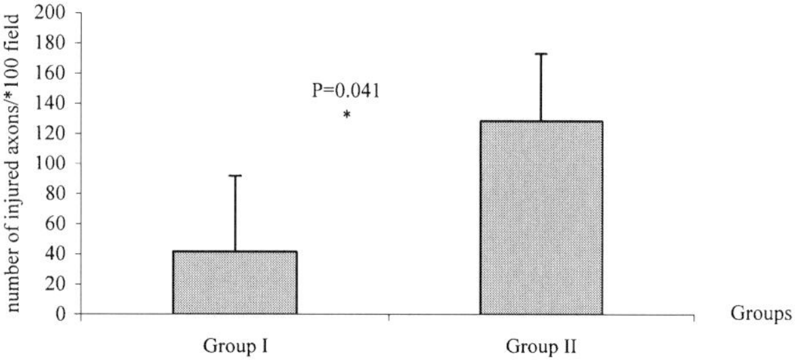

Fig. 3. Comparison of number of injured axons in right thalamus & basal ganglia region at four hours post-injury. Group I was for injury only group, Group II was for the group with injury followed by acute hyponatraemia (Mann-Whitney U Test)

Table 2. *Animal Groups*

Groups	Histopathological observation		Water content measurement	
	4 hr	1 day	4 hr	1 day
Control	5	–	5	5
Group I	6	5	5	6
Group II	6	5	5	5

* Group I represented injury only group, Group II represented the group with injury followed by acute hyponatraemia.

each brain. The water content was expressed as the percentage of water: $100 \times$ (wet wt. − dry wt.)/wet wt. %. Data were expressed as mean $\pm$ standard deviation, and evaluated by Mann-Whitney U test (SPSS 8.0™). A p value of less than 0.05 was considered as significant.

Results

At severe TBI, cortical contusion was observed at the projection-impacted site. When combined with acute hyponatraemia, the cortical contusional volume at 4 hr post-injury was significantly increased, as shown in Fig. 2.

Widespread diffuse axonal injury detected by β-APP immunohistochemical staining in the corpus callosum, thalamus & basal ganglia and pyramidal tracts was present in all injured objects. The extent of axonal injury in the right thalamus & basal ganglia region of Group II was significantly increased as shown in Fig. 3.

The contusional cortex of Group I showed edema formation at four hours post-injury, compared with control groups ($79.39 \pm 0.58\%$ vs. $78.28 \pm 0.72\%$, $P = 0.032$). At one day post-injury, there were significant increases of water content in thalami & basal

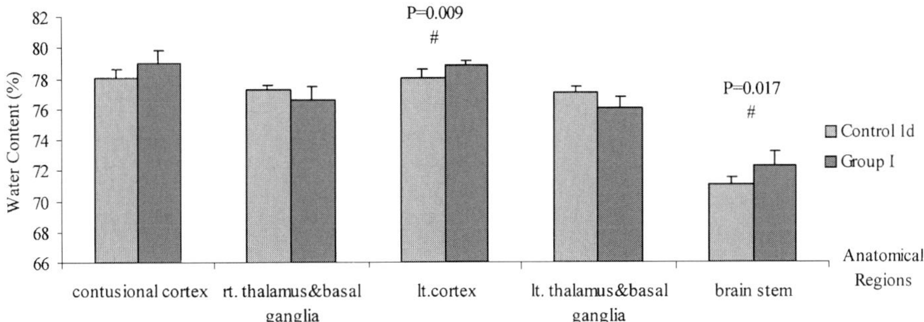

Fig. 4. Comparison of water content between control group and injury group at 1 day post-injury. Group I represented the injury only group. "rt." was for right, "lt." was for left

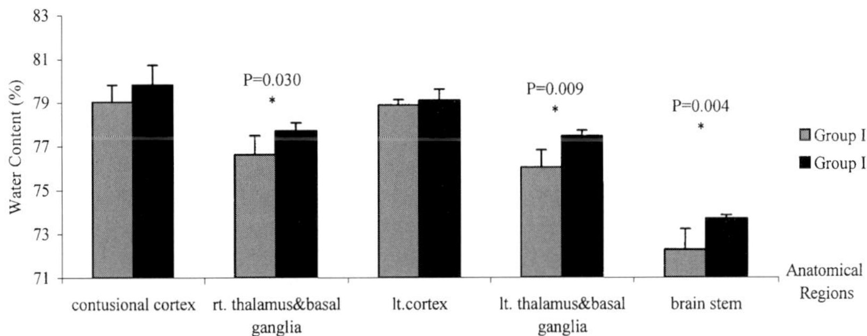

Fig. 5. Comparison of water content between group I and group II at 1 day post-injury. Group I was for the injury only group, Group II was for the injury followed by acute hyponatraemia. Abbreviations were the same as before

ganglia and brain stem of Group II, as shown in Figs. 4, 5.

Discussion

The present findings indicate that even a relatively short period of hyponatraemia (several hours) can increase the extent of severe TBI. A recent study showed that chronic hyponatraemia reduced the survival of involved magnocellular neurons with damaged axons [6]. The increased contusional volume in our study suggests that the survival of cortical neurons with damaged axons in the corpus callosum is exacerbated by the superimposed acute hyponatraemia. Since cellular mechanism of the traumatic injury is similar to ischemia, the adaptive processes to acute hyponatraemia (increased activity of Na^+-K^+- ATPase and decreased amiloride-sensitive sodium uptake) of the injured neurons could be severely impaired [9]. This may give rise to more neuronal swelling when the injury is followed by acute hyponatraemia. Secondly, brain acid buffering, ameliorating the intracellular acidosis, could also be impaired by acute hyponatraemia [1]. These adverse metabolic changes caused by acute hyponatraemia potentiate further neuronal death in the contusional area.

Acute hyponatraemia also increased the numbers of injured axons in the right (ipsilateral) thalamus & basal ganglia region at four hours post-injury. The time for the development of secondary axotomy (more than four hours) and axonal swelling (3–6 hrs post-injury) [8] was consistent with the time of increased axonal swelling and retraction balls in our study (four hours post-injury). This time point was also within the duration of induced experimental acute hyponatraemia. Thus, it was likely that acute hyponatraemia increased the axonal injury mainly through the increase of secondary axotomy and axonal swelling.

In the injury only group, the contusional cortex (at four hours), left cortex and the brain stem regions (at one day) showed oedema formation when compared with the control group. When severe TBI was combined with acute hyponatraemia, two less-involved cerebral regions (thalami and basal ganglia, not showing oedema formation in Group I) and brain stem showed significantly increased water content. In the contusional cortex and left cortex, even when accounting for the increased osmolar gradient between the blood and brain caused by acute hyponatraemia, the further increase in water content is not significant due to the pre-existing oedematous condition after TBI. However, the brain stem showed different trends: not only was oedema formation documented at the injury only level, but also a further significant increase of water content was observed when injury was followed by acute hyponatraemia. Therefore, it could be considered that the brain stem was more susceptible to the change of osmolarity resulting from acute hyponatraemia, compared with cerebral regions. The underlying mechanism of this phenomenon needs to be studied further.

Acknowledgment

We thank Kenny C. H. Ho, Rocky L. K. Ho and Ernest C. W. Chak from the Surgical Laboratory; also David S. Y. Lo and Hardy C. W. Ko from the Histopathological Laboratory of Dept. of Anatomical & Cellular Pathology for their technical assistance in this study.

References

1. Adler S, Verbalis JG, Williams D (1993) Effect of acute and chronic hyponatraemia on brain buffering in rats. Am J Physiol 264: F968–F974
2. Atchison JW, Wachendorf J, Haddock D, Mysiw WJ, Gribble M, Cornigan JD (1993) Hyponatraemia-associated cognitive impairment in traumatic brain injury. Brain Inj 7: 347–352
3. Auer RN, Kalimo H, Olsson Y, Siesjö BK (1985) The temporal evolution of hypoglycemic brain damage. I. Light- and electron-microscopic findings in the rat cerebral cortex. Acta Neuropathol (Berl) 67: 13–24
4. Dila CJ and Pappius HM (1972) Cerebral water and electrolytes. An experimental model of inappropriate secretion of antidiuretic hormone. Arch Neurol 26: 85–90
5. Dóczi T, Tarjányi J, Huszka E, Kiss J (1982) Syndrome of inappropriate secretion of antidiuretic hormone (SIADH) after head injury. Neurosurgery 10: 685–688
6. Dohanics J, Hoffman GE, Verbalis JG (1996) Chronic hyponatremia reduced survival of magnocellular vasopressin and oxytocin neurons after axonal injury. J Neurosci 16: 2373–2380
7. Marmarou A, Foda MAA, van den Brink W, Campbell J, Kita H, Demetriou K (1994) A new model of diffuse brain injury in rat: part I: pathophysiology and biomechanics. J Neurosurg 80: 291–300
8. Maxwell WL, Povlishock JT, Graham DL (1997) A mechanistic analysis of non disruptive axonal injury: a review. J Neurotrauma 14: 419–440
9. Vexler ZS, Ayus JC, Roberts TPL, Fraser CL, Kucharczk J, Arieff AI (1994) Hypoxic and ischemic hypoxia exacerbate brain injury associated with metabolic encephalopathy in laboratory animals. J Clin Invest 93: 256–264
10. Yang GY, Betz AL, Chenevert TL, Brunberg JA, Hoff JT (1994) Experimental intracerebral hemorrhage: relationship between brain edema, blood flow and blood-brain barier permeability in rats. J Neurosurg 81: 93–102

Correspondence: Dr. Wai S. Poon, Neurosurgical Unit, Department of Surgery, Prince of Wales Hospital, The Chinese University of Hong Kong. Shatin, N.T., Hong Kong.

Acta Neurochir (2000) [Suppl] 76: 409–413

Validation of a Closed Head Injury Model for use in Long-Term Studies

G. De Mulder[1], **K. Van Rossem**[2], **J. Van Reempts**[2], **M. Borgers**[2], and **J. Verlooy**[1]

[1] Department of Neurosurgery, University of Antwerp, Belgium
[2] Department of Life Sciences – Neuropathology, Janssen Research Foundation, Beerse, Belgium

Summary

To study pharmacotherapy of traumatic brain injury in rats, a modified closed head injury model was used that expresses clinically relevant features including intracranial hypertension and morphological alterations. Long-term survival under ethically acceptable conditions would greatly improve its clinical relevance. To ensure this goal with great reproducibility, the experimental protocol was adapted, in particular the impact-acceleration kinetics. Variations in impact-acceleration conditions were obtained by modifying the stiffness of the impact site and changing the height of a 400 g weight dropped from 51.5 to 31.5 cm (51.5/400; 31.5/400). Impact and acceleration were measured with a force sensor incorporated in a rigid dummy-rat and an accelerometer mounted on the platform onto which the animals are positioned. Significant correlation was shown between impact and acceleration. Accelerations obtained in rats were significantly lower than those in the dummy. Unlike the 51.5/400 group, in the 31.5/400 group no mortality or cranial fractures were observed. In both groups intracranial pressure rose to pathological values immediately after trauma and remained elevated longer than 24 h. Diffuse axonal injury developed in all groups and remained present for at least 7 days.

By reducing the impact-acceleration conditions, post-traumatic complications were diminished, while the clinically important features were maintained.

Keywords: Traumatic brain injury; histology; intracranial pressure; experimental model.

Introduction

Primary brain injury due to blunt head trauma results in focal or diffuse brain damage. This initial brain damage can be aggravated by secondary events such as hypoxia, ischemia, free radical production or intracranial hypertension. The substantial impact of diffuse brain injury on the outcome of head injured-patients has already been highlighted in various publications [1, 4, 6, 7, 8, 9, 11, 14]. Diffuse axonal injury is considered to be the principal morphological alteration and, depending on the extend to which it spreads and its location, is a determinant for the degree of morbidity [2, 3, 12]. Improvement of the long-term recovery of brain injured patients is of great importance to their social and economic rehabilitation. In addition, the reduction of mortality after traumatic brain injury would be more beneficial if accompanied by a significant reduction of morbidity. Investigation of the effect of pharmacotherapy on the convalescence of disabled patients would require long-term studies. To examine the pathophysiology and histopathology of traumatic brain injury a modified closed head injury (CHI) model was used that expresses several clinically relevant features, including intracranial hypertension, cellular (cytotoxic) and vasogenic oedema, neuronal necrosis and diffuse axonal injury [5, 10, 13]. The traditional impact-acceleration condition (a weight of 400 g dropped from a height of 70 cm) is well suited for acute experiments with anesthetized animals. However, detailed examination of the head of the rat after CHI occasionally revealed skull fractures, even remote from the impact site. This is considered a drawback for long-term studies. The aim of this study was to validate new conditions of impact and acceleration in the CHI model and evaluate the effects on their applicability and relevance with respect to long-term survival of the animals.

Materials and Methods

Trauma Device

The trauma device and original CHI conditions have been described in detail previously [5]. The trauma device consists of a horizontal platform mounted on four springs and a stabilizer to allow a vertical downward acceleration upon impact. The platform is placed under a vertical hollow Perspex© column containing a 400 g steel cylinder. The impact site of the cylinder is covered with a silicon disc 9 mm in diameter and 2 mm thick. The rat is firmly fixed onto the platform and impact is oriented to the bregma with the inter-aural line as a reference co-ordinate. Subsequently, the cylinder is dropped onto the unprotected head of the anesthetized rat, the respiration is checked, the skull carefully inspected and palpated and the airways cleared.

Adaptations

The impact-acceleration kinetics were adapted by modification of the stiffness of the impact site and alteration of the height from which the weight falls. The silicon disc at the tip of the weight was removed and the skull was exposed by retraction of the scalp. The impact-acceleration conditions were changed so that the weight of 400 g was dropped from a height of either 31.5 cm (31.5/400) or 51.5 cm (51.5/400).

To study the impact-acceleration kinetics of the apparatus in different conditions, a rigid teflon dummy rat was used and the weight and height were increased progressively.

Measurements of Impact and Acceleration

Impact and acceleration characteristics were measured respectively by means of a force sensor (type 9173, Kistler Instruments AG Winterthur, Switzerland) incorporated into a rigid, incompressible dummy rat and an accelerometer (type 8002, Kistler Instruments AG Winterthur, Switzerland) mounted on the stabilizer in the platform. The time course of force at impact and acceleration was displayed on an oscilloscope (Tektronix TDS 210, Beaverton, USA). Peak values were read from the display.

When animals underwent trauma, only the resulting acceleration was measured.

Animal Treatment and Preparation

Animal housing and treatment complied with European Union Directive for Animal Welfare. The study was carried out with 119 male Sprague-Dawley rats, weighing between 390 g and 420 g. Anesthesia was induced with 4% isoflurane in a mixture of 30% oxygen and 70% nitrous oxide, which was administered for 5 minutes. Subsequently, the rats were intubated and anesthesia was maintained at 2% isoflurane during further instrumentation. The head of the rat was fixed into a stereotaxic frame (Kopf Instruments, Düsseldorf) and the frontal and parietal bones of the skull were exposed by a 2 cm midline incision of the scalp and removal of the periost. Next the animal was positioned on the movable platform. A pointer indicating the correct position of the head ensured an impact at the bregma. The trachea tube was disconnected from the gas circuit and the weight was promptly dropped onto the skull. If skull fractures, apnea or convulsions occurred, the animals were excluded from the study and immediately killed with an overdose of pentobarbital. After induction of the trauma, the rat was repositioned in the stereotaxic apparatus for either intracranial pressure (ICP) measurements or closure of the scalp. A total of 26 and 81 animals were subjected to a CHI under conditions 31.5/400 and 51.5/400, respectively, and 12 sham-operated rats underwent anesthesia and surgical preparation but were not subjected to trauma. A total of 23 rats in the 31.5/400 group and 47 animals in the 51.5/400 group were used for ICP monitoring. ICP was measured either 15 min or 24 hours after trauma. A burr hole was made 2 mm caudal to the coronal suture and 4 mm from the midline in the right parietal plate of the skull. The microsensor probe (ICP Neuro microsensor, Codman & Shurtleff Inc. Randolph), mounted on a micromanipulator (DKI, Kopf Instruments, Düsseldorf) was inserted into the cortex of the right hemisphere. After a stabilization period of 15 minutes ICP was read from the recorder (Yokogawa, Europe B.V., Amersfoort).

Neuropathology

Rats used for histological studies were sacrificed 24 hours or 7 days after CHI. Fixation of the brain tissue was obtained by transcardial perfusion with a 4% formalin solution for 5 minutes at room temperature. Prior to perfusion, 0.2 ml of heparin (5000 IU/ml) was injected into the left ventricle, after which the descending aorta was clamped and the right atrium was opened. After transcardial perfusion the brains were immersion-fixed in situ in a 4% formalin solution for at least 24 hours. Coronal vibratome sections (300 μm) were prepared under stereotaxic guidance. The medial cingulum was considered the area of interest and was embedded in Epon. Histological evaluation was carried out with 2 μm sections stained with toluidine blue.

Statistical Analysis

Results were evaluated for statistical significance using a two-sided Wilcoxon-Mann-Whitney rank sum test. P-values of less than 0.05 were considered statistically significant.

Results

Impact Acceleration Kinetics

Table 1 shows accelerations obtained from the in vivo experiments and force and accelerations obtained with the dummy rat under the same conditions. Acceleration was reduced 80- to 100-fold when the weight

Table 1. *Impact and Acceleration Measurements*

		Impact ($kg.m/s^2$)		Acceleration (m/s^2)	
		31.5 cm/400 g	51.5 cm/400 g	31.5 cm/400 g	51.5 cm/400 g
Dummy	median	3860	5220	58.1×10^3	87×10^3
	range	3420–3910	4440–5220	54.2×10^3–60.5×10^3	75.7×10^3–95.2×10^3
Rats	median			680	900
	range			440–1210	620–1270

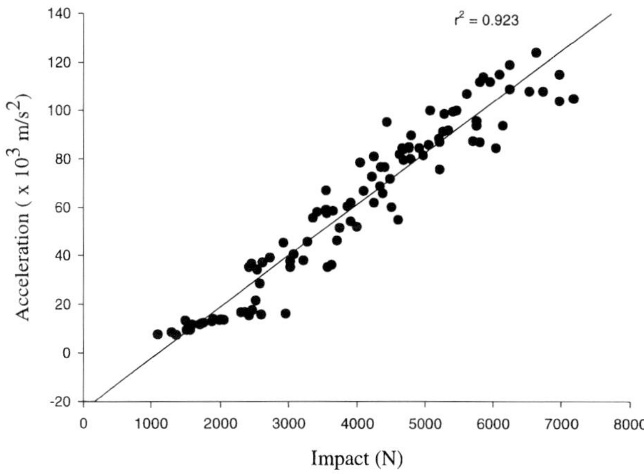

Fig. 1. Scatter plot with linear fit showing the linear correlation ($r^2 = 0.923$) between force upon impact and acceleration. These results were obtained using the dummy rat. Weight and height were gradually increased (20 cm/100 g up to 80 cm/500 g)

was dropped onto the rat skull. As shown in Fig. 1, a linear correlation was found between force at impact and the resulting acceleration of the movable platform ($r^2 = 0.923$).

ICP Measurements

In all impact-acceleration conditions ICP was significantly higher than in sham animals. There was a statistical difference in ICP between the 31.5/400 and the 51.5/400 group at 24 hours after trauma ($p = 0.03$), whereas no difference was shown after 15 minutes ($p = 0.25$) (Fig. 2).

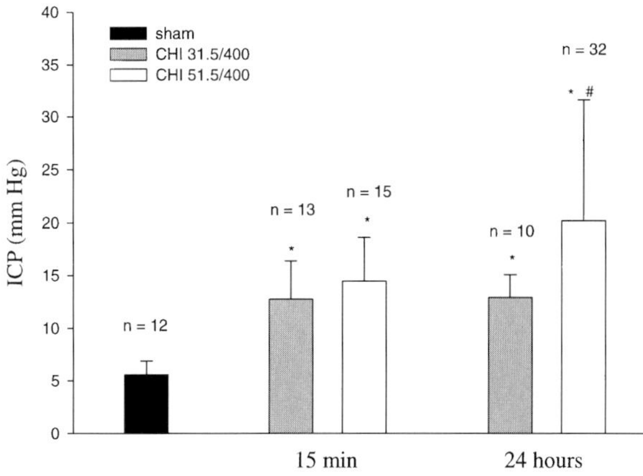

Fig. 2. Intracranial pressure in sham-injured rats and rats that underwent head trauma (51.5/400 and 31.5/400). ICP was obtained either 15 min or 24 hours after trauma. Values are mean ± SD. *$p < 0.001$ in comparison with sham rats; #$p = 0.03$ in comparison with the 31.5/400 condition after 24 hours (Wilcoxon-Mann-Whitney rank sum test)

Table 2. *Post-Traumatic Complications*

Complications	31.5 cm/400 g n = 26	51.5 cm/400 g n = 81
Skull fractures	0	12
Apnea	0	5
Convulsions	0	2
Asfyxia	0	4

Neuropathological Findings

The principal complication after closed head injury consists of skull fractures. Unlike in the 51.5/400 group, in the 31.5/400 group no mortality, nor cranial fractures, nor other complications were observed (Table 2).

Macroscopic evaluation of the rat brains revealed sporadic subdural hematomas and intraventricular hemorrhages in the 51.5/400 group only.

In sham-injured rats no histological damage was observed (Fig. 3a). Histological changes in the 51.5/400 group included cellular or perivascular edema and neuronal shrinkage with nuclear pycnosis (Fig. 3b). These were not present in the 31.5/400 group. Cortical contusions were sporadically seen in the severe condition, progressively evolving to a hemorrhagic infarction surrounded by a penumbra region (Fig. 3c). Diffuse axonal injury was observed in both groups 24 hours after CHI and was still present on the seventh day after the primary event. In contrast to sham-animals, axonal profiles in traumatized rats revealed a disorganized aspect (Figs. 3a, 4). At 24 hours after CHI, damage in the white matter was mainly characterized by axonal ballooning accompanied by densification of several axonal profiles in the 51.5/400 group (Figs. 4a, 4c). Six days later the latter damage was less pronounced while axonal swelling was still present (Figs. 4b, 4d). The alterations were more pronounced in the 51.5/400 group.

Discussion

In this study impact and acceleration were evaluated under various weight-drop conditions. A linear correlation between impact and acceleration was found through the use of a rigid dummy rat. This suggests that within the applied range of weights and heights the springs act in their linear range. When a true rat was used, the resulting acceleration was largely re-

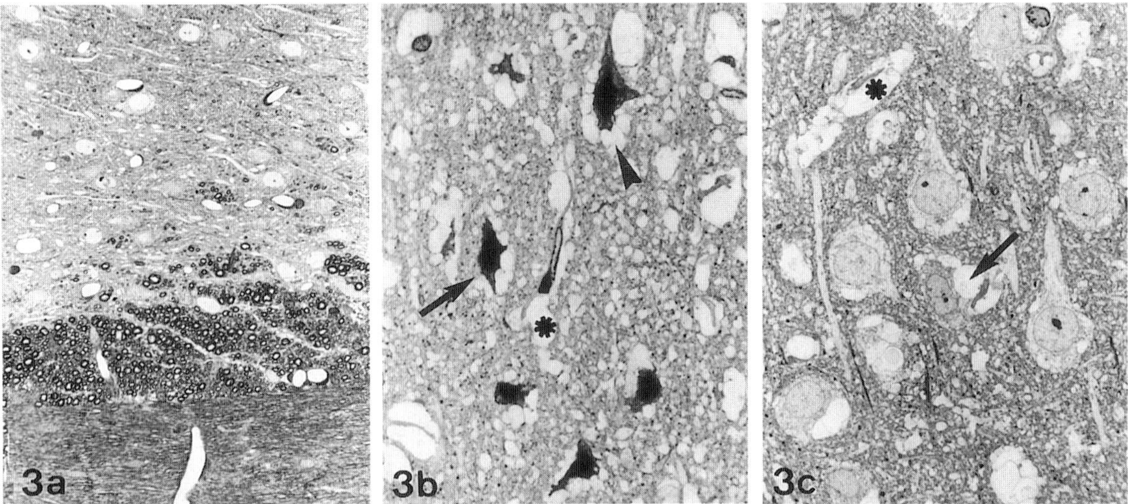

Fig. 3. Light microscopic picture of the cingulum in a sham-injured rat (a) and the cingulate cortex in rats that survived 24 hours after closed head injury (51.5/400) (b and c). (a) White and grey matter show a normal morphological aspect and normal structural organisation. (b) At the site of impact cortical neurons are shrunken and show nuclear pycnosis (arrow). Perineuronal (arrowhead) as well as the perivascular (asterisk) astroglia are swollen. (c) Around hemorrhagic contusions the tissue has a penumbra-like aspect. Micro-vessels are collapsd (asterisk), glial processes are swollen (arrow) but neurons are structurally preserved (2 μm epon section; toluidine blue-stained, a: × 280; b, c: × 580)

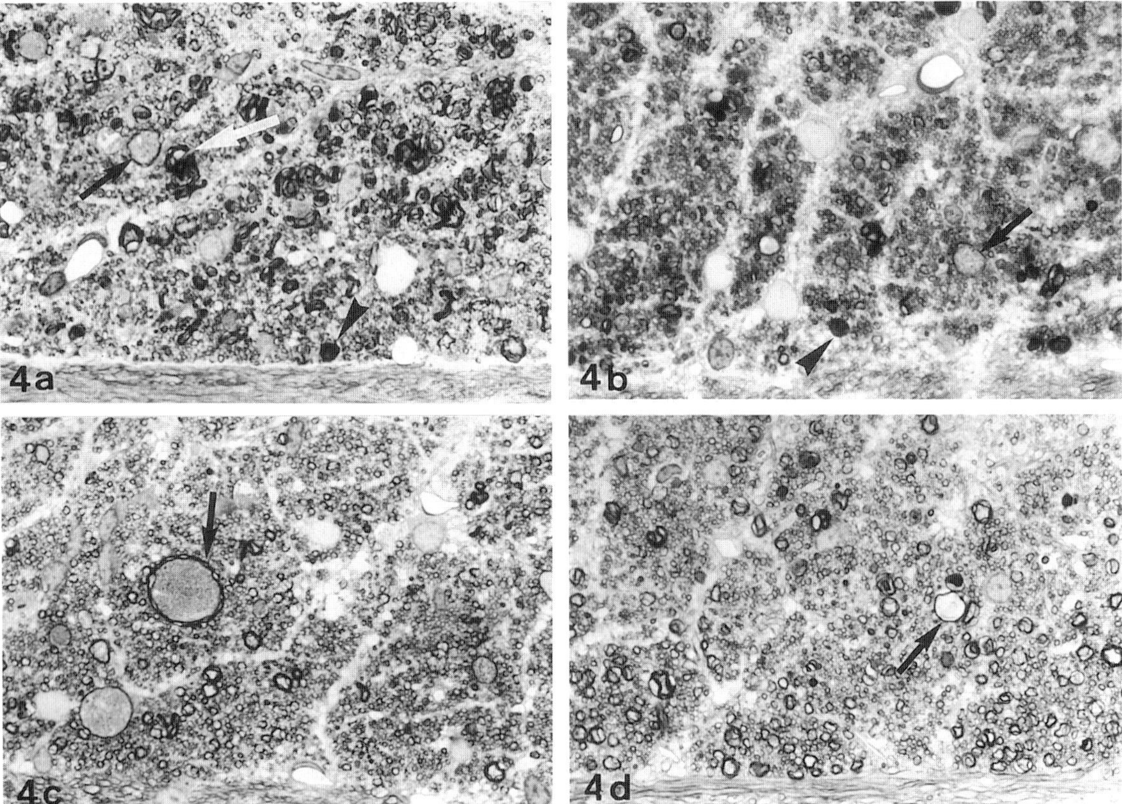

Fig. 4. Light microscopic aspect of the cingulum in rats that suffered from either a 51.5/400 (a and b) or a 31.5/400 trauma (c and d) and that survived either 24 hours (a and c) or 7 days (b and d). (a) In addition to pronounced disorganisation of the white matter, part of the axons show ballooning (arrow), myelin disintegration (white arrow) or densification of the axoplasm (arrowhead). (b) Seven days later axonal ballooning (arrow) and densification of axonal profiles (arrowhead) are still present. (c) Myelin disintegration, axonal swellings (arrow) and disorganisation are less pronounced after moderate head trauma. (d) Although to a lesser extend, axonal ballooning (arrow) and densification may persist at least for seven days (2 μm epon section; toluidine blue-stained, ×800)

duced indicating extensive energy absorption by the head of the rat.

Two impact-acceleration conditions were tested in rats with respect to their relevance and applicability in long-term studies of diffuse brain injury. In this scheme, the weight was kept constant at 400 g, the stiffness of the impact site remained unchanged, but the height was set at 31.5 cm or 51.5 cm. Both impact-acceleration conditions produced a pathologically elevated ICP and this was significantly higher in the 51.5/400 group 24 hours after trauma. In the 31.5/400 group there was no evidence of focal brain damage. The presence of such localized injuries in the 51.5/400 group might explain the more elevated ICP. Such injuries could induce secondary events with progressively developing edema around the lesion. Diffuse axonal injury, the major morphological alteration in diffuse brain injury, was present in both groups 24 hours after trauma and this change persisted for at least 1 week. In the 31.5/400 group no animals were excluded due to skull fractures, convulsions or apnea. We conclude that intracranial hypertension and diffuse axonal injury are consistent findings in the two conditions, whereas the impact-acceleration in the 31.5/400 group significantly reduces the post-traumatic complications. This moderate head trauma appears to be an appropriate and ethically acceptable paradigm for long-term hemodynamic, morphological and neurological studies of diffuse brain injury.

References

1. Adams JH, Graham DI, Murray LS, Scott G (1982) Diffuse axonal injury due to non-missile head injury in humans: an analysis of 45 cases. Ann Neurol 12: 557–563
2. Adams JH (1992) Head injury. In: Greenfield's neuropathology, 4th edn. In: JH Adams, LW Duchen (eds) Edward Arnold, London, pp 123–134
3. Blumbergs PC, Scott GT, Manavis J, Wainwright H, Simpson DA, McLean A (1995) Topography of axonal injury as defined by amyloid precursor protein and the sector scoring method in mild and severe closed head injury. J Neurotrauma 12(4): 565–572
4. Christman CW, Grady MS, Walker SA, Holloway KL, Povlishock JT (1994) Ultrastructural studies of diffuse axonal injury in humans. J Neurotrauma 11: 173–186
5. Engelborghs K, Verlooy J, Van Reempts J, Van Deuren B, Van De Ven M, Borgers M (1998) Temporal changes in intracranial pressure in a modified experimental model of closed head injury. J Neurosurg 89: 796–806
6. Gennarelli TA, Thibault LE, Adams JH, Graham DI, Thompson CJ, Marcincin RP (1982) Diffuse axonal injury and traumatic coma in the primate. Ann Neurol 12: 564–574
7. Gennarelli TA (1997) The pathobiology of traumatic brain injury. Neuroscientist 3: 73–81
8. Graham DI, Adams JH, Nicoll JA, Maxwell WL, Gennarelli TA (1995) The nature, distribution and causes of traumatic brain injury. Brain Pathol 5(4): 397–406
9. Graham DI, Gennarelli TA (1997) Trauma. Greenfield's neuropathology, vol. 1. 6th edn. In: DI Graham, PL Lantos (eds) Edward Arnold, London, pp 197–262
10. Marmarou A, Montasser A, Foda A-E, Van Den Brink W, Campbell J, Kita H, Demetriadou K (1994) A new model of diffuse brain injury in rats. Part I: pathophysiology and biomechanics. J Neurosurg 80: 291–300
11. Maxwell WL, Povlishock JT, Graham DI (1997) A mechanistic analysis of non) disruptive axonal injury: a review. J Neurotrauma 14: 419–440
12. Meaney DF, Ross DT, Winkelstein BA, Brasko J, Goldstein D, Bilston LB, Thibault LE, Gennarelli TA (1994) Modification of the cortical impact model to produce axonal injury in the rat cerebral cortex. J Neurotrauma 11: 599–612
13. Montasser A, Foda A-E, Marmarou A (1994) A new model of diffuse brain injury in rats. Part II: Morphological characterisation. J Neurosurg 80: 301–313
14. Shigemori M, Kikuchi N, Tokutomi T, Ochiai S, Kuramoto S (1992) Coexisting diffuse axonal injury (DAI) and outcome of severe head injury. Acta Neurochir [Suppl] (Wien) 55: 37–39

Correspondence: Gert De Mulder, M.D., University Hospital Antwerp, Department of Neurosurgery, Wilrijkstraat 10, B-2650 Edegem, Belgium.

Acta Neurochir (2000) [Suppl] 76: 415–418

Diffuse Axonal Injury with or Without an Evacuated Intracranial Hematoma in Head Injured Patients. Are They Different Lesions?

S. Lubillo[1], **J. Bolaños**[1], **J. A. Cardeñosa**[1], **F. Robaina**[2], **P. Ponce**[3], **J. Morera**[2], and **J. L. Manzano**[1]

[1] Intensive Care Unit, Hospital del Pino.C/Angel Guimerá, Las Palmas, Canary Islands, Spain
[2] Neurosurgery Department, Hospital del Pino.C/Angel Guimerá, Las Palmas, Canary Islands, Spain
[3] Radiology Department, Hospital del Pino.C/Angel Guimerá, Las Palmas, Canary Islands, Spain

Summary

The general classification of head injury proposed by Marshall *et al.*, based on admission CT scan findings, might mask a group of patients who have Diffuse Brain Injury (DI) in addition to intracranial haematomas. The aim of this study was to assess possible differences in outcome with respect to the level of intracranial pressure (ICP) and cerebral perfusion pressure (CPP) between a group of patients with DI: III–IV (Marshall's classification) after the evacuation of an intracranial haematoma (group A) and another group with DI: III–IV in the absence of a mass lesion (group B). We prospectively studied 129 patients with isolated and closed severe head injury (GCS < 9). In *group A* ($n = 61$), the median percentage of hours with ICP > 20 mmHg and CPP < 70 mmHg was 42.8 and 18, respectively and 17 (28%) survived with GOS 4–5. In *group B* ($n = 68$), median values of 20 and 5.5 hours were obtained for ICP > 20 and CPP < 70 respectively, whilst 39 (57.3%) survived with favourable outcomes. When we analysed the effects of the DI: III–IV in both groups of patients, we found that the differences in percentage of time with ICP > 20 and CPP < 70 were statistically significant ($p < 0.01$) and patients in group A had a higher morbidity and mortality ($p < 0.05$). This study has demonstrated that the levels of ICP, morbidity and mortality in patients with DI: III–IV and an evacuated mass lesion were higher than in patients with DI: III–IV without a mass lesion.

Keywords: Head injury; diffuse brain damage; intracranial pressure; outcome.

Introduction

The categorisation of severe head injuries on the basis of computerised tomography (CT) has proved useful in identifying subsets of patients at different risk for developing raised intracranial pressure (ICP) and further neurological deterioration [1, 4, 5, 8, 15–17]. Marshall's classification [11] allows a better prediction of the final outcome than previous classifications, separating traumatic injuries into the broader categories of diffuse versus focal or mass lesions, and is now widely accepted. However, this classification has significant limitations in terms of prognosis, because it has been based solely on the analysis of initial CT scans. As traumatic brain damage is a dynamic process, it is also important to document intracranial pathological changes that develop during the acute post-traumatic period, by analysis of a repeat CT scan. Thus, patients who have undergone craniotomy for the evacuation of an intracranial haematoma, who also have diffuse brain injury (DI) on their early post-operative CT Scan, and patients with DI: I–II on their admission scan, may develop "swelling" or new lesions on repeat CT Scans. Such patients are at risk from raised ICP and may have a high mortality, but they cannot be reclassified in the Trauma Coma Data Bank.

For this purpose, we analysed prospectively the differences in outcome with respect to the level of ICP and Cerebral Perfusion Pressure (CPP) between patients with DI: III–IV on post-operative CT scans after evacuation of a mass lesion, and those with DI: III–IV, but without a mass lesion, during the acute post-traumatic period.

Material and Methods

We have prospectively studied 129 patients with severe head injury admitted to our Intensive Care Unit (ICU) at the Hospital Universitario del Pino, over a period of four years (1994–1998). All patients had isolated and closed severe head injury (Glasgow Coma Score (GCS) [14] ≤ 8 points post-resuscitation), and were admitted during the first 6 hours after trauma. ICP and CPP were continuously measured and in all of them a repeat CT scan was performed within 24 hours of the admission CT scan. The best motor GCS (mGCS) and pupil reactions after resuscitation were obtained at the scene or immediately after admission to our hospital. The patients were classified in two groups depending on whether their best mGCS was greater or less than 3. With respect to the pupillary response, patients were classified as having 1 or 2 reactive pupils. Pre-hospital arterial hypotension was defined as one or more recordings of a systolic blood pressure lower than 90 mmHg.

On admission, all patients were classified as having focal lesions requiring evacuation (Marshall V) and Diffuse Injury (Marshall I–IV). On the CT Scan on admission, we also evaluated associated intracranial injuries (including the presence of intraventricular haemorrhage, intracerebral haematoma, cerebral contusions less than 25 cc and subarachnoid haemorrhage). A second CT Scan (the repeat scan) was performed in all patients within 24 hours of admission. Although following their original categorisation, patients with an evacuated mass lesion cannot be re-classified, for the purposes of this study, we re-allocated them to a diffuse brain injury category, on the basis of their immediate post operative (2–12 hours) CT scan. The patients were divided in two groups; the first group (A) included DI: III–IV after evacuation of a intracranial hematoma, and the second group (B) included DI: III–IV without a mass lesion. In the postoperative patients (Group A), patients with residual or recurrent mass lesions greater than 25 c were excluded from the study.

We studied the percentage of time that the ICP was higher than 20 mmHg and CPP lower than 70 mmHg applying this formula: 100 times the number of hours with ICP $>$ 20 or CPP $<$ 70 divided by total hours of monitoring of ICP/CPP gathered from the nurse chart.

Patients were scored on the 5 point Glasgow Outcome Scale [7] after six months of follow up and for statistical purposes, favourable (good recovery and moderate disability) and non-favourable (severe disability, vegetative state or deceased) outcome groups were considered.

All patients were managed by a standard regimen that emphasised prevention of secondary insults to the brain. It included: head up position 30°, maintenance of normovolemic state, normothermia and normoglycemia, ventilation to maintain a paO2 of at least 100 mmHg and paCO2 about 35 mmHg and insertion of pulmonary artery catheters when necessary. Intracranial pressure was continuously monitored, usually by ventriculostomy, and a pressure higher than 20 mmHg was treated with sedation, paralysis, cerebrospinal fluid drainage and mannitol. Hyperventilation with paCO2 lower than 30 mmHg and barbiturates were used only if ICP $>$ 20 was refractory to the above regimen, after ruling out a new intracranial space occupying lesion. Mean arterial blood pressure (MAP) was continuously monitored and fluids and inotropes were given to maintain a level of CPP of at least 70 mmHg.

Discrete variables were compared using chi-square analysis or Fisher's exact test. Continuous variables were compared using Wilcoxon's test. Differences at the 0.05 level were considered statistically significant. The statistical software package used was SPSS.

Results

We have followed 129 patients with isolated and closed severe head injury who were admitted to our ICU. Their age ranged from 16–81 years (median 35.3 $\pm$ 17.6) and their median GCS was 5 points (range 3–8). The overall hospital mortality was 37% (47 patients). All of the 82 patients who survived were followed up and their outcome 6 months after discharge from hospital was as follows: 56 patients (43.4%) had a favourable outcome (good recovery or moderate disability) and 26 had an unfavourable outcome, of whom 19 were severely disabled or vegetative and 7 had died.

There were no statistical differences in age, median GCS, percentage of patients with unreactive pupils, mGCS, pre-hospital hypotension and associated intracranial lesions on admission CT scan, between patients in group A (Diffuse Injury III–IV after the evacuation of an intracranial haematoma), and those in group B (Diffuse Injury III–IV without an intracranial mass lesion; Table 1).

In the sixty one patients in group A, the median percentage of hours with ICP $>$ 20 and CPP $<$ 70 was 42.8% and 18% respectively and 17 (28%) survived with favourable outcomes (good recovery or moderate disability). In the sixty eight patients in group, the median percentage of hours with ICP $>$ 20 and CPP $<$

Table 1. *Admission Characteristics of Patients with Diffuse Injury III–IV "with" and "Without" an Evacuated Mass Lesion*

Diffuse injury III–IV			
Admission characteristics	With evacuated mass lesion (N = 61p)	Without evacuated mass lesion (N = 68p)	p value
AGE (mean $\pm$ SD)	37.6 $\pm$ 17.2	33.8 $\pm$ 16.4	NS*
median GCS	5	5	NS*
Motor GCS $\leq$ 3p	38 (62%)	40 (58.8%)	NS**
Unilateral unreactive pupil	17 (27.9%)	11 (16.4%)	NS**
Bilateral unreactive pupils	24 (39.3%)	18 (26.4%)	NS**
Assoc. intracranial lesions	45 (73.8%)	50 (73.5%)	NS**
Pre-hospital hypotension	26 (42.6%)	20 (29.4%)	NS**

* Wilcoxon's Test. ** Chi Square Analysis.

Table 2. *Diffuse Injury III–IV "with" and "Without" an Evacuated Mass Lesion. Percentage of Time (Hours) of ICP > 20 mmHg and CPP < 70 mmHg and Outcome*

Diffuse injury III–IV				
	With evacuated mass lesion (N = 61p)	Without evacuated mass lesion (N = 68p)	p value	Odds ratio (95%) CI[2]
ICP > 20 mmHg (P50[1])	42.8	20	0.001[3]	–
CPP < 70 mmHg (P50[1])	18	5.5	0.001[3]	–
Favourable outcome	17 (28%)	39 (57.3%)	0.001[4]	1.98 (1.28–3.1)
Mortality	32 (52.5%)	22 (32.3%)	0.05[4]	2.30 (1.13–4.72)

[1] Median; [2] Confidence interval; [3] Wilcoxon's Test; [4] Chi square analysis.

70 mmHg was 20% and 5.5% respectively, and 39 patients (57.3%) survived with favourable outcomes.

When we compared the median percentage of hours with ICP > 20 and CPP < 70 mmHg in the two group of patients, we found that the differences were statistically significant ($p < 001$). In addition, in group A, there were fewer patients with favourable outcomes, ($p < 0.001$, OR = 1.98 (1.29–1.31)) and there was a significantly higher mortality than in group B ($p < 0.005$, OR = 2.30 (1.13–4.72; Table 2).

Discussion

Computerised tomography scanning is indispensable in the diagnosis and serial evaluation of patients suffering from severe head injury and has been used as a tool for assessing outcome in such patients. The classification proposed by Marshall *et al.* [11], based on CT findings on admission, uses the status of the mesencephalic cisterns, the degree of midline shift, and the presence or absence of focal lesions to categorize the patients into different prognostic groups. In our series, of the 43 patients in group A with patent basal cisterns on admission, 28 had compressed or absent cisterns and 6 had persistent midline shift > 5 mm on their post-surgical CT scans. Seven patients with initial effacement of the basal cisterns, had normal cisterns after surgical evacuation. In our study, group A patients underwent emergency surgery to evacuate the traumatic haematoma and of course may have subsequent injury. In twenty two patients with DI: II on admission in the absence of mass lesions or associated underlying contusions (group B), the second CT showed DI: III or IV within 24 hours of trauma. These data, that might reflect the dynamic process of brain damage after traumatic injury, are similar to those obtained by Lobato *et al.* [9]. They analysed changes in intracranial pathology, by comparing the initial and repeat CT scans, and 51% of the patients in their series were subsequently reassigned to a different diagnostic category.

Intracranial hypertension (ICP > 20) is a frequent finding in patients who have an abnormal CT scan. Eisenberger at al [4] in a National Institute of Health TCDB study and Narayan *et al.* [13], reported that the incidence of intracranial hypertension was higher than 50% in such patients. In our study, 109 patients (84%) had at least one episode of elevated ICP (> 20); 59 patients (97%) in group A (with an evacuated mass lesion) and 50 patients (84.5%) in group B (without mass lesion), but in the latter group, patients responded satisfactorily to therapy and had a shorter period of time with ICP > 20 and CPP < 70. Our most interesting finding was that the morbidity and mortality of patients with DI: III–IV and an evacuated mass lesion was higher than that of patients with the same diagnostic category of diffuse injury and admission characteristics, but without a mass lesion on admission.

Like other studies [5, 6, 12, 18], a fall was the most frequent mechanism of injury in group A, whereas in group B it was a road traffic accident. Our data might imply the involvement of different pathophysiological mechanisms in the evolution of traumatic brain damage. However, there is not always a strict separation in patients who suffer head trauma between those with diffuse injury and those with a haematoma. These lesions may co-exist, and their combined effects may explain why patients with mass lesions, and underlying diffuse injury have a worse outcome. It is likely that the presence of an intra-axial or extra-axial mass lesion might be the most severe form of diffuse injury, and when it is evacuated, the remaining lesions are similar to those found in cases without a mass. Other factors, such as re-perfusion brain oedema after evacuating an intracranial hematoma, and alteration of the blood brain barrier in remote areas from impact, have been implicated, but their relative contribution remains controversial [2, 3, 10].

In summary, the findings of this study suggest that there are different types of diffuse injury in patients with or without an evacuated mass lesion. Patients with DI: III–IV after an evacuated mass lesion had higher levels of ICP, morbidity and mortality than patients with DI: III–IV without a mass lesion.

References

1. Clifton Gl, Grossmann RG, Makela ME, Miner ME, Handel S, Sadhu V (1980) Neurological course and correlated computerised tomography findings after severe closed head injury. J Neurosurg 52: 611–624
2. Delzoppo GJ (1994) Microvascular changes during cerebral ischemia and reperfusion. Cerebrovasc Brain Cir Rev: 6: 47–96
3. Dodson BA (1995) Normal perfusion pressure breakthrough syndrome: Entity or excuse? J Neurosurg Anesth 7: 203–207
4. Eisenberger HM, Gary HE, Aldrich FE *et al* (1990) Initial CT findings in 753 patients with severe head injury. A report from NIH Traumatic Coma Data Bank. J Neurosurg 73: 688–699
5. Gennarelli TA, Speilman GM, Langfitt TW, Gildenberg PL, Harrington T, Jane JA, Marshall LF, Miller JD, Pitts LH (1982) Influence of the type of intracranial lesion on outcome from severe head injury. J Neurosurg 56: 26–32
6. Gennarelli *et al* (1993) Mechanism of head injury. J Emerg Med [Suppl] 11: 11–15
7. Jennet B, Bond M (1975) Assessment of outcome after severe brain damage. A practical scale. Lancet 1: 480–484
8. Lobato RD, Rivas JJ, Cordobes JJ, De la Fuente M, Montero A, Barcena A, Perez C, Cabrera A, Lamas E (1983) Outcome from severe head injury related to the type of intracranial lesion. A computerised tomography study. J Neurosurg 59: 762–774
9. Lobato RD, Gomez PA, Alday R, Rivas JJ, Dominguez J, Cabrera a, Turanzas FS, Benitez A, Rivero B (1997) Sequential computerized tomography changes and related final outcome in severe head injury patients. Acta Neurochir (Wien) 139: 385–391
10. Long DM (1982) Traumatic brain edema In: Weiss MH (ed) Clin Neurosurg 29: 174–202
11. Marshall LF, Marshall SB, Flauber MR *et al* (1991) A new classification of head injury based on computerized tomography. J Neurosurg 75: S15–S20
12. Miller JD, Becker DB (1982) Principles and pathophysiology of head injury. In: Youmans JR (ed) Neurological surgery, 2nd edn. WB Saunders Co, Philadelphia PA 4: 1896–1937
13. Narayan RK, Kishore PRS, Becker OP, Ward JD, Enas GG, Greenberg RP, Domingues Da, Silva A, Lipper MH, Choi SC, Mayhall CG, Lutz HA, Young HF (1982) Intracranial pressure: to monitor or not to monitor? A review of our experience with severe injury. J Neurosurg 56: 650–659
14. Teasdale G, Jennett B (1974) Assessment of coma and impaired consciousness. A practical scale. Lancet 2: 81–84
15. Teasdale E, Cardoso E, Galbraith S, Teasdale G (1984) CT scan in severe head diffuse injury: physiological and clinical correlations. J Neurol Neurosurg Psychiatry 47: 600–603
16. Turazzi S, Bricolo S, Pasut L, Formenton A (1987) Changes produced by CT scanning in the outlook of severe head injury. Acta Neurochir (Wien) 85: 87–95
17. van Dongen KJ, Braakman R, Gelpke GJ (1983) The prognostic value of computerized tomography in comatose head injury patients. J Neurosurg 59: 951–957
18. Wollner DG, Torner JC, Eisenberg HM, Marshall LF (1991) Age and outcome following traumatic coma: why do older patients fare worse? J Neurosurg 75: S37–S49

Correspondence: S. Lubillo, M.D. C/TTE Coronel Castillo Olivares, 26, 17A2, Las Palmas GC, 350011 Canary Islands, Spain.

Acta Neurochir (2000) [Suppl] 76: 419–421

Increased Adrenomedullin in Cerebrospinal Fluid After Traumatic Brain Injury in Children: A Preliminary Report

C. L. Robertson[1,5], **N. Minamino**[6], **R. A. Ruppel**[1,5], **K. Kangawa**[6], **P. D. Adelson**[3,5], **T. Tsuji**[7], **S. R. Wisniewski**[4,5], **H. Ohta**[7], **K. L. Janesko**[5], and **P. M. Kochanek**[1,2,5]

[1] Department of Anesthesiology and Critical Care Medicine, University of Pittsburgh, Pittsburgh, Pennsylvania
[2] Department of Pediatrics, University of Pittsburgh, Pittsburgh, Pennsylvania
[3] Department of Neurological Surgery, University of Pittsburgh, Pittsburgh, Pennsylvania
[4] School of Public Health, University of Pittsburgh, Pittsburgh, Pennsylvania
[5] Safar Center for Resuscitation Research, and the Brain Trauma Research Center, University of Pittsburgh, Pittsburgh, Pennsylvania
[6] National Cardiovascular Center Research Institute, Osaka, Japan
[7] Diagnostic Science Division, Shionogi & Co., Osaka, Japan

Summary

Adrenomedullin is a recently discovered 52-amino-acid peptide that is a potent vasodilator. Infusion of adrenomedullin increases regional cerebral blood flow and reduces infarct volume after vascular occlusion in rats. Adrenomedullin may represent an endogenous neuroprotectant since it is increased after focal brain ischemia. Cerebral hypoperfusion is present after traumatic brain injury (TBI) in children. We hypothesized that adrenomedullin levels would be increased in children with severe TBI. Total adrenomedullin concentrations were measured using a radioimmunometric assay. Thirty-six samples of ventricular cerebrospinal fluid (CSF) from 10 pediatric patients were collected during the first 10 days after severe TBI (GCS < 8). Control CSF was obtained from 5 children undergoing lumbar puncture, who had normal CSF parameters and no evidence of central nervous system infection. Patients underwent standard neuro-intensive care, including cerebrospinal fluid drainage. Data were analyzed using a univariate regression model. Adrenomedullin concentration was markedly elevated in CSF of children following TBI versus control (mean level 10.65 vs 1.51 fmol/ml, $p = 0.006$). All 36 case samples had an adrenomedullin concentration above the median value for the controls (1.52 fmol/ml). We conclude adrenomedullin is elevated in the CSF of children following severe TBI. We speculate that it participates in the endogenous response to cerebral hypoperfusion after TBI.

Keywords: Adrenomedullin; traumatic brain injury (TBI); cerebral blood flow; pediatrics.

Introduction

Adrenomedullin is a vasoactive peptide that was recently identified in human pheochromocytoma tissue [8]. It consists of 52 amino acids, and has slight structural homology to the calcitonin gene-related peptide (CGRP), which also has potent vasoactive properties. Adrenomedullin mRNA has been isolated in a number of peripheral tissues and in the central nervous system [9]. Its mRNA is constitutively expressed in both vascular endothelial and smooth muscle cells [13, 14]. Increases in plasma and tissue adrenomedullin concentrations occur in various disease states in humans, including hypertension [5], chronic renal failure [5], congestive heart failure [6], septic shock [11] and myocardial infarction [10]. Following central nervous system insults, Kikumoto *et al.* report increases in plasma adrenomedullin concentrations in patients with subarachnoid hemorrhage [7], and other studies document enhanced cerebral production of adrenomedullin after cardiopulmonary bypass [4]. In addition, adrenomedullin mRNA expression is upregulated after focal cerebral ischemia in the rat [15]. An endogenous cerebroprotective role for adrenomedullin in defense of the brain after ischemia has been suggested [3].

Following traumatic brain injury (TBI), patients experience a variety of pathophysiologic alterations in cerebral blood flow (CBF). In children, Adelson et al. reported that posttraumatic cerebral ischemia is strongly associated with poor outcome [1]. We hypothesized that CSF adrenomedullin concentrations would be increased (versus control) after severe TBI in children.

Materials and Methods

Collection of cerebrospinal fluid samples from patients was approved by the Children's Hospital of Pittsburgh Institutional Review Board, and the need for informed consent was waived. Samples were collected from the output of a ventricular catheter used to monitor intracranial pressure (ICP) and drain CSF, as part of standard neuro-intensive care of severely head-injured patients. Samples were collected during the first 10 days after injury. After collection, samples were centrifuged for 5–10 minutes and the supernatant was removed and stored at −70 °C until analysis. A total of 36 samples from 10 patients were collected and sent for analysis.

Total adrenomedullin concentration was measured by investigators blinded to patient identification using an immunoradiometric assay, as described by Ohta, *et al.* [12]. This method utilizes monoclonal antibodies against portions of the adrenomedullin molecule. It measures total adrenomedullin concentration in samples, including the amidated (active) and non-amidated (inactive) forms. This method is highly sensitive and specific, and has a lower detection limit of approximately 1 fmol/ml.

Control CSF was obtained from children undergoing lumbar puncture as part of an evaluation for meningitis or encephalitis. All control samples were culture negative and had normal CSF chemistries and cell counts.

Results

CSF samples were collected in 10 pediatric patients during the first 10 days after injury from July of 1997 to June of 1998. Patients ranged in age from 1.5 months to 10 years, with admission GCS range of 3–12. Head injury resulted from a variety of insults, including motor-vehicle accidents, falls, and suspected child abuse.

Adrenomedullin concentration was markedly elevated in CSF of children following TBI versus control (Fig. 1). The mean concentration in injured children was 10.65 fmol/ml versus 1.51 fmol/ml for controls. Also, all 36 CSF samples from head-injured children had a total adrenomedullin concentration that was greater than the median value for controls (1.52 fmol/ml).

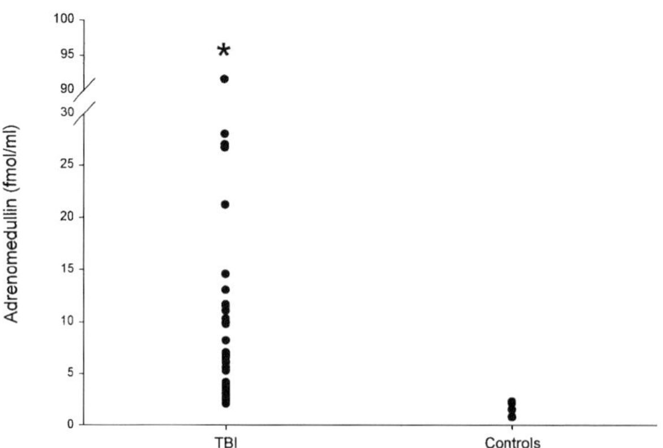

Fig. 1. Adrenomedullin concentration (fmol/ml) in children after severe TBI (left) versus controls (right). $^{*}p = 0.006$ for TBI vs control

Discussion

Increase in tissue or plasma adrenomedullin concentrations have been widely reported, especially after systemic insults [4–5, 8–9]. In these studies, adrenomedullin is felt to play a role as a vasoactive regulator. Its role in the brain is less well-defined. Kikumoto, *et al.* reported increased plasma adrenomedullin concentrations after subarachnoid hemorrhage (SAH) in adult patients (vs controls), and the higher concentrations correlated with more severe neurologic deficit on the first two days after the onset of SAH [7]. Dogan, *et al.* reported a neuroprotective effect of adrenomedullin infusion following middle cerebral artery occlusion (MCAO) in spontaneously hypertensive rats, with a 19.5% reduction in lesion volume at 24 hours after MCAO [3]. In addition, there was a dose-dependent increase in regional CBF in rats without affecting the systemic blood pressure [3]. Adrenomedullin also produced vasodilation of major cerebral arteries in dogs in vivo [2]. Wang *et al.* found similar dilation of rat pial vessels and canine basilar arteries with the application of adrenomedullin and showed upregulation of adrenomedullin mRNA in the ischemic cortex following rat MCAO, which remained elevated for up to 15 days [15]. However, while systemic (i.v.) or intracerebroventricular (i.c.v.) infusion of physiologic doses of adrenomedullin produced only modest improvements in infarct volume or percent swelling (versus vehicle), injection of pharmacologic doses (8 nmol) of adrenomedullin via the i.c.v. route resulted in a 30% increase in infarct volume [15].

In this study, we report the first evidence of increases in adrenomedullin in response to human TBI. Children demonstrated marked increases in CSF levels of adrenomedullin following TBI. This is consistent with the above experimental studies showing elevations of adrenomedullin following episodes of cerebral ischemia. Early after TBI children often demonstrate cerebral hypoperfusion, especially in the first few hours after trauma. After 24 hours, CBF becomes very heterogeneous, with regions of hyperemia as well as regions of persistent hypoperfusion. We reported that global cerebral ischemia (CBF < 20 ml/100 g/min) was strongly associated with poor outcome in children [1]. Consistent with the CBF trends, we found most of the increases in adrenomedullin concentrations tended to be on the first 1–2 days after injury. However, some patients had persistently elevated levels on days 6–10 after injury. This may represent ongoing cerebral hypoperfusion in these patients, or may reflect early (first few hours) upregulation of adrenomedullin mRNA, which has been shown to persist in experimental models of cerebral ischemia as late as 15 days post-insult [15].

We speculate that elevation of adrenomedullin CSF concentration represents a putative cerebroprotective response to the hypoperfusion seen after TBI. It may play a role as an endogenous neuroprotectant after head injury, attempting to counteract ischemia by promoting cerebral vasodilation. The specific clinical role of adrenomedullin after head injury, as well as its mechanisms of biological activity, will require further investigation.

References

1. Adelson PD, Clyde B, Kochanek PM, Wisniewski SR, Marion DW, Yonas H (1997) Cerebrovascular response in infants and young children following severe traumatic brain injury: a preliminary report. Pediatr Neurosurg 26: 200–207
2. Baskaya MK, Suzuki Y, Anzai M, Seki Y, Saito K, Takayasu M, Shibuya M, Sugita K (1995) Effects of adrenomedullin, calcitonin gene-related peptide and amylin on canine cerebral circulation in dogs. J Cereb Blood Flow Metab 15: 827–834
3. Dogan A, Suzuki Y, Koketsu N, Osuka K, Saito K, Takayasu M, Shibuya M, Yoshida J (1997) Intravenous infusion of adrenomedullin and increase in regional cerebral blood flow and prevention of ischemic brain injury after middle cerebral artery occlusion in rats. J Cereb Blood Flow Metab 17: 19–25
4. Inoue S, Hayashi Y, Ohnishi, Kikumoto K, Minamino N, Kangawa K, Matsuo H, Furuya H, Kuro M (1999) Cerebral production of adrenomedullin after hypothermic cardiopulmonary bypass in adult cardiac surgical patients. Anesth Analg 88: 1030–1035
5. Ishimitsu T, Nishikimi T, Saito Y, Kitamura K, Eto T, Kangawa K, Matsuo H, Omae T, Matsuoka H (1994) Plasma levels of adrenomedullin, a newly identified hypotensive peptide, in patients with hypertension and renal failure. J Clin Invest 94: 2158–2161
6. Jougasaki M, Wei CM, McKinley LJ, Burnett JC jun (1995) Elevation of circulating and ventricular adrenomedullin in human congestive heart failure. Circulation 92: 286–289
7. Kikumoto K, Kubo A, Hayashi Y, Minamino N, Inoue S, Dohi K, Kitamura K, Kangawa K, Matsuo H, Furuya H (1998) Increased plasma concentration of adrenomedullin in patients with subarachnoid hemorrhage. Anesth Analg 87: 859–863
8. Kitamura K, Kangawa K, Kawamoto M, Ichiki Y, Nakamura S, Matsuo H, Eto T (1993) Adrenomedullin: a novel hypotensive peptide isolated from human pheochromocytoma. Biochem Biophys Res Commun 192: 553–560
9. Kitamura K, Sakata J, Kangawa K, Kojima M, Matsuo H, Eto T (1993) Cloning and characterization of cDNA encoding a precursor for human adrenomedullin. Biochem Biophys Res Commun 194: 720–725
10. Miyao Y, Nishikimi T, Goto Y, Miyazaki S, Daikoku S, Morii I, Matsumoto T, Takishita S, Miyata A, Matsuo H, Kangawa K, Nonogi H (1998) Increased plasma adrenomedullin levels in patients with acute myocardial infarction in proportion to the clinical severity. Heart 79: 39–44
11. Nishio K, Akai Y, Murao Y, Doi N, Ueda S, Tabuse H, Miyamoto S, Dohi K, Minamiuo N, Shoji H, Kitamura K, Kangawa K, Matsuo H (1997) Increased plasma concentrations of adrenomedullin correlate with relaxation of vascular tone in patients with septic shock. Crit Care Med 25: 953–957
12. Ohta H, Tsuji T, Asai S, Tanizaki S, Sasakura K, Teraoka H, Kitamura K, Kangawa K (1999) A simple immunoradiometric assay for measuring the entire molecules of adrenomedullin in human plasma. Clin Chim Acta 287: 131–143
13. Sugo S, Minamino N, Kangawa K, Miyamoto K, Kitamura K, Sakata J, Eto T, Matsuo H (1994) Endothelial cells actively synthesize and secrete adrenomedullin. Biochem Biophys Res Commun 201: 1160–1166
14. Sugo S, Minamino N, Shoji H, Kangawa K, Kitamuia K, Eto T, Matsuo H (1994) Production and secretion of adrenomedullin from vascular smooth muscle cells: augmented production by tumor necrosis factor – α. Biochem Biophys Res Commun 203: 719–726
15. Wang X, Yue T, Barone FC, White RF, Clark RK, Willette RN, Sulpizio AC, Aiyar NV, Ruffolo RR Jr, Feuerstein GZ (1995) Discovery of adrenomedullin in rat ischemic cortex and evidence for its role in exacerbating focal brain ischemic damage. Proc Natl Acad Sci 92: 11480–11484

Correspondence: Patrick M. Kochanek, M.D., Safar Center for Resuscitation Research, 3434 Fifth Avenue, Pittsburgh, PA 15260.

Head Injury: Monitoring

In this important section new data are presented on monitoring of head injured patients with microdialysis by several different groups (a total of 292 patients with severe head injury are described). It has confirmed the importance of ischaemia in the trauma which is so important in the various types of diffuse and focal brain injury. All 4 reports (Alexandris *et al.*, Hutchinson *et al.*, Gopinath *et al.*, Reinert *et al.*) tend to reinforce each other's findings in that glucose was low and glutamate was high especially in patients with poor outcomes. Lactate levels were not always increased and did not correlate as well with outcome or severity of injury.

Autoregulation and CPP management remains controversial in this group of patients. No class I evidence was presented but observations by Jackson *et al.*, Schmidt *et al.* and Sahuquillo *et al.* have shed further light on this difficult area and they have suggested that we should be trying to measure autoregulation thresholds in individual patients. Fernandes *et al.* showed that high ICP with spontaneous ICH in 62 patients correlated with death and that high ICP is reduced following surgery. Juul *et al.* made the important point that the use of neuromuscular blocking agents in patients with severe head injury resulted in higher levels of ICP for longer periods than in control patients.

Monitoring with transcranial Doppler (TCD) is proposed as a useful index by Ng *et al.* and Czosnyka *et al.*, particularly with regard to the evaluation of autoregulation in individual head injured patients. Sahuquillo *et al.* include CBF monitoring in the evaluation of the autoregulatory status of head injuries. Monitoring with the objective of measuring compliance in head injury is reported by Piper *et al.*

Acta Neurochir (2000) [Suppl] 76: 425–430

Low Extracellular (ECF) Glucose Affects the Neurochemical Profile in Severe Head-Injured Patients

B. Alessandri, M. Reinert, H. F. Young, and **R. Bullock**

Medical College of Virginia, Division of Neurosurgery, Richmond, USA

Summary

Glucose (Gluc) is the main energy source for the brain. After severe head-injury energy demand is massively increased and supply is often decreased. In pilot microdialysis studies, many patients with severe head-injury had undetectable glucose concentrations, probably reflecting changes in metabolism and/or reduced supply. We therefore investigated whether patients with low ECF glucose (criterion: <50 μM for ≥ 5 hrs), LOWgluc, differ from patients with higher glucose levels (NORMALgluc) We also tested the interrelationships between other parameters such as lactate, glutamate, K+, brain O_2 and CO_2, ICP, CPP, and CBF in these two groups.

We found that patients with low ECF glucose, LOWgluc, have significantly lower lactate concentrations than patients with "normal" glucose, NORMALgluc, levels do. Spearman correlations between glucose and most other parameters were similar in both patient groups. However, glutamate correlated positively with glucose, lactate, brain CO_2 and negatively with brain O_2 in the NORMALgluc patient group, whereas glutamate did not significantly correlate with any of these parameters in the LOWgluc group. There was also no correlation between outcome and the dialysate glucose. The results indicate that low ECF glucose is almost always present in severe head-injury. Moreover, the lack of correlation between low glucose and outcome, however, suggests that other energy substrates, such as lactate, are important after TBI.

Keywords: Microdialysis; severe head-injury; glucose; energy metabolism.

Introduction

Glucose is the primary energy source of the human brain and it therefore occupies a central role in maintaining energy metabolism in the brain. A large portion of the total energy available in the brain has been calculated to be used for maintenance of ionic balance at physiological condition [16, 17]. Massive ionic fluxes such as increased extracellular potassium, intracellular sodium and calcium, are well documented following traumatic brain injury (TBI). Such ionic shift impose metabolic demands upon both neurons and glial cells, to restore ion homeostasis. Metabolic demand is additionally created by the release and reuptake of excitatory amino acids such as glutamate which has been reported in several animal models of TBI [2], and in severely head-injured patients [9, 12]. Released glutamate has recently been linked to hyperglycolysis, and the massive production of lactate [3, 24]. Hypermetabolism, a logical consequence of high energy demand, has been consistently found in animal models of brain injury [34]; Hovda, 1992 #40; Kawamata, 1992 #1005; Kawamata, 1995 #30; Yoshino, 1991 #1007; Inglis, 1990 #46; Inglis, 1992 #390], and in head-injured patients [5, 6, 13, 29, 32, 33]. A consequence of increased substrate demand, and impaired delivery to the brain (due to reduced CBF), may be a decrease of ECF glucose, even to undetectable levels, as reported in animal studies [1, 4, 27], and human head-injury [19, 26]. Unavailable or massively reduced glucose may impair the ability of cells to restore ionic homeostasis (with the provision of ATP, for the Na+/K+ ATPase pumps for instance), and thus regulate cell volume. Therefore, we investigated the effect of low ECF glucose in TBI patients on the relationship between neurochemical parameters und 3-month outcome.

Method

Microdialysis

As previously described [9, 12], custom-made, commercially produced microdialysis probes (CMA/20, 10 mm active membrane) were inserted into cortex, either at craniotomy, or via a ventriculostomy twist drill site [9–11, 14, 35, 36]. After placement, the probes were perfused with sterile 0.9% saline at 2 μL/min, and 60 μL fractions were collected into sealed glass vials, which were immediately analyzed or stored at −20 deg. Celsius until analysis.

Table 1. *Mean (±s.d.) Values of Neuro-Parameters in the LOWgluc and NORMALgluc Group*

Group	Gluc	Lac	Glu	ICP	CPP	K^+	pO_2	pCO_2
$NORMAL_{gluc}$ (n = 50)	626 ± 474	1312 ± 951	11.4 ± 26.7	14.5 ± 4.3	78.5 ± 18.7	1.42 ± 0.69	29.9 ± 12.2	49.5 ± 6.9
LOW_{gluc} (n = 50)	125*** ± 161	739* ± 865	24.4 ± 53.0	16.0 ± 7.9	82.0 ± 11.7	1.50 ± 1.14	36.1 ± 21.6	50.4 ± 17.9

Gluc, Lac given in μM. Potassium (K^+) given in mM. ICP, CPP, brain tissue O_2 and CO_2 (pO_2, pCO_2) are given in mmHg.

Neurochemical Analysis

Dialysates were analyzed for glucose (Gluc), lactate (Lac), glutamate (Glu), aspartate (Asp), threonine (Thr), using a Yellow Spring Enzymatic Analyzer (YSI 2700 Select (Gluc, Lac) or high pressure liquid chromatography (HPLC (Gluc, Lac, Glu, Asp, Thr).

Potassium

Potassium was measured using a flame photometer as described in this issue by Reinert *et al.*

Brain O_2 and CO_2 Tension

For the measurement of tissue oxygen (pO_2) and carbon dioxide tension (pCO_2) a multiparameter, minimally invasive sensor (Paratrend 7 or Neurotrend; Diametrics Medical, USA), described in detail elsewhere (Reinert *et al.*, this issue), has been used in a subset of patients.

Outcome (GOS)

For analysis the *Glasgow Outcome Scale* (GOS) assessed 3 months after injury was taken. Due to the small group size the outcomes were divided into *good outcome* (GOS 0–2) and *poor outcome* (GOS 3–4).

Patient and Grouping

One hundred (100) patients with severe head-injury were selected for this study. Patients were divided into two groups based on the glucose level in dialysates. If 10 or more consecutive half-hour samples showed glucose levels lower than 50 μM glucose, patients were assigned to the low glucose group, LOW_{gluc} (n = 50; mean = 125.3 ± 161 μM). All other patients were put into the normal glucose group, $NORMAL_{gluc}$ (n = 50; mean = 626 ± 474 μM). The groups did not differ in mean values for age (40.0 vs. 39.1 yrs.), GCS (median = 5), MABP (101 ± 10 vs. 97 ± 11).

Statistics

The difference in the n's in each analysis is due to the fact that not all brain chemistry analyses were performed at the same time in every patient. Mean values were compared using non-parametric statistics (Mann-Whitney U-Test; Chi-square test). To study the inter-relationship of parameters, the Spearman rank coefficient ("rho-value") was calculated *for each patient*. Contrary to the comparisons of mean values, the *intra-patient* relationship (positive or negative) between parameters is preserved. The significance of these relationships ("rho-values") was tested using a simple t-test and plotted as frequency histograms. Differences were considered significant at a p-level < 0.05.

Results

Mean Values of Monitoring Parameters

The LOWgluc and NORMALgluc group differed significantly in their mean glucose ($p < 0.001$) and lactate value ($p < 0.05$). The groups did not differ significantly in mean values for all other parameters (Table 1).

CBF and Substrate Delivery

As shown in Fig. 1, regional as well as global CBF was similar in both groups. The glucose-oxygen correlation data (Fig. 1b) indicates that in more than 70% of all cases brain tissue oxygen tension was above threshold levels for tissue hypoxemia (20 mmHG O_2). Similarly, even when tissue oxygen tension was adequate, glucose was low in 70% of observations.

Changes in Extracellular Glucose Over Time

The time-course of glucose in the LOW_{gluc} group showed mainly two distinct patterns: Half of the patients had low glucose throughout the microdialysis period, whereas the other half had initially high glucose levels which dropped to often undetectable levels for several hours. In most cases the glucose level did not recover with time. Many LOW_{gluc} patients had initially high glucose levels, with a mean level of 442.34 ± 490 μM, dropping thereafter to 6.62 ± 10.6 μM. The individual high glucose period in these LOWgluc patients ranged from 18 to 66% (mean: 38 ± 4%) of the whole microdialysis sampling period. None of the patients assigned to the $NORMAL_{gluc}$ group had any short episode of sub-threshold $Gluc_{dial}$, as defined.

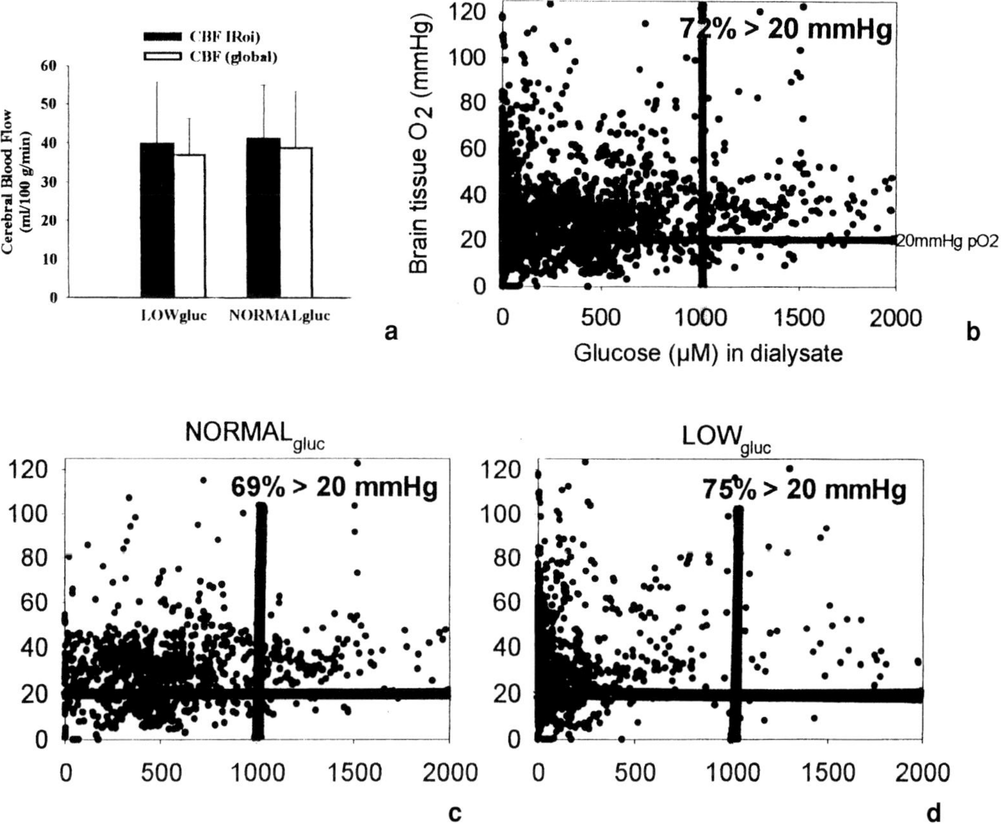

Fig. 1. (a) Cerebral blood flow (CBF; mL/100 g/min) assessed by stable Xenon CT. Calculations were made for whole brain CBF (global) and in the area around the brain monitoring (Roi, region of interest). (b) Plot of all glucose-oxygen pairs for both groups, and for the NORMAL-gluc (c), and the LOWgluc (d) group. The vertical line marks the hypoxic threshold (20 mmHg). The horizontal line indicates the estimated physiological value for glucose measured by microdialysis. Note: More than 80% of all glucose values are below the expected normal value

Relationship Between Parameters

A Spearman correlation analysis between glutamate or lactate and several other parameters showed marked differences in the profile of relationships between parameters in the two groups (Table 2A, B; Fig. 2).

Outcome

Although there was a higher percentage of patients with a more favorable outcome in the $NORMAL_{gluc}$ group than in the LOW_{gluc} group (65.1% vs. 55.3%, respectively), a Chi-square test did not indicate a significant effect of low glucose on the outcome of patients after severe head-injury.

Table 2. *Significance Levels of Correlation Between Glutamate (A) or Lactate (B) and Several Biochemical Parameters for the LOWgluc and NORMALgluc. Group + Indicates a Positive and – a Negative Correlation (n.s = Not Significant)*

(A) Group	*Glutamate vs.* Lactate	K^+	PCO_2	pO_2
$NORMAL_{gluc}$	$p < 0.001+$	$p < 0.005+$	$p < 0.01+$	$p < 0.005-$
LOW_{gluc}	n.s.+	$p < 0.02+$	n.s.–	n.s.
(B) Group	***Lactate vs.* Glu**	**K+**	**PCO_2**	**ICP**
$NORMAL_{gluc}$	$p < 0.001+$	$p < 0.004+$	n.s.	n.s.
LOW_{gluc}	n.s.	$p < 0.02+$	n.s.	$p < 0.02-$

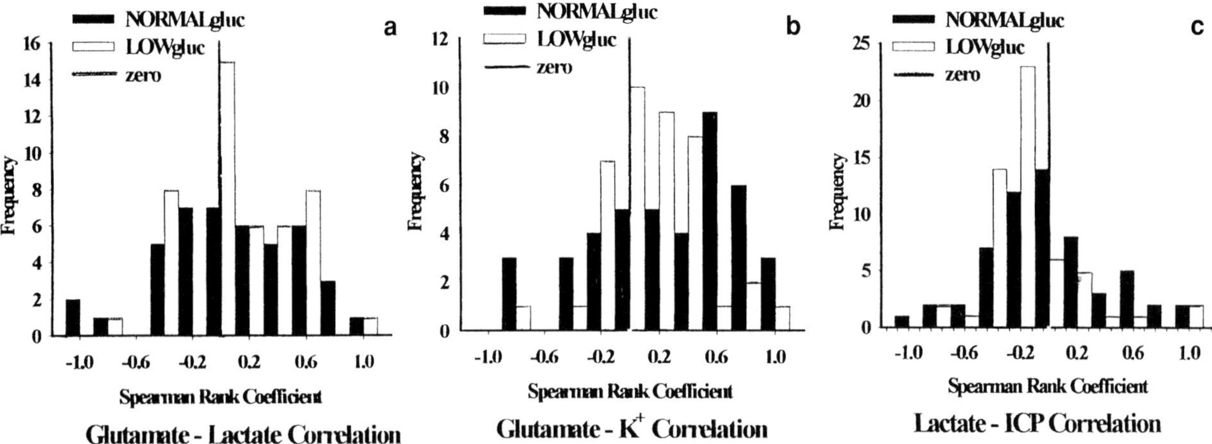

Fig. 2. Histograms showing the distribution of the Spearman rank correlation coefficients (rho) for the correlations between glutamate and lactate (a), glutamate and potassium (b), and lactate and ICP (c). For significance levels see Table 2

Discussion

The most important finding in this large study, was that low dialysate glucose was seen, in absence of tissue hypoxia (Fig. 1) or ischemia. This could be due to increased consumption, reduced transport to the tissue, or reduced delivering (i.e. low CBF). Hovda *et al.* [6] have shown increased early glycolysis in at least 35% of severe head-injured patients, in the first week after injury. They have also shown increased, not decreased activity of the GLUT1 transporter system, after human TBI. Our own data suggest ischemia, and thus reduced glucose delivery, maybe important in about 20–25% of patients with low dialysate glucose.

Low or undetectable dialysate glucose levels have already been reported by other groups using microdialytic monitoring in patients following severe head-injury [19] and subarachnoidal hemorrhage (SAH) [26], and have been associated with unfavorable outcome [26]. Our data do not support this trend. This study shows that ECF glucose values are in more than 80% of all cases below expected physiological values of ECF glucose when measured by microdialysis at 2 μL/min (800–1000 μM in dialysate). Very low glucose in the dialysate (<50 μM for at least 5 hrs.) of head-injured patients was not accompanied by massive differences in the mean values of most other measured parameters. However, the relationship between these parameters was strongly affected by low ECF glucose, indicating differences in biochemical processes initiated after TBI. Despite these changes due to massively reduced glucose availability in the ECF, there was apparent effect upon outcome, between the two study groups. The assumption that periods of low glucose reflect mainly compromised substrate availability for brain cells, and therefore may adversely influence the clinical outcome of patients could not be supported by our data. We speculate that the increased ECF concentration of lactate might become the major energy substrate for neurons.

All these studied patients were intensively treated in order to maintain a low ICP, high CPP, and physiological values for blood gases and glucose. The two groups did not differ in their local and global CBF, mean ICP, and CPP. Table II and figure 2 also show that more than 70% of all glucose values were associated with non-hypoxic brain O_2 values. These data suggest that the substrate delivery to the brain was comparable for both groups and most likely not the cause of low ECF glucose. However, it must be noted that Bouma *et al.* [7, 8] have shown early reductions of CBF to ischemic levels after trauma in 34% of patients, causing possible restrictions in substrate delivery (glucose, O_2), and our group also reported early low brain O_2 (<20 mmHg) in severely head-injured patients (e.g. [36]. Whether or not such early events had a significant effect on later ECF glucose levels as documented in this study, is not yet clear. It might be speculated that ultra-early events could cause changes in glucose transporters in the vessel walls or on neurons and astrocytes [23, 31], or that transient ischemia can cause later hyperglycolysis, to correct ionic inbalance.

Based on these observations, hypermetabolism after TBI seems the most prominent explanation for the generally low glucose values in all patients. Glutamate has been shown to be a key factor for stimulating hyperglycolysis in astrocytes [24, 25]. Glutamate in the NORMALgluc group showed strong correlations with lactate, potassium, tissue O_2 and CO_2. These correlations are consistent with finding that glutamate uptake into astrocytes stimulates glycolysis and concomitant lactate production [15, 20–22, 24, 25]. This increased metabolism consumes more oxygen and yields more CO_2.

The strong correlation between glutamate and potassium in this study are in accordance with previous findings by Katayama *et al.* in rat TBI [18] and Valadka *et al.* in patients [30]. This may suggest that agonist-operated ionic flux is important. In the LOWgluc group, however, a more positive glutamate-potassium correlation was seen. Since lactate is much lower in this group, this may imply that the tissue energy need is extremely high. This idea is supported by the fact that many studies have shown that lactate can be used as an energy substrate in neurons [28]. This could partially explain the lack of correlation between the low ECF glucose and the outcome in this study. If astrocytes rapidly take up glucose from the blood stream, producing lactate and pyruvate as end-products of glycolysis, and mainly release lactate into the ECF, only little glucose will appear in the ECF, to be detected by microdialysis. Under extremely high metabolic rates, the lactate produced also disappears quickly from the ECF, reducing the mean lactate levels in the LOWgluc group. This leads to the speculation that patients with very low glucose combined with low lactate will have poor outcome.

The data presented here suggests that the measurement of glucose and other parameters in the brain by microdialysis can be used to indirectly assess TBI-induced hypermetabolism. Clearly, studies with PET, to measure glucose utilization together with microdialysis, are needed to verify this hypothesis. The disturbed relationship between glutamate and other parameters together with reduced lactate and glucose values might point towards extremely high metabolic rates.

Acknowledgment

The study was supported by NIH grant #NS12587. We are grateful for the valuable suggestions of Dr. S. Choi of the Department of biostatistics of the Medical college of Virginia. Ross Bullock was supported by the Reynolds Foundation. Beat Alessandri was partially supported by the Swiss Academy of Medical Sciences.

References

1. Alessandri B, Basciani R, Langemann H, Lyrer P, Pluess D, Landolt H, Gratzl O (1999) Chronic effects of an aminosteroid on microdialytically measured parameters after experimental middle cerebral artery occlusion in the rat. J Clini Neurosci (accepted for publication)
2. Alessandri B, Bullock R (1998) Glutamate and its receptors in the pathophysiology of brain and spinal cord injuries. In: Ottersen OP, Langmoen I, Gjerstad L (eds) Progress in brain research. Elsevier Science, Amsterdam, pp 301–311
3. Alessandri B, Doppenberg E, Woodward J, Bullock R (1997) Evidence for time-dependent glutamate-mediated glycolysis in head-injured patients: a microdialysis study. In: Bullock Rea (ed) Neurochemical monitoring, Satellite Symposium of the 10th International Symposium on Intracranial Pressure . . . , vol. in press. Williamsburg, VA USA, pp PO-2-076
4. Alessandri B, Langemann H, Lutz TW, Basciani R, Fuhrer B, Lyrer P, Landolt H, Gratzl O (1999) Acute effects of an aminosteroid on microdialytically measured parameters after experimental middle cerebral artery occlusion in the rat. J Clini Neurosci 6 in press
5. Beck T, Goller HJ, Wree A (1995) Chronic depression of glucose metabolism in postischemic rat brains. Stroke 26: 1107–1113
6. Bergsneider M, Hovda DA, Shalmon E, Kelly DF, Vespa PM, Martin NA, Phelps ME, McArthur DL, Caron MJ, Kraus JF, Becker DP (1997) Cerebral hyperglycolysis following severe traumatic brain injury in humans: a positron emission tomography study. J Neurosurg 86: 241–251
7. Bouma GJ, Muizelaar JP (1995) Cerebral blood flow in severe clinical head injury. New horizons. http://www.biomednet.com/db/medline/96056618 3: 384–394
8. Bouma GJ, Muizelaar JP, Stringer WA, Choi SC, Fatouros P, Young HF (1992) Ultra-early evaluation of regional cerebral blood flow in severely head-injured patients using xenon-enhanced computerized tomography [see comments]. J Neurosurg http://www.biomednet.com/db/medline/92373299 77: 360–368
9. Bullock R, Zauner A, Myseros JS, Marmarou A, Woodward JJ, Young HF (1995) Evidence for prolonged release of excitatory amino acids in severe human head trauma. Ann NY Acad Sci 765: 290–297
10. Bullock R, Zauner A, Tsuji O, Woodward J, Young H, Marmarou A (1994) Excitatory amino acid releases after severe head trauma: Effect of intracranial pressure and cerebral perfusion pressure changes. In: Nagai H, Kamiya K, Ishii S (eds) Ninth International Symposium on Intracranial Pressure. Nagoya, Japan, pp 264–267
11. Bullock R, Zauner A, Tsuji O, Woodward JJ, Marmarou AT, Young HF (1995) Patterns of excitatory amino acid release and ionic flux after severe human head trauma. In: Tsubokawa T, Marmarou AT, Robertson C, Teasdale G (eds) Neurochemical monitoring in the intensive care unit. Springer, Berlin Heidelberg New York, Tokyo, pp 64–71
12. Bullock R, Zauner A, Woodward J, Young HF (1995) Massive persistent release of excitatory amino acids following human occlusive stroke. Stroke 26: 2187–2189
13. Dietrich WD, Alonso O, Busto R (1993) Moderate hyperglycemia worsens acute blood-brain barrier injury after forebrain ischemia in rats. Stroke 24: 111–116
14. Doppenberg EMR, Zauner A, Bullock R, Woodward J, Young HF (1996) Evidence for glutamate-medicated anerobic glycolysis, after human head injury? A microdialysis study. J Neurotrauma 13: 597

15. Fray AE, Boutelle M, Fillenz M (1997) Extracellular glucose turnover in the striatum of unanaesthetized rats measured by quantitative microdialysis [In Process Citation], J Physiol (Lond) 504: 721–726
16. Katayama Y, Becker DP, Tamura T, Hovda DA (1990) Massive increases in extracellular potassium and the indiscriminate release of glutamate following concussive brain injury. J Neurosurg 73: 889–900
17. Katayama Y, Kawamata T, Kano T, Tsubokawa T (1992) Excitatory amino acid antagonist adminstered via microdialysis attenuates lactate accumulation during cerebral ischemia and subsequent hippocampal damage. Brain Res 584: 329–333
18. Kawamata T, Katayama Y, Hovda DA, Yoshino A, Becker DP (1995) Lactate accumulation following concussive brain injury: the role of ionic fluxes induced by excitatory amino acids. Brain Res 674: 196–204
19. Langemann H, Mendelowitsch A, Landolt H, Alessandri B, Gratzl O (1995) Experimental and clinical monitoring of glucose by microdialysis. Clin Neurol Neurosurg 97: 149–155
20. Magistretti PJ, Pellerin L (1996) Cellular mechanisms of brain energy metabolism. Relevance to functional brain imaging and to neurodegenerative disorders. Ann NY Acad Sci 777: 380–387
21. Magistretti PJ, Pellerin L (1997) Metabolic coupling during activation. A cellular view. Adv Exp Med Biol 413: 161–166
22. Magistretti PJ, Sorg O, Naichen Y, Pellerin L, de Rham S, Martin JL (1994) Regulation of astrocyte energy metabolism by neurotransmitters. Ren Physiol Biochem 17: 168–171
23. McCall AL, Van BAM, Nipper V, Moholt Siebert M, Downes H, Lessov N (1996) Forebrain ischemia increases GLUT1 protein in brain microvessels and parenchyma. J Cereb Blood Flow Metab 16: 69–76
24. Pellerin L, Magistretti PJ (1994) Glutamate uptake into astrocytes stimulates aerobic glycolysis: a mechanism coupling neuronal activity to glucose utilization. Proc Natl Acad Sci USA 91: 10625–10629
25. Pellerin L, Magistretti PJ (1996) Excitatory amino acids stimulate aerobic glycolysis in astrocytes via an activation of the Na+/K+ ATPase. Dev Neurosci 18: 336–342
26. Persson L, Valtysson J, Enblad P, Warme PE, Cesarini K, Lewen A, Hillered L (1996) Neurochemical monitoring using intracerebral microdialysis in patients with subarachnoid hemorrhage. J Neurosurg 84: 606–616
27. Qian Y-Z, Di X, Chen T, Bullock R (1998) Lactate/glucose dynamics after rat fluid percussion injury. J Neurotrauma 15: 903
28. Schurr A, Payne RS, Miller JJ, Rigor BM (1997) Brain lactate, not glucose, fuels the recovery of synaptic function from hypoxia upon reoxygenation: an in vitro study. Brain Res 744: 105–111
29. Sutton RL, Hovda DA, Adelson PD, Benzel EC, Becker DP (1994) Metabolic changes following cortical contusion: relationships to edema and morphological changes. Acta Neurochir [Suppl] (Wien) 60: 446–448
30. Valadka AB, Goodman JC, Gopinath SP, Uzura M, Robertson CS (1998) Comparison of brain tissue oxygen tension to microdialysis-based measures of cerebral ischemia in fatally head-injured humans. J Neurotrauma, http://www.biomednet.com/db/medline/98337311 15: 509–519
31. Vannucci SJ, Seaman LB, Vannucci RC (1996) Effects of hypoxia-ischemia on GLUT1 and GLUT3 glucose transporters in immature rat brain. J Cereb Blood Flow Metab 16: 77–81
32. Yamaki T, Imahori Y, Ohmori Y, Yoshino E, Hohri T, Ebisu T, Ueda S (1996) Cerebral hemodynamics and metabolism of severe diffuse brain injury measured by PET [see comments]. J Nucl Med 37: 1116–1170
33. Yamaki T, Yoshino E, Fujimoto M, Ohmori Y, Imahori Y, Ueda S (1996) Chronological positron emission tomographic study of severe diffuse brain injury in the chronic stage. J Trauma 40: 50–56
34. Yao H, Ginsberg MD, Eveleth DD, LaManna JC, Watson BD, Alonso OF, Loor JY, Foreman JH, Busto R (1995) Local cerebral glucose utilization and cytoskeletal proteolysis as indices of evolving focal ischemic injury in core and penumbra. J Cereb Blood Flow Metab 15: 398–408
35. Zauner A, Bullock R, Kuta AJ, Woodward J, Young HF (1996) Glutamate release and cerebral blood flow after severe human head injury. Acta Neurochir [Suppl] (Wien) 67: 40–44
36. Zauner A, Doppenberg E, Woodward JJ, Allen C, Jebraili S, Young HF, Bullock R (1997) Multiparametric continuous monitoring of brain metabolism and substrate delivery in neurosurgical patients. Neurol Res 19: 265–273

Correspondence: Dr. B. Alessandri, Medical College of Virginia, Division of Neurosurgery, P.O. Box 980683, 1225 E. Marshall Street, Richmond, VA 23298, USA.

Acta Neurochir (2000) [Suppl] 76: 431–435

On-Line Monitoring of Substrate Delivery and Brain Metabolism in Head Injury

P. J. A. Hutchinson, P. G. Al-Rawi, M. T. O'Connell, A. K. Gupta, L. B. Maskell, D. B. A. Hutchinson, J. D. Pickard, and **P. J. Kirkpatrick**

Academic Department of Neurosurgery, Department of Neuroanaesthesia and Medical Research Council Centre for Brain Repair, University of Cambridge, UK

Summary

Head injury is associated with complex pathophysiological changes in metabolism. The objective of the study was to investigate these changes by applying on-line bedside monitoring of cerebral metabolism using microdialysis. Following approval by the Local Ethics Committee and consent from the next of kin, a microdialysis catheter was inserted into the frontal cortex of patients with severe head injury. Twenty-one patients were studied for 102.3 ± 26.9 hours (mean ± 95% confidence interval; total 89.4 patient monitoring days). The overall cerebral glucose (mean of means) was 1.63 ± 0.31 mM with periods of undetectable glucose recorded. The cerebral lactate and lactate/pyruvate ratio were 4.69 ± 0.61 mM and 29.9 ± 3.73 respectively. Patients who died (n = 4) or who were severely disabled (not proceeding to rehabilitation, n = 5) had a tendency towards lower glucose (1.39 ± 0.35 mM), higher lactate (5.10 ± 1.02 mM) and higher lactate/pyruvate ratios (35.5 ± 7.67) compared to patients with good outcome (home or proceeding to rehabilitation, n = 12, glucose 1.80 ± 0.49 mM, lactate 4.38 ± 0.85 mM, lactate/pyruvate ratio 27.9 ± 4.33). Trends in these metabolic parameters relating to outcome were identifiable. In the majority of patients, cerebral glutamate levels (overall mean of means 9.47 ± 4.59 μM) were initially high and then declined to stable levels. Patients in whom the glutamate level remained elevated or in whom secondary rises in glutamate were seen had a poor outcome. The application of bedside analysis of microdialysis enables the progress of the patient to be monitored on-line. In addition to establishing trends of improving and deteriorating metabolism, the technique has the potential to monitor the effects of therapeutic manoeuvres on the biochemistry.

Keywords: Head injury; microdialysis; brain metabolism.

Introduction

Following head injury there are a number of potentially preventable secondary insults including hypoxia, hypotension, intracranial hypertension and seizures which increase mortality and disability. Such insults are accompanied by complex pathophysiological changes in metabolism. Multi-modality monitoring of patients with severe head injury aims to detect these adverse events, enabling expeditious treatment to be initiated. Various techniques are available including intra-cranial pressure monitoring, jugular venous saturation monitoring, trans-cranial doppler and near-infrared spectroscopy [12]. Recently, intra-parenchymal probes have been applied to monitor cerebral metabolism directly. These probes include multi-parameter (oxygen, carbon dioxide, pH, and temperature) sensors and microdialysis catheters [1, 4, 7, 8, 13, 15, 18, 19, 23].

Microdialysis monitors the chemistry of the extracellular space directly [2, 5, 17]. The principle is to mimic the function of a capillary blood vessel by placing a fine catheter lined with dialysis membrane into the tissue. The catheter is perfused with a physiological solution at ultra-low flow rates (0.1–2 μl/min). Molecules (e.g. glucose, lactate, pyruvate, and glutamate) diffuse across the membrane into the solution which is then collected for analysis. The objective of the study was to apply microdialysis monitoring to patients with severe head injury, with on-line analysis using a bedside analyser.

Patients and Methods

Patient Selection

The study was approved by the Cambridge Local Research Ethics Committee. Patients admitted to the Neuro Critical Care Unit with a diagnosis of head injury requiring ventilation and intracranial pressure monitoring were enrolled. Exclusion criteria were patients under the age of 16 years and those with deranged coagulation. Consent was obtained from the next of kin.

Microdialysis Technique

The microdialysis catheter (CMA70, membrane length 10 mm, diameter 0.6 mm, CMA, Stockholm, Sweden) was introduced into

Table 1. *Summary of Microdialysis Results. Comparison of Cerebral 10 mm Catheter with Results from Cerebral and Subcutaneous 30 mm Catheters*

	Cerebral 10 mm catheter N = 21		Cerebral 30 mm catheter n = 11		Subcut 30 mm catheter n = 14	
	Mean	95% CI	Mean	95% CI	Mean	95% CI
Glucose mM	1.63	0.31	1.95	0.68	6.95	1.39
Lactate mM	4.69	0.61	8.27	1.31	3.36	1.17
Pyruvate μM	158	16.1	299	30.9	170	44.5
Glutamate μM	9.47	4.59	28.8	17.8	11.9	4.21

the frontal cortex of the brain in conjunction with an intracranial pressure monitor (Codman, Raynham, MA, USA) and multi-parameter sensor (Para- or Neurotrend, Diametrics, High Wycombe, UK) using a specially designed triple lumen bolt. CT scans were performed in all patients after insertion of the bolt. The microdialysis catheters were perfused with Ringer's solution at a rate of 0.3 μl/min using a CMA106 pump and the collecting vials were changed every 60 minutes. The analysis of the microdialysate was performed on-line using the bedside CMA600 microdialysis analyser (glucose, lactate, pyruvate, and glutamate). This is a purpose designed clinical microdialysis analyser based on the principle of enzyme spectrophotometry. We have calculated the in-vivo recovery (extrapolation to zero method) for these catheters (0.3 μl/min) to be 65–75%. The microdialysate from vials following catheter insertion was not included in the final analysis to exclude insertion artefact.

Results

Patient Population

21 patients (male:female = 15:6, mean age 36.8, range 17–68 years) with severe head injury were studied. Microdialysis monitoring commenced 26.3 ± 6.6 hours (mean ± 95% confidence limits) after injury (range 7.0–62.5 hours) and continued for 102.3 ± 26.8 hours (range 11.5 hours to 10 days). The total period of monitoring was 89.4 patient days. CT scanning following bolt insertion showed that the catheters were in the region of contusions in four patients. No complications were associated with the monitoring.

Microdialysis Analysis

The overall cerebral microdialysis results are shown in Tables 1 and 2. The cerebral glucose was low compared to subcutaneous adipose glucose with periods of undetectable glucose. The cerebral lactate was high compared to peripheral lactate. Patients who died (n = 5) or who were severely disabled (n = 4, not proceeding to rehabilitation) were classified as poor outcome (total n = 9, initial GCS 4.9 ± 1.7, mean ICP 18.5 ± 6.3 mmHg, Table 2). These patients had a tendency to lower mean glucose, and higher levels of lactate/pyruvate ratio compared to patients who were discharged home or proceeding to rehabilitation (classified as good outcome, n = 12, initial GCS 7.8 ± 2.3, mean ICP 13.2 ± 3.1 mmHg, Table 2). For individual patients, periods of improving (increasing glucose, decreasing lactate/pyruvate ratio) and deteriorating (decreasing glucose, increasing lactate/pyruvate ratio) metabolism were clearly identifiable (Fig. 1).

Glutamate levels were initially high and then declined to stable levels in the majority of patients. This pattern applied to all the patients in the good outcome group and was also observed in the poor outcome group. However, in patients in whom the glutamate remained elevated, and patients with secondary rises in glutamate, the outcome was poor (Fig. 2).

Correlation between the microdialysis parameters demonstrated good correlation between lactate and pyruvate levels during periods of uneventful monitoring (mean r = 0.74). Overall there was a moderate

Table 2. *Comparison of Good and Poor Outcome Groups. Data is Presented as the Mean (±95% Confidence Intervals) of the Individual Patient Means for Each Group*

	Good outcome	Poor outcome
N	12	9
Male:female	8:4	7:2
Age	35.0 ± 7.4	39.7 ± 15.5
Initial GCS	7.8 ± 2.3	4.9 ± 1.7
Time between injury and monitoring hrs	24.8 ± 6.1	28.1 ± 13.4
Duration of monitoring hrs	115.5 ± 44.3	89.4 ± 35.1
ICP mmHg	13.2 ± 3.1	18.5 ± 6.3
CPP mmHg	81.3 ± 5.6	74.5 ± 6.6
Glucose mM	1.80 ± 0.49	1.39 ± 0.35
Lactate mM	4.38 ± 0.85	5.10 ± 1.02
Lactate/pyruvate ratio	27.9 ± 4.33	35.5 ± 7.67
Glutamate μM	6.69 ± 2.24	13.7 ± 12.1

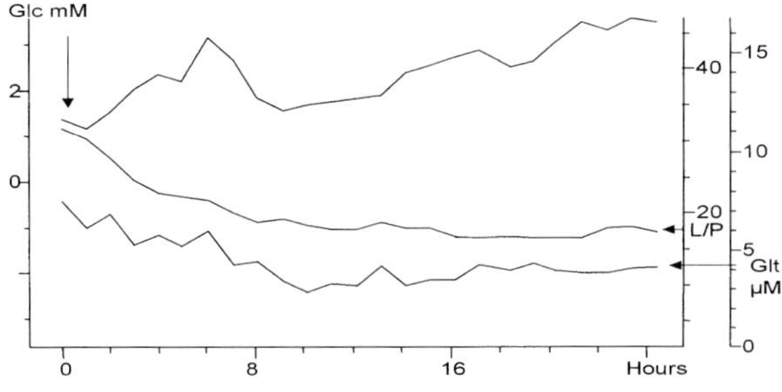

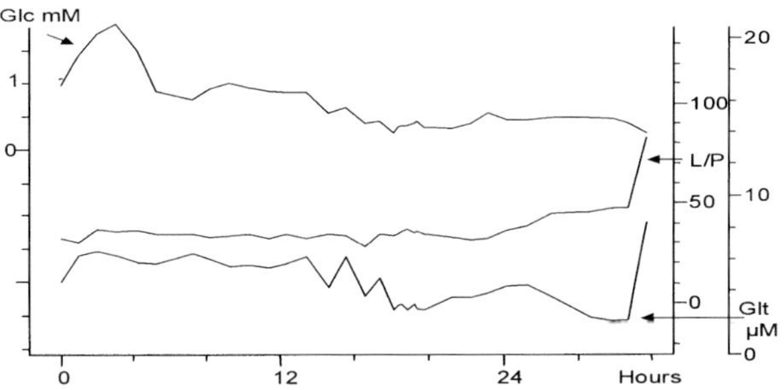

Fig. 1. Examples of improving and deteriorating metabolism monitored with on-line microdialysis. The upper graph shows improving chemistry in a patient (increasing glucose – glc – left vertical axis, decreasing lactate/pyruvate ratio – L/P – right vertical axis and decreasing glutamate – glt – separate right vertical axis). The lower graph shows deteriorating metabolism (decreasing glucose, increasing lactate/pyruvate ratio with a terminal rise in glutamate)

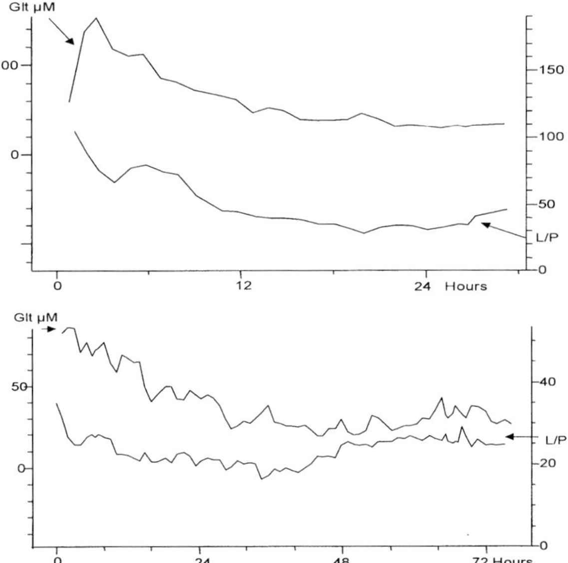

Fig. 2. Elevated glutamate levels in patients with poor outcome. The upper graph shows an initial rise in glutamate followed by a decline to stable but high levels (minimum 40 μM). The lactate/pyruvate ratio mirrors the glutamate trace. The lower graph also shows a decline in glutamate followed by a rise associated with a rise in the lactate/pyruvate ratio. The glutamate level is always above 20 μM in contrast to the patients with good outcome

correlation between the lactate/pyruvate ratio and glutamate (mean $r = 0.48$), with episodes of raised glutamate related to increases in the lactate/pyruvate ratio.

Discussion

Monitoring of the human brain with microdialysis catheters has been applied to patients with head injury [3, 6, 14, 18, 19, 23], subarachnoid haemorrhage [1, 9, 15, 16] and epilepsy [4]. The combination of the measurement of glucose, lactate, pyruvate and glutamate enables monitoring of substrate delivery, metabolite production and potential excitatory amino acid toxicity. The insertion of these catheters may lead to complications in terms of haemorrhage, infection, local tissue damage and artefactual recordings. No complications occurred as a result of catheter placement into the brain parenchyma. Neuropathology studies in animals and humans have shown that these fine sterile catheters do not disrupt the architecture and the blood brain barrier remains intact [2, 11, 20, 21].

The introduction of bedside analysis of microdialysate represents a major advance in the application of microdialysis and is essential if the technique is to be applied clinically to assist in the management of patients. By using the CMA600 microdialysis analyser, four substances can be monitored simultaneously and the effect of therapeutic manoeuvres on brain biochemistry can be monitored. The analyser was operated by the nursing staff on the Neuro Critical Care Unit and was found to be reliable. Validation using High Performance Liquid Chromatography is currently in progress. The preliminary results demonstrate good correlation between bedside and laboratory analysis.

The microdialysis concentration represents the dialysate concentration and not the true extracellular concentration. However, by using long membranes (10 mm) and slow flow rates (0.3 μl/min), high (70% of the true concentration) recovery rates can be obtained.

The findings of low cerebral glucose and high cerebral lactate correspond to the high metabolic activity of the brain. Our previous study, using the CMA60 30 mm catheter in the brain, has shown that brain glucose is lower, and lactate and pyruvate higher compared to subcutaneous adipose tissue [10]. The periods of undetectable cerebral glucose confirm the findings of other studies [22]. Although there was a tendency for lower glucose and a higher lactate/

pyruvate ratio in the poor outcome compared to the good outcome group, this did not achieve statistical significance when comparing the means and further investigation is required. Other factors related to outcome, particularly patients with multiple injuries and catheter location in normal cortex in patients with basal ganglia/brainstem injury require consideration. However, trends in these parameters related to outcome were clearly identifiable with reduction in glucose and elevation in the lactate/pyruvate ratio culminating in poor outcome. The trend as opposed to the absolute values may be more useful in interpreting the biochemical changes for individual patients. The findings confirm raised glutamate levels following head trauma [3, 14, 19]. The pattern of initial increase followed by decrease to stable levels occurred in patients with both good and poor outcomes. However, if the glutamate level remained elevated or if there were secondary rises in glutamate, this was a poor prognostic sign.

In this study, the catheter was placed in the frontal cortex. In four patients the catheter was in the region of contusions. Currently the microdialysis catheters are not visible on CT scans although their approximate location can be determined from the bolt and radio-opaque ICP transducer. No attempt was made to target the catheters to a particular area. Other studies have demonstrated higher glutamate levels in the region of contusions [3]. The combination of on-line monitoring with directed catheter placement has the potential to assist in the management of patients with contusions.

In conclusion, the results demonstrate that the application of microdialysis to patients with severe head injury on a Neuro Critical Care Unit is feasible and safe. On-line analysis of the dialysate at the bedside enables patterns of improving and deteriorating metabolism to be identified. Further investigation of the effects of interventions, for example, hyperventilation and hypothermia is in progress.

Acknowledgments

We wish to acknowledge the support and collaboration of Professor R Bullock, Dr L Hillered, Professor L Persson and Professor U Ungerstedt. We thank the nursing staff on the Neuro Critical Care Unit and Mr S Piechnik for assistance with data downloading. Mr P Hutchinson is supported by a Royal College of Surgeons' of England Research Fellowship and British Brain and Spine Foundation Research Fellowship.

References

1. Bachli H, Langemann H, Mendelowitsch A, Alessandri B, Landolt H, Gratzl O (1996) Microdialytic monitoring during cerebrovascular surgery. Neurol Res 18: 370–376
2. Benveniste H (1989) Brain microdialysis. J Neurochem 6: 1667–1679
3. Bullock R, Zauner A, Woodward J, Myseros JS, Choi SC, Ward JD, Marmarou A, Young HF (1998) Factors affecting excitatory amino acid release following severe human head injury. J Neurosurg 89: 507–518
4. During MJ, Spencer DD (1993) Extracellular hippocampal glutamate and spontaneous seizure in the conscious human brain. The Lancet 341: 1607–1610
5. Editorial (1992) Microdialysis. Lancet 339: 1326–1327
6. Goodman JC, Gopinath SP, Valadka AB, Narayan RK, Grossman RG, Simpson-RK J, Robertson CS (1996) Lactic acid and amino acid fluctuations measured using microdialysis reflect physiological derangements in head injury. Acta Neurochir [Suppl] (Wien) 67: 37–39
7. Gupta AK, Hutchinson PJ, Al RP, Gupta S, Swart M, Kirkpatrick PJ, Menon DK, Datta AK (1999) Measuring brain tissue oxygenation compared with jugular venous oxygen saturation for monitoring cerebral oxygenation after traumatic brain injury. Anesth Analg 88: 549–553
8. Hoffman WE, Charbel FT, Edelman G, Hannigan K, Ausman JI (1996) Brain tissue oxygen pressure, carbon dioxide pressure and pH during ischemia. Neurol Res 18: 54–56
9. Hutchinson PJA, Al-Rawi PG, O'Connell MT, Gupta AK, Maskell LB, Hutchinson DBA, Pickard JD, Kirkpatrick PJ (1999) Monitoring of brain metabolism during aneurysm surgery using microdialysis and brain multiparameter sensors. Neurol Res 21: 352–358
10. Hutchinson PJA, O'Connell MT, Al-Rawi PG, Gupta AK, Maskell LB, Gupta S, Hutchinson DBA, Pickard JD, Kirkpatrick PJ (1998) Intracerebral monitoring in severe head injury – intracranial pressure. Paratrend sensor and microdialysis using a new triple bolt. Br J Neurosurg 12: 87P
11. Hutchinson PJA, O'Connell MT, Al-Rawi PG, Maskell LB, Gupta AK, Hutchinson DBA, Pickard JD, Kirkpatrick PJ, Wharton SB (1999) Neuropathological findings after microdialysis catheter implantation. NeuroReport 10(3): i
12. Kirkpatrick PJ, Czosnyka M, Pickard JD (1996) Multimodality monitoring in neurointensive care. J Neurol Neurosurg Psychiatry 60: 131–139
13. Meyerson BA, Linderoth B, Karlsson H, Ungerstedt U (1990) Microdialysis in the human brain: extracellular measurements in the thalamus of Parkinsoinan patients. Life Sci 46: 301–308
14. Persson L, Hillered L (1992) Chemical monitoring of neurosurgical intensive care patients using intracerebral microdialysis. J Neurosurg 76: 72–80
15. Persson L, Valtysson J, Enblad P, Warme P-E, Cesarini K, Lewen A, Hillered L (1996) Neurochemical monitoring using intracerebral microdialysis in patients with subarachnoid haemorrhage. J Neurosurg 84: 606–616
16. Säveland H, Nilsson OG, Boris-Möller F, Wieloch T, Brandt L (1996) Intracerebral microdialysis of glutamate and aspartate in two vascular territories after aneurysmal subarachnoid haemorrhage. Neurosurgery 38: 12–20
17. Ungerstedt U (1991) Microdialysis-principles and applications for studies in animals and man. J Intern Med 230: 365–373
18. Valadka AB, Goodman JC, Gopinath SP, Uzura M, Robertson CS (1998) Comparison of brain tissue oxygen tension to microdialysis-based measures of cerebral ischemia in fatally head-injured humans. J Neurotrauma 15: 509–519

19. Vespa PM, Prins M, Ronne-Engstrom E, Caron M, Shalmon E, Hovda DA, Martin NA, Becker DP (1998) Increase in extracellular glutamate caused by reduced cerebral perfusion pressure and seizures after human traumatic brain injury: a microdialysis study. J Neurosurg 89: 971–982
20. Whittle IR (1990) Intracerebral microdialysis: a new method in applied clinical neuroscience research. Br J Neurosurg 4: 459–462
21. Whittle IR, Glasby M, Lammie A, Ball H, Ungerstedt U (1998) Neuropathological findings after intracerebral implantation of microdialysis catheters. Neuro Report 9: 2821–2825
22. Zauner A, Doppenberg EM, Woodward JJ, Allen C, Jebraili S, Young HF, Bullock R (1997) Multiparametric continuous monitoring of brain metabolism and substrate delivery in neurosurgical patients. Neurol Res 19: 265–273
23. Zauner A, Doppenberg EM, Woodward JJ, Choi SC, Young HF, Bullock R (1997) Continuous monitoring of cerebral substrate delivery and clearance: initial experience in 24 patients with severe acute brain injuries. Neurosurgery 41: 1082–1093

Note Added in Proof

Since submission of this manuscript patient recruitment continues. The outcome data ($n = 26$) indicates that the means ($\pm 95\%$ Confidence Interval). For the good outcome group are glucose 1.6 ± 0.69 mM, lactate 4.2 ± 1.1 mM, lactate pyruvate 26.6 ± 5.5, glutamate 7.9 ± 3.6 μM, and the means ($\pm 95\%$ confidence Interval). For the poor outcome group are glucose 1.7 ± 0.61 mM, lactate 5.2 ± 0.67 mM, lactate/pyruvate 36.4 ± 10.4, glutamate 16.7 ± 9.5 μM. The lactate/pyruvate ratio is significantly different between the two groups ($p < 0.05$).

Correspondence: P. J. A. Hutchinson, Academic Department of Neurosurgery, University of Cambridge, Box 167, Addenbrooke's Hospital, Cambridge, UK, CB22QQ.

Acta Neurochir (2000) [Suppl] 76: 437–438

Extracellular Glutamate and Aspartate in Head Injured Patients

S. P. Gopinath, A. B. Valadka, J. C. Goodman, and **C. S. Robertson**

Department of Neurosurgery, Baylor College of Medicine, Houston, Texas

Summary

Eighty-six patients in coma from a severe head injury underwent monitoring of extracellular concentrations of glutamate and aspartate by a microdialysis technique during the first few days after injury. The median value for glutamate was 7.4 μM (interquartile range 3.6–18.8 μM). The median value for aspartate was 2.4 μM (interquartile range 1.1–5.0 μM). Average values for the dialysate concentrations of glutamate and aspartate, were closely related to outcome ($p < .001$ and $p = .002$, respectively). Patients who died of their head injury had significantly higher dialysate glutamate and aspartate concentrations compared to patients who recovered to a Glasgow Outcome Score of good recovery or moderate disability. Dialysate glutamate and aspartate levels were also significantly related to type of injury ($p = .008$ and $p = .004$, respectively). The highest values were found in patients with gunshot wounds, followed by patients with evacuated and unevacuated mass lesions. Patients with diffuse injuries had the lowest values of glutamate and aspartate. These results suggest that excitatory amino acids may play a role in the evolution of injury to the brain after trauma.

Keywords: Glutamate; aspartate; traumatic brain injury.

Introduction

Excitatory amino acids (glutamate and aspartate) may play a role in the damage to the brain that occurs following traumatic brain injury. In experimental models, excitatory amino acids are transiently elevated in the brain after trauma in proportion to the severity of injury, but rapidly normalize [4, 5]. However, elevated levels of excitatory amino acids have been observed following human head injury for much more prolonged periods of time [1, 2, 6]. The purpose of this study was to examine the clinical factors that are related to excitotoxic amino acid release following human traumatic brain injury using a microdialysis technique.

Methods

Demographic Characteristics

Eighty-six head-injured patients who had a Glasgow Coma Score (GCS) ≤ 8 on admission or who deteriorated to a GCS ≤ 8 within 48 hours of admission were studied between April 1993 and August 1998. The research protocol was approved by the Baylor Institutional Review Board and informed consent was obtained from each patient's nearest relative for participation in the study. The average age of the patients was 35.5 ± 17.1 years. Seventy-five of the patients were male and 11 were female. The median GCS in the emergency department was 7 (range 3–11). The type of brain injury classified by the Traumatic Coma Data Bank computerized tomography (CT) scan system [3] included an evacuated mass lesion in 46 patients, unevacuated mass lesion in 5 patients, diffuse brain injury in 29 patients, and gunshot wound in 6 patients.

Microdialysis

Microdialysis probes were placed in the brain parenchyma of the 86 patients. An area of brain in the fronto-temporal region that appeared injured but not clearly necrotic was targeted for the probe placement, either by direct vision at surgery ($n = 49$) or by CT scan in the ICU ($n = 37$). The position of the probe was noted on follow-up CT scans when possible. The probes were perfused at 2 μl/min with normal saline and samples were collected every 30 minutes. Amino acids were measured in every 5th sample during time periods where the patients were stable and, in addition, in all samples surrounding clinical events.

From the 86 patients a total of 1905 microdialysate samples (average 22/patient) were analyzed. Concentrations of amino acids were determined by pre-column phenylisothiocyanate (PITC) derivatization, reverse phase gradient separation, and absorbance detection (Waters PICO-TAG). Amino acid concentrations were calculated by the peak area integration method using norleucine as the internal standard.

Results

Distribution of Glutamate and Aspartate Values in the Microdialysis Samples

The median value for glutamate was 7.4 μM (interquartile range 3.6–18.8 μM). Thirty-five percent of the values were less than 5 μM, and 60.2% of the values were less than 10 μM. The median value for aspartate was 2.4 μM (interquartile range 1.1–5.0 μM). Seventy-four percent of the values were less than 2.5 μM and 84.1% of the values were less than 5 μM.

Relationship of Glutamate and Aspartate to Demographic and Injury Characteristics of the Patients

Average values for the excitatory amino acids, glutamate and aspartate, were closely related to outcome. Patients who died of their head injury had a dialysate glutamate concentration of 29.5 μM (9.1–147.0 μM) compared to 7.2 μM (4.4–12.0 μM) in patients who recovered to a Glasgow Outcome Score of good recovery or moderate disability and to 7.6 μM (5.7–17.2 μM) in patients who were severely disabled or vegetative at 6 month after injury ($p < .001$). Dialysate aspartate concentrations were similarly elevated in patients who died of their injury, 5.7 μM (2.8–22.1 μM) compared to 3.4 μM (2.3–4.3 μM) and 2.3 μM (1.7–4.4 μM), respectively ($p = .002$).

Microdialysate glutamate and aspartate levels were also significantly related to type of injury ($p = .008$ and $p = .004$, respectively). The highest values were found in patients with gunshot wounds, followed by patients with evacuated and unevacuated mass lesions. Patients with diffuse injuries had the lowest values of glutamate and aspartate.

Microdialysis glutamate and aspartate concentrations were not significantly related to the initial injury severity judged by measures such as emergency room or best day 1 GCS, pupillary reactivity, presence of prehospital hypoxia or hypotension.

Discussion

The results suggest that excitatory amino acids are an important mediator damage to the brain after traumatic injury. The levels of excitatory amino acids observed during the first few days after injury were elevated and the concentrations were closely related to long-term neurological outcome. The microdialysis technique is a convenient method for monitoring excitatory amino acids in head injured patients and may allow insight into mechanisms of brain damage after trauma which are amenable to therapy.

References

1. Baker AJ, Moulton RJ, MacMillan VH, Shedden PM (1993) Excitatory amino acids in cerebrospinal fluid following traumatic brain injury in humans [see comments]. J Neurosurg 79: 369–372
2. Brown JIM, Baker AJ, Konasiewicz SJ, Moulton RJ (1998) Clinical significance of CSF glutamate concentrations following severe traumatic brain injury in humans. J Neurotrauma 15: 253–263
3. Marshall LF, Marshall SB, Klauber MR, van Berkum Clark M, Eisenberg HM, Jane JA, Luerssen TG, Marmarou A, Foulkes MA (1991) A new classification of head injury based on computerized tomography. J Neurosurg 75: S14–S20
4. Nilsson P, Hillered L, Ponten U, Ungerstedt U (1990) Changes in cortical extracellular levels of energy-related metabolites and amino acids following concussive brain injury in rats. J Cereb Blood Flow Metab 10: 631–637
5. Palmer AM, Marion DW, Botscheller ML, Swedlow PE, Styren SD, De KS (1993) Traumatic brain injury-induced excitotoxicity assessed in a controlled cortical impact model. J Neurochem 61: 2015–2024
6. Zauner A, Bullock R, Kuta AJ, Woodward J, Young HF (1996) Glutamate release and cerebral blood flow after severe human head injury. Acta Neurochir [Suppl] (Wien) 67: 40–44

Correspondence: Dr. Shankar P. Gopinath, Department of Neurosurgery, Baylor College of Medicine, Houston, Texas.

Acta Neurochir (2000) [Suppl] 76: 439–444

Substrate Delivery and Ionic Balance Disturbance After Severe Human Head Injury

M. Reinert[1], **B. Hoelper**[2], **E. Doppenberg**[2], **A. Zauner**[2], and **R. Bullock**[2]

[1] Department of Neurosurgery, Inselspital, Bern, Switzerland
[2] Division of Neurosurgery Medical College of Virginia, Virginia Commonwealth University, Richmond, Virginia

Abstract

The most important early pathomechanism in traumatic brain injury (TBI) is alteration of the resting membrane potential. This may be mediated via voltage, or agonist-dependent ion channels (e.g. glutamate-dependent channels). This may result in a consequent increase in metabolism with increased oxygen consumption, in order to try to restore ionic balance via the ATP-dependent pumps. We hypothesize that glutamate is an important agonist in this process and may induce an increase in lactate, potassium and brain tissue CO2, and hence a decrease in brain pH. Further we propose that an increase in lactate is thus not an indicator of anaerobic metabolic conditions as has been thought for many years.

We therefore analyzed a total of 85 patients with TBI, Glasgow Coma Scale (GCS) < 8 using microdialysis, brain tissue oxygen, CO2 and pH monitoring. Cerebral blood flow studies (CBF) were performed to test the relationship between regional cerebral blood flow (rCBF) and the metabolic determinants.

Glutamate was significantly correlated with lactate ($p < 0.0001$), potassium ($p < 0.0001$), brain tissue pH ($p = 0.0005$), and brain tissue CO2 ($p = 0.006$). rCBF was inversely correlated with glutamate, lactate and potassium. 44% of high lactate values were observed in brain with tissue oxygen values, above the threshold level for cell damage.

These results support the hypothesis of a glutamate driven increase in metabolism, with secondary traumatic depolarization and possibly hyperglycolysis. Further, we demonstrate evidence for lactate production in *aerobic* conditions in humans after TBI. Finally, when reduced regional cerebral blood flow (rCBF) is observed, high dialysate glutamate, lactate and potassium values are usually seen, suggesting ischemia worsens these TBI-induced changes.

Keywords: Traumatic brain injury; glutamate; ion balance disturbance, lactate.

Introduction

Secondary brain injury with brain swelling is the major cause for bad outcome after severe TBI. The exact causes leading to the secondary events are however not fully understood. Nevertheless continuing efforts in traumatic brain injury research have brought new insight into the pathophysiologic cascades after TBI. For example, it has been shown that TBI leads to generalized electrical activation, also described as traumatic depolarization [6, 14, 15]. As a consequence, brain oxygen consumption may be briefly increased early after TBI, thereafter followed by a period of reduced oxygen consumption [9], suggesting mitochondrial aerobic metabolism failure. The concept of compartmentalization of the metabolic events after TBI, has lead to the hypothesis of glutamate driven glycolysis in astrocytes [16]. However it is not known whether glutamate drives glycolysis by a direct mechanism in astrocytes, or if it is the consequence of mitochondrial dysfunction, as can be hypothesized through increased calcium influx and activation of the mitochondrial permeability transition pore [4, 10]. Nevertheless Pellerin and Magistretti as well as other groups have demonstrated experimentally, that glutamate "drives" glycolysis, and thus leads to an increase in extracellular fluid (ECF) lactate. This has been attributed to posttraumatic hyperglycolysis, which has been demonstrated in PET studies in patients after TBI [1, 2]. Furthermore potassium is increased extracellularly after TBI as can be demonstrated in a fluid percussion injury model as well as in cortical impact and impact-acceleration models [5, 21]. This posttraumatic increase in extracellular potassium can be explained by a sudden neuronal discharge, and by activation of voltage-gated K+ channels, as well as by the activation of ligand gated ion channels, e.g. through excitatory aminoacids such as glutamate [5, 6].

This brief early increase in oxygen consumption, and hyperglycolysis possibly in response to ionic fluxes implies transient increased metabolism early after trauma. However if substrate delivery cannot satisfy this demand, brain tissue will fail to establish ionic homeostasis. Cerebral blood flow (CBF) as an indicator of substrate delivery, has been shown to be reduced early after trauma in 34% of cases. Therefore when these two phenomena occur together, in failure to re-establish ionic homeostasis, may be especially likely, and will generate high ICP.

In this study we therefore test the hypothesis that after trauma, increased glycolytic metabolism due to generalized activation via excitatory aminoacids, such as glutamate, leads to increased lactate production, and increase in extracellular potassium.

Patients and Methods

All studies were approved by the Committee for conduct of Human Research, at the Virginia Commonwealth University.

Patients

A total of 85 patients, admitted to the Neuroscience Intensive Care Unit at the Medical College of Virginia (MCV), older than 16 years, with severe head injury, and a Glasgow Coma Score of 8 or less, were studied. All patients received intensive intracranial pressure (ICP)-directed management, according to a standard protocol at MCV. There were no significant differences found regarding distribution of sex or age. Patients who were brain dead or close to brain death on admission or for whom informed consent could not be obtained, were excluded from this study.

Cerebral Blood Flow Measurements

Stable xenon enhanced computed tomography (Xe CT Enhancer 300 DPP Inc. Houston, TX) was used for measuring cerebral blood flow in all patients. This was performed by repeated CT scanning during the inhalation of a gas mixture containing 30% xenon, 30–60% oxygen and room air. Regional CBF (rCBF) was calculated, using a 20 mm^2 region of interest, at the site where the microdialysis probe was placed. Attention was given to keep end tidal CO_2 as near as possible to 30 mm Hg, in order to optimize comparison between patients.

Measurement of Brain Tissue pO_2, pCO_2

Two different multiparameter, minimally invasive sensors (Paratrend or Neurotrend, Diametrics Medical Inc., Roseville, MN, USA) were used for continuous measurements of brain pH, brain CO_2 and brain O_2. In the Paratrend, an electrochemical Clark type pO_2 sensor is used, while the Neurotrend operates with a photochemical optical oxygen sensor. The pH sensor contains a phenol red indicator and as acidity increases, the indicator changes absorption. For brain CO_2 measurement, a pH sensitive dye and appropriate buffer are encapsulated by a CO_2 permeable membrane, which can then be used to calculate the pCO_2.

Microdialysis

A custom-built 51 mm flexible microdialysis probe (CMA Microdialysis, Acton, MA) with an external diameter of 0.5 mm, and a molecular weight cutoff of 20,000 Daltons was used to monitor extra-cellular cortical levels of glutamate and lactate. The probe was placed in a standard fashion through a custom-built triple lumen bolt in the right frontal cortex or alongside a ventriculostomy catheter. In some cases the microdialysis probe was inserted through the craniotomy. The microdialysis probe was perfused at two μl per minute using sterile 0.9% saline. Sixty μl dialysates were collected every half hour into sealed glass tubes using a refrigerated (4 °C) automated collector system (BAS Honeycomb). The time between the start of collection of dialysate or performance CBF measurements was at least one hour in each patient. The microdialysis probe was saved after removal for in vitro calibration. Glutamate and lactate were measured using high performance liquid chromatography (HPLC) and with the Yellow Spring YSI, respectively. Throughout the manuscript, extracellular glutamate, extracellular lactate, extracellular potassium are referred to as glutamate, lactate and potassium, unless otherwise specified. In vitro recovery for glucose, lactate an potassium were 35%, 42% and 65% respectively.

Potassium Measurements

Potassium measurements were done using the IL 943 Automatic Flame Photometer, Instrumentation Laboratory Inc. Lexington MA.

Statistical Analysis

Not all brain chemistry analyses could be performed at the same time in every patient, resulting in different n's for different correlations.

Microdialysis measurements for potassium, obtained 6 hours before until 6 hours after the cerebral blood flow study, were averaged and compared with the rCBF results. Regression analysis and Spearman Rank tests were used to test the interrelationships between these parameters.

To study the relationships between glutamate-lactate, glutamate-brain pH, glutamate-brain CO2, and glutamate-potassium, the regression coefficients ("r-values") *for each patient* were calculated. In this way the "nature" (positive or negative) of the relationship could be determined. For this analysis the software package Microsoft Access was used where glutamate was correlated with the corresponding values (time of glutamate ± 30 min) for lactate, potassium, pH and CO2. This was followed by a one-sample *t*-test over these r-values to test the significance of these regression results. Results are given as mean ± SEM unless otherwise specified.

Results

Glutamate and its Relationship with Lactate

For the analysis between glutamate and lactate, the regression coefficient of each patient was calculated. The mean r-value of the 85 patients with simultaneous glutamate and lactate analysis was calculated as 0.274 ± 0.044. The one sample t-test over the r-values was significant ($p<0.0001$). The histogram for the r-distribution is shown in Fig. 1A. Demonstrating a strong positive correlation between glutamate and lactate.

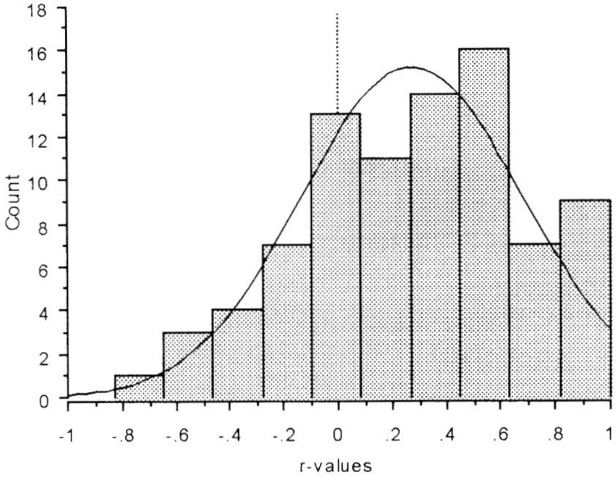

A) Glutamate – Lactate (n=85; r = 0.274 ; p<0.0001)

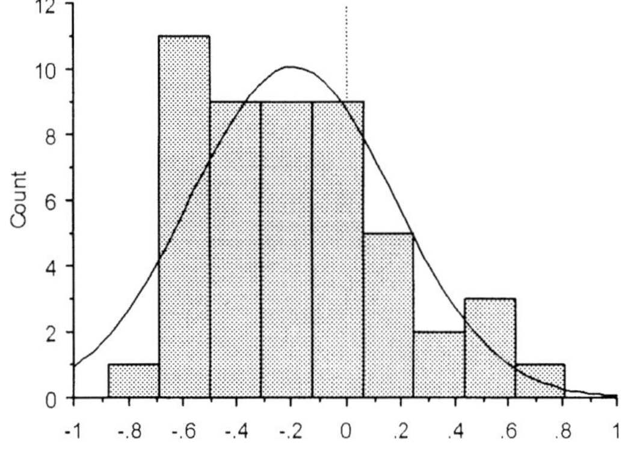

B) Glutamate – brain pH (n=50; r = -0.196 p=0.0005)

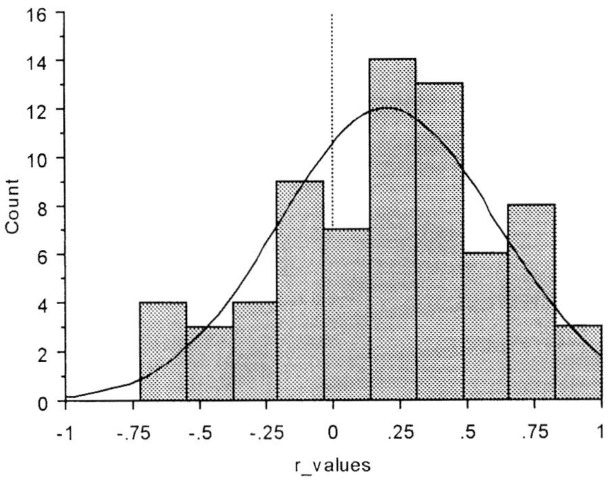

C) Glutamate – Potassium (n=72; r = 0.206 ; p<0.0001)

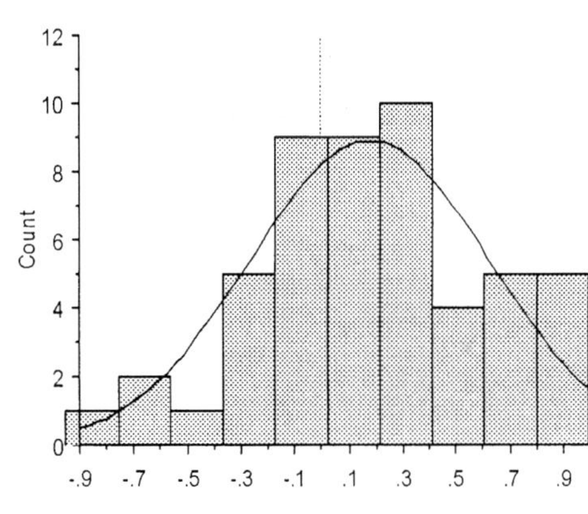

D) Glutamate – brain CO_2 (n=53; r = 0.179 ; p=0.006)

Fig. 1. Histograms: (A) Showing the distribution of the r-values for the correlation between glutamate and lactate of each patient ($n = 85$; mean $r = 0.274$; $p<0.0001$ (one sample t-test)). (B) Showing the distribution of the r-values for the correlation between glutamate and brain tissue pH of each patient ($n = 50$; mean $r = -0.196$; $p = 0.0005$). (C) Showing distribution of the r-values of the correlation between glutamate and potassium of each patient ($n = 72$; $r = 0.206$; $p<0.0001$). (D) Showing distribution of the r-values of the correlation between glutamate and brain tissue CO_2 of each patient ($n = 53$; $r = 0.179$; $p = 0.006$)

Glutamate and its Relationship with Brain Tissue pH

For the analysis between glutamate and brain pH the regression coefficient for each patient was calculated. The mean r-value of the 50 patients with simultaneous glutamate and brain pH analysis was -0.196 ± 0.052. The one sample t-test over the r-values was significant ($p = 0.0005$). The histogram of the r-distribution is shown in Fig. 1B, demonstrating a negative correlation between glutamate and brain tissue pH.

Glutamate and its Relationship with Potassium

For the analysis between glutamate and potassium the mean r-value of the 72 patients with simultaneous analysis of potassium and glutamate was 0.206 ± 0.04. The one sample t-test over the r-values was significant ($p<0.0001$). The histogram of the r-distribution is shown in Fig. 1C, demonstrating a positive correlation between glutamate and potassium.

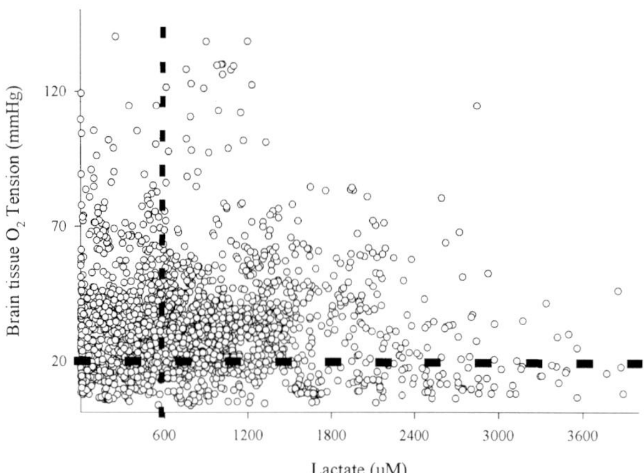

Fig. 2. Distribution of the values of lactate in relation to brain tissue oxygen. 44% of the values demonstrate increased brain lactate (>600 μmol) in presence of supra-ischemic brain tissue oxygen levels (20 mmHg)

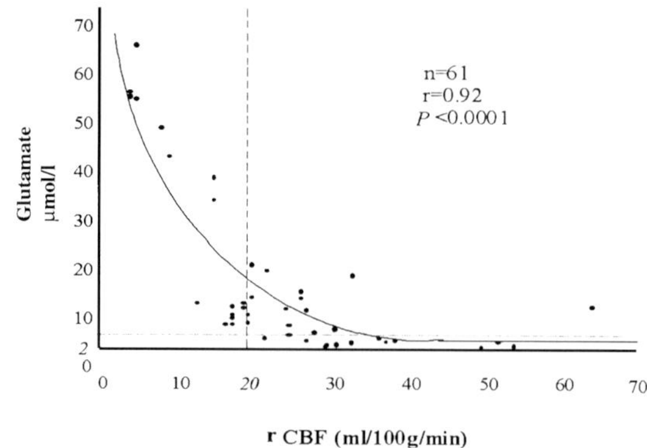

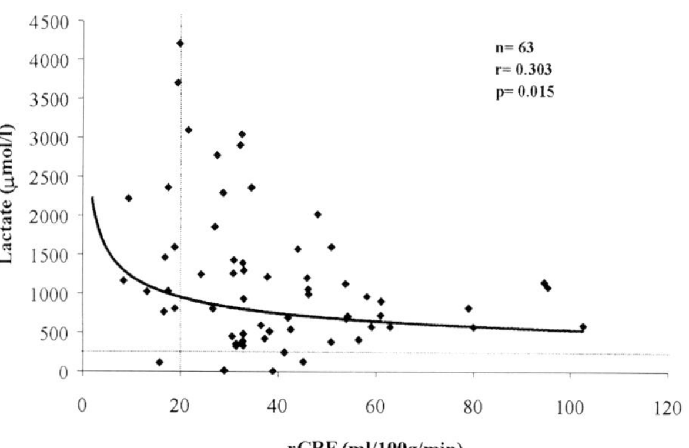

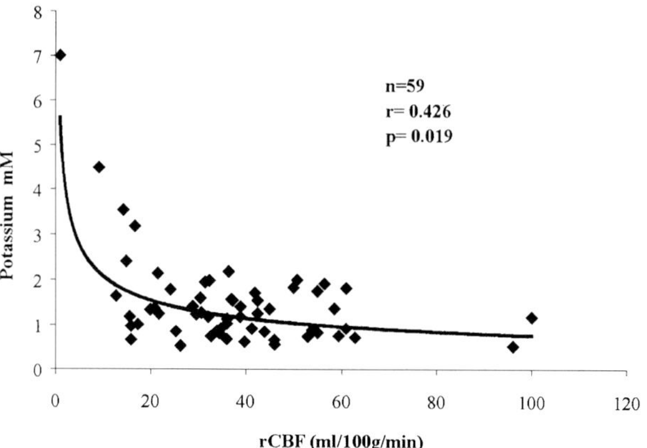

Fig. 3. (A) Showing inverse relationship between glutamate and rCBF. (B) Showing inverse relationship between Lactate and rCBF. (C) Showing inverse relationship between potassium and rCBF

Glutamate and its Relationship with Brain Tissue CO_2

The mean r-value of the 51 patients analyzed was 0.179 ± 0.062. The one sample t-test over the r-values was significant $p = 0.006$. The histogram of the r-distribution is shown in figure 1D, demonstrating a positive correlation between glutamate and brain tissue pCO_2.

Lactate and its Relationship with Brain Tissue O_2

Figure 2 demonstrates the distribution of the values of lactate in relation to brain tissue oxygen, where 44% of the values demonstrate increased brain lactate in presence of brain tissue oxygen levels above or high above the ischemic threshold around 20 mmHg, as measured by the paratrend-neurotrend.

Cerebral Blood Flow and its Relationship with Potassium, Glutamate and Lactate

In 59 patients, rCBF was compared with potassium values at the time of the Xe-CBF study (± 1 hour). The Spearman Rank Correlation was significant ($p = 0.019$) demonstrating an inverse relationship between potassium and cerebral blood flow ($r = -0.426$) (Fig. 3a).

In 61 patients, rCBF was compared with glutamate values at the time of the Xe-CBF study (± 1 hour). The Spearman Rank Correlation was significant ($p<0.0001$) demonstrating an inverse relationship between glutamate and cerebral blood flow ($r = -0.92$) (Fig. 3b).

In 63 patients, rCBF was compared with lactate values at the time of the Xe-CBF study (± 1 hour). The Spearman Rank Correlation was significant ($p<0.01$) demonstrating an inverse relationship between lactate and cerebral blood flow ($r = -0.303$) (Fig. 3c).

Discussion

The relationship between glutamate and lactate in the patients with severe TBI in this study showed a significant positive correlation. In accordance with these results, brain tissue pH was also negatively correlated with glutamate and thus lactate. The positive correlations between glutamate and potassium, seen in this study, were in accordance with the previous findings seen in the fluid percussion studies of Katayama *et al.* as well as the clinical studies of Valadka *et al.* [6, 23]. The new data shown here demonstrates that the regression analysis between glutamate and brain tissue CO_2 was positive and may thus reflect a glutamate driven increase in metabolism.

Advances in brain trauma research have put forward new concepts in the cascade of the pathophysiologic events, namely the compartmentalization between astrocytes and neurons. Pellerin and Magistretti and other groups have demonstrated in vitro, a new role for astrocytes. They may be responsible for lactate production, driven by glutamate even in aerobic conditions [12, 16, 24]. Furthermore several recent publications on brain metabolism have now demonstrated the importance of lactate as the preferred cerebral substrate over glucose [3, 7, 8, 13, 19, 20, 22, 25]. Schousboe *et al.* and Pellerin and Magistretti *et al.* demonstrated a selective lactate transporter between astrocytes and neurons [11, 17, 18]. A further important finding was that lactate dehydrogenase is expressed in different isoformes which are unevenly distributed in astrocytes and neurons. LDH-5 which is present in astrocytes converts pyruvate to lactate, whereas LDH-1 in neurons converts lactate to pyruvate. Lactate could thus be preferentially used by neurons and be shuttled into the tricarboxylic-acid (TCA) cycle [3, 25].

Altogether this date may reflect the well known excitotoxic effect of glutamate, worsening traumatic depolarization, and activating glycolysis and thus increasing lactate and decreasing pH. Further, brain tissue CO_2 is positively correlated with glutamate and decreased pH, suggesting a glutamate driven increase in metabolism. The second major finding in this study is that cerebral blood flow was inversely related to dialysate glutamate, lactate and potassium values. These results may be interpreted in different ways. Secondary cell swelling, as a response to massive ionic shift and cytotoxic edema, may lead to a compromise of the microcirculation, as has been shown previously. Alternatively, low CBF, may lead to ischemic release of glutamate, potassium and lactate. Our results however, cannot be used to favor either hypothesis. Nevertheless it can be clearly stated that after TBI, massive increase in glutamate, lactate or potassium is often accompanied by reduced rCBF. Cerebral tissue may go into a consumption-delivery mismatch situation, then further brain ischemia results with swelling, and the point of no return is reached. However, it is important to note that the lactate-brain tissue oxygen relationship (Fig. 2.) revealed a very important fact; namely that increased lactate production occurred both in anaerobic as well as aerobic conditions. For many years it has been accepted that elevated tissue lactate concentrations signaled the presence of hypoxia, and anaerobic energy metabolism. The results presented here however support the recent hypothesis proposed by different groups, that lactate is a crucial energy substrate that enables neurons to endure activation [19, 20, 24]. This new insight into brain metabolism after TBI may be helpful in aiming future therapy directions, against secondary brain injury.

Acknowledgments

We are grateful for the valuable suggestions of Dr. S. Choi of the Department of Biostatistics, of the Medical College of Virginia.

Ross Bullock was supported by the Reynolds Foundation. Michael Reinert was supported by the NIH Grant NS 12687, Novartis Foundation, and Swiss National Foundation.

References

1. Andersen B, Marmarou A (1992) Post-traumatic selective stimulation of glycolisis. Brain Res 585(1–2): 184–189
2. Bergsneider M, Hovda D, Shalmon E, Kelly D, Vespa P, MArtin N, Phelps M, McArthur D, Caron M, Kraus J, Becker D (1997) Cerebral hyperglycolisis following severe traumatic brain injury in humans: a positron emission tomography study. J Neurosurg 86(2): 241–251
3. Bittar P, Charnay Y, Pellerin L, Bouras C, Magistretti P (1996) Selective distribution of lactate dehydrogenase isoenzymes in neurons and astrocytes of human brain. J Cereb Blood Flow Metab 16: 1079
4. Friberg H, Ferrand-Drake M, Bengtsson F, Halestrap A, Wieloch T (1998) Cyclosporin A, but not FK 506, protects mitochondria and neurons against hypoglycemic damage and implicates the mitochondrial permeability transition in cell death. J Neurosci 18(4): 5151–5159
5. Katayama Y, Becker D, Tamura T, Hovda D (1990) Massive increases in extracellular potassium and the indiscriminate release of glutamate following concussive brain injury. J Neurosurg 73(6): 889–900
6. Katayama Y, Maeda T, Koshinaga M, Kawamata T, Tsubokawa T (1995) Role of excitatory amino acid-mediated ionic fluxes in traumatic brain injury. Brain Pathol 5(4): 427–435

7. Larrabee M (1995) Lactate metabolism and its effect on glucose metabolism in an excised neural tissue. J Neurochem 64: 1734–1741
8. Larrabee M (1996) Partitioning of CO2 production between glucose and lactate in excised sympathetic ganglia with implications for brain. J Neurochem 67: 1726–1734
9. Levasseur J, Alessandri B, Reinert M, Bullock M, Povlishock J, Kontos H (1999) Fluid percussion injury transiently increases then decreases brain oxygen consumption in the rat. J Neurotrauma (in submission)
10. Li P, Uchino H, Elmer E, Siesjo B (1997) Amelioration by Cyclosporin A of brain damage following 5 or 10 min of ischemia in rats subjected to preischemic hyperglycemia. Brain Res 753: 133–140
11. Magistretti P, Sorg O, Yu N, MArtin J, Pellerin L (1993) Neurotransmitters regulate energy metabolism in astrocytes: implications for the metabolic trafficking between neural cells. Dev Neurosci 15: 306–312
12. Magistretti P, Pellerin L, Rothman D, Shulman R (1999) Energy on demand. Science 283: 495–497
13. Maran A, Cranston I, Macdonald I, Amiel S (1994) Protection by lactate of cerebral function during hypoglycemia. Lancet 343: 16
14. Mayevsky A, Manor T, Meilin S, Doron A, Ouankine G (1998) Real-time multiparametric monitroing of the injured human cerebral cortex- a new approach. Acta Neurochir [Suppl] (Wien) 71: 78–81
15. Obrenovitch T, Urenjak J (1997) Is high extracellular glutamate the key to excitotxicity in traumatic brain injury. J Neurotrauma 14(10): 677–698
16. Pellerin L, Magistretti P (1994) Glutamate uptake into astrocytes stimulates aerobic glycolisis: A mechanism coupling neuronal activity to glucose utilization. Neurobiology 91(22): 10625–10629
17. Pellerin·L, Pellegri G, Bittar P, Charnay Y, Bouras C, Stella N, Magistretti P (1998) Evidence supporting the existence of an activity-dependent astrocyte-neuron lactate shuttle. Development Neurosci 20: 291–299
18. Schousboe A, Westergaard N, Waagepetersen H, Larsson O, Bakken I, Sonnewald U (1997) Trafficking between glia and neurons of TCA cycle intermediates and related metabolites. Glia 21: 99–105
19. Schurr A, West C, Rigor B (1988) Lactate supported synaptic function in the rat hippocampal slice preparation. Science 240: 1326–1328
20. Schurr A, Miller J, Payne R, Rigor B (1999) An increase in lactate output by brain tissue serves to meet the energy needs of glutamate-activated neurons. J Neurosci 19(1): 34–39
21. Tomita Y, Stiefel M, Marmarou A (1999) Ionic dysfunction accompanying traumatic brain injury in rats. Poster program, American Association of Neurological Surgeons. Poster 1417: 239
22. Tscaopoulos M, Magistretti P (1996) Metabolic coupling between Glia and Neurons. J Neurosci 16(3): 877–885
23. Valadka A, Goodman J, Gopinath S, Uzura M, Robertson C (1998) Comparison of brain tissue oxygen tension to microdialysis-based measures of cerebral ischemia in fatally head injured patients. J Neurotrauma 15(7): 509–519
24. Vega C, Poitry-Yamate C, Jirounek P, Tsacopoulos M, Coles J (1998) Lactate is released and taken up by isolated rabit vagus nerve during aerobic metabolism. J Neurochem 71(1): 330–337
25. Waagepetersen H, Bakken I, Larsson O, Sonnewald U, Schousboe A (1998) Metabolism of lactate in cultured GABAergic neurons studied by 13C nuclear magnetic resonance spectroscopy. J Cereb Blood Flow Metab 18(1): 109–117

Correspondence: Dr. Michael Reinert, Division of Neurosurgery Medical College of Virginia, Virginia Commonwealth University, Richmond, Virginia.

Acta Neurochir (2000) [Suppl] 76: 445–449

Assessment of the Variation in Cerebrovascular Reactivity in Head Injured Patients

S. A. Jackson[1], **I. Piper**[1], **L. Dunn**[1], **C. Leffler**[2], and **M. Daley**[3]

[1] Institute of Neurological Sciences, Southern General Hospital, Glasgow
[2] University of Tennessee, Memphis
[3] University of Memphis, Tennessee

Summary

Several indices have been reported which correlate with autoregulatory function [2, 3]. However, before critical thresholds for targeting therapy can be defined, a better understanding of the inherent variability of cerebrovascular reactivity as measured by these indices is required. In this study, patients had BP, ICP and bilateral MCA TCD velocity monitored before, during and after BP and CO2 challenges, applied in a random order, with measurements taken within 48 hours of injury. Four indices of reactivity were calculated: the PRx, the CORRx and the FV_{react} & ICP_{react}.

At 48 hours post-injury inter-patient variation in cerebrovascular reactivity, as measured by these indices, is large and injury specific factors remain important determinants of the variance. Within patient analysis has identified instances where the combined monitoring of the PRx and the CORRx may provide information about the function of pressure autoregulation and further study of the combined use of these two indices of reactivity is warranted.

Keywords: Intracranial pressure; pressure autoregulation; method assessment.

Introduction

A continuous measure of the state of cerebrovascular autoregulation would be useful in the intensive care management of head injured patients. Information on autoregulatory function would provide key information for targeting therapy for raised intracranial pressure (ICP) in brain injured patients. For example, indications for the use of arterial pressors as a means of improving cerebral perfusion pressure (CPP) are critically dependent upon whether pressure autoregulation is intact. With lost or severely impaired pressure autoregulation, increasing systemic arterial pressure (BP) will only cause a pressure passive increase in ICP with no net improvement in CPP.

Several indices have been reported which correlate with autoregulatory function. Czosnyka *et al.* [2] have reported an index, the PRx, which is a measure of the correlation of slow wave changes in mean BP and ICP. The PRx has been shown to be correlated with admission GCS and 6 month outcome as measured by the 5 point Glasgow Outcome Scale (GOS). Daley *et al.* [3] have used an auto-correlation/cross-correlation time-series method to study the correlation between the BP and ICP signals. Daley's index, the CORRx, has been shown to increase significantly under conditions which cause cerebral vasodilation. The CORRx is a measure of the correlation between the BP and ICP signal over all frequencies of the pressure waveforms, which is in contrast to the PRx which is chiefly a measure of the slow ICP wave activity.

It is not clear to what degree these two indices measure the same physiological mechanisms underlying pressure autoregulation. Also, an improved understanding of the inherent variability of cerebrovascular reactivity, as measured by these two indices, is required before clinically relevant treatment thresholds can be defined. The primary aim of this study was to assess the inherent variation in the PRx and the CORRx indices within head injured patients by studying the variation in responses to two controlled physiological challenges. The secondary aim was to compare the indices within individual patients to assess to what degree they measure similar mechanisms.

Patients and Methods

The study design and patient consent form were passed by the local Ethics committee. Consented patients had BP measured by an optimally damped external strain gauge catheter–transducer system

Table 1. *Distribution of Demographics for Patients when Classified as Autoregulating or Non-Autoregulating at their First Measurement Within 48 Hours of Injury According to the ARindex*

ARindex	N	AR value	Age mean ± SD	GCS mean ± SD	%PaCO2 mean ± SD	%BP mean ± SD
+	10	1.42	29 ± 13	7 ± 2	23 ± 3	19 ± 7
–	7	−22.9	28 ± 12	6 ± 3	25 ± 11	22 ± 7

placed into a radial artery. ICP was measured using the Camino intraparenchymal probe. Bilateral MCA TCD velocity was monitored using a SciMed QVL Doppler system. All parameters were monitored continuously before, during and after BP and CO2 challenges, applied in a random order. Patients were sedated (morphine, midazolam, propofol) and ventilated according to a standardised protocol. PaCO2 was increased by 1 kPa by adding known concentrations of CO2 into the inspired gas mixture. BP was increased by 25% from pre-challenge levels by IV infusion of noradrenalin (0.05 µg/kg/min). Arterial blood samples were taken before during and after each challenge. For each patient the standard demographic details (Age, Sex, GCS on Admission, Primary CT Scan Classification) were recorded. For all patients, the first measurements were taken within 48 hours of injury. Where possible, measurements were repeated daily until the ICP probe was removed.

Autoregulation Indices

As an index for classification of autoregulatory status, we used the "ARindex" described by Bouma and Muizelaar [1]. The ARindex = %Change in CPP/% Change in CVR which was calculated as follows: CVR = CPP/CBF_{fv} (MCA). CBF_{fv} is the cerebral blood flow velocity in the middle cerebral artery. Autoregulation was defined as intact if the ARindex was positive and <= 2.0.

Two further indices of "reactivity" were also calculated:

i) Fvreact = %Change in CBF_{fv}/mmHg of BP or CO2 Challenge
ii) ICPreact = %Change in ICP/mmHg of BP or CO2 Challenge

PRx and CORRx Indices

The methodology underlying calculation of these indices has been previously described [2, 3]. Briefly, the PRx is calculated from the correlation of 40 consecutive 5 second averages of BP and ICP. PRx ranges from −1 → 1 where 1 is a perfect positive correlation. Values significantly greater than 0 are interpreted to be indicative of a pressure passive state. The PRx describes only slow-wave activity of less than 0.1 Hz. The CORRx is based upon an auto-correlation/crosscorrelation time-series method which provides a measure of how well correlated the BP and ICP signals are over the whole frequency range of the recorded pressure waves. Similar to the PRx, the CORRx ranges from −1 → 1 with 1 being a perfect correlation.

Statistical Analysis

As a measure of variation of the indices the coefficient of variation (CV) was calculated. CV = (Standard Deviation of Samples/Mean of Samples) ×100%. Analysis of variance (ANOVA) was used to test for differences in indices between autoregulating and non-autoregulating groups. A general linear model (GLM) was used to model the effects of patient and injury specific factors upon the measured responses to physiological challenge.

Results

Seventeen severely head injured patients were recruited into the study. Age ranged from 14–49 years (mean = 29, median 27). Admission GCS ranged from 3–12 (mean = 6, median = 7). Admission CT-Scans showed the primary diagnosis as diffuse injury in 5 patients, subdural haematoma in 4 patients and unilateral or bilateral contusions in 8 patients.

Table 1 shows the distribution of demographics for patients when classified as autoregulating or non-autoregulating at their first measurement within 48 hours of injury according to the ARindex. Ten patients were autoregulating and seven were classified as *not* autoregulating. There were no significant differences between the two classes in terms of Age, GCS, percent change in PaCO2 or percent change in BP resulting from the physiological challenges.

Table 2 summarises the data for the reactivity indices before and in response to the physiological chal-

Table 2. *Reactivity Indices (mean ± SD) Before and in Response to a BP and CO2 Challenge when Classified into Two Groups (AR+, AR−) by the ARindex*

ARindex	PRx	CORRx	ΔPRx BP CO2	ΔCORRx BP CO2	ΔTCD BP CO2	ΔICP BP CO2
+	0.189 ± 0.22	0.638 ± 0.16	0.066 ± 0.34 *0.39 ± 0.29*	−0.041 ± 0.07 *0.124 ± 0.09*	0.194 ± 0.24* *0.674 ± 0.85*	−0.147 ± 0.14 *3.10 ± 2.95*
–	0.212 ± 0.45	0.668 ± 0.18	−0.119 ± 0.33 *0.496 ± 0.38*	−0.002 ± 0.06 *0.069 ± 0.23*	0.411 ± 0.11 *0.927 ± 1.5*	0.02 ± 0.19 *2.98 ± 3.5*

* $p < 0.05$ ANOVA.

Table 3. *Relative Variation in the Reactivity Indices (Coefficient of Variation: CV%) when Classified Between the AR+ and AR− Groups*

ARindex	PRx	CORRx	ΔPRx BP CO2	ΔCORRx BP CO2	ΔTCD BP CO2	ΔICP BP CO2
+	114%	25%	515%	168%	122%	94%
			73%	*75%*	*126%*	*95%*
−	214%	265%	280%	2,800%	26%	990%
			77%	*327%*	*163%*	*117%*

lenges when classified into the two groups (AR+, AR−) by the ARindex. The only index which showed a significant difference between the AR+ and AR− groups was the change in TCD flow velocity resulting from the physiological challenge. This, however, is to be expected as the flow velocity measurement is part of the ARindex classifier. There were no significant differences in either the pre-challenge values of the PRx and CORRx or the change in PRx and CORRx with challenge when classified into the AR+ and AR− group.

Table 3 summarises the relative variation in the indices (using the coefficient of Variation: CV) when classified between the AR+ and AR− groups. It can be seen that the variation in the reactivity indices between patients is very high and the CV ranges from 25% to greater than 2500%. The large inter-patient variability in these indices was modelled using a general linear model (GLM) procedure. Table 4 shows the resulting deviance and residual deviance of the GLM model which relates the TCD reactivity index to five factors: ARindex, primary CT-Diagnosis, Age, GCS and time to first measurement. It can be seen that the greatest variability in the data can be explained by the primary CT diagnosis which explains greater than 50% of the deviance in the model.

Figure 1 shows within patient data which demonstrates that the two indices the PRx and the CORRx may provide complementary information about the autoregulatory state of the patient. Figure 1a shows a segment of the ICP waveform taken from a 15 year old male patient with diffuse head injury. Note how the ICP waveform has a large pulse amplitude (>10 mmHg) with a shape which is similar to an arterial pressure waveform. In this patient, both the PRx and the CORRx have relatively high values which could be interpreted to indicate a pressure passive loss of autoregulatory tone. In contrast, Figure 1b, shows a segment of the ICP waveform taken from a 32 year old male patient with a subdural haematoma. Note the ICP waveform has a smaller amplitude and with a more rounded configuration. In this patient, the PRx remains high but the CORRx is low. This combination of indices could be interpreted to indicate a state of cerebrovascular vasodilation resulting from an active autoregulatory process.

Table 4. *GLM Output Sources of Variation in Model: TCDvariation = AR_Factor + CT.diag + Age + GCS + Time.to.First.Measure*

Factor	Deviance	Residual deviance
NULL		0.7678
AR Factor	0.1905	0.5773
CT Diag	0.4519	0.1253
Age	0.0005	0.1248
GCS	0.0117	0.1130
Time to first measure	0.0893	0.0237

Figure 2a shows PRx and CORRx data from a 32 year old patient with a subdural haematoma measured daily for 4 consecutive days. In this patient, PRx decreased from a large positive value at 24 hours post-injury to lower values and eventually to a negative PRx on days 2–4 post-injury. The CORRx did not change significantly, over time, remaining at a value around 0.3. These data might be interpreted to indicate a patient with intact autoregulatory tone which is actively dilated during the first 24 hours with a subsequent increase in vascular tone by days 2–4 post-injury. Figure 2b, shows ICP and PRx data trended on a minute by minute basis at two different time segments taken from a 16 year old male patient with diffuse injury. The early segment is taken when the patient was having raised ICP but before aggressive ICP therapy was applied. Note the relatively stable PRx values centred at high positive values. Following treatment with intravenous thiopentone, the ICP initially dropped but continued to show instability, eventually returning to pre-treatment levels. Note the large variability in the PRx during this period of ICP instability.

Discussion

A continuous measure of pressure autoregulation would prove helpful in the daily intensive care management of brain injured patients. In the past, autoregulation has been assessed through analysing the change in global volume cerebral blood flow (CBF) resulting from a physiological challenge. The inert

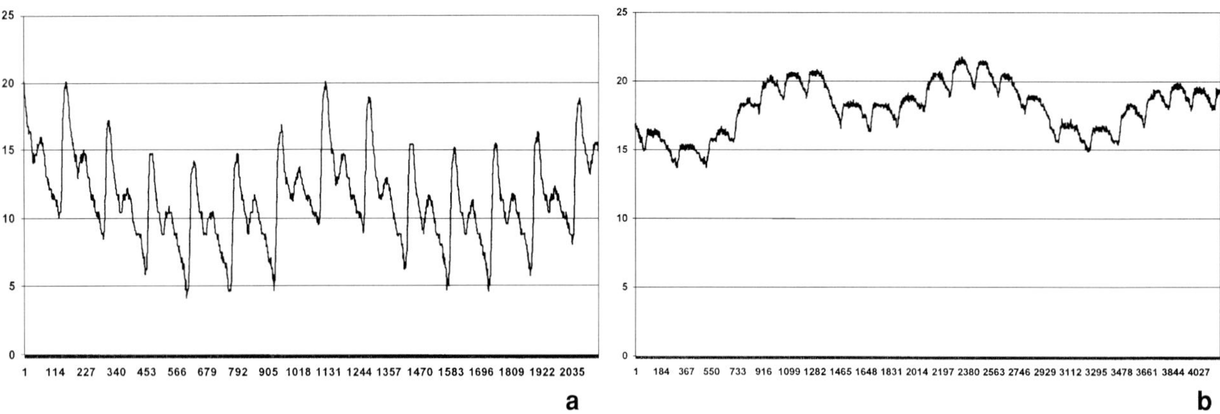

Fig. 1 (a) A segment of the ICP waveform taken from a 15 year old male patient with diffuse head injury. Note how the ICP waveform has a large pulse amplitude (>10 mmHg) with a shape which is similar to an arterial pressure waveform. In this patient, both the PRx and the CORRx have relatively high values which could be interpreted to indicate a pressure passive loss of autoregulatory tone. PRx = 0.80, CORRx = 0.83. (b) A segment of the ICP waveform taken from a 32 year old male patient with a subdural haematoma. Note the ICP waveform has a smaller amplitude and with a more rounded configuration. In this patient, the PRx remains high but the CORRx is low. PRx = 0.69, CORRx = 0.32

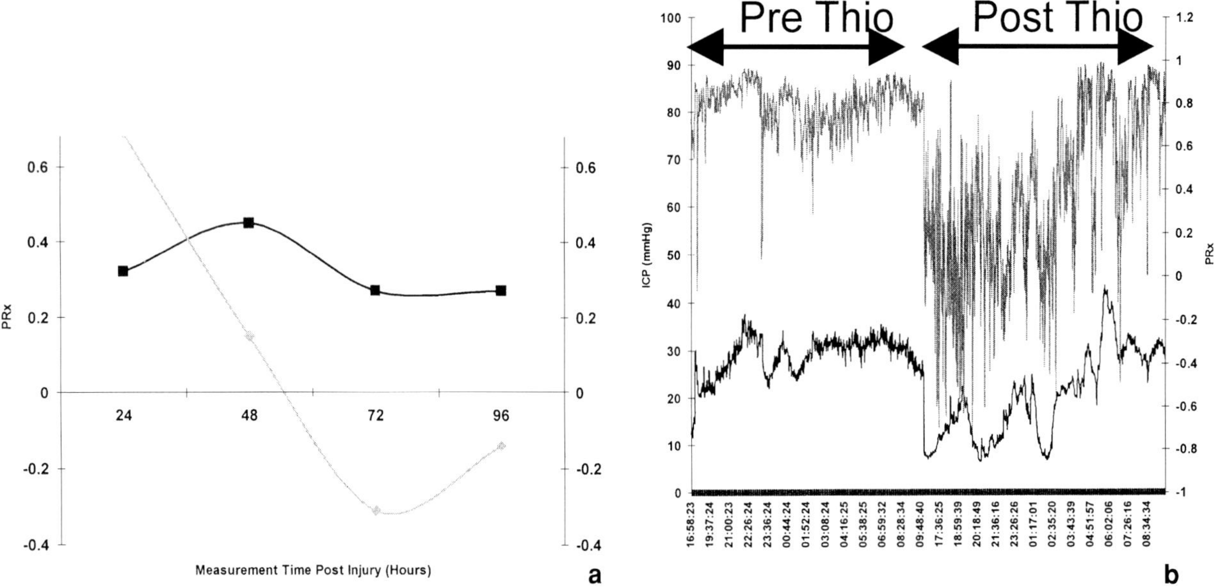

Fig. 2 (a) PRx and CORRx data from a 32 year old patient with a subdural haematoma measured daily for 4 consecutive days. In this patient, PRx decreased from a large positive value at 24 hours post-injury to lower values and eventually to a negative PRx on days 2–4 post-injury. The CORRx did not change significantly, over time, remaining at a value around 0.3. -■- CORRx, ◆ PRx, (b) ICP and PRx data trended on a minute by minute basis at two different time segments taken from a 16 year old male patient with diffuse injury. The early segment is taken when the patient was having raised ICP but before aggressive ICP therapy was applied. Note the relatively stable PRx values centred at high positive values. Following treatment with intravenous thiopentone, the ICP initially dropped but continued to show instability, eventually returning to pre-treatment levels. Note the large variability in the PRx during this period of ICP instability. — ICP_mean, ··· PrX_Corr

tracer methods used for these studies, generally prevented more than 2 to 3 assessments per day. The advent of transcranial Doppler ultrasound (TCD) has increased the practicality of more frequent autoregulatory assessment. However, despite improvements in the design of ultrasound probe fixation devices, the TCD method remains exquisitely sensitive to minor probe movements. Routine nursing and medical care of the patient, are not always readily compatible with maintaining a stable probe position.

Several methods have been reported which attempt to derive indirect information on the state of pressure autoregulation based upon the pressure transmission characteristics of the cerebrovascular bed derived from measurement of the BP and ICP waveforms. Two of the more recent methods which show promise are the PRx method as reported by Czosnyka [2] and the CORRx method reported by Daley [3]. This study has assessed in a group of head injured patients, the inherent variability in these indices across patients and within patients over time. The very large inter-patient variability found with these measures of autoregulation demonstrate that cerebrovascular pressure transmission remains highly variable within 48 hours of injury. Injury specific factors can explain a large proportion of the variability across patients observed in the measured pressure transmission. In the light of the critical dependence of the absolute and relative changes in these measures of autoregulation on injury specific factors, it is unlikely that specific target thresholds will be readily identified. However, from the stand point of targeting therapy for raised ICP, it may not be enough to know whether the cerebrovascular bed is dilated, it is perhaps more important to know if the vascular bed was dilated due to the action of an active autoregulatory mechanism or due to an impaired autoregulatory mechanism exhibiting a passive loss of vascular tone. This study has shown through within patient analysis, some preliminary evidence that the combined measurement of CORRx and the PRx may provide information towards differentiating these two conditions. Further study into the combined monitoring of both the PRx and the CORRx in brain injured patients is warranted.

References

1. Bouma G, Muizelaar JP, Bandoh K, Marmarou A (1992) Blood pressure and intracranial pressure-volume dynamics in severe head injury: relationship with cerebral blood flow. J Neurosurg 77: 15–19
2. Czosnyka M, Smielewski P, Kirkpatrick P, Raing RJ, Menon D, Pickard JD (1997) Continuous assessment of the cerebral vasomotor reactivity in head injury. Neurosurgery 41: 11–19
3. Daley M *et al* (1998) Intracranial pressure monitoring: Use of correlation analysis. Acta Neurochir (Wien) 71: 285–288

Correspondence: Ian Piper, Department of Clinical Physics, Institute of Neurological Sciences, Southern General Hospital, 1345 Govan Road, Glasgow, G51 4TF.

Acta Neurochir (2000) [Suppl] 76: 451–452

Non-Invasive Cerebral Perfusion Pressure (nCPP): Evaluation of the Monitoring Methodology in Head Injured Patients

E. A. Schmidt[1,2], **M. Czosnyka**[1], **B. F. Matta**[3], **I. Gooskens**[1], **S. Piechnik**[1], and **J. D. Pickard**[1]

[1] Wolfson Brain Imaging Centre and Academic Neurosurgery, Addenbrooke's Hospital, Cambridge, UK
[2] Neurosurgical Department, CHRU, Clermont-Ferrand, France
[3] Department of Anaesthesiology, Addenbrooke's Hospital, Cambridge, UK

Abstract

The method of direct calculation of cerebral perfusion pressure (CPP) as the difference between mean arterial pressure and intracranial pressure (ICP) produces a number, which not always adequately expresses brain perfusion. We investigated an alternative non-invasive method, based on waveform analysis of Transcranial Doppler blood flow velocity in Middle Cerebral Arteries (MCA).

25 consecutive head injured patients, paralysed, sedated and ventilated were studied. Intracranial pressure (ICP) arterial blood pressure (ABP) were monitored continuously. The left and right MCAs were insonated daily (116 measurements) using a purpose-built transcranial Doppler monitor (Deltex Ltd, Chichester, U.K.) with software capable of the non-invasive estimation of CPP. Time averaged values of ABP, mean and diastolic flow velocities (FVm, FVd) were calculated and CPPe was computed as: ABP*FVd/FVm + 14.

An absolute difference between real CPP and CPPe was less than 10 mm Hg in 82% of measurements and less than 13 mm Hg in 90% of measurements. The method demonstrated a high potential to detect both short-term and long-term changes in CPP. The method is of potential benefit for the intermittent measurement and continuous monitoring of changes in brain perfusion pressure in situations where the direct measurement of CPP is not available or its reliability is in question.

Keywords: Cerebral perfusion pressure; head injury; transcranial Doppler; non-invasive; monitoring.

Introduction

Direct measurement of cerebral perfusion pressure (CPP) as the difference between mean arterial pressure and intracranial pressure (ICP) produces a number which is not always adequate to express the brain perfusion. In fact, CPP should rather be understood as a condition for cerebral blood flow than a definite number. Therefore, an alternative method, based on waveform analysis of Transcranial Doppler blood flow velocity in basal cerebral arteries may sometimes be more useful.

Using this methodology, the prototype bi-lateral TCD machine with built-in algorithm to assess CPP using externally measured value of ABP has been designed (Deltex Ltd, Chichester, U.K). The prototype has been used in a prospective study to address the questions about an accuracy of CPP estimation, an advantage of day-by-day examination.

Material and Method

Twenty five consecutive patients admitted to Addenbrooke's Hospital suffering from head injury were studied (June–October 1998). There were 21 males and 4 females, the mean age was 36 (range 18 to 76).

All patients were sedated, analgesed, paralysed and ventilated to reach an adequate oxygenation and a mild hypocapnia. CPP was maintained above 70 mm Hg by means of intravenous fluids and inotropic support. ICP was kept below 25 mm Hg by vigorous management. Intracranial pressure (ICP) was monitored continuously with a microtransducer inserted intraparenchymally. Arterial pressure (ABP) was monitored directly. The left and right Middle Cerebral Arteries were insonated daily using a purpose-built transcranial Doppler device (Neuro Q^{TM}, Deltex Ltd.) with the software capable to the non-invasive estimation of CPP [1] Time averaged values of ABP, mean and diastolic flow velocities (FVm, FVd) were calculated using waveform epochs of 8 seconds, and CPP was estimated as: CPPe = ABP*FVd/FVm + 14. Estimated CPP was compared to the direct measurement: CPP = ABP − ICP in external laptop computer.

Results

An absolute difference between calculated and estimated CPP was in 82% of measurements less than 10 mm Hg (116 day-by-day measurements were stored – see Fig. 1). Correlation between averaged CPP and CPPe was significant ($R = 0.61$; $N = 22$; $p < 0.003$).

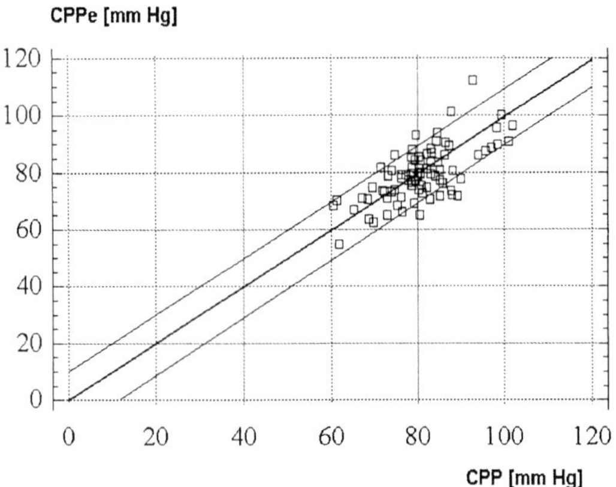

Fig. 1. 116 day-by-day measurement points of estimated CPP (*CPPe*) versus calculated CPP. Thin diagonal lines show the ±10 mm Hg margins of error

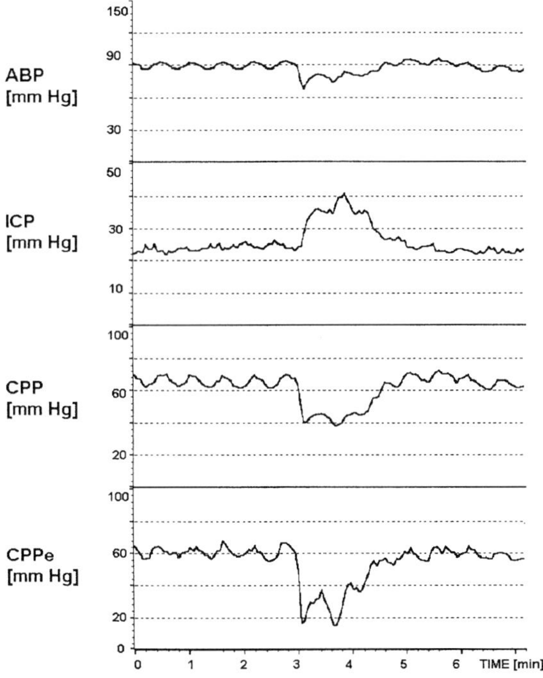

Fig. 2. Time plot of arterial pressure (*ABP*), intracranial pressure (*ICP*), blood flow velocities in left and right MCAs (*Fvleft, Fvright*) calculated CPP (*CPP = ABP – ICP*) and estimated CPP during recorded plateau wave of CPP

The method demonstrated a high potential to detect changes in CPP occurring in time (Fig. 2) or day-by-day variations in CPP (Fig. 3).

Conclusion

In our trial, an overall accuracy of this estimation occurred to be surprisingly good. Taking TCD machine to the bedside, the operator may expect that in 80% of cases the error will be less than 10 mm Hg and in 90% of cases less than 13 mm Hg. Apart from a value of nCPP estimating a 'number CPP' he can assess conditions for brain perfusion visually from TCD waveform and detect a gross a symmetry. Confounding factors in CPP estimation using nCPP have been identified previously [1] as change in arterial blood CO2 concentration, hyperaemia, and, probably, vasospasm.

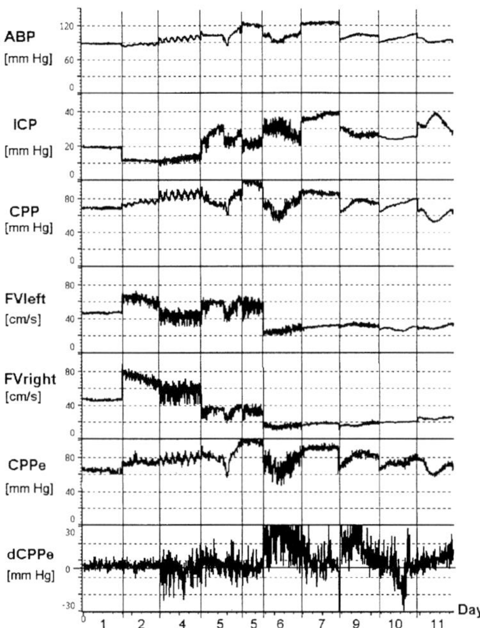

Fig. 3. 11 day recording of patient who died following head injury. Arterial pressure (*ABP*), intracranial pressure (*ICP*), blood flow velocities in left and right MCAs (*Fvleft, Fvright*) calculated CPP (*CPP = ABP – ICP*), estimated CPP (*CPPe*) and left-to-right difference in CPP were recorded. Note increasing difference between left and right estimates of CPP (*dCPPe*)

Our study confirmed previous findings [7] that with a non-invasive methodology, dynamic phenomena as 'B waves' and plateau waves or other transitional changes in CPP are reliably picked up by a reading of Neuro Q^{TM} monitor. This is of potential benefit for the continuous monitoring of changes in real brain perfusion pressure over time in situations where the direct measurement of CPP is not readily available.

Reference

1. Czosnyka M, Matta BF, Smielewski P, Kirkpatrick P, Pickard JD (1998) Cerebral perfusion pressure in head-injured patients: a noninvasive assessment using transcranial Doppler ultrasonography. J Neurosurg 88 [5]: 802–808

Correspondence: Dr. Eric A. Schmidt, Neurosurgical Department, CHRU, 63000 Clermont-Ferrand, France.

Acta Neurochir (2000) [Suppl] 76: 453–456

A Study of the Effects of Using Different Cerebral Perfusion Pressure (CPP) Thresholds to Quantify CPP "Secondary Insults" in Children

S. Jackson, I. R. Piper, A. Wagstaff, and **M. Souter**

Institute of Neurological Sciences, Southern General Hospital, Glasgow

Summary

Little is known about the incidence of secondary insults, particularly cerebral perfusion pressure insults, in children. The objectives of this study were to assess the duration of CPP insults at three different thresholds in children and to relate CPP insults to outcome.

Eighteen children (age < 16, median & mean 8 years) admitted to the Neurointensive Care Unit who had ICP, MAP and CPP continuously monitored were studied. Using the Edinburgh secondary insult analysis program, data was scanned for CPP insults at three different thresholds: CPP < 70 mmHg, <60 mmHg and <50 mmHg. Outcome was assessed using the Glasgow Outcome Scale.

Thirty percent of the time CPP was between 60 and 70 mmHg, 21% of the time CPP was between 50 and 60 mmHg and 8% of the time the CPP was less than 50 mmHg. Compared with adults, there was more than twice the incidence of CPP insults in all threshold groups.

BP remained relatively stable above 70 mmHg across all three CPP threshold groups. However, ICP increased slightly on average from about 13 → 17 mmHg when CPP decreased from the <70 to <60 mmHg group ($p < 0.001$). There was a marked increase in ICP to greater than 30 mmHg on average in the CPP < 50 mmHg group ($p < 0.001$).

CPP insults less than 70, 60 and 50 mmHg do occur commonly in children, a larger dataset and possibly longer term follow up measures will be needed to identify potentially treatable physiological factors most effecting the outcome of children.

Keywords: Secondary insults; children; head injury.

Introduction

Both early (pre-hospital) and late (ICU) secondary insults occur commonly in adult head injured patients and have been shown to be associated with patient morbidity and mortality [1, 4]. In adults, arterial hypotension, as a cause of CPP insults is common in the first 48 hours of intensive care whereas by days 2–5 post-injury an increasing proportion of CPP insults are due to raised ICP [2]. Less is known, however, about the incidence of secondary insults, particularly cerebral perfusion pressure insults, in children. There is also uncertainty about the critical threshold for maintaining CPP in the paediatric population. The threshold of 70 mmHg for treating reduced CPP in adults is not routinely used for managing children, where a threshold of 50–60 mmHg is often used.

The objectives of this study were to assess the incidence of CPP insults at three different thresholds (<70, <60 and <50 mmHg) in children and to study the proportion of CPP insults due to raised ICP with those due to arterial hypotension.

Patients and Methods

Eighteen children (age < 16) who were admitted to the Neurointensive Care Unit who had ICP, MAP and CPP continuously monitored were studied. All had BP measured by an optimally damped external strain gauge catheter–transducer system placed into a radial artery. ICP was measured using the Camino intraparenchymal probe. Minute by minute physiological data was downloaded to an intensive care data server (HP – DocVu System) before being automatically exported and archived on a networked research server. Data was scanned manually to remove obvious artifactual data in the BP and ICP channels. Using the Edinburgh secondary insult analysis program [3], data was scanned for CPP insults at three different thresholds: CPP < 70 mmHg, <60 mmHg and <50 mmHg. Insults had to be beyond the threshold for 5 minutes duration or longer to be defined as an insult. The secondary insult software used, also was configured to extract the mean ICP and BP value which was associated with each CPP insult episode. Outcome was assessed using the 5 point Glasgow Outcome Scale.

Statistical Analysis

In addition to the absolute CPP insult duration in minutes, the CPP insult duration was also normalised to the percentage of valid CPP monitoring time, where the valid CPP monitoring time was calculated as the total CPP monitoring time – the invalid or artifactual CPP monitoring time. Analysis of Variance (ANOVA) was used to test for differences between CPP threshold groupings.

Table 1. *Comparison of Age Distributions of Study Sample and Whole Population Admitted to Unit*

Age range	Sample with BP, ICP & CPP monitoring (n = 18)	Whole population of 79 children
<2 years	2	10
<6 years	5	24
<9 years	3	20
<13 years	6	20
<16 years	2	5

Outcome Assessment

The 5 point Glasgow Outcome Scale was used which was assigned by experienced research staff based upon using a specially modified structured 5-page questionnaire completed by parents.

Results

Seventy-nine children with head injury were admitted to the unit since April 1997. Eighteen of these children had BP, ICP and CPP data monitored and collected. Ten patients were male and 8 were female. The duration of monitoring ranged from 8 hours to 11 days with a mean monitoring time of 2.5 days (median = 1.9 days). Table 1 summarises the age distribution of the sample set with BP, ICP and CPP monitoring compared with the complete set of 79 children admitted to the unit. It can be seen from Table 1 that the age distribution in the sample set is representative of the larger population.

Figure 1a is a plot of the absolute duration of CPP insults at the three thresholds. CPP insults occurred at all thresholds with significantly fewer insults in the CPP < 50 mmHg group compared with the CPP < 70 mmHg group ($p < 0.001$). Figure 1b is a plot of the percentage of valid CPP monitoring time spent below each threshold. On average, 30% of the time CPP was between 60 and 70 mmHg, 21% of the time CPP was between 50 and 60 mmHg and finally, approximately 8% of the time the CPP was less than 50 mmHg. Compared with adults, there was more than twice the incidence of CPP insults in all threshold groups (Adults: CPP < 70 = 14%, CPP < 60 = 3% and CPP < 50 mmHg = 3%).

Figures 2a and 2b are plots of the mean BP and ICP associated with each CPP insult category. BP remained relatively stable above 70 mmHg across all three CPP threshold groups (Figure 2a). However, ICP increased slightly from about 13 → 17 mmHg when CPP decreased from the <70 to <60 mmHg group ($p < 0.001$). There was a marked increase in ICP to greater than 30 mmHg on average in the CPP < 50 mmHg group ($p < 0.001$).

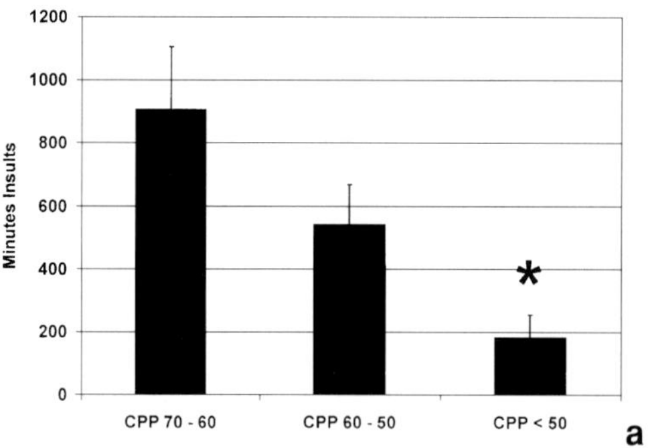

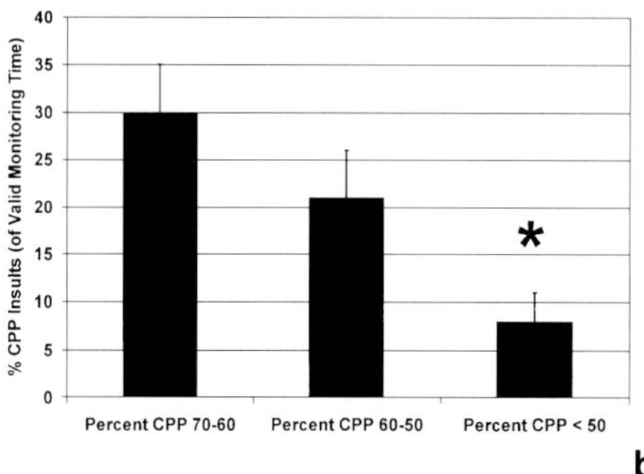

Fig. 1 (a) Plot of the absolute duration of CPP insults at the three thresholds. CPP insults occurred at all thresholds with significantly fewer insults in the CPP < 50 mmHg group compared with the CPP < 70 mmHg group ($p < 0.001$). (b) Plot of the % of valid CPP monitoring time spent below each threshold. Compared with adults there is twice the incidence of insults in the CPP < 70 and < 50 mmHg groups and more than 5 times the incidence of CPP insults in the CPP < 60 mmHg group. *$p < 0.001$

Six-month outcome data was available for 11 children. Two children died, 1 was coded as having severe disability, 4 with moderate disability and 4 made a good recovery. The small sample size precluded a formal outcome analysis, however, Fig. 3 compares the distribution of associated BP (Fig. 3a) and ICP (Fig. 3b), classed by GOS, in the CPP less than 50 mmHg analysis. There is no clear relationship between the occurrence of raised ICP seen with the CPP < 50 mmHg group and the outcome category.

Discussion

CPP insults less than 70, 60 and 50 mmHg do occur commonly in children. Compared with adults there is twice the incidence of insults in the CPP < 70 and < 50 mmHg groups and more than 5 times the incidence of CPP insults in the CPP < 60 mmHg group.

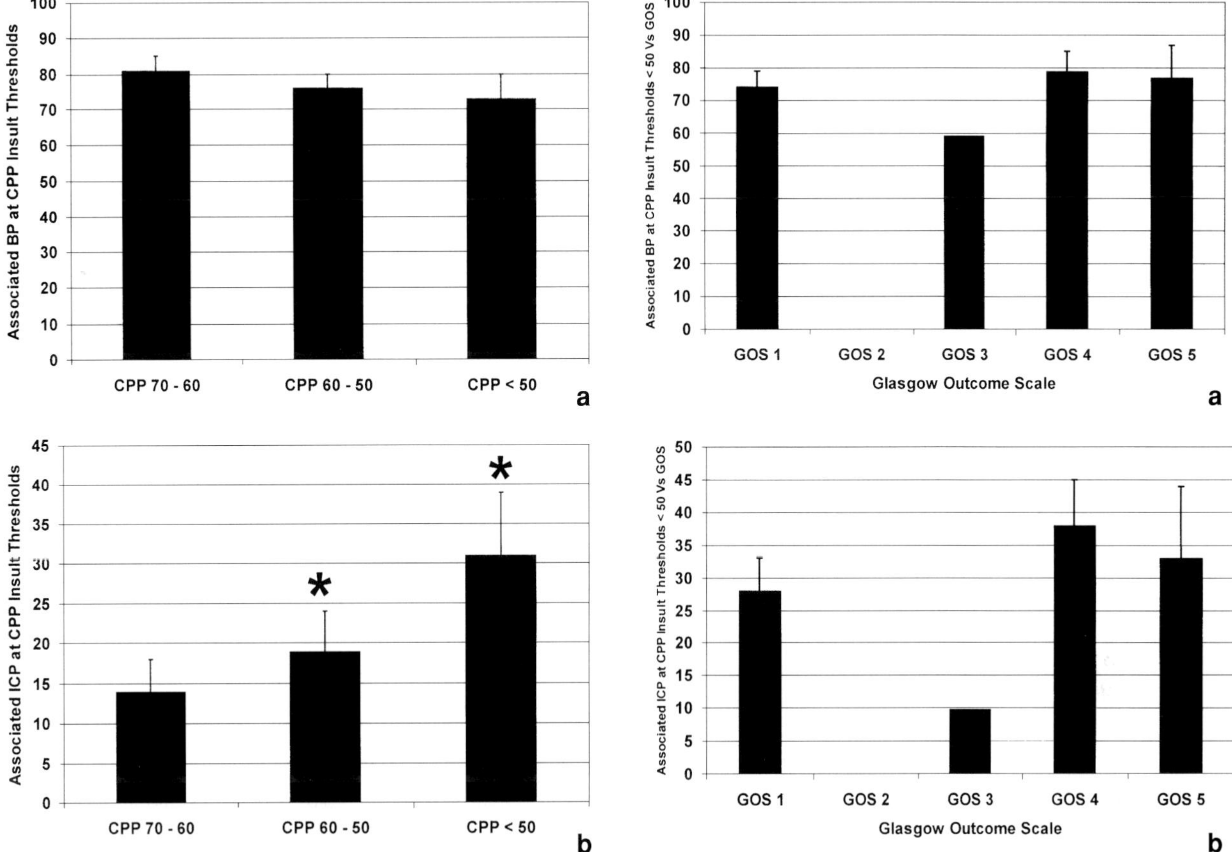

Fig. 2 (a) Plot of mean BP associated with each CPP insult category. BP remained relatively stable above 70 mmHg across all three CPP threshold groups. (b) Plot of mean ICP associated with each CPP insult category. ICP increased slightly on average from about 13 → 17 mmHg when CPP decreased from the < 70 to < 60 mmHg group ($p < 0.001$). There was a marked increase in ICP to greater than 30 mmHg on average in the CPP < 50 mmHg group ($p < 0.001$). $^{*}p < 0.001$

Fig. 3 (a) Plot of the distribution of associated BP when CPP was less than 50 mmHg classed by GOS. (b) Plot of the distribution of associated ICP when CPP was less than 50 mmHg classed by GOS. There is no clear relationship between the occurrence of raised ICP seen with the CPP < 50 mmHg group and the subsequent outcome category

Although, in this study, the average duration of monitoring for children is less than that reported by Jones *et al.* for adults [4], the cause of reduced CPP within the first 48 hours of monitoring was entirely due to raised ICP. This result may be in keeping with the underlying mechanism of brain injury, which, in this dataset, was predominantly one of diffuse head injury.

A significantly elevated ICP above 20 mmHg was only present in the analysis using a CPP threshold of less than 50 mmHg. Although this may indicate the presence of some active process (perhaps cerebrovascular vasodilation) which would support a critical CPP threshold in this region, the raised ICP could also be the result of non-vascular mechanisms as well.

The low numbers of patients in this study precludes any formal statistical outcome analysis, however, it is interesting to report on one case in this dataset which was evaluated as having a "Good Outcome" (GOS: 5), despite being managed in ICU for 18 days which included 21 hours of monitoring time when CPP was less than 40 mmHg, 17 hours when BP was less than 50 mmHg and 11 hours when ICP was greater than 40 mmHg. Such a case raises concern as to the adequacy of either our knowledge of cerebrovascular physiology in children, or of the sensitivity of our outcome assessment measure.

To identify critical CPP target thresholds in children, a larger dataset will be needed and due to the small numbers of children managed by any one neurosurgical unit, argues in favour for the design of a multi-centre trial. The question of whether our current outcome measures for children are optimal should be addressed. It may not be sufficient to assess the outcome of children at a single time point only, but may require us to follow their development over 2 to 3 years in order to quantify rates of progression as end points for children.

References

1. Chesnut RM, Marshall SB, Piek J, Blunt BA, Klauber MR, Marshall LF (1993) Early and late systemic hypotension as a frequent and fundamental source of cerebral ischaemia following severe brain injury in the traumatic coma data bank. Acta Neurochir [Suppl] (Wien) 59: 121–125
2. Cortbus F, Jones PA, Miller JD, Piper IR, Tocher JL (1994) Cause, distribution and significance of episodes of reduced cerebral perfusion pressure following head injury. Acta Neurochir (Wien) 130: 117–124
3. Piper IR, Lawson A, Dearden NM, Miller JD (1991) A microcomputer based research data collection system in head injury intensive care. Brit J Intensiv Care 1(2): 73–78
4. Jones PA, Andrews PJD, Midgley S, Auderson SI, Piper IR, Tocher JL, Housley AM, Corvie JA, Seattery J, Dearden NM (1994) Measuring the burden of secondary insults in head-injured patients during intensive care. J Neurosurg Anaesthesiol 6: 4–14

Correspondence: Ian Piper, Department of Clinical Physics, Institute of Neurological Sciences, Southern General Hospital, 1345 Govan Road, Glasgow, G51 4TF.

Acta Neurochir (2000) [Suppl] 76: 457–462

Does an Increase in Cerebral Perfusion Pressure Always Mean a Better Oxygenated Brain? A Study in Head-Injured Patients

J. Sahuquillo[1], S. Amoros[2], A. Santos[2], M. A. Poca[1], H. Panzardo[2], L. Domínguez[3], and S. Pedraza[4]

[1] Department of Neurosurgery, Vall d'Hebron University Hospitals, Barcelona, Spain
[2] Neurotraumatology Research Unit, Vall d'Hebron University Hospitals, Barcelona, Spain
[3] Neurotraumatology Intensive Care Unit, Vall d'Hebron University Hospitals, Barcelona, Spain
[4] Department of Neuroradiology, Vall d'Hebron University Hospitals, Barcelona, Spain

Abstract

The adequate management of cerebral perfusion pressure (CPP) continues to be a controversial issue in head-injured patients. The purpose of our study was to test two hypotheses. The first was that in patients with a CPP below 70 mm Hg, oxygen delivery is compromised and that therefore signs of tissue hypoxia would be reflected in low $PtiO_2$ measurements. The second hypothesis was that manipulating mean arterial blood pressure to increase CPP improves oxygen delivery, particularly in patients with a CPP below 70 mm Hg. Twenty-five moderately or severely head-injured patients were included in the study. In all of them $PtiO_2$ was monitored in the non-injured hemisphere using the Licox system (GMS, Kiel-Mielkendorf, Germany). Arterial hypertension was induced with phenylephrine 29 times. To quantify the effect of increasing mean arterial blood pressure (MABP) on oxygen delivery to the brain, the $PtiO_2$-BP index was calculated ($PtiO_2$-BP index $= \Delta PtiO_2/\Delta MABP$). In 16 tests (55%) baseline CPP was above or equal to 70 mm Hg and in the remaining 13 (45%) it was below 70 mm Hg. Mean increase in MABP after phenylephrine was 23.7 ± 10.2 mm Hg. Mean $PtiO_2$ was 29.5 ± 14.7 mm Hg in patients with a basal CPP of below 70 mm Hg and 28.9 ± 10.6 mm Hg in patients in the high CPP group. These differences being not statistically significant. The $PtiO_2$-BP index was 0.29 ± 0.23 in patients with a basal CPP of below 70 mm Hg and in patients with a CPP of above 70 mm Hg this index was 0.16 ± 0.11 Hg. These differences were not statistically significant (Student's t-test, $P = 0.09$). In our study a low $PtiO_2$ was not observed in patients with marginally low CPPs (48–70 mm Hg) and readings below 15 mm Hg were observed in cases with both normal or supranormal CPPs. We conclude that episodes of low $PtiO_2$ could not be predicted on the basis of CPP alone. On the other hand, raising CPP did not increase oxygen availability in the majority of cases, even if the CPP was markedly improved.

Keywords: Cerebral perfusion pressure; head injury; brain tissue oxygen.

Introduction

In the last decade, an influential concept underlying the management of head injuries has been that CPP should be maintained above the threshold of 70 mm Hg [3]. Some authors have even proposed so-called *CPP management* as a therapeutic strategy directed towards controlling ICP through stimulating what is known as the vasoconstrictory cascade [10]. The main rationale behind this treatment is the hypothesis that the upper and lower thresholds for autoregulation are usually preserved but are shifted to the right in patients after severe head trauma. Some authors have suggested that to induce the physiological vasoconstrictory cascade, MABP should be increased above supranormal levels by inotropic support or by vasoactive drugs [9]. However, for many, autoregulation is a very sensitive property of the cerebrovascular bed that is impaired or abolished in many patients after severe head injury [5].

Although increasing MABP in these situations sometimes produces an immediate increase in both CPP and CBF, the increased MABP can in the long-term overcharge microcirculation, facilitating edema. In contrast, a different approach for managing CPP in these patients has been suggested in papers from the University of Lund [1]. The *Lund concept* is based on the control or even the reduction of MABP in order to reduce capillary pressure and consequently to avoid brain edema. The most appropriate way to manage CPP in these patients is still open to debate.

The recent availability of probes which can measure oxygen partial pressure directly in the brain parenchyma ($PtiO_2$), has given us the opportunity to test how oxygen availability is modified in the injured brain when CPP is increased to supranormal levels.

The purpose of our study was to manipulate MABP in order to increase CPP and to observe the consequent changes, if any, in oxygen availability in patients with a moderate or severe head injury. There were two hypotheses to be tested. The first was that in patients with a low CPP (below 70 mm Hg) oxygen delivery is compromised and therefore signs of tissue hypoxia would be reflected in a reduced $PtiO_2$. The second was that manipulating MABP to increase CPP does improve oxygen delivery in patients after severe head injury, particularly in those with a CPP below 70 mm Hg.

Clinical Material and Methods

Between November 1997 and December 1998 we included in our study 25 consecutive patients with a moderate or severe head injury admitted to the Neurotraumatology Intensive Care Unit (NICU) of the Vall d'Hebron University Hospitals. The protocol of study was approved by the Institutional Ethical Committee on Human Research of the Vall d'Hebron University Hospitals (Protocol number TR-51/1995).

Continuous Physiological Monitoring

ICP was monitored with the Camino V420 monitor and an intraparenchymatous probe (manufactured by Camino Laboratories, San Diego, California, USA). Mean arterial blood pressure (MABP), cerebral perfusion pressure (CPP) and arterial oxygen saturation (SaO_2) were routinely monitored. SjO_2 was continuously monitored using the Oximetrix-3 system with a Opticath No 5.5 F fiberoptic catheter (Supplied by Abbot Laboratories, S.A, Madrid). In all the tests performed, jugular blood samples, not measurements given by the oximeter, were used to calculate $AVDO_2$. Arterio-jugular oxygen differences ($AVDO_2$) were calculated by the following equation: $AVDO_2 = 1.34 \times Hb \times (SaO_2 - SjO_2/100)$, where Hb is arterial oxyhemoglobin content in gr/dl and SaO_2 and SjO_2 are the percentage of saturated oxyhemoglobin in the arterial and jugular blood respectively. $AVDO_2$ were expressed in μmol/milliliter.

Methodology for Brain $PtiO_2$ Monitoring

In all patients, brain tissue oxygen partial pressure ($PtiO_2$) was continuously monitored using the LICOX monitor and either a CC1 or CC1.SB catheter (Revoxode© probes and monitor manufactured by GMS, Kiel-Mielkendorf, Germany). Catheter probes were always introduced in the frontal white matter of the non-injured hemisphere and always in the same position (12 cm from the nasion and 3 cm from midline). After $PtiO_2$ monitoring had been terminated, the probes were evaluated for zero drift and sensitivity error following the procedures defined by Dings *et al.* [4].

Methodology Used to Increase CPP

In every patient a CPP manipulation test was performed within the first 96 hours after injury. CPP was increased by augmenting MABP with the same methodology used by our group to test autoregulation, which has been published elsewhere [11]. In summary, the methodology used was as follows. As a first step, the ventilator settings were manipulated to change the basal arterial pCO_2. These settings were changed in order to increase or decrease arterial pCO_2 toward the 'normoventilation range'. After waiting for 15–30 minutes, basal arterial and jugular blood samples were extracted to establish baseline values for arterial pCO_2 (pCO_{2B}), arterial pO_2, oxyhemoglobin saturation in the jugular bulb (SJO_{2B}), arterial oxyhemoglobin saturation (SaO_2), hemoglobin content (Hb), and basal arterio-jugular differences of oxygen ($AVDO_{2B}$). Basal intracranial pressure (ICP_B), mean arterial blood pressure ($MABP_B$), and cerebral perfusion pressure (CPP_B) were also determined. In every case, MABP was measured directly through a catheter introduced into the radial artery and zeroed to the foramen of Monro level. In patients with stable hemodynamics, phenylephrine was used to gradually increase MABP by about 20–30%. Arterial and jugular blood samples to calculate $AVDO_2$ were again obtained 15–20 minutes after a steady state of MABP had been achieved and each basal variable was again measured. Changes in global CBF after inducing hypertension were estimated from repeat measurements of $1/AVDO_2$ [12]. The percent change in estimated CBF (%ECBF) relative to the resting value (not corrected for pCO_2) was calculated according to the following equation: $\%ECBF = [(1/AVDO_{2H} - 1/AVDO_{2B})/(1/AVDO_{2B})]*100$, where $AVDO_{2B}$ are the basal arterio-jugular differences of oxygen and $AVDO_{2H}$ the arterio-jugular differences of oxygen after raising MABP with phenylephrine. The $PtiO_2$-BP index was calculated as the increase in $PtiO_2$ divided by the change in MABP ($PtiO_2\text{-BP index} = \Delta PtiO_2/\Delta MABP$). This index was used to quantify the effect of increasing MABP on oxygen delivery to the brain.

Statistical Analysis

The assumption that data came from a normal distribution was tested using the Shapiro-Wilks test. In normally distributed data, the mean ± SD was used to summarize the variables. Differences in variables before and after increasing MABP with phenylephrine were compared by the Student's paired t-test for normally distributed data and the Wilcoxon rank-sum test for paired data, which did not have a normal distribution. Statistical analysis was performed with the SAS statistical package version 6.12 (Supplied by SAS Institute Inc., Cary, NC, USA). The level of statistical significance was established at $P \leq 0.05$.

Results

Twenty-five patients were included in our study. In these 25 cases, CPP manipulations were performed 29 times. In the 4 patients in whom the CPP test was performed twice, the time between tests was at least 24 hours. The mean age in our series was 38 ± 17 years, ranging from 16 to 69 years. Eighteen patients were male (72%) and 7 female (28%). The causes of injury were motor-vehicle related in 17 cases (68%), falls in 7 (28%) and work-related in 1 patient (4%). Analysis of the post-resuscitation Glasgow Coma Scale score recorded on admission, showed that 19 patients (76%) scored equal to or below eight points and 6 patients (24%) scored above eight and below or equal to 13 points. According to the Traumatic Coma Data Bank classification, thirteen patients (52%) were included in the diffuse injury II category, 6 cases in the diffuse in-

Table 1. *Basal Physiological Variables Before Testing Autoregulation in the 29 Tests Performed in the 25 Patients Included in the Study*

	Mean ± SD	Range
Hb (grs/dl)	11.4 ± 1.6	8–14
ICP (mm Hg)	21 ± 10	−1–38
MABP (mm Hg)	94.0 ± 16	71–135
CPP (mm Hg)	74 ± 19	48–117
PCO_2 (mm Hg)	36 ± 4.6	25–46
SjO_2 (%)	76 ± 8	52–91
$AVDO_2$ (μ mol /ml)	1.5 ± 0.6	0.4–3.0
$PTiO_2$ (mm Hg)	29 ± 12	6.5–66.4

jury III (24%), 2 patients in the diffuse injury IV (8%), 3 in the evacuated mass lesion category (12%) and only 1 in the non-evacuated mass lesion subgroup (4%).

Basal Systemic and Cerebral Hemodynamic Variables

A summary of the systemic and cerebral hemodynamic variables before increasing MABP is presented in Table 1. In 16 of the 29 tests (55%), basal CPP was above or equal to 70 mm Hg at the moment of the test. In the remaining 13 cases (45%) CPP was below 70 mm Hg.

$PtiO_2$ and CPP

Mean $PtiO_2$ was 29.5 ± 14.7 mm Hg in the group of patients whose CPP was below 70 mm Hg at the moment of testing (Fig. 1). In the 16 patients in whom basal CPP was above or equal to 70 mm Hg immediately before testing, mean $PtiO_2$ was 28.9 ± 10.6 mm Hg (Fig. 1). Differences in mean $PtiO_2$ between both groups were not significant (Student's t-test, $P = 0.91$).

When basal and post-phenylephrine data were grouped together, no linear or non-linear correlation between $PtiO_2$ and CPP was found when both variables were scatterplotted with CPP considered as the independent variable (Fig. 2). The lowest CPP reading observed in our study was 48 mm Hg. Only 1 of the 13 patients with a CPP below 70 mm Hg and 2 in the high CPP group, had a $PTIO_2$ below 15 mm Hg. In these 3 patients SJO_2 and $AVDO_2$ measurements did not show any indication of global hypoperfusion. Hypoperfusion was not detected by global measurements even in the patient in whom $PtiO_2$ was 6.5 mm Hg (SJO_2 78% and $AVDO_2$ 1.24 μmol/ml).

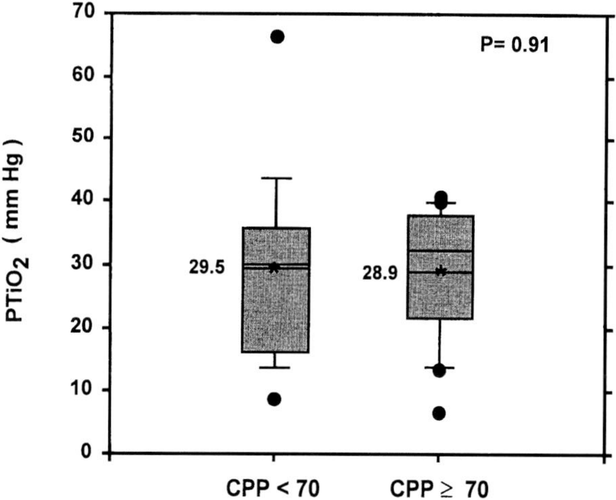

Fig. 1. Box-and-whisker plots in which the distribution of $PtiO_2$ readings in groups with low and high basal CPP are shown. The line inside the box represents the median for the whole distribution while the mean is written outside each box-plot and is represented inside the box by the line with an asterisk. The Student t-test showed no statistically significant difference between the two $PtiO_2$ means ($P = 0.91$)

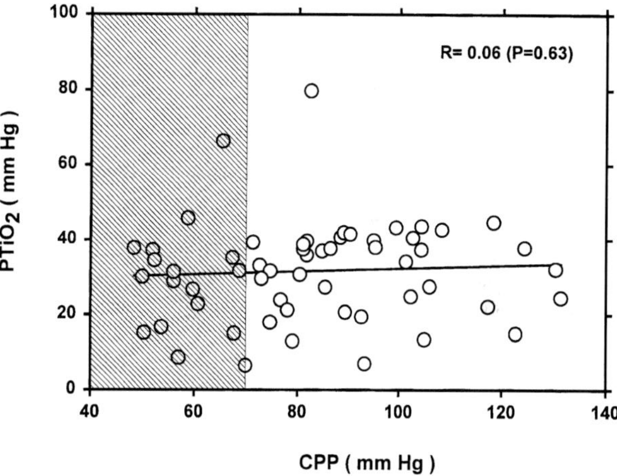

Fig. 2. Graph showing both basal and post-phenylephrine $PtiO_2$ and CPP plotted for the 58 matched readings obtained from the 29 tests performed. In this analysis, we did not find any linear or non-linear correlation between $PtiO_2$ and CPP (Pearson's correlation coefficient $R = 0.06$, $P = 0.63$). This was also the case when separating the whole data set in the two CPP groups. The shadowed area on the left of the graph, delimits the 70 mm Hg CPP threshold

Effects of Increasing MABP on $PtiO_2$

The mean increase in MABP in the 29 tests after phenylephrine was given was 23.7 ± 10.2 mm Hg. This increase in MABP induced an increase in CPP of 19.6 ± 9.2 mm Hg. The basal $PtiO_2$ in the 29 tests

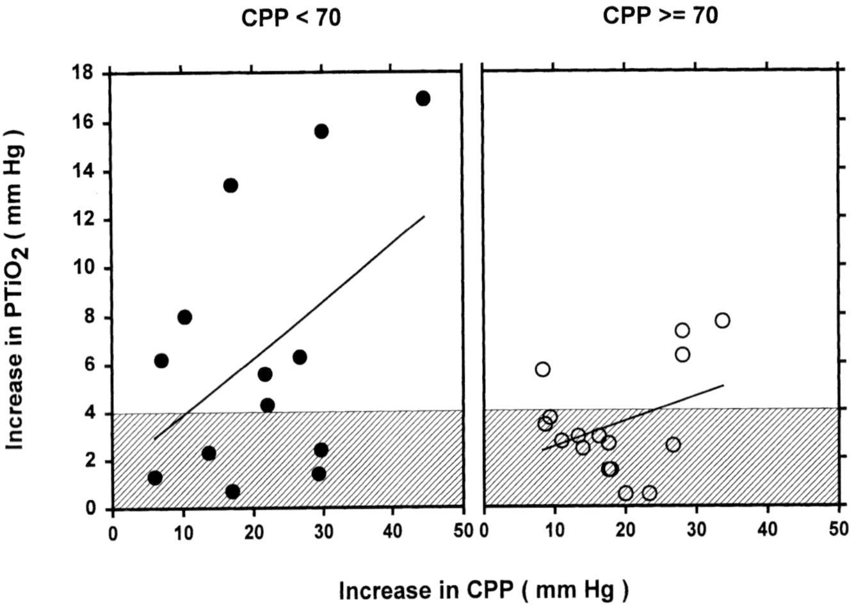

Fig. 3. Chart showing the induced increase in CPP plotted against the observed increase in $PtiO_2$. In the left panel, data are shown for the group of patients with a basal CPP of below 70 mm Hg while on the right panel the same plot is shown for patients with a basal CPP of 70 mm Hg or above. Spearman's R_s for the left panel was 0.38 (P = 0.20) and for the right panel $R_s = 0.02$ (P = 0.95)

was 29.2 ± 12.4 which increased modestly to 34.7 ± 14.9 mm Hg after hypertension had been induced (Wilcoxon matched pairs test, $P \leq 0.001$). The $PtiO_2$-BP index for the 29 tests was 0.20 mm Hg $PtiO_2$/mm Hg MABP with a lowest value of 0.017 and a highest value of 0.79. The mean index was 0.29 ± 0.23 in patients with a basal CPP below 70 mm Hg and was 0.16 ± 0.11 in patients with a CPP above 70 mm Hg. These differences were not statistically significant (Student's t-test, P = 0.09). When plotting the induced increase in CPP against the observed increase in $PtiO_2$ (Fig. 3), there was no evidence of an association between the two variables for the whole group (Spearman's rank correlation coefficient, Rs = 0.18, P = 0.32) or for the two subgroups of CPP. In the 3 cases where significant increases in $PtiO_2$ were observed (shown in the panel on the left in Fig. 3, basal $PtiO_2$ was always above 15 mm Hg (15.1, 26.7 and 66.4 mm Hg respectively). In the 3 cases in whom a low $PtiO_2$ was detected, the induced MABP hypertension did not modify $PtiO_2$ to a significant level (above 15 mm Hg).

Discussion

Assumptions about optimal CPP are generally based on indirect evidence, analysis of surrogate variables and what is known as class III evidence (retrospective studies, case reports etc.). The rationale behind the 70 mm Hg threshold is based on the concept that the normal autoregulatory curve is shifted to the right in severely head-injured patients and that therefore patients with a CPP below this threshold are in the rising part of the autoregulatory curve where CBF is passively dependent on CPP. In this situation, covert tissue hypoxia may be present or the brain can maintain tissue oxygenation at the expense of increasing the rate of oxygen extraction from the oxyhemoglobin. In these patients, either tissue hypoxia or a reduced saturation of the oxyhemoglobin in the jugular bulb, or both, may be present and should be detected by adequate monitoring methods. In our study we could not prove the hypothesis that in patients with a CPP below 70 mm Hg, oxygen delivery is compromised and that therefore signs of tissue hypoxia would be reflected in lower $PtiO_2$ measurements. No differences in mean $PtiO_2$ were observed when comparing high and low CPP groups. Only in one case in whom CPP was below 70 mm Hg, was $PtiO_2$ below 15 mm Hg. On the other hand, two patients with a high CPP, had low $PtiO_2$. Furthermore, no relationship was found between CPPs and $PtiO_2$ when scatterplotting both variables within the range of CPPs studies (Fig. 2). A paradoxical finding was that in cases with a low $PtiO_2$

(below 15 mm Hg), tissue hypoxia was not identifiable by global parameters of ischemia such as SjO_2 or $AVDO_2$. To gain insight into the clinical significance of these paradoxical findings, further studies of these variables should be performed. Possible interpretations of regional tissue hypoxia in situations where global monitoring methods suggest a normal or hyperemic brain are multiple. Some of the possible explanations are high affinity of the Hb for the oxygen and alterations in oxygen diffusion through the BBB among others. These multiple options should be considered and studied for a better understanding of the physiopathology of head injury.

Although our findings should be considered preliminary and only valid for the range of CPPs studied (above 48 mm Hg) and for morphologically "normal" brain tissue, our observations raise several points. The first, and perhaps the most controversial, is that it may be possible that in some patients, marginally low CPPs (50–70 mm Hg) can be well tolerated in the less injured regions of the brain without these patients showing any signs of global or regional ischemia. Vespa *et al.* have recently observed that extracellular glutamate increases in some patients with CPPs below 70 mm Hg but not in others, with a similar reduction in CPP [14]. To interpret our findings, four hypotheses may be proposed. The first is that autoregulation is intact in these patients and that its lower threshold is not shifted to the right. Therefore, reductions in CPP are adequately compensated and CBF is maintained within the normal range by a decrease in cerebrovascular resistance. However, this situation would not be desirable because cerebral blood volume is also increased and therefore either compliance is reduced or ICP is more difficult to control. A second possibility is that even if the patients are below the lower limit of autoregulation with a CPP below 70 mm Hg, the cerebral extraction rate of oxygen is increased enough to compensate for the reduction in CPP and CBF. This seems not to be the case in our group where global measurements did not detect an increase in the cerebral extraction rate of oxygen. A third hypothesis is that $CMRO_2$ is so reduced in these patients that moderately reduced CPP and CBF may be enough to maintain adequate oxygen supply to the brain tissue. In these cases, a marginally reduced CPP may be sufficient to maintain a decreased $CMRO_2$. The final possibility which should be considered is that cytochromes could be inhibited in the injured brain. In this situation, a normal $PtiO_2$ could mask tissue hypoxia (histotoxic hypoxia). Distinguishing between the different possibilities in these patients requires further studies in which anaerobic metabolism should be monitored. Using microdialysis to measure the lactate/pyruvate index would be the best method to determine which of the above mentioned hypothesis is the most reasonable. From a clinical point of view, the importance of elucidating this issue is fundamental in order to enable the clinician to rationalize the treatment of some patients with a diffuse brain injury and high ICP. If a marginally low CPP were acceptable in some of these patients, high ICP could be better controlled, as has been suggested by the Lund group [1].

Another finding of our study is that it is not enough to know only the CPP in order to predict episodes of low $PtiO_2$. In our data, $PtiO_2$ measurements below 15 mm Hg were observed in cases with normal or even supranormal CPPs. Our findings are in agreement with those of Härtl *et al.* [6] who suggested that patients with a CPP above 60 mm Hg can have $PtiO_2$ below 15 mm Hg and that an optimum CPP does not exclude an hypoxemic brain. Our data also disprove our second hypothesis that manipulating MABP to increase CPP above supranormal levels would improve oxygen availability to the brain, particularly in the patients with a CPP below 70 mm Hg. In the group with a high CPP, increasing MABP had slight and non-significant effects on $PtiO_2$. A mean increase of 0.16 mm Hg of $PtiO_2$ for each mm Hg of increase in MABP was found in this high CPP group. In the group with low CPP (<70 mm Hg), the mean $PtiO_2$-BP index, although higher (0.29 mm Hg), was not significantly different from the index observed in the low CPP group. If we accept that $PtiO_2$ is the best parameter to evaluate tissue oxygenation, because it offers a direct quantitative assessment of oxygen availability to the cell, our data did not suggest that, in general, increasing CPP above supranormal levels improves the oxygen availability in the macroscopically non-injured brain. This lack of correlation between Δ $PtiO_2$/Δ CPP has also been observed by Bauhuf *et al.* in patients in whom autoregulation was tested by inducing hypotension [2]. Our findings are also close to the observations of Kiening *et al.* who found that a CPP of 60 mm Hg is usually enough to maintain normal oxygenation in the injured brain and that increasing CPP above 60 mm Hg, does not significantly improve the delivery of oxygen to the brain [7]. However, we cannot disregard the fact that the macrocopically injured brain can respond very differently to the manipulation of arterial blood pressure as has been suggested by Stocchetti *et al.* [13].

When manipulating MABP, the increase in oxygen delivery to the brain depends on the autoregulatory status of the cerebrovascular bed. It is well accepted that, within the upper and lower limits of autoregulation, changes in CPP should induce negligible changes in CBF and consequently in brain tissue oxygen delivery. It is therefore essential to know the status of autoregulation in order to determine which of the options for improving oxygen delivery is the best in those patients with a detected or suspected brain hypoxia. In those with impaired or abolished autoregulation, increasing CPP can sometimes significantly increase CBF and therefore $PtiO_2$. However, in these patients the benefits of improving $PtiO_2$ have to be balanced against the risk of overloading microcirculation, a situation that would facilitate brain edema.

The most important limitation of our study, apart from the reduced number of patients included, is that the response to increased MABP was only evaluated in the morphologically "normal" brain tissue (according to CT scan criteria). Because of this, we cannot disregard the fact that the injured brain can respond very differently to manipulation of MABP. Also, we have to take into consideration that, even among the same patients, different regions of the brain may have a distinct metabolic response to reduced CPP. However, we think the findings of this study are valid for patients with a diffuse brain injury. An additional consideration is that we have analyzed only moderately reduced CPPs (always above 48 mm Hg) and for that reason our findings cannot be extrapolated to patients with CPPs below this level. Although it is difficult to draw definitive conclusions from our data, we consider that the acceptable lower limit of autoregulation in the head-injured patient should be redefined. To do this, adequate and reliable monitoring is required. As suggested by Maas *et al.*, monitoring $PtiO_2$ could be a very valuable tool for indicating, in each particular patient, the critical perfusion pressure below which the brain is at risk of ischemia [8].

Acknowledgments

The authors gratefully acknowledge the assistance of Gail Craigie in translating the manuscript. This work was supported by *Grant 98/1385* from the Fondo de Investigación Sanitaria (FIS) and *Grant 1031/97* from the Marato de TV3 to Dr. J. Sahuquillo.

References

1. Asgeirsson B, Grände PO, Nordström CH (1995) The Lund concept of post-traumatic brain oedema therapy. Acta Anaesthesiol Scand 39: 103–106
2. Bauhuf C, Hofmann R, Steinmeier R, Fahlbusch R (1998) Monitoring of cerebral O2 metabolism-comparison of local tissue pO2 and jugular-bulb oxygen saturation (abstract). Acta Neurochir [Suppl] (Wien) 71: 392
3. Bullock R, Chesnut RM, Clifton G, Ghajar J, Marion D, Narayan R, Newell D, Pitts L, Rosner M, Wilberger J (1996) Guidelines for the management of severe head injury. J Neurotrauma 13: 641–734
4. Dings J, Meixensberger J, Roosen K (1997) Brain tissue pO2-monitoring: catheterstability and complications. Neurol Res 19: 241–245
5. Enevoldsen EM, Cold G, Jensen FT, Malmros R (1976) Dynamic changes in regional CBF, intraventricular pressure, CSF pH and lactate levels during the acute phase of head injury. J Neurosurg 44: 191–214
6. Härtl R, Bardt T, Unterberg A, Sarrafzadeh AS, Kiening K, Schneider GH, Lanksch W (1998) PO_2-monitoring in traumatic brain injury: are ICP and CPP indicators of brain tissue hypoxia? (abstract). Acta Neurochir [Suppl] (Wien) 71: 420
7. Kiening KL, Unterberg AW, Bardt TF, Schneider GH, Lanksch WR (1996) Monitoring of cerebral oxygenation in patients with severe head injuries: brain tissue PO2 versus jugular vein oxygen saturation. J Neurosurg 85: 751–757
8. Maas AIR, Fleckenstein W, De Jong DA, Wolf M (1993) Effect of increased ICP and decreased cerebral perfusion pressure on brain tissue and cerebrospinal fluid oxygen tension. In: Avezaat CJJ, Van Eijndhoven JHM, Maas AIR, Tans JTJ (eds) Intracranial pressure VIII. Springer, Berlin Heidelberg New York Tokyo, pp 233–237
9. Rosner MJ, Rosner SD (1994) Cerebral perfusion pressure management of head injury. In: Avezaat CJJ, Van Eijndhoven JHM, Maas AIR, Tans JTJ (eds) Intracranial pressure VIII. Springer, Berlin Heidelberg New York Tokyo, pp 540–543
10. Rosner MJ, Rosner SD (1994) CPP management. I: Results. In: Nagai H, Kamiya K, Ishii S (eds) Intracranial pressure IX. Springer, Berlin Heidelberg New York Tokyo, pp 218–221
11. Sahuquillo J, Poca MA, Ausina A, Baguena M, Gracia RM, Rubio E (1996) Arterio-jugular differences of oxygen ($AVDO_2$) for bedside assessment of CO2-reactivity and autoregulation in the acute phase of severe head injury. Acta Neurochir (Wien) 138: 435–444
12. Schmidt JF, Waldemar G, Vorstrup S, Andersen AR, Gjerris F, Paulson OB (1990) Computerized analysis of cerebral blood flow autoregulation in humans: validation of a method for pharmacologic studies. J Cardiovasc Pharmacol 15: 983–988
13. Stocchetti N, Chieregato A, De Marchi M, Croci M, Benti R, Grimoldi N (1998) High cerebral perfusion pressure improves low values of local brain tissue O2 tension (PtiO2) in focal lesions [In Process Citation]. Acta Neurochir [Suppl] (Wien) 71: 162–165
14. Vespa P, Prins M, Ronne-Engstrom E, Caron M, Shalmon E, Hovda DA, Martin NA, Becker DP (1998) Increase in extracellular glutamate caused by reduced cerebral perfusion pressure and seizures after human traumatic brain injury: a microdialysis study. J Neurosurg 89: 971–982

Correspondence: Dr. Juan Sahuquillo, Osona 6, 2–4, 08023 Barcelona, Spain.

Acta Neurochir (2000) [Suppl] 76: 463–466

Continuous Monitoring of ICP and CPP Following ICH and its Relationship to Clinical, Radiological and Surgical Parameters

H. M. Fernandes[1], **S. Siddique**[1], **K. Banister**[2], **I. Chambers**[2], **T. Wooldridge**[1], **B. Gregson**[1], and **A. D. Mendelow**[1]

[1] Department of Neurosurgery, University of Newcastle upon Tyne, UK
[2] Department of Medical Physics, University of Newcastle upon Tyne, UK

Summary

Sixty-two patients with a spontaneous supratentorial haemorrhage had continuous Intracranial Pressure (ICP) and Cerebral Perfusion Pressure (CPP) monitoring. In addition to the recordings of physiological data their past medical history, presenting neurological state, Computed Tomograph (CT) findings, daily Glasgow Coma Score (GCS) and outcome were noted. The mean age was 57.6 years (sd 13.3). Onset of recording, after ictus was at a mean of 32.6 hours (sd 26.0). Average length of recording was 62.0 hours (sd 39.8). Thirty-one patients had evacuation of haematoma, 6 insertion of External Ventricular Drain (EVD).

Preoperative measures of ICP were significantly related to delayed neurological deterioration, death within three days and Glasgow Outcome Scale (GOS) at neurosurgical discharge. No such relationships existed with preoperative measures of CPP and neither ICP nor CPP was related to outcome at 6 months.

Post-operative measures of both ICP and CPP demonstrated a significant relationship with death within three days of ictus and GOS at neurosurgical discharge. Again no relationship existed with these parameters and outcome at six months.

Surgical evacuation of haematoma acted to significantly reduce ICP and improve CPP. Given that these factors seem to be related to deterioration, death and early outcome, it would seem that surgery could play a role in reducing mortality and improving outcome following Intra cerebral Haemonhage (ICH).

Keywords: Intracerebral haemorrhage; intracranial pressure; cerebral perfusion pressure; surgery; outcome.

Introduction

The deleterious effect of raised Intracranial Pressure (ICP) following Head Injury is well known [1, 2]. The relationship of CPP to outcome after head injury has been extensively studied and several investigators hold the view that CPP is the critical parameter that determines outcome [3, 4]. Little is known about the relationship between outcome and ICP after spontaneous Intracerebral Haemorrhage (ICH) [5, 6, 2, 7] and there have been no previous reports about the relationship between Cerebral Perfusion Pressure (CPP) and outcome with ICH.

Materials and Methods

Patients admitted to Newcastle General Hospital with a spontaneous supratentorial ICH haemorrhage who underwent a period of intracranial pressure monitoring, during their hospital admission, were included in this study. All patients were monitored using the Camino OLM fibreoptic intracranial pressure monitor which was inserted under aseptic conditions in the frontal area ipsilateral to the intracerebral haematoma. A computerised system was used to continuously record ICP at 1-minute intervals. In some cases ($n = 18$), however, the computerised equipment was not available and in these instances the attending nursing staff recorded end hour 'spot' values of ICP.

All patients also had concurrent monitoring of systolic and diastolic blood pressure, and thus the cerebral perfusion pressure (CPP) could be calculated. Many patients had non-invasive cuff recordings of blood pressure at 1 to 4 hourly intervals in which case 'spot' values of CPP could be calculated but for those patients with an arterial line computerised recordings at one minute intervals were taken.

For each patient, in addition to the physiological data, the past medical history including hypertension, presenting neurological state, CT findings, daily GCS and outcome assessments were recorded.

For the purposes of time series analysis the recorded data was 'smoothed' using in house software to produce a rolling average of hourly-recorded data. Each data point generated was an average of data recorded 30 minutes before and 30 minutes after. Patients included in the study fell into 4 groups: (i) those patients with pre and post-operative recordings, (ii) those who did not have an operation, (iii) those patients who had post-operative recordings only and a small group of 3 patients that had only (iv) pre-operative data. Operation included craniotomy for evacuation of haematoma and/or insertion of external ventricular drain. Non-parametric statistical methods were used for data analysis.

Results

In total 62 patients, following a spontaneous supratentorial intracerebral haemorrhage underwent a pe-

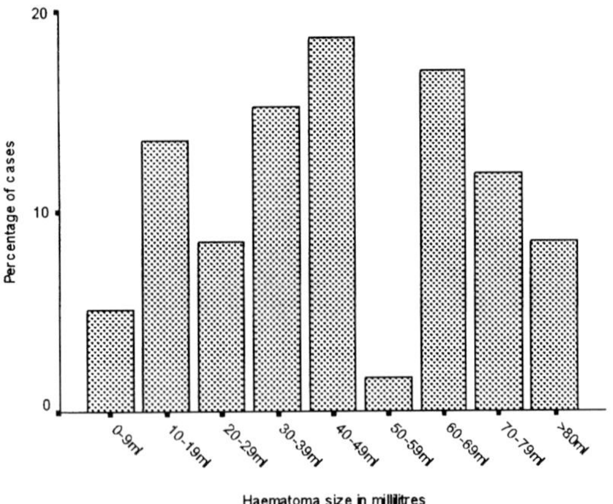

Fig. 1. Bar chart to show haematoma volume

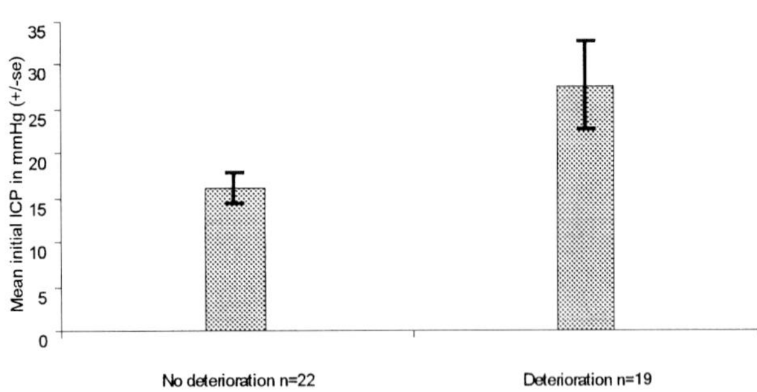

Fig. 2. Mean initial preoperative ICP for patients that did and did not deteriorate p = 0.017

riod of intracranial pressure monitoring. The mean age for the group was 57.6 (sd 13.3).

Onset of recording varied between 4 and 107 hours post ictus with a mean of 32.6 hours (sd 26.0). Actual hours of recording ranged from 1 to 191, with a mean of 62.0 (sd 39.8). Thirty-six of the monitored patients went on to have an operation (58.1%). Thirty-one had craniotomy and evacuation of haematoma and six insertion of external ventricular drain (EVD). One patient had both procedures.

At presentation just over a quarter of patients (25.8%) were Glasgow Coma Score (GCS) 15, 8% GCS 13, 33.9% GCS 11 and 14.5% GCS 9. Almost a fifth (17.8%) were in coma. Nearly half of the ICH were located in the basal ganglia (47.7%, 28 cases) with a further 8 (13.7%) described as frontal, 17 (27.4%) tempero-parietal and 6 (10.3%) occipital. For those haematomas located in the basal ganglia most were putaminal in location (32.2%).

The size in millilitres for each haematoma was recorded in 10 ml bands and is shown in Fig. 1. Intraventricular haemorrhage (IVH) was recorded as being present in 34 (56.7%) of the cases but only 13 cases (21.7%) were noted to have enlarged ventricles. Midline shift was present in 45 cases (75%).

Analysis of ICP and CPP Data

For the purposes of statistical analysis of the data patients were grouped together on the basis of whether or not they underwent surgery and the timing of physiological monitoring in respect to this. Group A contains data from the pre-operative period in 41 patients; Group B contains data from the postoperative period in 33 patients; Group C are those patients who had recordings made both pre and postoperatively (12 in number). All patients in this group had surgical evacuation of haematoma by craniotomy.

Group A: Pre-Operative

Delayed Neurological Deterioration. A delayed neurological deterioration (DND) (fall in best daily GCS of 2 points or single point in motor score) was recorded in 19 patients (46.3%). This occurred at a mean of 2.73 days (sd 2.9) post ictus. Of the physiological variables initial ICP, maximum ICP and mean ICP were significantly related to DND ($p = 0.017$, 0.001 and 0.004 respectively). Essentially the higher the ICP (initial, maximum and mean) the more likely the patient was to experience a DND (Fig. 2). No relationship was found between deterioration and CPP.

Death Within Three Days. Three patients in this preoperative group died within three days of ictus (7.3%). Death within this time period was significantly associated with maximum ICP ($p = 0.002$) (Fig. 3) and mean ICP ($p = 0.008$). No relationship was found with any of the CPP variables.

Outcome on Neurosurgical Discharge. Outcome (GOS) was recorded at the point of discharge from Neurosurgery. Patients stayed an average of 11.7 days (sd 8.6) and for 7 (17.1%) patients discharge took the form of death. Maximum ICP was the only variable that showed a relationship with outcome at this point ($p = 0.004$) (Fig. 4). No relationship however with any recorded variable (ICP, CPP) was seen with outcome (GOS) at 6 months

Group B: Post-Operative

Death Within Three Days. Four patients within this post-operative group died within three days of ictus

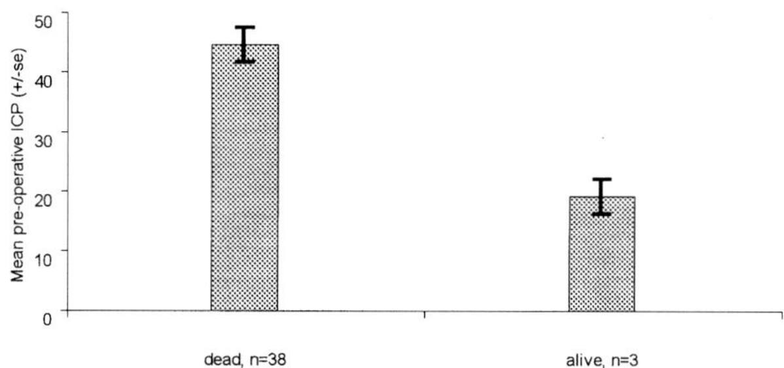

Fig. 3. Maximum preoperative ICP for those patients that died within three days of ictus and those that did not p = 0.002

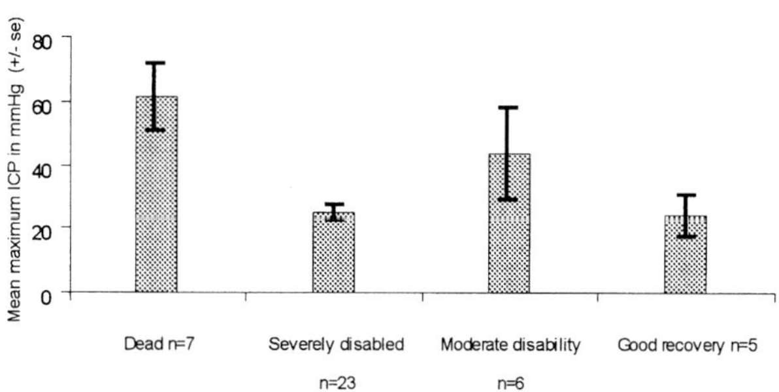

Fig. 4. Graph to show mean maximum pre-operative ICP for patients according to their GOS at Neurosurgical Discharge, p = 0.004

(12.1%). Death within this time period was significantly associated with initial ICP (p = 0.001) and mean ICP (p = 0.018). Post-operative CPP variables, unlike those pre-operatively, were associated with death. Mean CPP (p = 0.009) and minimum CPP (p = 0.009) both showed a significant relationship. Both initial post-operative ICP and CPP further showed no significant relationship (not surprisingly) to any variables recorded from the presenting CT scan.

Outcome on Neurosurgical Discharge. Mean CPP (p = 0.035) (Fig. 5) and minimum CPP (p = 0.047) were the only variables that showed a significant association with outcome (GOS) at discharge from Neurosurgery. For this group discharge took the form of death in 11 (33.3%) patients. No relationship was seen for any of the parameters measured and outcome at six months.

Group C: Comparison of pre and post-Operative

Values recorded in the pre and post-operative period were compared to assess the effect of surgery. Initial ICP was significantly reduced (p = 0.002) and initial CPP was increased (p = 0.033). Mean ICP was also significantly reduced post-operatively (p = 0.016).

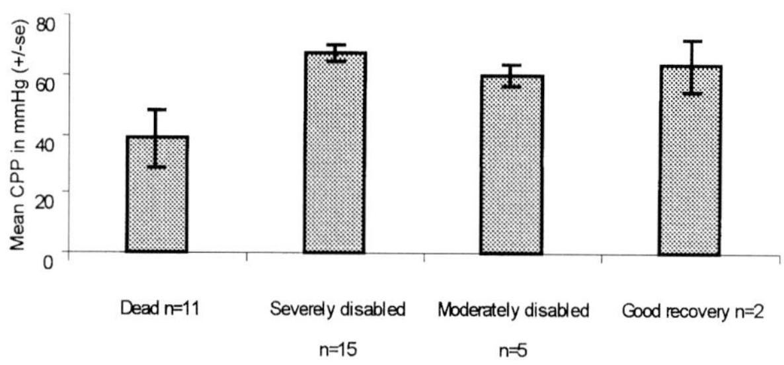

Fig. 5. Graph to show mean post-operative CPP for patients according to their GOS at Neurosurgical Discharge, p = 0.035

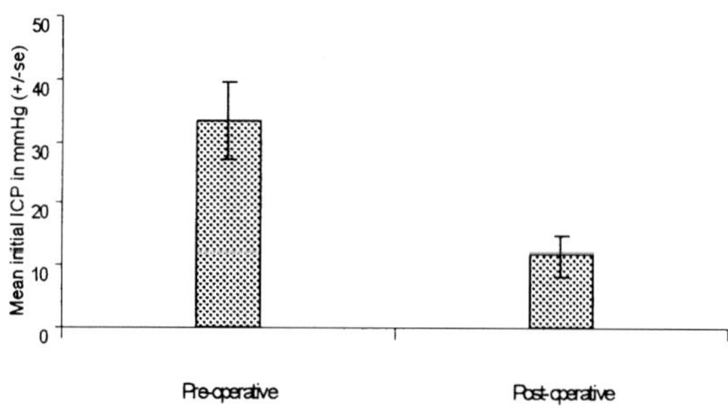

Fig. 6. Bar chart to show initial ICP before and after surgery p = 0.002

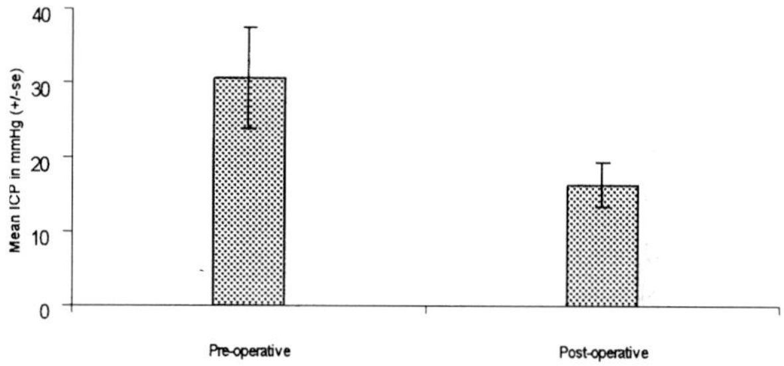

Fig. 7. Bar chart to show mean ICP before and after surgery p = 0.016

Surgical evacuation of haematoma did not however significantly alter the maximum ICP and minimum CPP (p = 0.530, p = 0.638 respectively). Neither was the mean CPP for each period affected (p = 0.136) (Figs. 6 to 8).

Discussion

Pre-operative measures of ICP demonstrate a number of significant relationships with DND, death within three days of ictus and outcome as measured on the GOS at neurosurgical discharge. Pre-operative CPP was not related to these endpoints. By contrast, during

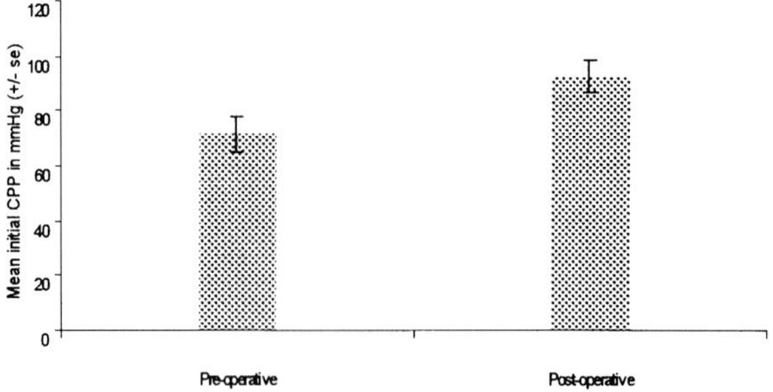

Fig. 8. Bar chart to show mean CPP before and after surgery $p = 0.033$

the post-operative period, CPP demonstrated significant relationships with death within three days and outcome at neurosurgical discharge. No relationship was seen between any of the parameters measured and outcome at 6 months. Surgical evacuation of haematoma resulted in significant improvement in both ICP and CPP. Given these factors are significantly related to DND, early death and outcome, it would seem that surgery could have a beneficial effect on both mortality and morbidity after spontaneous ICH. Also these data suggest that the effect of surgery may be greater on mortality than disability. Previous studies on the effect of surgery have failed to resolve the question of whether or not surgery improves outcome [8]. The ongoing Surgical Trial in Intracerebral Haemorrhage (STICH) should resolve this issue.

Acknowledgments

This work has been made possible with grants from the Stroke Association, the Northern Brainwave Appeal, the Royal College of Surgeons of England and the UK Medical Research Council.

References

1. Miller J, Becker DP, Ward JD, Sullivan HG, Adams WE, Rosner MJ (1977) Significance of intracranial hypertension in severe head injury. J Neurosurgery 47: 503–516
2. Janny P, Papo I, Chazal J, Colnet G, Barretto LC (1982) Intracranial hypertension and prognosis of spontaneous intracerebral haematomas. A correlative study of 60 patients. Acta Neurochir (Wien) 61 (1–3): 181–186
3. Rosner M, S Daughton (1990) Cerebral perfusion pressure. J Trauma 30: 933–941
4. Robertson CS *et al* (1998) Prevention of secondary ischaemic insults after severe head injury. J Neurosurg
5. Duff TA, Ayeni S, Levin AB, Javid M (1981) Nonsurgical management of spontaneous intracerebral haemorrhage. Neurosurgery 9: 387–393
6. Ropper AH, RB King (1984) Intracranial pressure monitoring in comatose patients with cerebral haemorrhage. Arch Neurol 41: 725–728
7. Papo I, Janny P, Caruselli G, Coluet G, Luongo A (1979) Intracranial pressure time course in primary intracerebral haemorrhage. Neurosurgery 4: 504–511
8. Hankey GJ, Hon C (1997) Surgery for primary intracerebral hemorrhage. Stroke 28: 2126–2132

Correspondence: Dr. H. M. Fernandes, Clinical Trials Office, Ward 31 North Wing, Newcastle General Hospital, Westgate Road, Newcastle-upon-Tyne, NE4 6BE, UK.

Acta Neurochir (2000) [Suppl] 76: 467–470

Neuromuscular Blocking Agents in Neurointensive Care

N. Juul[1,2], **G. F. Morris**[1], **S. B. Marshall**[1], and **L. F. Marshall**[1]

[1] Division of Neurosurgery, University of California San Diego, San Diego, USA
[2] Department of Anaesthesia, Aarhus University Hospital, Aarhus, Denmark

Summary

Introduction. Intensive care treatment of patients with severe head injury is aimed at preventing secondary injury. One of the cornerstones in this treatment is sedation and ventilation. Use of Neuromuscular Blocking Agents (NBA) has gained widespread use as part of the protocol for maintaining normal intracranial pressure values, without class 1 evidence for the efficacy of the treatment.

Methods. We examined data of the use of NBA as infusion during ventilator treatment, and IntraCranial Pressure (ICP) measurements in the database from the international multicenter randomized double blind trial of the NMDA receptor antagonist Selfotel. No specific mode of sedation was recommended in the study protocol.

Results. Of the 427 patients enrolled in the study 326 had a full data set, 138 received NBA during their stay in the ICU. There were no statistical difference in demographic data between the two groups. During their stay in the ICU, patients who received NBA had a median of 13.5 hours with a recorded ICP above 20 mm Hg, patients who did not receive NBA had a median of 6.5 hours with ICP above 20 mm Hg ($p < 0.05$).

Conclusion. Our data challenges the concept of using NBA as part of a routine sedation strategy in treatment of patients with severe head injury.

Keywords: Head injury; neuromuscular blocking agents; intensive care unit; intracranial pressure control.

Introduction

Intensive care treatment of patients with severe head injury is aimed on preventing secondary injury. The main goal is to control Intracranial Pressure (ICP), delivery of oxygen and energy to the brain and to ensure adequate perfusion of the brain. Use of Neuromuscular Blocking Agents (NBA) to facilitate artificial ventilation of patients in neurointensive care units (ICU) is controversial, and little is known of the true prevalence of its use. Two editorials in 1995 advocate opposing opinions; one said: NBA is used rarely in the ICU [9], the other that NBA's are used frequently [3]. Concern about long term use of NBA in the ICU setting has been brought forward in the last years with an increasing number of publications on prolonged motor weakness after the use of NBA [5]. Furthermore Hsiang *et al.*, analysing data from the Traumatic Coma Databank, showed that the use of NBA was corelated with increased incidence of pneumonia and longer stay in the ICU [2].

Neuromuscular Blocking Agents has over the years been recommended in the treatment of patients with intracranial hypertension and the use is included in many treatment protocols [1, 6, 7], despite the fact that there is no class 1 evidence, proving these drugs' abilities to lower raised ICP in the intensive care setting.

The present analysis of data from a multicenter trial of patients with severe head injury, examines the relationship of recordings of raised ICP with the use of Neuromuscular Blocking Agents given as infusion during ventilator treatment in the ICU.

Materials and Methods

Selfotel Database

Data was prospectively collected in a double-blind randomized trial of the novel pharmacological agent Selfotel. This drug is an antagonist to the excitatory amino acid glutamate N-methyl-D-aspartate receptor. The multicenter international trial was carried out in 52 centres worldwide, which were selected based on their dedication to the treatment of patients with traumatic brain injuries. Patients with a post-resuscitation GCS of 4–8 (inclusively), one reactive pupil, and abnormal initial CT-scan were included. Victims of gunshot wounds and children were excluded. Therapy included emphasis on the prevention of secondary injury, reduction of ICP and maintenance of a cerebral perfusion pressure > 60 mm Hg. All the patients were initially sedated and mechanically ventilated, use of Neuromuscular Blocking Agents was left to the discretion of the treating physician. Clinical data were collected prospectively hourly during the first five days of hospital stay, or to the time of discharge from the ICU. Data collected included ICP, arterial pressure and computed cerebral perfusion pressure.

Statistical Analysis

Data management was performed at the trial coordinating centre at the University of California San Diego, in collaboration with Ciba-Geigy Pharmaceuticals. The commercial computer program SPSS version 7.0 (Statistical Package for Social Sciences, Chicago, IL), was used for data processing and analysis. Outcome analysis was performed using the Glasgow Outcome Scale (GOS) score modified with special reference to favourable outcome (good or moderate on the GOS scale) and death. Dependent on data characteristics Mann-Whitney rank test, Chi-square or Fishers exate test was used for statistical analysis. The 5% level was used for statistical significance.

Results

Of the 427 patients included in the original study 101 were excluded in the present analysis for the following reasons; no 6 month follow-up 18, insufficient ICP/ICU data 50, and start of muscle relaxant treatment >24 hours after injury 33. Thus 326 patients were analysed. The excluded patients did not differ in demographic data from the analysed group. Evaluation of Selfotel has been reported elsewhere [10], because no significant differences between the vehicle and treatment groups were detected in the trial, the groups were combined for the present analysis. Treatment with NBA in addition to sedation was started during the first 24 hours after admission to hospital on 138 patients (42%). Pancuronium was used in the treatment of 42% of the 138 patients receiving NBA, 34% received Vecuronium and 24% Atracurium.

Demographic analysis revealed no significant differences between the two groups (Table 1). Median duration of stay in the ICU was 13 days and the patients were mechanically ventilated for 8.6 days (Table 2).

Table 1. *Demographic Data*

	All	Relax	No relax	p
N	326	138	188	
Median age (years)	28	29	27	NS
Male	77%	78%	77%	NS
Hypoxia	6%	9%	4%	NS
Shock	14%	10%	16%	NS
Median GCS on arrival*	6	6	6	NS
Pupil blown	23%	22%	24%	NS
CT class 1-4 #	68%	65%	70%	NS
CT class 5-6 #	32%	35%	30%	NS

*GCS, Glasgow Coma Scale. # CT Computed tomographic classification after traumatic Coma Data Bank data. *NS* Not significant.

ICP was recorded hourly for 5 days or to time of discharge from the ICU. Increased ICP (ICP $\geq$ 20 mm Hg) was recorded for a median of 14 hours in the group of patients treated with NBA, patients who did not receive NBA had 7 hours with increased ICP ($p < 0.05$) (Table 2). The difference was even more pronounced looking at patients with more severe injuries, categories 3 and 4 in the classification based on data from the national Traumatic Coma data Bank (4). Patients who were treated with NBA had a median of 24 hours with increased ICP, patients who did not get NBA had 8 hours with increased ICP ($p < 0.05$). No significant differences were found in the use of either barbiturates, inotropes or mannitol (Table 2).

Discussion

Until the pathophysiological mechanisms that occur at the time of and following head injury are better elu-

Table 2. *Data Collected in the Intensive Care Unit*

	All	Relax	No relax	p
N	326	138	188	
Median ICU days	13	13	12	NS
Median ventilator days	8.6	8.9	8.4	NS
Favourable outcome	58%	56%	60%	NS
Mortality	25%	28%	23%	NS
Intracerebral surgery	29%	35%	26%	NS
Inotropes*	53%	54%	51%	NS
Pentobarbital	29%	33%	27%	NS
Mannitol	68%	73%	54%	NS
Hours with ICP $\geq$ 20 #	8 (0–112)	14 (0–108)	7 (0–112)	$p < 0.05$

*Dopamine, Dobutamine, Epinephrine and Norepinephrine. #Hourly recordings with IntraCranial Pressure $\geq$20 mm Hg. *NS* Not significant.

cidated, and more specific medical treatment that enables us to shorten the length of stay in the ICU has been developed, we must protect the patient from secondary injury during this extended stay.

The present analysis indicates that neither survival nor ICP control is enhanced with use of NBA in neurointensive care (Table 2). Surprisingly the present analysis showed that patients who received NBA had a higher number of recordings with ICP > 20 mm hg (Table 2). We do not have data about the indication for use of NBA on every patient so it is impossible for us to know if the patients treated with NBA got the medication because they had intracranial hypertension or if it was part of a routine for the treating physician.

Little is known of the true prevalence of use of NBA in intensive care. In Scandinavia, where most ICUs are run by anaesthesiologists, NBA's are seldom used to facilitate mechanical ventilation [11]. In other parts of the world the prevalence of use is presumably higher, but opinions differ [3, 9].

Current treatment protocols recommend that patients with an initial GCS < 9 are being sedated and ventilated. In most protocols use of NBA is included as part of the routine sedation strategy [1, 6, 7], regardless of the fact that no class 1 evidence exists proving that use of NBA in addition to sedation reduces ICP to a level that leads to increased survival.

All the registered neuromuscular blocking agents with intermediate or long lasting effect have been tested for the ability to raise ICP, and all have been found to have no influence on ICP when given as bolus doses. In a study by Werba *et al.* [12] it was shown that vecuronium and atracurium given prior to tracheobronchial suction kept ICP unchanged, but the observation time was short, the drugs were given as bolus doses and there is no information on the degree of sedation. There are several serious concerns about using NBA in neurointensive care.

When patients are paralysed, it is impossible to perform repeated neurological examinations. Symptomes of progressive enlargement of intracranial mass lesions or areas of swelling will be manifested only as ICP elevations or pupillary changes. Furthermore Hsiang *et al.* concluded that early, routine, long-term use of NBA in the treatment of patients with severe head injury leads to prolongation of their ICU stay and to increased extracranial complications (2). In the recent years increasing numbers of publications on prolonged motor weakness after use of NBA have been published [5]. It has been estimated that each patient with prolonged muscle weakness was associated with an increase in ICU and hospital stay, continued mechanical ventilation, and disproportionate healthcare expenditures in excess of US$66,000 [8].

The use of additional drugs known for their ability to reduce ICP, pentobarbital and mannitol, was not lower in the group of patients who received NBA. We did not have data describing the type or amount of sedatives used, neither on the degree of sedation. If the patients who did not receive NBA were sedated deeper, one could expect a greater use of dopamine and other inotrophic drugs. In our data there was no significant difference on the use of inotrophic agents. There may be an advantage in using NBA in a subpopulation of head injured patients who needs either much sedation to accept the situation or high concentrations of inotrophic agents to keep an adequate perfusion pressure. Further controlled trials must elucidate this.

Conclusion

Our data challenges the concept of using NBA as part of a routine sedation strategy in treatment of patients with severe head injury. There might be a beneficial effect of the drugs used on a subpopulation of patients with very severe head injury, but further controlled blinded trials must show if neuromuscular blocking agents have a place in modern treatment of traumatic brain injury.

References

1. Cooper PR (1993) Head injury, 3rd edn. Williams & Wilkins, Baltimore, pp 234–235
2. Hsiang JK, Chesnut RM, Crisp CB, Klauber MR, Beunt BA, Marshall LF (1994) Early, routine paralysis for intracranial pressure control in severe head injury: is it necessary? Crit Care Med 22: 1471–1476
3. Lee C (1995) intensive care unit syndrome? Anesthesiology 83: 237–240
4. Marshall LF, Marshall SB, Klauber MR *et al* (1991) A new classification of head injury based on computerized tomography. J Neurosurg 75: S14–S20
5. Prielipp RC, Coursin DB (1995) Sedative and neuromuscular blocking drug use in critically Ill patients with head injuries. New Horizons 3(3): 456–468
6. Robertson CS, Contant CF, Gokaslan ZL *et al* (1992) Cerebral blood flow, arteriovenous oxygen difference and outcome in head injured patients. J Neurol Neurosurg Psychiatry 55: 594–603
7. Rosner MJ, Rosner SD, Johnson AH (1995) Cerebral perfusion pressure: management and clinical results. J Neurosurg 83: 949–962
8. Rudis MI, Guslits BJ, Peterson EL, Hathaway SJ, Angus E, Beis S, Zarowitz BJ (1996) Economic impact of prolonged motor

weakness complicating neuromuscular blockade in the intensive care unit. Crit Care Med 24: 1749–1755
9. Sladen RN (1995) Neuromuscular blocking agents in the intensive care unit: a two-edged sword. Crit Care Med 23: 423–428
10. Trembly B (1995) Neuroprotective agents: clinical and experimental aspects. New York Academy of Sciences, New York, pp 262–271
11. Viby-Mogensen J (1993) Monitoring neuromuscular function in the Intensive Care Unit. Intensive Care Med 19: S74–S79
12. Werba A, Klezl M, Schramm W, Langenecker S, Muller C, Gosch M, Spiss CK (1993) The level of neuromuscular block needed to supress diaphragmatic movement during tracheal suction in patients with raised intracranial pressure: a study with vecuronium and atracurium. Anaesthesia 48: 301–303

Correspondence: Niels Juul, Department of Anaesthesia, Aarhus University Hospital, Aarhus kommunehospital, 8000 Aarhus C, Denmark.

Acta Neurochir (2000) [Suppl] 76: 471–473

The Role of Nitric Oxide in Reoxygenation Injury of Brain Microvascular Endothelial Cells

T. Nagashima, S. Wu, K. Ikeda, and **N. Tamaki**

Department of Neurosurgery, Kobe University School of Medicine, Japan

Summary

Object. The role of nitric oxide (NO) in reperfusion injury of the brain is still controversial. The authors demonstrate that NO injures the brain capillary endothelial cells in a reoxygenation state by the formation of peroxynitrite.

Materials and Methods. 1) Rat brain capillary endothelial cells (BCECs) were isolated by a two-step enzymatic purification method. The BCECs were identified by the presence of factor VIII. 2) Anaerobic cell preparations were achieved by purging under nitrogen gas with 0.5% CO2 at 37 °C for 20 minutes and then reoxygenating in an incubator. To ascertain the degree of BCEC injury after anoxia and reoxygenation, lactate dehydrogenase (LDH) release was measured. The production of NO was measured by the Griess method. 3) The cell-protective effects of superoxide dismutase (SOD), NG-nitro-L-arginine (L-NAME), and S-Methyl-ITU (i-NOS blocker) were studied.

Results. 1) Both L-NAME and SOD protected the cells from reoxygenation injury. The protective effect of L-NAME was dose-dependent. S-Methyl-ITU did not protect the cells. 2) The NO production after anoxia/reoxygenation was blocked by L-NAME.

Conclusion. NO from the BCEC can injure the cells themselves through the formation of peroxynitrite under anoxia/reoxygenation conditions. Increased NO production after anoxia can be attributed to the induction of e-NOS.

Keywords: Nitric oxide; endothelial cells; reoxygenation injury; brain ischemia.

Introduction

The role of nitric oxide (NO) in reperfusion injury of the brain is still controversial. Previous in vitro and in vivo studies of the effects of nitric oxide synthase inhibition in the brain have yielded conflicting results. The effect of the inhibition of NO synthase on cerebral ischemic damage may vary depending on the timing of the inhibition relative to the induction of ischemia. The administration of L-NAME 3 h after the induction of ischemia has been shown to reduce the neocortical infarct size [9]. In contrast, NO production by cerebral vascular endothelial cells may be neuroprotective in the area of focal ischemia by increasing blood flow to ischemic penumbra [5].

In the present study, the authors demonstrated that NO produced by brain capillary endothelial cells (BCECs) injures the cells themselves during anoxia/reoxygenation.

Materials and Methods

Isolation and Culture of Brain Microvascular Endothelial Cells

Rat brain capillary endothelial cells were isolated by a two-step enzymatic purification method from ten male Sprague-Dawley rats as reported elsewhere [7]. Briefly, 10 rats brain cortices were cleared of meninges and overlying vessels. The tissues were incubated at 37 °C in 20 ml of Dulbecco-medium (D-MEM) (Nissui, Tokyo, Japan) with 0.5% dispase (Boehringer Mannheim, Indianapolis, Indiana) for 3 hours, then suspended in 80 ml of D-MEM containing 13% dextran (M.W. 70,000. Sigma Chemical, St. Louis, Mo). The microvessels were separated from the brain tissue by centrifugation at 5,800 g for 10 minutes. The tissues were then passed through a 300 mm nylon mesh, and treated with 1 mg/ml collagenase/dispase in 5 ml of medium for 6 hours. The pellets of cells were layered over 7-ml Percoll gradients containing 50% Percoll in MEM. The band containing mainly endothelial cells was removed and seeded onto a collagen-coated dish (diameter of 60 mm, Falcon, Lincoln Park, New Jersey).

Serial passage was accomplished at a subculture ratio of 1:2. The culture medium, which consisted of MEM with 20% fetal bovine serum, 2 mM glutamine, 100 U/ml penicillin G, 100 mg/ml streptomycin sulfate, and 0.08% heparin was changed, and bovine pituitary fibroblast growth factor (1 mg/ml) (Takarashuzo, Tokyo, Japan) was added every other day. Capillary endothelial cell was identified based on the presence of Factor VIII-related antigen.

Experimental Protocol

The BCECs were seeded into a 24 well plate for the experiment. After the confluent conditions were obtained, we added the NO synthase inhibitor NG-nitro-L-arginine methyl ester (L-NAME) (20, 50, 100 mM), specific i-NOS inhibitor S-Methyl-ITU (20, 50,

100 mM) into the medium to evaluate the cytoprotective effect. To assess the relative effects of superoxide on A/R injury, we applied the specific scavenger SOD (2000 U/ml) to the medium. All reagents were applied to Ca^{2+}-free, glucose-free PBS without growth factors or serum 2 hours before the study. The control group was anoxia/reoxygenated BCECs without any protective reagents.

The anaerobic cellular preparations were placed in an air-tight chamber under a continuous flow of nitrogen gas with 5% CO_2 and were maintained at 37 °C for 20 minutes, followed by reoxygenation achieved by incubation in 5% CO_2-95% air at 37 °C with 90% relative humidity for 3 hours. The normoxia preparation was incubated in an atmosphere consisting of 95% air and 5% CO_2 with D-PBS.

The A/R injury of the BCECs was assessed by measurement of the release of intracellular LDH. After A/R injury, the LDH concentration in the medium was measured with a spectrophotometer. The LDH release is expressed as a percentage of the total intracellular LDH, which was calculated by the following equation: (LDH in medium/(LDH in medium + LDH in cells)) × 100%. The production of NO was measured by the Griess method.

Results

1) The BCECs produced a significantly larger amount of NO after anoxic stress than under the normoxic conditions. This increase was blocked by L-NAME (100 mM). The L-NAME treatments both before and after the anoxia decreased NO production (Fig. 1), indicating that NO production continues during anoxia/reoxygenation.

2) Both L-NAME and SOD protected the brain microvascular endothelial cells from reoxygenation injury. SOD protected the cells more significantly than L-NAME (paired t test, $p < 0.01$). The protective effect of L-NAME occurred in a dose-dependent manner (Fig. 2).

3) S-Methyl-ITU did not protect the cells as compared to the control (paired t test, $p < 0.01$).

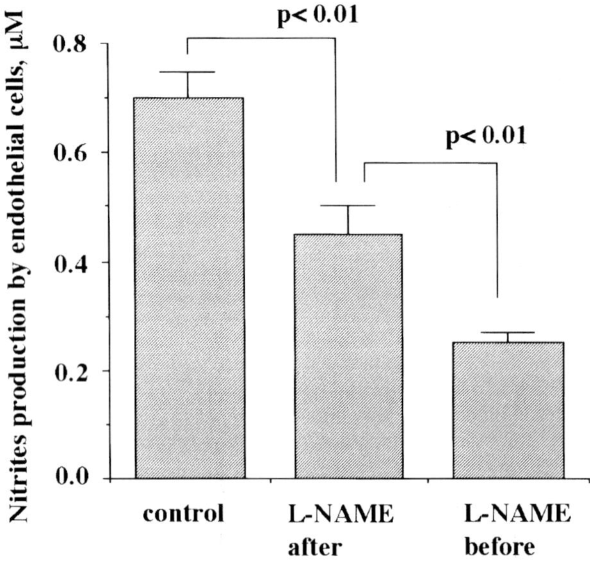

Fig. 1. Nitric oxide production by endothelial cells. The control conditions include 20 minutes anoxia and 3 hours reoxygenation. L-NAME (100 mM) added before and after anoxia significantly suppressed nitric oxide production ($p < 0.01$)

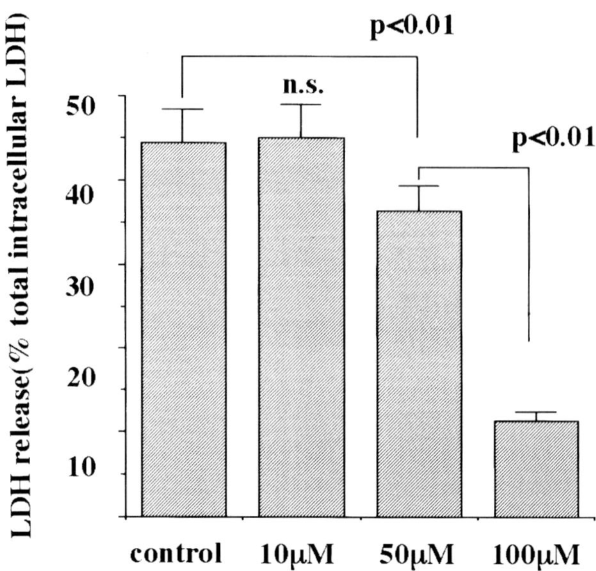

Fig. 2. L-NAME suppressed LDH release from the brain microvascular endothelial cells dose dependently. LDH was measured after 20 minutes anoxia followed by 3 hours reoxygenation

Discussion

Nitric Oxide Production During Anoxia/Reoxygenation

The production of NO in the ischemic brain is a dynamic, time-dependent and spatially heterogeneous process. The NO signal of EPR spectra increases rapidly after the onset of focal ischemia and continued over 60 minutes in an MCA occlusion model [6]. The administration of L-NAME significantly decreases plasma nitrate/nitrite as well as nitrite level at 30 min of reperfusion after 2 h of MCA occlusion [3]. The endothelial NOS in the cerebral vessels is upregulated at 1 hour after the induction of ischemia throughout the ischemic region [8]. This induction of endothelial NOS progressively increases for up to 24 hours of ischemia. The rapid and intense expression of endothelial NOS in the ischemic lesion indicates a role for endothelial NOS in ischemic cell damage. The present study showed increased NO production in the brain microvascular endothelial cells in response to 20 minutes anoxia followed by 3 hours reoxygenation as well as decreased NO production in response to administration of L-NAME.

Toxicity of NO in Anoxia/Reoxygenation

The direct toxicity of NO is modest but is greatly enhanced by reacting with superoxide to form peroxynitrite. Peroxynitrite reacts relatively slowly with most biological molecules and modifies tyrosine in proteins to create nitrotyrosines. The nitration of structural proteins, including actin, can disrupt filament assembly [2]. Kumura *et al.* have shown that the L-arginine-NO synthase pathway is activated during reperfusion after focal cerebral ischemia, indicating the involvement of a reaction between NO and superoxide during early reperfusion [4]. Azuma has reported that agonist-stimulated NO production but not basal production in endothelial cells can be cytotoxic [1]. The present results indicate that NO from brain microvascular endothelial cells can injure the cells themselves through the formation of peroxynitrite under anoxia/reoxygenation conditions by reacting with superoxide.

In contrast, L-Arginine treatment decreases the infarct size in rats subjected to distal middle cerebral arterial occlusion in spontaneously hypertensive rats [5]. Therefore, NO production by cerebral vascular endothelial cells may be neuroprotective in the area of focal cerebral ischemia by increasing blood flow to marginally ischemic tissue [5]. However, the effects of the inhibition of NO synthesis on focal cerebral ischemic damage are time-dependent [9]. We should be careful in our interpretation of the experimental results because the ischemic phenomenon depends on the time course, the spatial arrangement of individual cell types, the local blood flow, and the removal of metabolites. The present results indicate the toxic effect of NO in the acute phase of anoxia/reoxygenation in a simple experimental model with a single cell type. The clinical implications of these results are that the use of an NO donor in the treatment of focal cerebral ischemia may exacerbate endothelial cell damage in the acute reperfusion phase. The role of NO in the whole process of cerebral ischemia should be considered as a summation of reactions of different cell types.

iNOS activity is significantly induced in the infarct lesion more than 24 hours after MCA occlusion and peaks at day 2 [4]. The protective effect of aminoguanidine (iNOS inhibitor) is time-dependent and occurs only when the drug is administered for longer than 2 days after the induction of ischemia [10]. NO formation in neurons is triggered by the activation of the NMDA receptor and is involved in the process leading to glutamate neurotoxicity [4]. The present study shows that S-Met-ITU (iNOS blocker) does not ameliorate endothelial cell damage during the acute phase of anoxia/reoxygenation. The results indicate that the increased production of NO from endothelial cells during the acute phase of anoxia/reoxygenation is not caused by iNOS.

References

1. Azuma T, Fujii K, Yuge O (1996) Self-limiting enhancement of nitric oxide of oxygen free radical-induced endothelial cell injury: evidence against the dural action of NO as hydroxyl radical donor/scavenger. Br J Pharmacol 119: 455–462
2. Beckman JS, Koppenol WH (1996) Nitric oxide, superoxide and peroxynitrite: the good, the bad, and the ugly. Am J Physiol 271: C1424–1437
3. Kumura E, Kosaka H, Shiga T, Yoshimine T, Hayakawa T (1994) Elevation of plasma nitric oxide end products during focal cerebral ischemia and reperfusion in the rat. J Cereb Blood Flow Metab 14: 487–491
4. Kumura E, Yoshimine T, Iwatsuki KI, Yamanaka K, Tanaka S, Hayakawa T, Shiga T, Kosaka H (1996) Generation of nitric oxide and superoxide during reperfusion after focal cerebral ischemia in rats. Am J Physiol 270: C748–752
5. Morikawa E, Huang Z, Moskowitz MA (1992) L-arginine decreases infarct size caused by middle cerebral arterial occlusion in SHR. Am J Physiol 263: H1632–1635
6. Sato S, Tominaga T, Ohnishi T, Ohnishi T (1994) Role of nitric oxide in brain ischemia. Ann NY Acad Sci 17, 738: 369–373
7. Wu S, Tamaki N, Nagashima T, Yamaguchi M (1998) Reactive oxygen species in reoxygenation injury of rat brain capillary endothelial cells. Neurosurgery 43(3): 577–583
8. Zhang ZG, Chopp M, Zaloga C, Pollock JS, Forstermann U (1993) Cerebral endothelial nitric oxide synthase expression after focal cerebral ischemia in rats. Stroke 24: 2016–2021
9. Zhang F, Xu S, Iadecola C (1995) Time dependence of effect of nitric oxide synthase inhibition on cerebral ischemic damage. J Cereb Blood Flow Metab 15(4): 595–601
10. Zhang F, Iadecola C (1998) Temporal characteristics of the protective effect of aminoguanidine on cerebral ischemic damage. Brain Res 17, 802(1–2): 104–110

Correspondence: Dr. T. Nagashima, 7-5-1, Kusunokicho, Chuo-ku, Kobe, Japan 650-0012.

Acta Neurochir (2000) [Suppl] 76: 475–478

The Use of Decompressive Craniectomy for the Management of Severe Head Injuries

U. Meier, F. S. Zeilinger, and **O. Henzka**

Department of Neurosurgery, Unfallkrankenhaus Berlin, Germany

Summary

The aim of Neurosurgical care is to minimise the secondary brain damage that occurs after a severe head injury. This includes the evacuation of an intracranial space occupying haematoma, the reduction of intracranial volume, external ventricular drainage with hydrocephalus, and conservative therapy to reduce intracranial pressure (ICP) and to maintain tissue oxygen $p(ti)O_2$. When conservative treatment fails, a decompressive craniectomy might be successful in lowering ICP. From September 1997 until April 1999 we operated on 128 patients with severe head injuries. 19 patients (15%) were treated by means of a decompressive craniectomy.

The prognosis after decompression depends on clinical signs and symptoms on admission, patients' age and the existence of major extracranial injuries. Our guidelines for decompressive craniectomy after failure of conservative intervention and evacuation of space occupying hematomas included: a patient's age below 50 years without multiple trauma or a patient's age below 30 years in the presence of major extracranial injuries; severe brain swelling on CT scan (primary brainstem injuries were excluded). In 8 patients conservative ITU treatment had failed.

Keywords: Severe head injury; brain oedema; decompressive craniectomy; intracranial pressure.

Introduction

Bergmann described in 1880 a decompressive craniectomy and Cushing published in 1908 a case report about a subtemporal decompressive craniectomy for relief of intracranial pressure. There is still a controversy about the value of operative decompression after severe head injuries with traumatic brain oedema [1, 2, 5, 6].

The aim of neurosurgical care after severe head injuries is the minimisation of the secondary brain damage. General principles of neurosurgical therapy are the evacuation of space occupying hematomas, the reduction of intracranial volume, respectively the drainage of hydrocephalus, and conservative therapy focused on intracranial pressure (ICP), cerebral perfusion pressure (CPP) and brain tissue pO_2. In intractable intracranial hypertension which is refractory to conservative interventions, a decompressive craniectomy is indicated in a few patients. Indications for decompressive craniectomy, course of disease, and prognostic criteria are analysed and compared with the literature [16, 17, 18].

Patients and Methods

One hundred and twenty eight patients with severe head injuries were operatively treated in the Department of Neurosurgery of the Unfallkrankenhaus Berlin between September 1997 to April 1999. The average age of the 89 male and 20 female patients was 39,1 years. Nineteen patients (15%) underwent decompressive craniectomy. In 11 patients a decompressive craniectomy was performed with removal of a space-occupying mass (subdural or epidural hematoma or contusion) because intraoperatively generalised brain oedema was evident. The second group included 8 patients in whom conservative treatment on the intensive care unit remained therapy-resistant at neuromonitoring with ICP-, CPP-, MAP- and $p(ti)O_2$-measurements. The average age of the group of patients who were decompressed was 31,7 years and the male/female ratio was 5:1 (16 male, 3 female). In 17 patients we performed a unilateral craniectomy (right side 6, left side 11), and in 2 patients a bilateral craniectomy was necessary.

Results

In accordance with the results of other groups [16] the majority of head injuries with indication for craniectomy was due to motor vehicle accidents (53%), followed by falls (12%), attempted suicide (12%) and violence (6%). The primary diagnoses that underwent craniectomy are illustrated in Fig. 1. Fifty eight percent had a craniectomy because of a diffuse brain injury, 21 percent after an acute subdural hematoma and 16 percent with an open head injury. In patients with a diffuse brain injury the primary operative intervention was for evacuation of a space occupying contusion.

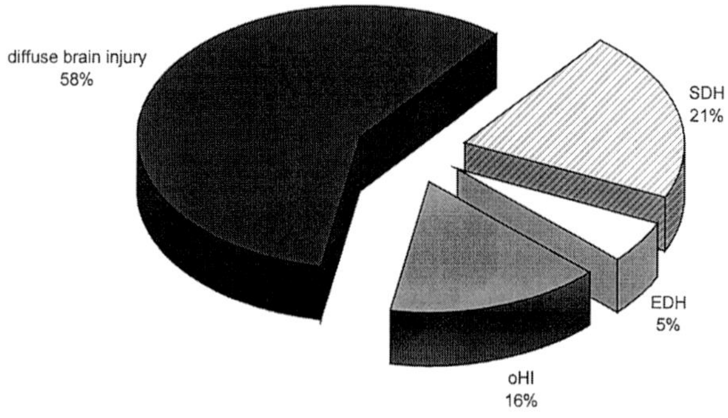

Fig. 1. Diagnoses of patients who underwent a decompressive craniectomy (n = 19)

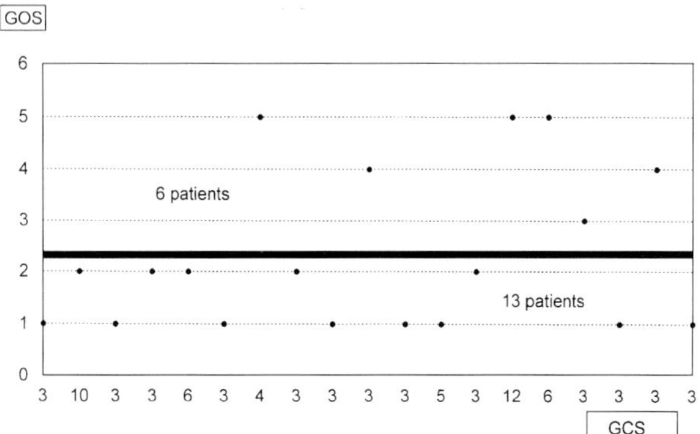

Fig. 2. Course of disease versus admission status

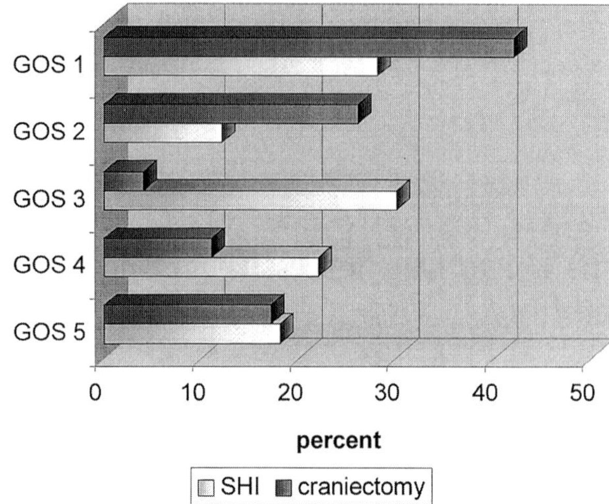

Fig. 3. Outcome after Craniectomy, SHI versus craniectomy

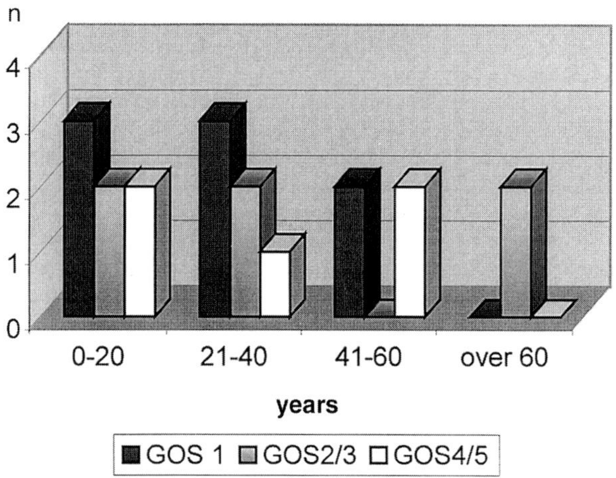

Fig. 4. Outcome after Craniectomy, GOS versus patients age

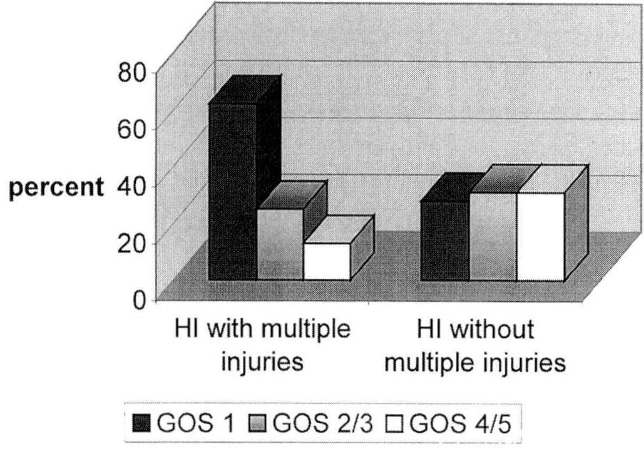

Fig. 5. Outcome after decompressive craniectomy, GOS versus multiple injuries (n = 19)

Fig. 2 summarises the dependency of outcome on the admission GCS. Eight patients (43%) died despite decompression, 5 patients (26%) remained in a vegetative state, 1 patient (5%) had a persistent severe neurological deficit, and 5 patients (26%) reached a GOS of 4 or 5. The comparison of the course of disease between patients with a severe head injury and those who were decompressed is illustrated in Fig. 3. It is evident that patients with a decompressive craniectomy had a poorer outcome.

It is not appropriate to compare the postoperative results because of the small number of patients (Fig. 4). Nevertheless, patients younger than 40 years had a better prognosis than the older ones. Also in the fourth and fifth decade, satisfactory results were obtainable in 50 percent. According to our results a decompression is less favourable in patients over 60 years of age and our two patients in this group remained in a vegetative state.

There is evidence of an important influence on the outcome of major extracranial injuries in contrast to isolated head injury (Fig. 5). We found an increased mortality of 63 percent when there was a multiple trauma in contrast to 27 percent with an isolated head injury.

Discussion

The prognosis after severe head injuries depends on the clinical status on admission, the intracranial lesions, the patient's age and the existence of accompanying injuries. Patients with epidural hematomas and open head injuries have a better prognosis than those with acute subdural hematomas. A poor prognosis is associated with brain contusions, diffuse brain injuries, traumatic injuries of the sinuses, less than 8 points on the Glasgow Coma Scale as well as advanced age [16, 17, 18].

Decompressive craniectomy changes the pressure-volume relationship and causes an increase in compliance and therefore a shift to the right of the pressure-volume curve [1, 2, 6, 8, 9, 15].

In animal experiments it was found by other groups [1, 2, 4, 10] that after decompression the injured brain exhibits an ICP decrease and an increase of the pressure-volume-index (PVI) and furthermore a decrease of the interstitial fluid accumulation. There are contradictory statements in the literature concerning an improvement of the regional cerebral blood flow (rCBF) and of the cerebrovascular resistance [8, 10, 24]. In clinical studies with PET, Xenon-CT and MR-spectroscopy Yamakami *et al.* [24] and Yoshida *et al.* [25] found an rCBF increase and an increase in cerebral metabolism after the craniectomy as compared to the preoperative results. This required an early decompression and the craniotomy was wide enough and included an opening of the dura. The craniectomy should be performed when conservative treatment fails to influence an ICP between 25 up to 40 mmHg and before cerebral perfusion is irreversibly disturbed [2].

There are different methods described in the literature. Clark *et al.* [3] prefers a circumferential cranioestomy and other groups [13, 20, 23] advise a bifrontal craniotomy, Gerl *et al.* [6] recommend a bilateral craniotomy, and Gaab *et al.* [5, 12] recommend a wide unilateral or bilateral frontotemporoparietal craniectomy with dura opening and dura patch plasty. According to the recommendations of Gaab *et al.* [5, 12] we performed a wide frontotemporoparietal craniectomy with dura plasty for which we used the temporal muscle and its fascia or a Neuropatch (Braun, Melsungen, Germany) as a graft. In 17 patients we made a unilateral decompression over the affected hemisphere and in one patient a frontal and in another patient a bilateral craniectomy. The bone flap was preserved by implantation subcutaneously into abdominal fat or by storage under sterile conditions at −80 °C.

Besides decompression in patients with diffuse brain injuries (Fig. 1) we performed a craniectomy primarily more often in patients with acute subdural hematomas when the development of cerebral oedema appeared during the operation and was resistant to conservative interventions.

The course of disease after craniectomy depends on the clinical status on admission (Fig. 2) and this was also found by other authors [5, 12, 21, 22]. In the literature between 11 and 71 percent died despite the decompression; 8 to 27 percent were in a vegetative state; 8 to 27 percent survived with severe neurological deficits; 0 to 21 percent survived with mild neurological deficits and 0 to 41 percent had a good recovery [5, 6, 7, 11, 12, 14, 20]. In a large analysis Guerra *et al.* [12] found 49 percent of patients had died, 13 percent survived with severe neurological deficits (corresponding to a GOS of 2 and 3) and 32 percent had a favourable outcome with a GOS score of 4 and 5. Our results are similar to those reported above but we had slightly more patients in the vegetative state.

The influence of the patient's age on the outcome after severe head injuries and craniectomy (Fig. 4) was also found by other authors [5, 12, 14, 20, 21]. According to like Karlen *et al.* [11] the prognosis was worse when there were major extracranial injuries present (Fig. 5). Under the influence of the results of Gaab *et al.* [5, 12, 21] we used the following guidelines for decompressive craniectomy after severe head injuries:

1. Patients age below 50 years without multiple trauma.
2. Patients age below 30 years in the presence of major extracranial injuries.
3. Severe brain swelling on CT scan.
4. Exclusion of a primary brainstem lesion/injury.
5. Intervention before irreversible brainstem damage.
6. ICP increase up to 40 mmHg and unsuccessful conservative therapy.
7. Primarily for space-occupying hematomas with hemispheric brain oedema.
8. Secondarily while monitoring ICP and $p(ti)O_2$ in an interval up to 48 hours after the accident before irreversible brainstem damage or generalised brain damage has occurred.

References

1. Burkert W (1985) Zeitlicher Verlauf des posttraumatischen Hirnödems nach Ultraschalleinwirkung – Experimentelle Untersuchungen und Modellvorstellungen zum Zeitpunkt der operativen Dekompression und zur Größe der Trepanationsfläche. Dissertation B, Martin-Luther-Universität Halle
2. Burkert W, Plaumann H (1989) Der Wert der großen druckentlastenden Trepanation beim therapieresistenten Hirnödem. Tierexperimentelle Untersuchungen, erste klinische Ergebnisse. Zentralbl Neurochir 50: 106–108
3. Clark K, Nash TM, Hutchison GC (1968) The failure of circumferential craniotomy in acute traumatic cerebral swelling. J Neurosurg 29: 367–371
4. Cooper PR, Hagler H, Clark WK, Barnett P (1979) Enhancement of experimental cerebral edema after decompressive craniectomy: implications for the management of severe head injuries. Neurosurgery 4: 296–300
5. Gaab MR, Rittierodt M, Lorenz M, Heissler HE (1990) Traumatic brain swelling and operative decompression: a prospective investigation. Acta Neurochir [Suppl] (Wien) 51: 326–328
6. Gerl A, Tavan S (1980) Die bilaterale Kraniektomie zur Behandlung des schweren traumatischen Hirnödems. Zentralbl Neurochir 41: 125–138
7. Gower DJ, Lee KS, Mc Whorter JM (1988) Role of subtemporal decompression in severe closed head injury. Neurosurgery 23: 417–422
8. Grände PO, Asgeirsson B, Nordström CH (1997) Physiologic principles for volume regulation of a tissue enclosed in a rigid shell with applications to the injured brain. J Trauma 42: 23–30
9. Hase U, Reulen HJ, Meinig G, Schürmann K (1978) The influence of the decompressive operation on the intracranial pressure and the pressure-volume relation in patients with severe head injuries. Acta Neurochir (Wien) 45: 1–13
10. Hatashita S, Hoff JT (1987) The effect of craniectomy in the biomechanics of normal brain. J Neurosurg 67: 573–578
11. Karlen J, Stula D (1987) Dekompressive Kraniotomie bei schwerem Schädelhirntrauma nach erfolgloser Behandlung mit Barbituraten. Neurchirurgia 30: 35–39
12. Kleist-Welch Guerra W, Gaab MR, Dietz H, Mueller JU, Piek J, Fritsch MJ (1999) Surgical decompression for traumatic brain swelling: indications and results. J Neurosurg 90: 187–196
13. Kjellberg RN, Prieto A Jr (1971) Bifrontal decompressive craniotomy for massive cerebral edema. J Neurosurg 34: 488–493
14. Kunze E, Meixensberger J, Janka M, Sörensen N, Roosen K (1998) Decompressive craniectomy in patients with uncontrollable intracranial hypertension. Acta Neurochir [Suppl] (Wien) 71: 16–18
15. Meier U (1985) Computertomographische Untersuchungen zum generalisierten Hirnödem nach Schädel-Hirn-Trauma und Subarachnoidalblutung. Dissertation A, Humboldt-Universität Berlin
16. Meier U, Gärtner F, Knopf W, Klötzer R, Wolf O (1992) The traumatic dural sinus injury – a clinical study. Acta Neurochir (Wien) 116: 91–93
17. Meier U, Heinitz A, Kintzel D (1994) Operationsergebnisse nach schwerem Schädel-Hirn-Trauma im Kindes- und Erwachsenenalter – Eine Vergleichsstudie. Unfallchirurgie 97: 406–409
18. Meier U, Zeilinger F, Kintzel D (1996) Prognose und Ergebnisse der operativen Versorgung von schweren Schädel-Hirn-Traumen. Akt Traumatol 26: 1–5
19. Pasaoglu A, Kurtsoy A, Koe RK, Konts O, Akdemir H, Öktem IS, Selcuklu A, Kavuncu IA (1996) Cranoplasty with bone flaps preserved under the scalp. Neurosurg Rev 19: 153–156
20. Polin RS, Shaffrey ME, Bogaev CA, Tisdale N, Germanson T, Bocchicchio B, Jane JA (1997) Decompressive bifrontal craniectomy in the treatment of severe refractory posttraumatic cerebral edema. Neurosurgery 41: 84–94
21. Rittierodt M, Gaab MR, Lorenz M (1991) Decompressive craniectomy after severe head injury: Useful therapy in pathophysiologically guided indications. In: Bock WJ *et al* (eds) Advances in neurosurgery, vol 19. Springer, Berlin Heidelberg New York Tokyo, pp 265–273
22. Shigemori M, Syojima K, Nakayama K, Kojima T, Watanabe M, Kuramoto S (1979) Outcome of acute subdural haematoma following decompressive hemicraniectomy. Acta Neurochir [Suppl] (Wien) 28: 195–198
23. Venes JL, Collins WF (1975) Bifrontal decompressive craniectomy in the management of head trauma. J Neurosurg 42: 429–433
24. Yamakami I, Yamaura A (1993) Effects of decompressive craniectomy on regional cerebral blood flow in severe head trauma patients. Neurol Med Chir 33: 616–620
25. Yoshida K, Furuse M, Izawa A, Iizima N, Kuchiwaki H, Inao S (1996) Dynamics of cerebral blood flow and metabolism in patients with cranioplasty as evaluated by ^{133}Xe CT and ^{31}P magnetic resonance spectroscopy. J Neurol Neurosurg Psychiatry 61: 166–171

Correspondence: Privat-Dozent Dr. med. Ullrich Meier, Department of Neurosurgery, Unfallkrankenhaus Berlin, Rapsweg 55, 12683 Berlin.

Acta Neurochir (2000) [Suppl] 76: 479–482

Transcranial Doppler Ultrasonography (TCD) in Ventilated Head Injured Patients: Correlation with Stable Xenon-Enhanced CT

S. C. P. Ng[1], **W. S. Poon**[1], **M. T. V. Chan**[2], **J. M. K. Lam**[1], **W. Lam**[3], and **C. Metreweli**[3]

[1] Division of Neurosurgery, Department of Surgery, Prince of Wales Hospital, The Chinese University of Hong Kong, Hong Kong
[2] Department of Anaesthesia and Intensive Care, Prince of Wales Hospital, The Chinese University of Hong Kong, Hong Kong
[3] Department of Diagnostic Radiology & Organ Imaging, Prince of Wales Hospital, The Chinese University of Hong Kong, Hong Kong

Summary

Disturbance of cerebral vasomotor regulation has been shown to be associated with the severity of traumatic brain injury (TBI). The transient hyperaemic response (THR) test is a test of the pressure autoregulatory response in terms of cerebral blood flow velocity after a brief carotid artery compression. Correlating with the test of cerebral vascular reactivity (CVR) to carbon dioxide by means of passive hyperventilation suggested that the THR test is a simple clinical test for the assessment of cerebral haemodynamic status in head-injured patients.

Keywords: Cerebral blood flow velocity; transient hyperaemic response; regional cerebral blood flow; cerebral vascular reactivity.

Introduction

The status of cerebrovascular autoregulation and carbon dioxide (CO_2) motor reactivity have been shown to be affected by head injury and correlate with the neurological condition and clinical outcome. Dissociation between the two is a common phenomenon. Therefore, it is important to measure cerebrovascular responses for the assessment of cerebral haemodynamic status in head-injured patients.

Transcranial Doppler ultrasonography (TCD) is a non-invasive and potentially reliable method for its assessment. By employing the transient hyperaemic response (THR) test with TCD measurement to assess the blood flow velocity (BFV) response of the middle cerebral artery (MCA) to a brief compression of the ipsilateral carotid artery provides a simple method for repeated assessment of cerebrovascular autoregulatory reserve [3]. The cerebral vascular reactivity (CVR) test with CO_2 challenge using stable xenon-enhanced computed tomographic (XeCT) cerebral blood flow (CBF) measurement technique to evaluate CO_2 vascular reactivity after TBI is well documented [2]. However, the relationship between these two tests has not been carried out systematically.

The aim of this study was to validate the THR test using TCD BFV measurement against the CVR test using regional CBF measurement by stable XeCT in determining the cerebral haemodynamic status of ventilated head-injured patients.

Materials and Methods

Thirteen patients (10 males and 3 females; mean age: 34.8 years, range: 5 to 65 years) with moderate to severe head injury defined as admission post-resuscitation Glasgow Coma Scale (GCS) score less than or equal to 12 points (median: 7 points) were included in the study. After surgical treatment, all patients were managed by a standard protocol including artificial ventilation with sedation and muscle paralysis.

The THR Test

Blood flow velocities in both MCA were determined by TCD. Figure 1 shows an example of MCA BFV recording in the THR test. After a stable baseline, the ipsilateral carotid artery was manually occluded by compression. The compression was accepted only if there was at least 30% reduction in baseline BFV. During the period of carotid artery compression, intact autoregulation would be associated with vasodilatation due to the fall in perfusion pressure in the MCA distribution. Once the compression was released, a transient increased in BFV due to reactive hyperaemia would result. Normally there should be more than a 10% increase [3] in systolic flow velocity. The THR ratio was defined as the percentage change in the systolic flow velocity after carotid release. Cerebral pressure autoregulation was considered lost if this ratio was less than 10%.

The CVR Test

Cerebral Blood Flow at two levels of CO_2 concentration (normocapnia and moderate hyperventilation) were evaluated using XeCT on days 1, 3 and 5 after head injury. During each CBF measurement,

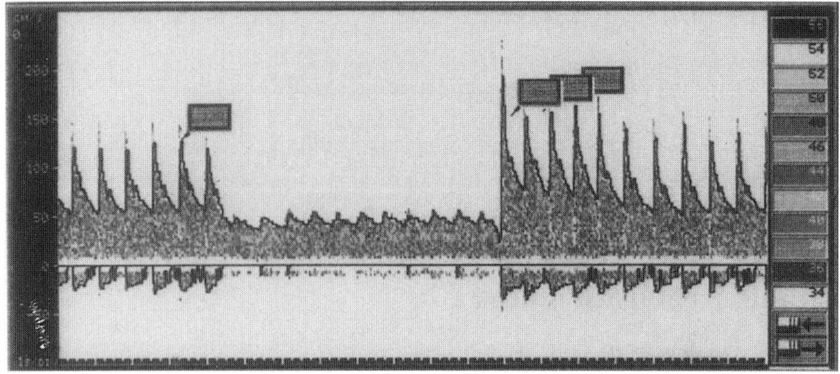

Fig. 1. TCD spectrum showing the transient hyperaemic response *(THR)* of elevated MCA blood flow velocity *(BFV)* after carotid artery compression release

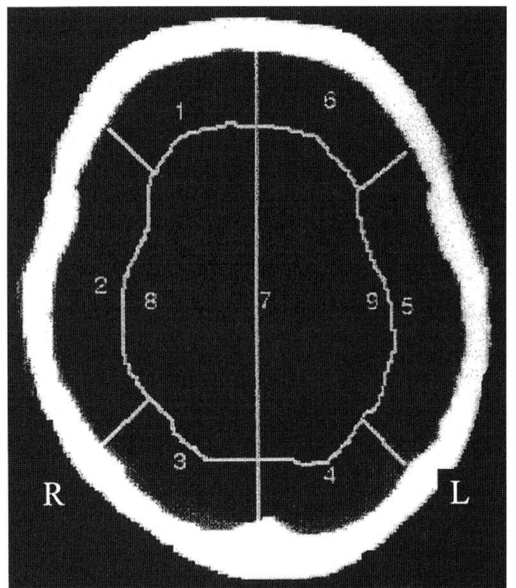

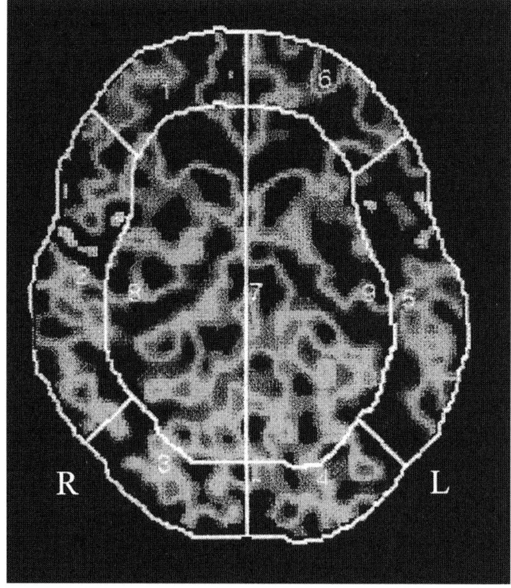

Fig. 2. (Left) A representative axial CT scan showing the regions of anterior, middle and posterior cerebral arteries territories. (Right) The corresponding XeCT cerebral blood flow map

a mixture of 30% stable xenon and 40% oxygen was administered for 4.5 minutes. Three axial brain scans were used for each measurement. Figure 2 shows an axial brain scan and the corresponding XeCT CBF map. The lines were drawn by XeCT CBF software based on the anatomical landmark showing the regions of anterior, middle and posterior cerebral arteries territories. In this study, the regions of interest were both MCA territories. The CVR ratio was defined as the percentage change in CBF after CO_2 variation per unit change in mmHg end-tidal CO_2 concentration. CO_2 motor reactivity was considered to be impaired if this ratio was less than 2%/mmHg [1].

Table 1. *Table Showing the Mean, Standard Deviation and Range of MCA Blood Flow Velocity (BFV), Cerebral Blood Flow (CBF) at MCA Territories, the Transient Hyperaemic Response (THR) Ratio and Cerebral Vascular Reactivity (CVR) Ratio*

	Mean	S.D.	Range
BFV (cm/s)	86.1	31.2	32.0–170.0
CBF (ml/100 g/min)	55.5	30.4	4.1–119.0
THR ratio (%)	13.4	11.1	−3.5–46.6
CVR ratio (%/mmHg)	6.0	8.6	−6.9–34.5

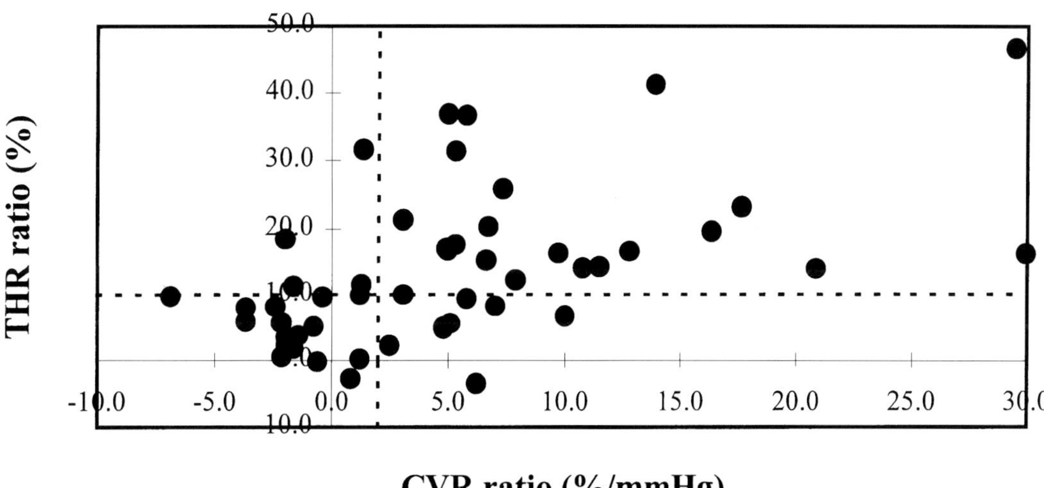

Fig. 3. Graph plotting transient hyperaemic response *(THR)* ratio versus cerebral vascular reactivity *(CVR)* ratio. The horizontal dotted line represents the THR ratio cut-off point of 10% and the vertical dotted line represents the CVR ratio cut-off point of 2%/mmHg

Table 2. 2 × 2 *Table for Evaluating Sensitivity and Specificity of the Transient Hyperaemic Response (THR) Test and the Cerebral Vascular Reactivity (CVR) Test*

	CVR test	
THR test	Impaired	Intact
Lost	16	9
Intact	4	25

Results

Thirteen patients underwent 54 pairs of THR and CVR tests. Table 1 summaries the findings of studies parameters. Both values of BFV and CBF seemed to be within normal range despite some abnormalities in terms of THR and CVR ratios.

Correlation coefficients of BFV/CBF and THR/CVR ratios were 0.38 ($p = 0.01$) and 0.40 ($p = 0.01$) respectively. Figure 3 shows the scatter plot of THR ratio versus CVR ratio. The cut-off point of THR ratio is 10%. 25 out of 54 THR ratios were below 10% at which cerebral autoregulation was considered to be lost. The cut-off point of CVR ratio is 2%. 20 out of 54 CVR ratios were below 2% at which CO_2 vascular response was considered to be impaired.

Table 2 shows a 2 × 2 table for evaluating sensitivity and specificity of the THR test for the CVR test. Sensitivity was 80%, specificity was 74%, predictive values for a positive test and a negative test were equal to 64% and 86% respectively.

Discussion

Previous studies have shown that impairment of the cerebral vasomotor regulation occurs after head injury. This impairment takes the form of disturbances in cerebrovascular autoregulation and CO_2 motor reactivity.

Cerebrovascular autoregulation is more sensitive to brain damage, whereas the CO_2 response is less sensitive to brain damage. By correlating the transient hyperaemic response, THR, test for cerebrovascular autoregulation assessment to the cerebral vascular reactivity, CVR, test for cerebrovascular response to CO_2 determination, this study showed absolute BFV and CBF measurements did not provide adequate information on the cerebral haemodynamic status of this group of ventilated head-injured patients. Although the CVR test provides an important index for determining a patient's CO_2 motor reactivity, this very involved test is not suitable to be performed daily. With good satisfactory sensitivity and specificity to CVR ratio, this study suggested that the THR test is reliable in the daily assessment of cerebral haemodynamic status in ventilated head-injured patients.

References

1. Enevoldsen EM, Jensen FT (1978) Autoregulation and CO_2 responses of cerebral blood flow in patients with acute severe head injury. J Neurosurg 48: 689–703
2. Marion DW and Bouma GJ (1991) The use of stable xenon-enhanced computed tomographic studies of cerebral blood flow

to define changes in cerebral carbon dioxide vasoresponsivity cased by a severe head injury. Neurosurgery 29: 869–873

3. Smielewski P, Czosnyka M, Kirkpatrick P, McEroy H, Rutkowska H, Pickard JD (1996) Assessment of cerebral autoregulation using carotid artery compression. Stroke 27: 2719–2203

Correspondence: Wai Poon, Division of Neurosurgery, Department of Surgery, Prince of Wales Hospital, The Chinese University of Hong Kong, Hong Kong.

Acta Neurochir (2000) [Suppl] 76: 483–484

Continuous Assessment of Cerebral Autoregulation – Clinical Verification of the Method in Head Injured Patients

M. Czosnyka[1], **P. Smielewski**[1], **S. Piechnik**[1], **E. A. Schmidt**[2], **H. Seeley**[1], **P. Al-Rawi**[1], **B. F. Matta**[1], **P. J. Kirkpatrick**[1], and **J. D. Pickard**[1]

[1] Academic Neurosurgical Unit & Wolfson Barain Imaging Centre, Department of Anaesthesiology, Addenbrooke's Hospital, Cambridge, UK
[2] University Hospital, Clermont Ferrand, France

Summary

Previously, using transcranlal Doppler ultrasonography, we investigated whether the hemodynamic response to spontaneous variations in cerebral perfusion pressure (CPP) provides reliable information about cerebral autoregulatory reserve. In the present study we have verified this method in 166 patients after head trauma. Waveforms of intracranial pressure (ICP), arterial pressure and transcranial Doppler flow velocity (FV) were captured daily over 0.5–2.0 hour periods. Time-averaged mean flow velocity (FV) and CPP were resolved. The correlation coefficient indices between FV and CPP (Mx) were calculated over 3 minutes epochs, and averaged for each investigation. An index of CBF (flow velocity diastolic to mean ratio) was calculated independently for each investigation. Mx depended on CPP ($p < 0.0001$) increasing to positive values when CPP decreased below 60 mm Hg. This threshold coincided with an averaged breakpoint for autoregulation, expressed by the index of CBF. Mx depended on outcome following head injury stronger than the Glasgow Coma Score on admission (ANOVA, F values 18 and 15 respectively; $N = 166$). In patients who died, cerebral autoregulation was disturbed during the first two days following injury. These results indicate an important role for the continuous monitoring of autoregulation following head trauma.

Keywords: Autoregulation; doppler ultrasonography; head injury.

Introduction

Disturbed cerebral autoregulation is believed to associate with an unfavourable outcome following head injury. Previously, using transcranial Doppler ultrasonography, we investigated whether hemodynamic response to spontaneous variations in cerebral perfusion pressure (CPP) provides reliable information on cerebral autoregulatory reserve [1]. In the present study we have verified this method in a large group of patients after head trauma.

Material and Method

One hundred and seventy five head injured sedated and ventilated patients were studied daily. All patients were paralysed, sedated and ventilated to achieve mild hypocapnia (3.5–4 kPa). Alternating colloid and normal saline infusions, with the addition of inotropic agents (infusion of dopamine at a rate of 2–15 μg/kg per minute), were used selectively to prevent arterial hypotension leading to a reduction of cerebral perfusion pressure (CPP) below 60 mm Hg. Boluses of mannitol (200 ml of 20%, over a period of 20 min or longer) were given to manage episodes of intracranial pressure above 25 mm Hg. Outcome was assessed 6 months or more after injury using the Glasgow Outcome Scale.

Arterial pressure (ABP) was monitored directly in the radial or dorsalis pedis artery (System 8000, S&W Vickers Ltd, Sidcup, UK). Intracranial pressure (ICP) was monitored continuously using a fibre-optic transducer (Camino Direct Pressure Monitor, Camino Laboratories, San Diego, CA or Codman Microsensors ICP Transducer, Codman & Shurtlef Inc., Randolph, MA). The catheter tip was inserted into the right frontal region intraparenchymally.

The middle cerebral artery (MCA) blood flow velocity was measured using PCDop 842 Doppler Ultrasound Unit (Scimed, Bristol, UK) or Neuroguard (Medasonics, Fremont, CA) transcranial ultrasonographs) daily for a period from 20 minutes to 4 hours starting from the day of admission until discharge. The recordings were undertaken during periods of stable respiration undisturbed by physiotherapy. Periods of tracheal suction or other nursing interventions were eliminated from recordings before further analysis.

Waveforms of intracranial pressure (ICP), arterial pressure and transcranial Doppler flow velocity (FV) were captured over a half to two hour periods. Time averaged mean flow velocity (FV) and CPP were resolved. The correlation coefficient indices between FV and CPP (Mx) was calculated over 3 minutes epochs, and averaged for each investigation. A positive correlation signifies passive dependence of blood flow on CPP, i.e. disturbed autoregulation. Zero or negative correlation characterises good autoregulation, that is blood flow independent of changes in CPP. Index of CBF (flow velocity diastolic to mean ratio) was calculated independently for each investigation.

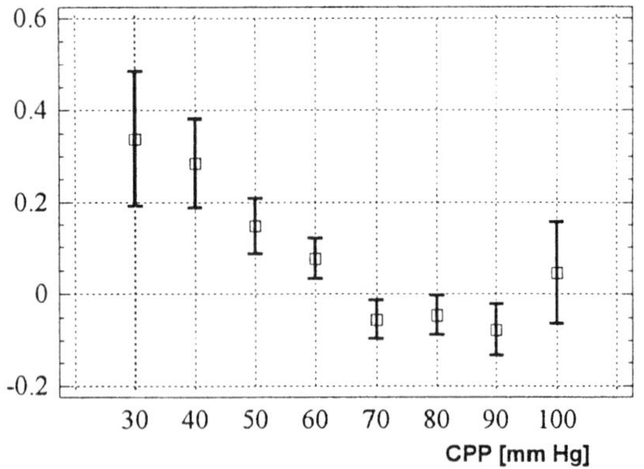

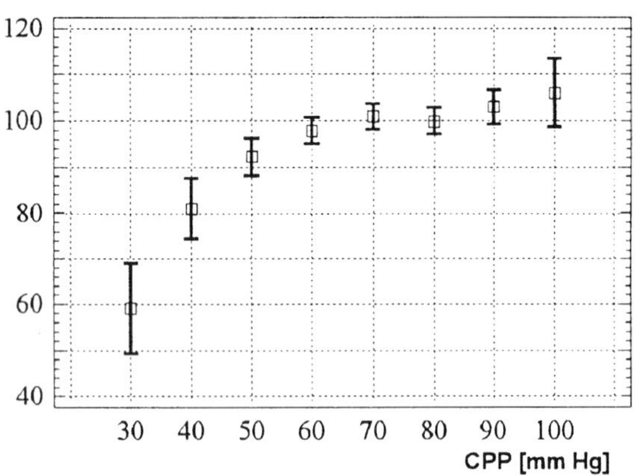

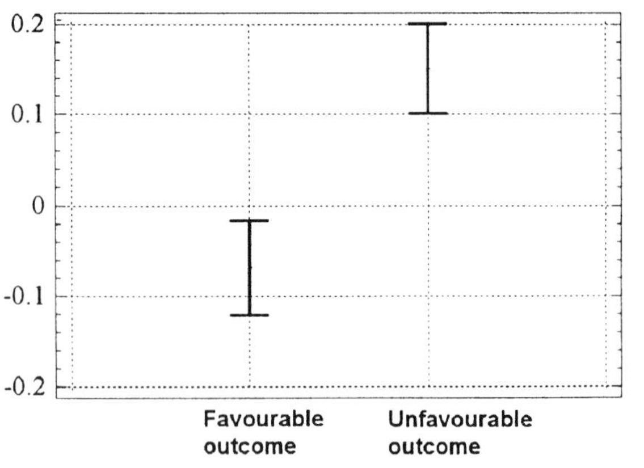

Fig. 1. Relationship between index of autoregulation (a) and index of CBF (b) and cerebral perfusion pressure (ANOVA; $p < 0.0001$). Autoregulation fails when Mx becomes significantly positive (CPP= 60 mm Hg) which coincides with the beginning of gradual decrease in CBF. Significantly positive mean value of Mx ($p < 0.001$) is seen in patients with unfavourable outcome following head injury (c)

Results

Mx depended on CPP (ANOVA; $p < 0.0001$) increasing to positive values when CPP decreased below 60 mm Hg. This threshold coincided with the averaged breakpoint for autoregulation, expressed by the index of CBF (see Fig. 1). Mx depended on outcome following head injury to a greater extent than the Glasgow Coma Score on admission (ANOVA, F values 17 and 15 respectively; $N = 175$). In patients who died, cerebral autoregulation was more severely disturbed (mean Mx value above 0.3; $p > 0.05$) during initial period (first two days) following injury.

Conclusion

Positive values of the index of autoregulation, expressing positive association between slow waves of CPP and blood flow velocity, indicate disturbed autoregulation. This index correlates with low CPP, a lower limit of autoregulation and unfavourable outcome following head injury. It seems to be suitable for monitoring autoregulation-oriented therapy in the neuro-intensive care unit. Similar methods utilising slow vasocycling seen in blood flow velocity, ICP and ABP for continuous monitoring of cerebral autoregulation are becoming popular in clinical practice [2–6].

References

1. Czosnyka M, Smielewski P, Kirkpatrick P, Menon DK, Pickard JD (1996) Monitoring of cerebral autoregulation in head-injured patients. Stroke 27: 829–834
2. Diehl RR, Linden D, Lucke D, Berlit P (1998) Spontaneous blood pressure oscillations and cerebral autoregulation. Clin Autonom Res 8: 7–12
3. Hu H, Kuo TB, Wong WJ, Luk YO, Chern CM, Hsu LC, Sheng WY (1999) Transfer function analysis of cerebral hemodynamics in patients with carotid artery stenosis. J Cereb Blood Flow Metab 19: 460–465
4. Harper AM (1966) Autoregulation of cerebral blood flow: influence of arterial blood pressure on blood flow through the cerebral cortex. J Neurol Neurosurg Psychiatry 29: 398–403
5. Panerai RB, White RP, Markus HS, Evans DH (1998) Grading of cerebral dynamic autoregulation from spontaneous fluctuations in arterial blood pressure. Stroke 29(11): 2341–2346
6. Steinmaier R, Bauhuf C, Hubner U, Baure RD, Fahlbush R, Laumer R, Bondar I (1996) Slow rhythmic oscillations of blood pressure, intracranial pressure, microcirculation and cerebral oxygenation: Dynamic interrelation and time course in humans. Stroke 27: 2236–2243

Correspondence: Dr. Marek Czosnyka, Academic Neurosurgical Unit, Box 167 Addenbrooke's Hospital, Cambridge CB2 2QQ, U.K.

Acta Neurochir (2000) [Suppl] 76: 485–490

False Autoregulation (Pseudoautoregulation) in Patients with Severe Head Injury. Its Importance in CPP Management

J. Sahuquillo[1], S. Amoros[2], A. Santos[2], M. A. Poca[1], H. Valenzuela[2], M. Báguena[3], and A. Garnacho[3]

[1] Department of Neurosurgery, Vall d'Hebron University Hospitals, Barcelona, Spain
[2] Neurotraumatology Research Unit, Vall d'Hebron University Hospitals, Barcelona, Spain
[3] Neurotraumatology Intensive Care Unit, Vall d'Hebron University Hospitals, Barcelona, Spain

Summary

False autoregulation has been described as an alteration of autoregulation in which the apparent maintenance of a constant cerebral blood flow (CBF) when increasing cerebral perfusion pressure (CPP) is due to an increase in brain tissue pressure. The objective of our study was to investigate how often false autoregulation occurred in patients with a severe head injury. In forty-six patients with a moderate or severe head injury autoregulation was studied using arterio-jugular differences of oxygen ($AVDO_2$) to estimate changes in CBF after inducing arterial hypertension with phenylephrine. Changes in mean arterial blood pressure (MABP), intracranial pressure (ICP), cerebral perfusion pressure (CPP) and $AVDO_2$ were calculated before and after inducing hypertension. Ninety-five episodes of provoked hypertension were studied in 46 patients. In 28 tests (29.5%) a constant or even reduced CBF was detected simultaneously with a median increase in parenchymal ICP of 8.5 mm Hg (false autoregulation). In this group the median of the induced increase in MABP was 20.6 mm Hg with a median increase in CPP of 11.5 mm Hg. From our data we can conclude that false autoregulation is frequently found in patients after a severe head injury. Increasing MABP to obtain a better CPP in these patients is not beneficial because CBF is not modified or may even be reduced.

Keywords: Cerebral perfusion pressure; head injury; autoregulation.

Introduction

Autoregulation is defined as the brain's capacity to maintain an almost constant cerebral blood flow in spite of changes in cerebral perfusion pressure (CPP). Autoregulation has been extensively studied in the human kidney and brain [3]. One common characteristic of both organs is that they are enclosed in a rigid container, the brain in the skull and the kidney in its capsule. In such enclosed organs, tissue pressure can play an important role in regulating blood flow through their microcirculation. The relationship between tissue pressure and flow in such organs can mimic a normal autoregulatory response, even though autoregulatory mechanisms are severely impaired or abolished. This phenomenon has been called *false autoregulation* or *pseudoautoregulation*.

One of the most controversial issues in the management of severe head injuries concerns whether or not autoregulation is impaired, abolished or preserved in these patients. The main importance of this question is that many of the therapeutic options used in their management are based upon assumptions about the status of autoregulation. The rationale behind what is known as *CPP management* is that autoregulation is preserved after injury but that its upper limit and lower limit are shifted to the right and that therefore higher CPPs are necessary to maintain an optimum cerebral blood flow (CBF) and cerebral blood volume (CBV) [9, 10]. In contrast, the recently introduced *Lund approach* to the treatment of severe head injury is based upon the concept that autoregulation is impaired after head trauma and that blood brain barrier (BBB) permeability is altered [6].

In previous studies we used arteriojugular differences of oxygen ($1/AVDO_2$) to test autoregulation in severely head injured patients. In some of these tests, paradoxical stability in estimated changes in CBF was observed in some patients in whom increasing mean arterial blood pressure induced significant increases in intracranial pressure (ICP). In these cases, the changes observed were similar to what has been described as *pseudoautoregulation*. The purpose of our study was to evaluate autoregulation in a group of patients with a moderate or severe head injury and to determine the frequency of false autoregulation. The early detection of this pattern would be very useful when attempting to rationalize the management of ICP and CPP in this heterogeneous and physiopathologically complex group of patients.

Material and Methods

Between January 1994 and October 1996, we studied CO_2-reactivity and autoregulation in 46 patients with a moderate or severe head injury (best post-resuscitation Glasgow coma scale score below or equal to 12), admitted to the Neurotraumatology Intensive Care Unit (NICU) of the Vall d'Hebron University Hospitals. In this study, we included only patients with a diffuse brain injury type II or III according to Marshall's classification. Cerebrovascular response to changes in pCO_2 and autoregulation were tested in all patients within the first 72 hours after injury. The study protocol was approved by the Institutional Ethical Committee on Human Research of Vall d'Hebron University Hospitals (Protocol numbers TR-113/1994 and TR-51/1995). In these 46 patients, 119 tests were performed with a minimum interval of 18 hours between them. Twenty-one of these tests were discarded because spontaneous changes in arterial pCO_2 after increasing MABP were above ± 5 mm Hg or because of technical deficiencies. The remaining 95 tests were the object of this study.

Continuous Physiological Monitoring

In all patients ICP was monitored with the Camino V420 monitor and an intraparenchymatous device (Model 110-4B manufactured by Camino Laboratories, San Diego, CA, USA). Mean arterial blood pressure (MABP), cerebral perfusion pressure (CPP) and arterial oxygen saturation (SaO_2) were routinely monitored. SjO_2 was monitored using the Oximetrix-3 system with a No 5.5 F fiberoptic catheter (Opticath, 5.5 Fr. catheter and Oximetrix-3 monitor supplied by Abbot Laboratories, S. A, Madrid). The catheter for continuous SjO_2 monitoring is always placed in the side which shows the highest ICP increase after alternately compressing both jugular veins. X-ray verification of the catheter position was obtained in all patients before extracting jugular blood samples and once a day thereafter. In all the tests performed, jugular blood samples, not measurements of the oximeter, were used to calculate $AVDO_2$. Blood gases were analyzed on a BGM Instrumentation Laboratory analyzer, model 1312 (Supplied by Medical Europe, Milan, Italy). Arterio-jugular differences of oxygen ($AVDO_2$) were calculated by the following equation: $AVDO_2 = 1.34 \times Hb \times [SaO_2 - SjO_2]/100$, where Hb is arterial oxyhemoglobin content in gr/dl and SaO_2 and SjO_2 are respectively the percentage of saturated oxyhemoglobin in the arterial and jugular blood. $AVDO_2$ were expressed in µmol/milliliter.

CO_2-Reactivity and Autoregulation Studies

The methodology used for testing CO_2-reactivity has been previously published and is based on the measured changes in $1/AVDO_2$ induced by changes in ventilator parameters [12]. CO_2-reactivity was tested in each patient immediately before performing the autoregulation test. Assuming a constant $CMRO_2$ during tests, changes in $AVDO_2$ reflect inverse changes in global CBF. In every case, absolute CO_2-reactivity (CO_2R_{ABS}) was calculated as the change in $AVDO_2$ divided by the measured change in $pCO_2 : \Delta\ AVDO_2/\Delta\ pCO_2$. The results were expressed as µmol/mm Hg pCO_2. To test autoregulation, changes in global CBF were also estimated from repeated measurements of $1/AVDO_2$ after increasing MABP by about 20–30% using phenylephrine. In every patient, to prevent pCO_2 from influencing the autoregulatory response, the ventilator settings were manipulated when necessary to obtain a baseline pCO_2 in the normoventilation range (35–45 mm Hg). MABP was measured directly through a catheter introduced into the radial artery and zeroed to the foramen of Monro level. Arterial and jugular blood samples to calculate $AVDO_2$ were obtained at baseline and 15–20 minutes after a steady state of MABP was achieved. $AVDO_2$ values were corrected for spontaneous changes in pCO_2 using the CO_2R_{ABS}. Theoretically, changes in CBF should be negligible if autoregulation is intact and therefore $1/AVDO_2$ should not change significantly when increasing MABP. The percentage of estimated change in CBF relative to the resting value (corrected for pCO_2) was calculated according to the following equation: $\%ECBF = [(1/AVDO_{2B} - 1/AVDO_{2H})/(1/AVDO_{2B})] * 100$, where $AVDO_{2B}$ are the basal arterio-jugular differences of oxygen and $AVDO_{2H}$ are the arterio-jugular differences of oxygen after raising MABP. Changes in percentage of ECBF were considered significant when changes in that parameter was above or below the limits of error for repeated measurements of $1/AVDO_2$. This limit was established at $\pm 20\%$ and was obtained in a study performed in our Unit (unpublished results). Therefore we assumed that changes in $1/AVDO_2$ above or below 20% reflected true changes in CBF while changes within the $\pm 20\%$ range were considered nonsignificant. Using these limits and a modification of the model proposed by

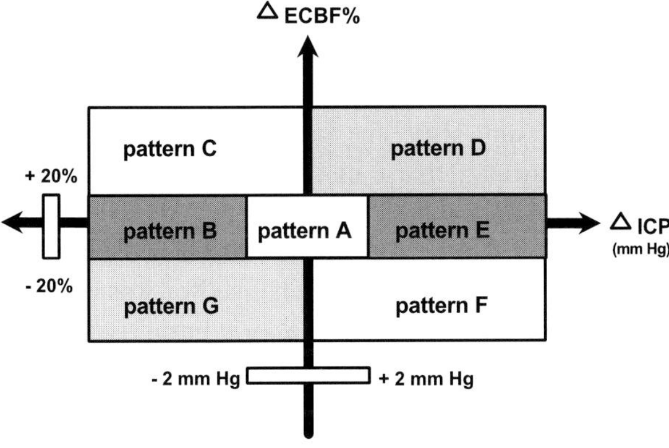

Fig. 1. In this graph the 7 possible patterns that can be defined by taking into consideration the observed changes both in ICP and in estimated CBF after inducing hypertension with phenylephrine are shown. Patients with no changes in estimated CBF (±20%) and in ICP (±2 mm Hg) are considered to have intact autoregulation (*Pattern A*). In *pattern B*, all patients with a reduced ICP and no significant changes in CBF are included. In *pattern C*, ICP decreases while estimated CBF increases. In *pattern D*, both ICP and estimated CBF increase. *Patterns E and F* are characterized by a significant increase in ICP (above 2 mm Hg), while estimated CBF is unchanged (*Pattern E*) or even reduced (*Pattern F*). Patients who show patterns E and F were considered to have false autoregulation. Patients included in *pattern G* exhibit a reduction in estimated CBF and a significant decrease in ICP. The horizontal bar represents the range of non-significant changes in ICP and the vertical bar the non-significant changes in estimated CBF

Enevoldsen and Jensen [2], which we had used in a previous study [11], we differentiated among 7 possible autoregulatory patterns (A to F) taking into account both estimated changes in CBF and observed changes in ICP. Changes in ICP were arbitrarily considered as non significant when they were within a range of ±2 mm Hg. This model is summarized and explained in Fig. 1. Patients with no changes in estimated CBF and ICP after hypertension had been induced were considered to have an intact autoregulation (*Pattern A*). Patients included in patterns E and F were considered to show the phenomenon of *false autoregulation*. These patterns were characterized by a significant increase in ICP (above 2 mm Hg), while estimated CBF was not modified (*Pattern E*) or even reduced (*Pattern F*).

Statistical Analysis

The assumption that data came from a normal distribution was tested using the Shapiro-Wilks test. In normally distributed data, the mean ± SD was used to summarize variables. In non-normally distributed data, the median and the lowest and highest values were reported. Statistical analysis was performed with the SAS statistical package version 6.12 (Supplied by SAS Institute Inc., Cary, NC, USA).

Results

Description of the Sample and CT Scan Findings

The mean age in our series of 46 patients was 29.7 ± 11 years (mean ± SD) with a range from 15 to 59 years. Thirty-seven of the patients were male (80%) and 9 female (20%). Of the 46 patients, 34 (74%) had been injured in a road accident. Analysis of the post-resuscitation Glasgow Coma Scale Score recorded on admission, showed that 37 patients (80%) scored equal to or below 8 points and nine patients (20%) scored above 8 and below 13 points. Twenty-one patients presented a Diffuse injury type II (46%) on admission and 25 a Diffuse Injury type III (54%) according to Marshall's classification.

Patterns of Autoregulation

In the 46 patients, 95 autoregulation tests were performed. Baseline variables in the 28 tests showing autoregulation are summarized in Table 1. Of the seven described patterns, Pattern A was observed in 8 of the 95 tests (8.4%), Pattern B in 7 tests (7.4%), Pattern C in 8 (8.4%), Pattern D in 40 (42.1%), Pattern E in 19 (20%), Pattern F in 9 (9.5%) and Pattern G in 4 tests (4.2%) (Fig. 2). Therefore, what we considered to be false autoregulation was observed in 28 of the 95 tests performed (29.5%). In total, these 28 patterns were detected at least once in 19 of the 46 patients.

Table 1. *Basal Physiological Variables in the 28 Tests Performed in Which the Pattern of Pseudoautoregulation was Observed*

	Mean ± SD	Range
Hb (grs/dl)	11.7 ± 1.7	9–15
ICP (mm Hg)	23.6 ± 13.9	4–54
MABP (mm Hg)	92.6 ± 13.5	70–127
CPP (mm Hg)	68.9 ± 14	38–99
PCO_2 (mm Hg)	37.5 ± 5.6	20–50
SjO_2 (%)	78.9 ± 7.5	60–90
$AVDO_2$ (μmol/ml)	1.3 ± 0.6	0.4–3.0

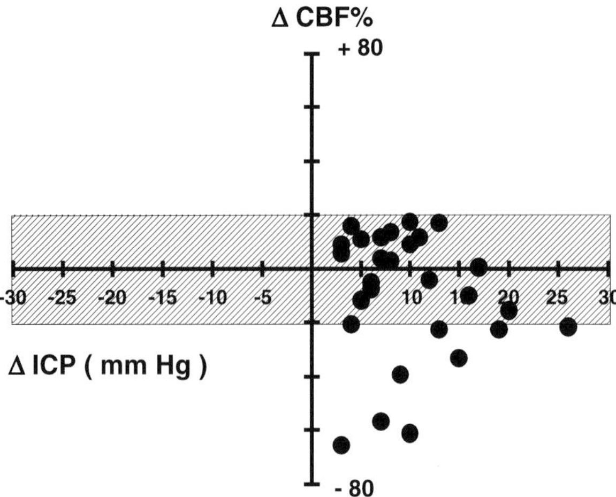

Fig. 2. In this chart the percent change in estimated CBF is plotted against changes in ICP (in mm Hg) for each of the 28 tests that exhibited false autoregulation. Observe the important reduction in estimated CBF in some of the cases in which ICP also increased. The shadowed area represents the $\pm 20\%$ range in estimated CBF change. Changes within this range were considered to be within the range of error measurement and therefore non-significant

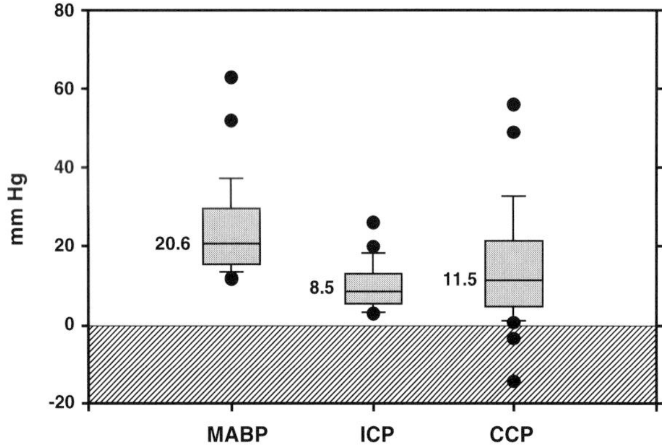

Fig. 3. Box-and-whisker plot in which the distribution of the change in the 3 variables of interest is shown after inducing hypertension with phenylephrine in the 28 tests that showed false autoregulation. In the x-axis mean arterial blood pressure (*MABP*), intracranial pressure (*ICP*) and cerebral perfusion pressure (*CPP*) are shown. The number at the left side of the box represents the median. For the sake of clarity, the cases plotted within the shadowed area are those in whom CPP decreased in spite of an increase in MABP

Changes in Cerebral Hemodynamics Induced by Testing Autoregulation

In twelve of the 28 tests showing false autoregulation, basal ICP was below or equal to 20 mm Hg (42.9%) while in 16 (57.1%) ICP was above 20 mm Hg. The median of the induced change in MABP was 20.6 mm Hg (11.6–63 mm Hg). As shown in Fig. 3, the changes in CPP induced by increasing MABP were very variable. In the whole group, inducing hypertension caused a change in median CPP of 11.5 mm Hg (−14 to 56 mm Hg). The increase in MABP did not induce a linear increase in CPP because of a parallel increase in ICP, which varied from 3 to 36 mm Hg (median of 8.5 mm Hg). As shown in Fig. 3, in some patients CPP was actually unchanged or was even reduced by increasing MABP because brain tissue pressure simultaneously increased. In some cases in whom MABP was increased by more than 25 mm Hg, $AVDO_2$ showed an important decrease in CBF. The most extreme cases showed a reduction of more than 50% in estimated CBF.

Discussion

The elastic property of tissues is an important variable involved in the regulation of flow in any organ enclosed in a rigid fluid-filled container [8]. According to the model proposed by Riley *et al.*, knowledge of arterial pressure, venous pressure and even arteriolar resistance alone is not enough to predict blood flow through and organ when tissue pressure is affected by an increase in arterial pressure [8]. In those cases, a paradoxical constant flow can be maintained in spite of a severe impairment of autoregulation.

The fact that increases in both arterial blood pressure and in CPP are sometimes not accompanied by a parallel increase in CBF in the injured and non-autoregulating brain, was observed by Miller *et al.* in 1975 in an experimental model of cryogenic injury in primates [4]. These authors suggested that tissue pressure may play an important role in these situations. For some, tissue pressure could even be the normal controlling factor in autoregulation. Although this view is only maintained by a few authors, it is generally accepted that in the presence of impaired or abolished autoregulation, tissue pressure plays a very important role in controlling flow in organs enclosed in a rigid container. When autoregulation is impaired or abolished, the protective vasoconstriction of arterioles is partially or completely lost and therefore increases in MABP are freely transmitted to the capillary bed. Increased pressure in microcirculation might, to a variable extent, increase extravascular pressure and might therefore increase the resistance of microcirculation [5]. In the brain, an increase in interstitial brain water due to increased filtration though the BBB, could compress capillaries reducing or maintaining flow at a relatively constant level in spite of impaired autoregulation [3].

Using changes in $AVDO_2$ to evaluate autoregulation is a reliable method if the cerebral metabolic rate of oxygen ($CMRO_2$) is maintained constant during tests. The advantage of this method lies in its simplicity and in that it allows useful information about autoregulation to be obtained at the bedside. If autoregulation is intact, either no changes in estimated CBF or only very small ones, are expected when increasing MABP within the limits of the autoregulatory curve.

One of the difficulties of interpreting the results of any method of testing autoregulation lies in the fact that in patients with an impaired or abolished vasoconstrictory response to increased CPP, increasing MABP induces parallel and variable changes in cerebral blood volume (CBV) and a variable increase in water filtration through the BBB. These changes always induce an increase in ICP. When this happens, although the net CPP may be increased, this increase is obtained at the expense of ICP being reset to a higher value. For this reason, using the traditional approach of characterizing autoregulation according to cerebrovascular resistance (CPP/CBF ratio) can be misleading when autoregulation is impaired or abolished because of the mathematical coupling of the variables involved in the calculations. The changes in CBF induced by an increase in MABP in these patients is unpredictable because tissue pressure often increases in parallel. Consequently, we believe that to better characterize autoregulatory impairment, the use of changes in both observed ICP and in estimated CBF is necessary.

The paradoxical decrease in CBF when increasing MABP in patients with impaired or abolished autoregulation has been described in different types of brain lesions [7]. The hypothesis of false autoregulation in head injury was first proposed by Miller and was subsequently elaborated by Enevoldsen and Jensen [1, 2], who observed the paradoxical fact that in some patients, autoregulation appeared to be preserved in the most injured regions of the brain, such as in areas where the brain tissue was severely lacerated [2]. Another unexpected finding was that autoregulation became progressively impaired as the patients recovered but that it was preserved during clinical deterioration [2]. These authors hypothesized that in patients with apparently preserved autoregulation, CBF was maintained constant by an increase in interstitial pressure in a microcirculatory bed devoid of the protective mechanisms of the arteriolar vasoconstriction.

If we accept that tissue pressure is important in defining flow in the microcirculation and that vasogenic edema is enhanced in patients with impaired autoregulation when MABP is increased, the optimal CPP in the management of these patients should be obtained, as suggested by Miller *et al.* at the lowest level of MABP and the lowest level of ICP. In our study we frequently observed false autoregulation. In such patients, ICP is immediately increased after inducing arterial hypertension. As a consequence, therapeutic measures directed to reduce capillary hydrostatic load may help to control high ICP. According to this reasoning, when patients have a predominantly diffuse brain injury and exhibit the phenomenon of false autoregulation, what is known as the *Lund approach* may be an option worth considering. The use of permissive low CPPs in these patients, if brain oxygen supply is adequately monitored, could be helpful in controlling increased ICP.

Although autoregulation is a global phenomenon its impairment can be different in different regions of the brain. In patients with predominantly focal lesions, it is possible that the affected areas can have a different autoregulatory response than that predicted by global measurements. In this situation, no test of autoregulation can accurately reflect the true situation in specific regions of the brain. This problem has been observed in patients with brain tumors in whom autoregulation was lost within the brain tumor and was preserved in normal and edematous peritumoral tissue [13]. Although this possibility is, in our opinion, unlikely in patients with a diffuse injury, it should be considered a potential pitfall when using global methods of monitoring autoregulation. In our series, all of the patients tested had a diffuse brain injury and therefore global autoregulation measurements were likely to be representative of the whole brain autoregulatory status.

The wide variation in autoregulatory status in patients with a severe head injury makes treatment based on targeting CPP difficult to use. In order to decide the best approach in different patients with different lesions, we need reliable multimodality monitoring that can easily be integrated at the bedside. The application of different treatment strategies and fine-tuning the management of increased ICP can only be rationally applied if therapeutic decisions are based on a better knowledge of the autoregulatory status of the patient.

Acknowledgments

The authors gratefully acknowledge the assistance of Gail Craigie in translating the manuscript. This work was supported by Grant 98/1385 from the Fondo de Investigación Sanitaria (FIS) and Grant 1031/97 from the Marató de TV3 to Dr. J. Sahuquillo.

References

1. Enevoldsen EM, Jensen FT (1977) "False" autoregulation of cerebral blood flow in patients with acute severe head injury. Acta Neurol Scand [Suppl] 64: 514–515
2. Enevoldsen EM, Jensen FT (1978) Autoregulation and CO2 responses of cerebral blood flow in patients with acute severe head injury. J Neurosurg 48: 698–703
3. Johnson PC (1964) Review of previous studies and current theories of autoregulation. Circ Res [Suppl] 1: I2–I9
4. Miller JD, Garibi J, North JB, Teasdale GM (1975) Effects of increased arterial pressure on blood flow in the damaged brain. J Neurol Neurosurg Psychiatry 38: 657–665
5. Milnor WR (1990) Regional circulations. In: Milnor WR (ed) Cardiovascular physiology. Oxford University Press, New York, pp 387–428
6. Nordström CH, Grände PO (1998) The "Lund Concept" in neurointensive care. In: von Wild KRH, Nordström CH, Hernández-Meyer F (eds) Pathophysiological principles and controversies in neurointensive care. W. Zuckschwerdt Verlag, München Bern Wien New York, pp 67–74
7. Olesen J (1973) Quantitative evaluation of normal and pathologic cerebral blood flow regulation to perfusion pressure. Changes in man. Arch Neurol 28: 143–149
8. Riley RL, Permutt S, Bromberger-Barnea B (1962) Elastic properties of tissues and autoregulation of blood flow. Physiologist 5: 203
9. Rosner MJ (1987) Cerebral perfusion pressure: Link between intracranial pressure and systemic circulation. In: Wood JH (ed) Cerebral blood flow. Physiological and clinical aspects. McGraw-Hill Company, New York, pp 425–448
10. Rosner MJ, Daughton S (1990) Cerebral perfusion pressure management in head injury. J Trauma 30: 933–941
11. Sahuquillo J, Munar F, Báguena M, Poca MA, Pedraza S, Rodriguez-Baeza A (1998) Evaluation of cerebrovascular CO2-reactivity and autoregulation in patients with post-traumatic diffuse brain swelling (diffuse injury type III). Acta Neurochir [Suppl] (Wien) 71: 233–236
12. Sahuquillo J, Poca MA, Ausina A, Baguena M, Gracia RM, Rubio E (1996) Arterio-jugular differences of oxygen ($AVDO_2$) for bedside assessment of CO2-reactivity and autoregulation in the acute phase of severe head injury. Acta Neurochir (Wien) 138: 435–444
13. Tomura N, Kato T, Kanno I, Shishido F, Inugami A, Uemura K, Higano S, Fujita H, Mineura K, Kowada M (1993) Increased blood flow in human brain tumor after administration of angiotensin-II: demonstration by PET. Comput Med Imaging Graph 17: 443–449

Correspondence: Dr. Juan Sahuquillo, Osona 6, 2–4, 08023 Barcelona, Spain.

Acta Neurochir (2000) [Suppl] 76: 491–494

Multi-Centre Assessment of the Spiegelberg Compliance Monitor: Preliminary Results

I. Piper[1], **L. Dunn**[1], **C. Contant**[2], **Y. Yau**[3], **I. Whittle**[3], **G. Citerio**[4], **K. Kiening**[5], **W. Schvning**[5], **S. Ng**[6], **W. Poon**[6], **P. Enblad**[7], **P. Nilsson**[7], and **Brain-IT Group**

[1] Institute of Neurological Sciences, Glasgow, Scotland, UK
[2] Department of Neurosurgery, Baylor College of Medicine, Houston
[3] Department of Clinical Neurosciences, University of Edinburgh, Scotland, UK
[4] Ospedale San Gerardo, Monza, Italy
[5] Department of Neurosurgery, Virchow Hospital, Berlin, Germany
[6] Chinese University of Hong Kong, Department of Neurosurgery, Hong Kong
[7] University Hospital, Uppsala, Sweden

Summary

Acute brain injury states (eg. head injury, subarachnoid haemorrhage) show clear inverse relationships of ICP vs compliance, with ICP instability at times of lower compliance states. Variance in compliance values is large in hydrocephalus where ICP is relatively lower and compliance higher. Nonetheless, early experience shows that compliance data influence decisions on CSF diversion treatments. Future work will focus on the ability of intracranial compliance to predict ensuing ICP instability and methodological refinement for monitoring patients who have higher compliance states.

Keywords: Intracranial pressure; craniospinal compliance; monitoring evaluation.

Introduction

A multi-centre collaborative group (*Brain-IT Group*) has recently been formed and consists of basic scientists and clinicians with a specific interest in the development and assessment of new forms of intensive care monitoring for use in Brain Injured Patients. Each member of the group contributes data to a common database collected according to a standard protocol [1]. A Web-Page has been set up which describes the guidelines and procedures of the group: http://i-www.brainit.gla.ac.uk. Currently the group is focused on assessing the Spiegelberg Compliance Monitor. Raised intracranial pressure (ICP) remains a significant clinical problem in patients with brain trauma, mass lesions and disturbances to cerebrospinal fluid (CSF) dynamics. Measurement of craniospinal compliance offers the potential of earlier identification of processes which lead to raised ICP. In addition to predicting ICP, a measure of compliance in combination with other features of the ICP signal may aid in clinical decisions concerning definitive measures for CSF diversion. A new method for measurement of compliance on a continuous basis has been developed [2] and we report on analyses focused on studying the relationship between compliance and ICP data from the first 41 patients monitored with the Spiegelberg device.

Methods

The Spiegelberg compliance monitor calculates intracranial compliance ($C = \Delta V/\Delta P$) from a moving average of small ICP perturbations (ΔP) resulting from a sequence of up to 200 pulses of added volume ($\Delta V = 0.1$ ml, total $V = 0.2$ ml) made into a double lumen intraventricular balloon catheter. Once a stable average has developed, the device produces a minute by minute measure of intracranial compliance. Neurointensive care data collected from 6 centres (Glasgow, Edinburgh, Monza, Berlin, Uppsala and Hong Kong) have been recruited to date which include a total of 55000 minutes (38 days) of paired ICP and compliance values. Collected data was grouped by patient type into 4 groups: a) Head Injury (HI) $n = 11$ patients, b) Hydrocephalus (HYDRO) $n = 18$ patients, c) Post-Operative tumour (TUMOUR) $n = 10$ patients, d) Post-Subarachnoid Haemorrhage (SAH) $n = 2$ patients. Summary statistics were produced for compliance data when grouped into 6 ICP bands and classed by patient type. A mixed model ANOVA was used

Table 1. *Associated Mean Compliance (±Median Absolute Deviation) Classed into 6 ICP Bands (mmHg)*

	0–10	10–20	20–30	30–40	40–50	50+
HI	0.89	0.77	0.61	0.41	0.42	0.30
(n = 11)	±.40	±.32	±.35	±.26	±.32	±0.42
SAH	1.07	0.810	0.62	0.36	—	—
(n = 2)	±.51	±.22	±.23	±.02	—	—
Tumour	0.88	0.79	0.64	0.63	0.57	—
(n = 10)	±.37	±.34	±.21	±.21	±.21	—
Hydroceph	0.87	0.74	0.80	0.83	—	.73
(n = 18)	±.36	±.32	±.26	±.14	—	.11

to test for differences in slopes of the ICP/Compliance relationship between patient groups. All analyses were performed with S-Plus 4.0.

Results

TABLE 1 summarises the associated mean compliance (±median absolute deviation) classed into 6 ICP bands. Both the HI and SAH groups show a clear inverse relationship between compliance and ICP whereas there was no clear relationship found with ICP for the hydrocephalus group (Fig. 1a). The post-operative tumour group compliance shows a more subtle relationship with ICP. Figure 2a shows the relative distribution of ICP between the patient groups and shows high ICP was predominantly found in the Head Injury and Tumour groups whereas there was proportionally very little raised ICP within the hydrocephalus group. Figure 2b shows the relative distribution of Compliance between the patient groups, which demonstrates, as expected, that the lowest compliance was observed predominantly in the Head injury group. However, Fig. 2b also demonstrates all groups showed episodes of lower compliance (<= 0.5 ml/mmHg) which can, in the case of the hydrocephalus group, occur in the absence of significantly raised ICP. Figure 1b shows data from a single patient where data equal to or above 20 mmHg is classed by compliance greater or less than 0.5 ml/mmHg. It can be observed from figure 1b that there is a 10 fold higher deviation in ICP about the mean in the class with compliance less than 0.5 ml/mmHg. This shows that, in this patient, compliance bordering 0.5 ml/mmHg is a threshold for the presence of ICP instability, possibly indicating a patient at risk of raised ICP. Using a mixed model ANOVA, the slope of the relationship between compliance and ICP was also found to be significantly different between head injured and hydrocephalus patients (p = 0.0018). With the current device, with high compliance values (>1.0 ml/mmHg) associated with low ICP (<10 mmHg) the variance in measured compliance is large, as would be expected for methodolog-

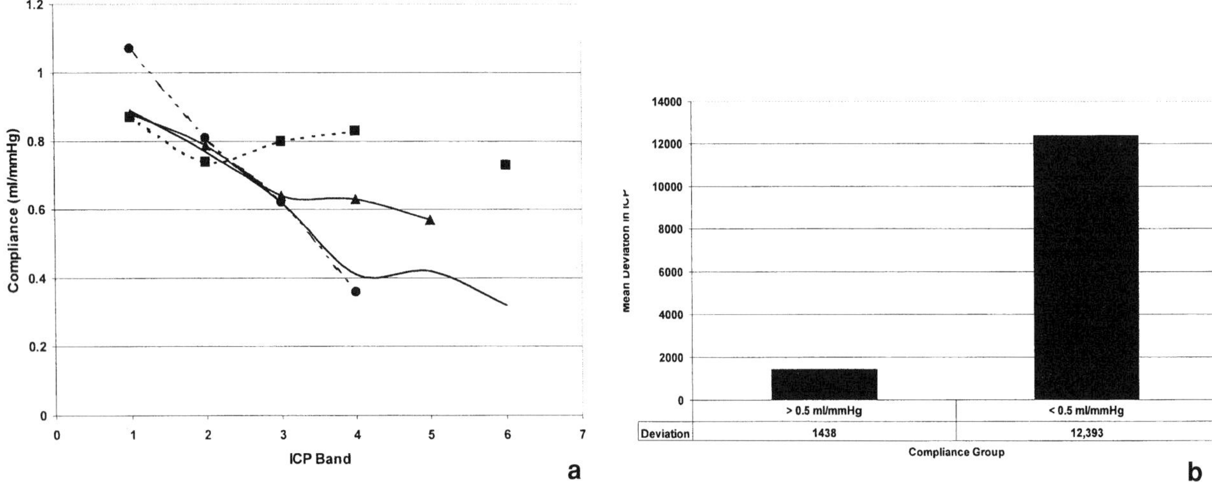

Fig. 1. (a) Line plot of the change in mean compliance Vs ICP band (0–10, 10–20, 20–30, 30–40, 40–50, >50 mmHg). Both the HI and SAH groups show a clear inverse relationship between compliance and ICP whereas there was no clear relationship found with ICP for the hydrocephalus group. The post-operative tumour group compliance shows a more subtle relationship with ICP. (b) Bar chart showing data from a single head injured patient where ICP data equal to or above 20 mmHg is classed by compliance greater or less than 0.5 ml/mmHg. It can be observed that there is a 10 fold higher deviation in ICP about the mean in the class with compliance less than 0.5 ml/mmHg. This shows that compliance bordering 0.5 ml/mmHg is a threshold for the presence of ICP instability in this patient, possibly indicating a patient at risk of raised ICP. —— HI, —●- SAH, —▲— Tumour, - ■- - Hydro

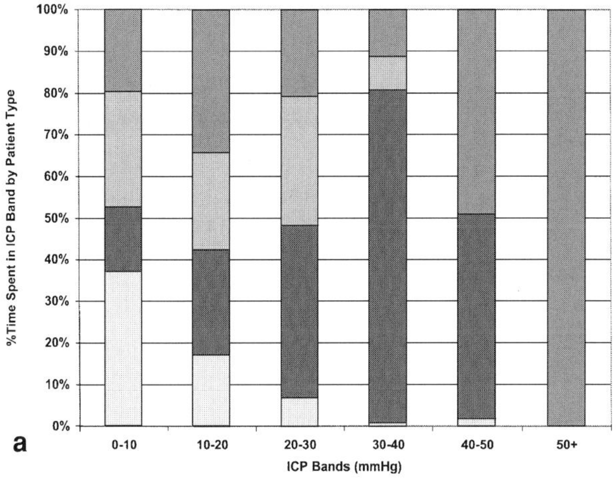

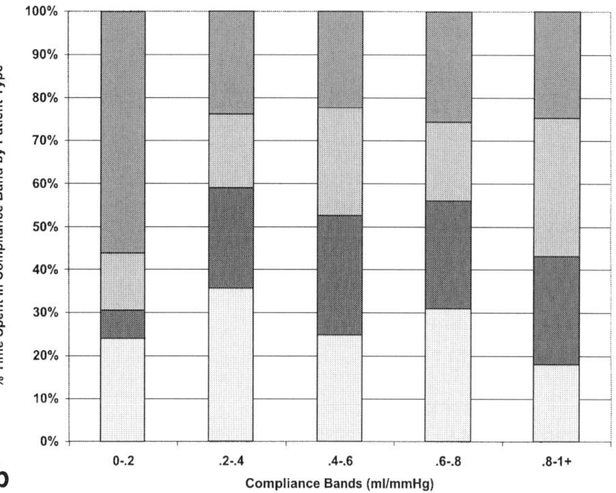

Fig. 2. (a) Bar chart showing the relative distribution of ICP between the patient groups and shows high ICP was predominantly found in the Head Injury and Tumour groups whereas there was proportionally very little raised ICP within the hydrocephalus group. (b) Bar chart showing the relative distribution of compliance between the patient groups, which demonstrates, as expected, that the lowest compliance was observed predominantly in the Head injury group. Note, that all patient groups showed episodes of lower compliance (<= 0.5 ml/mmHg) which can, in the case of the hydrocephalus group, occur in the absence of significantly raised ICP. ■ HI, ■ SAH, ■ Tumour, □ Hydroceph

ical reasons, however, further research to improving the stability of the device within this range of compliance is warranted.

Case Studies: Hydrocephalus

HYDRO1, HYDRO2 are two patients with enlarged ventricles and gait deterioration (Fig. 3a,b). ICP values and significant pressure waves in the trace for HYDRO1 was enough to suggest shunting was required. A month after shunting, HYDRO1 was walking independently having been wheelchair-bound preoperatively. HYDRO2 had much lower ICP values and less convincing evidence of pressure waves and on this basis alone, shunting would not have been offered. However, significant periods of time when compliance was reduced (<0.5 ml/mmHg) provided additional information in favour of shunting. The time for a 10-metre walk was halved one week after insertion of the shunt and standing balance was much improved.

Case Studies: Subarachnoid Haemorrhage

SAH1 & SAH2 are patients suffering subarachnoid haemorrhage with associated hydrocephalus who required temporary external ventricular drainage of CSF (Fig. 3c,d). A comparison is given of ICP and compliance values during initial drainage and later during trial clamping of the external drain. Tracings are on day of drain clamping. For SAH1, the amount of time compliance values were at low levels (<0.5 ml/mmHg) decreases and suggests an overall improvement in CSF dynamics from the time of initial drainage until trial clamping. External drainage was successfully removed and SAH1 has had no further problems from symptomatic hydrocephalus. For SAH2, compliance values fell and the amount of time compliance was low increased when the drainage was clamped suggesting that CSF dynamics were still impaired. SAH2 deteriorated after drain removal and required further external CSF drainage.

Conclusions

In patient groups known to exhibit "tight brains", intracranial compliance, as measured continuously with the Spiegelberg device, shows the expected inverse relationship with ICP. All patient groups show significant periods of lower compliance (<0.5 ml/mmHg) which, in the case of patients with hydrocephalus, are not necessarily associated with raised ICP. In individual patients compliance data can add pivotal information to routine ICP monitoring in the clinical decision to undergo CSF diversion. Future analyses will focus on time-series methods assessing to what degree compliance change predicts subsequent periods of ICP instability within different patient populations.

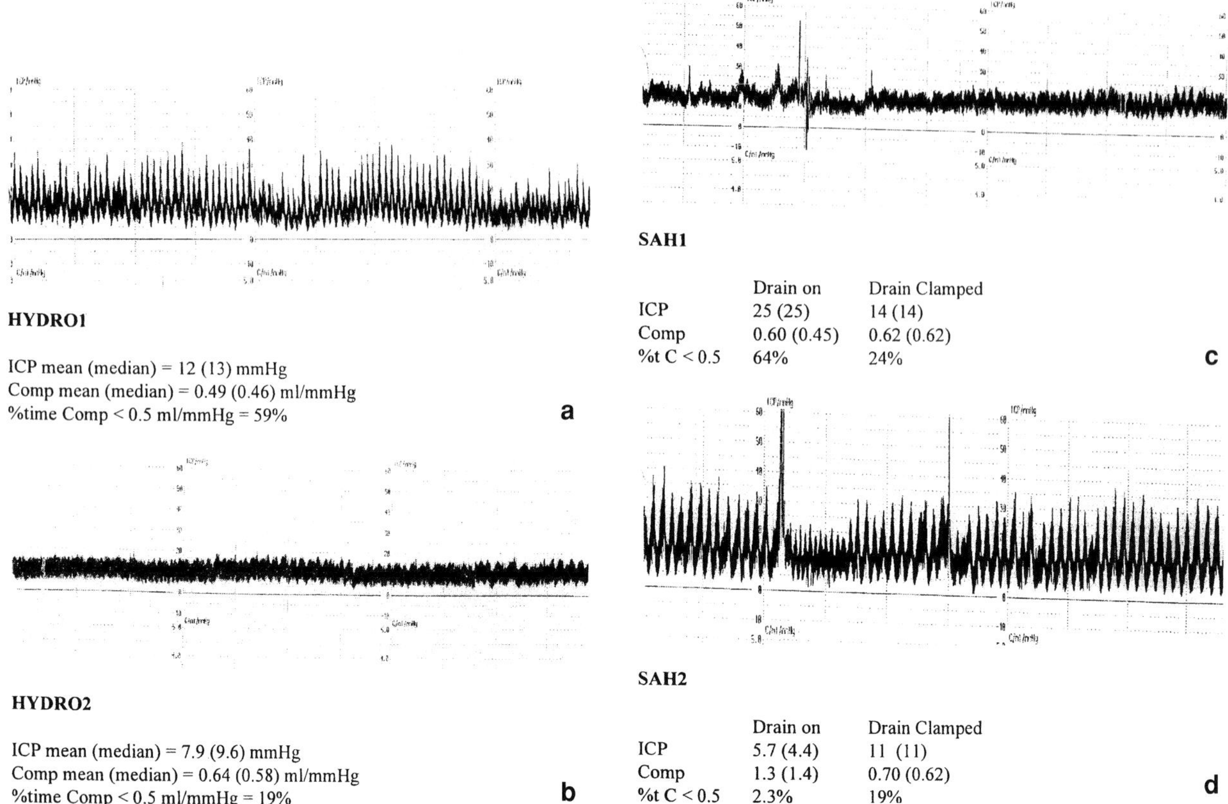

Fig. 3. (a) ICP trace from a patient with hydrocephalus showing moderate ICP values and significant pressure wave activity. The ICP trace alone was enough to suggest shunting was required. (b) ICP trace from a patient with hydrocephalus with much lower ICP values and less convincing evidence of pressure waves on the ICP trace and on this basis alone, shunting would not have been offered. However, the significant periods of time that the compliance was reduced (<0.5 ml/mmHg) was additional information in favour of shunting. (c) ICP trace from a patient suffering aneurysmal subarachnoid haemorrhage with associated hydrocephalus requiring temporary external drainage of CSF. Comparison is given for the ICP and Compliance values during initial drainage and later trial clamping of the external drainage. Mean ICP and Compliance values in the usual units are quoted with the median values in brackets. In this patient time spent with lower compliance decreases suggesting an overall improvement in the CSF dynamics from the time of initial drainage until trial clamping of drainage occurs. (d) ICP trace from a patient suffering aneurysmal subarachnoid haemorrhage with associated hydrocephalus requiring temporary external drainage of CSF. Comparison is given for the ICP and Compliance values during initial drainage and later trial clamping of the external drainage. Mean ICP and Compliance values in the usual units are quoted with the median values in brackets. In this patient time spent with lower compliance increases suggesting an overall deterioration in the CSF dynamics from the time of initial drainage until trial clamping of drainage occurs. This may indicate that this patient will require permanent measures of CSF diversion

References

1. Piper I, Contant C (1999) Results of a survey of 11 centres on multi-modality monitoring: influence on the design of a multi-centre database. (Abstract) Brit J Neurosurg 13: 101–118
2. Piper I, Spiegelberg A, Whittle I, Mascia L, Signorini D, Miller JD (1999) A comparative study of the spiegelberg compliance device with a manual volume-injection method: a clinical evaluation in patients with hydrocephalus. Brit J Neurosurg 13(6): 581–586

Correspondence: Ian Piper Department of Clinical Physics Institute of Neurological Sciences, Southern General Hospital, 1345 Govan Road, Glasgow, G51 4TF.

Stroke, Subarachnoid and Intracerebral Haemorrhage

A clinical trial of monitoring in stroke patients has suggested that outcome was better in those patients who were monitored than in those who were not (Davis *et al.*).

Experimental models of intracerebral haemorrhage [ICH] have contributed to our understanding of this disorder and a new 500 ul ICH model in the rabbit is reported by Holtmanspotter *et al.* who found that the oedema fluid around the ICH drains into the subarachnoid and ventricular cerebrospinal fluid [CSF]. Xi *et al.* described the Ann Arbour rat ICH model with special reference to the role of thrombin. Ogihara *et al.* from the Jackson group reported that Oxyhaemaglobin induced necrosis but not apoptosis in rat aortic smooth muscle cells.

In clinical cases of ICH Siddique *et al.* showed that CBF measured with Single Photon Emission Computerised Tomography (SPECT) was reduced initially in the penumbra around the clot, but, with surgical evacuation, CBF improved while with non-operative treatment CBF decreased. Mendelow *et al.* summarized the progress of the multicentre International STICH trial (Surgical Trial in Intracerebral Haemorrhage), which sets out to discover if surgical removal of the ICH improves outcome compared with initial conservative treatment.

Acta Neurochir (2000) [Suppl] 76: 497–499

Intracranial Hypertension Influences the Resolution of Vasogenic Brain Edema Following Intracerebral Hemorrhage

M. Holtmannspötter[1], **A. Schoch**[1], **A. Baethmann**[2], **H.-J. Reulen**[1], and **E. Uhl**[1]

[1] Department of Neurosurgery, Klinikum Großhadern, University of Munich, Germany
[2] Institute for Surgical Research, Klinikum Großhadern, University of Munich, Germany

Summary

Aim of the current study was to investigate the influence of intracranial hypertension on the resolution of vasogenic brain edema following intracerebral hemorrhage. An intracerebral hematoma was induced by 500 µl of blood injected into the left frontal lobe of rabbits (n = 25). Na^+-fluorescein (MW376) and Texas-Red-albumin (MW67.000) were administered intravenously as edema markers. By using a closed cranial window for superfusion of the brain surface and a ventriculo-cisternal perfusion the clearance of both fluorescence markers was measured in the CSF-effluates up to 8 hours using spectrophotometry. ICP was adjusted between 2–6 mmHg (low pressure, n = 10), 8–12 mmHg (moderate pressure, n = 10) or 14–20 mmHg (high pressure, n = 5). In all groups Na^+-fluorescein started to accumulate at 60 min after induction of the hematoma in the subarachnoid space, while at 90 min in the ventricular system. In the low intracranial pressure group Na^+-fluorescein (mean ± SEM) in the ventricular system amounted to 1.47 ± 0.42 nmol as compared to 1.34 ± 0.41 nmol in the moderate, or 0.38 ± 0.11 nmol in the high intracranial pressure group. In the subarachnoid space the marker reached 1.96 ± 0.57 nmol, 4.15 ± 1.28 nmol, or 0.96 ± 0.32 nmol, respectively. In conclusion, the data demonstrate that vasogenic edema induced by an intracerebral hematoma is cleared into both CSF compartments, albeit with delay into the ventricular system. Edema resorption occurred earlier and to a higher extent into the subarachnoid space as compared to the ventricular system. Further, edema resorption is influenced by the actual intracranial pressure, with marked inhibition by a high intracranial pressure.

Keywords: Vasogenic brain edema; intracerebral haemorrhage; intracranial pressure; edema clearance.

Introduction

It has been shown that vasogenic brain edema resolves via drainage through various pathways including uptake by astrocytes [1], reabsorption through the vascular system [2], and resolution via bulkflow into the ventricular system [4] and the subarachnoid space [3, 5]. This was concluded from previous experiments utilizing an edema infusion model. In this model vasogenic brain edema was induced by direct infusion of artificial edema fluid into the cerebral white matter [2, 4, 5]. Purpose of the present study was to investigate the influence of an increased intracranial pressure on resolution of vasogenic brain edema in a clinically oriented model of intracerebral hemorrhage.

Method

Details of the model have been previously described [5]. Male New Zealand white rabbits (n = 25, b.w. 2.5–3.0 kg) were used as experimental animals. Anesthesia was induced with thiopental i.v. (3 mg as bolus) and continued with alpha-chloralose (50 mg/kg i.v.) Polyethylene catheters were inserted into the femoral artery and vein for continuous monitoring of the arterial blood pressure, blood sampling, and infusion of anesthetics and fluorescent dyes. 20 mmol/l Na^+-fluorescein was used as a small-molecular weight edema marker (Sigma Chemical, St. Louis, MO, USA, MW: 376 D), while 0.2 mmol/l Texas-Red-albumin as high-molecular weight marker (MoBiTec GmbH, Göttingen, Germany, MW: 67.000 D). Following relaxation by pancuronium bromide (initial bolus of 4 mg, followed by continuous infusion of 1.2 mg/h) and analgesia with piritramid (bolus of 7.5 mg i.v.) the animals were mechanically ventilated ($PaCO_2$ 36–40 mmHg, PaO_2 100–120 mmHg). Arterial blood samples were obtained every hour for the measurement of blood gases, blood pH and base excess (BE). The rectal temperature was continuously controlled and maintained at 38.0 ± 0.6 °C using a feed-back controlled heating pad (Effenberger, Pfaffing, Germany). For surgical preparation the skull of the rabbits was immobilised by a stereotactic holder (Model 9000, David Knopf Inc., Tujunga, CA, USA), and the scalp was cut in the midline. For induction of the intracerebral hematoma a cannula (20 gauge) was inserted into the white matter of the left frontal lobe according to stereotactic coordinates (5 mm rostral of bregma and 5 mm lateral of sutura sagittalis, depth 3.5 mm from dura). A second cannula for measurement of the intracranial pressure and serving as inflow for the ventriculo-cisternal perfusion (3 ml/h) was implanted into the right lateral ventricle. The outflow cannula was introduced into the cisterna magna after preparation of the atlanto-occipital membrane. By changing the height of the outflow catheter the intracranial pressure (ICP) was adjusted to the desired ICP-level of the different groups (low

ICP: 2–5 mmHg (n = 10), moderate ICP: 8–12 mmHg (n = 10) and high ICP: 14–20 mmHg (n = 5). For superfusion of the brain surface in the subarachnoid space (3 ml/h) a closed cranial window was implanted over the left parietal cortex. After surgical preparation the ventriculo-cisternal perfusion and the superfusion of the left parietal cortex were started simultaneously (each 3 ml/h). After stabilisation for half an hour, 500 µl of arterial non-heparinised blood, taken from the femoral artery was injected into the white matter of the left frontal lobe using an infusion pump (10 ml/h). Immediately thereafter the edema markers Na^+-fluorescein (continuous infusion 1 ml/h b.w.) and Texas-Red-albumin (one bolus of 6 ml) were intravenously infused. CSF and blood samples were collected after induction of the hematoma every 30 min for 8 hours. The concentration of the edema markers in the cisternal and subarachnoid perfusates as well as in the blood samples was measured by fluorescence spectrophotometry (Fluorolite 1000, Dynatech, Denkendorf, Germany) using two different filter sets. The total amount of fluorescent markers in each sample was calculated with respect to the volume of the sample. The total amount of fluorescence markers in each sample was calculated by accumulation of the individual samples. The concentration of the fluorescent dyes in the blood was measured to check whether a constant level was attained by the intravenous infusion of the edema markers throughout the experiment. After termination of the experiment the animals were sacrificed by perfusion with 0.9% NaCl solution. The brain was carefully removed, and deep frozen (−80 °C) for later examination.

Results

Data are presented as mean ± SEM. The ICP equilibrated at 4.1 ± 1.3 mmHg in the low ICP group, at 9.7 ± 2.2 mmHg in the moderate ICP group, and at 15.2 ± 3.8 mmHg in the group with high ICP (Table 1). In all groups Na^+-fluorescein started to accumulate at 60 min in the subarachnoid space, while at 90 min in the ventricular system. In the low-pressure group Na^+-fluorescein (mean ± SEM) amounted to 1.47 ± 0.42 nmol in the ventricular system as compared to 1.34 ± 0.41 nmol in the moderate and 0.38 ± 0.11 nmol in the high-ICP group. In the subarachnoid space the marker accumulated to 1.96 ± 0.57 nmol, 4.15 ± 1.28 nmol, or 0.96 ± 0.32 nmol, respectively (Table 1). The high-molecular weight marker Texas-Red-albumin could not be detected in the subarachnoid space or in the ventricular system. The concentration of both fluorescent dyes in the blood remained stable at 0.36 ± 0.1 mmol/l for Na^+-fluorescein and 0.24 ± 0.4 µmol/l for Texas-Red-albumin throughout the experiment.

Discussion

For the present study we have developed a new model to assess quantitatively the reabsorption of vasogenic brain edema fluid into the subarachnoid space and the ventricular system following intracerebral hemorrhage with special consideration of the influence of different intracranial pressure levels. The model is based on previous studies on infusion of edema fluid as described by Uhl *et al.* [5] and was modified for stereotactic induction of an intracerebral hematoma. Fluorescent markers of different molecular weight and different excitation- and emission spectra served as edema markers and indicators of blood-brain barrier damage. In accordance with Ohata and Marmarou [3] and Wrba *et al.* [6] the results confirm that vasogenic brain edema is cleared via both CSF compartments. In contrast to the results of Wrba *et al.* [6], however, resorption of edema fluid occurred to a higher extent into the subarachnoid space in the current experiments on intracerebral hemorrhage. Most likely this might be attributed to the different distances between the lesion and the reabsorption site. Furthermore, only the small-molecular weight marker Na^+-fluorescein was recovered in the samples collected by ventricular perfusion or superfusion of the brain surface, whereas the high-molecular marker Texas-Red albumin could not be detected. This may indicate that intracerebral hemorrhage opens the blood-brain barrier for small molecules only – at least during the first

Table 1. *Recovery of i.v. Administered Na^+-Fluorescein of Animals with Low (2–5 mmHg, n = 10), Moderate (8–12 mmHg, n = 10) or High (14–20 mmHg, n = 5) Intracranial Pressure (ICP) in the Subarachnoid Space (SAS) or Ventricular System (VS). The Marker is Given as the Accumulated Total Amount [nmol] Found at the Given Time of Sampling (Mean ± SEM)*

ICP-level	Recovery [nmol]	Time					
		60 min	120 min	210 min	300 min	390 min	480 min
Low	SAS	0.06 ± 0.03	0.39 ± 0.18	0.89 ± 0.30	1.33 ± 0.39	1.72 ± 0.49	1.96 ± 0.57
	VS	0.00 ± 0.00	0.27 ± 0.19	0.53 ± 0.23	0.83 ± 0.28	1.18 ± 0.35	1.47 ± 0.42
Moderate	SAS	0.04 ± 0.02	0.40 ± 0.11	1.33 ± 0.35	2.33 ± 0.65	3.44 ± 1.02	4.15 ± 1.28
	VS	0.00 ± 0.00	0.14 ± 0.06	0.45 ± 0.15	0.78 ± 0.24	1.10 ± 0.36	1.34 ± 0.41
High	SAS	0.03 ± 0.01	0.29 ± 0.12	0.63 ± 0.22	0.81 ± 0.23	0.91 ± 0.28	0.96 ± 0.32
	VS	0.00 ± 0.00	0.10 ± 0.01	0.25 ± 0.05	0.35 ± 0.08	0.35 ± 0.11	0.38 ± 0.11

hours after bleeding. Finally, we had expected to observe a similar correlation between the resolution of the vasogenic brain edema into the CSF-compartments and the actual ICP-level as shown in the edema infusion model [6]. Yet, the current results show that edema reabsorption was at maximum in the moderate ICP group when studying clearance into the subarachnoid space. The degree of edema resorption into the ventricles was similar in animals with low or moderately increased ICP. Nevertheless, clearance of edema fluid fell to a minimum in animals with the highest ICP. While the present data are preliminary and the study is not yet completed, we conclude that under clinical conditions a lower intracranial pressure facilitates resolution of vasogenic brain edema, while intracranial hypertension impedes this potentially lifesaving mechanism.

Acknowledgment

This work was supported by the "BMBF-Verbund 'Neurotrauma' Munich", FKZ01K09704.

References

1. Klatzo I, Miquel J, Otenasek R (1962) The application of fluorescein labeled serum proteins (FLSP) to the study of vascular permeability in the brain. Acta Neuropathol 2: 144–160
2. Marmarou A, Hochwald G, Nakamura T, Tanaka K, Weaver J, Dunbar J (1944) Brain edema resolution by CSF pathways and brain vasculature in cats. Am J Physiol 267: H514–520
3. Ohata K, Marmarou A (1992) Clearance of brain edema and macromolecules through the cortical extracellular space. J Neurosurg 77: 387–396
4. Reulen HJ, Tsuyumu M, Tack A, Fenske AR, Prioleau GR (1978) Clearance of edema fluid into cerebrospinal fluid. A mechanism for resolution of vasogenic brain edema. J Neurosurg 48: 754–764
5. Uhl E, Wrba E, Nehring V, Chang RCC, Baethmann A, Reulen H-J (1999) Technical note: A new model for quantitative analysis of brain edema resolution into the ventricles and the subarachnoid space. Acta Neurochir (Wien) 141: 89–92
6. Wrba, E, Nehring V, Baethmann A, Reulen HJ, Uhl E (1998) Resolution of experimental vasogenic brain edema at different intracranial pressures. Acta Neurochir [Suppl] (Wien) 71: 313–315

Correspondence: Eberhard Uhl, M.D., Department of Neurosurgery, Klinikum Großhadern, Ludwig-Maximilians-University, Marchioninistr. 15, 81377 Munich, Germany.

Acta Neurochir (2000) [Suppl] 76: 501–505

Induction of Colligin may Attenuate Brain Edema Following Intracerebral Hemorrhage

G. Xi, Y. Hua, R. F. Keep, and **J. T. Hoff**

Department of Surgery (Neurosurgery), University of Michigan, Ann Arbor, MI, USA

Summary

Brain edema plays an important role in the secondary brain injury following intracerebral hemorrhage (ICH). Edema formation after ICH has been linked to thrombin toxicity. Therefore, the induction of endogenous serine protease inhibitors, which inhibit thrombin prior to ICH may limit edema formation. This study examines whether injection of a low dose of thrombin upregulates such inhibitors and induces tolerance to subsequent ICH. Rats received intracerebral infusions of either one unit thrombin or saline into the right caudate nucleus. After seven days, the rats were either (A) used to examine colligin (a serine protease inhibitor) induction by Western blot analysis, immunohistochemistry and immunofluoresent double labeling, (B) to determine brain water content, or (C) they received a second injection of 50 μL blood and brain edema was determined one day later. Intracerebral infusion of thrombin caused a marked upregulation of colligin, a serine protease inhibitor, in the ipsilateral basal ganglia. Immunocytochemistry and immunofluorescent double labeling showed that colligin was induced in astrocytes. Infusion of this dose of thrombin alone did not affect brain water content but it significantly attenuated subsequent ICH-induced brain edema (79.0 ± 0.5 vs. $81.4 \pm 0.9\%$, $P < 0.01$). Our results demonstrate that low doses of thrombin upregulate brain colligin levels and attenuate edema formation induced by ICH.

Keywords: Brain edema; intracerebral hemorrhage; colligin; thrombin.

Introduction

Intracerebral hemorrhage (ICH) is a common and often fatal subtype of stroke and may produce severe neurologic deficits in survivors [9]. Although death may occur acutely after an ICH, delayed neurologic deterioration, which may be related to brain edema formation, often occurs in patients with large hematomas. At present, there is no effective treatment that improves long-term outcome in ICH. We have demonstrated that thrombin, a serine protease and an essential component in the coagulation cascade, is responsible for early brain edema formation after ICH [14, 15, 29]. In addition, direct intracerebral thrombin infusion causes inflammation and gliosis in rat brain [20]. However, we have found that intracerebral injections of a low dose of thrombin (thrombin preconditioning, TPC) can reduce the edema formation from a subsequent injection of a large dose of thrombin given 7 days later [28]. This study is part of an examination of whether the low dose of thrombin might be upregulating serine protease inhibitors (serpins) in the brain. Serpins are a superfamily of proteins which inhibit serine proteases such as thrombin. This study focuses on colligin, a collagen binding serpin which was first found in parietal endoderm cells [11] and then detected as glycoprotein 46 (gp46) in myoblasts [2] and as heat shock protein 47 (HSP47) in chick fibroblasts [18]. Colligin localizes in the lumen of the endoplasmic reticulum [8] and is induced in microglia and astrocytes after cerebral ischemia [7] and subarachnoid hemorrhage [24]. In this study, we examined whether intracerebral injection of thrombin upregulates colligin, and whether such induction of colligin prior to ICH may reduce ICH-induced brain edema.

Materials and Methods

Animal Preparation and Experimental Protocols

Adult male Sprague-Dawley rats (Charles River Laboratories, Portage, MI) weighing 300–400 g were used for all experiments. Rats were anesthetized with sodium pentobarbital (40 mg/kg, i.p.). The right femoral artery was catheterized for blood gases, blood pressure, blood glucose and hematocrit monitoring. Rat rectal temperature was maintained at 37.5 °C using a feedback-controlled heating pad. Thrombin, autologous blood or saline was infused stereotactically into the right basal ganglia (coordinates: 0.2 mm anterior, 5.5 mm ventral and 4 mm lateral to the bregma) at a rate of 10 μL/min with the use of a microinfusion pump (Harvard Apparatus Inc.).

Rats received intracerebral infusions of either one unit thrombin or the same volume of saline in right basal ganglia or no infusion and were used for a three part study seven days later. In the first part, the rat brain was used to examine colligin induction with Western blot analysis, immunohistochemistry and immunofluorescent double labeling; in the second part, brain was sampled for brain edema determination; and in the third part, rats received a second infusion of 50 μL autologous blood after 7 days and brain water and ion contents were measured 24 hours later.

Brain Water, Sodium, and Potassium Content Measurements

Brain water and ion contents were performed as described in our previous studies [27, 29]. Briefly, brain samples were weighed using and electronic analytical balance and dried at 100 °C for 24 hours in a gravity oven. Water contents were expressed as a percentage of wet weight. The brain water content was calculated as (Wet Weight–Dry Weight)/Wet Weight. The dehydrated samples were digested in 1 mL of 1 mol/L nitric acid and brain sodium and potassium contents were measured with a flame photometer seven days later. Sodium and potassium ion contents were expressed in milliequivalents per kilogram of dry brain tissue (mEq/kg dry wt).

Western Blot Analysis

Rats were anesthetized with pentobarbital (60 mg/kg, i.p.) and underwent intracardiac perfusion with saline. A coronal brain slice (≈3 mm thick) 4 mm from the frontal pole was obtained and the brain slice was dissected into four samples (ipsilateral cortex, ipsilateral basal ganglia, contralateral cortex and contralateral basal ganglia). Western blot analysis was performed as described previously [28]. Briefly, the protein was run on SDS-PAGE gel and transferred to hybond-C pure nitrocellulose membrane (Amersham). The membranes were probed with mouse anti-colligin monoclonal antibody (StressGen) followed by peroxidase-linked anti-mouse Ig G antibody (Amersham). Finally, the antigen-antibody complexes were visualized with the ECL chemiluminescence system (Amersham) and exposed to Kodak X-OMAT film. The relative densities of the protein bands were analyzed with a public domain NIH Image program (NIH Image Version 1.61).

Immunohistochemistry for Colligin

Rats were anesthetized with pentobarbital (60 mg/kg, i.p.) and perfused with 4% paraformaldehyde in 0.1 M pH 7.4 phosphate-buffered saline (PBS). Removed brains were kept in 4% paraformaldehyde for six hours, then immersed in 25% sucrose for three to four days at 4 °C. The brains were embedded in O.C.T compound (Sakura Finetek U.S.A Inc.) and sectioned on a cryostat (18 μm thick). Sections were incubated overnight with 1:800 dilution of mouse anti-colligin monoclonal antibody. Normal mouse IgG was used as a negative control. After three washes in PBS, sections were incubated for 90 min with 1:1000 dilution of biotinylated second antibody. After another three PBS washes, brain sections were incubated with avidin-biotinylated horseradish peroxidase (Vector Laboratories) for 90 min. Brain sections were re-washed three times in PBS and then incubated with diaminobenzidine and hydrogen peroxide (Stable DAB, Research Genetics, Inc.). The sections were then washed in water for five minutes, dehydrated and covered with a coverslip for microphotography.

Immunofluorescent Double Labeling

Mouse anti-colligin or goat anti-glial fibrillary acidic protein (GFAP) antibody (Chemicon, 1:100 dilution) was incubated overnight at 4 °C. Fluorescein isothiocyanate (FITC) or rhodamine labeled second antibody was incubated with sections for 2 hours at room temperature. The double labeling was analyzed by a fluorescence microscope (Nikon Microphoto-SA) using a rhodamine filter and a FITC filter.

Statistical Analysis

All data in this study are shown as mean ± SD and analyzed by ANOVA with a Scheffe's multiple comparisons test. Differences are considered significant at the $p < 0.05$ level.

Results

Physiological variables (blood gases, blood pH, blood glucose, mean arterial blood pressure and hematocrit) were measured at the time of intracerebral infusion. There were no significant differences among groups.

Western Blot Analysis for Colligin

Western blot analysis showed that colligin immunoreactivities were increased significantly in the ipsilateral basal ganglia after intracerebral infusion of one unit thrombin (12-fold increase versus uninjected normal rats and 4-fold increase versus saline-injected controls; Fig. 1a). No colligin immunoreactivity was detected in the contralateral basal ganglia by Western blotting. No marked upregulation of colligin immunoreactivity was found by Western blot analysis in either the ipsilateral or contralateral cortices.

Brain Water, Sodium and Potassium Ion Contents

Rats received either no injection (normal controls) or intracerebral infusions of either 50 μL saline (saline controls) or one unit thrombin (thrombin preconditioning, TPC) into right caudate nucleus. After seven days, the rats received a second injection of 50 μL autologous blood and brain water, sodium ion and potassium ion contents were determined 24 hours later. Thrombin preconditioning, which markedly upregulates colligin in the brain, significantly attenuated brain edema formation ipsilateral basal ganglia 24 hours after intracerebral hemorrhage (Fig. 1b). Attenuations of brain edema after ICH by thrombin pretreatment were associated with reductions of sodium ion accumulation (214 ± 5 *versus* 333 ± 19 mEq/kg dry wt. in normal control, $p < 0.01$). No

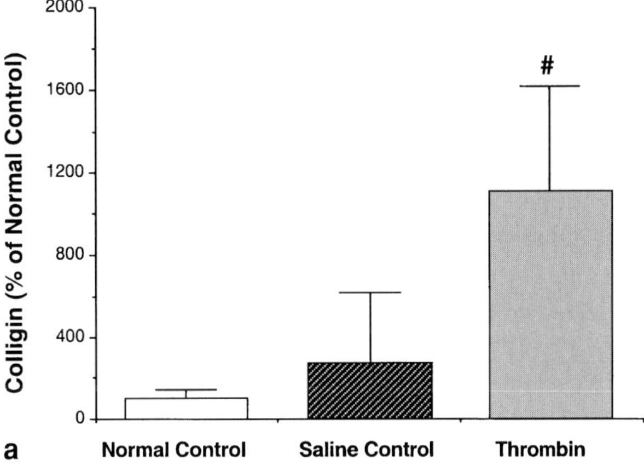

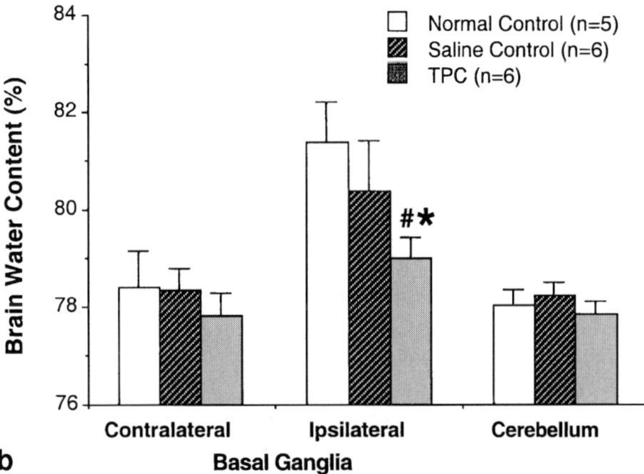

Fig. 1. Colligin upregulation and ICH-induced brain edema. (a) Colligin immunoreactivity (Western blot analysis) in ipsilateral basal ganglia 7 days after intracerebral infusion of either 50 μL saline or 50 μL thrombin (one unit, n = 3). Normal rat brain was used as normal control. Values shown are mean ± SD. # $p < 0.01$ vs. other groups. (b) Brain water contents 24 hours after intracerebral infusion of 50 μL autologous blood. The brains had been infused with either nothing (normal controls), 50 μL saline (saline controls) or 1 unit thrombin (50 μL, thrombin preconditioning, TPC) seven days before the blood infusion. Values are expressed as means ± SD, * $p < 0.05$ versus saline control. # $p < 0.01$ versus normal control

significant potassium loss was found in all three groups.

Immunohistochemistry and Immunofluorescent Double Labeling

Intracerebral infusion of thrombin induced colligin immunoreactivity in the brain. Immunohistochemistry showed that colligin immunoreactivity was induced in ipsilateral basal ganglia seven day after thrombin pretreatment. Only a few colligin positive cells were found in ipsilateral cortex. Most of the colligin immunoreactivity appeared to be found in glia (Fig. 2a). No colligin immunoreactivity was detected in the contralateral basal ganglia and cortex (Fig. 2b). Immunofluorescent double labeling confirmed that colligin positive cells were astrocytes, i.e. they were also GFAP positive.

Discussion

The present study shows that colligin is an inducible serine protease inhibitor in the brain and that upregulation of colligin is associated with attenuation of brain edema formation after ICH. These results suggest that induction of brain serine protease inhibitors such as colligin may reduce ICH-induced brain edema.

Thrombin is a serine protease formed immediately around a hematoma after ICH and has been linked to brain edema formation [14, 15, 29]. The concentration of prothrombin in plasma is about 1 to 5 μM and a 50-μL clot can produce 8 to 10 units thrombin. This suggests thrombin concentrations could reach very high levels around a hematoma or after severe blood-brain barrier breakdown. Thrombin-induced brain edema results partly from a direct opening of the blood-brain

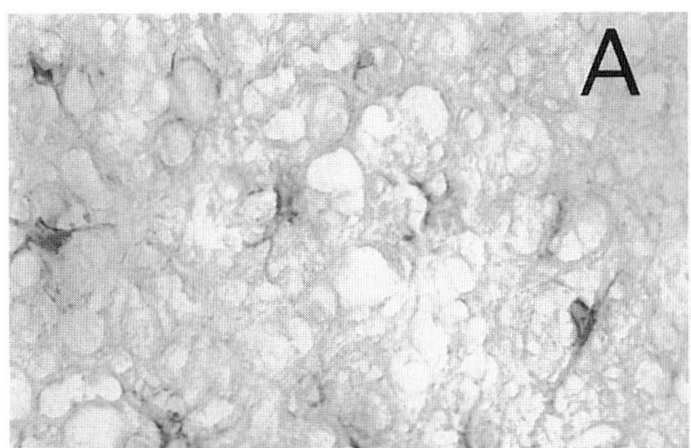

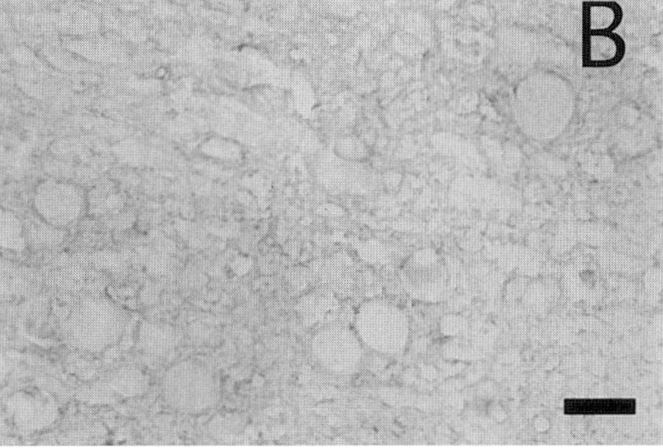

Fig. 2. Colligin immunoreactivities seven days after thrombin preconditioning (one unit thrombin intracerebral infusion) in the rat caudate nucleus. (A) Ipsilateral caudate nucleus. (B) Contralateral caudate nucleus. Scale bar is 20 μm

barrier [16] and disruption of the blood-brain barrier may in turn cause more thrombin production.

The mechanisms of colligin upregulation attenuating ICH-induced brain edema are unclear. Colligin expression may directly or indirectly inhibit the effects of thrombin. Colligin, one of the serpins, may directly inhibit thrombin (a serine protease). The sequence of colligin is about 25% identical to that of protease nexin-1 (PN-1, a major thrombin inhibitor in the brain). On the other hand, the effects of colligin against thrombin may develop through restructuring the extracellular matrix rather than direct protease inhibition. Colligin is an essential factor for procollagen formation in the endoplasmic reticulum and prevents abnormal procollagen secretion [17]. Procollagen is secreted to the extracellular space and forms collagen, a primary component of extracellular matrix. The extracellular matrix has been suggested as an important factor that regulates thrombin toxicity [4]. In vitro, cells attached to an extracellular matrix were not killed by thrombin, but cells not attached to an extracellular matrix died with the same concentration of thrombin [4].

Thrombin-induced colligin upregulation may be related to thrombin receptor activation. Carney and Cunningham identified thrombin receptors on cell surfaces in 1978 [1]. The thrombin receptor cDNA was cloned in 1991 [22, 25]. Based on these studies, we know that thrombin receptor is a seven transmembrane G protein-coupled receptor that is activated by proteolytic cleavage rather than by ligand binding. Three protease-activated receptors (PARs), PAR-1, PAR-3 and PAR-4, have been identified as thrombin receptors [3, 5]. Thrombin receptor-activated peptides are able to mimic many cellular activities of thrombin and expression of thrombin receptor mRNA is found in neurons and astrocytes [19, 26].

We find that colligin is induced in glia by thrombin pretreatment (Fig. 2). That astrocytes can produce colligin has been confirmed by immunofluorescent double labeling. Colligin induction in glia and tolerance to edema in the brain indicate cellular interactions may be important factors in brain tolerance. Plumier *et al.* has suggested that astrocytes may be involved in neuroprotection [21]. Astrocytes protect neurons from hydrogen peroxide-induced death [6], regulate extracellular pH and potassium ion concentration in the brain [13] and maintain glutathione level in neurons [23]. Largo *et al.* found that glia dysfunction may cause neuronal death in the ischemic penumbra [12]. Furthermore, cortical spreading depression by the application of potassium chloride induced ischemic tolerance [10] and expression of heat shock protein in astrocytes [21].

In conclusion, our study shows induction of colligin, an endogenous serine protease inhibitor, attenuates ICH-induced brain edema. We suggest that colligin upregulation which reduces perihematomal edema may be related to direct or indirect thrombin inhibition.

Acknowledgment

This work was supported by grant NS-17760 from the National Institutes of Health.

Reference

1. Carney DH, Cunningham DD (1978) Role of specific cell surface receptors in thrombin-stimulated cell division. Cell 15: 1341–1349
2. Cates GA, Brickenden AM, Sanwal BD (1984) Possible involvement of a cell surface glycoprotein in the differentiation of skeletal myoblasts. J Biol Chem 259: 2646–2650
3. Chinni C, de Niese MR, Tew DJ, Jenkins AL, Bottomley SP, Mackie EJ (1999) Thrombin, a survival factor for cultured myoblasts. J Biol Chem 274: 9169–9174
4. Cunningham DD, Donovan FM (1997) Regulation of neurons and astrocytes by thrombin and protease nexin-1. Relationship to brain injury. Adv Exp Med Biol 425: 67–75
5. Dery O, Corvera CU, Steinhoff M, Bunnett NW (1998) Proteinase-activated receptors: novel mechanisms of signaling by serine proteases. Am J Physiol 274: C1429–1452
6. Desagher S, Glowinski J, Premont J (1996) Astrocytes protect neurons from hydrogen peroxide toxicity. J Neurosci 16: 2553–2562
7. Higashi T, Takechi H, Uemura Y, Kikuchi H, Nagata K (1994) Differential induction of mRNA species encoding several classes of stress proteins following focal cerebral ischemia in rats. Brain Res 650: 239–248
8. Hughes RC, Taylor A, Sage H, Hogan BL (1987) Distinct patterns of glycosylation of colligin, a collagen-binding glycoprotein, and SPARC (osteonectin), a secreted Ca^{2+}-binding glycoprotein. Evidence for the localisation of colligin in the endoplasmic reticulum. Eur J Biochem 163: 57–65
9. Kase CS, Caplan LR (1994) Intracerebral hemorrhage. Butterworth-Heinemann, Boston
10. Kobayashi S, Harris VA, Welsh FA (1995) Spreading depression induces tolerance of cortical neurons to ischemia in rat brain. J Cereb Blood Flow Metab 15: 721–727
11. Kurkinen M, Taylor A, Garrels JI, Hogan BL (1984) Cell surface-associated proteins which bind native type IV collagen or gelatin. J Biol Chem 259: 5915–5922
12. Largo C, Cuevas P, Herreras O (1996) Is glia disfunction the initial cause of neuronal death in ischemic penumbra? Neurol Res 18: 445–448
13. Largo C, Cuevas P, Somjen GG, Martin del Rio R, Herreras O (1996) The effect of depressing glial function in rat brain in situ on ion homeostasis, synaptic transmission, and neuron survival. J Neurosci 16: 1219–1229

14. Lee KR, Betz AL, Kim S, Keep RF, Hoff JT (1996) The role of the coagulation cascade in brain edema formation after intracerebral hemorrhage. Acta Neurochir (Wien) 138: 396–400
15. Lee KR, Colon GP, Betz AL, Keep RF, Kim S, Hoff JT (1996) Edema from intracerebral hemorrhage: the role of thrombin. J Neurosurg 84: 91–96
16. Lee KR, Kawai N, Kim S, Sagher O, Hoff JT (1997) Mechanisms of edema formation after intracerebral hemorrhage: effects of thrombin on cerebral blood flow, blood-brain barrier permeability, and cell survival in a rat model. J Neurosurg 86: 272–278
17. Nagata K (1996) Hsp47: a collagen-specific molecular chaperone. TIBS 21: 22–26
18. Nagata K, Yamada KM (1986) Phosphorylation and transformation sensitivity of a major collagen-binding protein of fibroblasts. J Biol Chem 261: 7531–7536
19. Niclou S, Suidan HS, Brown-Luedi M, Monard D (1994) Expression of the thrombin receptor mRNA in rat brain. Cell Mol Biol 40: 421–428
20. Nishino A, Suzuki M, Ohtani H, Motohashi O, Umezawa K, Nagura H, Yoshimoto T (1993) Thrombin may contribute to the pathophysiology of central nervous system injury. J Neurotrauma 10: 167–179
21. Plumier JC, David JC, Robertson HA, Currie RW (1997) Cortical application of potassium chloride induces the low-molecular weight heat shock protein (Hsp27) in astrocytes. J Cereb Blood Flow Metab 17: 781–790
22. Rasmussen UB, Vouret-Craviari V, Jallat S, Schlesinger Y, Pages G, Pavirani A, Lecocq JP, Pouyssegur J, Van Obberghen-Schilling E (1991) cDNA cloning and expression of a hamster alpha-thrombin receptor coupled to Ca^{2+} mobilization. FEBS Lett 288: 123–128
23. Sagara JI, Miura K, Bannai S (1993) Maintenance of neuronal glutathione by glial cells. J Neurochem 61: 1672–1676
24. Turner CP, Panter SS, Sharp FR (1999) Anti-oxidants prevent focal rat brain injury as assessed by induction of heat shock proteins (HSP70, HO-1/HSP32, HSP47) following subarachnoid injections of lysed blood. Mol Brain Res 65: 87–102
25. Vu TK, Hung DT, Wheaton VI, Coughlin SR (1991) Molecular cloning of a functional thrombin receptor reveals a novel proteolytic mechanism of receptor activation. Cell 64: 1057–1068
26. Weinstein JR, Gold SJ, Cunningham DD, Gall CM (1995) Cellular localization of thrombin receptor mRNA in rat brain: expression by mesencephalic dopaminergic neurons and codistribution with prothrombin mRNA. J Neurosci 15: 2906–2919
27. Xi G, Keep RF, Hoff JT (1998) Erythrocytes and delayed brain edema formation following intracerebral hemorrhage in rats. J Neurosurg 89: 991–996
28. Xi G, Keep RF, Hua Y, Xiang JM, Hoff JT (1999) Attenuation of thrombin-induced brain edema by cerebral thrombin preconditioning. Stroke 30: 1247–1255
29. Xi G, Wagner KR, Keep RF, Hua Y, de Courten-Myers GM, Broderick JP, Brott TG, Hoff JT (1998) The role of blood clot formation on early edema development following experimental intracerebral hemorrhage. Stroke 29: 2580–2586

Correspondence: Guohua Xi, M.D., R5550 Kresge I, University of Michigan, Ann Arbor, Michigan 48109-0532, USA.

Acta Neurochir (2000) [Suppl] 76: 507–510

Oxyhemoglobin Produces Necrosis in Cultured Smooth Muscle Cells

K. Ogihara, A. Y. Zubkov, A. D. Parent, and **J. H. Zhang**

Department of Neurosurgery University of Mississippi Medical Center, Jackson, Mississippi

Summary

Object. Myonecrosis in the tunica media, which is defined morphologically, is one of the most striking alterations in the cerebral arterial wall following subarachnoid hemorrhage (SAH). In this study, oxyhemoglobin (OxyHb) was added to cultured rat aortic smooth muscle cells to determine the pattern of cell death by morphological and biochemical techniques.

Methods. Confluent rat aortic smooth muscle cells were treated with OxyHb in a concentration- and time-dependent manner. Cell density was assayed by counting the number of cells that attached to the culture dishes after exposed to OxyHb. To identify cell death pattern, DNA analysis, electron microscopy, and Western blotting using poly (ADP-ribose) polymerase (PARP) antibody were performed.

Conclusions. OxyHb decreased cell density in a concentration- and time-dependent manner. DNA analysis showed a smear pattern characteristic of cell necrosis. Transmission electron microscopy demonstrated disintegration of cell membrane and destruction of cell organelles. No apoptotic changes, such as condensation of chromatin or apoptotic bodies were observed. Western blotting using PARP antibody revealed that 116 kDa PARP was not cleaved to 85 kDa, an apoptosis-related fragment. These results demonstrated morphologically and biochemically that OxyHb induced necrosis, not apoptosis, in cultured smooth muscle cells.

Keywords: Necrosis; oxyhemoglobin; smooth muscle cell; vasospasm.

Introduction

The pathophysiology of cerebral vasospasm following subarachnoid hemorrhage (SAH) is unclear, in spite of the intensive clinical and experimental investigations in the past years. Morphological changes after SAH in human or in animal cerebral arteries include necrotic changes in smooth muscle cells in cerebral arteries demonstrated by intracytoplasmic vacuoles and dense bodies, degeneration of mitochondria, condensed lysosomes, dissolution of nuclear substance, and appearance of cell debris [1].

Although multiple factors are proposed to be involved in cerebral vasospasm, oxyhemoglobin (OxyHb), the main component of erythrocytes, is probably the principal causative agent [4, 6]. OxyHb produced not only progressive cell contraction but also ultrastructural changes resembling myonecrosis in cultured aortic smooth muscle cells [2]. The mechanism of smooth muscle cell death induced by oxyhemoglobin, however, remains a matter of discussion. Recent investigation showed apoptosis, as an important factor of atherosclerosis, restenosis, and hypertension, was induced by free radical in cultured smooth muscle cells [3]. The purpose of this study was to investigate the pattern of cell death induced by OxyHb in cultured rat aortic smooth muscle cells by using not only morphological but also biochemical techniques, such as DNA analysis and Western blotting using poly (ADP-ribose) polymerase (PARP) antibody.

Materials and Methods

Cell Culture

Rat aortic smooth cells were kindly provided by Drs. Corinne Gajdusek and Marc R. Mayberg (University of Washington, Seattle, Washington). Cells were cultured in Waymouth's MB 752/1 Medium supplemented with 100 units/ml penicillin, 100 μg/ml streptomycin, and 10% fetal bovine serum (FBS). Cultures were incubated at 37 °C in 5% CO_2. In this study, cells were used from passages 5–10.

Preparation of OxyHb

OxyHb was prepared as described previously [5].

Cell Density Study

The cytotoxic effect of OxyHb was determined by measuring the cell density [11].

Analysis of DNA-Fragmentation (DNA Ladder)

DNA-fragmentation analysis was assessed following modifications of previously described methods [12].

Transmission Electron Microscopy

Confluent smooth muscle cells (100 mm dish) were incubated with 100 μM OxyHb or saline in serum free media for 24 hours. The cells were then scraped and collected by centrifugation at 500× g for 5 minutes at 4 °C. The cells were fixed with 2.5% gluteraldehyde in 0.1 M Na phosphate buffer pH 7.4, dehydrated in graded ethanol and embedded in Epon. Ultrathin sections were stained with uranyl acetate and lead citrate and examined with transmission electron microscopy (LEO 906, LEO, Thornwood, NY).

Western Blotting

Western blotting was performed following modifications of previously described methods [1].

Data Analysis

Data are expressed as mean ± SD. Statistical differences between the control and other groups were compared using one-way analysis of variance (ANOVA) and Scheffé's method (95% lower and upper confidence interval) if significant variance was found. A value of $P < 0.05$ was considered statistically significant.

Results

Cell Density

OxyHb produced a decrease in cell density in a concentration- and time-dependent manner in cultured smooth muscle cells. Although the cell density did not change in serum free medium within 24 hours (data not shown), to evaluate the possibility that serum free conditions may damage DNA, we used 24 hours saline treated cells as a control. OxyHb (100 μM), after 24 hours incubation, reduced significantly ($p < 0.05$) the number of cells attached to the culture dishes. Lower concentration of OxyHb failed to reduce markedly the cell adherence in 24 hours.

DNA Analysis

DNA analysis showed nondescript smear pattern characteristic of necrosis in smooth muscle cells induced by OxyHb. There was no ladder pattern of DNA fragments, which is a biochemical hallmark of apoptosis, in any kind of treatments. The effect of OxyHb-induced DNA degradation was in a dose-dependent, but not in a time-dependent fashion. Time course study revealed that 100 μM of OxyHb induced DNA degradation within 3 hours, and further incubation (6, 12, and 24) with 100 μM of OxyHb did not increase DNA degradation.

Transmission Electron Microscopy

As shown in Fig. 1, ultrastructural analysis of smooth muscle cells incubated with OxyHb (100 μM)

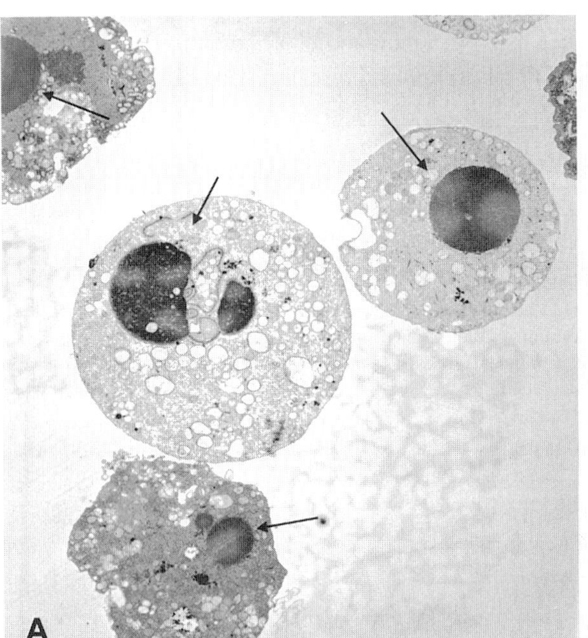

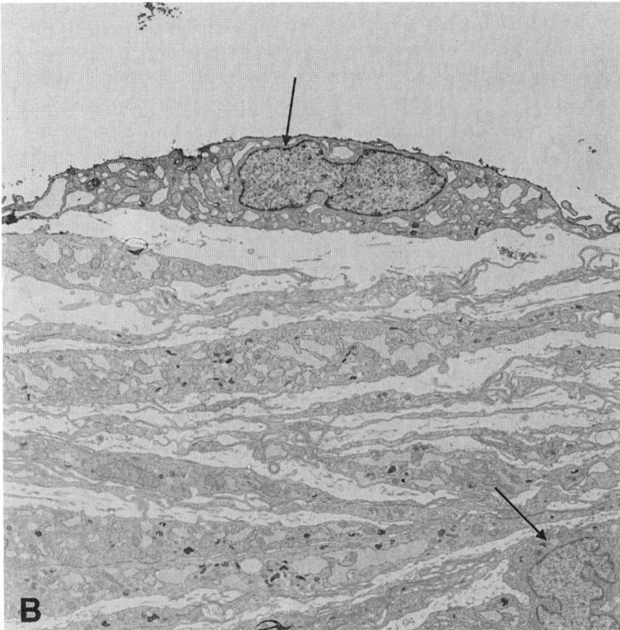

Fig. 1. Ultrastructural analysis of smooth muscle cells incubated with OxyHb (100 μM) for 24 hours revealed morphologic changes of smooth muscle cells. (A) Endothelial cells treated with oxyhemoglobin demonstrated condensation of chromatin (arrows), condensation of cytoplasm, vacuolization of cytoplasm. (B) In smooth muscle cells oxyhemoglobin caused necrotic changes, characterized by cell swelling, disintegration of cellular membranes, without condensation of chromatin (arrows)

for 24 hours revealed morphologic changes. Endothelial cells treated with oxyhemoglobin showed characteristic apoptotic changes (Fig. 1A). In contrast, OxyHb induced irregularity, or disintegration, of plasma and nuclear membrane and loss of complex internal structure (Fig. 1B). We did not observe typical apoptotic changes, such as condensation of nuclei or apoptotic body.[17]

Western Blotting

Cleavage of PARP from the native 116 kDa to 85 kDa is now widely accepted as a biochemical hallmark of apoptosis. Strong 116 kDa bands were observed in both OxyHb treatment and saline treatment in smooth muscle cells, although there were very weak 85 kDa bands in both lanes. Cleavage from 116 kDa to 85 kDa was not observed after cells were exposed to OxyHb (100 μM) for 24 hours.

Discussion

The present studies demonstrate 1) OxyHb induced a concentration- and time-dependent decrease in cell density. 2) DNA analysis showed nondescript smear pattern characteristics of necrosis induced by OxyHb. The effect of OxyHb-induced DNA degradation was in a dose-dependent, but not in a time-dependent fashion. 3) OxyHb induced irregularity, or disintegration, of plasma and nuclear membrane and loss of complex internal structure 4) OxyHb did not induce PARP clevage. These results show morphological, and biochemical evidence of necrosis, not apoptosis, induced by OxyHb in cultured rat aortic smooth muscle cells.

Detachment of endothelial cells and necrotic changes in the smooth muscle cells of the tunica media are the most striking histological alterations after SAH [1]. OxyHb, the main component of erythrocytes, produced direct cytotoxicity in smooth muscle or endothelial cells. In feline cerebral arteries, OxyHb caused myonecrosis, transformation of nerve endings, invasion of myointimal cells into the tunica intima, changes in endothelial cell basement membrane, and the detachment of endothelial cells [8]. In a double SAH model, the number of smooth muscle cells on the crossline of the coronal section in canine basilar artery was significantly decreased (10.8 ± 1.9 to 7.6 ± 1.6 layers/tunica media) 14 days after the initial SAH [7] Our cell density study demonstrated 78% of cells attached after 24 hours incubation with 100 μM of OxyHb. The number of detached cells in our study was somewhat more than that was seen in an acute spastic artery from an animal model. This may be due to direct application of OxyHb to smooth muscle cells.

The mechanism of smooth muscle cell death induced by OxyHb remains a matter of discussion. OxyHb exerts its cytotoxic effect on freshly isolated rat basilar smooth muscle cells by generation of free radicals, chiefly hydroxyl radicals [10] So far, we do not have a good explanation for the different cell death pattern between their results and ours. It is possible that some unidentified factors other than free radical generation may play a role for necrosis induced by OxyHb in cultured smooth muscle cells.

DNA analysis demonstrated that 100 μM of OxyHb induced DNA degradation within 3 hours, and further incubation with 100 μM of OxyHb did not increase DNA degradation. Therefore, the substance responsible for toxic effect to DNA induced by OxyHb diminished within 3 hours in our experimental condition. It was reported that the content of OxyHb, which was prepared with the same method as ours, was shown to be rapidly reduced to approximately 10% at 3 hours [13] Repeated application of OxyHb may cause further cell death. However, enough smooth muscle cells in the spastic artery may survive to maintain arterial constriction, even though a high concentration of OxyHb (27.6 μM to 537 μM in CSF, 50 ± 20 μM in perivascular) is released continuously from subarachnoid blood clot in patients and animals with SAH [9]. These controversial findings require further investigation.

Conclusion

This study showed that necrosis induced by OxyHb was identified not only by morphological but also biochemical methods in cultured smooth muscle cells. The mechanism underlying necrosis in smooth muscle cells is unclear and needs further elucidation.

Acknowledgments

This work was supported in part by a grant-in-aid to J.H.Z. from the American Heart Association and the Robert R. Smith Fellowship at the University of Mississippi Medical Center to K.O. The authors thank Mr. Glenn Hoskins for the support in electron microscopy. Electron microscope (LEO 906) is supported by grants 1S10RR11321-01A1 from National Institutes of Health. The authors thank Drs. Corinne Gajdusek and Marc R. Mayberg for providing the cultured smooth muscle cells.

References

1. Findlay JM, Weir BK, Kanamaru K, Espinosa F (1989) Arterial wall changes in cerebral vasospasm. Neurosurgery 25: 736–745
2. Fujii S, Fujitsu K (1988) Experimental vasospasm in cultured arterial smooth-muscle cells. Part 1: contractile and ultrastructural changes caused by oxyhemoglobin. J Neurosurg 69: 92–97
3. Li PF, Dietz R, von Harsdorf R (1997) Differential effect of hydrogen peroxide and superoxide anion on apoptosis and proliferation of vascular smooth muscle cells. Circulation 96: 3602–3609
4. Macdonald RL, Weir BK (1991) A review of hemoglobin and the pathogenesis of cerebral vasospasm. Stroke 22: 971–982
5. Martin W, Villani GM, Jothianandan D, Furchgott RF (1985) Selective blockade of endothelium-dependent and glyceryl trinitrate-induced relaxation by hemoglobin and by methylene blue in the rabbit aorta. J Pharm Exp Ther 232: 708–716
6. Mayberg MR, Okada T, Bark DH (1990) The role of hemoglobin in arterial narrowing after subarachnoid hemorrhage. J Neurosurg 72: 634–640
7. Oka Y, Ohta S, Todo H, Kohno K, Kumon Y, Sakaki S (1996) Protein synthesis and immunoreactivities of contraction-related proteins in smooth muscle cells of canine basilar artery after experimental subarachnoid hemorrhage. J Cereb Blood Flow Metab 16: 1335–1344
8. Okada H, Endo S, Kamiyama K, Suzuki J (1980) Oxyhemoglobin-induced cerebral vasospasm and sequential changes of vascular ultrastructure. Neurol Med Chir 20: 573–582
9. Pluta RM, Afshar JK, Boock RJ, Oldfield EH (1998) Temporal changes in perivascular concentrations of oxyhemoglobin, deoxyhemoglobin, and methemoglobin after subarachnoid hemorrhage. J Neurosurg 88: 557–561
10. Steele JA, Stockbridge N, Maljkovic G, Weir B (1991) Free radicals mediate actions of oxyhemoglobin on cerebrovascular smooth muscle cells. Circ Res 68: 416–423
11. Takenaka K, Kassell NF, Foley PL, Lee KS (1993) Oxyhemoglobin-induced cytotoxicity and arachidonic acid release in cultured bovine endothelial cells. Stroke 24: 839–845
12. Tsukada T, Eguchi K, Migita K, Kawabe Y, Kawakami A, Matsuoka N, Takashima H, Mizokami A, Nagataki S (1995) Transforming growth factor beta 1 induces apoptotic cell death in cultured human umbilical vein endothelial cells with downregulated expression of bcl-2. Biochem Biophys Res Comm 210: 1076–1082
13. Yoshimoto Y, Kim P, Sasaki T, Kirino T, Takakura K (1995) Functional changes in cultured strips of canine cerebral arteries after prolonged exposure to oxyhemoglobin. J Neurosurg 83: 867–874

Correspondence: John H. Zhang, M.D., Ph.D., Department of Neurosurgery, University of Mississippi Medical Center, 2500 North State Street, Jackson, Mississippi 39216.

Acta Neurochir (2000) [Suppl] 76: 511–515

Thrombin Preconditioning, Heat Shock Proteins and Thrombin-Induced Brain Edema

G. Xi, R. F. Keep, Y. Hua, and **J. T. Hoff**

Department of Surgery (Neurosurgery), University of Michigan, Ann Arbor, MI, U.S.A.

Summary

Intracerebral injections of high concentrations of thrombin cause brain edema but, in vitro, low concentrations of thrombin may be neuroprotective. This study investigated whether a low dose of thrombin might induce tolerance to subsequent large doses of thrombin (thrombin preconditioning; TPC) in a manner analogous to ischemic preconditioning. The study involved five parts. The first tested the effect of intracerebral infusion of a small dose (1 U) of thrombin on brain water content. In the second part, the effect of such a small dose of thrombin on subsequent edema formation from a large dose of thrombin (5 U) was evaluated. The time course of TPC was examined in the third part. In the fourth part, heat shock protein (HSP) 27, HSP32 and HSP70 were quantitated by Western blotting analysis while the fifth identified the cell types expressing HSPs.

Injection of a low dose of thrombin alone did not cause brain edema. However, TPC significantly attenuated the edema induced by a subsequent injection of a large dose of thrombin. This effect of TPC was abolished by co-injection of a thrombin inhibitor, hirudin. The maximal effect of TPC on edema formation was seven days after pretretment. This time course was similar to that for a marked up-regulation in astrocytic HSP27. TPC also induced HSP32, but this effect occurred earlier than the effect on edema formation. TPC had no effect on HSP70. These results suggest that thrombin-induced brain tolerance may be related to HSP27 induction.

Keywords: Thrombin; brain edema; heat shock proteins (HSPs); preconditioning.

Introduction

Brain edema after intracerebral hemorrhage (ICH) exacerbates brain injury. The coagulation cascade, especially thrombin formation, plays an important role in brain edema formation after ICH [14, 23]. However, recent studies indicate that low concentrations of thrombin may actually protect neurons and astrocytes from cell death induced by hypoglycemia and 'ischemia' in vitro [19, 21].

The term ischemic preconditioning was first introduced by Murry *et al.* in 1986 [16]. They found brief episodes of ischemia (ischemic preconditioning) reduced infarct size by subsequent lethal ischemia in dog hearts (ischemic tolerance). Several years later, ischemic tolerance was found in the brain [10, 11]. As in ischemic preconditioning in the heart, there are two windows for preconditioning-induced tolerance in the brain, an immediate (minutes to hours) and a delayed (days) window. The mechanisms of induced ischemic tolerance are not well understood. One mechanism may be by induction of heat shock proteins (HSPs). These are a class of proteins induced by various stresses, such as hyperthermia, heavy metals, toxins, and ischemia. Mounting evidence suggests that HSPs protect the brain against a variety of harmful injuries [20].

In this study, we have examined whether cerebral thrombin preconditioning can attenuate thrombin-induced brain edema and whether thrombin-induced brain tolerance is associated the induction of HSPs.

Materials and Methods

Experimental Model and Groups. Male Sprague-Dawley rats (Charles River Laboratories), weighing among 300–400 g, were used in this study. Rats were anesthetized with pentobarbital (40 mg/kg, i.p.) and the right femoral artery was catheterized for blood pressure monitoring and blood sampling. Arterial blood was obtained for analysis of blood pH, blood gases, hematocrit and blood glucose. The rectal temperature was maintained at 37.5 °C using a feedback-controlled heating pad. Thrombin or saline was infused into the right caudate nucleus stereotactically at a rate of 10 μL/min through a 26-gauge needle (coordinates: 0.2 mm anterior, 5.5 mm ventral, and 4.0 mm lateral to the bregma) using a microinfusion pump. The needle was removed and the skin incision was closed with suture following infusion. This study was performed in five parts.

Part 1. This part examined whether intracerebral infusion of small dose thrombin induced brain edema. Three groups of five rats each were examined. In the first group, rats received 50-μL saline infusion. In the second and third groups, rats received 1 U rat thrombin

(Sigma) in 50 μL saline. Rats were sacrificed at 24 hours for the first and second group and at seven days for the third group to determine brain water and ion contents.

Part 2. In this part, three groups of five rats each were used to examine whether TPC reduced thrombin-induced brain edema. The first group had 50 μL saline infusion, the second group received 1 U thrombin in 50 μL saline and the third group had 1 U thrombin plus 1 U hirudin (Sigma) in 50 μL saline. Rats in these three groups received a second infusion (5 U thrombin in 50 μL saline) seven days later. Rats were killed 24 hours after the second infusion for brain water and ion content measurements.

Part 3. In this TPC time course study, five groups of five or six rats each were tested. The first group of rats had 5 U thrombin. Rats in the second to fifth group were pretreated with 1 U thrombin, then received a second infusion (5 U thrombin in 50 μL saline) at either 3, 7, 14 or 21 days later. All rats were killed 24 hours after the second infusion to determine brain water and ion contents.

Part 4. Six groups of three rats each in this part were used for Western blot analysis. The first group of rats received intracerebral infusion of 50 μL saline and were killed seven days later. The other groups received 1 U thrombin, then were killed at either 1, 3, 7, 14 or 21 days.

Part 5. Eight rats were used for immunohistochemistry and immunofluorescent double staining in this part. Rats had 1U thrombin ($n = 5$) or 50 μL saline ($n = 3$) intracerebral infusion and were killed seven days later.

Brain Water and Sodium Contents

Rats were killed under pentobarbital anesthesia (60 mg/kg). The brain was removed and a coronal brain slice (about 3-mm thick) was cut 4-mm from the frontal pole. The brain slice was divided into two hemispheres along the midline; each hemisphere was dissected into cortex and basal ganglia. The cerebellum was used as control. Brain samples were weighed and dried at 100 °C for 24 hours. Water contents were expressed as a percentage of wet weight [22]. Sodium contents were measured using by flame photometer and expressed in milliequivalents per kilogram of dehydrated brain tissue (mEq/kg dry wt).

Western Blotting Analysis

Rats were anesthetized and killed at different time points. Rats underwent intracardiac perfusion with saline and brain tissues were sampled as described in the preceding paragraph. For Western blot analysis, proteins were separated by SDS-PAGE gel and transferred to hybond-C pure nitrocellulose membrane (Amersham). The antigen-antibody complexes were visualized with the ECL chemiluminescence system (Amersham) and exposed to a Kodak X-OMAT film. The relative densities of HSP27 (also called HSP25 in mouse), HSP32 and HSP70 protein bands were analyzed with an image program (NIH Image Version 1.61). The primary antibodies (rabbit anti-mouse HSP25, rabbit anti-rat HSP32 and mouse anti-rat HSP70) were purchased from StressGen Biotechnologies Corp.

Immunohistochemistry and Immunofluorescent Double Labeling

Rats were anesthetized with pentobarbital (60 mg/kg, i.p.) and underwent intracardiac perfusion with 4% paraformaldehyde in 0.1 M pH 7.4 phosphate-buffered saline (PBS). Brain immunohistochemistry and immunofluorescent double labeling were performed on unfixed cryostat sections. For immunohistochemistry, four primary antibodies (rabbit anti-mouse HSP25, rabbit anti-rat HSP32, or mouse anti-rat HSP70, StressGen; goat anti-GFAP, Santa Cruz Biotech) were used.

Six combinations of primary antibodies were used for immunofluorescent double labeling: 1, 2) mouse anti-glial fibrillary acidic protein (GFAP) monoclonal antibody (Chemicon) and rabbit anti-Hsp25 or anti-HSP32 polyclonal antibody (StressGen); 3, 4) mouse anti-neuron specific enolase (NSE) monoclonal antibody (Chemicon) and rabbit anti-Hsp25 or anti-HSP32 antibody; 5, 6) mouse anti-rat OX-42 antibody (Serotec) and rabbit anti-Hsp25 or anti-HSP32 antibody. The immunofluorescent double labeling was examined by a fluorescence microscope (Nikon).

Statistical Analysis. Data from different groups in this study were presented as mean ± SD and were analyzed with analysis of variance (ANOVA) with a Scheffé F-test. Statistical significance was accepted at $p < 0.05$.

Results

Low dose thrombin and brain edema. Intracerebral infusion of 1 U of thrombin did not significantly affect brain water and ion contents at either one or seven days ($p > 0.05$). The water contents of the ipsilateral basal ganglia were 78.6 ± 0.3, 79.8 ± 1.3 and 78.7 ± 0.4% in one day saline control, one day 1 U thrombin and 7 days 1 U thrombin groups, respectively.

TPC and thrombin-induced brain edema. Large dose thrombin (5 U) infusion caused a marked increase of water content at 24 hours (84.0 ± 0.3 vs. 78.6 ± 0.3% in saline control, $p < 0.001$). Intracerebral infusion of 1 U thrombin (TPC) seven days prior to infusion of 5 U thrombin significantly reduced edema formation compared to a group in which saline was infused seven days prior to the 5 U of thrombin infusion (Fig. 1), it also significantly attenuated an increase in brain sodium content that occurs following 5 U of thrombin infusion ($p < 0.01$). The protective effect of TPC on brain edema and brain sodium was abolished by co-infusion of 1 U thrombin with 1 U of hirudin, a thrombin inhibitor (Fig. 1).

TPC time course. The optimal interval between TPC and the second thrombin (5 U) infusion for reducing the formation of brain edema was tested. Brain water and sodium contents were measured 24 hours after the second infusion following TPC and the second thrombin infusion intervals of 3, 7, 14, or 21 days. All these time intervals showed a protective effect on brain edema; the maximal protective interval was 7 days (brain water content 79.2 ± 0.4 and 82.6 ± 0.8% in TPC and saline control rats, respectively, $p < 0.001$).

Western blot analysis. The concentrations (density of protein band) of HSP27, HSP32 and HSP70 were semi-quantitated by Western blot seven days after intracerebral infusion of 1 U thrombin since our brain edema data showed this was the most effective interval for TPC. The concentrations of HSP27 and HSP32 in the ipsilateral basal ganglia were, respectively, about

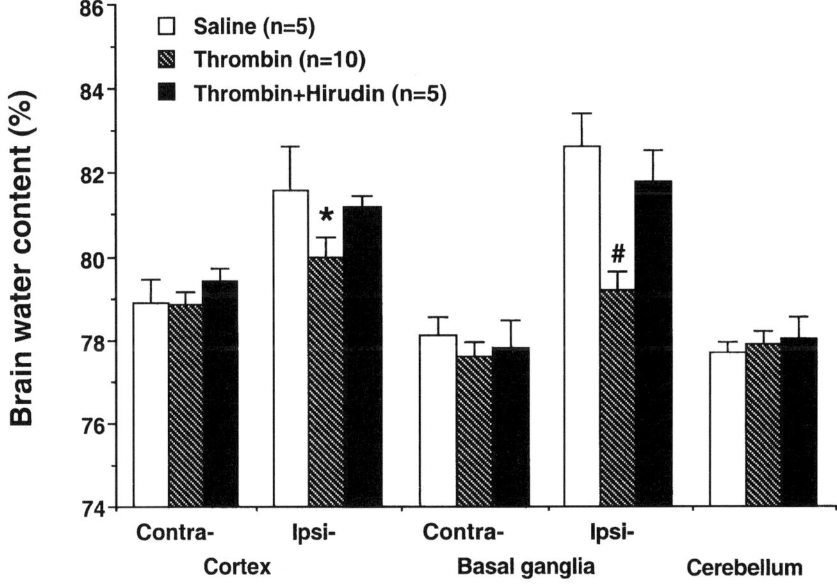

Fig. 1. Brain water contents 24 hours after intracerebral thrombin (5 U) infusion. The rat brains had been pretreated with either saline, 1 U thrombin or 1 U thrombin + 1 U hirudin seven days prior to 5 U thrombin infusion. Values are expressed as mean ± SD. *$p < 0.05$ vs. the other groups; #$p < 0.01$ vs. the other groups

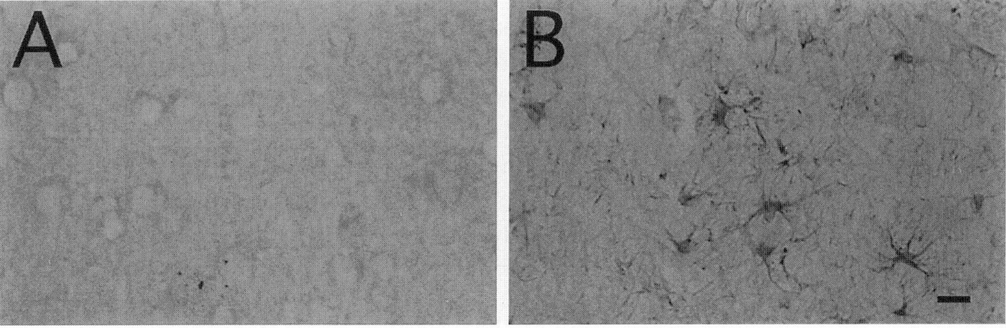

Fig. 2. HSP27 immunoreactivity in the caudate nucleus seven days after one unit thrombin pretreatment. (A) contralateral caudate nucleus. (B) ipsilateral caudate nucleus. Scale bar = 20 μm

10-fold and 3-fold higher than that of the control group. HSP70 was not detected. The time courses of HSP induction after TPC showed that HSP27 immunoreactivity increased gradually, reached a peak between 7 and 14 days (5-fold increase vs. the first day). In contrast to HSP27, HSP32 immunoreactivity reached a peak on the first day and then declined progressively. HSP70 was undetectable at any time point after TPC.

Immunohistochemistry and Immunofluorescent double labeling. Immunohistochemistry also demonstrated the induction of HSP27 and HSP32 immunoreactivity after TPC. Seven days after TPC, HSP27 immunoreactivity was observed in all ipsilateral basal ganglia, but was only observed in part of the ipsilateral cortex (Fig. 2B). HSP27 immunoreactivity was not observed in the contralateral hemisphere (Fig. 2A). HSP32 immunoreactivity was also detected in the ipsilateral and not the contralateral hemisphere. HSP70 immunoreactivity was only observed around the needle track. The morphological appearance of HSP27 and HSP32 positive cells was similar to that of astrocytes. In saline injection control rats, the immunoreactivities of HSP27, HSP32 and HSP70 were only detected around the needle track.

Seven days after TPC, we found that HSP27-positive cells in the ipsilateral caudate nucleus were also GFAP-positive. HSP32 immunoreactive cells were also GFAP positive using double staining. Neither neurons nor microglia were detected as HSP27-positive or HSP32-positive in the present study.

Discussion

This study demonstrates that an intracerebral injection of a low dose of thrombin can markedly reduce the edema formation that results from a subsequent injection of a large dose of thrombin. The most effective tolerance against thrombin-induced edema appears seven days after thrombin pretreatment. This time delay for tolerance induction suggests that new proteins may be synthesized. The HSP27 Western blot time course showed that the upregulation of HSP27 also reaches a peak about 7 to 14 days after TPC, suggesting that thrombin-induced tolerance is associated with HSP27 upregulation.

In a number of tissues, HSP27 confers protection against a variety of stresses such as heat shock [12]. The protective effects of HSP27 against heat shock [13] and oxidative stress [7] may be through stabilization of actin filaments. Such stabilization is related to activation of the p38 mitogen-activated protein kinase (p38 MAP kinase) signal transduction pathway that induces resistance to stress-induced actin fragmentation [7]. Activation of p38 MAP kinase activates MAP kinase-activated protein kinase 2 (MAPKAP kinase-2) which, in turn, causes HSP27 phosphorylation [6]. Heat shock protein 27 then modulates the cytoskeleton by altering actin dynamics.

There is evidence, in vitro, that thrombin modulates the cytoskeleton of astrocytes and neurons as demonstrated by changes in cell shape [3]. The regulation of actin filament dynamics by thrombin is abolished by SB203580 (a pyridinyl imidazole) that can inhibit p38 MAP kinase specifically. The actin cytoskeleton is necessary for thrombin-induced protection from hypoglycemia in astrocytes since cytochalasin D (an actin filament assembly inhibitor) can diminish thrombin-induced protection [4]. Moreover, thrombin can activate p38 MAP kinase [5] and MAPKAP kinase-2 [2]. These findings lead us to speculate that upregulation of HSP27, which is not detectable in normal adult rat cerebrum and cerebellum [18], may also participate in the protective effects of TPC in vivo by stabilizing actin.

We found that HSP27 immunoreactivity at seven days after TPC was related to increased GFAP immunoreactivity in the ipsilateral basal ganglia. Immunofluorescent double staining demonstrated that HSP27 positive cells were also GFAP positive. HSP27 expression in glial cells has been correlated with ischemic tolerance [9]. Recently, Plumier *et al.* [17] found that cortical application of potassium chloride triggered HSP27 in astrocytes suggesting that expression of HSP27 might increase resistance to ischemic injury. Furthermore, the overexpression of HSP27 through an adenovirus vector protests ischemic cardimyocyte injury, whereas lowering HSP27 with an adenoviral vectors expressing antisense HSP27 aggravates ischemic injury [15].

HSP32, also called heme oxygenase 1 (HO-1), is a stress protein and the rate-limiting enzyme in the heme degradative pathway. Recent studies suggest that HSP32 plays an important role in cytoprotection against oxidative injury as well as heme- and hemoglobin-induced toxicity [1]. Our present data show that intracerebral TPC induces HSP32 immunoreactivity. However, in contrast to HSP27, the time course for the upregulation of HSP32 (peak at the first day) is faster than our observed effects of TPC on edema formation (seven days).

Heat shock protein 70 expression may be responsible for ischemic tolerance through the preconditioning process [20]. Overexpression of HSP70 by gene transfer therapy protects the brain against injury induced by ischemia and systemic kainic acid administration induced seizure [24]. In addition, inhibition of HSP70 gene expression causes thermosensitivity [8]. Our Western blot analysis data, however, demonstrates that HSP70 induction did not occur at any time points in thrombin preconditioning. With immunohistochemistry, some HSP70 immunoreactive cells were found, but these were only localized around the needle track. Interestingly, Yoshida *et al.* [25] found that another form of pharmacological preconditioning, exposure of rabbit hearts to monophosphoryl lipid, also did not induce HSP70 expression.

In conclusion, our present study finds TPC attenuates thrombin-induced brain edema, which may be related to HSP27 expression.

Acknowledgment

This study was supported by grant NS-17760 from the National Institutes of Health.

References

1. Abraham NG, Lavrovsky Y, Schwartzman ML, Stoltz RA, Levere RD, Gerritsen ME, Shibahara S, Kappas A (1995) Transfection of the human heme oxygenase gene into rabbit coronary microvessel endothelial cells: protective effect against heme and hemoglobin toxicity. Proc Natl Acad Sci USA 92: 6798–6802
2. Brophy CM, Woodrum D, Dickinson M, Beall A (1998) Thrombin activates MAPKAP2 kinase in vascular smooth muscle. J Vascular Surg 27: 963–969
3. Cavanaugh KP, Gurwitz D, Cunningham DD, Bradshaw RA

(1990) Reciprocal modulation of astrocyte stellation by thrombin and protease nexin-1. J Neurochem 54: 1735–1743
4. Donovan FM, Cunningham DD (1998) Signaling pathways involved in thrombin-induced cell protection. J Biol Chem 273: 12746–12752
5. Guay J, Lambert H, Gingras-Breton G, Lavoie JN, Huot J, Landry J (1997) Regulation of actin filament dynamics by p38 map kinase-mediated phosphorylation of heat shock protein 27. J Cell Sci 110: 357–368
6. Huot J, Houle F, Marceau F, Landry J (1997) Oxidative stress-induced actin reorganization mediated by the p38 mitogen-activated protein kinase/heat shock protein 27 pathway in vascular endothelial cells. Circulation Res 80: 383–392
7. Huot J, Houle F, Spitz DR, Landry J (1996) HSP27 phosphorylation-mediated resistance against actin fragmentation and cell death induced by oxidative stress. Cancer Res 56: 273–279
8. Johnston RN, Kucey BL (1988) Competitive inhibition of hsp 70 gene expression causes thermosensitivity. Science 242: 1551–1554
9. Kato H, Liu Y, Kogure K, Kato K (1994) Induction of 27-kDa heat shock protein following cerebral ischemia in a rat model of ischemic tolerance. Brain Res 634: 235–244
10. Kirino T, Tsujita Y, Tamura A (1991) Induced tolerance to ischemia in gerbil hippocampal neurons. J Cereb Blood Flow Metab 11: 299–307
11. Kitagawa K, Matsumoto M, Tagaya M, Hata R, Ueda H, Niinobe M, Handa N, Fukunaga R, Kimura K, Mikoshiba K, *et al* (1990) 'Ischemic tolerance' phenomenon found in the brain. Brain Res 528: 21–24
12. Landry J, Chretien P, Lambert H, Hickey E, Weber LA (1989) Heat shock resistance conferred by expression of the human HSP27 gene in rodent cells. J Cell Biol 109: 7–15
13. Lavoie JN, Lambert H, Hickey E, Weber LA, Landry J (1995) Modulation of cellular thermoresistance and actin filamant stability accompanies phosphorylation-induced changes in the oligomeric structure of heat shock protein 27. Mol Cell Biol 15: 505–516
14. Lee KR, Colon GP, Betz AL, Keep RF, Kim S, Hoff JT (1996) Edema from intracerebral hemorrhage: the role of thrombin. J Neurosurg 84: 91–96
15. Martin JL, Mestril R, Hilal-Dandan R, Brunton LL, Dillmann WH (1997) Small heat shock proteins and protection against ischemic injury in cardiac myocytes. Circulation 96: 4343–4348
16. Murry CE, Jennings RB, Reimer KA (1986) Preconditioning with ischemia: a delay of lethal cell injury in ischemic myocardium. Circulation 74: 1124–1136
17. Plumier JC, David JC, Robertson HA, Currie RW (1997) Cortical application of potassium chloride induces the low-molecular weight heat shock protein (Hsp27) in astrocytes. J Cereb Blood Flow Metab 17: 781–790
18. Plumier JC, Hopkins DA, Robertson HA, Currie RW (1997) Constitutive expression of the 27-kDa heat shock protein (Hsp27) in sensory and motor neurons of the rat nervous system. J Comp Neurol 384: 409–428
19. Reiser G, Breder J, Reymann KG, Striggow F (1998) The protease thrombin is involved in neuroprotection again ischemia-induced cell death. Soc Neurosci Abstr 24: 2144
20. Sharp FR, Massa SM, Swanson RA (1999) Heat-shock protein protection. TINS 22: 97–99
21. Vaughan PJ, Pike CJ, Cotman CW, Cunningham DD (1995) Thrombin receptor activation protects neurons and astrocytes from cell death produced by environmental insults. J Neurosci 15: 5389–5401
22. Xi G, Keep RF, Hoff JT (1998) Erythrocytes and delayed brain edema formation following intracerebral hemorrhage in rats. J Neurosurg 89: 991–996
23. Xi G, Wagner KR, Keep RF, Hua Y, de Courten-Myers GM, Broderick JP, Brott TG, Hoff JT (1998) The role of blood clot formation on early edema development following experimental intracerebral hemorrhage. Stroke 29: 2580–2586
24. Yenari MA, Fink SL, Sun GH, Chang LK, Patel MK, Kunis DM, Onley D, Ho DY, Sapolsky RM, Steinberg GK (1998) Gene therapy with HSP72 is neuroprotective in rat models of stroke and epilepsy. Ann Neurol 44: 584–591
25. Yoshida K, Maaieh MM, Shipley JB, Doloresco M, Bernardo NL, Qian YZ, Elliott GT, Kukreja RC (1996) Monophosphoryl lipid A induces pharmacologic 'preconditioning' in rabbit hearts without concomitant expression of 70-kDa heat shock protein. Mol Cell Biochem 159: 73–80

Correspondence: Guohua Xi, M.D. R5550 Kresge I, University of Michigan, Ann Arbor, Michigan 48109-0532 U.S.A.

Acta Neurochir (2000) [Suppl] 76: 517–520

Changes in Cerebral Blood Flow as Measured by HMPAO SPECT in Patients Following Spontaneous Intracerebral Haemorrhage

M. S. Siddique[1], **H. M. Fernandes**[1], **N. U. Arene**[1], **T. D. Wooldridge**[1], **J. D. Fenwick**[2], and **A. D. Mendelow**[1]

[1] Department of Surgery (Neurosurgery), University of Newcastle, Newcastle-upon-Tyne, UK
[2] Regional Medical Physics Department, Newcastle General Hospital, Newcastle-upon-Tyne, UK

Summary

Lack of an effective treatment for spontaneous intracerebral haemorrhage (ICH) is partly because the mechanism of neuronal damage in ICH is not fully understood. Animal experiments have shown that there is a zone of ischaemia and oedema around the haematoma which can be reduced by early evacuation of the mass lesion. We set out to study Cerebral Blood Flow (CBF) changes in patients with ICH. We present data on 13 patients (mean age 60). SPECT scans were performed within 48 hours of ictus and 4–7 days later. Four patients had surgical evacuation of the clot; 9 were managed conservatively. The ratio of uptake of the isotope in the cerebral hemisphere containing the haematoma to the isotope uptake in the contra-lateral (un-affected) cerebral hemisphere was taken as an index of perfusion of the affected cerebral hemisphere. The perfusion index of the affected hemisphere improved between the first and the second scans in all the surgically treated patients; in the conservatively managed group, it was worse in 6 patients, the same in 1 and very slightly better in 2. There was an overall mean improvement of 3.87% in the surgical group, and an overall mean deterioration of 3.61% in the medical group. This data suggests that surgical evacuation of the clot may improve perfusion in the ipsilateral cerebral hemisphere in ICH. It underlines the importance of a prospective randomised trial to assess the value of surgery in patients with ICH. The Surgical Trial in Intracerebral Haemorrhage (STICH) is currently underway worldwide. We also describe the application of Difference Based Region Growing (DBRG) to SPECT image analysis. This method overcomes the difficulties posed by 1) the presence of a mass lesion and 2) surgical evacuation of haematoma.

Keywords: Intracerebral haemorrhage; Cerebral Blood Flow; Penumbra; Surgery.

Introduction

Spontaneous Intracerebral Haemorrhage (ICH) accounts for about 10–30% of all strokes [2, 10] but has the highest mortality of all stroke sub-types. Some 62% of patients die and up to a half of the survivors are left severely disabled [1, 3, 7, 8]. Despite the enormous evolution of medical knowledge and the growing recognition of "Evidence Based Medicine", the treatment of intracerebral haemorrhage, at the turn of the millennium remains anecdotal and inconsistent [11]. At present, we do not know of any medical or surgical intervention that could save the enormous amount of brain surrounding an intracerebral bleed that is initially possibly viable but is eventually destroyed in the course of the illness.

An important reason for this unsatisfactory situation is a poor understanding of the underlying mechanism of neurological damage in this illness.

Animal models of intracerebral haemorrhage have shown that blood is irritating to the parenchyma, and that there is an area of oedema, ischaemia and haemorrhagic necrosis at the margin of the clot (ischaemic penumbra) [4, 5]. The volume of this ischaemic brain may exceed the volume of the haemorrhage several times. Experimental studies in animals have suggested that early removal of the mass lesion can reduce the ischaemic damage [12].

We set out to study the changes in cerebral blood flow (CBF) in human ICH, with particular reference to the region surrounding the haematoma by means of ^{99m}Technetium hexamethyl propylene amine oxime (^{99m}Tc-HMPAO) (Amersham International plc) Single Photon Emission Computed Tomography (SPECT).

Materials and Methods

We report data from thirteen patients admitted to the Neurosurgical Unit at Newcastle General Hospital with spontaneous supratentorial ICH. Patients with underlying vascular abnormalities

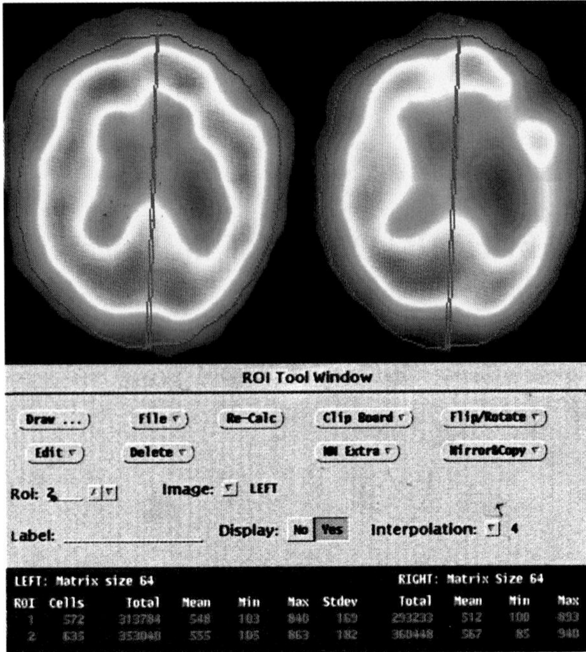

Fig. 1. Drawing regions of interest around each hemisphere. The axial slices with the largest defect from a patient with a left hemisphere clot, managed conservatively. The scan on the left is the earlier one. Visual inspection suggests deterioration in the perfusion of the left hemisphere with time. This is confirmed by the isotope counts calculated by the computer software

were not included. There were 8 males and 5 females. The median age of the group was 60. CBF was studied in these patients by performing ^{99m}Tc-HMPAO SPECT scans. These scans were performed twice during the course of the illness. The first scan was performed within 48 hours of ictus. The second scan was performed 4 to 7 days later. Some of these patients were randomised in the Surgical Trial in Intracerebral Haemorrhage (STICH). Four patients underwent surgical evacuation of their clots. Nine were managed conservatively. In the case of surgically treated patients, the second scans were post-operative.

SPECT Methodology

500 MBq of ^{99m}Tc-HMPAO was injected approximately 10 minutes prior to acquisition of data. Data was acquired by means of IGE CamStar single head gamma camera, with high resolution collimator. Data was processed on a Hermes Nuclear Diagnostics workstation. The axial slice showing the maximal deficit on the initial scan and the corresponding slice on the second scan were chosen for comparison in all cases. Regions of Interest (ROI) were drawn around each cerebral hemisphere separately (Fig. 1). The isotope count in each ROI was accurately calculated by the computer software. The ratio of uptake of the isotope in the cerebral hemisphere containing the haematoma to the isotope uptake in the contra-lateral (un-affected) cerebral hemisphere was taken as an index of perfusion of the affected cerebral hemisphere.

Hemisphere Perfusion Index

$$= \frac{\text{Isotope count in the affected cerebral hemisphere}}{\text{Isotope count in the un-affected cerebral hemisphere}} \times 100$$

Table 1. *Results*

Hemisphere Perfusion Index of the affected hemisphere			
Surgical patients		Medical patients	
First scan	Second scan	First scan	Second scan
91.3	94.7	89.4	90.4
97.8	98.0	84.4	81.7
91.7	100.0	97.2	97.6
93.3	95.6	96.8	81.2
		92.1	83.3
		98.6	98.6
		98.9	97.6
		98.2	94.9
		92.0	91.6
MEAN = 93.5	MEAN = 97.1	MEAN = 94.2	MEAN = 90.8

Results

Patients were divided into two groups; those managed conservatively and those treated surgically. Data for the two groups was analysed separately. The Hemisphere Perfusion Index (HPI) of the affected hemisphere in the initial and subsequent scans is given for all patients in Table 1. These results are plotted in the form of a line chart in Fig. 2. The perfusion index of the hemisphere containing the haematoma was higher in the second scan compared to the first scan in all the surgically treated patients; in the conservatively managed group, it was worse in 6 patients, the same in 1 and very slightly better in 2. There was an overall mean improvement of 3.87% in the perfusion index of

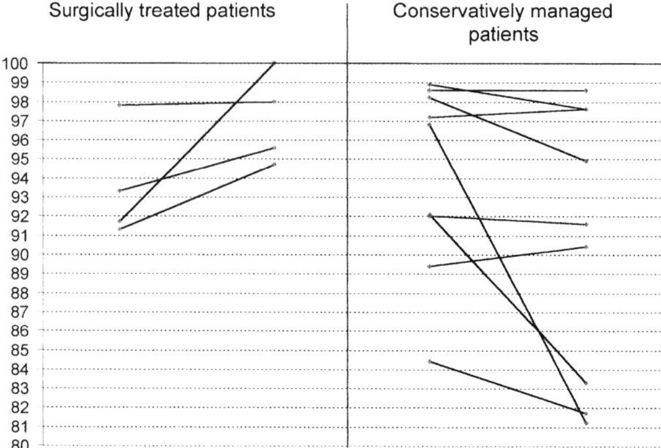

Fig. 2. Results. The hemisphere perfusion index of the affected hemisphere from all the scans plotted in the form of a line chart. The trend of improvement in the surgical group and deterioration in the medical group between the first and the second scans is obvious

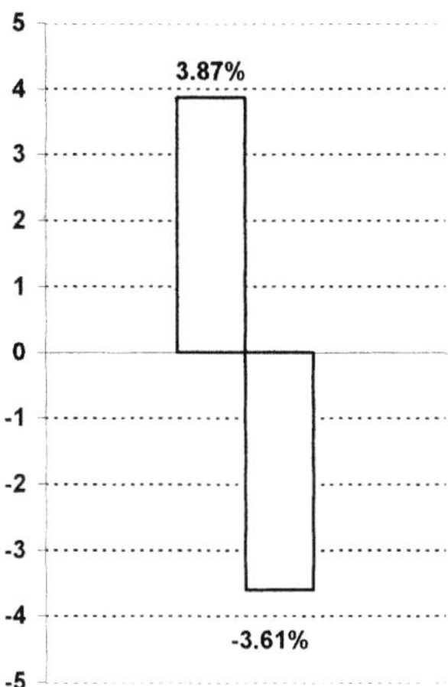

Fig. 3. Results. Mean Overall % change in the perfusion index of the affected hemisphere between the first and second scans in the two groups. 3.87% improvement in the surgical group and 3.61% deterioration in the medical group

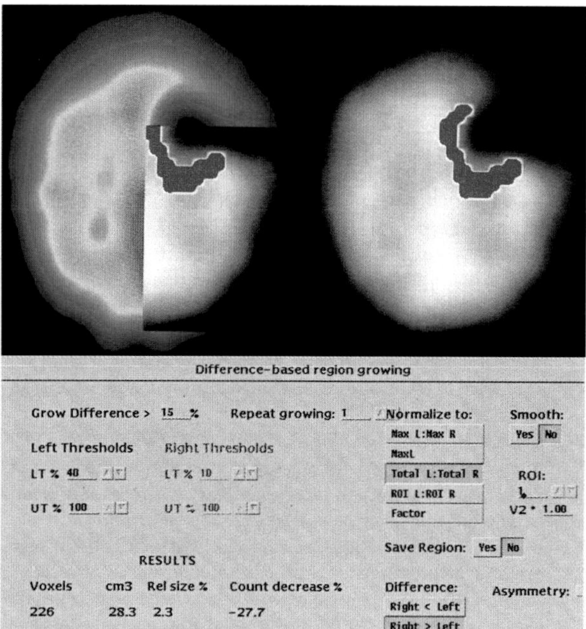

Fig. 4. Difference based region growing. Axial slices from the pre (left) and post-operative (right) scans of a patient who had her left hemisphere clot evacuated surgically. The volume of brain which is receiving at least 15% more isotope on the post-op scan compared with the pre-op scan has been calculated (28.3 cm^3). Areas of brain taking up less than 40% isotope have been excluded from analysis. This excludes the haematoma and all CSF spaces

the affected hemisphere in the surgical group, whereas in the conservative management group there was an overall mean deterioration of 3.61% (Fig. 3).

Discussion

This data suggests that surgical evacuation of the clot may improve perfusion in the ipsilateral cerebral hemisphere in ICH. This finding is in keeping with the results of animal experiments [4, 5]. It underlines the importance of a prospective randomised trial to assess the value of surgery in patients with ICH (STICH).

The images obtained with SPECT are relative and there is no generally accepted method of obtaining quantitative cerebral blood flow values [9, 13]. Analysis of SPECT data is usually performed by comparison of isotope uptake in a region of interest (ROI) against counts either in the cerebellum [6, 13] or other parts of the brain [13]. The presence of space occupying lesions (e.g. ICH) complicates this form of quantitative analysis because of midline shift and distortion of intracranial anatomy [13]. We applied Difference Based Region Growing (DBRG) (Hermes, Nuclear Diagnostics) to serial SPECT image analysis in patients with ICH. This method overcomes the difficulties posed by the presence of a mass lesion and defines the zone of perilesional ischaemia in a manner which is quantifiable, consistent and reproducible (Fig. 4). In comparing two temporally separated scans in the same patient, it is possible to measure volumes of brain which may be taking up more or less isotope by a percentage that can be specified. In addition the defect caused by the clot, the ventricles and other CSF spaces can be excluded from analysis by specifying a threshold of isotope uptake. All areas on the scan absorbing isotope below that threshold are excluded from the analysis. It thus makes it easier to compare scans from patients whose clots may have been removed to those who are managed conservatively and the clot is still physically present in the subsequent scans. We believe that this method of SPECT image analysis can enhance our understanding of the pathophysiology and natural history of this devastating illness. In addition, it may be helpful in assessing the efficacy of any therapeutic interventions aimed at reducing the neurological damage caused by ICH.

Acknowledgments

This work was made possible by the financial support of The Stroke Association and The Medical Research Council (MRC) UK.

References

1. Anderson CS, Jamrozik KD, Burvill PW, Chakera TM, Johnson GA, Stuart-Wynne EG (1993) Determining the incidence of different subtypes of stroke: results from the Perth Community Stroke Study, 1989–1990. Med J Austral 158: 85–89
2. Anonymous (1993) Epidemiology of cerebrovascular disease in Korea – A Collaborative Study, 1989–1990. Korean Neurological Association. J Korean Med Sci 8: 281–289
3. Bamford J, Sandercock P, Dennis M, Burn J, Warlow C (1990) A prospective study of acute cerebrovascular disease in the community: the Oxfordshire Community Stroke Project – 1981–86. 2. Incidence, case fatality rates and overall outcome at one year of cerebral infarction, primary intracerebral and subarachnoid haemorrhage. J Neurol Neurosurg Psychiatry 53: 16–22
4. Bullock R, Mendelow AD, Teasdale GM, Graham DI (1984) Intracranial haemorrhage induced at arterial pressure in the rat. Part 1: description of technique, ICP changes and neuropathological findings. Neurol Res 6: 184–188
5. Bullock R, Brock-Utne J, van Dellen J, Blake G (1988) Intracerebral hemorrhage in a primate model: effect on regional cerebral blood flow. Surg Neurol 29: 101–107
6. Costa DC, Ell PJ (1991) Brain blood flow in neurology and psychiatry. Churchill Livingstone, Edinburgh London Melbourne New York, pp 39–51
7. Coull BM, Brockschmidt JK, Howard G, Becker C, Yatsu FM, Toole JF, Mcleroy KR, Feibel J(1990) Community hospital-based stroke programs in North Carolina, Oregon, and New York. IV. Stroke diagnosis and its relation to demographics, risk factors, and clinical status after stroke. Stroke 21: 867–873
8. Fogelholm R, Nuutila M, Vuorela AL (1992) Primary intracerebral haemorrhage in the Jyvaskyla region, central Finland, 1985–89: incidence, case fatality rate, and functional outcome. J Neurol Neurosurg Psychiatry 55: 546–552
9. Friedman AH, Drayer BP, Jaszczak RJ (1996) Single photon tomography, 2nd eds. McGraw-Hill Health Professions Division, New York, pp 271–273
10. Klimo H, Kaste M, Halita M (1997) Greenfield's Neuropathology, 6th edn. Arnold, London Sydney Auckland, pp 321
11. Masdeu JC, Rubino FA (1984) Management of lobar intracerebral haemorrhage: medical or surgical. Neurology 34: 381–383
12. Nehls DG, Mendelow AD, Graham DI Teasdale GM (1990) Experimental intracerebral hemorrhage: early removal of a spontaneous mass lesion improves late outcome. Neurosurgery 27: 674–682
13. Wyper DJ (1993) Functional neuroimaging with single photon emission computed tomography (SPECT). Cerebrovasc Brain Metabolism Rev 5: 199–217

Correspondence: Prof. A. D. Mendelow, Departments of Neurosurgery, Regional Neurosciences Centre, Newcastle General Hospital, Newcastle upon Tyne, NE4 6BE UK.

Acta Neurochir (2000) [Suppl] 76: 521–522

Surgical Trial in Intracerebral Haemorrhage (S.T.I.C.H)

A. D. Mendelow on behalf of the investigators

Department of Surgery (Neurosurgery), University of Newcastle, England, UK

Summary

The International Surgical Trial in Intracerebral haemorrhage has been set up to determine the role of surgery in spontaneous supratentorial intracerebral haemorrhage. This is an interim report as the results will remain blinded until all patients have been recruited and followed up.

Keywords: Intracerebral haemorrhage; stroke; surgery; craniotomy.

Introduction

There is clinical uncertainty about the need for surgical evacuation of spontaneous supratentorial intracerebral haemorrhage (ICH). Previous trials have yielded conflicting results. Meta-analysis of existing trials has revealed that there is no significant benefit from surgery [1]. Two subsequent trials have also failed to reveal a conclusive result one way or the other [2, 3]. Experimental studies have shown that removal of a mass lesion designed to simulate a haematoma resulted in less ischaemic neuronal damage and a smaller volume of ischaemic tissue [4]. Clinical studies with Single Photon Emission Tomography (SPECT) in patients with ICH have confirmed some of these experimental findings in that the area of ischaemia is much larger than the haematoma itself [5]. There are some clear-cut reasons for operation: for example, a young patient with a superficial right-sided lobar haematoma who deteriorates from an initially orientated state of consciousness would need surgery in the opinion of most UK neurosurgeons [6]. There are also some patients where most neurosurgeons would agree that no operation is required either because the patient is too ill or because he or she is too well. There are patients between these limits in whom there is uncertainty about the need for surgery. This uncertainty creates the circumstances for undertaking another formal randomised controlled trial with sufficient power to resolve the issue.

The Trial

The STICH trial has set out to discover if "early surgical removal" of the clot is better than "initial conservative treatment". The trial was funded by the UK Stroke Association initially and is now funded by the Medical Research Council. The power calculations indicate that a total of 1000 patients will be required allowing for cross-overs which occur most frequently from the "initially conservative group" to later surgery. The primary outcome measure is the Glasgow Outcome Score at 6 months using a postal questionnaire. Other secondary outcome measures include the modified Rankin Score, the Barthel index, mortality, length of hospital stay and an economic analysis.

Progress to Date

So far (August 1999) there have been 208 patients randomised from 65 Centres. Recruitment will continue until the target has been reached or until the Data Monitoring and Ethics committee stop the trial because one group is doing significantly better than the other. Analysis of pooled results has indicated that the randomised patients have a median age of 63 years and that there are more males than females. The majority are randomised within the first 24 hours of ictus and that the Glasgow Coma Score ranges between 5 and 15 with half of the patients being greater than 10. Preliminary analysis of the pooled data has revealed that the number of patients with a "favourable outcome" on

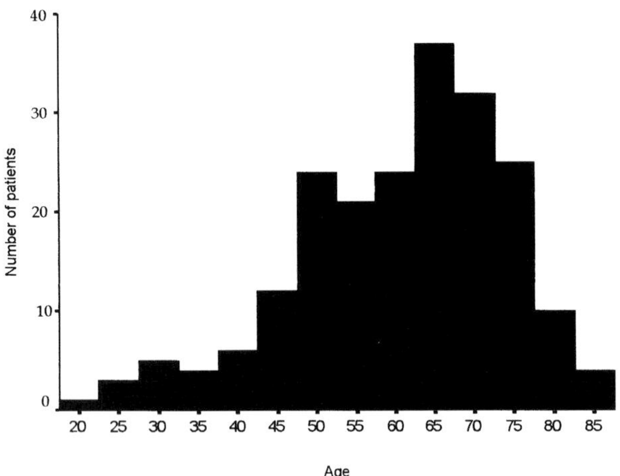

Fig. 1. Age of randomised patients

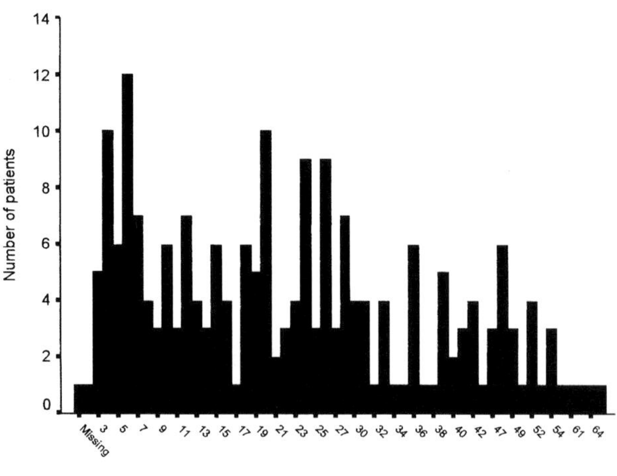

Fig. 3. Time from ictus to randomisation

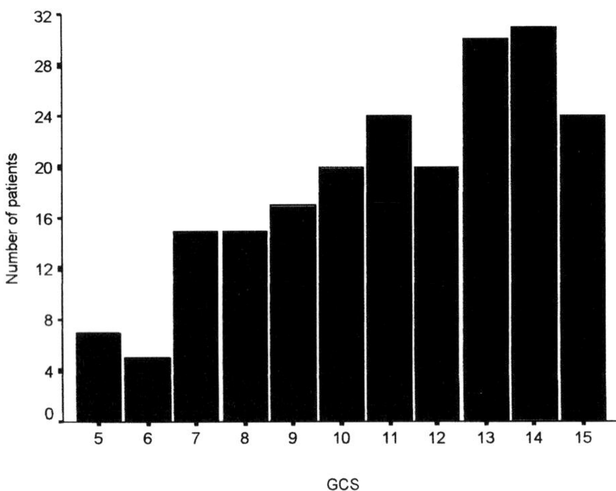

Fig. 2. Glasgow Coma Score in randomised patients

the Glasgow Outcome Scale is less than 15%. If this trend continues, then the power calculations may need to be revised. Active recruitment is continuing.

Contact with the STICH group in Newcastle can be made through STICH@ncl.ac.uk.

References

1. Hankey GJ, Hon C (1997) Intracerebral haemorrhage. Stroke 28: 2126–2132
2. Chen X, Yang H, Cheng Z (1992) The comparative study of the total medical and surgical treatment of hypertensive intracerebral haemorrhage. Acta Acad Med Shanghai 19: 234–240
3. Morgenstern LB, Frankowski RF, Shadden P, Pasteur W, Grotta JC (1998) Surgical treatment for intracerebral hemorrhage (STICH). Neurol 58: 1359–1363
4. Nehls DG, Mendelow AD, Graham DI, Teasdale GM (1990) Experimental intracerebral hemorrhage – early removal of a spontaneous mass lesion improves late outcome. Neurosurgery 674–682
5. Siddique, Mendelow AD (1999) SPECT in ICH. Acta Neurochir (Wien) (in press)
6. Fernandes H, Mendelow A (1997) Spontaneous intracerebral haemorrhage: a snapshot of UK Neurosurgical Management. Br J Neurosurg 11–464

Correspondence: A. D. Mendelow on behalf of the investigators, Department of Surgery (Neurosurgery), University of Newcastle, England, UK.

Thermal Effects

This section addresses the response of the nervous system to changes in temperature. The effect of hyperthermic injuries on the brain is discussed by Sharma *et al.* They address the effects of selective alteration of calcitonin gene related peptide (CGRP) following hyperthermia. Heat stress has the ability to influence this gene related peptide immunoreactivity and the distribution of the peptide is somehow associated with the molecular mechanisms of thermal information that occur with heat stress. The authors discuss the significance of these findings and their application to the clinical setting. The documentation that histamine is involved in the pathophysiology of heat stress and induces brain dysfunction is further demonstrated by these authors when they analyse the effects of heat stress by blocking histamine H-2 receptors. The effect of hypothermia on the brain is discussed as well. Nago *et al.* present the protective effects of mild hypothermia on symptomatic vasospasm in the clinical setting. They report a favourable outcome in some patients with the employment of mild hypothermia (brain temperature of 32–34 C). The implications of this with reference to creating a window in treatment to employ other forms of therapy are discussed by the authors. To analyse the effect at a cellular level of hypothermia, Nimasu *et al.* discuss the effects of post ischemic hypothermia on apoptotic cell death in transient focal ischemia models. By employing an experimental model, the authors demonstrate reduced numbers of apoptotic cells in the animals submitted to post ischemic hypothermia.

The protective potential of moderate hypothermia, confirmed by a host of studies on brain trauma and ischaemia, was assessed by Mueller *et al.* as to whether it interferes with cell volume control, or glial swelling, respectively from lactacidosis, or cytotoxic mediator agents. Surprisingly, mild and moderate hypothermia (32 deg., 27 deg. C) itself led to swelling of glial cells invitro, which could be prevented by omission of Na+-ions from the medium, or attenuated by blocking of the Na+/H+-antiporter. Moreover, hypothermia did not afford protection against the acidosis-, arachidonic acid-, or glutamate-induced cell swelling. It was, therefore, concluded that neuroprotection by hypothermia can obviously not be attributed to an inhibition of cytotoxic brain oedema.

Acta Neurochir (2000) [Suppl] 76: 525–527

Postischemic Hypothermia Attenuates Apoptotic Cell Death in Transient Focal Ischemia in Rats

J. Inamasu, S. Suga, S. Sato, T. Horiguchi, K. Akaji, K. Mayanagi, and **T. Kawase**

Department of Neurosurgery, Keio University School of Medicine, Tokyo, Japan

Summary

Hypothermia confers potent neuroprotection against ischemic injury. Attenuation of apoptosis by hypothermia can be one of the responsible mechanisms. In this study, in situ DNA nick-end labeling (TUNEL) and immunostaining of Bax protein were performed to evaluate the effect of postischemic hypothermia on apoptotic cell death, employing rodent transient focal ischemia. Animals received 1 hour of transient focal ischemia. Brain temperature was maintained at 37.5 ± 0.5 °C during ischemia. Immediately after reperfusion, animals were assigned to either a normothermic or hypothermic group. In hypothermia, animals were cooled and brain temperature was lowered to 34.5 ± 1.0 °C. Prolonged hypothermia was maintained for 16 hours and animals rewarmed. In both groups, TUNEL and immunostaining of Bax was performed. In normothermia, the number of TUNEL positive cells reached the peak at 2 days after ischemia and decreased gradually. In hypothermia, the peak was shifted to 3 days after ischemia. The number of TUNEL positive cells in hypothermia was persistently below that of normothermia. Similarly, in hypothermia, immunostaining of Bax showed attenuated immunoreactivity compared with that in normothermia. In conclusion, postischemic hypothermia reduced both the number of TUNEL positive cells and immunoreactivity of Bax, which may be one of the responsible mechanisms with which hypothermia exerts neuroprotection.

Keywords: Apoptosis; Bax; postischemic hypothermia; TUNEL (In situ DNA nick-end labeling).

Introduction

It has been proved that hypothermia has potent neuroprotective effects against ischemic injury through a variety of mechanisms [4]. Since apoptotic cell death is involved in the progression of ischemic neuronal death [3, 5, 6], the authors speculate that hypothermia may decrease the number of apoptotic cells following ischemia, which results, at least in part, in an attenuation of ischemic neuronal damage. Hypothermia during the ischemic period (intraischemic hypothermia) has been reported to attenuate the apoptotic cell death following ischemia [9], but few experiments have been undertaken concerning the efficacy of hypothermia after the ischemic period (postischemic hypothermia). In situ DNA nick-end labeling (TUNEL) and immunostaining of Bax protein, one of the products of bcl-2 gene family and a major determinant in proapoptotic cascade, were performed to evaluate the effect of postischemic hypothermia on apoptotic cell death compared with that of normothermic ischemia.

Materials and Methods

Animal Preparation

40 male Wistar rats, 300–350 g in weight, were employed. Animals received 1 hour of left middle cerebral artery occlusion, using intraluminal suture method. During the surgical procedure, animals were anesthetized with 1.0–2.0% halothane and a mixture of nitrous oxide-oxygen (70:30%). Brain and rectal temperature was monitored with a telemetry system, and maintained at 37.5 ± 0.5 °C using a heating lamp. Immediately after reperfusion, animals were randomly assigned to either a normothermic or hypothermic group. In the normothermic group, no further manipulation for temperature control was done. In the hypothermic group, animals were cooled transferring them into the cold room (inner temperature; 4 °C) and brain temperature was lowered to 34.5 ± 1.0 °C within 30 min. Prolonged hypothermia was maintained for 16 hours and thereafter, rewarmed gradually. After rewarming, animals were returned to their cage. All surgical procedures and handling of the animals were performed according to the institutional guideline for animal care.

In Situ DNA Nick-End Labeling (TUNEL)

In both groups, animals were sacrificed at 1, 2, 3, 5 and 7 days following ischemia by intraperitoneal injection of pentobarbital (n = 3–4 in each time point). 20 μm coronal slices in the level of the frontoparietal cortex were prepared using cryostat. TUNEL was performed with a commercially available detection kit (Apokit, Takara, Tokyo), and the number of the TUNEL positive cells were

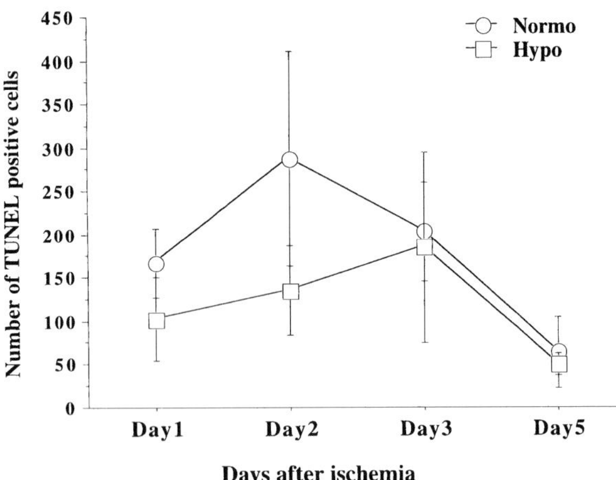

Fig. 1. Temporal profile of the number of TUNEL (In situ DNA nick-end labeling) positive cells in ischemic cortex. In normothermia (circle), the number of TUNEL positive cells reached its peak 2 days after ischemia, and decreased gradually thereafter. In hypothermia (square), peak number was at 3 days after ischemia, one day later as compared with normothermia. The number in hypothermia was persistently below that of normothermia, although statistic analysis with ANOVA failed to show a significant difference between the two groups

counted microscopically: the number in one high power field (×100 magnification) per animal was counted in a blinded fashion.

Immunohistochemistry

In both groups, animals were sacrificed at 1, 2, 3, 5 days following ischemia (n = 3–4 in each time point). Similarly, 20 μm coronal slices in the level of the frontoparietal cortex were prepared. Immunostaining of Bax protein was performed using a rabbit polyclonal antibody to Bax protein (P19, Santa Cruz, CA), and observed microscopically (×50–100 magnification).

Results

The temporal profile of the number of TUNEL positive cells was plotted and indicated (Fig. 1). In both groups, TUNEL positive cells were identifiable in the ischemic cortex at one day after ischemia. In the normothermic group, the number of TUNEL positive cells reached its peak at 2 days after ischemia, and decreased gradually thereafter. In the hypothermic group, the peak of the number of positive cells was attained 3 days after ischemia, one day later as compared with the normothermic group. The number of positive cells in the hypothermic group was persistently below that of the normothermic group, although statistic analysis with ANOVA failed to show a significant difference between the two groups. Few cells were TUNEL positive in the contralateral hemisphere in both groups at any time point measured.

Immunostaining of Bax demonstrated that in the normothermic group, immunoreactivity was clearly identified in the ischemic cortex at one day after ischemia and became strongest at two days. Immunoreactivity began to fade at three days, and was hardly recognizable at five days after ischemia. In the hypothermic group, immunoreactivity was only weakly recognized at one day after ischemia. At two days, immunoreactivity became evident and gradually faded from three days. Immunoreactivity to Bax protein was stronger in the normothermic group than in the hypothermic group at any time point measured (Fig. 2). In the contralateral cortex, few cells were immunopositive to Bax in both groups.

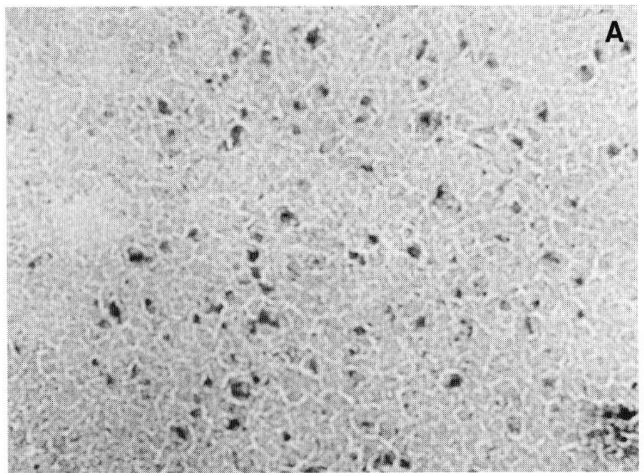

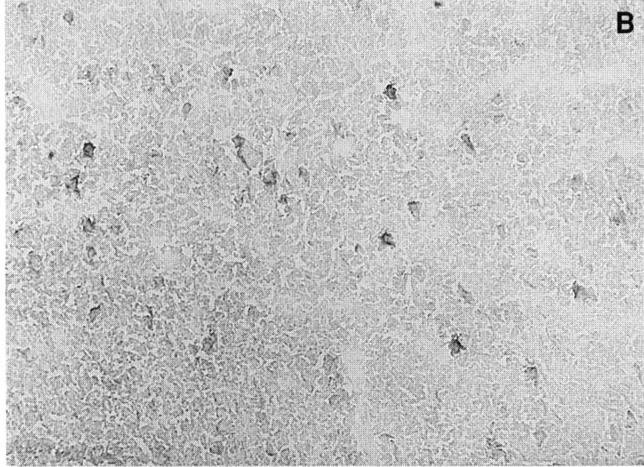

Fig. 2. Representative photomicrographs of the ischemic cortex immunochemically stained with polyclonal antibody to Bax. Both sections were taken from animals two days after one hour of transient focal ischemia. Normothermic animal (A) has more potent immuno-reactivity compared with hypothermic animal (B). Original magnification: ×80

Discussion

Hypothermia confers potent neuroprotection against ischemic insult through various mechanisms including reduction of metabolic demand, attenuation of production of noxious excitatory amino acids/free radicals, and earlier recovery of cerebral blood flow in reperfusion phase [4]. Since some population of neuron dies in a fashion similar to apoptosis following ischemia, it can be considered that one of the protective effects of hypothermia is attributable to the attenuation of apoptotic cell death. Maier *et al.* [9] reported that *intraischemic* hypothermia reduced the number of TUNEL positive cells following transient focal ischemia in rats. Similarly, the authors demonstrated in this study that the number of TUNEL positive cells was reduced in *postischemic* hypothermia. Although the precise mechanism by which hypothermia attenuates apoptotic cell death remains to be elucidated, there is a possibility that hypothermia modifies the apoptotic cell death cascade by affecting the expression of many apoptosis-related genes. The authors showed in this study that following ischemia, the expression of Bax protein was attenuated in hypothermia. Since Bax has been demonstrated to play a crucial role in favor of apoptotic cell death in the upstream of the cascade [1, 2, 10], it can be speculated that the attenuation of Bax in hypothermia can lead to attenuation of apototic cell death, contributing to neuroprotection. Bax forms a heterodimer with a bcl-2 family apoptosis-suppressor gene product [2], and the ratio of Bax to Bcl-2/Bcl-X_L can be a major determinant in the regulation of apoptotic cell death [7]. Therefore, it should be investigated whether the expression of Bcl-2, a potent cell death repressor, has a change in hypothermia. Moreover, it remains unsolved whether the expression of caspases, final common executioners situated in the downstream of the apoptotic cell death cascade [8], is modified by hypothermia.

In conclusion, postischemic hypothermia following normothermic ischemia attenuated both apoptotic cell death and the expression of Bax protein. Further study is warranted to evaluate whether the expression of many other apotosis-related genes is affected by hypothermia.

References

1. Chen J, Zhu RL, Nakayama M, Kawaguchi K, Jin K, Stetler RA, Simon RP, Graham SH (1996) Expression of the apoptosis-effector gene, *Bax*, is up-regulated in vulnerable hippocampal CA1 neurons following global ischemia. J Neurochem 67: 64–71
2. Ferre I, Pozas E, Lopez E, Ballabriga J (1997) Bcl-2, Bax, and Bcl-x expression following hypoxia-ischemia in the infant rat brain. Acta Neuropathol 94: 583–589
3. Gillardon F, Lenz C, Waschke KF, Krajewski S, Reed JC, Zimermann M, Kuschinsky W (1996) Altered expression of Bcl-2, Bcl-x, Bax, and c-Fos colocalizes with DNA fragmentation and ischemic cell damage following middle cerebral artery occlusion in rats. Mol Brain Res 40: 254–260
4. Ginsberg MD, Sternau LL, Globus MYT, Dietrich WD, Busto R (1992) Therapeutic modulation of brain temperature: relevance to ischemic brain injury. Cereb Brain Metab Rev 4: 189–225
5. Hara A, Iwai T, Niwa m, Uematsu T, Yoshimi N, Tanaka T, Mori H (1996) Immunohistochemical detection of Bax and Bcl-2 proteins in gerbil hippocampus following transient forebrain ischemia. Brain Res 711: 249–253
6. Honkaniemi J, Massa SM, Breckinridge, Sharp FR (1996) Global ischemia induces apoptosis-associated genes in hippocampus. Mol Brain Res 42: 79–88
7. Krajewski S, Mai JK, Krajewska M, Sikorska M, Mossakowski MJ, Reed JC (1995) Upregulation of Bax protein levels in neurons following cerebral ischemia. J Neurosci 15: 6364–6376
8. MacManus JP, Linnik MD (1997) Gene expression induced by cerebral ischemia: an apoptotic perspective. J Cereb Blood Flow Metab 17: 815–832
9. Maier CM, Ahern KvB, Cheng ML, Lee JE, Yenari MA, Steinberg GK (1998) Optimal depth and duration of mild hypothermia in a focal model of transient cerebral ischemia: Effect on neurologic outcome, infarct size, apoptosis, and inflammation. Stroke 29: 2171–2180
10. Niwa M, Hara A, Iwai T, Sassa T, Mori H, Uematsu T (1997) Expression of Bax and cl-2 protein in the gerbil hippocampus following transient forebrain ischemia and its modification by phencyclidine. Neurol Res 19: 629–633

Correspondence: Joji Inamasu, M.D., Department of Neurosurgery, Keio University School of Medicine, Shinanomachi 35, Shinjuku-ku, Tokyo 160-8582, Japan.

Acta Neurochir (2000) [Suppl] 76: 529–533

Effects of Hypothermia on Intracranial Hemodynamics and Ischemic Brain Damage-Studies in the Rat Acute Subdural Hematoma Model

N. Kawai, T. Nakamura, M. Okauchi, and **S. Nagao**

Department of Neurological Surgery, Kagawa Medical University, Kagawa, Japan

Summary

Brain ischemia is the leading pathophysiological mechanism in the development of secondary brain damage after subdural hematoma (SDH). Hypothermia has been used as the effective neuroprotective treatment in clinical and laboratory studies of ischemic brain injury. In this study, we have examined the rat acute SDH model to assess the effect of hypothermia upon intracranial hemodynamics and also upon ischemic brain injury 4 hours after the induction of hematoma. Moderate hypothermia (32 °C) did not affect the intracranial pressure nor cerebral perfusion pressure, and it significantly reduced cortical brain edema formation underneath the hematoma ($80.88 \pm 0.17\%$; $p < 0.01$) compared with the normothermic control group ($81.65 \pm 0.52\%$). This reduction in brain edema formation was comparable to the result of MK-801 (2 mg/kg) treatment ($80.95 \pm 0.35\%$; $p < 0.01$). Ischemic brain damage detected by H-E staining was also significantly reduced in the hypothermia and MK-801 treated groups (59.1 ± 12.3 mm^3 and 66.4 ± 13.8 mm^3; $p < 0.01$ and $p < 0.05$) compared with the normothermic control group (86.6 ± 20.7 mm^3). In conclusion, the present study demonstrates that hypothermia is a potent neuroprotective method and an inhibition of the glutamate excitotoxic process may contribute the protective mechanism of hypothermia in this rat acute SDH model.

Keywords: Brain ischemia; hypothermia; intracranial pressure; glutamate.

Introduction

Acute subdural hematoma (SDH) is the most common mass lesion in severe head injury and secondary brain damage following direct brain injury is an important underlying pathophysiological process in patients with SDH. Brain ischemia has been regarded as the leading mechanism in the development of secondary brain damage after acute SDH.

The rat SDH model reveals consistent ischemic damage within the hemisphere beneath the hematoma [7]. Studies on this model have demonstrated that acute SDH induces massive release of the excitatory amino acids in the cortex under the hematoma [1], suggesting that an "excitotoxic" process could contribute to the ischemic damage observed in this model.

Hypothermia has been employed as an effective neuroprotective treatment in clinical and laboratory studies [4, 6] on ischemic brain injury. Despite extensive experimental studies on glutamate antagonist drugs [2], the effects of hypothermia on acute SDH have not yet been elucidated. In this study, we attempted to evaluate the effects of hypothermia on the intracranial hemodynamics and also on ischemic brain injury at 4 hours after induction of the hematoma using a rat SDH model.

Materials and Methods

Adult male Sprague-Dawley rats weighing 280 to 370 grams were divided into five experimental groups, as follows: (a) control group (normothermia, 37 °C), (b) mild hypothermia group (34 °C), (c) moderate hypothermia group (32 °C), (d) hyperthermia group (39 °C), and (e) MK-801 group (2 mg/kg, i.p.).

Intracranial Pressure and Brain Temperature Monitoring

A 3-mm burr hole was drilled on the right parietal calvaria. After a small incision in the dura, a Codman MicroSensor^{TM} intracranial pressure transducer (Johnson & Johnson Prof. Inc., Raynham, MA) was inserted and advanced anteriorly into the subdural space.

A thermocouple probe of 0.05 mm in diameter was inserted to a depth 5 mm in the left frontal cortex, and continuous measurements were made using a digital thermometer (model CT-1300, Custom Corp., Tokyo).

Induction of Acute Subdural Hematoma

A burr hole of 3 mm in diameter was drilled at 3 mm to the left of the sagittal suture and 5 mm posterior to the coronal suture. Under an operating microscope, the dura was incised and a blunt J-shaped 23-gauge needle was carefully inserted into the subdural space over the left parietal cortex. Cyanoacrylate glue was employed to seal the burr hole and secure the needle in position. The hematoma was induced by slowly injecting 0.4 ml of non-heparinized autologous blood into the subdural space over a period of 8 minutes.

Brain Temperature Modulation

Hypothermia was induced by external body cooling using a cold-water circulating blanket above and below the animal starting at 30 minutes before the induction of SDH. The brain temperature was maintained at 34 °C and 32 °C in the mild and moderate hypothermia groups, respectively, by a combination of the water blanket and heating system.

Ischemic Brain Damage

The rats were sacrificed by decapitation at 4 hours after the induction of SDH. The cortex was cut into frontal and parietal cortices. The tissue samples were immediately weighed on an electronic analytical balance to obtain the wet weight (WW). The tissue was then dried in an oven at 110 °C for 24 hours and weighed again to obtain the dry weight (DW). The formula (WW – DW)/WW*100 was employed to calculate the water content expressed as a percentage of the WW.

In another set of experiment, the area of cerebral infarction was quantified by hematoxylin and eosin (H&E) staining at 4 hours after the induction of SDH. The brain were removed, and six coronal slices at 2, 4, 6, 8, 10, and 12 mm distal from the frontal pole were stained by H&E. The extent of ischemic damage was defined in each brain section and the measured with an image-analyzing computer (NIH image 1.61). The total volume of infarction was calculated by integrating the area in each section and multiplying by the distance between section (2 mm).

Results

The hematomas were typically 1 mm thick and largest over the posteroparietal convexity, expanding to midparietal to frontal convexities, and rarely over the contralateral convexity.

Intracranial Pressure and Cerebral Perfusion Pressure

Baseline ICP values were similar and within normal range in all groups. The peak ICP values by hematoma induction did not differ significantly between the five groups (63 to 70 mmHg). ICP then declined to values two or three times above baseline by the 40-minute time point in all groups. The hypothermia-treated animals had a significant reduction in ICP within 60 minutes after the hematoma induction when a comparison was made with the hyperthermia-treated group but not with the control group (Fig. 1a). CPP decreased to 10 to 17 mmHg by hematoma induction

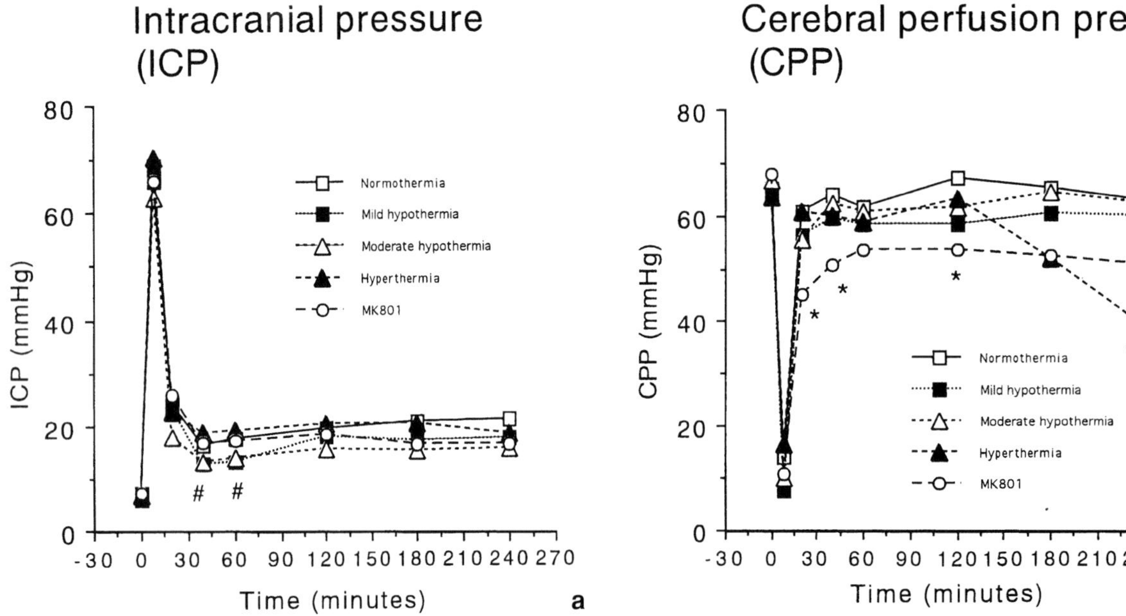

Fig. 1. The intracranial hemodynamic parameters for each group. (a) Hypothermic animals exhibited a significantly lowered ICP when comparison was made with the hyperthermia group at 40 and 60 minutes at the $p < 0.05$ (#) level. (b) The CPP was significantly lower from 20 to 120 minutes in the MK-801 group as compared to the controls at the $p < 0.05$ (*) level

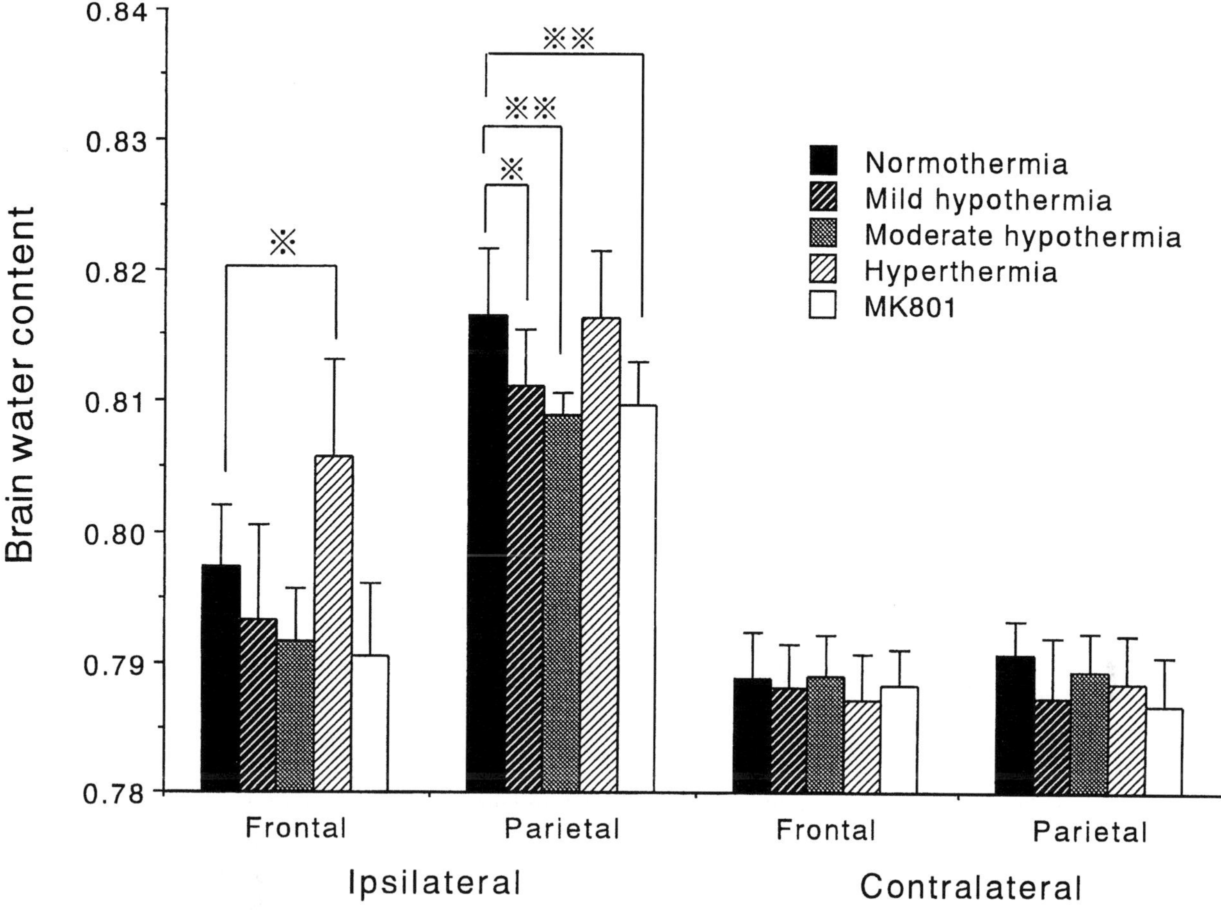

Fig. 2. The brain water content in the frontal and parietal corticies at 4 hours after induction of the hematoma. The values are from ipsi- and contralateral to the site of the hematoma. Values are mean $\pm$ S.D. * and ** indicate significant differences from the control group at the $p < 0.05$ and $p < 0.01$ levels, respectively

despite of a mild vasopressor response and increase in blood pressure, and then returned to the preinduction value by the 20-minute time point except for the MK-801 treated animals. Administration of MK-801 significantly decreased MABP without an ICP change and therefore CPP was significantly lower at 20- to 120-minute time points after hematoma induction in comparison with the control group. Hyperthermia also decreased MABP and a significantly lowered CPP was observed in animals at the final time point of the observation (Fig. 1b).

Ischemic Brain Damage (Brain Edema Formation and Cerebral Infarction)

Brain water content in contralateral hemispheres did not differ by brain temperature modulation or MK-801 treatment. In the parietal cortex, a marked increase in brain water content was noted in the normothermic controls ($81.65 \pm 0.52\%$). Mild and moderate hypothermia significantly lowered the brain water content in the parietal cortex as compared to the normothermic controls ($81.09 \pm 0.46\%$; $p < 0.05$ and $80.88 \pm 0.17\%$; $p < 0.01$, respectively) (Fig. 2). Treatment with MK-801 also significantly decreased the brain water content in the parietal cortex ($80.95 \pm 0.35\%$; $p < 0.01$) which was comparable in value to that following hypothermic treatment.

The moderate hypothermia group showed a significantly smaller volume of infarction (59.1 ± 12.3 mm^3) as compared to the normothermic controls (86.6 ± 20.7 mm^3; $p < 0.05$). Treatment with MK-801 also significantly decreased the volume of infarction (66.4 ± 13.7 mm^3; $p < 0.05$) which was comparable in value to that following hypothermic treatment (Fig. 3).

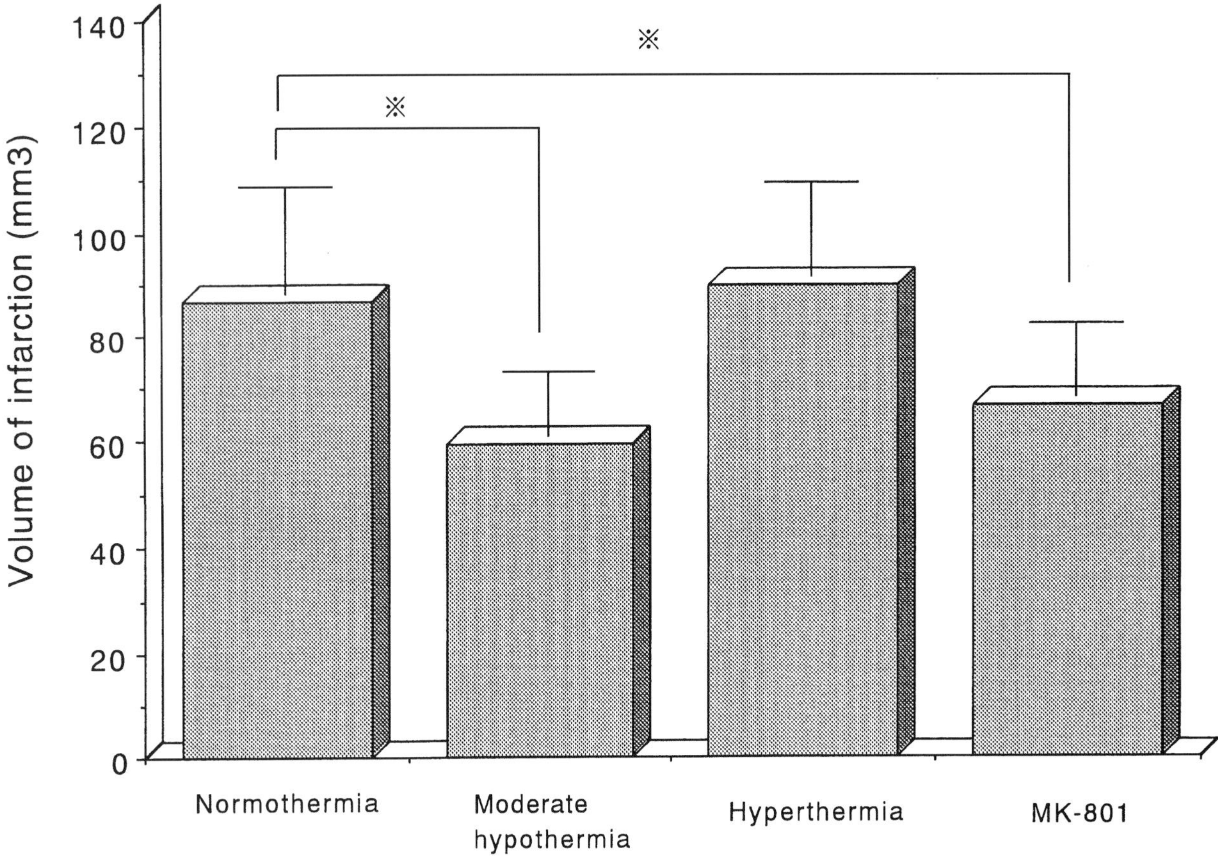

Fig. 3. The cerebral infarct volume at 4 hours after induction of the hematoma. Values are mean ± S.D. * indicates a significant difference from the control group at the $p < 0.05$ level

Discussion

There is strong evidence to suggest that the "excitotoxic" process plays a leading role in the development of ischemic damage in this model. A massive release of excitatory amino acids (EAAs) and a concomitant marked reduction of local CBF have been observed in the cortex underlying the hematoma [1]. Glucose hypermetabolism has also been demonstrated at the margins of the severely ischemic area under the subdural hematoma [5]. In rat focal cerebral ischemia, a similar pattern of glucose hypermetabolism has been reported in the peri-ischemic areas, and in areas where glutamate-induced hyperactivation of the cerebral tissue was noted. Although the local CBF was not measured in our study, we postulate that the increase in ICP following SDH induction would have been sufficient to cause a marked reduction in CBF and consequent global cerebral ischemia, resulting in transient marked increases in EAAs. We postulate therefore that the brain edema formation occurring in this model could be mainly cytotoxic involving glutamate-mediated cell damage mechanisms adjacent to the hematoma. Cerebroprotective effects of hypothermia in traumatic brain injury have been demonstrated both clinically and experimentally [4, 6]. Several mechanisms of hypothermic cerebroprotection have been suggested in cerebral ischemia. A reduction in brain metabolism has been long viewed as a primary mechanism of hypothermic protection. However, recent evidence has indicated that temperature variations may also influence many of the pathophysiological events associated with brain injury. Busto *et al.* [3] demonstrated that hypothermia attenuated the post-injury glutamate release, as well as free radical productions in their ischemic study. Although further studies are needed to establish clearly that hypothermia influences the concentration of EAAs in this acute SDH model, we speculate that one of the most important mechanisms of hypothermic cerebroprotection could derive from a reduction in the accumulation of EAAs.

References

1. Bullock R, Butcher SP, Chen MH, Kendall L, Mcculloch J (1991) Extracellular glutamate concentration correlates with the extent of blood flow reduction after subdural hematoma in the rat. J Neurosurg 74: 794–802
2. Bullock R, Fujisawa H (1992) The role of glutamate antagonists for the treatment of CNS injury. J Neurotrauma 9: S443–462
3. Busto R, Globus MY-T, Dietrich WD, Martines E, Valdes I, Ginsberg MD (1989) Effect of mild hypothermia on ischemia-induced release of neurotransmitters and free fatty acids in rat brain. Stroke 20: 904–910
4. Clifton GL, Jiang JY, Lyeth BG, Jenkins LW, Hamm RJ, hayes RL (1991) Marked protection by moderate hypothermia after experimental traumatic brain injury. J Cereb Blood Flow Metab 11: 141–121
5. Kuroda Y, Inglis, FM, Miller JD, Mcculloch J, Graham DI, Bullock R (1992) Transient glucose hypermetabolism after acute subdural hematoma in the rat. J Neurosurg 76: 471–477
6. Marion DW, Obrist WD, Carlier PM, Penrod LE, darby J (1993) The use of moderate therapeutic hypothermia for patients with severe head injuries: a preliminary report. J Neurosurg 79: 354–362
7. Miller JD, Bullock R, Graham DI, Chen M-H, Teasdale GM (1990) Ischemic brain damage in a model of acute subdural hematoma. Neurosurgery 27: 433–439

Correspondence: Nobuyuki Kawai, M.D., Department of Neurological Surgery, Kagawa Medical University, 1750-1 Ikenobe, Miki-cho, Kita-gun, Kagawa 761-0793, Japan.

Acta Neurochir (2000) [Suppl] 76: 535–539

Blockade of Histamine H_2 Receptors Attenuate Blood-Brain Barrier Permeability, Cerebral Blood Flow Disturbances, Edema Formation and Cell Reactions Following Hyperthermic Brain Injury in the Rat

R. Patnaik[1,2], **S. Mohanty**[3], and **H. S. Sharma**[1]

[1] Laboratory of Neuroanatomy, Department of Medical Cell Biology, Biomedical Centre, Uppsala University, Uppsala, Sweden
[2] Department of Biomedical Engineering, Institute of Technology, Banaras Hindu University, Varanasi, India
[3] Department of Neurosurgery, Institute of Medical Sciences, Banaras Hindu University, Varanasi, India

Summary

Role of histamine H_2 receptors in blood-brain barrier (BBB) disturbances, cerebral blood flow (CBF), brain edema formation, and cell injury caused by heat stress in a rat model was examined using the pharmacological approach. Blockade of histamine H_2 receptors by cimetidine or ranitidine significantly attenuated the BBB permeability to Evans blue albumin and ^{131}I-sodium extravasation, brain edema formation and cell injury following 4 h heat stress in rats at 38 °C. These drug treatments also restored the CBF to near normal values. These beneficial effects in heat stress were most marked in rats treated with ranitidine compared to cimetidine given in identical dosage. Our observations suggest that blockade of histamine H_2 receptor is beneficial in hyperthermic brain injury and indicates that histamine is involved in the pathophysiology of heat stress induced brain dysfunction. Our study strongly suggests further need to develop more specific and sensitive histaminergic H_2 receptor blockers for the treatment of neurological ailments.

Keywords: Histamine; brain edema; histamine H_2 receptor antagonists; cerebral blood flow.

Introduction

The mechanisms behind breakdown of the blood-brain barrier (BBB) in hyperthermia is not well understood [5, 14, 16, 17]. The BBB is a physiologically dynamic barrier [1, 3]. The physicochemical properties of the barrier is very similar to that of an extended plasma membrane [3, 4]. The BBB mainly resides within the endothelial cell of cerebral vessels which are connected with tight junctions [1, 3, 4, 17]. The cerebral endothelial cells also lack vesicular transport [3, 4]. The BBB remains very tight under normal conditions [1, 16, 17]. However, in several pathological conditions, the BBB becomes leaky and extravasation of serum proteins will take place into the brain extracellular compartment [1, 3, 4, 16, 17] resulting in vasogenic edema and adverse cell reaction [4, 14].

The cerebral endothelium contains receptors of several neurochemicals which are known mediators of the BBB permeability and brain edema formation [1, 4, 11]. Release of several neurochemicals occur in hyperthermia which may act on the cerebral endothelium to induce a receptor mediated breakdown of the BBB permeability and consequently cerebral edema formation [14, 16, 17]. Previous reports from our laboratory suggest that serotonin, prostaglandin and opioids are involved in the mechanisms of BBB breakdown in hyperthermic injury [14]. However, apart from these neurochemicals histamine is also liberated from mast cells or histaminergic neurons which can also influence the BBB function [10, 18]. Both histamine H_1 and histamine H_2 receptors are located within the endothelium [11] and histamine H_2 receptors are known to be involved in the BBB disruption following trauma or intracarotid histamine infusion [9, 11–13].

Histamine is a neurotransmitter in the central nervous system (CNS) and histaminergic neurons are present in large numbers in the brain [18]. The projections of histaminergic neurons are distributed throughout the CNS [4, 18]. In spite of a dense and widespread presence of histaminergic neurons, there are only few previous reports which indicate that the amine is involved in the central mechanisms of thermoregulation [2]. However, its involvement in hyperthermic brain injury is still not well known. Traumatic injuries to the brain will induce an increase in plasma and brain histamine levels and the amine is involved in the pathogenesis of brain edema in various traumatic or hypoxic injuries of the CNS, probably via histamine H_2 receptors [10]. Since hyperthermia has the capacity to induce leakage of the BBB [17], a possibility exists that endogenous histamine will contribute to some of these changes [13].

The present investigation was carried out to understand the involvement of histamine in the pathophysiology of hyperthermic brain injury by blockade of histamine H_2 receptors using two potent H_2 receptor antagonist cimetidine and ranitidine [8, 9]. Since histamine is known to influence vasomotor tone of the cerebral microvessels, influence of histamine H_2 receptor antagonists on the CBF was also examined.

Materials and Methods

Animals

Experiments were carried out on male Wistar rats (90–100 g, age 8–9 weeks) housed at controlled room temperature ($21 \pm 1\,°C$) with 12 h light and 12 h dark schedule. Rat feed and tap water were supplied ad libitum before the experiments.

Heat Exposure

Animals were exposed to heat stress in a biological oxygen demand incubator (BOD, wind velocity 20–26 cm/sec; relative humidity 50–55%) maintained at 38 °C for 4 h [12]. This experimental condition is approved by the Ethical Committee of Uppsala University, Uppsala, Sweden; Lund University, Lund, Sweden and Banaras Hindu University, Varanasi, India. Rats kept at room temperature were used as controls.

Treatment with Cimetidine and Ranitidine

In separate groups of rats, two prototypes of histamine H_2 receptor antagonists, cimetidine or ranitidine (Sigma Chemical Co., USA) were administered (10 mg/kg, i.p.) 30 min before the onset of heat stress [12, 16, 17].

Stress Symptoms

In all animals subjected to heat stress, the rectal temperature, behavioural salivation, prostration and occurrence of gastric ulceration in the stomach was measured as indices of stress response [17].

Blood-Brain Barrier Permeability

The blood-brain barrier (BBB) permeability was measured using Evans blue albumin and ^{131}I-sodium [16, 17] according to the standard protocol.

Cerebral Blood Flow

The CBF was measured using carbonised microsphere (15 ± 0.6 μm diameter) labelled with ^{125}Iodine as described earlier [12, 13].

Brain Edema

The water content of the brain was measured to determine brain edema [4]. For this purpose brain samples were taken and weighed immediately. Thereafter the wet samples were placed in an oven maintained at 90 °C for 72 h to obtain dry weight of these samples. The brain water content was calculated from the differences in the dry and wet weight of the samples.

Cell Injury

In separate groups of rats cell injury in the cerebral cortex was determined using standard light and electron microscopy as described earlier [14].

Statistical Analysis

Student's unpaired t-test was used to evaluate the statistical significance of the data obtained. A p-value less than 0.05 was considered to be significant.

Results

Effect of Cimetidine and Ranitidine on Stress Symptoms

Pretreatment with cimetidine or ranitidine did not influence stress symptoms in general. However, a mild but significant reduction in hyperthermia was evident in these drug treated rats compared to the untreated stressed group (Fig. 1). The occurrence of gastric haemorrhages, was significantly attenuated by cimetidine and ranitidine treatment. The drug treatments alone, however, did not influence these parameters in normal rats.

Effect of Cimetidine and Ranitidine on the BBB Permeability

Subjection of rats to 4 h heat stress resulted in a marked increase in the permeability of Evans blue and radioactive iodine in several brain regions. Pretreatment with cimetidine or ranitidine significantly reduced the extravasation of these tracers in the brain following heat stress (Fig. 1). The effect of ranitidine was most pronounced in attenuating the BBB permeability to these tracers in heat stress.

Effect of Cimetidine and Ranitidine on the Brain Edema Formation

Pretreatment with ranitidine or cimetidine significantly attenuated brain edema formation following 4 h heat exposure in rats (Fig. 1). This effect was most

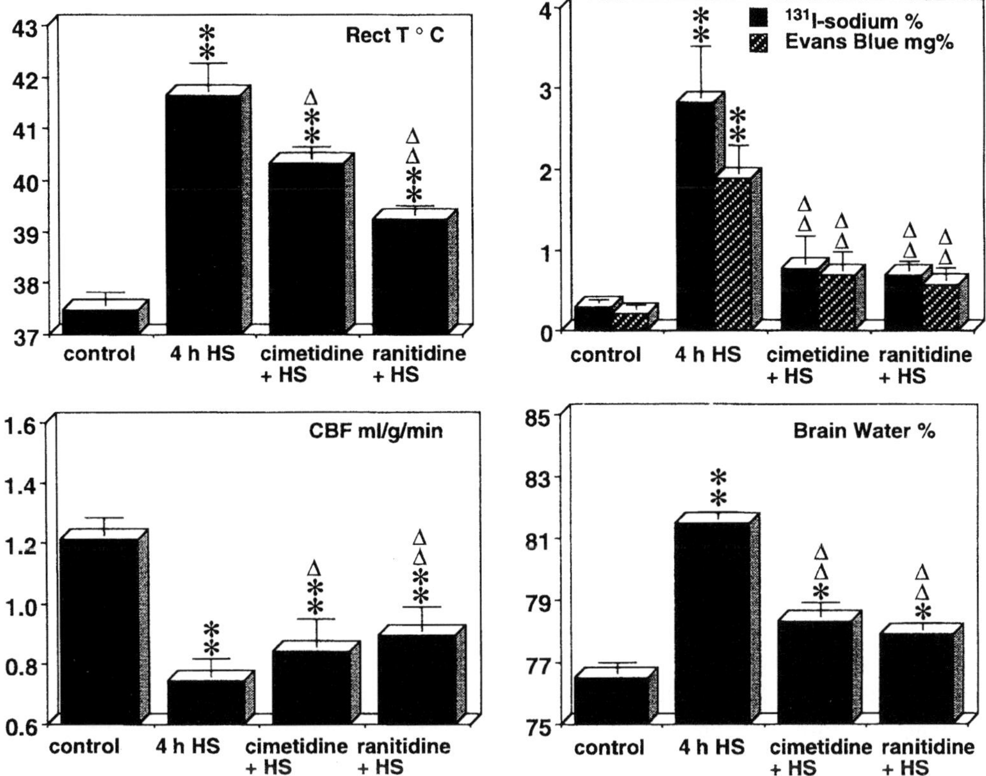

Fig. 1. Effects of cimetidine and ranitidine on heat stress induced changes in rectal temperature (upper panel, left); blood-brain barrier (*BBB*) permeability (upper panel, right); cerebral blood flow (*CBF*) (lower panel, left) and brain water content (lower panel right). * $P < 0.05$; ** = $P < 0.01$ compared to control; ΔΔ = $P < 0.01$ compared to 4 h heat stress (HS); Student's unpaired t-test. Values are mean ± SD

pronounced in rats which received ranitidine as pretreatment compared to the cimetidine treatment. Normal rats received ranitidine or cimetidine, however, did not exhibit any significant alterations in the brain water content.

Effect of Cimetidine and Ranitidine on CBF

At the end of 4 h heat stress, the CBF declined by 30% from the control value (Fig. 1). Pretreatment with cimetidine or ranitidine significantly attenuated ischemia caused by heat stress. Thus the CBF was restored near normal values in drug treated heat stressed animals. Ranitidine seems to be more effective in restoring CBF values compared to cimetidine. On the other hand, treatment of ranitidine or cimetidine in normal rats did not influence the CBF significantly.

Effect of Cimetidine and Ranitidine on Cell Injury

Heat stress induces marked neuronal, glial and axonal changes in the cerebral cortex of rats. Thus, distortion of the nerve cells, swollen glial cells, membrane disruption, edema and myelin vesiculation were quite frequent in untreated heat stressed rats. Pretreatment with ranitidine or cimetidine markedly reduced cell injury following heat stress.

Discussion

These present results show that blockade of histamine H_2 receptors seems to be beneficial in the pathophysiology of brain injury caused by heat stress. This indicates the use of histamine H_2 receptor antagonists as a suitable therapeutic tool in neurological diseases, a feature which however, requires additional investigation. The salient new findings of the present investigation further show that the effects of ranitidine given in identical doses is far superior than cimetidine in attenuating heat stress induced hyperthermia, BBB dysfunction, brain edema, CBF changes and cell injury. This observation suggests that ranitidine is more effective than cimetidine. Previously, ranitidine pretreatment significantly attenuated hypertension induced breakdown of the BBB permeability [9]. Our results for the first time show that ranitidine is also capable to reduce microvascular permeability disturbances in heat stress. The probable mechanisms behind superior effects of ranitidine over cimetidine is not known. It seems likely that ranitidine is more specific to histamine H_2 receptors and may cross the normal BBB more effectively than cimetidine [8]. However, further research is needed to explore this point.

Involvement of histamine in the mechanisms of thermoregulation is not well known. It seems likely that histamine is released from cerebral mast cells, histaminergic nerve fibres or from other peripheral sources [19]. An increased level of histamine in heat stress will induce a breakdown of the BBB permeability probably by stimulating histamine H_2 receptors. A breakdown of the BBB permeability will contribute to vasogenic edema formation which in turn may induce cell injury. Increased histamine concentrations in the plasma or brain may act on local microvessels to influence the local cerebral blood flow [18]. Since histamine in large doses mainly accounts for vasoconstriction, a reduction in the CBF is quite likely following histamine elevation in the circulation or its release through various sources.

The above hypothesis is well supported by our observations using two potent histamine H_2 receptor antagonists cimetidine and ranitidine. Cimetidine is known to reduce brain edema caused by a focal incision of the cerebral cortex [10]. Thus, the mechanisms of brain edema formation following a focal lesion or hyperthermia appears quite similar to that of brain injury. In the brain injury model, a significant increase in plasma and brain histamine was found following 5 h after lesion, indicating that trauma has the capacity to induce histamine increase in the brain and plasma [10]. It may be that histamine level in circulation will also increase in hyperthermia. To further confirm this hypothesis, measurements of the plasma and brain histamine in heat stress are needed.

Histamine has the capacity to induce brain edema [11]. Thus, intracarotid histamine infusion induces brain edema and disrupts the BBB permeability [18]. Blockade of histamine H_2 receptors with high doses of cimetidine reduces irradiation induced brain edema indicating involvement of histamine [9–11]. Our observations with histamine H_2 receptor antagonists in heat stress are in good agreement with these findings and further show that histamine H_2 receptor antagonists are also able to reduce the magnitude of cell injury caused by hyperthermia. A reduction in cell injury by blockade of histamine H_2 receptors may be due to the ability of a reduction in the BBB permeability, cerebral blood flow and brain edema. A reduction of these factors alone or in combination will result in significant neuroprotection [17].

Furthermore, our observations suggest that histamine H_2 receptor antagonists attenuate hyperthermia following heat stress. A reduction in the magnitude of hyperthermia may induce less release of neurochemicals or histamine thereby influencing neuroprotection. A significantly less rise in the body temperature following heat stress in drug treated rats clearly suggests that the amine is involved in the pharmacology of thermoregulation at high ambient temperature. However, further research is needed to clarify this point.

Histamine may also exert some direct effects on the cerebral endothelial cells to influence nitric oxide formation probably via histamine H_2 receptors. Thus, cimetidine and ranitidine inhibits nitric oxide induced endothelial relaxation in the cerebrovascular bed [6]. Since nitric oxide is a potential contributor of the BBB breakdown, brain edema and cell injury, blockade of NO by these drug treatments may also induce neuroprotection [17]. To further confirm this point, NOS upregulation in cimetidine or ranitidine treated animals in heat stress are needed.

In conclusion, our observations suggest that histamine is involved in the pathophysiology of the BBB permeability, brain edema formation and cerebral circulatory disturbances in heat stress and histamine H_2 receptors play an important role in the pathophysiology of hyperthermic brain injury.

Acknowledgments

This investigation is supported by grants from Swedish Medical Research Council nrs. 02710 (JW, HSS); Göran Gustafsson Stiftelse (HSS), Sweden; and The University Grants Commission (HSS), New Delhi, India. The technical assistance of Kärstin Flink, Kerstin Rystedt, Inga Hörte, Ulla Johansson and Secretarial assistance of Gun-Britt Lind and Aruna Sharma are highly appreciated with thanks.

References

1. Black KL (1995) Biochemical opening of the blood-brain barrier. Adv Drug Del Rev 15: 37–52
2. Blatteis C (1997) Thermoregulation: recent progress and new frontiers. Ann NY Acad Sci 813: 1–865
3. Bradbury MWB (1992) Physiology and pharmacology of the blood-brain barrier. Handb Exp Pharmacol 103: 1–450, Springer, Berlin Heidelberg New York Tokyo

4. Cervós-Navarro J, Ferszt R (1980) Brain edema: pathology, diagnosis and therapy. Raven Press, New York. Adv Neurol 20: 1–450
5. Hanin I (1996) The Gulf War, stress and a leaky blood-brain barrier (news & views). Nature Med 2: 1307–1308
6. Hunter RP, Short CR, McClure JR, Koch CE, Keowan ML, Vansteenhouse JL, Dees AA (1999) Cimetidine inhibits nitric oxide associated nitrate production in a soft-tissue inflammation model in the horse. J Vet Pharmacol Ther 22: 136–147
7. Malamud N, Haymaker W, Custer RP (1946) Heat stroke. A clinicopathological study of 125 fatal cases. Milit Surg 99: 397–449
8. Martinez C, Albet C, Agundez JAG, Herrero E, Carrillo JA, Marquez M, Benitez J, Ortiz JA (1999) Comparative in vitro and in vivo inhibition of cytochrome P450 CYP1A2, CYP2D6, and CYP3A by H_2 receptor antagonists. Clin Pharmacol Ther 65: 396–376
9. Mayhan WG (1996) Role of nitric oxide in histamine-induced increase in permeability of the blood-brain barrier. Brain Res 743: 70–76
10. Mohanty S, Dey PK, Sharma HS, Chansouria JPN, Olsson Y (1989) Role of histamine in traumatic brain edema. An experimental study in the rat. J Neurol Sci 90: 87–97
11. Schilling L, Wahl M (1994) Opening of the blood-brain barrier during cortical superfusion with histamine. Brain Res 653: 289–292
12. Sharma HS, Cervós-Navarro J (1991) Role of histamine in the pathophysiology of heat stress. Recent Perspectives in Histamine Research. In: Timmermann H, van der Groot (eds) Birkhauser, Basel. Agents Actions [Suppl] 33: 97–102
13. Sharma HS, Nyberg F, Cervós-Navarro J, Dey PK (1992) Histamine modulates heat stress induced changes in blood-brain barrier permeability, cerebral blood flow, brain oedema and serotonin levels: An experimental study in conscious young rats. Neuroscience 50: 445–454
14. Sharma HS, Westman J, Nyberg F (1998) Pathophysiology of brain edema and cell changes following hyperthermic brain injury. Prog Brain Res 115: 351–412
15. Sharma HS, Westman J (1998) Brain function in hot environment. Prog Brain Res 115: 1–520
16. Sharma HS, Westman J, Cervós-Navarro J, Dey PK, F. Nyberg F (1998) Blood-brain barrier in stress: a gateway to various brain diseases. New frontiers of stress research: modulation of brain function. In: Levy A, Grauer E, Ben-Nathan D, de Kloet ER (eds) Harwood Academic Publishers Inc, Amsterdam, pp 259–276
17. Sharma HS (1999) Pathophysiology of blood-brain barrier, brain edema and cell injury following hyperthermia: New role of heat shock protein, nitric oxide and carbon monoxide. An experimental study in the rat using light and electron microscopy. Acta Universitatis Upsaliensis 830: 1–94
18. Timmerman H, van der Groot H (1991) New perspectives in histamine research. Agents Actions [Suppl] 33: 1–434
19. Zhuang X, Silverman AJ, Silver R (1996) Brain mast cell degranulation regulates blood-brain barrier. J Neurobiol 31: 393–403

Correspondence: Hari Shanker Sharma, Ph.D., Laboratory of Neuroanatomy, Department of Medical Cell Biology, Box 571, Biomedical Centre, Uppsala University, S-75123 Uppsala, Sweden.

Acta Neurochir (2000) [Suppl] 76: 541–545

Selective Alteration of Calcitonin Gene Related Peptide in Hyperthermic Brain Injury. An Experimental Study in the Rat Brain Using Immunohistochemistry

H. S. Sharma[1], **J. Westman**[1], and **F. Nyberg**[2]

[1] Laboratory of Neuroanatomy, Department of Medical Cell Biology, Department of Pharmaceutical, Uppsala, Sweden
[2] Department of Pharmaceutical Biosciences, Division of Biological Research on Drug Dependence, Biomedical Centre, Uppsala University, Uppsala, Sweden

Summary

The possibility that calcitonin gene related peptide (CGRP) participates in the pathophysiology of hyperthermic brain injury was examined in a rat model. The CGRP immunoreactivity was examined in several brain regions of control and 4 h heat stressed rats using immunohistochemistry. Subjection of animals to heat stress in a biological oxygen demand (BOD) incubator at 38 °C for 4 h resulted in a marked redistribution of CGRP immunoreactivity. Thus, in cerebral cortex, hippocampus, cerebellum, medulla and spinal cord the CGRP immunoreactivity was profoundly increased following heat stress. On the other hand in brain stem and pons, the CGRP activity is downregulated. These observations suggest that heat stress has the capacity to influence CGRP immunoreactivity and this redistribution of the peptide is somehow associated with the molecular mechanisms of thermal information processing system of the CNS in heat stress, not reported earlier.

Keywords: Heat stress; CGRP; thermal information processing; brain injury.

Introduction

Heat stress and associated hyperthermia is known to induce central nervous system (CNS) dysfunction in a relatively short period of time [2, 11]. Depending on the magnitude and severity of the primary heat stimulus, disturbances in brain function may range from delirium, mental confusion to coma and unconsciousness [11, 15]. Death may rapidly ensue in these heat stress victims if hyperthermia exceeds beyond 42 °C [11]. Sporadic post-mortem reports of heat injured victims show marked neuronal damage associated with profound microhaemorrhages and brain edema [2, 11]. Uncontrolled volume swelling of the brain in a closed cranium together with rise in intracranial pressure will induce severe compression on the brain including vital centres resulting in instantaneous death of the victims [16].

The mechanisms of cell death following hyperthermia may be due to a direct damage of the cell membranes or cellular enzymes due to increased brain and circulating blood temperatures [2, 11, 15, 16]. However, release of several secondary injury factors in hyperthermia leading to pathophysiology of cell injury is also likely [15]. Increased release of neurochemicals will result in breakdown of the blood-brain barrier (BBB) permeability, vasogenic brain edema formation and cell injury [3, 17]. Our laboratory has been engaged since the last two decades to understand the basic mechanisms of cell injury in hyperthermia in a rat model. Our results clearly show that serotonin, prostaglandins and histamine play important roles in the pathological mechanisms of BBB disruption, brain edema formation and cell injury [14, 16, 17]. High dose of naloxone, a potent opioid receptor antagonist, pretreatment attenuates breakdown of the BBB permeability, brain edema and cell injury [17]. This indicates that opioid peptides are somehow involved in hyperthermia induced brain damage. However, involvement of other neuropeptides which are either involved in primary sensory mechanisms or are able to influence neurotransmission of serotonin, prostaglandins and nitric oxide in pathophysiology of hyperthermic brain injury is not yet known. Thus, involvement of several neuropeptides in thermal brain injury is a new subject and requires further investigation.

Calcitonin gene related peptide (CGRP) is a well known neuropeptide found in neurons and in dendrites in the CNS of several mammalian species [9]. Peripheral nerve lesion, stress or thermal stimulation are known to cause redistribution of CGRP in the CNS

[9, 13]. Recent observations suggest that CGRP is involved in thermal sensation [6, 9, 13]. Thus, thermal stimulation of hind paw is associated with upregulation of CGRP in the dorsal horn neurons. However, effect of systemic heat exposure on CGRP expression in the CNS is still not known and the functional significance of this peptide in cell injury or cell survival is unclear.

The present investigation was undertaken to find out whether systemic heat exposure influences CGRP immunostaining in the rat brain and if so, whether the altered immunoreactivity of the peptide is somehow related with hyperthermia induced cell injury in the brain.

Materials and Methods

Animals

Experiments were carried out on 20 Sprague Dawley male rats (100–150 g) housed at controlled room temperature 21 ± 1 °C with 12 h light and 12 h dark schedule. The rat food pellets and tap water were supplied ad libitum before the experiments.

Heat Exposure

Rats (8–9 weeks) were exposed to a 4 h heat stress in a biological oxygen demand (BOD) incubator (relative humidity 50–55%, wind velocity 20–25 cm/sec) [14]. This experimental condition is approved by the Ethical Committee of Uppsala University, Uppsala, Sweden; Lund University, Lund, Sweden and Banaras Hindu University, Varanasi, India. Normal rats kept at room temperature served as controls.

Stress Symptoms

Rectal temperature, behavioural salivation, prostration and occurrence of gastric haemorrhage in the stomach were used as indices of heat stress [14, 17].

Physiological Variables

The changes in mean arterial blood pressure (MABP), arterial pH and blood gases were recorded using standard protocol as physiological variables after heat stress as described earlier [17].

CGRP Immunohistochemistry

The CGRP immunohistochemistry was examined using monoclonal antibodies on free floating 40 μm thick vibratome sections obtained from several brain regions of the rats exposed to heat stress according to the commercial protocol [9]. In brief, after *in situ* fixation of the brain with 4% paraformaldehyde selected tissue pieces from the cerebral cortex and brain stem reticular formation were dissected out. About 40 μm thick multiple vibratome sections were cut and processed for CGRP immunostaining according to the standard protocol. Rats kept at room temperature (21 °C) served as controls. Both control and experimental sections were processed for CGRP immunohistochemistry in parallel.

The immunostaining of CGRP was examined independently by two independent observers and photographed. The CGRP positive cells in different regions of the brain were counted per section from each animal and were used to semiquantitative analysis.

Statistical Significance

Unpaired Student's t-test was used to analyse the statistical significance of the data obtained. A p-value less than 0.05 was considered to be significant.

Results

CGRP Immunostaining in Heat Stress

Only a few CGRP immunostained neurons, nerve fibres and terminals were present in the brain stem and cerebral cortex of normal rats. Subjection of rats to 4 h heat stress significantly altered the CGRP immunoreactivity in several brain regions examined. Thus marked increase in the CGRP immunoreactivity was noted in regions such as cerebral cortex, hippocampus, cerebellum, medulla and spinal cord (Fig. 1). On the other hand a significant downregulation was noted in the brain stem and pons regions. In general, the decrease in CGRP immunostaining was most pronounced in the nerve fibres and in dendrites (Fig. 2). In some brain regions loss of CGRP immunoreactivity in nerve cell was also noticed in the brain stem pontine regions (Fig. 2). On the other hand, in most cases, increase in CGRP immunoreactivity was seen in the nerve terminals and nerve fibres in several brain regions following heat stress (Figs. 1 and 2).

The semiquantitative analyses showed that CGRP positive nerve cells and nerve fibres are distributed

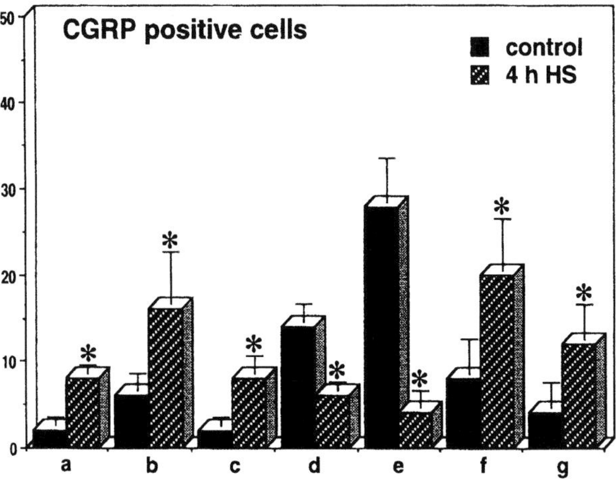

Fig. 1. Semiquantitative data on CGRP positive cells in different regions of the CNS in control and in heat stressed rats. * = $P < 0.001$, Student's unpaired t-test (*a* cortex; *b* hippocampus; *c* cerebellum; *d* brain stem; *e* pons; *f* medulla; *g* spinal cord)

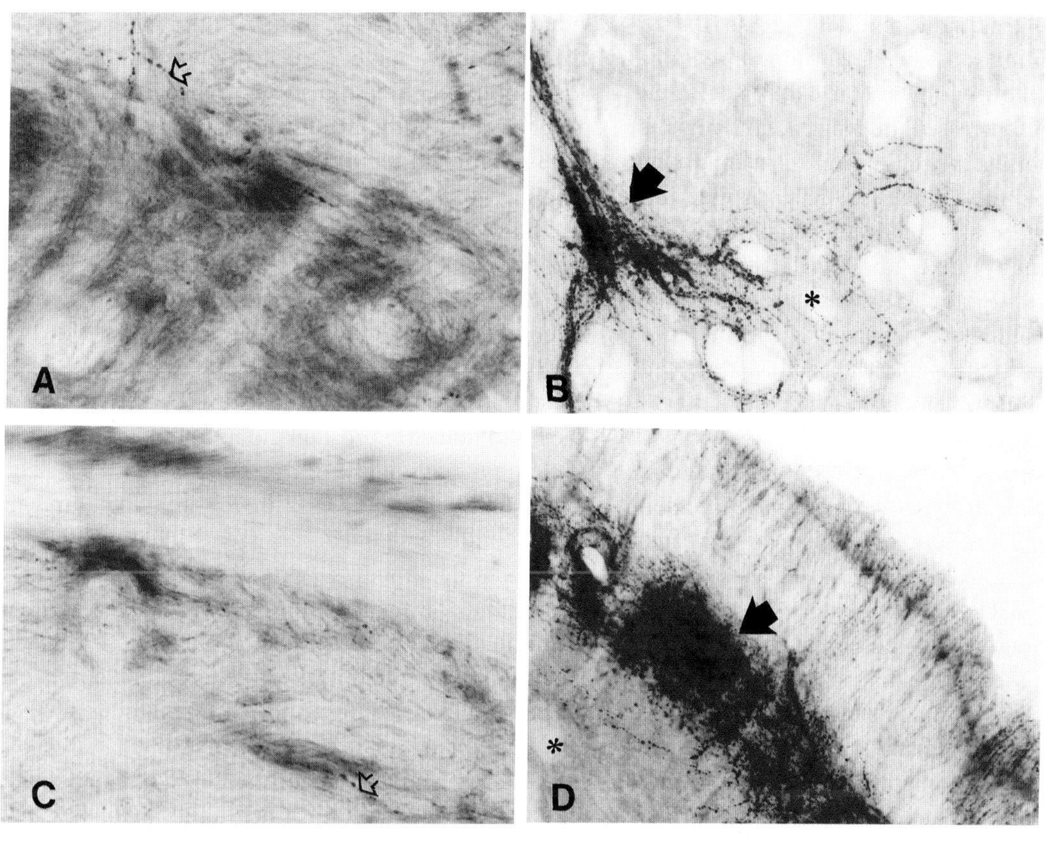

Fig. 2. A representative example of CGRP immunostaining in the thalamus and brain stem reticular formation in control (A, C) and following heat stress (B, D) respectively. In control animal, few CGRP stained nerve fibres and terminals are clearly visible (blank arrows). In heat stress CGRP immunostained bundles of nerve fibres and terminals (filled arrows) are clearly visible. Specific distribution of CGRP immunostained nerve fibres and terminals can be seen around the edematous nerve cells (*) (bar = 50μm)

sporadically throughout the brain of the heat stressed rats. A semiquantitative analysis of CGRP positive cells in some brain regions during heat stress is shown in Fig. 1. As apparent from the figure, CGRP positive cells increased significantly in many brain regions whereas a significant decrease in CGRP immunostaining was also noted in these animals. Many CGRP positive nerve fibres and terminals are located in areas of thermal sensation such as reticular activating system and thalamus. However, the distribution of CGRP in nerve fibres and terminal markedly varied from one region to the other brain region.

Stress Symptoms and Physiological Variables

Heat stress significantly increased the rectal temperature from 37.0 ± 0.23 to 41.68 ± 0.23 ($P < 0.001$) after 4 h exposure. Stressed rats showed profound signs of salivation and behavioural prostration during heat exposure. The MABP was reduced significantly in stressed rats (74 ± 4 Torr) compared to the control group (110 ± 6, $P < 0.001$). The PaO_2 values increased whereas $PaCO_2$ values showed a mild decline, however the arterial pH did not change significantly from the control group.

Discussion

The present results for the first time demonstrate that hyperthermic brain damage caused by systemic heat exposure induces marked redistribution of CGRP in several brain regions. This indicates that CGRP is involved in the molecular mechanisms of thermal sensation and hyperthermia induced brain injury.

The immunohistochemistry of CGRP in nerve cells, terminals and nerve fibres seen in normal rats is in good agreement with the previous observations of CGRP mapping obtained on fresh frozen sections in the rat CNS [9]. This indicates that our method to detect CGRP immunostaining on vibratome sections is also valid. Following hyperthermia, CGRP immunoreactivity is decreased in many brain regions which is seen in both nerve cells as well as in dendrites. This observation suggest a release of the peptide following hyperthermia in other brain regions. On the other hand, in many areas, the CGRP immunoreactivity is increased and can be seen in several axonal bundles, nerve terminal not normally seen in control animals. This suggests that CGRP is activated at synapses to influence neuronal communication in hyperthermia, not reported earlier.

A direct relationship between CGRP upregulation and cell injury following hyperthermia is not evident in our investigation. Thus, in many regions of the brain which show edematous swelling and cell injury are associated with CGRP downregulation. On the other hand, in several brain regions the peptide upregulation in nerve terminals or nerve fibres was related with cell injury. These observations suggest that CGRP is involved in the thermal information processing system or the peptide influence sensory thermal pathways. However, this is a new subject and requires further investigation.

In cell culture studies, addition of CGRP tightens the BBB (Paul Fraser, Personal communication). Keeping this view in consideration, it seems likely that a decrease in CGRP in some regions is related with massive increase in the BBB permeability in that area. However, to further confirm this point, mapping of regional BBB disturbances using endogenous serum protein extravasation and CGRP immunoreactivity in the CNS of heat stressed rats is needed.

CGRP is often co-localised with serotonin and Subtance P [6, 13]. Since serotonin levels are increased in hyperthermia which is related with the edema formation and cell injury [14], a possibility exists that CGRP may influence serotonergic neurotransmission in heat stress. Since CGRP is known to influence vasomotor tone of the microvessels [7, 10], a redistribution of the peptide may have some influence on the local cerebral circulation. There are reports that CGRP mediates vascular reaction through mechanisms involving nitric oxide [10]. Nitric oxide synthase (NOS), the enzyme responsible for nitric oxide (NO) synthesis is upregulated in several brain regions in heat stress [16, 17]. Thus a possibility exists that CGRP may influence NOS activity in different brain regions. NOS occurs in three different isoforms, namely, constitutive (cNOS), inducible (iNOS) and endothelial (eNOS). Expression of all isoforms of NOS are not injurious to the cell. Activation of eNOS seems to be beneficial. Thus, it is plausible that CGRP activates different isoforms of NOS in different regions of the brain in hyperthermia to influence neuronal communication. It is not certain whether CGRP activates all isoforms of NOS or its specificity is more directed towards eNOS or iNOS. Further studies using co-localisation of CGRP with different isoforms of NOS in heat stress are needed to clarify this point.

Apart from its interaction with NO, the peptide is known to influence prostaglandins and its synthesising enzyme cyclooxygenase (COX-1 and COX-2) [18]. The role of COX-1 and COX-2 in cell injury or survival is still controversial. Thus, it seems likely CGRP influences wide range of neurochemicals or enzymes responsible for their synthesis in order to exert its action in the CNS. Whether the effects of CGRP in the CNS are mediated via specific receptors located on the nerve cells is not clear and certainly require further investigation.

CGRP is a sensory neuropeptide [1] and CGRP receptors are located on the nerve cells, axons as well as on the astrocytes [4, 12]. There are evidences that CGRP concentration is altered in spinal trauma [8] or following trimethyltin induced poisoning in the hippocampus [4]. The peptide concentration is increased following trauma above the lesion site and decreased below the injury level [8]. However, in trimethyltin poisoning, the peptide content showed good relation with cell injury [12]. Thus the functional significance of CGRP in cell injury is still controversial. There are indications that local accumulation of growth factors, cytokines, hormones and other neuropeptides may influence CGRP activity [4, 5, 7, 8, 10, 18]. It appears that during heat stress, the thermal sensory pathways in several brain regions could be different and depending on the activation of a particular region, the up- and down-regulation of CGRP is possible depending on the local neurochemical metabolism.

In conclusion, our results show that CGRP immunoreactivity is altered remarkably following hyperthermic brain damage. The regional redistribution of CGRP in the CNS of hyperthermic animals depends on many other local neurochemical or injury factors which require additional investigation. To further understand the role of CGRP in cell injury following heat stress, effect of neuroprotective drugs on CGRP immunoreactivity and biochemical measurement of the peptide using radioimmunoassay are needed, which is currently being investigated in our laboratory.

Acknowledgments

This study is supported by grants from Swedish Medical Research Council nrs. 02710 (JW/HSS), Göran Gustafsson Stiftelse (HSS), and The University Grants Commission (HSS), New Delhi, The Indian Council of Medical Research (HSS), New Delhi, India. The technical assistance of Kärstin Flink, Katjya Deparade, Ingamarie Olsson and secretarial assistance of Angela Ludwig, Gun-Britt Lind and Aruna Sharma are highly appreciated.

References

1. Ai XB, MacPhedran SE, Hall AK (1998) Depolarization stimulates initial calcitonin gene-related peptide expression by embryonic sensory neurons in vitro. J Neurosci 18: 9294–9302
2. Austin MG, Berry JW (1956) Observation on one hundred case of heatstroke. JAMA 161: 1525–1529
3. Bradbury MWB (1992) Physiology and pharmacology of the blood-brain barrier. Springer, Berlin Heidelberg New York Tokyo Handb Exp Pharmacol 103: 1–450
4. Bulloch K, Sadamatsu M, Patel A, McEwen BS (1999) Calcitonin gene-related peptide immunoreactivity in the hippocampus and its relationship to cellular changes following exposure to trimethyltin. J Neurosci Res 55: 441–457
5. Hu CP, Li YJ, Deng HW (1999) The cardioprotective effects of nitroglycerine preconditioning are mediated by calcitonin gene-related peptide. Eur J Pharmacol 369: 189–194
6. Hökfelt T, Elde R, Johansson O, Ljungdahl Å, Schultzberg M, Fuxe K, Goldstein M, Nilsson G, Pernow B, Terenius L, Ganten D, Jeffocate SL, Rehfeld J, Said S (1978) Distribution of peptide containing neurons. In: Lipton MA, DiMascio A, Killam KF (eds) Psychopharmacology: A Generation of Progress. Raven Press, New York, pp 39–66
7. Jansen GB, Torkvist L, Lofgren O, Raud J, Lundberg T (1999) Effects of calcitonin gene-related peptide on tissue survival, blood flow and neutrophil recruitment in experimental skin flaps. Br J Plast Surg 52: 299–303
8. Krenz NR, Weaver LC (1996) CGRP expression increase in the ventral horn rostral to spinal cord transection. Neuro Report 7: 2859–2862
9. Kruger L, Mantyh PW, Sternini C, Brecha NC, Mantyh CR (1988) Calcitonin gene-related peptide (CGRP) in the rat central nervous system: patterns of immunoreactivity and receptor binding sites. Brain Res 463: 223–244
10. Lu LF, Fiscus RR (1999) Calcitonin gene-related peptide causes long-term inhibition of contraction in rat thoracic aorta through a nitric oxide-dependent pathway. Neuropeptides 33: 145–154
11. Malamud N, Haymaker W, Custer RP (1946) Heat stroke. A clinicopathological study of 125 fatal cases. Milit Surg 99: 397–449
12. Morara S, Wimalawansa SJ, Rosina A (1998) Monoclonal antibodies reveal expression of the CGRP receptor in Purkinje cells, interneurons and astrocytes of rat cerebellar cortex. Neuro Report 9: 3755–3759
13. Nyberg F, Sharma HS, Wisenfeld-Hallin Z (1995) Neuropeptides in the spinal cord. Progress in Brain Research, vol 104. Elsevier, Amsterdam, pp 1–430
14. Sharma HS, Dey PK (1987) Influence of long-term acute heat exposure on regional blood-brain barrier permeability, cerebral blood flow and 5-HT level in conscious normotensive young rats. Brain Research 424: 153–162
15. Sharma HS, Westman J (1998) Brain functions in hot environment. Progress in Brain Research, vol 115. Elsevier, Amsterdam, pp 1–516
16. Sharma HS, Westman J, Nyberg F (1998) Pathophysiology of brain edema and cell changes following hyperthermic brain injury. Brain functions in hot environment. In: Sharma HS, Westman J (eds) Prog Brain Res 115: 351–412
17. Sharma HS (1999) Pathophysiology of blood-brain barrier, brain edema and cell injury following hyperthermia: new role of heat shock protein, nitric oxide and carbon monoxide. An experimental study in the rat using light and electron microscopy, Acta Universitatis Upsaliensis 830: 1–94
18. Tang Y, Han C, Wang X (1999) Role of nitric oxide and prostaglandins in the potentiating effects of calcitonin gene-related peptide on lipopolysaccharide-induced interleukin-6 release from mouse peritoneal macrophages. Immunology 96: 171–175

Correspondence: Hari Shanker Sharma, Ph.D., Laboratory of Neuroanatomy, Department of Medical Cell Biology, Box 571, Biomedical Centre, Uppsala University, S-75123 Uppsala, Sweden.

Acta Neurochir (2000) [Suppl] 76: 547–550

Protective Effect of Mild Hypothermia on Symptomatic Vasospasm: A Preliminary Report

S. Nagao, K. Irie, N. Kawai, K. Kunishio, T. Ogawa, T. Nakamura, and **M. Okauchi**

Department of Neurological Surgery, Kagawa Medical University, Kagawa, Japan

Summary

Mild hypothermia (32–34 °C of brain temperature) was used for brain protection in patients with progressive ischemic neurological deficits associated with severe cerebral vasospasm and who did not respond to medical treatment or intravascular angioplasty. Results showed that 2 of 3 patients in Hunt & Kosnik grade I to III and 2 patients who underwent delayed operation on day 5 and 9 each and had ischemic neurological deficits made good recovery with this treatment. Favourable outcome was obtained in 4 of 9 patients in grade IV and V. Mild hypothermia is thought to provide brain protection in critical ischemia due to severe cerebral vasospasm and can lengthen therapeutic time to employ angioplasty and intraarterial Papaverin infusion.

Keywords: Subarachnoid hemorrhage; cerebral vasospasm; cerebral ischemia; mild hypothermia.

Introduction

Cerebral vasospasm associated with subarachnoid hemorrhage (SAH) remains a significant cause of morbidity and mortality following ruptured aneurysm. An essential pathology of cerebral vasospasm is focal or diffuse cerebral ischemia. In order to ameliorate cerebral ischemia secondary to vasospasm, hypertension, hypervolemia and hemodilution therapy, administration of Ca^{2+} antagonists, intraarterial Papaverine infusion and angioplasty have been employed. Some patients, however, show progressive ischemic neurological deficit (PIND) following these treatments. Recent experimental and clinical studies show that mild hypothermia provides significant beneficial effects following ischemic cerebral injury [1–9]. In the present study, we employed mild hypothermia (32–34 °C of brain temperature) in patients with severe vasospasm who showed PIND and assessed the effectiveness of this particular treatment on critical cerebral ischemia due to cerebral vasospasm.

Patients and Methods

The hypothermic therapy was undertaken in three groups as follows (Fig. 1): 1) in Hunt and Kosnik grade I–III, 3 patients underwent emergency clipping of aneurysm and revealed PIND even after medical and intravascular treatments; 2) in grade IV and V, 9 patients received emergency clipping [7] or aneurysm coiling [2] and mild hypothermia during or immediately after operation; 3) 2 patients who were admitted on Day 5 and 9 after SAH and had PIND also received clipping under hypothermia.

The patients were anesthetized by neuroleptics (droperidol and fentanyl), paralyzed by pancuronium and artificially ventilated, and then maintained with fentanyl, midazolam, and bechronium chloride. The brain temperature was monitored with a thermistor placed in the internal jugular bulb. The body temperature was reduced by the use of hypothermic cooling water blankets (5 °C) until the brain temperature decreased to 32–34 °C within 3 hours. The mild hypothermia was maintained for 5 to 14 days. Rewarming was carried out in a stepwise manner from 0.5 to 1.0 °C a day by assessing internal jugular oxygen saturation (SjO_2), ICP and serial CT scan. As patients were sedated, cerebral circulation and metabolism were monitored using SjO_2, measurement of flow velocity of the middle cerebral artery with transcranial Doppler sonogram and ^{99m}Tc-ECD SPECT.

Results

In grade I to III, 2 of 3 patients showed good recovery but 1 was severely disable on Glasgow Outcome Scale (GOS).

Case 1

A 46 year old female who suffered from SAH from ruptured aneurysm of the left middle cerebral artery was diagnosed as having Hunt and Kosnik grade III and Fisher group 3 hemorrhage on CT scan. She underwent emergency clipping on day 1 and showed good recovery until day 13. On day 14, she gradually developed right hemiparesis and aphasia due to severe

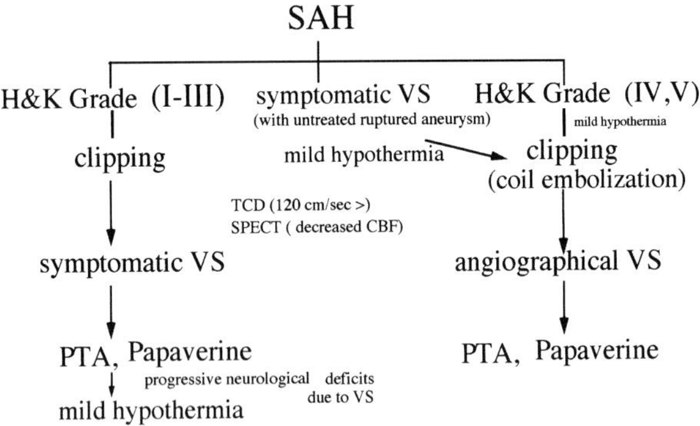

Fig. 1. Strategy of hypothermia therapy in patients with subarachnoid hemorrhage

vasospasm predominantly at the left middle cerebral artery. She received intraarterial infusion of Papaverine hydrochloride (total 200 mg) on day 15, resulting in transient improvement. On day 16, her condition deteriorated again, so that mild hypothermia was employed for brain protection.

Mild hypothermia was maintained for 10 days and rewarming was started on day 26. She had no neurological deficits and was judged as having good recovery on discharge. Figure 2 shows serial measurements of CBF using ^{99m}Tc-ECG SPECT. Before onset of neurological deterioration (Day 12), mean CBF was well preserved with a lowerflow in the left cerebral hemisphere. On day 16, mean CBF decreased even after intraarterial administration of Papaverine hydrochloride. During hypothermic treatment, CBF remained at a critical low value, around 33 ml/100 g/min, and before rewarming increased up to 38ml /100 g/min.

In grade IV and V on GOS, 3 patients showed good recovery, 1 moderate disability and 5 died. In 4 of the 5 deceased patients, the main cause was presumed to be primary brain injury associated with SAH. Two patients who underwent delayed aneurysm clipping with PIND on day 5 and 9 each showed good recovery.

Case 2

A 47 year old male who was referred to our clinic with chief complaints of headache and left hemiparesis. He had a severe headaches 10 days prior to admission. Angiography revealed an aneurysm and severe cerebral vasospasm of the right middle cerebral artery. He underwent aneurysm clipping under mild hypothermia on day 10 and hypothermia was continued until day 19. He made full recovery.

Figure 3 demonstrates changes in CBF before and during mild hypothermia in this patient. During hypothermia, mean CBF remained at a critical low value of 30.7 ml/100 g/min. Angioplasty and intraarterial administration of Papaverine hydrochloride (total 160 mg) on day 15 resulted in an increase of mean CBF to 42.7 ml/100 g/min.

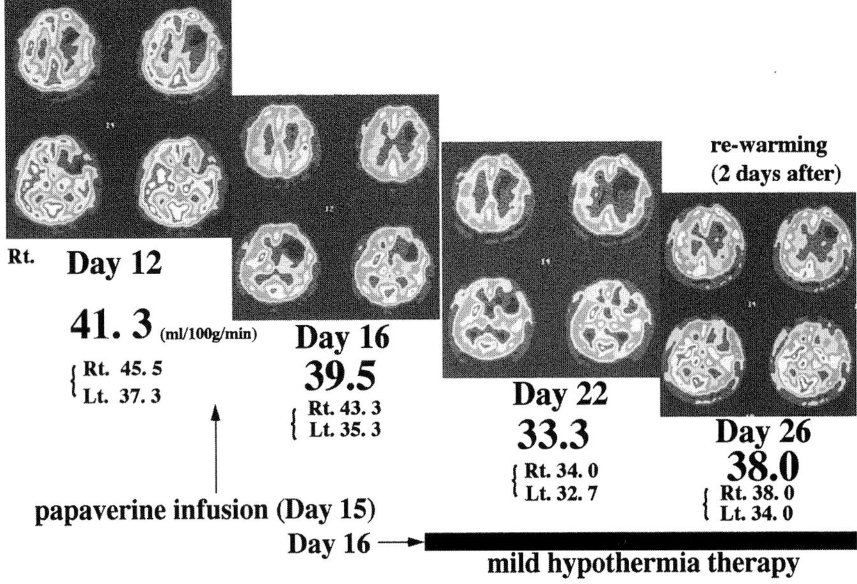

Fig. 2. Serial changes in cerebral blood flow (*CBF*) measured by ^{99m}Tc-ECD SPECT in a patient with severe cerebral vasospasm (case 1). CBF remained at low values during mild hypothermia therapy

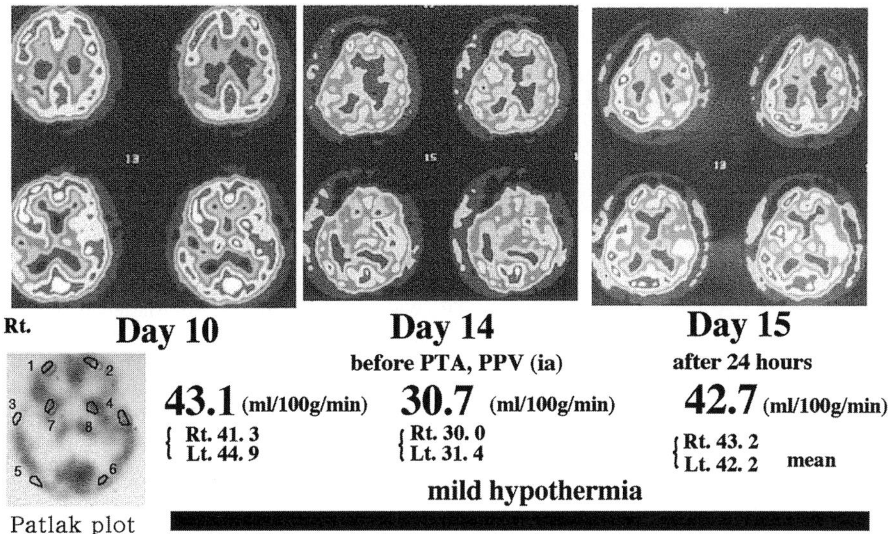

Fig. 3. Serial changes in cerebral blood flow (*CBF*) measured by ^{99m}Tc-ECD SPECT in a patient with delayed operative intervention and progressive neurological deterioration (case 2). Angioplasty and intraarterial Papaverine administration on day 15 produced a significant increase in CBF under mild hypothermia

Discussion

Experimental studies have shown that mild hypothermia (32–34 °C of brain temperature) may have beneficial effects on cerebral ischemia. The main mechanisms of hypothermic brain protection is presumed to be by suppression of neurotoxic glutamate release and reduction of intracellular Ca^{+2} accumulation [1, 4], prevention of free radical production [5], tissue acidosis [2], suppression of energy metabolism [2], and protection of blood brain barrier [3]. Hypothermia has been shown to markedly reduce the size of infarction produced by the middle cerebral artery occlusion in rats [7, 9]. Hypothermia in patients has been shown to decrease intracranial pressure due to a reduction of cerebral edema in severe head injury [6] and an unproved outcome after cerebral embolism [8]. An essential component of the pathophysiology of cerebral vasospasm is progressive focal and/or global cerebral ischemia, which then results in neurological deterioration. In some patients, the progression of cerebral ischemia due to vasospasm cannot be controlled with medical and intravascular treatments.

In the present study, we applied mild hypothermia in progressive cerebral ischemia for neuronal protection. In Hunt and Kosnik grades I–III, 2 out of 3 patients and 2 patients with delayed operative intervention and neurological deterioration, made a good recovery. In these 4 patients, poor outcome was predicted employing "conventional" treatments. Thus, mild hypothermia appears to exert sufficient protective effect on ischemic brain especially at the critical blood flow threshold of 30 ml/100 g/min. In the patient with delayed aneurysm clipping with PIND, use of mild hypothermia was considered to be appropriate to reduce progression of cerebral vasospasm by operative manipulation and to institute aggressive antispasm treatment. Mild hypothermia may have given a longer therapeutic window and opportunity to employ angioplasty and intraarterial administration of Papaverine hydrochloride by its brain protective effect. In grade IV and V cases, a favourable outcome was obtained only in half of the patients indicating the limitation of this treatment. One must be aware of the harmful effects of mild hypothermia which include impairment of the cardiocirculatory system, infection, serum electrolyte abnormalities and abnormal coagulopathy, especially seen in prolonged hypothermia.

In conclusion, the results of the present study warrant further study of this form of therapy for patients with uncontrollable cerebral vasospasm following SAH.

References

1. Busto R, Globus MYT, Dietrich WD, Martinez E, Valdés I, Ginsberg MD (1989) Effect of mild hypothermia on ischemia-induced release of neurotransmitters and free fatty acids in rat brain. Stroke 20: 904–910

2. Chopp M, Kuight R, Tidwell CD, Helpern JA, Brown E, Welch KMA (1989) The metabolic effects of mild hypothermia on global cerebral ischemia and recirculation in the cat: Comparison to normothermia and hyperthermia. J Cereb Blood Flow Metab 9: 141–148
3. Dietrich WD, Busto R, Halley M, Valdes I (1990) The importance of brain temperature in alterations of the blood-brain barrier following cerebral ischemia. J Neuropath Exp Neurol 49: 486–497
4. Ginsberg MD, Sternau LL, Globus MYT, Dietrich WD, Busto R (1992) Therapeutic modulation of brain temperature: relevance to ischemic brain injury. Cerebrovasc Brain Metab Rev 4: 189–225
5. Kil HY, Zhang J, Piantadosi CA (1996): Brain temperature alters hydroxyl radical production during cerebral ischemia/reperfusion in rats. J Cereb Blood Flow Metab 16: 100–116
6. Marion DW, Obrist WD, Carlier PM, Penrod LE, Darby JM (1993) The use of moderate therapeutic hypothermia for patients with severe head injuries: a preliminary report. J Neurosurg 79: 354–362
7. Morikawa E, Ginsberg MD, Dietrich WD, Duncan RC, Kraydich S, Globus MYT, Busto R (1992) The significance of brain temperature in focal cerebral ischemia: Histopathological consequences of middle cerebral artery occlusion in the rat. J Cereb Blood Flow Metab 12: 380–389
8. Naritomi H, Shimizu T, Oe H, Kinugawa H, Sawada T, Hirata T (1996) Mild hypothermia therapy in acute embolic stroke: A pilot study. J Stroke Cerebrovascul Diss 6: 193–196
9. Rindenour TR, Warner DS, Todd MM, McAllister AC (1992) Mild hypothermia reduces infarct size resulting from temporary but not permanent focal ischemia in rats. Stroke 23: 733–738

Correspondence: Dr, Seigo Nagao, 1750-1, Miki-cho, Kita-gun, Kagawa 761-0793, Japan.

Acta Neurochir (2000) [Suppl] 76: 551–555

Influence of Hypothermia on Cell Volume and Cytotoxic Swelling of Glial Cells in Vitro

E. Mueller, J. Wietzorrek, F. Ringel, S. Guretzki, A. Baethmann, and **N. Plesnila**

Institute for Surgical Research, Ludwig-Maximilians-Universität, Munich, Germany

Summary

In view of the increasing significance of mild hypothermia (32 °C) as an efficient procedure of neuroprotection, the present study was performed to examine the influence of this level of hypothermia on the volume of glial cells under physiological as well as under pathological conditions.

The influence of mild (32 °C) and moderate (27 °C) hypothermia on cell volume and cell viability of C6 glioma cells was studied for 60 minutes in vitro. Cells were suspended in an incubation chamber under continuous control of temperature, pH and pO_2. Cell volume was measured by an advanced Coulter system. Hypothermia itself was causing significant cell swelling in a dose-dependent manner, which could be prevented by omission of Na^+-ions from the suspension medium, while the replacement of Cl^--ions failed to prevent cell swelling from hypothermia. Inhibition of the Na^+/H^+-antiporter with EIPA (5N-ethyl-n-isopropyl-amiloride, 50 μM) was significantly reducing the hypothermia induced cell swelling, indicating activation of the Na^+/H^+-antiporter.

Conversely, mild or moderate hypothermia failed to prevent cell swelling from lactic acid, arachidonic acid or glutamate, i.e. agents which are mediating the development of cytotoxic brain edema in vivo in cerebral trauma, ischemia and other acute insults. The findings indicate that cerebral protection by hypothermia in vivo is most likely not attributable to an inhibition of cytotoxic brain edema. Further investigations, however, are required in vivo and in vitro to elucidate the hypothermia-induced swelling of glial cells in more detail, e.g. as to the role of the Na^+/H^+-antiporter.

Keywords: Hypothermia; cell swelling; glial cells; Na^+/H^+-antiporter.

Introduction

Stroke and severe traumatic brain injury are associated with secondary sequelae in the brain, which exacerbate the primary lesion. The development of intracranial hypertension from the formation of ischemic or traumatic brain edema is one of the most important manifestations as well as cause of *secondary brain damage.* The currently available therapeutical options, however, are limited and often fail to lower the increased intracranial pressure. In recent years, hypothermia has regained interest for the treatment or prevention of secondary brain damage from acute cerebral insults [2, 3, 4]. Yet, underlying mechanisms as well as the most effective level of hypothermia affording cerebral protection while exerting minimal side effects at the cellular level are poorly understood so far. The present studies were carried out to shed more light on the influence of hypothermia on maintenance of the physiological cellular volume and its therapeutical potency on cell swelling from lactacidosis, arachidonic acid, or glutamate, respectively, which are known to mediate the development of cytotoxic brain edema in vivo.

Movements of ions across cell membranes are well known to be temperature-dependent. The purpose of the current experiments was, therefore, to study the effect of hypothermia *per se* on the glial cell volume including activation of membrane transporters, as for example the Na^+/H^+-antiporter under these circumstances. In further experiments, the protective therapeutical potential of mild hypothermia was assessed on glial cell swelling, which was elicited in vitro by mediator compounds of cytotoxic brain edema as for example lactic- or arachidonic acid.

Material and Methods

The experimental model has been described previously [9, 13]. In brief, C6 glioma cells were cultured as monolayers under standard conditions (humidified room air, 5% CO_2, 37 °C, pH 7.4, DMEM + 10% FCS + 100 IU/ml Penicillin + 50 μg/ml Streptomycin). Subcultivation was carried out daily. The cells were harvested upon reaching confluency (0.5% trypsin/0.02% EGTA in PBS) and suspended in serum-free bicarbonate-buffered (25 mM) DMEM at a density of 2–3 × 10^6 cells/ml. The cell-suspension was then trans-

Table 1. *Hypothermia-Induced Swelling of Glial Cells. Contribution of Na^+ and Cl^-*

Medium	Temperature [°C]	Cell volume at 30 min [% baseline]	Cell volume at 60 min [% baseline]
Physiological (bicarbonate buffered)	37	100.6 ± 0.6	100.8 ± 0.6
	32	110.2 ± 2.9	111.3 ± 2.9
	27	112.2 ± 2.9	113.5 ± 1.9
Na^+-free (substituted by choline)	32	99.5 ± 0.8	98.0 ± 1.2
Cl^--free (substituted by gluconate)	32	105.9 ± 0.9	109.0 ± 1.1
EIPA – Na^+/H^+-exchange inhibitor (50 μM)	32	106.3 ± 0.5	100.4 ± 1.6

Omission of Na^+-ions prevented the hypothermia-induced swelling, while omission of Cl^--ions failed to prevent the volume increase to an altered ambient temperature. Inhibition of the Na^+/H^+-antiporter by EIPA significantly inhibited cell swelling from hypothermia; Mean ± SEM.

Table 2. *Effect of Hypothermia on Cytotoxic Swelling of Glial Cells*

	Temperature [°C]	Cell Volume at 30 min [% baseline]	Cell Volume at 60 min [% baseline]	Cell Volume at 90 min [% baseline]
Glutamate [1 mM]	37	110.0 ± 0.2		122.8 ± 1.2
	32	113.3 ± 1.9		121.5 ± 3.1
Arachidonic Acid [0.3 mM]	37	106.1 ± 0.2	104.6 ± 0.7	
	32	108.5 ± 0.7	104.9 ± 0.3	
				Recovery (pH 7.4)
Lactacidosis pH 6.2	37	117.8 ± 2.2		106.0 ± 1.4
	32	118.9 ± 0.6		102.3 ± 0.1

Cell volume (mean ± SEM) of glial cells exposed to glutamate [1 mM], arachidonic acid [0.3 mM] and lactacidosis [6.2] at normo- [37 °C] and hypothermia [32 °C]. Mild hypothermia did neither prevent cell swelling from glutamate or arachidonic acid nor from exposure to lactacidosis.

ferred to a temperature-controlled incubation chamber furnished with a membrane-oxygenator to supply the suspension with a physiological mixture of CO_2, O_2 and N_2. The temperature and medium pH were continuously monitored. The cell volume was assessed by using an advanced flow cytometry system according to the Coulter principle, affording detection of changes of no more than 1–1.5%. Calibration was performed using Latex beads of known size. For each measurement, the volume of $1–2 \times 10^4$ cells was determined. The cell volume of the first three measurements served as baseline value. Cell viability was assessed by Trypan blue exclusion. Following a control period at 37 °C, the ambient temperature in the chamber was lowered to either 32 or 27 °C for 60 min. These temperature levels were reached within 5 min. Subsequently, the temperature was normalized to 37 °C for another 30 min. Cell volume was measured every 5 min.

A similar protocol was used to study the cell volume response to hypothermia utilizing Na^+-ion or Cl^--ion-free suspension medium. These ions were replaced by choline or gluconate, respectively, maintaining isotonicity. In another experimental group, the amiloride derivative EIPA (5N-ethyl-n-isopropyl-amiloride, 50 μM) was added 15 min prior to induction of hypothermia of 32 °C. For control measurements, the cells were suspended in bicarbonate-buffered medium. In further experiments, the therapeutical influence of hypothermia was analysed on cytotoxic glial swelling induced by either lactacidosis of pH 6.2 (addition of isotonic lactic acid), exposure to 0.3 mM arachidonic acid, or 1.0 mM glutamate. In these studies, lactic acid, arachidonic acid, or glutamate was added simultaneously with induction of hypothermia of 32 °C. Respective experiments carried out at normothermia served as control.

Results

As observed earlier [12], the incubation of the C6 glioma cells in standard medium at 37 °C did neither affect the cell volume (100.8 ± 0.6% at baseline, mean ± SEM) nor the cell viability during the entire experimental period. Induction of mild hypothermia (32 °C), however, resulted in significant cell swelling of 111.3 ± 2.9% baseline within 60 min ($p < 0.05$ vs. 37 °C). Upon lowering the medium temperature to 27 °C, the swelling response was further increased to 113.5 ± 1.9%. Both levels of hypothermia were characterized by typical swelling kinetics, beginning with a rapid volume increase during the first 5 min, reaching a plateau within 20 or 40 min, at 27 or 32 °C, respectively.

To investigate the significance of the cellular net-influx of Na^+-ions in the hypothermia-induced swelling process, the cells were suspended in Na^+-ion-free medium at 32 °C. The omission of Na^+-ions from the medium was completely preventing the hypothermia-induced cell swelling ($p < 0.008$ vs. control). Rather, some cell shrinking to a volume of 98.0 ± 1.2% baseline was observed at 60 min. Yet, the hypothermic exposure of the cells in Na^+-free medium was reducing cell viability to 70% at 60 min as compared to 90% viable cells found in control studies using normal, Na^+-ion containing medium. Suspension of the glial cells in Cl^--free medium, however, did not have any significant effect on the hypothermia-induced cell swelling.

In order to examine the role of the Na^+/H^+-antiporter in the hypothermia-induced swelling, the specific inhibitor EIPA (5N-ethyl-n-isopropyl-amiloride, 50 μM) was added to the medium 15 min prior to lowering of the ambient temperature to 32 °C. During baseline conditions, neither the cell volume nor the cell viability were affected by EIPA. However, the procedure was significantly ($p < 0.016$ vs. control) attenuating the swelling response of the glial cells to hypothermia indicative of an activation of the antiporter in the swelling process.

To study the *therapeutical* potential of hypothermia on glial cell swelling caused by cytotoxic agents, as isotonic lactic acid, arachidonic acid or glutamate these compounds were added to the cell suspension. The pathophysiological significance of an elevated glutamate or arachidonic acid level in the brain and of brain tissue lactacidosis is well known from the literature [11, 12]. Administration of a high glutamate concentration (1 mM) to the medium was associated with a significant increase of the glial cell volume, which was not inhibited during hypothermic exposure of the cells (32 °C). Further, exposure of the cell suspension to arachidonic acid led also to a rapid and significant volume increase without significant differences of the swelling response between normo- and hypothermia. Hence, hypothermia did not attenuate the cell volume response to arachidonic acid. With regard to the volume response to lactacidosis (pH 6.2) hypothermia appeared to afford only some enhancement of the volume recovery upon neutralization of the medium to pH 7.4 after lactacidosis of pH 6.2. During this experimental phase, a cell volume of $102.3 \pm 0.1\%$ baseline was attained by hypothermia as compared to $106.0 \pm 1.4\%$ as observed in the glial cells of the normothermic group. Nevertheless, hypothermia did not affect the swelling response of the glial cells to lactacidosis.

Discussion

Hypothermia is attracting renewed interest for neuroprotection. A number of experimental and clinical studies on *mild* hypothermia indicate beneficial properties in severe head injury and cerebral ischemia [2, 3, 5, 10]. Nevertheless, only limited information is available, on how the procedure protects brain parenchyma, particularly whether hypothermia is inhibiting the development of cytotoxic brain edema.

C6 glioma is a useful experimental model cell line to characterize the cell biological mechanisms of cell swelling and cell damage in vitro. Important physiological parameters, such as the ambient temperature pH and pO_2 were continuously monitored during the present experiments and adjusted if necessary. The cell volume was measured by an advanced flowcytometric system utilizing electrical temperature compensation. The present findings demonstrate that mild (32 °C) and moderate (27 °C) hypothermia cause significant swelling of C6 glioma cells. Upon lowering of the temperature from normal (37 °C) to e.g. 27 °C, the cell volume was immediately increasing, reaching a plateau after 20 min (32 °C), or 40 min (27 °C), which apparently was temperature-dependent. Further investigations revealed a comparable volume response to hypothermia of suspended rat astrocytes, which were obtained from primary culture.

The dose-dependency of the swelling response to the different levels of hypothermia indicates that both active and passive control processes are involved in the cellular volume regulation, which might be differently affected by mild and moderate hypothermia.

Na^+-ions are representing the most important osmotically active solutes in the extracellular compartment. The normal extra-/intracellular Na^+-concentration gradient is fueling a variety of transmembrane transport processes. This gradient is actively maintained by the Na^+/K^+-ATPase, requiring metabolic energy made available by the cell [5]. Most likely, the inhibition of the cellular energy metabolism by hypothermia is contributing to the breakdown of the transmembrane Na^+-concentration gradient due to the shortage of ATP required to fuel the Na^+/K^+-ATPase. The resulting Na^+-ion accumulation – for osmotic reasons – together with water would thereby represent the final step of the hypothermia induced cell swelling. The experiments carried out under omission of Na^+-ions in the medium indicate that the availability of this ion species is mandatory for the cell swelling from hypothermia. Accordingly, during the Na^+-free experimental conditions inhibition of the energy metabolism by the low temperature could not induce a net-flux of Na^+-ions into the glial cells as final mechanism of cell swelling. The choline ions, which were replacing Na^+-ions do not penetrate the cellular membrane.

The current findings on administration of EIPA, a selective inhibitor of the Na^+/H^+-exchanger indicate that the antiporter was obviously involved in the cell swelling from hypothermia, while in the studies on Cl^--ion-free suspension medium significant alterations of the volume response to hypothermia were not observed. Thereby, these findings confirm again the central role of the net-influx of Na^+-ions in cell swelling. Nevertheless, information is still limited on the complexity of the cellular volume control during hypothermia.

On the basis of these findings, it is not surprising that mild hypothermia did not prevent cell swelling from conditions inducing cytotoxic brain edema in vivo, such as lactacidosis, or accumulation of glutamate or arachidonic acid. The mechanisms which are underlying cell swelling from e.g. lactacidosis, glutamate or arachidonic acid exposure are quite well understood [1, 8, 9, 11]. Briefly, exposure of glial cells to higher than normal glutamate levels is activating high-affinity glutamate transporters in the cell membrane affording clearance of glutamate from the extracellular compartment by a downhill co-transport of Na^+-ions and, thus, water for osmotic reasons. Due to the steep intra- to extracellular glutamate concentration gradient, the clearance of glutamate by the cell is an uphill process, therefore dependent on the downhill co-transport of Na^+-ions from the extra- to the intracellular compartment. The resulting osmotic load of the cell causing swelling is the prize which is paid to normalize the interstitial, i.e. low glutamate concentration as a requirement of a normal neuronal function.

On the other side, cell swelling induced by arachidonic acid is more reflecting a cytotoxic process secondary to the activation of a variety of pathophysiological mechanisms. One is the resulting intracellular acidification with activation of the Na^+/H^+-antiporter, another is the formation of O_2-derived free radicals and lipid peroxides from metabolization of arachidonic acid as the mechanism, which directly injures the cell membrane [13]. Obviously, these mechanisms causing cell swelling from glutamate or arachidonic acid were not therapeutically affected by hypothermia. The same is true for the lactacidosis induced cell swelling, whereby the medium pH was lowered to 6.2. The mechanisms of the lactacidosis-induced cell swelling have also been extensively studied [8, 11, 13]. It is known that exposure of cells to lactic acid causes formation of CO_2 from bicarbonate buffering, resulting in an intracellular acidification upon diffusion of carbon dioxide into the cell. Subsequently, H^+-ions generated in the cell are exchanged from activation of the Na^+/H^+-antiporter against extracellular Na^+-ions, which together with Cl^--ions and water induce an osmotic load of the cell as factor underlying the acidosis induced cell swelling. As seen, hypothermia again was failing to prevent these complex mechanisms underlying the acidosis induced cell swelling. Yet, it appeared to afford a somewhat more rapid normalization of the cell volume after neutralization of the suspension medium, while the extent of the acidosis induced swelling was not affected.

Taken together, both mild and moderate hypothermia are causing a temperature-dependent increase of the volume of suspended glial cells in vitro. Although further details are not explored yet, it is quite likely that hypothermia is affecting the balance of Na^+-ion fluxes into and out of the cell. Thereby, cell swelling ensued from a gradual net-accumulation of Na^+-ions in the cell. This mechanism most likely was supported by activation of the Na^+/H^+-antiporter, which quite obviously is dependent on an intact extra- to intracellular not-concentration gradient. The important role of the net-influx of Na^+-ions can also be concluded from the results obtained during suspension of the glial cells under hypothermic conditions in Na^+-ion-free medium, which was completely inhibiting the hypothermia-induced cell swelling. With regard to the powerful neuroprotection afforded by moderate hypothermia in both trauma and ischemia of the brain in vivo under clinical and experimental conditions, the current findings clearly indicate that this therapeutical potential is not based on an inhibition of cytotoxic brain edema. Rather, cell swelling elicited by hypothermia must be considered an important side effect of this promising therapeutical method.

Acknowledgments

The secretarial and technical assistance of H. Kleylein and I. Kölbl is gratefully acknowledged.

References

1. Baethmann A, Staub F, Kempski O, Plesnila N, Chang RCC, Schneider GH, Eriskat J, Stoffel M, Ringel F (1997) Glutamate enhances brain damage from ischemia and trauma. In: Ito U *et al* (eds) Maturation phenomenon in cerebral ischemia II. Springer, Berlin Heidelberg New York Tokyo

2. Clifton GL, Allen S, Berry J, Koch SM (1992) Systemic hypothermia in treatment of brain injury. J Neurotrauma 9: S487–495
3. Clifton GL, Allen S, Barrodale P, Plenger P, Berry J, Koch SM, Fletcher J. Hayes RL, Choi SC (1993) A phase II study of moderate hypothermia in severe brain injury. J Neurotrauma 10: 263–271
4. Dietrich WD, Busto R, Globus MYT, Ginsberg MD (1996) Brain damage and temperature: cellular and molecular mechanisms. Adv Neurol 71: 177–194
5. Ginsberg MD, Sternau L, Globus MYT, Dietrich WD, Busto R (1992) Therapeutic modulation of brain temperature: relevance to ischemic brain injury. Cerebrovasc Brain Metab Revs 4: 189–225
6. Huang R, Shuaib A, Hertz L (1993) Glutamate uptake and glutamate content in primary cultures of mouse astrocytes during anoxia, substrate deprivation and simulated ischemia under normothermic and hypothermic conditions. Brain Res 618: 346–351
7. Karibe H, Zarow G, Graham S, Weinstein P (1994) Mild intraischemic hypothermia reduces postischemic hyperperfusion, delayed postischemic hypoperfusion, blood-brain barrier disruption, brain edema, and neuronal damage volume after temporary focal cerebral ischemia in rats. J Cereb Blood Flow Metab 14: 620–627
8. Karibe H, Zarow GJ, Weinstein PR (1995) Delayed induction of mild hypothermia to reduce infarct volume after temporary middle cerebral artery occlusion in rats. J Neurosurg 83: 93–98
9. Kempski O, Chaussy L, Gross U, Zimmer M, Baethmann A (1992) Swelling of C6 glioma cells and astrocytes from glutamate, high K+ concentrations or acidosis. Prog Brain Res 94: 69–75
10. Marion DW, Penrod LE, Kelsey SE, Obrist WD, Kochanek PM, Palmer AM, Wisniewski SR, DeKoskey ST (1997) Treatment of traumatic brain injury with moderate hypothermia. N Eng J Med 336: 540–546
11. Siesjö BK (1981) Cell damage in the brain: a speculative synthesis J Cereb Blood Flow Metab 1: 155–185
12. Staub F, Baethmann A, Peters J, Weigt H, Kempski O (1990) Effects of lactacidosis on glial cell volume and viability. J Cereb Blood Flow Metab 10: 866–876
13. Staub F, Winkler A, Peters J, Kempski O, Kachel V, Baethmann A (1994) Swelling, acidosis, and irreversible damage of glial cells from exposure to arachidonic acid in vitro. J Cereb Blood Flow Metab 14: 1030–1039

Correspondence: Nikolaus Plesnila, M.D., Stroke and Neurovascular Regeneration Laboratory, Massachusetts General Hospital, Harvard Medical School, 149 13th St., CNY 6403, Charlestown, MA 02129, USA.

Hydrocephalus

Hydrocephalus and the implications of movement of CSF and tissue water in the clinical setting are presented in this section. Zeilinger *et al.*, describe the treatment of normal pressure hydrocephalus with reference to endoscopic ventriculostomy, as well as clinical testing, to document the need for surgical treatment. They state in their presentation that pathologically increased resistance to CSF outflow in the lumbar infusion test indicates that a shunt placement is necessary. For those patients who have an outflow resistance increase in the ventricular infusion test (Meier *et al.*) accompanied by a physiological lumbar infusion test, endoscopically assisted ventriculostomy is indicated. The authors postulate a functional aqueduct stenosis in these patients. For those patients requiring a shunt procedure, the authors discuss the various valve options. The advantages and disadvantages of the different valves with reference to the horizontal position and the upright position are reported.

Acta Neurochir (2000) [Suppl] 76: 559–562

Clinical Experiences with the Dual-Switch Valve in Patients with Normal Pressure Hydrocephalus

F. S. Zeilinger[1], **T. Reyer**[2], **U. Meier**[1], and **D. Kintzel**[2]

[1] Department of Neurosurgery, Unfallkrankenhaus Berlin mit berufsgenossenschaftlicher Unfallklinik, Germany
[2] Department of Neurosurgery, Krankenhaus im Friedrichshain, Germany

Summary

In patients with normal pressure hydrocephalus (NPH) we compared the postoperative results reference to the implanted valve type.

In 117 patients diagnosed with normal pressure hydrocephalus there was placement of 47 Cordis Standard valves (CSV), 20 Cordis Orbis Sigma valves type I (OSV) and 50 Miethke Dual-switch valves (DSV). Ninety-five patients (36/19/40) were re-evaluated. Normal pressure hydrocephalus was graduated according to the results of the intrathecal infusion test in an early and late stage. There were no statistical differences in mechanical and infective complications between the different valve types. We found significant differences in overdrainages and subdural hematomas. Two patients (6%) with a CSV, 3 patients (16%) with an OSV and 1 patient (3%) with a DSV developed clinical symptoms due to this.

The course of disease in patients with NPH is influenced by the stage of disease – degree of cerebral atrophy – and also by the implanted valve type. The great amount of overdrainage complications and subdural hematomas in the Cordis Orbis Sigma valve group may be an argument against this valve. Our clinical experiences with the Miethke Dual-switch valve show that this hydrostatic valve may be advantageous for patients with NPH.

Keywords: Normal pressure hydrocephalus; shunt operation; hydrostatic valve; overdrainage.

Introduction

Despite emerging knowledge in valve regulated shunt therapy for treatment of hydrocephalus internal, there are still biomechanical problems caused by an unphysiological construction of the valves. This is reflected in the high number of available devices with more than 195 different valves, which can be subdivided into three construction types. The first group, the so called differential pressure valves, have a fixed opening pressure which is related to the horizontal position of the patient. The programmable valves allow a non-invasive adjustment of the opening pressure but they also bear the problem that they do not take the posture of the patient into account. The third group are hydrostatic valves which aim to reduce the flow through the shunt when the patient moves into the upright position [1, 15, 16].

Conventional differential pressure valves have the disadvantage in patients with a normal pressure hydrocephalus (NPH) that they open abruptly when the patient moves into the upright position and therefore induce a negative pressure on the brain.

Patients and Methods

117 patients with normal pressure hydrocephalus were treated by a ventriculo-peritoneal shunt insertion in the Department of Neurosurgery of the hospital Berlin-Friedrichshain from May 1982 and in the Department of Neurosurgery of the Unfallkrankenhaus Berlin from September 1997 through March 1999. In 47 patients we implanted a Cordis-Standard valve, in 20 patients a Cordis-Orbis-Sigma valve type I, and in 50 patients a Miethke Dual-Switch valve (Fig. 1). Ninety-five of these patients (39/19/40) were thoroughly reinvestigated. The signs of each patient were classified according to the clinical grading of Kiefer and Steudel, and we compared the course of disease after surgery and catamnesia at an average of 7 months, with our created NPH-Recovery-Rate [13].

$$\text{NPH-R-R} = \frac{\text{Clinical grading preoperative–postoperative}}{\text{Clinical grading preoperative}} \times 10$$

Comparison of the internationally established Black grading scale for shunt assessment [2] and our NPH-Recovery-rate is illustrated in Table 1. The indication for shunt implantation was made according to the clinical signs and the results of the intrathecal infusion test with measurement of a pathological, increased resistance [7, 11, 12]. The resistance to cerebrospinal fluid outflow (R_{out}) is the main criterion for grouping patients into those with normal pressure hydrocephalus and those with cerebral atrophy. A further differentiation into early stage (NPH without atrophy) and late stage (NPH in association with atrophy) is made by measuring the compliance (C_P) – this being a secondary criterion (Fig. 1). Patients whose outflow resistance was in the physiological range were diagnosed for cerebral atrophy. The mathematical fundamentals, the standardized investi-

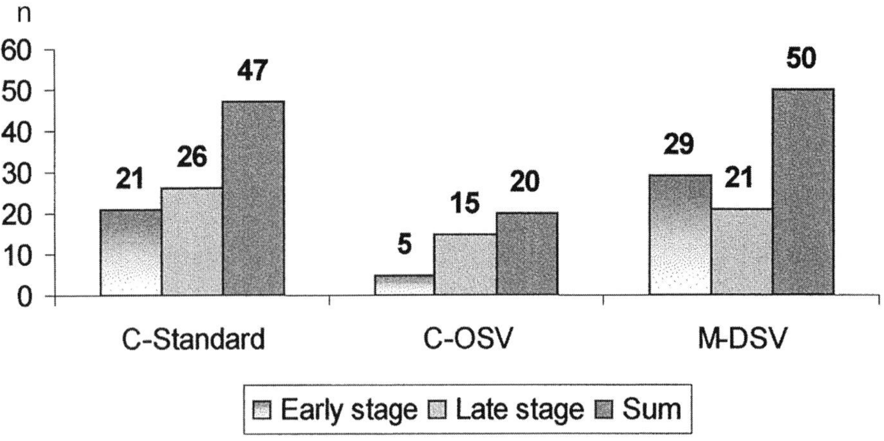

Fig. 1. Valve types versus NPH stage

Table 1. *Black Grading Scale for Shunt Assessment Versus NPH-Recovery-Rate*

Black grading scale for shunt assessment		NPH-recovery-rate
Grading	Description	More/same
Excellent	activity like before	7
Good	slight reduction	5
Fair	gradual improvement	3
Transient	temporary improvement	2
Poor	unchanged or worsened	less than 2

gation procedure, and the indications for the performance of a computer aided infusion test have been described previously [7–13].

Results

In the clinical follow up according to the NPH-Recovery-Rate and using the U-test of Mann-Whitney ($p < 0,01$), we have found a statistically significant improvement in patients with an implanted Miethke-Dual-Switch valve (*) and also catamnestia after a mean time interval of 7 months (**). While differentiating the operative and valve induced morbidity we found no difference in mechanical and infectious complications between the different valve types. Distinct differences exist in overdrainage complications and subdural hematomas (Fig. 3). Four patients (11%) with a Cordis-Standard valve, 5 patients (26%) with a Cordis-Orbis-Sigma valve type I and 2 patients (5%) with a Miethke-Dual-Switch valve had a reduction of ventricular width visualised in the CT scan or MRI. Of those, 2 patients (6%) with Cordis-Standard valve, 3 patients (16%) with a Cordis-Orbis-Sigma valve type I and 1 patient (3%) with a Miethke-Dual-Switch valve exhibited clinical signs. The 3 patients with a Cordis-Orbis-Sigma valve type I developed subdural hematomas and 2 (11%) of them had to be evacuated. One of these patients (5%) died due to a hematocephalus.

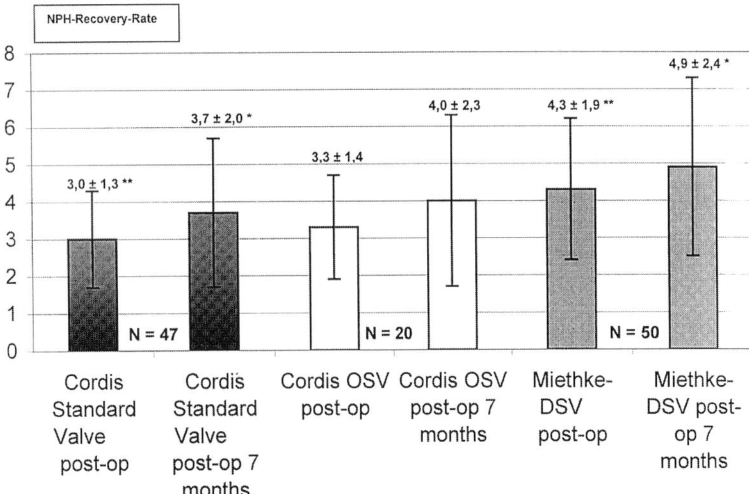

Fig. 2. NPH-recovery-rate versus valve types

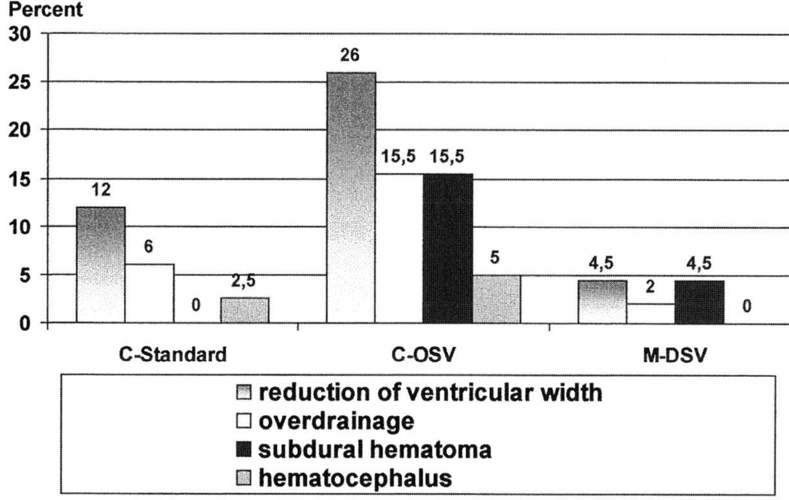

Fig. 3. Complications due to valve related overdrainages versus valve types

Two patients (5%) with a Miethke-Dual-Switch valve developed subdural hematomas, in one of these patients the subdural hematoma was resorbed without accompanying clinical symptoms within one month, and in the other patient we had to remove the shunt (Fig. 3).

Discussion

In patients with an early stage NPH there were 2 (6%) clinically relevant overdrainage complications after insertion of a Cordis-Standard valve (Fig. 3). Trost *et al.* [16] pointed out that many patients tolerate negative intraventricular pressure values which are a matter of fact of the physical characteristics of this valve type. In the Dutch multicentre study [3] there was a statistically significant better postoperative result obtainable with the implantation of low pressure differential pressure valves in comparison with medium pressure valves but this advantage was accompanied by a high overdrainage rate (71% versus 34%). The clinical relevance of the high overdrainage rate was not described in this study but in our opinion, this rate is too high. One reason for the implantation of differential valves is their low price but the costs for treatment of overdrainage complications are much higher. The reasons for the statistically significant better results after insertion of the Miethke-Dual-Switch valve (Fig. 2) are our subtle diagnostic procedures [7–13] and the construction of this valve which takes the changes of the patient's posture into account [14, 15, 16].

The Orbis-Sigma valve aims to regulate a constant flow which depends on the differential pressure acting on the system. This is very important in patients with a late stage NPH in order to avoid overdrainage complication. Unfortunately, we had altogether 5 overdrainages (26%) including 3 chronical subdural hematomas (16%) as complications with this valve type. Also Weiner *et al.* [17] reported about subdural hematomas in patients with NPH after insertion of an Orbis-Sigma valve. In contrast to Czosnyka *et al.* [4], Decq *et al.* [5] found a significantly lower overdrainage rate after Orbis-Sigma valve insertion in contrast to conventional differential pressure valves. These studies were not exclusively evaluating patients with NPH and therefore they cannot completely be compared with our results. According to our results the Orbis-Sigma valve is not appropriate for patients with NPH. The Cordis differential pressure valve bears the disadvantage in patients with a late stage NPH that they induce a suction effect on the brain when the patient moves into the upright position. An anti-siphon device can prevent this problem but the resistance of the system is then increased. In our patients we observed 3 overdrainages (8%) and 2 (6%) of these patients developed clinical signs with this valve type. The Miethke Dual-Switch valve [14] is the first construction which changes between two different valve chambers in parallel depending on the posture of the patient. Two of our patients (5%) with a Dual-Switch valve developed subdural hematomas and one of those exhibited no clinical signs. The more favourable results of the patients with the Dual-Switch valve are evident and are expressed in the criteria of the NPH-Recovery-Rate (Fig. 2).

The course of disease in patients with NPH is influenced by the stage of disease (NPH with or without cerebral atrophy) at the moment of therapy and of the implanted valve type. According to Lee *et al.* [6] an adequate shunt operation offers the chance for an improvement of cerebral blood flow and vasomotor reactivity in NPH patients. The low overdrainage rate with less than 5 percent and the good postoperative results in our opinion are the main aspects that the Miethke Dual-Switch valve represents at the present moment, the best valve in patients for NPH.

References

1. Aschoff A, Benesch C, Kremer P, Fruh K, Klank A, Kunze S (1995) Overdrainage and shunt-technology. A critical comparison of programmable, hydrostatic and variable-resistance-valve and flow-reducing devices. Childs Nerv Syst 11: 193–202
2. Benzell EC, Pelletier AL, Levy PG (1990) Communicating hydrocephalus in adults: Prediction of outcome after ventricular shunting procedures. Neurosurgery 26: 655–660
3. Boon AJW, Thans JThJ, Delwel EJ, Egeler-Peerdman SM, Hanlo PW, Wurzer JAL, Avezaat CJJ, Jong de DA, Gooskens RHJM, Hermans J (1997) Does CSF outflow resistance predict the resistance to shunting in patients with normal pressure hydrocephalus? In: Marmarou A, Bullock R, Avezaat C, Baethmann A, Becker D, Brock M, Hoff J, Nagai H, Reulen H-J, teasdale G (eds) Intracranial pressure and neuromonitoring in brain injury. Springer, Wien New York, pp 331–333
4. Czosnyka Z, Czosnyka M, Richards HK, Pickard JD (1998) Posture-related overdrainage: comparison of the performance of 10 hydrocephalus shunts in vitro. Neurosurgery 42: 327–334
5. Decq P, Barat JL, Duplessis E, Lequerinel C, Gendrault P, Keravel Y (1995) Shunt failure in adult hydrocephalus: flow controlled shunt versus differential pressure shunts – a cooperative study in 289 patients. Surg Neurol 43: 333–339
6. Lee EJ, Hung YC, Chang CH, Pai MC, Chen HH (1998) Cerebral blood flow velocity and vasomotor reactivity before and after shunting surgery in patients with normal pressure hydrocephalus. Acta Neurochir (Wien) 140: 599–605
7. Meier U, Reichmuth B, Knop W, Riederer A (1993) Intrathecal infusion test: An investigative method to treat malresorptive hydrocephalus by shunt operation. In: Lorenz R, Klinger M, Brock M (eds) Advances in neurosurgery 21. Springer, Berlin Heidelberg New York Tokyo, pp 125–129
8. Meier U, Reichmuth B, Zeilinger FS, Lehmann R (1996) The importance of xenon-computed tomography in the diagnosis of normal pressure hydrocephalus. Intern J Neuroradiology 2: 153–160
9. Meier U (1997) Der intrathekale Infusionstest als Entscheidungshilfe zur Shunt-Operation beim Normaldruckhydrozephalus. Akt Neurol 24: 24–35
10. Meier U, Zeilinger FS, Kintzel D (1997) Klinik und Krankheitsverlauf beim Normaldruckhydrocephalus im Vergleich zur Hirnatrophie. Schw Arch Neurol Psychiatr 147: 73–83
11. Meier U, Künzel B, Zeilinger FS, Riederer A, Kintzel D (1997) Die Diagnostik des Normaldruckhydrozephalus: Ein Berechnungsmodell zur Ermittlung der ICP-abhängigen Resistance und Compliance. Nervenarzt 68: 496–502
12. Meier U, Zeilinger FS, Kintzel D (1998) Pathophysiologie, Klinik und Krankheitsverlauf beim Normaldruckhydrocephalus. Fortschr Neurol Psychiatr 66: 176–191
13. Meier U (1999) Zur klinischen Graduierung des Normaldruckhydrocephalus. Akt Neurol 26: 127–132
14. Miethke C, Affeld K (1994) A new valve for the treatment of hydrocephalus. Biomed Tech 39: 181–187
15. Sprung C, Miethke C, Trost HA, Lanksch WR (1996) The dual-switch valve. Childs Nerv Syst 12: 573–581
16. Trost HA, Sprung C, Lanksch W, Stolke D, Miethke C (1998) Dual-Switch valve: clinical performance of a new hydrocephalus valve. Acta Neurochir [Suppl] (Wien) 71: 360–363
17. Weiner HL, Constantini S, Cohen H, Wisoff JH (1995) Current treatment of normal pressure hydrocephalus: Comparison of flow-regulated and differential-pressure shunt valves. Neurosurgery 37: 877–888

Correspondence: Dr. med. Frank S. Zeilinger, Department of Neurosurgery, Unfallkrankenhaus Berlin mit berufsgenossenschaftlicher Unfallklinik e.V., Rapsweg 55, 12683 Berlin, Germany.

Acta Neurochir (2000) [Suppl] 76: 563–566

Endoscopic Ventriculostomy Versus Shunt Operation in Normal Pressure Hydrocephalus: Diagnostics and Indication

U. Meier, F. S. Zeilinger, and **B. Schönherr**

Department of Neurosurgery, Unfallkrankenhaus Berlin, Germany

Summary

In contrast to shunt operation the indication for an endoscopic ventriculostomy in patients diagnosed for normal pressure hydrocephalus is not scientifically established. From September 1997 to March 1999 we operated on 36 patients diagnosed for normal pressure hydrocephalus. Diagnosis was established by means of the intrathecal lumbar or ventricular infusion test, the cerebrospinal fluid tap test and MRI-CSF flow studies pre- and post-operatively. In 30 patients (83%) we implanted a ventriculo-peritoneal shunt, and in 6 patients (17%) we performed the endoscopic assisted third ventriculostomy. With our created NPH recovery rate and use of the clinical grading for normal pressure hydrocephalus created by Kiefer and Steudel we compared the operative results of both patient groups. In patients with a pathologically increased resistance to CSF outflow in the lumbar infusion test a shunt implantation is indicated. Patients whose outflow resistance is increased in the ventricular infusion test but with a physiological lumbar infusion test are suspected for a functional aqueduct stenosis and should be treated by means of an endoscopic assisted ventriculostomy.

Keywords: Endoscopic ventriculostomy; normal pressure hydrocephalus; aqueduct stenosis; phase contrast MRI.

Introduction

In contrast to insertion of a ventriculo-peritoneal shunt, the indication for an endoscopic ventriculostomy in patients diagnosed for normal pressure hydrocephalus (NPH) is not scientifically established. Our prospective clinical study was designed as to find predictors for each operative method and to evaluate the long-term results.

Material and Method

Thirty-six patients with normal pressure hydrocephalus were surgically treated in the Department of Neurosurgery of the Unfallkrankenhaus Berlin between September 1997 and March 1999. Diagnosis of NPH was obtained by the intrathecal infusion test on a lumbar and/or ventricular route, the cerebrospinal fluid tap test, and MRI cerebrospinal fluid flow studies pre- and postoperatively. The signs of each patient were registered according to the clinical grading for normal pressure hydrocephalus by Kiefer and Steudel. We then compared the course of disease at a mean time interval of 7 months while using our created NPH recovery rate [12]:

$$\text{NPH recovery rate} = \frac{\text{clinical grading preoperative} - \text{postoperative}}{\text{clinical grading postoperative}} \times 10$$

The indication for shunt operation or endoscopic ventriculostomy was assessed by evaluating the clinical signs and the results of the intrathecal infusion test [8]. The outflow resistance is the main criterion for classifying patients into those with NPH and those with cerebral atrophy. A pathological increased outflow resistance in the intrathecal infusion test represents an indication for an operative intervention. Patients with a physiological outflow resistance and increased compliance were diagnosed for cerebral atrophy and not treated operatively [8]. The mathematical fundamentals, the standardized investigation procedure and the indications for the performance of a computer assisted infusion test as well as pathophysiological consideration. Clinical signs and the course of disease in NPH has been described previously [6–12].

Results

In 30 patients (83%) a ventriculo-peritoneal shunt with a Miethke Dual-Switch valve [13] was inserted, and in 6 patients (17%) we performed an endoscopic assisted third ventriculostomy. After evaluation of the clinical signs according to the clinical grading for normal pressure hydrocephalus, the lumbar infusion test was accomplished [12]. The indication for shunt operation was assessed by means of measuring the intracranial pressure and a baseline pressure within physiological limits, a hydrocephalus of all ventricles visualised in CT scan or MRI and a pathological increased outflow resistance in the lumbar infusion test.

Indication for Shunt Operation in NPH

MRI/CT:	hydrocephalus involving all ventricles
Baseline ICP:	within physiological limits
Lumbar infusion test:	*pathological resistance*
Ventricular infusion test:	pathological resistance

In patients with suspected aqueductal stenosis on MRI examinations and/or physiological outflow resistance in the lumbar infusion test, a ventricular infusion test was performed. With a pathological outflow resistance in the ventricular infusion test but physiological resistance in the lumbar infusion test a third ventriculostomy was favoured (Fig. 2).

Indication for Third Ventriculostomy in NPH

MRI/CT:	suspected aqueductal stenosis
Baseline ICP:	within physiological limits
Lumbar infusion test:	*physiological resistance*
Ventricular infusion test:	pathological resistance

Patients with an elevated baseline ICP in the horizontal position were classified as pressure hydrocephalus and excluded from this study. The complications of both operative methods were analysed regarding reoperation rate, operation related morbidity and mortality (Table 1). The comparison of the postoperative course of disease and catamnesis at a mean time interval of 7 months while using our own NPH recovery rate, allows no statistical evaluation due to the small number of patients where we have performed a third ventriculostomy (Fig. 1). Our experiences with shunt therapy and different valve types were published elsewhere [8, 9, 11]. From 1997 we exclusively inserted the Miethke Dual Switch valve [13, 14] in patients with NPH.

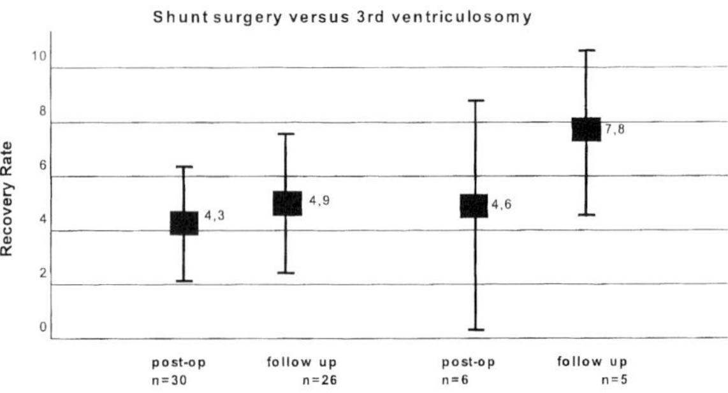

Fig. 1. NPH-Recovery-Rate according to the clinical grading for NPH of Kiefer

Table 1. *Complications*

Complications	Shunt-operation	Third ventriculostomy
Revisions complete	5	0
Infections	2	0
Insufficiency	1	0
Dislocation	1	0
SDH	2	0
Pneumatocepahlus	0	1
Morbidity	*20%*	*17%*
Morbidity OP-related	6	1
Lethality OP-related	0	0
Lethality independent	1	1

Discussion

Indications for an intracranial endoscopy, as agreed by different authors [1, 4, 5, 17], are obstructive hydrocephalus caused by intraventricular cysts and tumors. According to the Aachen workgroup [16] we favor the combination of neuronavigation and endoscopic techniques for an intraoperative quality assessment. The type of normal pressure hydrocephalus described as functional aqueduct stenosis by our own workgroup is established by measuring normal baseline ICP values in the horizontal position, and an increased outflow resistance in the ventricular infusion test. The reason for this phenomenon is, in our opinion, a valve like mechanism in the region of the stenosis, which causes a pathologically increased resistance, mostly at ICP values between 15 and 30 Torr, decreasing gradually at higher ICP values to normal range, due to the intrathecal infusion (volume-pressure-load) (Fig. 2). Pathophysiologically a reduced bulk flow of cerebrospinal fluid between third and fourth ventricle must be considered. This induces a dilatation of the lateral and third ventricle. When the intraventricular pressure exceeds the resistance of the stenosis, CSF can flow. The physiologial examination results of the lumbar infusion test prove that these patients have no disturbances in the extraventricular cerebrospinal fluid bulk flow.

According to Barlow and Ching [1] the ratio between patients with shunt operation and endoscopic ventriculostomy (150:30) is about 15 percent which is in accordance with our results (17 percent). These authors [1] conclude – based on their excellent clinical results after endoscopic third ventriculostomy – that ventriculostomy has the advantage of a reduced revision rate and reduced length of hospital stay, which is a relevant economic factor. Due to the small number of

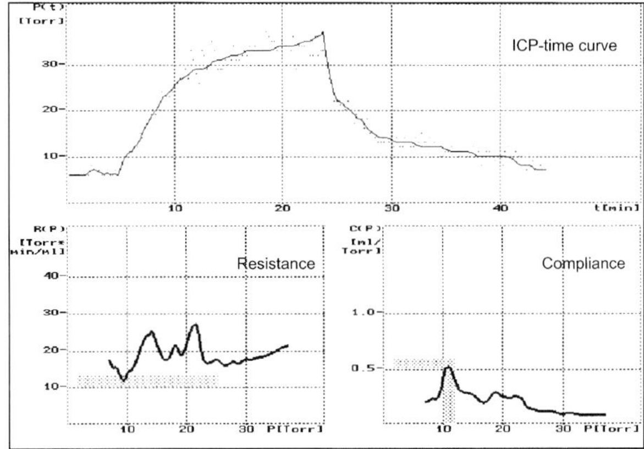

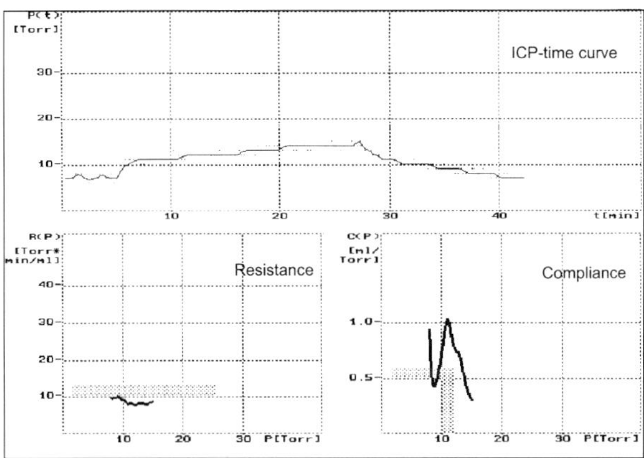

Fig. 2. Example of a patient with NPH in an early stage. Examination protocol of ventricular infusion test (above) with an elevated ICP-time curve; pathological increased outflow resistance (above left); physiological compliance (above right). Examination protocol of lumbar infusion test (below) with a flat ICP-time-curve; outflow resistance in the physiological range (below left) and compliance (below right)

patients in our study we cannot make a similar assumption. Regarding the complications in our patients we could not find significant differences with 20 percent after shunt insertion and 17 percent after third ventriculostomy. De Divitiis [2] reported complications in 11 percent, being mostly a temporary bleeding out of an external drainage after endoscopic ventriculostomy. In contrast to Mohanty *et al.* [15] who reported on acute sudural hematomas after endoscopic ventriculostomy, this did not occur in our patients. The operation related morbidity due to shunt operations has been discussed extensively in other reports [13]. The mortality rate due to operations was 0 percent, as also reported by other groups [2, 4].

Foroutan *et al.* [3] points out that aside of the improved clinical symptoms the postoperative functional MRI confirms the right indication and operative therapy of the endoscopic ventriculostomy. We can agree with this statement. In contrast to Schwartz *et al.* [17] we did not recognize a marked reduction of ventricular width in patients with NPH. Contrary to pressure hydrocephalus a reduction of ventricle width cannot be expected in normal pressure hydrocephalus in a chronic state because the bioplastic deformation decreases parenchymatous tissue. Therefore the determining factors for a restitution are accomplished by the intracranial compensating mechanisms and the quantity of undamaged structures [13]. Bearing this in mind, normal pressure hydrocephalus should be diagnosed at an early stage because disturbances of cerebral autoregulation take place in the late stage and therefore, the therapeutic results are worse after valve implantation or endoscopic ventriculostomy. Thus a delay in the diagnostic reduces the rehabilitational of the patients due to an irreversible disturbance of their cognitive potential.

We conclude that for patients diagnosed for NPH with findings of a pathological outflow resistance in the lumbar infusion test a shunt operation is indicated. Patients whose outflow resistance is pathologically increased in the ventricular infusion test as well as with physiological results in the lumbar infusion test and signs of an aqueduct stenosis in MRI, an endoscopic assisted third ventriculostomy is indicated. Postoperative a functional MRI with phase-contrast imaging is a way to visualize the operative result. Follow up examinations for a quality assessment of these endoscopic operation method, are still in progress.

References

1. Barlow P, Ching HS (1997) An economic argument in favour of endoscopic third ventriculostomy as a treatment for obstructive hydrocephalus. Minim Invasive Neurosurg 40: 37–39
2. De Divitiis O (1998) Provision of a neuroendoscopy service. The Southhampton experience. J Neurosurg Sci 42: 137–143
3. Foroutan M, Mafee MF, Dujovny M (1998) Third ventriculostomy, phase-contrast cine MRI and endoscopic techniques. Neurol Res 20: 443–448
4. Gaab MR, Schroeder HW (1998) Neuroendoscopic approach to intraventricular lesions. J Neurosurg 88: 496–505
5. Gangemi M, Maiuri F, Donati P, Sigona L, Iaconetta G, De Divitiis E (1998) Neuroendoscopy: Personal experience, indications and limits. J Neurosurg Sci 42: 1–10
6. Meier U, Michalik M, Reichmuth B (1987) Computertomographie und Infusionstest bei einem posttraumatischen Hydrocephalus. Psychiatry Neurol Med Psychol 39: 754–758
7. Meier U, Reichmuth B, Zeilinger FS, Lehmann R (1996) The Importance of Xenon-Computed Tomography in the Diagnosis of Normal Pressure Hydrocephalus. Intern J Neuroradiology 2: 153–160

8. Meier U (1997) Der intrathekale Infusionstest als Entscheidungshilfe zur Shunt-Operation beim Normaldruckhydrozephalus. Akt Neurologie 24: 24–35
9. Meier U, Zeilinger FS, Kintzel D (1997) Klinik und Krankheitsverlauf beim Normaldruckhydrozephalus im Vergleich zur Hirnatrophie. Schw Arch Neurol Psychiatry 147: 73–83
10. Meier U, Künzel B, Zeilinger FS, Riederer A, Kintzel D (1997) Die Diagnostik des Normaldruckhydrozephalus: Ein Berechnungsmodell zur Ermittlung der ICP-abhängigen Resistance und Compliance. Nervenarzt 68: 496–502
11. Meier U, Zeilinger FS, Kintzel D (1998) Pathophysiologie, Klinik und Krankheitsverlauf beim Normaldruckhydrozephalus. Fortschr Neurol Psychiatry 66: 176–191
12. Meier U (1999) Zur klinischen Graduierung des Normaldruckhydrozephalus. Akt Neurologie 26: 127–132
13. Meier U, Zeilinger FS, Reyer T, Kintzel D (2000) Klinische Erfahrungen mit verschiedenen Shuntsystemen beim Normaldruckhydrozephalus: Hydrostatische versus konventionelle Differentialdruckventile. Zent bl Neurochir 61 (in Druck)
14. Miethke C, Affeld K (1994) A new valve for the treatment of hydrocephalus. Biomed Tech 39: 181–187
15. Mohanty A, Anandh B, Reddy MS, Sastry KV (1997) Contralateral massive acute subdural collection after endoscopic third ventriculostomy – a case report. Minim Invasive Neurosurg 40: 59–61
16. Rodhe V, Reinges MH, Krombach GA, Gilsbach JM (1998) The combined use of image-guided frameless stereotaxy and neuroendoscopy for surgical managment of occlusive hydrocephalus and intracranial cysts. Br J Neurosurg 12: 531–538
17. Schwartz TH, Yoon SS, Cutruzzola FW, Goodman RR (1996) Third ventriculostomy: post-operative ventricular size and outcome. Minim Invas Neurosurg 39: 122–129

Correspondence: Privat-Dozent Dr. med. Ullrich Meier, Department of Neurosurgery, Unfallkrankenhaus Berlin, Rapsweg 55, 12683 Berlin, Germany.

Author Index

Index of Keywords

Antonio F. Germanò,
Francesco Tomasello

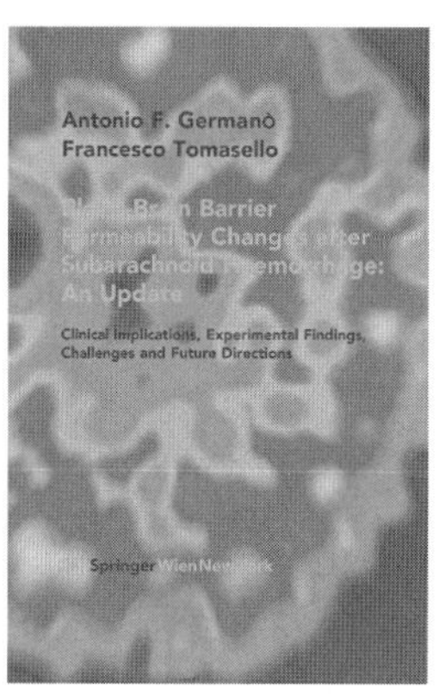

Blood-Brain Barrier Permeability Changes after Subarachnoid Haemorrhage: An Update

Clinical Implications, Experimental Findings,
Challenges and Future Directions

2001. Approx. 180 pages. Approx. 40 figures.
Hardcover DM 98,–, öS 686,–
(recommended retail price)
ISBN 3-211-83526-1
Due June 2001

This monograph constitutes a comprehensive overview of BBB permeability changes and related damaging sequelae asscociated with subarachnoid haermorrhage. Despite improvements in the surgical and clinical management patients still experience an unacceptably high morbidity and mortality linked to the presence of subarachnoid blood.

In this monograph, the authors have reviewed the historical basis of this problem, the anatomical substrates of the BBB, the occurrence and adverse consequences of barrier disruption following SAH, the related sequelae of oedema formation, ICP alteration and vasospasm discussed from both the basic science and clinical perspective, with the consideration of multiple clinical and laboratory investigative tools, including all aspects of modern imaging.

The text is supplemented by presenting key research publications in the field, focusing on the damaging consequences of subarachnoid blood, while attempting to explain the hierarchy of events in those progressive changes associated with blood-brain barrier perturbation, including vasospasm, ischaemia and elevated intracranial pressure.

Contents

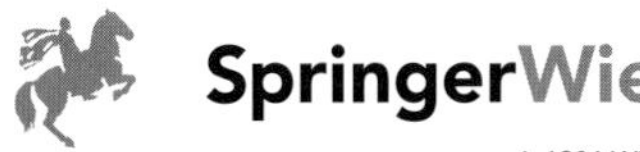

SpringerWienNewYork

A-1201 Wien, Sachsenplatz 4–6, P.O. Box 89, Fax +43.1.330 24 26, e-mail: books@springer.at, Internet: **www.springer.at**
D-69126 Heidelberg, Haberstraße 7, Fax +49.6221.345-229, e-mail: orders@springer.de
USA, Secaucus, NJ 07096-2485, P.O. Box 2485, Fax +1.201.348-4505, e-mail: orders@springer-ny.com
Eastern Book Service, Japan, Tokyo 113, 3–13, Hongo 3-chome, Bunkyo-ku, Fax +81.3.38 18 08 64, e-mail: orders@svt-ebs.co.jp

Springer-Verlag
and the Environment

WE AT SPRINGER-VERLAG FIRMLY BELIEVE THAT AN international science publisher has a special obligation to the environment, and our corporate policies consistently reflect this conviction.

WE ALSO EXPECT OUR BUSINESS PARTNERS – PRINTERS, paper mills, packaging manufacturers, etc. – to commit themselves to using environmentally friendly materials and production processes.

THE PAPER IN THIS BOOK IS MADE FROM NO-CHLORINE pulp and is acid free, in conformance with international standards for paper permanency.